Cancer and its Management

Cancer and its Management

Jeffrey Tobias

MA (Cantab), MD, FRCP, FRCR
Professor of Cancer Medicine
University College London
London, UK
and
Consultant in Clinical Oncology
Department of Oncology
University College Hospital
London, UK

Daniel Hochhauser

MA (Cantab), DPhil, FRCP
Kathleen Ferrier Professor of Medical Oncology
UCL Cancer Institute
University College London
London, UK
and
Consultant in Medical Oncology
UCLH Trust
London, UK

Seventh Edition

WILEY Blackwell

This edition first published 2015 © 2015 by John Wiley & Sons, Ltd.

© 2005, 2003, 1998, 1995, 1987, 1986 by R. Souhami and J. Tobias,

© 2010 J. Tobias and D. Hochhauser

Blackwell Publishing was acquired by John Wiley

Registered office: John Wiley & Sons, Ltd, The Atrium, Southern Gate, Chichester, West Sussex, PO19 8SQ, UK

Editorial offices: 9600 Garsington Road, Oxford, OX4 2DQ, UK
  The Atrium, Southern Gate, Chichester, West Sussex, PO19 8SQ, UK
  111 River Street, Hoboken, NJ 07030-5774, USA

For details of our global editorial offices, for customer services and for information about how to apply for permission to reuse the copyright material in this book please see our website at www.wiley.com/wiley-blackwell

Library of Congress Cataloging-in-Publication Data has been applied for.

ISBN 978-1-118-46873-9

A catalogue record for this book is available from the British Library.

Wiley also publishes its books in a variety of electronic formats. Some content that appears in print may not be available in electronic books.

Fluorescence microscopy of human endothelium highlighting cadherin (green) between cells. Image courtesy of Wikimedia Commons under the GNU Free Documentation License.

Typeset in 9.25/11.5pt MinionPro by Laserwords Private Limited, Chennai, India
Printed and bound in Malaysia by Vivar Printing Sdn Bhd

1   2015

To Susan and Jo, with love and thanks

Contents

Preface

In the 4 years that have elapsed since the previous edition of this book was published, we have been astonished by the number of changes made necessary by the introduction of newer treatments for cancer. Once again we can say without fear of contradiction that both our understanding of the biology, causation and natural history of many malignant tumours has continued to move forward. Equally and perhaps even more important, the outlook at least for some types of cancer has improved, in a number of cases, quite dramatically. Patients now have access to a far more integrated and seamless service, with multidisciplinary teams meeting regularly to discuss all aspects of patient management, resulting in a more balanced and expert approach to decision-making. They are increasingly managed by well-informed specialists with particular experience and expertise in their field of practice, and communication between general practitioners, hospital specialist and community services have continued to improve. Palliative care teams, which only 10 years ago were unevenly distributed even in economically developed parts of the world, have now become more fully accepted and much more widely available.

New chemotherapeutic agents and targeted therapies have appeared at a remarkably rapid rate, and in many cases have become fully established as part of standard treatment regimens – breast, lymphoma, colorectal cancer and melanoma are good examples. We noted this development in the Preface to this book when it last appeared in 2010, and these innovations have progressed still further since then. It seems hard to believe that targeted therapies, so widely used today, have been available for less than 20 years, the first of these, the monoclonal antibody rituximab, appearing and achieving licence for use as recently as 1997. As we have previously remarked, it remains an exciting time to be in cancer medicine, though it is profoundly important to remember that the human, pastoral and technical lessons of the past do not change. We have tried to stress this in the specific site-related chapters, particularly since increasing levels of specialization carry the real danger that tomorrow's specialists will so to speak 'know more and more about less and less'. Broadly speaking, we accept as so many others do that the benefits of site specialization clearly outweigh the disadvantages, but nonetheless it is as well to remember that most patients look to their specialist oncologist for far more than simply his or her technical expertise.

As we pointed out in the Preface to previous editions, a textbook limited to this size and designed to be widely comprehensible demands that only essential information can be presented. We have had to synthesize and abbreviate a variety of expert opinions and summarize interesting or unresolved controversies, which, in a larger text, would have been the subject of more detailed discussion. Nonetheless, we hope the result is an accessible text that avoids being too didactic in tone or synoptic in style. The aim of the book has not altered: it is to provide an introductory text for medical staff, nurses and other allied professionals, students and scientists interested in and challenged by the problems of cancer care.

Initially, we wrote this book because we were aware that many busy physicians, surgeons and gynaecologists, who are not themselves cancer specialists, may find it difficult to keep abreast in areas that are nonetheless of crucial importance in their professional lives. General surgeons, for example, spend a substantial portion of their time dealing with gastrointestinal and abdominal tumours, yet have little working knowledge of the non-surgical treatment of these conditions. Similarly, gynaecological surgeons need to know – in a fair degree of detail – about what the radiotherapist and medical oncologist can offer.

In many medical schools, the students' knowledge of the management of malignant disease is acquired from specialists whose main interest may not be related to cancer. Medical students should know more about the disease that, in many countries, is now both the largest cause of mortality and being regularly recognized by the public at large as the most feared of all diseases. Needless to say, we hope that postgraduate trainees in medicine, surgery and gynaecology will find the book of value, and that it will also be of help to those beginning a career in radiotherapy or medical oncology. Finally, we would like to think that general practitioners, all of whom look after cancer patients and who have such an important role in diagnosis, management and terminal care, will find this book helpful. If specialists in cancer medicine feel that it is a useful digest of current thought in cancer management, so much the better. However, this book is not intended primarily for them. There are several very large texts that give specialist advice. Although some of these details necessarily appear in our book, we do not regard it as a handbook of chemotherapy or radiotherapy. To some extent it is a personal view of cancer and its management today and, as such, it will differ in some details from the attitudes and approaches of our colleagues.

We have attempted to give a thorough working knowledge of the principles of diagnosis, staging and treatment of tumours and to do so at a level that brings the reader up to date. We have tried to indicate where the subject is growing, where controversies lie and from which direction future advances might come. In the first nine chapters, we have attempted to outline the essential mechanisms of tumour development, cancer treatment and supportive care. In the remaining chapters, we have given an account of the principles of management of the major cancers. For each tumour, we have provided details of the pathology, mode of spread, clinical presentation, staging and treatment with radiotherapy and chemotherapy. The role of surgery is of course outlined, but details of surgical procedure are beyond the scope of this book. Once again, the references that we have included in the text or for further reading have been chosen because they are either clear and authoritative reviews, historical landmarks or perhaps, most excitingly, represent the cutting edge of recent research.

Finally, a brief word about prevalence and mortality trends. In England alone, it is estimated that around 1.8 million people are currently living with and beyond a diagnosis of cancer, a figure that is increasing by over 3% annually giving a projected total figure of over 3 million by 2030. Despite the continuing fall in mortality from heart attacks and stroke, which has resulted in cancer now being the largest cause of death in the twenty-first century, we can be sure that cancer deaths have certainly fallen over this same period. Recent figures from Cancer Research, UK, show that cancer deaths in middle-aged people have fallen in recent years to a record low – a remarkable reduction of 40% from 1971, when over 21,300 people aged between 50 and 59 years died, compared with under 14,000 people in the latest survey. The improvement in children's cancers has continued as well, with overall 5-year survival improving from 67% in 1990 to 81% last year.

However, we now need to redouble our efforts in diseases such as lung cancer, which have stubbornly remained resistant to major improvements in mortality, a particularly tragic example of course, since this disease could very largely be prevented by a further fall in the number of smokers. In 2012, lung cancer alone was responsible for over 30,000 deaths (England and Wales) compared, for example, with ischaemic heart disease just over 40,000, breast cancer around 10,500 and prostate cancer approximately 9,500. In many parts of the developing world, with increasing rates of smoking fuelled by increasing affluence and the cynical efforts of tobacco manufacturers and companies, the problem becomes still more acute and death rates will inevitably rise still further. In more affluent parts of the world, obesity is becoming not only an increasingly important cause of ill-health from non-malignant condition that is also now well recognized as a causative factor for cancer. A recent UK-based survey showed that each year some 12,000 of the commonest cancer can be attributed to obesity and that if average BMI in the population continues to increase, there could be over 3500 extra cancers every year as a result.

Although acknowledging the enormous advances made in cancer treatment over the past 25 years, we must recognize that there is no room for complacency – we still have a very long way to go. Making the best of today's treatments available to *all* patients, by improving the quality of care across the board to the high standards set by centres of excellence, would at least be a pretty good start.

Jeffrey Tobias and Daniel Hochhauser
London 2014

Acknowledgements

We were greatly helped by the commissioning editor at Wiley-Blackwell, Thom Moore, and his team. We would like to thank him most sincerely for giving us the sustained encouragement that even the most seasoned authors need. In addition, we are particularly grateful to the development editor, Jon Peacock, and the project manager, Krupa Muthu, for all their help and input before and during the production stages of the book.

We acknowledge the assistance of Professor Martyn Caplin, Royal Free Hospital, London, with the chapter on neuroendocrine tumours (Chapter 15).

My (J.T.) personal thanks also go to my long-suffering secretary Jayshree Kara, who dealt with many alterations, reverses and inconsistencies with unfailing good cheer. Any inaccuracies or shortcomings are of course entirely the responsibility of the authors.

Jeffrey Tobias and Daniel Hochhauser
London 2014

Abbreviations

5-FU	5-fluorouracil	CNS	central nervous system
5-HIAA	5-hydroxyindoleacetic acid	CSF	cerebrospinal fluid
5-HT	5-hydroxytryptamine	CT	computed tomography
6-MP	6-mercaptopurine	CTV	clinical target volume
6-MPRP	6-mercaptopurine ribose phosphate	DCIS	ductus carcinoma *in situ*
6-TG	6-thioguanine	DHFR	dihydrofolate reductase
ACTH	adrenocorticotrophic hormone	DIC	disseminated intravascular coagulation
ADH	antidiuretic hormone	DPD	dihydropyrimidine dehydrogenase
AFP	α-fetoprotein	EBV	Epstein-Barr virus
AJCC	American Joint Committee on Cancer	ECOG	Eastern Cooperative Oncology Group
ALL	acute lymphoblastic leukaemia	EF	extended field
AML	acute myeloid leukaemia; acute myeloblastic leukaemia	EGF	epidermal growth factor
		EGFR	epidermal growth factor receptor
AMML	acute myelomonocytic leukaemia	EORTC	European Organization for Research and Treatment of Cancer
ANL	acute non-lymphocytic leukaemia		
APL	acute promyelocytic leukaemia	EpCAM	epithelial cell adhesion molecule
APUD	amine precursor uptake and decarboxylation	EPO	erythropoietin
		ER	estrogen receptor
ASCO	American Society for Clinical Oncology	ERCP	endoscopic retrograde cholangiopancreatography
ATRA	all -*trans*-retinoic acid		
BCG	bacille Calmette-Guérin	ESR	erythrocyte sedimentation rate
BCNU	bis-chloroethyl nitrosourea	FAP	familial adenomatous polyposis
BMI	body mass index	FDA	Food and Drug Administration
BMT	bone-marrow transplantation	FdUMP	5-fluoro-2-deoxyuridine monophosphate
BrdU	bromodeoxyuridine		
BTV	biological target volume	FIGO	International Federation of Gynecology and Obstetrics
CALLA	common acute lymphoblastic leukaemia antigen		
		FISH	fluorescence *in situ* hybridization
CCNU	*cis*-chloroethyl nitrosourea	FIT	faecal immunochemical test
CEA	carcinoembryonic antigen	FOBT	faecal occult blood test
CGL	chronic granulocytic leukaemia	FSH	follicle-stimulating hormone
CHART	continuous hyperfractionated accelerated radiotherapy	G6PD	glucose 6-phosphate dehydrogenase
		G-CSF	granulocyte colony-stimulating factor
CI	confidence interval	GFR	glomerular filtration rate
CIN	cervical intraepithelial neoplasia	GH	growth hormone
CLL	chronic lymphocytic leukaemia	GIST	gastrointestinal stromal tumour
CMF	cyclophosphamide, methotrexate and 5-fluorouracil	GM-CSF	granulocyte/macrophage colony-stimulating factor
CMI	cell-mediated immunity	GSH	glutathione
CML	chronic myeloid leukaemia	GTV	gross tumour volume

HAART	highly active antiretroviral therapy
HBI	hemibody irradiation
HBV	hepatitis B virus
HCC	hepatocellular carcinoma
HCG	human chorionic gonadotrophin
HCL	hairy cell leukaemia
HCV	hepatitis C virus
HDI	HER dimerization inhibitor
HGPRT	hypoxanthine-guanine phosphoribosyltransferase
HHV	human herpesvirus
HIV	human immunodeficiency virus
HLA	human leucocyte antigen
HNPCC	hereditary non-polyposis colon cancer
HPV	human papillomavirus
HR	hazard ratio
HRT	hormone-replacement therapy
HTLV	human T-cell leukaemia/lymphotropic virus
HVA	homovanillic acid
IF	involved field
IGF	insulin-like growth factor
IL	interleukin
IMRT	intensity-modulated radiation therapy
INRG	International Neuroblastoma Risk Group
INSS	International Neuroblastoma Staging System
IPSID	immune proliferative small-intestine disease
IVU	intravenous urography
KGF	keratinocyte growth factor
KSHV	Kaposi's sarcoma herpesvirus
LAK	lymphokine-activated killer (cell)
LDH	lactate dehydrogenase
LET	linear energy transfer
LH	luteinizing hormone
LHRH	luteinizing hormone releasing hormone
LOH	loss of heterozygosity
LVEF	left ventricular ejection fraction
M-CSF	macrophage colony-stimulating factor
MDR	multidrug resistance
MDS	myelodysplastic syndrome
MEN	multiple endocrine neoplasia
MGMT	O^6-methylguanine-DNA methyltransferase
MGUS	monoclonal gammopathy of unknown significance
MHC	major histocompatibility complex
MIBG	meta-iodobenzylguanidine
MMP	matrix metalloproteinase

MRC	Medical Research Council
MRCP	magnetic resonance cholangiopancreatography
MRI	magnetic resonance imaging
MTI	malignant teratoma intermediate
mTOR	mammalian target of rapamycin
MTT	malignant teratoma trophoblastic
MTU	malignant teratoma undifferentiated
NCAM	neural-cell adhesion molecule
NCRI	National Cancer Research Institute
NF	neurofibromatosis
NHL	non-Hodgkin's lymphoma
NICE	National Institute for Health and Clinical Excellence
NK	natural killer (cell)
NLCN	North London Cancer Network
NSABP	National Surgical Adjuvant Breast Project
NSAID	non-steroidal anti-inflammatory drug
NSCLC	non-small-cell lung cancer
NWF	New Working Formulation
PAS	periodic acid-Schiff (stain)
PCI	prophylactic cranial irradiation
PCR	polymerase chain reaction
PDGF	platelet-derived growth factor
PDGFR	platelet-derived growth factor receptor
PEL	primary effusion lymphoma
PET	positron emission tomography
PKC	protein kinase C
PLAP	placental alkaline phosphatase
PMBL	primary mediastinal B-cell lymphoma
PNET	primitive neuroectodermal tumour
PR	progesterone receptor
PSA	prostate-specific antigen
PTH	parathyroid hormone
PTHrP	parathyroid hormone-related protein
PTV	planning target volume
REAL	revised European-American lymphoma (classification)
RPA	recursive partitioning analysis
RS	Reed-Sternberg (cell)
RSV	Rous sarcoma virus
RTOG	Radiation Therapy Oncology Group
RT-PCR	reverse-transcriptase polymerase chain reaction
SCLC	small-cell lung cancer
SEER	Surveillance, Epidemiology and End Results (program)
SNCC	small non-cleaved cell (lymphoma)
SVCO	superior vena caval obstruction

TBI	total-body irradiation	UV	ultraviolet
TCC	transitional cell carcinoma	VAIN	vaginal intraepithelial neoplasia
Tdt	terminal deoxynucleotidyltransferase	VAP	vincristine, doxorubicin and prednisone
TGF	transforming growth factor	VEGF	vascular endothelial growth factor
TIBC	total iron-binding capacity	VEGFR	vascular endothelial growth factor
TNF	tumour necrosis factor		receptor
TNI	total nodal irradiation	VIN	vulval intraepithelial neoplasia
TNM	tumour, node, metastasis	VIP	vasoactive intestinal polypeptide
TS	thymidylate synthase	VMA	vanillylmandelic acid
TSH	thyroid-stimulating hormone	WBC	white blood cell count
UICC	*Union Internationale Contre le Cancer*	WHO	World Health Organization

1 The modern management of cancer: an introductory note

Cancer is a vast medical problem. It is now the major cause of mortality, both in the UK and elsewhere in the Western world [1] (Figure 1.1), diagnosed each year in one in every 250 men and one in every 300 women. The incidence rises steeply with age so that, over the age of 60, three in every 100 men develop the disease each year (Figure 1.2a). It is a costly disease to diagnose and investigate, and treatment is time-consuming, labour-intensive and usually requires hospital care. In the Western world the commonest cancers are of the lung, breast, skin, gut and prostate gland [2,3] (Figures 1.2b and 1.3). The lifetime risk of developing a cancer is likely to alter sharply over the next decade because the number of cancer cases has risen by nearly one-third over the past 30 years. An ageing population, successes from screening and earlier diagnosis have all contributed to the rise. Present estimates suggest that the number of cases is still rising at a rate of almost 1.5% per annum. The percentage of the population over the age of 65 will grow from 16% in 2004 to 23% by 2030, further increasing the overall incidence [4].

For many years the main methods of treating cancer were surgery and radiotherapy. Control of the primary tumour is indeed a concern, since this is usually responsible for the patient's symptoms. There may be unpleasant symptoms due to local spread, and failure to control the disease locally leads to certain death. For many tumours, breast cancer, for example, the energies of those treating the disease have been directed towards defining the optimum methods of eradication of the primary tumour. It is perhaps not surprising that these efforts, while improving management, have not greatly improved the prognosis because the most important cause of mortality is metastatic spread. Although prompt and effective treatment of the primary cancer diminishes the likelihood of recurrence, metastases have often developed before diagnosis and treatment have begun. The prognosis is not then altered by treatment of the primary cancer, even though the presenting symptoms may be alleviated. Progress in treatment has been slow but steady. Worldwide, between 1990 and 2001, the mortality rates from all cancers fell by 17% in patients aged 30–69 years, but rose by 0.4% in those aged 70 years or older [1,5]. This may sound impressive at first reading, but the fall was lower than the decline in mortality rates from cardiovascular disease, which decreased by 9% in the 30–69 year age group (men) and by 14% in the 70 year (or older) age group. In the UK there has been a steady fall in mortality from cancer of about 1% a year since the 1990s (Figure 1.4), but with a widening gap in the differing socioeconomic groups. As the authors forcefully state [2]: 'Increases in cancer survival in England and Wales during the 1990s are shown to be significantly associated with a widening deprivation gap in survival'. In the USA, the number of cancer deaths has now fallen over the past 5 years, chiefly due to a decline in deaths from colorectal cancer, itself thought to be largely due to an increase in screening programmes. Interestingly, the

Cancer and its Management, Seventh Edition. Jeffrey Tobias and Daniel Hochhauser.
© 2015 John Wiley & Sons, Ltd. Published 2015 by John Wiley & Sons, Ltd.

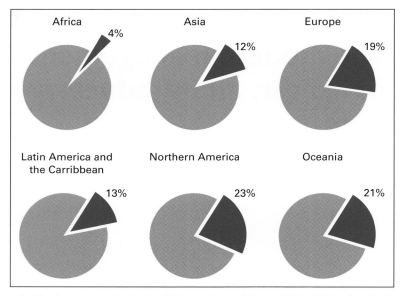

Figure 1.1 Percentage of all deaths due to cancer in the different regions of the world. Available at http://info.cancerresearchuk.org/cancerstats/geographic/world/mortality/?a=5441, accessed 10 September 2008. (© Cancer Research UK).

fall in mortality has also been paralleled by a reduction in incidence rates in the USA – for men since 1990 and for women since 1991 [6]. Nonetheless, cancer continues as the leading cause of death in the USA, under the age of 85 years [3].

Every medical speciality has its own types of cancer which are the concern of the specialist in that area. Cancer is a diagnosis to which all clinicians are alerted whatever their field and, because malignant disease is common, specialists acquire great expertise in diagnosis, often with the aid of techniques such as bronchoscopy and other forms of endoscopy. Conversely, the management of cancer once the diagnosis has been made, especially the non-surgical management, is not part of the training or interest of many specialists. This has meant that radiotherapists ('clinical oncologists') and medical oncologists are often asked to see patients who have had a laparotomy at which a tumour such as an ovarian cancer or a lymphoma has been found, but the abdomen then closed without the surgeon having made an attempt to stage the disease properly or, where appropriate, to remove the main mass of tumour. This poses considerable problems for the further management of the patient. More generally, lack of familiarity with the principles of cancer management, and of what treatment can achieve, may lead to inappropriate advice about outcome and a low level of recruitment into clinical

trials. An understanding of the principles of investigation and treatment of cancer has become essential for every physician and surgeon if the best results for their patients are to be achieved.

During the latter part of the last century, advances in the chemotherapy and radiotherapy of uncommon tumours such as Hodgkin's disease and germ-cell tumours of the testis, together with the increasing complexity of treatment decisions in more common tumours, led to a greater awareness of the importance of a planned approach to clinical management. This applies not only for the problems in individual patients, but also in the planning of clinical trials. For each type of cancer, an understanding of which patients can be helped, or even cured, can come only by close attention to the details of disease stage and pathology. Patients in whom these details are unknown are at risk from inappropriate over-treatment or from inadequate treatment, resulting in the chance of cure being missed. Even though chemotherapy has not on the whole been of outstanding benefit to patients with diseases such as squamous lung cancer or adenocarcinoma of the pancreas, it is clearly essential that clinicians with a specialized knowledge of the risks and possible benefits of chemotherapy in these and other diseases are part of the staff of every oncology department. Knowing when not to treat is as important as knowing when to do so.

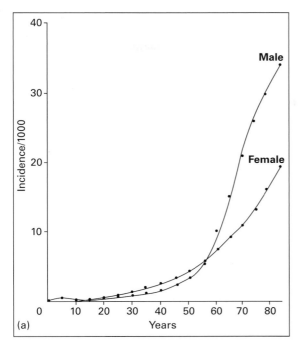

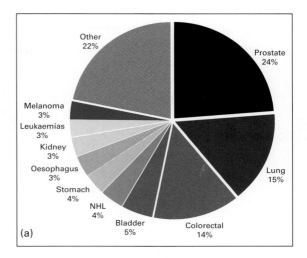

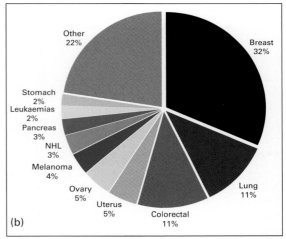

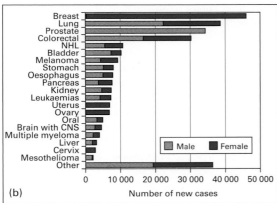

Figure 1.2 (a) Age-specific cancer incidence in England and Wales. (b) The 20 most commonly diagnosed cancers (excluding non-melanoma skin cancer) in the UK, 2005. NHL, non-Hodgkin's lymphoma. Available at http://info.cancerresearchuk.org/cancerstats/incidence/commoncancers/, accessed 10 September 2008. (© Cancer Research UK).

Figure 1.3 (a) The 10 most common cancers in males (excluding non-melanoma skin cancer) in the UK, 2005. Available at http://info.cancerresearchuk.org/cancerstats/incidence/males/, accessed 10 September 2008. (b) The 10 most common cancers in females (excluding non-melanoma skin cancer) in the UK, 2005. Available at http://info.cancerresearchuk.org/cancerstats/incidence/females/?a=5441, accessed 10 September 2008. NHL, non-Hodgkin's lymphoma. (© Cancer Research UK).

For many cancers, improvements in chemotherapy have greatly increased the complexity of management. Cancer specialists have a particular responsibility to validate the treatments they give, since the toxicity and dangers of many treatment regimens mean that the clinical indications have to be established precisely. In a few cases an imaginative step forward has dramatically improved results and the need for controlled comparison with previous treatment is scarcely necessary. Examples are the early studies leading to the introduction of combination chemotherapy in the management of advanced Hodgkin's disease, and the prevention of central nervous system relapse of leukaemia by prophylactic treatment. However, such clear-cut advances are seldom made (see,

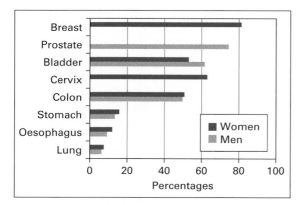

Figure 1.4 Cancer survival rates improved between 1999 and 2004. Available at http://www.statistics.gov.uk/cci/nugget .asp?id=861. (Reproduced under the terms of the Click-Use Licence).

Table 1.1 The 5-year relative survival percentage for adults diagnosed with major cancers during 1998–2001 and 1999–2003, England.

Cancer		1998–2001 survival (%)	1999–2003 survival (%)
Breast	Women	79.9	81.0
Colon	Men	49.4	49.6
	Women	50.2	50.8
Lung	Men	6.3	6.5
	Women	7.5	7.6*
Prostate	Men	70.8	74.4

*It was not possible to produce an age-standardized 5-year survival figure for lung cancer in women; therefore, this figure refers to the unstandardized estimate.
Source: Cancer survival increases in England. Available at http://www.statistics.gov.uk/pdfdir/ can0807.pdf. (Reproduced under the terms of the Click-Use Licence.)

e.g. Table 1.1, which outlines the modest improvement in survival for four major types of cancer between 1998 and 2003 in England). For the most part, improvements in treatment are made slowly in a piecemeal fashion and prospective trials of treatment must be undertaken in order to validate each step in management. Modest advances are numerically nonetheless important for such common diseases. Only large-scale trials can detect these small differences reliably. Collaboration on a national and international scale has become increasingly important, and the results of these studies have had a major impact on management, for example, in operable breast cancer. There is always a tendency in dealing with cancer to want to believe good news and for early, uncontrolled, but promising results to be seized upon and over-interpreted. Although understandable, uncritical enthusiasm for a particular form of treatment is greatly to be deplored, since it leads to a clamour for the treatment and the establishment of patterns of treatment that are improperly validated. There have been many instances where treatments have been used before their place has been clearly established: adjuvant chemotherapy in non-small-cell lung cancer, limb perfusion in sarcomas and melanoma, radical surgical techniques for gastric cancer and adjuvant chemotherapy for bladder cancer are examples. The toxicity of cancer treatments is considerable and can be justified only if it is unequivocally shown that the end-results are worthwhile either by increasing survival or by improving the quality of life.

The increasing complexity of management has brought with it a recognition that in most areas it has become necessary to establish an effective working collaboration between specialists. Joint planning of management in specialized clinics is now widely practised for diseases such as lymphomas and head and neck and gynaecological cancer. Surgeons and gynaecologists are now being trained to specialize in the oncological aspects of their speciality. In this way patients can benefit from a coordinated and planned approach to their individual problems.

Before a patient can be treated, it must be established that he or she has cancer, the tumour pathology must be defined, and the extent of local and systemic disease determined. For each of these goals to be attained, the oncologist must rely on colleagues in departments of histopathology, diagnostic imaging, haematology and chemical pathology. Patients in whom the diagnosis of cancer has not been definitely made pathologically but is based on a very strong clinical suspicion with suggestive pathological evidence, or where a pathological diagnosis of cancer has been made which, on review, proves to be incorrect, are often referred to oncologists. It is essential for the oncologist to be in close contact with histopathologists and cytologists so that diagnoses can be reviewed regularly. Many departments of oncology have regular pathology review meetings so that the clinician can learn of the difficulties which pathologists have with diagnosis and vice versa. Similarly, modern imaging techniques have led to a previously unattainable accuracy in preoperative and postoperative staging, although many of these techniques are only as reliable as the individuals using them (e.g. abdominal or pelvic ultrasound). The cancer specialist must be fully conversant with the uses and limitations of imaging methods. The techniques are expensive and the results must be interpreted in the light of other clinical information. The practice of holding regular meetings to review cases with specialists from the imaging departments has much to commend it. Modern cancer treatment often carries a substantial risk of toxicity. Complex and difficult treatments are best managed in a specialized unit with skilled personnel. The centralization of high-dependency care allows staff to become particularly aware of the physical and emotional problems of patients undergoing treatments of this kind. Additionally, colleagues from other departments such as haematology, biochemistry and bacteriology can more easily help in the investigation and management of some of the very difficult problems which occur, for example, in the immunosuppressed patient.

The increasingly intensive investigative and treatment policies which have been adopted in the last 25 years impose on clinicians the additional responsibility of having to stand back from the treatment of their patients and decide on the aim of treatment at each stage. Radical and aggressive therapy may be essential if the patient is to have a reasonable chance of being cured. However, palliative treatment will be used if the situation is clearly beyond any prospect of cure. It is often difficult to decide when the intention of treatment should move from the radical to the palliative, with avoidance of toxicity as a major priority. For example, while many patients with advanced lymphomas will be cured by intensive combination chemotherapy, there is no prospect of cure in advanced breast cancer by these means, and chemotherapy must in this case be regarded as palliative therapy. In this situation it makes little sense to press treatment to the point of serious toxicity. The judgement of what is tolerable and acceptable is a major task in cancer management. Such judgements can come only from considerable experience of the treatments in question, of the natural history of individual tumours and an understanding of the patient's needs and wishes.

Modern cancer management often involves highly technological and intensive medical care. It is expensive, time-consuming and sometimes dangerous. Patients should seldom be in ignorance of what is wrong with them or what the treatment involves. The increasingly technical nature of cancer management and the change in public and professional attitudes towards malignant disease have altered the way in which doctors who are experienced in cancer treatment approach their patients. There has been a decisive swing towards honest and careful discussion with patients about the disease and its treatment. This does not mean that a bald statement should be made to the patient about the diagnosis and its outcome, since doctors must sustain the patient with hope and encouragement through what is obviously a frightening and depressing period. Still less does it imply that the decisions about treatment are in some way left to the patient after the alternatives have been presented? Skilled and experienced oncologists advise and guide patients in their understanding of the disease and the necessary treatment decisions. One of the most difficult and rewarding aspects of the management of malignant disease lies in the judgement of how much information to give each particular patient, at what speed, and how to incorporate the patient's own wishes into a rational treatment plan.

The emotional impact of the diagnosis and treatment can be considerable for both patients and relatives. Above everything else, treating patients with cancer involves an awareness of how patients think and feel. All members of the medical team caring for cancer patients must be prepared to devote time to talking to patients and their families, to answer questions and explain what is happening and what can be achieved. Because many patients will die from their disease, they must learn to cope with the emotional and physical needs of dying patients and the effects of anxiety, grief and bereavement on their families. In modern cancer units management is by a team of healthcare professionals, each of whom has their own contribution to make. They must work together, participating in management as colleagues commanding mutual respect. The care and support of patients with advanced malignant disease and the control of symptoms such as pain and nausea have greatly improved in the last 10 years. This aspect of cancer management has been improved by the collaboration of many medical workers. Nurses who specialize in the control of symptoms of malignancy are now attached to most cancer units, and social workers skilled in dealing with the problems of malignant disease and bereavement are an essential part of the team. The development of hospices has led to a much greater appreciation of the way in which symptoms might be controlled and to a considerable improvement in the standard of care of the dying in general hospitals. Many cancer departments now have a symptom support team based in the hospital but who are able to undertake the care of patients in their own homes, giving advice on control of symptoms such as pain and nausea and providing support to patients' families.

There have been dramatic advances in cell and molecular biology in the last 20 years, with the result that our understanding of the nature of malignant transformation has rapidly improved. This trend will continue, placing many additional demands on oncologists to keep abreast of both advances in management and the scientific foundations on which they are based. The power of modern techniques to explore some of the fundamental processes in malignant transformation has meant that cancer is at the heart of many aspects of medical research, and has led to an increased academic interest in malignancy. This, in turn, has led to a more critical approach to many aspects of cancer treatment. Cancer, and its management, is unquestionably among the most complex and demanding disciplines within medicine, and many more healthcare workers now recognize that cancer medicine is a profoundly rewarding challenge. Standards of patient care have improved dramatically as a result of these welcome changes.

References

1 Danaei G, Vander Hoorn S, Lopez AD *et al.* Causes of cancer in the world: comparative risk assessment of nine behavioural and environmental risk factors. *Lancet* 2005; 366: 1784–93.

2 Coleman MP, Rachet B, Woods LM *et al.* Trends in socioeconomic inequalities in cancer survival in England and Wales up to 2001. *Br J Cancer* 2004; 90: 1367–73.

3 Parkin DM, Bray F, Ferlay J, Pisani P. Global cancer statistics, 2002. *CA Cancer J Clin* 2005; 55: 74–108.

4 Bray F, Moller B. Predicting the future burden of cancer. *Nat Rev Cancer* 2006; 6: 63–74.

5 Colditz GA, Sellers TA, Trapido E. Epidemiology: identifying the causes and preventability of cancer? *Nat Rev Cancer* 2006; 6: 75–83.

6 McCarthy M. Number of cancer deaths continues to fall in USA. *Lancet* 2007; 369: 263.

Further reading

Cavalli F. Cancer in the developing world: can we avoid the disaster? *Nat Clin Pract Oncol* 2006; 3: 582–3.

Department of Health. *NHS Cancer Plan: A Plan for Investment, a Plan for Reform.* London: The Stationery Office, 2000.

Lake RA, van der Most RG. A better way for a cancer cell to die. *N Engl J Med* 2006; 354: 2503–4.

National Audit Office. *NHS Cancer Plan: A Progress Report.* London: The Stationery Office, 2005.

Riberiro RC, Pui CH. Saving the children: improving childhood cancer treatment in developing countries. *N Engl J Med* 2005; 352: 2158.

Rosen R, Smith A, Harrison A. *Future Trends and Challenges for Cancer Services in England: A Review of Literature and Policy.* London: Kings Fund, 2006.

2 Epidemiology, cure, treatment trials and screening

The epidemiology of cancer, which concerns the study of the frequency of the disease in populations living under different conditions, has been illuminating in many ways. It has allowed the testing of theories about the cause of a cancer by correlating factors related to lifestyle, occupation or exposure to infection with the incidence of a cancer. It has suggested ways in which cancer might be prevented by changing the prevalence of a postulated aetiological agent, as shown by the decline of lung cancer in doctors who have given up smoking. It has provided a stimulus for research into the biological basis of the induction of cancer by these exposures. Finally, epidemiological evidence has proved invaluable in planning cancer services.

Terminology and methods in epidemiology

Prevalence means the proportion of a defined group having a condition at a single point in time. *Incidence* means the proportion of a defined population developing the disease within a stated time period. *Crude incidence* or *prevalence rates* refer to a whole population. *Specific rates* refer to selected groups, for example, a higher crude incidence of breast cancer in one population might be due to more postmenopausal women being in the population in question. *Standardized populations* should, therefore, be used when comparing incidence and prevalence.

In trying to find connections between a disease and a postulated causal factor, epidemiologists may construct either *case–control* or *cohort* studies. For example, to determine if there is a connection between dietary fat and breast cancer, a *case–control study* would compare the dietary intake of people with the disease (cases) and those without (controls). Choosing appropriate controls is vital to the study design. Case–control studies are also suitable for studies of rare tumours in which a group of people who are exposed to the putative aetiological agent are followed and the frequency of the disease is measured. The control group is unexposed, or exposed to a lesser extent. In the case of dietary fat and breast cancer, a *cohort study* would compare the incidence of the disease, over a given period of time, in those with,

---

Cancer and its Management, Seventh Edition. Jeffrey Tobias and Daniel Hochhauser.
© 2015 John Wiley & Sons, Ltd. Published 2015 by John Wiley & Sons, Ltd.

say, a high-fat and a low-fat diet. If the cancer incidence is low, as it usually is, large numbers of women will be followed over many years before an answer is obtained. Other variables must be allowed for, since eating habits, for example, are influenced by social class and ethnic origin and these may in turn be independently linked to the likelihood of developing breast cancer. Cohort studies take a long time, are very expensive and are unsuitable for studies of rare tumours.

There are considerable problems in the interpretation of data obtained from epidemiological studies. A possible relationship between a characteristic and a cancer may be discovered, but there are several considerations that should influence us in deciding whether a causal connection really exists.

1 *Is the relationship between the characteristic and the disease specific, or can a similar association be found with other diseases?* An association with other diseases does not necessarily invalidate a causal connection but may suggest that both the characteristic and the cancer are themselves associated with another factor. For example, both lung cancer and coronary artery disease are more

common in social classes 4 and 5. The problem is then to determine if these diseases are due to social class itself or to the higher frequency of cigarette smoking in these social groups.

2 *Is the relationship a strong one?* The likelihood of a causal connection is strengthened if, for example, the risk of cancer in the population showing the characteristic is increased 10-fold rather than doubled.

3 *Is the degree of risk correlated with amount of exposure?* This is the situation with lung cancer and cigarette smoking (Figure 2.1b) and with length of exposure to hormone replacement therapy and breast cancer (Figure 2.1a). Such a gradation greatly increases the likelihood of a causal connection.

4 *Is the association biologically plausible?* For example, it appears intuitively reasonable to accept an association between smoking and lung cancer, but the relationship between smoking and bladder cancer is at first more surprising. However, it may be difficult to assess the biological basis for an association since often we do not know the explanation for these events until further investigation, perhaps prompted by the discovery of an

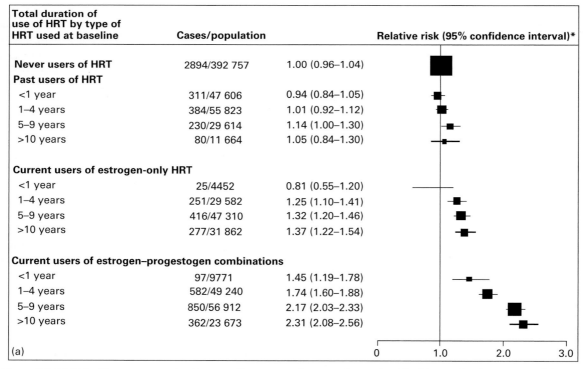

Total duration of use of HRT by type of HRT used at baseline	Cases/population	Relative risk (95% confidence interval)*	
Never users of HRT	2894/392 757	1.00 (0.96–1.04)	
Past users of HRT			
<1 year	311/47 606	0.94 (0.84–1.05)	
1–4 years	384/55 823	1.01 (0.92–1.12)	
5–9 years	230/29 614	1.14 (1.00–1.30)	
>10 years	80/11 664	1.05 (0.84–1.30)	
Current users of estrogen-only HRT			
<1 year	25/4452	0.81 (0.55–1.20)	
1–4 years	251/29 582	1.25 (1.10–1.41)	
5–9 years	416/47 310	1.32 (1.20–1.46)	
>10 years	277/31 862	1.37 (1.22–1.54)	
Current users of estrogen–progestogen combinations			
<1 year	97/9771	1.45 (1.19–1.78)	
1–4 years	582/49 240	1.74 (1.60–1.88)	
5–9 years	850/56 912	2.17 (2.03–2.33)	
>10 years	362/23 673	2.31 (2.08–2.56)	

(a)

Figure 2.1 (a) Risk of breast cancer related to use of hormone replacement therapy (HRT). (b) Mortality from cancer of the lung related to number of cigarettes smoked daily. (Data from Doll and Bradford Hill [2].)

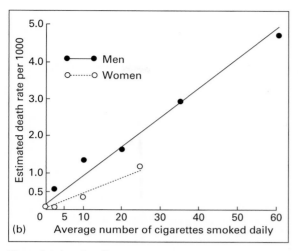

(b)

Figure 2.1 (*continued*)

Table 2.1 Geographical variation in cancer incidence.

Cancer type	Ratio high : low	High incidence	Low incidence
Oesophagus	200:1	Kazakhstan	Holland
Skin	200:1	Queensland	India
Liver	100:1	Mozambique	Birmingham
Nasopharynx	100:1	China	Uganda
Lung	40:1	Birmingham	Ibadan (Nigeria)
Stomach	30:1	Japan	Birmingham
Cervix	20:1	Hawaii, Colombia	Israel
Rectum	20:1	Denmark	Nigeria

association, reveals it. Animal models of the disease may help both in suggesting which environmental agents may be causal and in strengthening the conclusions of epidemiological investigations.

5 *Is there an alternative explanation for what has been found and do the findings fit with other epidemiological data?* The nature of epidemiological evidence is such that absolute proof that an association is causal may sometimes be impossible to obtain except by intervention studies in which the suspected factor is altered or removed to see if the incidence of cancer then falls. Such studies are difficult, expensive and time-consuming, especially if randomization is necessary. In some circumstances randomized intervention may be impossible (we cannot randomly allocate people to give up smoking or to continue!) and the epidemiological data derived from studies of the population provide the only possible information.

Geographical distribution of cancer

Clues to the aetiology of cancer have been obtained from studies of the difference in incidence of cancers in different countries, races and cultures. There are obvious difficulties in obtaining reliable data in some countries. Problems of different age distributions can to some extent be overcome by using age-standardized incidence and by restricting the comparison to the mature adult population aged 35–64 years. This age range excludes the ages where the figures are likely to be least reliable. A further difficulty lies in incomplete documentation of

histological type. Sometimes the registration refers to the whole organ – bone or lung – without specifying histological type.

Very large differences in incidence of various tumours between countries have been disclosed (Table 2.1). The very high incidence of liver cancer in Mozambique may be related to aflatoxin mould on stored peanuts, and the incidence is now falling since steps have been taken to store the peanuts under different conditions. In the Ghurjev region of Kazakhstan, carcinoma of the oesophagus is 200 times more common than in the Netherlands; and in the Transkei region the incidence of the disease appears to have increased greatly in the last 30 years. The high incidence of carcinoma of the stomach in Japan is in contrast to the UK and the USA where the incidence of the disease is falling [3]. Studies such as these provide strong evidence for environmental factors causing cancer, but there may be an interaction with genetic predisposition.

An analysis of the relative contributions of the environmental and genetic components can be made by studying cancer incidence in people who have settled in a new country and who have taken on a new way of life. Japanese immigrants in the USA, for example, have a similar incidence of colon cancer to native Americans but 5 times that of Japanese in Japan [4] (Table 2.2) and it is therefore clear that this difference in rates is not mainly genetic.

Temporal distribution of cancer

The incidence of cancer in a given community may change with time, providing further clues to aetiology.

Table 2.2 Cancer incidence (cases per 100 000 per year) in Japanese immigrants compared with country of origin and residents of adopted country.

	Japanese in Japan	USA (mostly Hawaii)	
		Japanese	White
Stomach	130	40	21
Breast	31	122	187
Colon	8.4	37	37
Ovary	5.2	16	27
Prostate	1.5	15	35

With rare tumours, this may be more dramatically apparent when a disease appears as a cluster in a given place at a given time. An example would be several cases of acute leukaemia occurring in close proximity in a town within a short space of time. Such clustering has indeed been observed in acute leukaemia [5] and has been suggested for Hodgkin's disease. Chance effects make analysis difficult. However, in the case of Burkitt's lymphoma, outbreaks in Uganda have been shown to spread from one part of a district to another in a way that cannot be attributed to chance but which fits well with an infective aetiology that is widespread in the community but produces cancer only in a few children. Stronger evidence of environmental factors comes from the change in cancer incidence with time. However, the interpretation of these changes with time may be made difficult by changes in registration methods, by shifts in diagnostic accuracy and by the long latent period of many cancers. The dramatic rise in lung cancer in the Western world can be attributed confidently to smoking but the fall in stomach cancer is of unknown cause.

Causes of cancer suggested by epidemiological studies

The realization that cancer might largely be preventable has gained more widespread acceptance in recent years. It seems probable that at least 50% of cancers could be avoided by lifestyle changes. Many substances present in the environment or in the diet have been shown to be carcinogenic in animals. The epidemiological approach has been used to investigate the link between human cancers and substances which in animals are known to be carcinogens, and to identify unsuspected carcinogens by

Table 2.3 Some aetiological factors.

Ionizing irradiation
Atomic bomb and nuclear accidents: acute leukaemia, breast cancer
X-rays (diagnostic and therapeutic): bone cancer, acute leukaemia, squamous cell carcinoma of skin
Ultraviolet irradiation: basal and squamous cell skin cancer; melanoma
Background irradiation: acute leukaemia

Inhaled or ingested carcinogens
Cigarette smoking: cancers of lung, larynx and bladder
Atmospheric pollution with polycyclic hydrocarbons: lung cancer
Asbestos: mesothelioma, bronchial carcinoma
Nickel: cancer of the lung and paranasal sinuses
Chromates: lung cancer
Arsenic: lung and skin cancer
Aluminium: bladder cancer
Aromatic amines: bladder cancer
Benzene: erythroleukaemia
Polyvinylchloride: angiosarcoma of the liver

Viral causes
Papillomavirus: cancers of the cervix and anus
HHV8: Kaposi's sarcoma
HTLV-1: T-cell lymphoma

HHV, human herpesvirus; HTLV, human T-cell leukaemia/lymphoma virus.

observations on human populations without reference to previous animal experiments. Some of the factors known, or strongly suspected, to be carcinogenic in humans are shown in Table 2.3.

It has been estimated that more than one in three of the 7 million annual cancer deaths worldwide are caused by nine potentially modifiable risk factors, many of which are listed in Table 2.3. Others include excess body weight and obesity (particularly for carcinomas of the uterus, rectum and colon and postmenopausal breast cancer), together with physical inactivity and inadequate dietary intake of fruit and vegetables. Alcohol use is clearly associated with hepatic and oesophageal cancers, together with those of the oral cavity and oropharynx. However, some of the important cancers including prostate, kidney and lymphoma, seem not to be attributable to any of these specific risks. Smoking alone is estimated to have caused about 21% of deaths from cancer worldwide, with alcohol use and low fruit and vegetable intake causing another 5% each.

Inhaled carcinogens

Cigarette smoking has been the subject of epidemiological investigation since the early work of Doll and Hill [2] demonstrated the relationship between smoking and lung cancer. All studies have shown a higher mortality for lung cancer in smokers. This mortality has a dose–response relationship with the number of cigarettes smoked and diminishes with time after stopping smoking. This relationship is discussed further in Chapter 12. Cigarette smoking has also been implicated in the development of carcinoma of the bladder, larynx, pancreas and kidney and is considered to be responsible for 35% of all cancer deaths.

Cigarette smoking is the major known cause of cancer. All other causes are quantitatively less important at present. Reversal of this public health hazard will do more to improve cancer mortality than any other single preventive measure.

Atmospheric pollutants such as chimney smoke and exhaust fumes have been widely suspected as a cause of lung cancer. Polycyclic hydrocarbons, such as 3,4-benzpyrene, are present in these fumes and are known to be carcinogenic in humans. The incidence of lung cancer in men in large cities is 2 or 3 times greater than in those living in the country. This increase is small compared with the increase in incidence in smokers compared with non-smokers.

Lifestyle and diet

Evidence is accumulating that diet and body weight are important determinants of cancer risk [6]. There is considerable concern about the rising levels of obesity in the UK population. The increase in weight affects all ages and social classes but to different degrees (Figure 2.2) [7].

The nature of the dietary factors in cancer causation, and the mechanisms involved in tumour production, are poorly understood. In countries where there is a high average daily fat intake the age-adjusted death rate of postmenopausal breast cancer and colon cancer is also high. However, those countries where dietary fat intake is high also tend to be the most heavily industrialized. Furthermore, the total caloric intake is higher in these nations, and a similar association exists for levels of dietary protein. Over-nutrition has been shown to increase the incidence of spontaneous tumours in animals. There is strong evidence that obesity is an

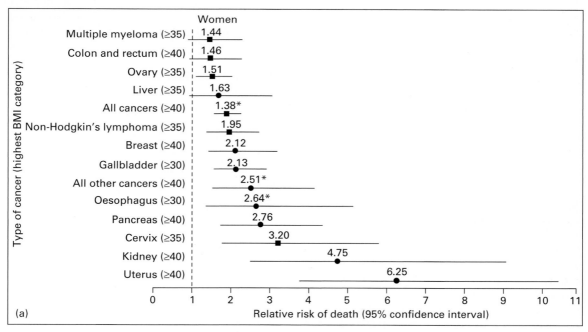

Figure 2.2 Obesity and cancer risk. (a) Relative risk of cancer death in obese versus normal-weight individuals. BMI, body mass index. (b) Percentage of men and women defined as obese 1993–2002. (c) Obesity in children related to neighbourhood deprivation. Key indicates socioeconomic class. (Data from Sproston and Primatesta [7].)

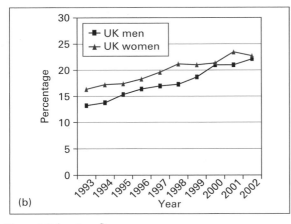

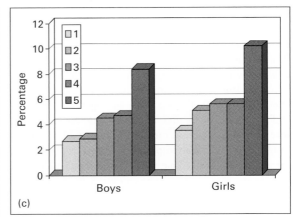

Figure 2.2 (*continued*)

aetiological factor in cancers of the breast, endometrium and gallbladder. Case–control studies relating dietary fat to cancer incidence have given conflicting results. A recent meta-analysis has attempted to provide an analysis of the risk but the methodological problems and the interpretation of the results present considerable difficulties. Rather than being causally linked to the cancer, it may be that these dietary constituents are associated with other factors that are themselves causal. Other dietary factors that may be associated with the development of cancer are dietary fibre, which may protect against the development of cancer of the large bowel, and vitamin A analogues (retinoids). However, no change in breast cancer risk has been shown in relation to dietary intake of vitamins C, E and A [8]. Two randomized trials of retinoids in patients at high risk of aerodigestive cancer have failed to demonstrate a protective effect of supplementation.

Ionizing irradiation

Ionizing irradiation has been well established as a human carcinogen. There has been an increased incidence of leukaemia and breast cancer in the survivors of the Nagasaki and Hiroshima atom bombs. Skin cancer frequently occurred on the hands of radiologists in the days before the significance of radiation exposure was understood. The internal deposition of radium (see Chapter 23) was a cause of osteosarcoma, as is external beam radiation. There is also an increased incidence of leukaemia in patients treated by irradiation for ankylosing spondylitis. Ultraviolet irradiation is responsible for the increased incidence of skin cancer on sites exposed to intense sunlight. Early intense exposure to sunlight is

associated with increased risk of melanoma in later life [9].

Background environmental radiation is at a much smaller dose in total, and is received at a much slower rate ($<10^{-8}$) compared with diagnostic X-rays. Diagnostic X-rays may account for about 0.6% of cumulative cancer risk [10]. For most cancers, background radioactivity appears to constitute a small risk at present, with the exception of lung cancer, where background radiation from radon is responsible for an increase in incidence [11].

Occupational factors

Aetiological factors in cancer, including occupational factors, are listed in Table 2.3. Asbestos inhalation is associated with two types of cancer: mesothelioma of the pleura and peritoneum, and bronchogenic carcinoma. Prolonged and heavy exposure is needed in the case of bronchogenic cancer, and cigarette smoking further increases the risk. In recent years, the incidence of mesothelioma has risen dramatically in both men and women [12]. This can be related to the widespread use of asbestos in postwar building and the number of cases will continue to rise for the next two decades. There is also an increased risk of lung cancer in workers in nickel refining and the manufacture of chromates, and a possible association with haematite mining and gold mining. Lung cancer has also been described in workers in a sheep-dip factory where there was a very high exposure to inhaled arsenic. These workers had signs of chronic arsenicalism, and the risk of lung cancer with lower levels of exposure is probably very small.

Other human carcinogens have been identified as a result of industrial epidemiological evidence. Aniline dye workers were shown to have a greatly increased incidence of bladder cancer, and this observation led to the demonstration, in animals, of the carcinogenic effect of 2-naphthylamine. Benzidine and 2-naphthylamine have also been implicated in the pathogenesis of bladder cancer in these workers and those in the rubber industry who are also exposed. Workers in the aluminium industry have been shown to have an increased incidence of bladder cancer. It has been estimated that about 4% of all cancers can be related to occupational factors.

Some epidemiologists attribute a large proportion of cancers to as yet unspecified industrial poisons and claim that there is an increase in cancer incidence which is unrelated to tobacco consumption. The figures are disputed, however, since there are the confounding variables of improved diagnosis and registration among the poorer sections of society during this period (see below). The issue is intensely political, and the prevention and control of industrial pollution potentially involve large sums of money.

Viral causes

Viral infection accounts for 10–15% of human cancer. The importance of viral infection as a cause has increased greatly since the onset of the AIDS epidemic because viral-induced malignancy is a common cause of death.

The mechanisms of viral-induced malignancy are discussed in Chapter 3. Epstein–Barr virus (EBV) and Kaposi's sarcoma herpesvirus (KSHV; human herpesvirus 8 or HHV8) and human papillomavirus are among the viruses most clearly associated with cancer [13,14]. EBV causes Burkitt's lymphoma and nasopharyngeal carcinoma in a small proportion of infected patients. The lymphoma occurs in sub-Saharan Africa in the malaria-endemic region. The virus itself is a ubiquitous gamma herpes virus that generally establishes lifelong symptomatic infection in memory B lymphocytes by mimicking cellular signalling pathways that regulate antigen-dependent B-cell differentiation. Disability appears to be due to the biological properties of a set of EBV-encoded proteins, expressed in both normal and transformed cells. It looks as though these EBV proteins are able to 'hijack' critical cellular pathways to promote the proliferation and survival of infected cells, while impairing antiviral immune responses. Kaposi's sarcoma has long existed in a similar distribution in sub-Saharan Africa and in the Mediterranean Jewish population. HHV8 is now known to be closely linked with the sarcoma in the endemic and AIDS-related disease as well as in multicentric Castleman's disease and primary effusion lymphoma. The prevalence of antibodies to HHV8 (KSHV) is higher in Italy and Africa than in the UK or the USA.

Papillomaviruses are the major causative factor in the development of cervical cancer (see Chapter 17). Of over 100 types of virus, types 16, 18, 31 and 33 are particularly high-risk types (6 and 11 being low risk).

Retroviruses are causes of human cancer, the best-defined example being human T-cell leukaemia virus (HTLV)-1, which is an endemic infection in southern Japan and the Caribbean, where the disease develops in a small proportion of those infected. The virus is transmitted from mother to child via the placenta and in breast milk and is also transmitted in semen.

Hepatitis B is a DNA virus transmitted by blood and sexual contact. It causes hepatitis and cirrhosis. Hepatocellular carcinoma is 100-fold more frequent in infected than non-infected individuals. *Hepatitis C* is an RNA virus that also causes chronic hepatitis with a greatly increased incidence of hepatocellular carcinoma. Both viruses have a worldwide distribution but are especially prevalent in China and Taiwan and among intravenous drug takers. The two viruses are responsible for the majority of liver cancer deaths worldwide.

Cancer statistics

Each year more than a quarter of a million people are newly diagnosed with cancer in the UK. The commonest four types – breast, lung, colorectal and prostate – account for over half of all new cases. More than one in three people will develop some form of cancer during their lifetime, with a striking age relationship such that, on a population basis, only one person in 27 will develop cancer under the age of 50. About two-thirds of all cases are diagnosed in people aged 65 and over, with over one-third of cases in people aged at least 75 years. Less than 1% of all cases occur in children (1400 cases diagnosed during childhood in 2003 in the UK). For older children the figure is slightly higher, with 1700 teenagers and young adults (15–24 years) diagnosed during 2003 in the UK.

Registries have been established in the UK and other countries to record the number of patients developing cancer. The registry is usually notified of new cancer cases by the hospital where the diagnosis is made. In addition, it receives copies of all death certificates of patients within the region where the diagnosis of cancer appears on a certificate. The quality of the data collected varies greatly between registries and countries. Incomplete information, changing patterns of registration and diagnosis, introduction of screening programmes and improved treatment – all these factors change the number of patients being registered as dying of the disease in a given area in a given time. Minor fluctuations or differences in incidence or mortality should, therefore, be viewed with caution, especially if comparisons are made between countries with widely differing rates of registration. Recent comparisons between mortality in different European countries are confounded by markedly different registration rates. Consistent trends over several years require investigation before it can be accepted that a change in the incidence or mortality of a disease is occurring.

However, more caution must be attached to any report that seeks to determine the impact of a particular treatment by examining cancer registry data. The relative merits of one treatment or another must be determined by prospective randomized trials.

Even the most complete registries may have histological confirmation of the diagnosis in less than 60% of cases, although the completeness of the records with respect to the primary site of the tumour is much greater. The incidence figures for tumours of a defined histological type or stage are therefore usually much less reliable than those which describe their site of origin.

Despite these reservations, an examination of the age-specific incidence of various tumours is revealing. For example, the figures for female genital cancer (Figure 2.3) show that cancers of the ovary and uterus follow a very similar pattern, the incidence rising sharply towards the end of the child-bearing years, reaching a peak after the menopause. An understanding of the causes of these cancers must clearly take into account these dramatic changes. This is not the pattern seen with all adenocarcinomas in women (Figure 2.4). Indeed, cancers of the ovary and uterus stand out as not showing the typical large increase in incidence from the age of 60 onwards which characterizes other adenocarcinomas such as bowel, stomach and pancreas.

Cancers of the cervix and of the vagina, chiefly squamous cell cancers, are quite unlike each other in age of onset, that of the cervix being a disease of young and middle-aged women, and that of the vagina a disease of elderly women. The impact of screening programmes for cervical cancer has meant that many of these cases are diagnosed at a very early stage, and study of the

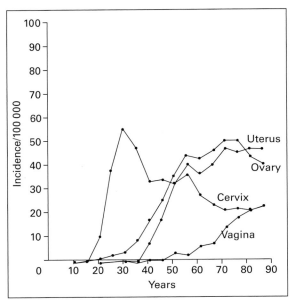

Figure 2.3 Age-specific incidence of female genital cancer. The figures for cervical cancer include carcinoma *in situ*, diagnosed by screening examination, which accounts for the majority of cases in young patients.

histology shows a large percentage of cases diagnosed *in situ*. Should we, therefore, conclude that the higher incidence of cervical cancer in young women is an artefact of early diagnosis and that these cancers would have been clinically apparent, if at all, only many years later? This problem is discussed in more detail in Chapter 17, but it serves to illustrate how cancer statistics may be dramatically altered by early diagnosis. Similarly, the introduction of prostate-specific antigen (PSA) testing has greatly increased the incidence of cancer of the prostate but without any change in mortality yet detectable as a result of treatment of these very early asymptomatic tumours (see Chapter 18). Prostate cancer is now the most commonly diagnosed cancer in UK males, with almost 32 000 cases diagnosed during 2003. Perhaps surprisingly, this is a significantly larger figure than for lung cancer in males (22 000 cases annually), partly of course a reflection of the falling incidence in lung cancer rates at least in males in the UK since the 1960s, due to a sharp decline in the prevalence of smoking (see also Chapter 12).

The figures for other adenocarcinomas in women (Figure 2.4) are revealing in another respect. The onset of cancer of the uterus and ovary is earlier than that of the gut and stomach, and does not increase in incidence

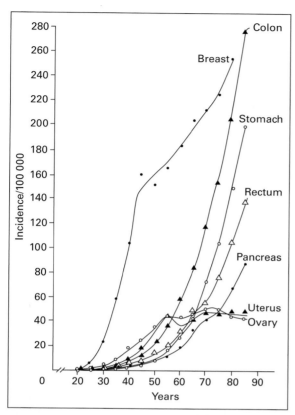

Figure 2.4 Age-specific incidence of female adenocarcinoma. The incidence of cancer of the breast increases rapidly in pre-menopausal women and then slows. This change is more marked with ovarian and uterine adenocarcinoma. By contrast, the incidence of gastrointestinal cancers shows no relation to menopause but increases markedly over the age of 60.

with old age. Conversely, cancer of the breast rises rapidly in incidence in early middle age, and then continues to rise in incidence after the menopause but at a slower rate compared with colonic cancer, so that the incidence at over 80 years of age is less than that of the colon, while at 40 years of age breast cancer occurs 14 times more frequently. The factors responsible for the origin and growth of breast cancer clearly differ from those giving rise to gastrointestinal malignancy.

Survival data and determination of cure in cancer

When results of cancer treatment are presented, a graph of survival is often shown, or the proportion of patients alive

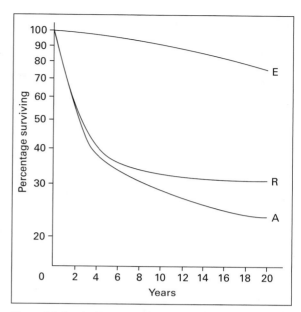

Figure 2.5 Survival in ovarian cancer. Curve A shows observed survival, curve E age-adjusted expected survival and curve R relative survival.

at, say, 5 or 10 years is stated. It is often difficult to decide whether the results mean that some patients are cured. An understanding of how survival figures are derived is therefore necessary for judging the effectiveness of treatment.

A *survival curve* is a plot of the proportion of patients surviving as a function of time. An example is shown in Figure 2.5, where curve A gives the survival up to 20 years for all cases of cancer of the ovary. A disease-free survival curve would be displayed in a similar manner but the *x*-axis would then represent the length of time before the disease reappears. Since some patients may be effectively treated on relapse, the information is not the same as that in a survival curve. This is especially true in a condition such as Hodgkin's disease where many patients can be cured on relapse.

Can we judge whether patients are cured by looking at survival curves? The general answer is that cure can be assumed if the group of patients returns to a rate of survival similar to those who have not had the same cancer. In the case of ovarian cancer, the comparison would be made with a large population of women with the same age distribution. The survival curve expected in such a population is the *age-adjusted expected survival curve*. In Figure 2.5 the data for ovarian cancer are shown

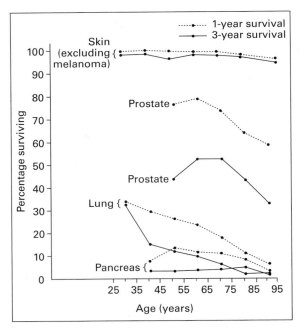

Figure 2.6 Age-related relative survival rates for several cancers. The data for the skin, lung and pancreas are for men, but are similar in both sexes.

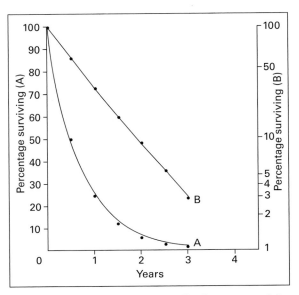

Figure 2.7 Survival in advanced small-cell carcinoma of the bronchus. There appears to be a flattening of the survival curve (curve A) but the rate of death is in fact exponential (curve B).

for a 20-year follow-up period. Curve A is the observed survival of the patients and curve E is the age-adjusted expected survival curve; it can be seen that A is approximately parallel to E at 15–20 years. The age-adjusted relative survival curve (R) is constructed by dividing the observed survival curve (A) by the expected curve (E). If there is no increased risk of dying due to the cancer, this curve will run parallel to the abscissa. A difficulty might arise if the ability to cure the cancer were dependent on age, for example, if young women were more easily cured than elderly women. The age distribution of survivors would then change with time and the age distribution of the control population would therefore have to be adjusted accordingly.

For many tumours, survival does depend on age: Figure 2.6 shows *age-related survival rates* at 1 and 3 years for a variety of common tumours. For most cancers, survival is worse in the elderly population at both 1 and 3 years.

In Figure 2.5 the survival curves are given for all cases of cancer of the ovary but they could be plotted for individual ages at presentation, or for the *different stages* of the disease. This may indicate that cure is being achieved only for certain age groups or stages of disease. In practice,

however, data on very large groups of patients (thousands) are needed to demonstrate cure with confidence.

A linear-scale plot of survival figures may suggest that a small proportion of patients are going to be long survivors. In Figure 2.7, for example, the survival figures for a large trial in small-cell lung cancer (SCLC) are shown on the linear scale. Curve A seems to flatten out at 2 years, which might be interpreted as showing that a proportion of patients are cured. However, on a logarithmic scale, curve B is shown to be a straight line (i.e. exponential), indicating that the rate of death has remained constant with time, the slope of the line giving the rate. This shows that up to the 3-year point there is no evidence of cure in the group in question.

Survival in clinical trials is often depicted as an *actuarial survival curve*. This may be thought of as a prediction of how the final survival curve will look if all the cases have similar survival characteristics to those which have been followed longest. In curve A in Figure 2.8, the survival curve up to 10 years is based on complete 10-year follow-up on all patients. Curve B is an actuarial survival curve. The curve is similar in shape to curve A for the first 2 years (when there are most observations) but appears to show improved survival thereafter. Such a conclusion would be unwise, however, because of the small number of observations between 2 and 4 years on which the curve is

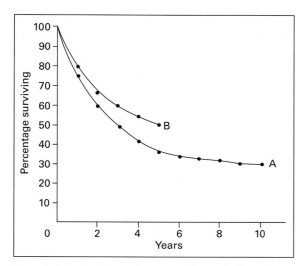

Figure 2.8 Survival in ovarian cancer (all stages). Curve A represents survival of a group of patients where all patients had been diagnosed at least 10 years previously. Curve B is an actuarial survival curve: none of these patients had been diagnosed more than 5 years previously and some had been diagnosed only 2 years previously (see text).

based. It would not need many deaths to occur to alter the shape of curve B to that of curve A. These curves are therefore less reliable in the 'tails' (i.e. at longer time intervals) because only a proportion of patients have been followed for a long time and for some cancers the number of late survivors is relatively small. This means that the tail of the curve is based on only a few events.

Assessment of results: trials of treatment

Many of the basic methods and techniques of treatment in cancer have been developed by experienced physicians and surgeons using their common sense. When the treatment has resulted in a clear improvement, as was the case, for example, when mastectomy was first introduced to treat patients with breast cancer, this approach has worked satisfactorily because it was clear that surgery was better than no treatment. When differences in treatment results have been less obvious, for example, in the case of simple mastectomy compared with lumpectomy, the benefits are smaller and, therefore, are more difficult to measure accurately.

The problem of assessment of results is made more complex by changing criteria for diagnosis and treatment during the period in question. For example, refined methods of detection of metastases at presentation, such as computed tomography (CT), may result in patients being rejected for a treatment which in earlier days they would have received. This means survival may alter as a result of a change in selection in the characteristics of the patients being included in the series being treated. This hidden change might then result in improved outcome being wrongly attributed to a treatment.

Randomized trials

It is now generally accepted that the only way to avoid these and other biases in assessing new treatments is to carry out a randomized prospective comparison of the new treatment with the best standard regimen, or in some cases with no treatment. In this way, hidden factors in case selection, such as histological subtypes, presence of occult metastases and site of tumour, will be randomly distributed in the two groups. Similarly, factors which are not known to be associated with prognosis at the start of the trial, but which are later shown to be so, do not bias the results since these factors will be equally represented in each of the randomly allocated groups, especially if the number of patients is large.

When an analysis of the effect of different treatments is made, the data may be examined for effect on survival or disease-free survival. The results are typically presented as actuarial survival or disease-free survival curves. There are several points to remember. The curves are actuarial curves: this means that not all the patients have been followed until relapse or death. If the number of long-term survivors is small, the tails of the curves may be unstable as discussed above. If a difference in outcome is suggested, the probability of this happening by chance can be assessed by statistical methods. The log-rank test is a convenient and commonly used method of comparing survival and disease-free survival curves. The test is especially appropriate for survival curves which separate to reveal a consistent survival difference (i.e. where the hazard ratio remains at the same proportion throughout the follow-up period). Other tests are more sensitive to early differences that become less apparent later. If a difference in disease-free survival is demonstrated, it represents a delay in onset of recurrence. As previously explained, this may not be reflected in improved survival. This apparent discrepancy may be because although there is a delay in onset of metastases or local recurrence in one of the groups leading to an improved disease-free survival, at the time of recurrence patients might benefit from other treatments so that the overall survival curves are less divergent. Early effects of this type on disease-free survival are often seen in cancer treatment. Delay of

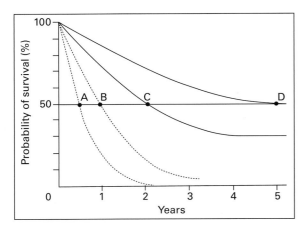

Figure 2.9 Median survival in cancer trials. Trial 1 (dotted lines) median survival: A, 6 months; B, 1 year. Trial 2 (continuous lines) median survival: C, 2 years; D, 5 years. The differences are reliable in trial 1 but less so in trial 2.

recurrence is certainly desirable but, for most treatments, improved survival is the real objective.

A commonly used method of presentation of results is to quote *median* survival, namely, the time from randomization at which 50% of the patients will be alive. These figures are unreliable unless the death rate in the 25–75% range is high and the number of patients in the study is large. This point is illustrated in Figure 2.9. *Mean* survival times are often misleading because they can be greatly affected by one or two long-term survivors. Analysis of the proportion surviving at a single point in time makes use of only part of the data available. A survival curve analysis is preferred because it makes use of the whole time-span of the study.

It should also be remembered that tests of significance merely provide estimates of the probability that an observed difference (or a more extreme one) could have arisen by chance. There are many considerations besides the probability level which should affect one's judgement about whether the difference is interesting or important, and whether or not it is solely the result of the treatment.

In designing a prospective randomized trial of treatment many factors must be taken into account, some of which may affect the value of the study.

1 *Can a single question be asked?* Wherever possible the hypothesis being tested should be as simple as possible. For example, can the study ask the question 'Is this treatment better than no treatment at all?' A simple study design is always preferable but sometimes not possible. Studies in which there is a 'cross-over' from one

treatment to another on relapse are sometimes hard to interpret. Studies that include several randomized groups will usually have to be very large if they are to detect realistic differences between the groups.

2 *Which patients will be included?* A precise statement must be made of the type of patient on which the treatments are to be tested.

3 *Are there known prognostic factors?* Patients with limited-stage small-cell lung cancer (SCLC) have a better prognosis than those with extensive disease. In trials of treatment in SCLC it is advisable to randomize limited and extensive category patients separately to ensure balanced numbers of each group in each arm of the study. This is termed *stratification*. Major prognostic criteria should be stratified, but too many stratifications can cause confusion and are unnecessary in a large trial.

4 *What is the end-point?* Some trials will be concerned with differences in survival, others with disease-free interval, others with local recurrence. In some studies differences in median survival may be shown without any change in the final long-term survival. An example is a trial of the treatment of advanced or metastatic cancer with cytotoxic drugs. Although all patients may die of the disease in both treated and untreated groups, death might be delayed by treatment. Such differences may be clinically worthwhile, especially if associated with symptomatic relief and minimal toxicity.

5 *Is the difference between the treatments in question likely to be large?* This is seldom the case in cancer, where if the effect of the therapy is dramatic, the trial would probably not be considered necessary or justified. To detect absolute differences in survival of 10% with a significance level of 0.05, between 160 and 500 patients will be needed per patient group, the numbers varying with the proportion surviving. It requires fewer patients to show a 10% survival difference between 10 and 20% (a doubling of survival) than between 40 and 50% (an increase of one-quarter). Figure 2.10(a) illustrates the basis of the calculations of sample size. It can be seen that the reliable detection of small survival differences, and a precise estimation of the size of the effect, require very large numbers of patients. Because of the very large numbers of patients necessary to detect even smaller differences with confidence, many cancer trials are collaborative efforts between different centres. Indeed, for rare diseases such as leukaemia or osteosarcoma, treatment trials are almost impossible without such collaboration.

6 *The difficulties of collaboration are considerable.* Investigators participating in the study must agree on what is the

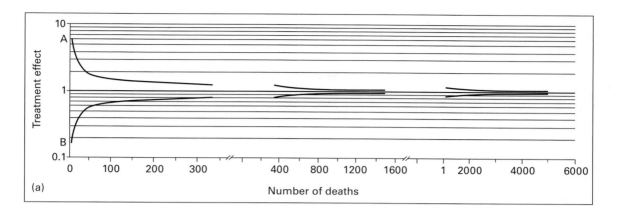

(a)

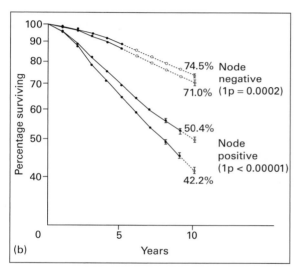

(b)

most important question to answer: how the treatment should be administered (including details of surgery, radiotherapy and chemotherapy); what the documentation should be and how it should be organized; who will pay for the study; who will analyse the data; and so on. In a disease like breast cancer, where the rate of death is low, the answers may not be available for 10 years or more. Physicians are usually, to put it kindly, 'individualistic' in their approach to treatment and large-scale trials sometimes acquire a design which proves an unsatisfactory compromise. Exceptionally intensive treatments cannot be carried out in every hospital and may not be of the same quality as when undertaken by a few specialized units. Such treatments may be 'watered down' in order to include more centres, possibly weakening the intention of the study.

7 *Even if the differences in survival are small, they may be clinically worthwhile.* Dramatic advances in treatment are rare. Large randomized studies are usually carried out where it is not clear if one treatment is better than another and differences are, therefore, likely to be small. However, a small difference may lead to a change in clinical practice. In breast cancer in postmenopausal women following local therapy, treatment with a drug such as tamoxifen improves survival by 8%. This is a major contribution to management because in 20 000 women, 1600 lives can be saved with negligible toxicity. Conversely, some might regard a 7% improvement achieved with cytotoxic chemotherapy as less compelling, due to the greater toxicity of the treatment (although most patients do not take this view). In Europe an 8% improvement in mortality in breast cancer would save 64 000 lives each year. This is a greater saving than that achieved by the successful treatment of diseases such as lymphoma or leukaemia.

Figure 2.10 (a) In a comparison between treatments A and B the darker line at 1 is the line of equivalence between the treatments. The curves represent the 95% confidence intervals for this line. For a result to be significantly different it must lie outside this line. Each horizontal line represents a relative difference of 20% between treatments. A difference of 30% in favour of B will be seen only if there are more than 300 deaths in the study; a difference of 5–10% will require several thousand deaths to be observed. (b) Results of treatment trials of adjuvant tamoxifen in operable breast cancer. An overview of analysis of many thousands of randomized patients allows a significant survival benefit to be demonstrated in the range of 4–8% with different treatments.

There is a growing awareness that our expectations of likely improvements in survival with cancer treatments need to be revised downwards. We cannot expect 20% absolute improvements in survival. We might expect 10–20% improvements in relative survival (from 40% to 44–48%) but such improvements require trials much larger in size than those which we have been accustomed to perform [15]. The reason is shown in Figure 2.10(a). Failure to achieve these numbers leads to false-negative results. Figure 2.10(b) shows the results of treatment trials of adjuvant chemotherapy and/or tamoxifen in breast cancer. The trials were usually small so the 95% confidence intervals overlapped with 'no effect' (see Figure 13.7). The combined dataset shows a clear difference with a reduction of relative risk of 22% (7% increase in 5-year survival) and the confidence intervals are separated from the point where no effect is observed. Trials designed to recruit thousands of patients need to be of simple design and execution, with flexible entry criteria, and must concern a widely practicable treatment. The organization and execution of these studies is a major task for cancer specialists.

Analysis of the results of randomized trials

Just as it is essential not to be too impressed by dramatic results from uncontrolled studies, it is important not to be intimidated by the authority which randomized clinical trials appear to possess. A critical approach is needed. Some points to watch out for include the following.

1 *Is it likely that a false-positive result (type I error) or false-negative result (type II error) has occurred?* False-positive errors are uncommon. False-negative errors are more common, but negative trials are not published as frequently as positive ones because journal editors tend to prefer 'positive' results. Does the trial accord with other studies addressing the same point?

2 *Were the treatments genuinely randomized?* Authors sometimes claim their study was randomized, but closer inspection of the method reveals it was not. These studies are nearly always misleading.

3 *Did one particular group of patients benefit?* This is an important matter because it allows treatment to be offered selectively and suggests future directions for study. However, it is almost impossible to draw firm conclusions about subgroups from a single study unless it contains thousands of patients.

4 *Have all the patients been included in the analysis?* If not, why not? Sometimes patients who cannot be evaluated are discarded from the report. One should be aware of this, particularly if it occurs for large numbers of patients. One reason sometimes given is that the patient only completed one part of the treatment before deteriorating. This practice will obviously greatly improve the apparent results because early failures are not included. It is a major error in the practice of clinical trials and means that the trial results are unreliable.

5 *Has the trial run for sufficient time to allow enough events (deaths, relapses) to have occurred?* What are the confidence intervals for the treatment difference? A statement of the 95% confidence limits for the treatment difference allows the reader to judge the result being presented and is more informative than a *P*-value from a significance test. A *P*-value indicates the level of statistical significance. What the clinician also needs to know is the degree of likely difference. If the confidence interval for the difference in survival between two treatments ranges from −4% to +15% with a point estimate of 7%, this will be regarded differently from an outcome where the confidence interval ranges from +4% to +20% with a point estimate of 11%. Although both results may be 'significant', the latter result is more compelling both because the difference is larger and the certainty of benefit greater since the confidence intervals do not cross zero, the point of equivalence.

A recent development, and one that causes some concern, is the introduction of 'stopping guidelines' and their use by data safety and monitoring committees. These are statistical methods for the detection of survival differences early in a trial. They were originally introduced to prevent early closure of studies because an effect appeared to be present. Unfortunately, these guidelines are sometimes used rigidly to stop trials when it has been shown that a treatment effect is present but result in uncertainty about the size of the effect since there are not enough events to make a precise estimate. This practice misses one of the central aims of trials, which is to provide convincing evidence of a clinically worthwhile effect if one is present. This means that the size of any difference must be estimated *with as much precision as possible*. This usually requires large numbers of patients to be followed over long periods.

Informed consent

Before starting any treatment most clinicians will want to discuss the benefits and problems of treatment and the possible different approaches that might be used. In a clinical trial, doctors also have to discuss the reason for the study, the meaning of randomization and the right of the patient not to be involved. This creates problems for both doctors and patient. Their relationship may be upset by these disclosures, especially the admission that the results of the treatments are not known with certainty. There may have to be discussion of failure rates in the disease. The patient may become confused, and the time necessary for explanation discourages entry into trials. Several studies have shown that patients find the concept of random allocation of treatment, for a disease as serious as cancer, to be a major factor in refusing to take part in trials.

Non-randomized studies of treatment

The difficulties of controlled trials of treatment have led many investigators to perform uncontrolled studies and to report survival with a given treatment in the hope that a clear advantage over the best current methods of treatment will be shown. There is an important role for well-conducted pilot studies, but the results are often misleading or wrong and must be interpreted cautiously.

A compromise has been sought between the cumbersome controlled trial and the unreliable uncontrolled study. This has involved the use of *historical controls* which compare a new treatment to patients treated in the past. An attempt is normally, but not always, made to match the controls for age, sex, site and stage of tumour, and other known prognostic factors such as histological grade and menopausal status. The problems are that staging methods are changing continually, that selection of control cases may not be impartial and that not all prognostic factors will be known.

These studies may sometimes point the way in management and indicate which questions should be asked in large-scale prospective studies. Another variant is the use of 'databases' containing results of treatment of very large numbers of patients. Such analyses have the same problems of selection bias and thus the same unreliability in deciding on the value of a treatment.

Screening for cancer

The aim of screening a population for cancer is to make the diagnosis early and thereby increase the cure rate. When a previously unscreened population undergoes screening, a relatively large number of *prevalence* cases are detected. When this same, previously screened, population undergoes subsequent screening procedures, the number of new, *incidence*, cases is much smaller and the cost per case detected therefore greater. The problem is simply summarized in Figure 2.11. The objective of

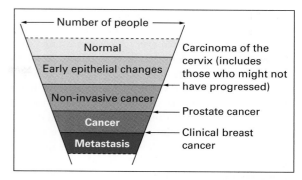

Figure 2.11 The later in the natural history, the fewer 'false positives', but there is less chance to alter the outcome.

screening is simple yet there are many problems and assumptions involved.

1 *What is the sensitivity of the test used?* Highly sensitive tests are essential if the disease is curable early and if the consequences of a false-positive test are not physically or psychologically serious for the patients. The Papanicolaou smear is a sensitive test for cervical cancer and the diagnosis can be easily confirmed on biopsy. Screening by ultrasound and serum CA-125 is much less sensitive but may prove to be of value for ovarian cancer. Plasma PSA is a sensitive test for prostatic carcinoma but the consequences for management of a positive result are not well defined [16].

2 *Is the disease curable if diagnosed early?* Carcinoma *in situ* or locally invasive carcinoma of the cervix is a curable disease. Earlier diagnosis of colorectal cancer using screening by flexible sigmoidoscopy or faecal occult blood testing may increase the cure rate [17]. Tumours such as colorectal cancer present late in their natural history. However, the limit of detection of an established cancer by screening may be only a little earlier than when the tumour would be clinically apparent. The question is, therefore, whether the potential for metastasis is significantly less at the time when such a tumour is detectable by screening methods compared with the stage at which it is clinically apparent.

3 *Is the disease common?* Cancer of the breast, prostate, cervix and lung are so common at certain ages and in certain groups that screening is a practical proposition. Screening a general population for a disease such as gastric carcinoma is less practicable in the UK, but is feasible in Japan where the disease is much more common. Clearly the incidence of the tumour has to be high enough to justify the screening programme.

4 *How frequently should the examination be undertaken, and in which population?* In some countries cervical smears are recommended every 3 years in women aged 20–65 years. In the UK, the recommendation is for all sexually active women to be screened every 5 years. It is not yet clear what recommendations should be made for other investigations such as pelvic or ultrasound examination (for ovarian and uterine cancer) and flexible sigmoidoscopy. The group at greatest risk from ovarian cancer includes nulliparous women over the age of 40 years; and for colorectal cancer, men and women over 50 years. Routine chest radiography, even in smokers, has failed to show any benefit in the early detection of lung cancer. A limited chest CT scan is much more sensitive but its clinical value is unproven.

Patients with a greatly increased genetic predisposition to certain cancers, for example, polyposis coli (see Chapter 16), should have regular checks by the appropriate specialist (Table 2.4). The definition of the populations to be screened will undergo considerable change if, as is likely, identification of genetic predisposition to increased risk becomes a practical proposition in common cancers. In breast cancer, for example, mutations in *BRCA1* and *BRCA2* clearly identify patients at high risk. However, these patients account only for a small proportion of all cases of breast cancer. Common polymorphisms of other genes may contribute to risk, accounting for many more cases. If this proves to be the case the patients at increased risk will clearly be those where more intensive screening is needed, while those women at very low risk might need much less intensive surveillance.

5 *What are the disadvantages of screening?* Routine screening examinations can produce anxiety in the mind of the public at large and in certain individuals, in particular. If applied to the whole population they would require a great expenditure of time and money. The benefits may be small and achieved at great expense. If the yearly incidence of breast cancer in women aged 50–70 years is taken to be 2 per 1000, by screening 10 000 women every 2 years, 40 new cases may be expected. If this is done by mammography and trained nurses in a clinic, the cost might be in the region of £50 per visit. If the cure rate were improved from 40% to 60% by this procedure, then eight lives would have been saved at a cost of £250 000 a year. Screening of this type is,

Table 2.4 Currently used screening methods. Several of these methods are still under investigation to determine their clinical value.

Cervical cancer (Chapter 17): cervical smear
Breast cancer (Chapter 13): mammography
Colorectal cancer (Chapter 16): faecal occult blood testing, rectal examination, flexible sigmoidoscopy
Ovarian and uterine cancer (Chapter 17): pelvic examination, pelvic ultrasound, CA-125
Skin cancers (Chapter 22): self-examination
Gastric cancer, Japan (Chapter 14): radiological and endoscopic examination
Prostate cancer (Chapter 18): prostate-specific antigen
Lung cancer (Chapter 12): chest radiography, spiral CT scan

therefore, more expensive, per life saved, than many high-technology procedures. For some cancers the case for screening is not primarily economic.

The longest established screening procedure in the Western world is the cervical smear for carcinoma of the cervix. Breast cancer screening has now been introduced in the UK and other European countries. There remain concerns as to its cost-effectiveness, and difficulties over the treatment to be recommended when early breast cancer is diagnosed (e.g. ductal carcinoma *in situ*). Screening procedures which have been proposed are shown in Table 2.4.

The most important outcome measure in a screening programme is mortality, which may require prolonged follow-up (e.g. in the case of breast cancer). The efficacy of the screening programme should also be demonstrated by a shift towards diagnosis at an earlier stage of the tumour.

Despite widespread enthusiasm for cancer screening, increasingly recognized as an important political opportunity, the potential advantages are increasingly being questioned. The absolute advantages are generally small, and the relatively frequent problem of a false positive, with the ensuing anxiety and possible further intervention, represent two of the commoner drawbacks. For example, Welch [18] describes the acute problem of ductal carcinoma *in situ* (DCIS), sometimes just a few millimetres across, a diagnosis over 10 times as common nowadays as in the 1970s. While the true natural history of DCIS remains uncertain, it is often treated as invasive cancer with regard to surgical options (see page 83 in ref. 18). However, most of the evidence suggests that what is diagnosed as DCIS is in fact a 'pseudo-disease', since most women whose DCIS is missed at biopsy do not go on to develop invasive breast cancer [19].

Secondary prevention of cancer

Some cancers arise in a 'field' of malignant change in which the tissue adjacent to a cancer has been subject to the same carcinogenic process that gave rise to the initial tumour. The clearest example of this is squamous carcinoma of the upper aerodigestive tract – mouth, pharynx, oesophagus and bronchi – which have been exposed to cigarette smoke. In the case of head and neck cancer, after successful therapy, 30–50% of patients develop local or regional recurrence and 10–40% a second primary tumour.

In recent years, it has been shown that vitamin A analogues are able to modulate the differentiation of epithelial cells, can cause regression of the lesions of leucoplakia and diminish the likelihood of developing squamous cancer as long as treatment continues. Isotretinoin (13-*cis*-retinoic acid), given as an adjuvant following treatment of head and neck cancer, greatly diminishes the risk of second cancers developing but does not diminish the likelihood of recurrence. This interesting finding opened the way to other secondary prevention. However, recent trials have shown a deleterious effect in lung cancer. The breast cancer overview [20] has shown a decreased risk of cancer in the contralateral breast in women taking tamoxifen as adjuvant therapy following surgery for breast cancer. This had led to randomized trials of tamoxifen as a primary preventive measure in women at high risk of developing breast cancer. The ATAC trial [21] has demonstrated a similar effect for aromatase inhibitors. One of the likely areas of use of immunotherapy in cancer, if effective methods can be found, is in the prevention of recurrence after the successful initial treatment of patients who are at high risk of relapse.

References

1 Million Women Study Collaborators. Breast cancer and hormone replacement therapy in the Million Women Study. *Lancet* 2003; 362: 419–27.

2 Doll R, Hill AB. A study of the aetiology of carcinoma of the lung. *Br Med J* 1952; 2: 1271–86.

3 Coleman MP, Estève J. Trends in cancer incidence and mortality in the United Kingdom. In: *Cancer Statistics: Registrations of Cancer Diagnosed in England and Wales.* Series MB1 no. 22. London: HMSO, 1989: 8–13.

4 Haenszel W, Kurihera M. Studies of Japanese migrants. 1. Mortality from cancer and other diseases among Japanese in the United States. *J Natl Cancer Inst* 1968; 40: 43–68.

5 Kinlen L, Doll R. Population mixing and childhood leukaemia: Fallon and other US clusters. *Br J Cancer* 2004; 91: 1–3.

6 Calle EE, Rodriguez C, Walker-Thurmond K, Thun MJ. Overweight, obesity, and mortality from cancer in a prospectively studied cohort of US adults. *N Engl J Med* 2003; 348: 1625–38.

7 Sproston K, Primatesta P, eds. *Health Survey for England 2002 vol. 1: The Health of Children and Young People.* London: The Stationery Office, 2003.

8 Bjelakovic G, Nikolova D, Simonetti RG *et al.* Antioxidant supplements for prevention of gastrointestinal cancers: a systematic review and meta-analysis. *Lancet* 2004; 364: 1219.

9 Armstrong BK, Kricker A. Epidemiology of sun exposure and skin cancer. *Cancer Surv* 1996; 26: 133–53.

10 de Gonzales AB, Darby S. Risk of cancer from diagnostic X rays: estimates for the UK and 14 other countries. *Lancet* 2003; 362: 1–8.

11 Darby S, Hill D, Auvinen A *et al.* Radon in homes and risk of lung cancer: collaborative analysis of individual data from 13 European case–control studies. *Br Med J* 2005; 33: 223.

12 Peto J, Hodgson JT, Matthews FE, Jones JR. Continuing increase in mesothelioma mortality in Britain. *Lancet* 1995; 345: 535–9.

13 Klein G. Epstein–Barr virus strategy in normal and neoplastic B cells. *Cell* 1994; 77: 791–3.

14 Martin JN, Ganem DE, Osmond DH *et al.* Sexual transmission and the natural history of human herpesvirus 8 infection. *N Engl J Med* 1998; 338: 948–54.

15 Yusuf S, Collins R, Peto R. Why do we need some large, simple randomized trials? *Stat Med* 1984; 3: 409–22.

16 Ganz PA, Litwin MS. Prostate cancer: the price of early detection. *J Clin Oncol* 2001; 19: 1587–8.

17 Hardcastle JD, Thomas WM, Chamberlain J *et al.* Randomised controlled trial of faecal occult blood screening for

colorectal cancer: results of the first 107,349 subjects. *Lancet* 1989; 1: 1160–4.

18 Welch HG. *Should I Be Tested for Cancer? Maybe Not and Here's Why*. Berkeley, CA: University of California Press, 2004.

19 Lagios MD, Margolin FR, Westdahl PR, Rose MR. Mammographically detected ductal carcinoma in situ: frequency of local recurrence following tylectomy and prognostic effect of nuclear grade on local recurrence. *Cancer* 1989; 63: 618–24.

20 Early Breast Cancer Trialist's Collaborative Group. Tamoxifen for early breast cancer: an overview of the randomized trials. *Lancet* 1998; 351: 1451–67.

21 ATAC Trialists' Group. Results of the ATAC (Animidex, Tamoxifen, Alone or in Combination) trial after completion of 5 years' adjuvant treatment for breast cancer. *Lancet* 2005; 365: 60–2.

Further reading

Collingridge D. Three countries – half the global cancer burden. *Lancet Oncol* 2014; 15: 483.

Goss PE, Strasser-Weippl K, Lee-Bychkovsky B *et al.* Challenges to effective cancer control in China, India, and Russia. *Lancet Oncol* 2014; 15: 489–538.

World Health Organization. Global status report on non-communicable diseases 2010. Chapter 4: Prevention. Chapter 5: Early detection of cancer. Geneva, W H O 2011. ISBN 978 92 4 068645 8 (PDF), 978 92 4 156422 9, (NLM classification: WT 500).

3 Biology of cancer

Several steps occur during the transformation of a normal cell into a cancer cell (Figure 3.1). The properties of cancer cells have been summarized in a classic article by Hanahan and Weinberg [1] subsequently updated [2] and are listed in Table 3.1. Some or all of these features apply to all cancers. An important property of cancer cells is genomic instability, which has critical implications for therapy as such instability allows the evolution of resistant clones. This chapter aims to give a brief summary of some of these events, especially from the point of view of their relevance to therapy. Readers are recommended to refer to a recent excellent text, which address these topics in detail [3].

Carcinogenesis: persistent genetic damage

Chemical carcinogens
It has long been known that cancers may arise from chemical causes. In 1775 Sir Percival Pott noticed an unusually large number of cases of cancer of the scrotum in chimney-sweeps. In 1895 Rehn pointed out the high frequency of bladder cancer in dye factory workers. Since that time many carcinogens have been identified in the environment and in food (Table 3.2). Cigarette smoke is by far the most important carcinogen. Some of the mechanisms of chemical carcinogenesis have now been elucidated.

Polycyclic hydrocarbons and inhaled carcinogens
These chemicals are among the products of combustion of carbon-containing materials. They are present in cigarette smoke, coal tar, car exhaust fumes and some cooked foods. Following the demonstration that benzanthracene was present in coal tar and was carcinogenic, 3,4-benzpyrene was isolated from coal tar and was also shown to be capable of inducing skin cancers in animals. Not all polycyclic hydrocarbons are carcinogens. It appears that the carcinogenic property resides in one region of the molecule, to which oxygen is added in a reaction catalysed by cellular enzymes. This portion of the molecule reacts with cellular DNA, especially with guanine bases. This reaction with DNA is probably responsible for its carcinogenic effect.

Nitrosamines
Dimethylnitrosamine was shown to cause liver cancer in animals when added to diet. Nitrites, which are present

Cancer and its Management, Seventh Edition. Jeffrey Tobias and Daniel Hochhauser.
© 2015 John Wiley & Sons, Ltd. Published 2015 by John Wiley & Sons, Ltd.

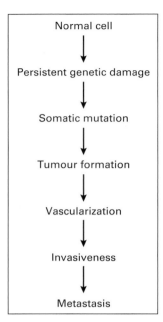

Figure 3.1 Steps in the development of a metastasizing cancer.

Table 3.1 Biological hallmarks of cancer.

Self-sufficient proliferation of growth
Refractory to inhibitory signals
Survival without survival signals
Unlimited replicative potential
Recruitment of blood supply
Invasion and metastasis
Loss of genomic stability

Source: Hanahan and Weinberg, 2000 [1]. Reproduced with permission from Elsevier.

Table 3.2 Some chemical carcinogens.

Polycyclic hydrocarbons: 3,4-benzpyrene
Nitrosamines: dimethylnitrosamine
Aromatic amines and azo dyes: α-naphthylamine, dimethylamino-azobenzene, benzidine
Plant products: aflatoxin, Senecis (producing pyrrolozidium)
Alkylating agents: nitrogen, melphalan, nitrosourea, etoposide
Inorganic chemicals: arsenic, nickel, asbestos, cadmium

---

in many foods, are converted to nitrous acid in the stomach and may then react with amines in food to produce nitrosamines. Thus a mechanism exists for the formation of a potential carcinogen from food. However, there is no conclusive evidence that the formation of nitrosamines is important in carcinogenesis in humans.

Aromatic amines and azo dyes

Following Rehn's original observation of the increased frequency of bladder cancer in aniline dye workers, the aniline derivatives α-naphthylamine and benzidine were shown to be carcinogens. Later, azo dye derivatives were also found to be carcinogenic, including dimethylamino-azobenzene (butter yellow) which was used to add colour to margarine. When ingested, these substances produce cancers at sites remote from the gut. They are first metabolized to an active form which is the carcinogen. For example, α-naphthylamine is hydroxylated to a carcinogen which is then glucuronated to an inactive water-soluble form in the liver and excreted in the urine. Glucuronidases in the bladder mucosa liberate the active carcinogen. The cancers develop only in those species that possess this bladder enzyme. The liberated aminophenol reacts directly with guanine bases in DNA and, as with polycyclic hydrocarbons, this is presumed to be the basis of their carcinogenic action. In humans there is a 20-year latent period between exposure and the development of bladder cancer. Cigarette smoke also contains 3-naphthylamine, and bladder cancer is associated with smoking.

Aflatoxin

This toxin is produced by *Aspergillus flavus*, which may contaminate staple foods. It is a carcinogen in hepatic cancer and there is an association between dietary aflatoxin and the high frequency of hepatic cancers, although direct proof is lacking. The hepatitis B virus (HBV) is involved in the development of a hepatoma, aflatoxin perhaps acting as a promoter (see below). The toxin is a complex molecule that is metabolized by the same pathway as polycyclic hydrocarbons, and the products react with DNA.

Cytotoxic drugs

Several drugs used in the treatment of cancer are also carcinogens and this is particularly the case with DNA-interactive agents. Alkylating agents bind directly to DNA and their use has been associated with the development of second malignancies, for example, acute myeloid leukaemia (AML) in patients successfully treated for Hodgkin's disease or ovarian cancer. The epipodophyllotoxin etoposide is also linked with a risk of secondary AML associated with the characteristic 11q23 translocation; this is related to the cumulative total dose. However, despite the widespread use of DNA-interactive agents, the overall incidence of secondary cancers is low and the benefits of these agents far outweigh the risks. However, these observations do emphasise the need for caution regarding long-term effects of the use of cytotoxic agents.

Ionizing and ultraviolet irradiation

Irradiation produces breaks in DNA strands and chromosomal abnormalities such as fragmentation, deletions and translocations. These abnormalities may lead to cell death in dividing cells but under certain circumstances may induce oncogenic effects. However, the mechanisms of carcinogenesis are poorly understood. Skin cancers and bone cancers are caused by therapeutic radiation. In the survivors of the atom bomb explosions at Hiroshima and Nagasaki there is a dose-related increase in acute and chronic myeloid leukaemia and in breast and thyroid cancer.

It is difficult to extrapolate from the high dose received after the atom bomb explosions to an assessment of the risks from the much smaller levels of background radiation. The average exposure as a result of toxic waste is 0.001 mSv (millisievert) with a maximum of 0.3 mSv. The average dose from clinical X-rays is 0.3 mSv (the same as from cosmic rays). The average annual total dose in the UK from all sources is about 2.5 mSv. Estimates now place the death rate at about three to five cases per 100 000 per millisievert of prolonged exposure. This would account for perhaps 2000 cancer deaths per year out of 160 000 annually in the UK. Radon gas is one of the most important sources of background radiation and increases the risk of lung cancer especially. Radiation exposure is a less important cause of cancer than cigarette smoking, and industrial exposure is the least important source of background radiation and increases the risk of lung cancer, especially in smokers. Sarcomas of bone and soft tissue may be caused from radiation, and represent one of many reasons for limiting the use of therapeutic radiation in treating cancers of children. This is discussed further in Chapter 23.

Ultraviolet (UV) light increases the likelihood of development of skin cancer (see Chapter 22). DNA absorbs photons, and alterations in thymine bases occur with the formation of dimers. In normal individuals these pyrimidine dimers are rapidly repaired by nucleotide excision repair. Faulty repair leads to base mismatch mutations. In xeroderma pigmentosum the DNA repair process is faulty, leading to an excess of UV-induced skin cancers (though not cancers at other sites).

Initiators and promoters in carcinogenesis

Some agents appear to act as 'initiators' (Figure 3.2): they produce a permanent change in the cells with which they come in contact but do not themselves cause cancer. This contact may result in a gene mutation. Other agents act as 'promoters', producing transient changes and causing cancer only when they are repeatedly in contact with cells that have been 'initiated' by another compound. From a clinical point of view, cancers are more likely to arise as a result of long-continued exposure to an agent, and removal of the agent may result in stabilization or even gradual reversal of the increased risk. The reduction in incidence of lung cancer following cessation of cigarette smoking is an example of how the risk of developing cancer can be reduced by removal of the stimulus.

Repair of damage to DNA induced by carcinogens

The action of chemical carcinogens leads to damage to DNA. The production of permanent DNA damage, and the development of the subsequent disorganization of chromosomal DNA that is the characteristic of an established cancer, depends on the nature of the chemical

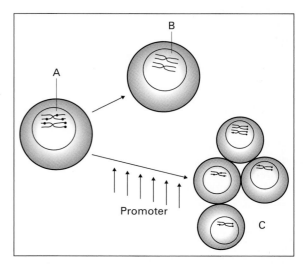

Figure 3.2 Initiators and promoters in carcinogenesis. In stage A, chromosomal damage is caused by an initiator. This might be repaired (as in B) or, under the influence of a promoter, give rise to neoplastic growth (stage C).

adduct, the duration of exposure and, importantly, on the efficiency of cellular repair processes. DNA repair is thus central to the process of carcinogenesis. Many of the hereditary cancer syndromes have been shown to be due to mutation in essential DNA repair genes, resulting in impaired repair over a lifetime. The process of repair is through several mechanisms. The processes are essential mechanisms for survival for all living cells. Actively transcribed genes are repaired more efficiently than inactive genes. In *base excision repair* the abnormal DNA base is excised enzymatically, first by endonucleases which cleave the DNA strand, then by exonucleases which remove the abnormal segment, followed by the action of a polymerase which resynthesizes the missing segment. This is then joined to the strand by a ligase. More complex chemical lesions, such as those made by alkylating agents and UV light, are repaired by *nucleotide excision repair* in which there is excision of a longer strand of DNA, the strand then being resynthesized by a DNA polymerase.

Radiation causes both single- and double-strand breaks in DNA. Specific processes repair these two types of lesion. The double-strand break is the lethal lesion responsible for the cell-killing effect, but the mechanism of radiation-induced carcinogenesis is less well understood.

Inherited defects involving DNA damage or repair processes that predispose to cancer

Genetic predisposition to cancer may be mediated through change in function of genes involved in many aspects of cell growth and division. Genes that control the stability and integrity of DNA are especially important, both in correcting damage that arises spontaneously during the life of the cell – for example, due to oxygen reacting with DNA – and during cell division, and in repairing the damage caused by external agents. Many of the inherited syndromes of cancer susceptibility are due to mutations in genes involved in the maintenance of DNA integrity.

• *Genes that regulate the conversion of potentially toxic agents to their active form, and their detoxification.* These are processes that are dependent on enzymes in organs such as the gut, kidney and liver. They are described in more detail in Chapter 6. Common polymorphisms of these genes may account for differences in susceptibility to DNA damage and thus to carcinogenesis.
• *Genes that repair mismatches of DNA base pairs.* Mutation in one of this family of genes causes hereditary

non-polyposis colorectal cancer, an autosomal dominant trait that accounts for 5% of all such cancers.
• *Genes that maintain the genetic stability of the cell.* The *p53* gene (see below) is a critical mediator of cell cycle progression following DNA damage. Activation of *p53* protein results in cell cycle arrest, which allows repair of damaged DNA or induction of apoptosis. Several hereditary cancer syndromes are due to defects in these genes (Li–Fraumeni syndrome due to *p53* mutation, retinoblastoma due to *Rb* gene mutation).
• *Genes that are directly involved in maintaining the structure of DNA and in repairing damage.* Hereditary non-polyposis colon cancer is due to mutations in mismatch repair genes. The gene mutation causing Bloom's syndrome impairs the normal maintenance of DNA structure. The *BRCA1* and *BRCA2* genes are involved in homologous recombination repair of DNA damage; carriers of mutations in these genes have a high incidence of breast and ovarian cancer following loss of the wild type allele. Other genes including *PALB2, CHEK2, ATM* and *BRIP1*, which interact with BRCA1 and BRCA2, also play a role in hereditary predisposition to these cancers [4].

Viral causes of cancer

In 1910, Peyton Rous showed that a cell-free filtrate made from avian sarcomas could induce sarcomas in chickens, and at the same time the disease avian myeloblastosis was shown to be viral in origin. Later it was realized that viruses might require a long latent period before the tumour appeared. However, it was not until the 1960s that it was appreciated that incorporation of viral DNA into the host genome could result in malignant transformation, and that the infectious virus might not be isolated from the cancer cell.

Two patterns of viral oncogenesis have been described. In both instances the viral genome is incorporated into the cellular DNA. In the first, the virus has genes, *oncogenes*, which transform the cell in culture and cause tumours *in vivo*. The action of the oncogene dominates the cell. In the second, the virus acts slowly and tumours take longer to appear. These viruses do not transform cells in culture.

RNA viruses

RNA viruses are implicated in the production of a wide variety of tumours in animals, notably lymphomas, leukaemias and sarcomas. The virus contains two identical RNA molecules within a glycoprotein envelope together with the duplex enzyme reverse transcriptase. Through the action of this enzyme the viruses are able to make the cell synthesize a sequence of DNA, complementary to their RNA, which is incorporated into the host DNA. The action of this incorporated DNA leads to the manufacture of new viral proteins, envelope and reverse transcriptase by the cell (Figure 3.3). They are, therefore, called *retroviruses*.

Some retroviruses (e.g. avian leukosis, feline and murine leukaemia) have only three genes and have a long incubation period before producing the tumour in animals. Others rapidly transform cells and are usually isolated from tumours in culture, an example being the Rous sarcoma virus (RSV). RSV has been shown to contain a gene (v-*src*) that appears to be the gene responsible for transformation of fibroblasts in culture. This gene codes for a protein kinase which phosphorylates tyrosine. It has become apparent that normal and malignant cells contain DNA sequences which are similar

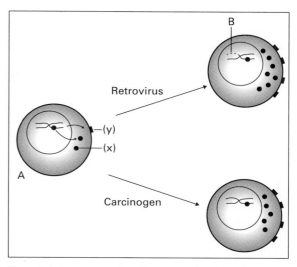

Figure 3.4 Oncogenes and malignant transformation. In stage A, a normal cell has a low level of proto-oncogene activity producing a growth factor (x), or a differentiation protein or a receptor (y). Carcinogens increase the activity of the proto-oncogene and give rise to neoplastic transformation. Alternatively, infection with a retrovirus leads to insertion of viral promoter sequences or oncogenes (B) and excess oncogene activity, also resulting in neoplastic transformation.

or identical to the oncogenic sequences of RNA tumour viruses. These are known as *cellular proto-oncogenes* (as distinct from viral oncogenes). It is postulated that these cellular oncogenes, when activated by DNA mutations, activate pathways resulting in malignant transformation (Figure 3.4). It has been suggested that retroviruses have incorporated these cellular genes into the viral genome during evolution.

The mechanisms of action of the products of gene activation produced by the viruses are now better understood. Examples of these mechanisms are the phosphokinase produced by *src* and other viral oncogenes; epidermal growth factor (EGF) receptor by the v-*erb*B gene; platelet-derived growth factor (PDGF) fragment by the v-*sis* gene; and a variety of nuclear-binding proteins by the avian leukaemia virus.

Viral oncogene products often differ from their normal cellular counterparts. They lack introns and may have structural differences. For example, the v-*erb* product is the homologue of the cellular receptor for EGF but lacks part of the extracellular domain including the EGF-binding site. Together with loss of a cytoplasmic site for autophosphorylation the virally coded receptor is permanently 'switched on'. Normal and malignant cells

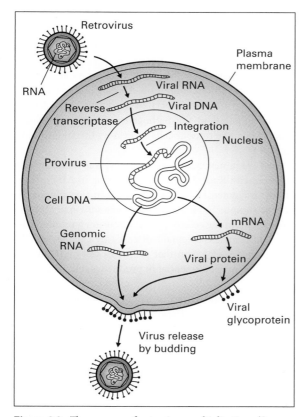

Figure 3.3 The process of retrovirus multiplication. (Source: Cancer Research UK 2006. Reproduced with permission.)

contain DNA sequences which are similar or identical to the oncogenic sequences of RNA tumour viruses. These cellular oncogenes, when over-expressed or activated by mutation, cause the events leading to malignant transformation (see Figure 3.4).

A virus may activate cellular processes by inserting a promoter or enhancer sequence adjacent to the region of a cellular growth-regulating oncogene, disturbing its normal process of control of transcription. This process of *insertional mutagenesis* may be very complex. An example is the insertion of a viral long terminal repeat (LTR) sequence. This DNA sequence may be able to initiate transcription in either direction on the DNA strand, allowing transcription of both viral and cellular genes. This occurs with the avian leukosis virus which is integrated next to c-*myc*, thereby activating it.

The first retrovirus to be definitely associated with malignancy was the human T-cell leukaemia virus (HTLV)-1, isolated from chronic cutaneous T-cell lymphoma. The virus is widely distributed, and transmitted sexually, by intravenous drug abuse and perinatally. It is prevalent in tropical countries, but in the USA seropositivity is 1 in 4000. In addition to the association with T-cell leukaemia, it is the cause of tropical spastic paraplegia. The risk of disease over 20 years of seropositivity is about 5%. One of the viral genes, *tax*, stimulates the cellular genes to produce interleukin (IL)-2 and IL-2 receptor, which stimulate T-cell division.

Retroviruses may be indirectly carcinogenic as shown by human immunodeficiency virus (HIV)-1, the cause of AIDS. HIV-1 infection is associated with cancers [5]. There are three types that are particularly frequent: intermediate or high-grade B-cell lymphoma; Kaposi's sarcoma, which is associated with a novel herpesvirus called Kaposi's sarcoma herpesvirus (KSHV), also known as human herpesvirus (HHV)8; and cervical carcinoma. Before the advent of effective therapy for HIV infection, about 40% of all patients infected developed a cancer. However, the relationship between the viral infection and the different cancers is complex and appears to be related to the chronic immune suppression, which allows other carcinogenic viruses to produce cancer. The lymphomas also have a complex pathogenesis since they are usually tumours of B cells. These are not infected by HIV-1. Other viruses such as Epstein–Barr virus (EBV) may be involved. Similarly, cervical cancer may be due to a second virus, such as human papillomavirus (HPV), in women who are immunosuppressed by HIV-1. The tumour appears to be particularly aggressive clinically in this situation.

Hepatitis C virus (HCV) is an RNA virus that is now clearly linked to the occurrence of hepatocellular carcinoma. The risk of the tumour arising is 100 times greater in infected persons. The mechanism of viral carcinogenesis is similar to that of HBV (see below) but there is a greater incidence of cirrhosis with HCV, which may be related to evasion of host immune responses. The risk of liver cancer is higher if there is co-infection with HBV. These two viruses infect almost one billion people worldwide.

DNA viruses

DNA viruses have also been implicated in carcinogenesis. The largest of the DNA viruses are those in the herpes group. EBV was first demonstrated in cultured cells from a patient with Burkitt's lymphoma. EBV causes continued proliferation of human B cells *in vitro*. Viral genes maintain the virus in these cells and drive cellular proliferation through activation of cellular growth-regulating genes (oncogenes).

In patients with Burkitt's lymphoma, antibody titres to viral capsid antigen and membrane antigen are higher than in controls. However, many African children are infected with EBV at some time but Burkitt's lymphoma develops in very few, so the mechanism of oncogenesis is not explained by the occurrence of viral infection alone. In addition, some non-African cases of Burkitt's lymphoma are not associated with the virus. EBV is also implicated in the pathogenesis of nasopharyngeal carcinoma, the tumour cells expressing the viral EBNA-1 antigen.

In 1994, a new herpesvirus, KSHV, was found in association with Kaposi's sarcoma occurring in AIDS. This is now designated HHV8 and is found in the spindle cells of the tumour in all cases of Kaposi's sarcoma. HHV8 is also found in the cells of primary effusion lymphoma and in multicentric Castleman's disease (see Chapter 26). The virus encodes a cyclin that promotes cell cycle progression. This may be essential in producing cellular proliferation.

HPVs are the cause of cutaneous warts and some benign papillomas. There are numerous subtypes that have a variable association with cancer. Most viral types produce limited cellular proliferation. Other types have a much greater propensity to cause malignant transformation. The high-risk types are 16, 18, 31 and 33. Over 90% of cases of *in situ* carcinoma of the cervix contain HPV genome sequences. The virus plays a causative role in the invasive and multiple squamous cancers of the skin that frequently occur in patients on long-term immunosuppressive therapy. There is integration of viral DNA into the cells of the basal epithelium. There are eight early and two late viral genes. The early genes E6 and E7 drive the cellular transformation by targeting the *p53* and retinoblastoma (*pRB*) genes, respectively. These genes are frequently inactivated in human cancers and abrogation of their function is associated with multiple tumorigenic events including increased apoptotic threshold and loss of cell cycle checkpoint inhibition.

HBV is associated with the development of hepatocellular carcinoma (see Chapter 15). The risk is 200 times greater than in non-infected persons. The pathways involved in HBV-induced carcinogenesis are complex and involve pathways including host–viral interactions as well as activation of oncogenes by insertion into the host genome. Repeated cycles of necrosis, inflammation and regeneration may contribute to accumulation of mutations and development of cancers. These molecular pathways have been well reviewed [6].

This brief summary shows that an essential mechanism of carcinogenesis is damage to DNA and the efficiency of its repair. The initial damage, if not repaired, is followed at a variable interval by increasing chromosomal instability and somatic mutation. Although many of these mutations will be lethal to the cell, others will not, and the malignant phenotype emerges with accumulation of increasing numbers of deleterious mutations. Our understanding of how this process works has greatly improved in recent years with increased knowledge of the control of the cell cycle and the discovery of key proteins that can halt cell division if the genome is damaged.

An initial mutation in a growth-regulating gene may not be sufficient to produce tumour progression, but a succession of such events will be. The important mutations will be activating mutations in genes that promote cell growth (oncogenes), disabling mutations in those genes that suppress growth (*tumour-suppressor genes*), and mutations in those genes that produce proteins responsible for ensuring that cell division does not take place if DNA is damaged. Successive mutations in several of these genes lead to increasing cellular disorganization and loss of control of cell growth. The next section describes the action of oncogenes and the essential features of the control of the cell cycle.

Cellular oncogenes

The discovery of the sequence homologies between viral oncogenes and DNA found in normal and cancer cells has led to a greater understanding of the growth regulatory mechanisms that may be abnormal in malignant cells.

These are not cancer genes but proliferation-inducing genes whose regulation may be disturbed in cancer and contribute to its development, including invasion and metastasis.

Genes have been identified by homology with retroviral genes by DNA transfer and by gene rearrangements. The mechanisms of activation of the genes are varied. In Burkitt's lymphoma there is reciprocal translocation of part of chromosome 8 with chromosomes 2, 14 or 22. The 8;14 translocation is commonest. The c-*myc* oncogene is adjacent to the part of chromosome 8 which is translocated, and the translocation is accompanied by reorganization of the c-*myc* gene. In chronic granulocytic leukaemia, the c-*abl* oncogene, with its translocation partner *bcr*, forms a fusion protein resulting in permanent expression of growth-inducing tyrosine kinase. Activation of a single proto-oncogene in this way does not often lead to malignancy. Indeed, in chronic myeloid leukaemia, the transformation to an aggressive leukaemia (blast phase) requires additional mutations. Increased expression of cellular oncogenes has been found in many human cancer cell lines, for example, c-*myc* in small-cell lung cancer and Burkitt's lymphoma, and N-*myc* in neuroblastoma. In gastrointestinal stromal tumours, the oncogene c-*KIT* is frequently mutated. This oncogene is the homologue of a viral oncogene (v-*KIT*) that was discovered in feline fibrosarcoma virus. The gene codes for a receptor tyrosine kinase and the mutation activates the kinase. The tyrosine kinase imatinib, developed to block the Abl kinase activated in chronic myeloid leukaemia, also inhibits c-*KIT* leading to tumour regression (Figure 3.5 and also see Chapter 28).

Figure 3.5 shows a simplified scheme of the events following binding of a growth factor to a membrane-associated receptor. The receptor activates a signal-transducing protein, which may in turn bind other molecules such as guanine nucleotides (when the signal transducer is then called a G protein). These molecules in turn may stimulate the activity of a second messenger such as adenosine 3′,5′-cyclic monophosphate (cyclic AMP). Alternatively, the internal component of the receptor may have tyrosine kinase activity leading to phosphorylation of tyrosines on intracellular proteins, some of which cause activation of cell growth and division.

Some oncogenes and their products are shown in Table 3.3. The oncoprotein ErbB1 (HER1, EGFR) is the receptor for EGF, which is a member of a family of tyrosine kinase receptors: HER2/neu (ErbB2), ErbB3 and ErbB4. Binding of EGF and other ligands to the receptor

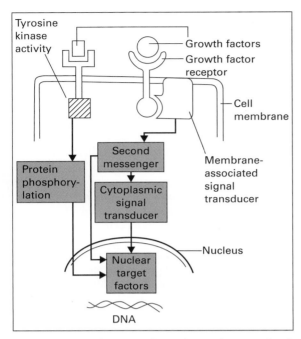

Figure 3.5 Mechanisms of signal transduction of cell membrane-associated receptors for a growth factor. The normal events are shown in this simplified diagram. Abnormal activation may contribute to tumour growth.

Table 3.3 Some oncogenes and their products associated with cancer in humans.

Oncogene	Activity	Association with human tumour
abl	Non-receptor tyrosine kinase	Chronic myeloid leukaemia, acute leukaemias, breast cancer
erbB1	EGF receptor	Breast cancer
erbB2	EGF receptor activity	Increased expression in breast cancer (comedo and *in situ*)
sis	Platelet-derived growth factor	?Breast cancer
ras	G protein	Adenocarcinoma of lung, prostate, large bowel

activates dimerisation and activation of tyrosine kinase activity, which leads to a cascade of protein phosphorylations in the cell. Over-expression or mutation of EGFR in cancer may lead to over-activation of receptor activity. The main pathways by which EGFR produces its effects are the ras-raf-MAP kinases, the protein kinase pathway Jak/Stat, and the phosphatidylinositol 3-kinase pathway. The receptor and the downstream pathways are now the targets of drugs that inhibit activity and antibodies that block receptor function. The pivotal discovery of mutations in the kinase domain of EGFR in a significant proportion of patients with non-small cell lung cancer (especially female, non-smokers, adenocarcinoma, Oriental ethnicity) demonstrated that there are cancers which are 'addicted' to this oncogene activation and derive major benefit from therapy with EGFR inhibitors [7].

Membrane proteins bind guanosine 5'-triphosphate (GTP) and also have GTPase activity which terminates the signal. Abnormal G proteins may be produced by mutated *ras* oncogenes, which have deficient GTPase activity and consequently lead to defective signal termination. The *ras* family consists of three members (H-*ras*-1, K-*ras*-2, N-*ras*) and other proteins which show partial homology (*rho*, R-*ras*, *ras*, *rab*). Activating *ras* mutations have been found in 40% of human colon cancers and 95% of pancreatic cancers. The Ras protein is capable of transforming fibroblasts in tissue culture, and its expression is associated with various stages of differentiation in embryonic life. Several malignancies are associated with a high prevalence of KRAS mutations, notably pancreatic cancer.

Tumour-suppressor genetic mechanisms in cancer development

Some genes result in abnormal growth regulation when they are deleted, namely, they act in a recessive manner with respect to the development of cancer. For a tumour-suppressor gene to be inactivated both alleles must usually be affected and for this reason these recessive mechanisms have been most clearly defined in inherited cancer syndromes where there is a germline mutation or deletion of one allele and the tumour is associated with deletion or mutation of the remaining allele in childhood or adult life. Table 3.4 lists some of the features distinguishing oncogenes and tumour-suppressor genes.

Retinoblastoma Li–Fraumeni syndrome and Wilms' tumour are among the best-studied tumours. Knudson suggested that retinoblastoma would arise as a two-step process in which germline allele loss would be followed

Table 3.4 Distinguishing features of tumour-suppressor genes and oncogenes.

Tumour-suppressor genes	Oncogenes
Recessive in effect	Dominant in effect
Often tissue-specific tumours, e.g. retinoblastoma	Tendency to broad specificity
Deletions promote cancer	Translocations increase activity
Germline inheritance in some cases	Both hereditary and non-hereditary forms

by loss of the other allele. It seems that loss of the second allele is usually by recombination or mitotic non-disjunction. Survivors of retinoblastoma have a 300 times greater risk of osteosarcoma. It is not known why the tumours are restricted to these sites (bone and eye). The *Rb* gene is located at chromosome 13q14. It is clear that there is a complexity in the tumour susceptibility effect of loss of Rb which is modulated by other genes [8].

The *p53* gene is a key tumour suppressor gene and is implicated in a multitude of cellular pathways including cell cycle arrest, apoptosis and angiogenesis. *p53* is frequently mutated in sporadic cancers of many types [9]. Germline mutation in the *p53* gene occurs in the Li–Fraumeni syndrome. Affected families are characterized by high incidence of sarcomas in probands during childhood, early onset of breast cancer in the mother or female siblings, and increased likelihood of cancer of the brain or adrenal gland or of leukaemia in other members. The breast cancer susceptibility genes *BRCA1* and *BRCA2* have the properties of tumour-suppressor genes. The germline mutation is carried on the maternal or paternal chromosomes 17 and 13, respectively. There is subsequently loss of the non-mutated allele leading to loss of activity. The BRCA1 protein is a ubiquitin ligase with multiple functions, including effects on cell cycle progression, DNA repair and transcriptional regulation. The BRCA2 protein is directly involved in homologous recombination and abrogation of function results in defects in DNA repair. Loss of activity leads to further genetic change, leading to malignancy. The male carriers of the mutated genes have a small increase in risk in prostate cancer.

Cell division

Prior to cell division there is a phase of cell growth (G_1) following which the cell moves to a phase of DNA synthesis (S phase) that results in two genetically identical copies of the chromosomal DNA. The duplicate chromosomes are termed sister chromatids. They appear as condensed chromosomes in the cell until mitosis begins. A phase of cell growth (G_2) occurs before entry into mitosis, which is initiated by proteins known as cyclin-dependent kinases (Figure 3.6). At the onset of mitosis, prometaphase, each member of the pairs attaches at its centromere to proteins that will form part of the mitotic spindle. Unattached chromatids issue a delaying signal until all are attached and the spindle formed (metaphase). The nuclear membrane disappears while this process is occurring. A second group of proteins assembles, the anaphase-promoting complex, which degrades proteins that prevent anaphase from beginning. In anaphase there is enzymic cleavage of the ties (cohesins) that bind the two sister chromatids and the two sets of chromosomes separate to opposite poles of the cell. The cell divides and the daughter cells pass into a prolonged resting phase (G_0) or into a first growth phase (G_1) that leads to a further cycle of DNA replication.

At each stage there are checks to ensure the fidelity of the process before it continues. Mitosis does not begin

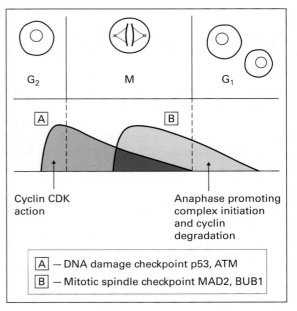

Figure 3.6 Diagrammatic representation of the process of mitosis and the checkpoints. The terms are explained in the text.

until the presence of DNA damage has been detected by proteins such as *p53* (see below), ATM and CHK2. The integrity of the mitotic spindle phase is checked by BUB1 and MAD proteins (see Figure 3.6). If these proteins are inactive, the chromosomes fail to segregate correctly.

Chromosomal instability is a hallmark of cancer where cells are often aneuploid. There are many ways in which such instability can be produced, bearing in mind the complexity of the mitotic process. Mutations in many of the genes maintaining normal mitosis have been described in cancer. For example, *p53* mutations are frequent in established cancers. The lack of functional *p53* protein that results allows cell division to occur in the presence of DNA damage, leading to further genetic changes and progression towards malignancy. Some of the protective proteins are targets for viral carcinogenesis. For example, HTLV-1 produces a protein (TAX) that degrades MAD1 and results in chromosomal instability. Numerous other proteins are involved in the regulation of mitosis, such as APC (mutated in adenomatous polyposis coli).

The instability of chromosomal structure, apart from contributing to the malignant phenotype (mobility, invasion and metastasis), also confers a susceptibility to genotoxic damage that accounts for the response of cancers to cytotoxic drugs. It is this susceptibility that results in lethal damage to cancer cells at doses of drugs that do not cause irrecoverable damage in the normal tissues.

Inheritance of cancer

There are numerous inherited genetic abnormalities which predispose to the development of malignancy. The major syndromes are shown in Table 3.5. There has been great progress in the isolation and cloning of genes involved in familial cancer syndromes. This is leading to an understanding of the molecular mechanisms of oncogenesis, which has a wider significance than the inherited disorder itself. As discussed several inherited cancer syndromes are due to mutations in genes that are important in DNA repair or in detecting damage to DNA. For example, in both xeroderma pigmentosum and ataxia telangiectasia the inherited abnormality is in a DNA-repair protein. The genetic defects in cancers of the breast, ovary and colon also involve DNA repair pathways.

In addition to single gene defects that carry a high risk of cancer, there are probably numerous polymorphisms that increase the cancer risk to a small degree [10]. These

may code for enzymes or proteins involved in detoxification of carcinogens, in DNA repair, or in growth factor signalling. Common polymorphisms, each carrying only a small increase in cancer risk, may, nevertheless, be of great quantitative importance in contributing to the total inherited cancer susceptibility of an individual. Screening for genes predicting an increased likelihood of developing cancer will have major implications for cancer screening and for counselling services.

Clonal origin, progression and growth of a cancer

Cancer cells are not fully responsive to the normal constraints in the parent tissue. The restriction point in the cell cycle marks the point at which cells are irreversibly committed to proceeding with DNA replication. This depends on the presence of exogenous nutrients and growth factors in normal cycling cells. An important property of cancer cells is their ability to continue the cell cycle in the presence of nutrient deprivation. Additionally, cancers always show a degree of anaplasia, which is a failure of the mechanism of cellular differentiation. Critically, cancers have the ability to metastasise, that is, the ability to spread from the site of origin to distant tissues.

While these features are present in most human cancers, some of these properties are not absolutely distinct from normal tissues. Thus it is true that the normal regulatory mechanisms controlling growth are defective in cancer, but there often remains a check or constraint on the pattern of growth of human neoplasms (see below). Similarly, although we regard the most anaplastic of cancers as 'undifferentiated' in the sense that they seem to have arisen from the more primitive precursors of the differentiated tissue, many cancers nonetheless do retain some of the functions of the mature tissues. Metastasis, however, is a property unique to cancer. Furthermore, it is metastasis which in most instances kills the patient, and understanding the biology of metastasis is one of the central problems of cancer research.

The following section is concerned with the events that follow the carcinogenic event and which lead to the development of an invasive, metastasizing malignancy.

Monoclonality and heterogeneity in cancer

It is probable that human neoplasms are monoclonal in origin. This means that the original oncogenic events affected a single cell and that the tumour is the result of growth from that one cell. There are two major lines of evidence which have led to this conclusion. First, certain women are heterozygotes for two forms of the enzyme

Table 3.5 Constitutional (inherited) genetic factors in cancer.

Abnormality	Cancer
Chromosomal abnormalities	
Trisomy 21 (Down's syndrome)	Acute leukaemia
47XXY (Klinefelter's syndrome)	Breast cancer
Mosaicism (45X0/46XY)	Gonadoblastoma
11p– (aniridia–Wilms' syndrome)	Wilms' tumour
13q– (multiple malformations)	Retinoblastoma
Inherited bowel disorders	
Polyposis coli (AD)	Carcinoma of colon
Gardner's syndrome (AD)	Carcinoma of colon
Peutz–Jeghers syndrome (AD)	Duodenal cancer
Tylosis palmaris (AD)	Oesophageal cancer
Neurological–cutaneous disorders	
Von Recklinghausen's neurofibromatosis (AD)	Sarcomas, glioma, acoustic neuroma
Retinal/cerebellar angiomatosis (von Hippel–Lindau syndrome) (AD)	Medullary thyroid cancer, phaeochromocytoma, hypernephroma
Tuberous sclerosis (AD)	Ependymoma, gliomas
Skin disorders (see Chapter 9, Tables 9.2 and 9.3)	
Breast and ovary	
BRCA1, BRCA2	Breast and ovary
Paediatric cancers (see Chapter 24)	
Immune deficiency disorders	
X-linked lymphoproliferative syndrome (XLR)	Lymphoma
Ataxia telangiectasia (AR)	Lymphoma, gastric cancer
Sex-linked agammaglobulinaemia (Bruton)	Lymphoma
Wiskott–Aldrich syndrome (XLR)	Lymphoma
IgA deficiency (S, AD, AR)	Adenocarcinomas
Miscellaneous syndromes	
Hemihypertrophy (AR)	Wilms' tumour, hepatoblastoma
Beckwith's syndrome (gigantism, macroglossia, mental retardation, visceromegaly) (S)	Wilms' tumour, hepatoblastoma
Multiple enchondromas (Ollier's syndrome) (S)	Chondrosarcoma
Bloom's syndrome (telangiectasia, short stature, chromosome fragility) (AR)	Leukaemias, numerous other cancers
Fanconi's anaemia (skeletal abnormalities, mental retardation, pigmented patches)	Acute leukaemia

AD, autosomal dominant; AR, autosomal recessive; S, sporadic; XLR, X-linked recessive.

glucose 6-phosphate dehydrogenase (G6PD). The gene for the enzyme is carried on the X chromosome and, in female heterozygotes, either the maternal or the paternal form is present on either one of the X chromosomes. In a female, each cell loses activity of one or other X chromosome and therefore, in a heterozygote for this enzyme, every cell in the body will have either one form of the enzyme or the other. In studies on haematological malignancies arising in heterozygotes for G6PD, the cancers are found to contain either the maternal or the paternal form of the enzyme, implying that the original cancer arose from one cell which either had one form of the enzyme or the other. In chronic granulocytic leukaemia, the restriction of enzyme expression is found in cells of the granulocyte series and, importantly, in red cells and platelets as well, implying that a stem cell is affected by the malignant process.

This technique is more difficult to apply to carcinomas. It is possible that some carcinomas arise from a 'field of change' in a tissue with many clones arising at the same time. An analysis of bladder cancer in women has shown the same pattern of suppression of the X chromosome in all cells in the tumour, while normal bladder cells showed random suppression of one or other of the two chromosomes. This strongly suggests a single clonal origin. In addition, there was the same pattern of allele deletion on 9q, while losses on 17p and 18q were variable, suggesting these were later events in the evolution of the tumour, showing that even if a tumour arises monoclonally, heterogeneity of genetic change may occur as the tumour progresses.

The second line of evidence pointing towards the monoclonal origin of cancer comes from lymphomas and other lymphoid malignancies in which it can be shown that the immunoglobulin produced by the lymphoid neoplasm (on its surface, or exported into the blood in the case of myeloma) is nearly always monoclonal, being of a single class and showing restriction of light chain expression (see Chapter 27).

The concept of monoclonality has sometimes led investigators to believe that there is a far greater uniformity of behaviour of cancer than is in fact the case. Despite the monoclonal origin of neoplasms, heterogeneity appears to arise during the course of development of the tumours. This has important implications for treatment and for understanding the nature of metastases.

How does heterogeneity arise if cancer is monoclonal? Malignant transformation is accompanied by genetic instability that causes phenotypic differences in clonogenic cells. Some cells with mutations survive and undergo still further changes, while others, depending on their ability to survive hormonal, biochemical or immunological adversity, die. The mature tumour can therefore be envisaged as being composed of cells that are monoclonal in origin, but diverse in capacity to metastasize and to resist cytotoxic drugs and immune attack.

A sequence of chromosomal alterations during the progression from colonic polyp to colonic cancer is illustrated in Figure 16.2. As the tumour progresses increasing genetic instability occurs with different cells within the same tumour showing a wide variety of chromosome breaks, deletions and reduplications. Studies in several neoplasms including colorectal cancer suggest increasing genetic instability during cancer progression [11].

Many cancers acquire mutations in the *p53* gene. This gene encodes a nuclear phosphoprotein that appears to act as a check to the cell cycle, arresting the cell in G_1 as a result of DNA damage. UV light and cytotoxic drugs induce a rapid increase in *p53* in normal cells due to stabilization of the protein after translation. Loss of *p53* function by mutation allows mitosis to proceed despite the presence of damaged DNA. The mutations in the *p53* gene that occur in cancer result in a conformational change in the protein, which may render it inactive, though some mutations have been found to activate specific oncogenic pathways in the cell. Thus, although *p53* is a tumour-suppressor gene, some mutant forms of the gene may have oncogenic pathways. *p53* function may be abrogated by deletion or by over-expression of the hDM2 gene which is amplified in some tumours and can degrade *p53* by ubiquitination. *p53* mutation may thus be an important step on the pathway of tumour progression where an already malignant cell is permitted to move into the cell cycle without time to repair damaged DNA. Further mutations can then occur.

Diversity within the cell population of a single tumour, therefore, occurs with regard to growth rate, cytoplasmic constituents, hormone receptor status, radiosensitivity and susceptibility to killing by cytotoxic agents. For example, in the case of small-cell carcinoma of the bronchus, different levels of cytoplasmic calcitonin, histaminase and L-dopa decarboxylase have been found in the primary tumour compared with a metastasis. Primary and secondary tumours may also show karyotypic differences.

It has become increasingly clear that cancers express significant molecular heterogeneity which may be an important barrier to effective therapy [12]. This has been known for decades in the haematological malignancies and with DNA deep sequencing these alterations are becoming more apparent in solid tumours such as kidney cancers. Expansion of distinct clones within different areas of the primary tumour as well as metastases may make the 'truncal' mutations driving cancers difficult to identify as targets for therapy [13]. Thus heterogeneity of neoplasms presents a formidable problem for therapy of cancer. Alterations in oxygenation within the tumour may result in altered gene expression patterns in hypoxic regions. Likewise, a single tumour may contain cells with wide variation in susceptibility to cytotoxic agents, and drug-resistant clones will predominate with repeated treatment. It will be of importance to define the pathways activated by these variable clones to optimise the use of novel targeted agents in treatment although resistance is clearly always likely to remain the major issue.

The growth of cancer

Normal tissues vary greatly in both the rate of cell division and the numbers of cells that are actively proliferating. Examples of rapidly proliferating cells are the intestinal mucosa, the bone marrow, the hair follicle cells and normal tissue regenerating after injury, for example, after surgical resection or infections.

An idealized representation of the way in which proliferation occurs in a normal tissue is shown in Figure 3.7. This figure shows the stem or progenitor cell supplying a proliferating pool of cells that follow a particular differentiation pathway. These become mature cells which are held to be incapable of further division and subsequently die. While this model may apply also to human cancers, it is possibly an oversimplification. Tumours probably do contain progenitor and mature cells but it is not clear whether cell renewal in a tumour comes from a small progenitor fraction. Nevertheless, the model is useful in explaining many aspects of tumour growth. While the progeny of stem cell division go through successive divisions, their number increases but the number of further divisions they are 'programmed' to make declines concomitantly. The stimulus to death, and its mechanism, is a programmed process under genetic control. Programmed cell death has been termed *apoptosis* (Figure 3.8). The morphological changes are condensation of the nucleus followed by pitting and explosion of the cytoplasm. The cell density rises, there

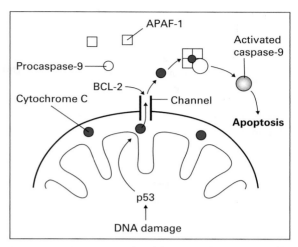

Figure 3.8 Apoptosis induced by DNA damage: (i) DNA damage and *p53* activation trigger cytochrome C release from mitochondria through a voltage-regulated anion channel in the outer mitochondrial membrane; (ii) cytochrome C causes an oligomer of apoptosis activating factor (APAF)-1, which binds procaspase-9 and activates it; (iii) activated procaspase-9 initiates apoptosis; (iv) BCL-2 blocks the voltage channel and is therefore anti-apoptotic. BAX enhances cytochrome release and is pro-apoptotic.

is endonuclease activation and the DNA is cleaved. The process involves the release of caspase enzymes from mitochondria. The cell may thus be switched to growth arrest, cell death or division by active processes. The *bcl*-2, *ras* and *LMP*-1 genes permit population expansion, while *p53* may prevent this.

When a tumour is treated with radiation or cytotoxic drugs it may shrink in size. This response may be entirely at the expense of later, non-self-renewing cells, in which case the tumour will regrow. To prevent regrowth it is probably essential to kill the progenitor or stem cells. The growth fraction of a tumour is the proportion of cells in active proliferation. Many cancer cells have long cycle times and calculations of the growth fraction may underestimate the proliferative capacity of the tumour. These slow-growing cells are probably less susceptible to chemotherapy, particularly using cycle-active agents.

A normal tissue grows and develops to a point when cell proliferation is balanced by cell loss and the tissue remains static in size, unless subjected to a changing environment, for example, the normal breast ductular tissue during the menstrual cycle or during pregnancy. In a cancer, on the other hand, the regulatory mechanisms are defective and the tumour gradually increases in size.

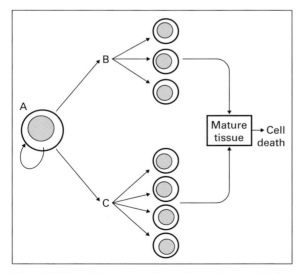

Figure 3.7 Normal tissue renewal. A produces cells committed to differentiation path B or C. Cellular proliferation leads to mature tissue and then to cell death.

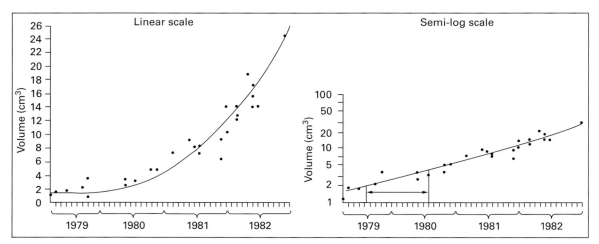

Figure 3.9 Growth of a squamous carcinoma. The patient had a peripheral squamous carcinoma, untreated because of dementia and hypertension. Over 4 years this almost spherical tumour increased slowly in size, exhibiting exponential growth with a doubling time of just over 1 year (horizontal arrows).

Normal somatic cell division is accompanied by loss of a repeating DNA sequence found at the tip of chromosomes called telomeres. When telomeres are lost all cell division ceases. Telomerase is an enzyme with reverse-transcriptase properties that catalyses telomere formation. It is over-expressed in many cancers and may be one mechanism for sustaining tumour growth.

Nevertheless, it must be emphasized that sustained growth does not necessarily mean rapid growth. Figure 3.9 shows the volume doubling time of an almost spherical squamous carcinoma. Slow exponential growth can be seen, with a volume doubling time of 1 year. During their growth, tumours undergo cell loss as well as cell renewal. This cell loss is partly due to the vascularization of tumours being defective. There is often inadequate nutrition when cells are more than 150 μm from a nutrient capillary. Sometimes the centres of human cancers are grossly necrotic where the tumour has clearly outstripped its blood supply. Other possible causes of cell loss are unsuccessful mitosis (possibly due to chromosomal aberrations), and death of tumours by immune or inflammatory attack as a result of both specific immunity and non-specific processes excited by the tumour.

In tissue culture the doubling times of human tumours show wide variation. It is not clear whether tumours exhibit a consistent rate of growth from the origin of the cancer to the time when the patient has a massive tumour and is about to die. Exponential growth can be observed in some human malignancies. In the case shown in Figure 3.9, if one were to extrapolate back to the origin of the tumour, it would prove to have arisen some 30 doublings (30 years) before the clinical presentation, if the growth had been exponential at the same rate throughout this time. We have no way of knowing whether spontaneously arising tumours grow faster when they are small and then slow down. For *visible* tumours, there is some evidence that a progressive slowing of the rate of growth may sometimes occur, a type of growth pattern known as Gompertzian (Figure 3.10). It is clear that, whether

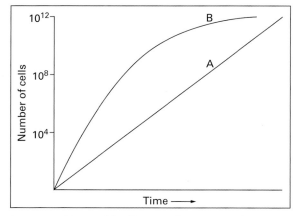

Figure 3.10 Two models of kinetics of tumour growth. In curve A the growth is exponential. In curve B there is progressive slowing of growth rate with increasing size, termed Gompertzian growth.

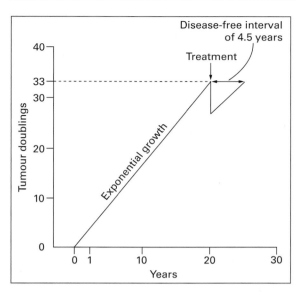

Figure 3.11 The lifespan of a tumour. The tumour is clinically apparent after 33 doublings. Treatment reduces the tumour mass, but the disease is again clinically detectable after 4.5 years.

growth changes during tumour development or not, a clinical cancer is late in its natural history by the time it presents (Figure 3.11), and this has implications for the possible success or failure of screening programmes to detect cancer early. Similarly, in a tumour with a volume doubling time of 70 days, a treatment which caused a reduction of 10 doublings would delay its reappearance for over 2 years if the growth rate was unchanged. This might lead to erroneous claims for the treatment if the follow-up time was short. These oversimplifications make the point that, in the treatment of clinically apparent tumours, the disease is already late in its natural history.

Differentiation in cancer

In a normal tissue the progeny of stem cells develop into the mature cells. During this process the cells acquire specialized structures, functions and biochemical properties, a process known as differentiation. Cellular differentiation continues progressively for several cell divisions after the stem cell.

Although cancer cells differ from their normal tissue counterparts in many respects, these differences are often those of degree. An *undifferentiated* tumour, indicates a lack of morphological resemblance with normal tissue. Some of the histological features will be present but the arrangement of cells appears chaotic and disorganized, with variation in nuclear size and shape. An *anaplastic*

carcinoma is one in which all the characteristic morphological appearances have disappeared, to the extent that the primary tissue of origin cannot be determined.

The term 'undifferentiated' often carries the implication that the neoplasm has somehow reverted to a more primitive state. However, it is possible that the oncogenic event has occurred early in the cell's differentiation pathway (e.g. in the stem cell) and that the neoplastic proliferation is occurring in a phase of cell development where the cell has not yet acquired the mature functional characteristics of the final tissue. The neoplastic counterpart might therefore be morphologically and functionally similar to the stage of cellular differentiation at the point where the malignant proliferation occurred.

Changes in cell surface properties are associated with the structural and functional alterations, with the acquisition of markers for various stages in the cell's differentiation pathway. Numerous cell surface proteins and glycolipids have been identified, some of which are differentiation-linked, and others that are expressed on the cell surface in increased amounts when the cell is undergoing division but which are not detectable in the resting phase.

Invasion, angiogenesis and metastasis

The malignant cell is one that has escaped to some degree from the normal control of growth. When normal tissues proliferate, they do so to the point where cell–cell contact exerts an inhibiting role on further mitosis. This inhibition is lost in malignancy. Tumours will grow and increase in size when planted subcutaneously in immunosuppressed mice, while normal tissues will not. The nature of the cell-surface glycoproteins differs from that of normal cells, with an increase in sialic acid content and alterations in the surface charge. The locomotor apparatus of cells (microfilaments and microtubules) becomes disorganized and the cells alter their shape and show membrane movement at sites of contact with normal cells.

At the same time the tumour cells become locally invasive, although the biochemical basis of this property is ill understood. Tumour cells may show decreased adhesiveness and attachment compared with normal cells. Secretion of enzymes is part of the mechanism of invasion. Several enzymes play a part in the proteolysis of the intracellular matrix that accompanies invasion by tumour cells. Among these is the family of matrix metalloproteinase (MMP) enzymes, which includes collagenases, gelatinases and stromelysins. They are secreted as inactive enzymes and are activated by disruption of the sulphydryl group which holds the metal atom (often zinc). This leads to a conformational change and activation of the enzyme. Tissue inhibitors of metalloproteinases terminate the activity. Certain tissues are characteristically resistant to invasion, for example, compact bone, large blood vessels and cartilage. Presumably some of these properties of cancer cells relate to normal processes of tissue remodelling and repair. However, the relation of the invasive phenotype to patterns of known genetic change in cancer is not understood.

As the tumour grows, tumour blood vessels proliferate under the influence of tumour angiogenesis factors, which stimulate capillary formation. The tumour vasculature offers a potential approach to treatment [14]. Tumour cells stimulate endothelial cell proliferation by production of angiogenic cytokines such as vascular endothelial growth factor (VEGF), PDGF and basic fibroblast growth factor. Endothelial cells can, in turn, stimulate tumour cell growth. A gram of tumour may contain 10–20 million endothelial cells that are not themselves neoplastic.

Antigens of normal endothelial cells, including procoagulant factors, may be upregulated in proliferating tumour endothelium. Apart from cytokines, hypoxia in the tumour circulation may also regulate production of VEGF and other factors. During angiogenesis, endothelial cells invade the stroma and divide to produce a capillary sprout, which later takes on a tubular form. As with cancer cells, this invasion may involve a complex interplay between MMPs, produced by the endothelial cells, and their natural inhibitors (see below).

One of the results of local invasion is that tumour cells can enter vascular and other channels of the body and metastasize. The sequence of events is shown in Figure 3.12. Lymphatic spread, which is particularly common with carcinomas, follows invasion of lymphatic channels, and the tumour cells grow in cords and clumps in the lymphatic vessels and lymph nodes. From there, spread to distal lymph nodes readily occurs. Haematogenous spread occurs after tumour cells have entered the vessels near the primary tumour or have been shed into the blood from the thoracic duct. Tumour cells are then trapped in the next capillary network, namely, in the lung or liver. Local anatomy is often important; for example, gastrointestinal cancers typically spread via the portal venous system to the liver. Tumours may also metastasize via a tissue space; for example, those arising in the peritoneal cavity may seed widely over the peritoneal space, and lung cancer may spread over

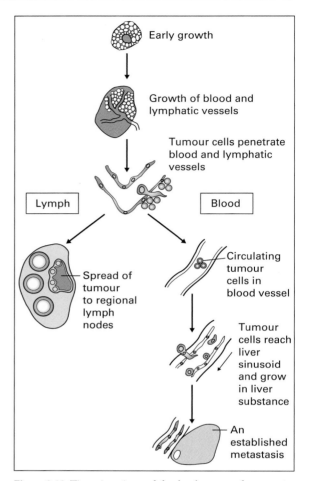

Figure 3.12 Tissue invasion and the development of metastasis.

the pleura. Certain tumours characteristically spread to some structures while others do not; for example, sarcomas typically metastasize to lungs, and breast cancer to the axial skeleton. The biological mechanisms for these preferences are not known.

Regional lymph nodes may form a barrier to further metastases from the primary site. It is not clear whether lymph nodes create a barrier to spread of tumour by virtue of specific immune mechanisms.

Having penetrated the vascular compartment, tumour cells must withstand the process of arrest in the capillary bed of an organ and then start to divide. At this site the tumour cell must leave the capillary bed of the new tissue. To do this the tumour cell must pass through the capillary endothelium and survive attack by host defence mechanisms such as phagocytic cells and so-called *natural killer* (NK) cells.

The capacity for invasion and colonization of distant tissues varies with different tumour types, presumably related to the pattern of gene expression associated with the tumour. With time most cancers acquire enough genetic change to become invasive and metastasizing, but this may take several years even after the tumour is clinically apparent. An example is low-grade lymphoma. Similarly, a tumour of the same type and degree of differentiation has a different tendency to metastasize in different individuals. This has led to a search for molecular markers that might relate to outcome more precisely than histopathological appearances alone (although this is by far the best single determinant). Within a single tumour there is heterogeneity in the metastatic potential of its constituent cells. Cloned sublines from a single tumour differ markedly in their ability to metastasize. The basis of this variability is not known.

It is apparent that the problems of tissue invasion, metastatic spread and tumour heterogeneity are among the most fundamental in cancer research and clinical management of cancer patients. The lack of homogeneity of tumours, the similarities between tumours and their parent tissue, and the lack of a single identifiable lesion in cancer cells that distinguishes them from normal together mean that many of our simple assumptions about tumour immunity and the mode of action of cytotoxic drugs must be looked at critically, particularly if they are derived from experiments using homogeneous tumours.

Tumour immunology

The idea that human tumours might be recognized as foreign to the host has obvious attractions because if an immune response to the tumour occurred as part of the disease or could be provoked artificially, there would be opportunities for using such an immune response diagnostically or therapeutically.

Immune responses to cancer

T-lymphocyte reactivity against human tumours is being reinvestigated now that it is possible to identify types of lymphocyte reliably, using antibodies (usually monoclonal, see below) to lymphocyte surface antigens that relate to function. Thus subpopulations of T cells with cytotoxic, helper and suppressor function can be identified in blood, lymph nodes and the infiltrates

in tumours. T cells can be separated from NK cells in cytotoxicity experiments. T-cell killing will take place only if there is genetic identity between the effector T cells and the targets.

T cells from blood, draining lymph nodes or, better still, from tumours, can now be isolated, expanded in number and cloned, allowing a more precise definition of their properties and target specificity. Carcinoma cells usually express class I major histocompatibility complex (MHC) antigens on their surface, but not class II. Cellular proteins are degraded in the cell to peptides that can bind to class I MHC. These are potential recognition targets for specialized antigen-presenting cells to stimulate a T-cell response. Recent research has attempted to identify the nature of the peptides which are tumour-derived, and to determine whether they differ from cellular peptides of normal cells and whether they can be presented in such a way as to provoke an antitumour response.

Until tumour antigens are defined and the nature of the immune response to them, if any, is elucidated, active specific immunity to cancer remains an elusive goal for many tumours. However, recent identification of melanoma-associated peptides has led to the first trials of tumour vaccines based on defined antigens. The clinical responses observed in a minority of patients with melanoma is encouraging but it is still unclear how generally applicable this approach might be. In other tumours, in the absence of knowledge of the antigens to which a specific and effective immune response could be generated, attempts have been made to provoke immunity to modified, widely distributed, epithelial membrane antigens. Nevertheless, immunization to protect against recurrence is an attractive therapeutic strategy if it can be realized.

Vaccines to viral antigens of HBV, EBV or HPV may prove to be a practical approach for immunization to prevent cancer in high-risk groups, but tumour-associated antigens are not sufficiently defined for this to be a practical proposition.

Treatment with non-specific immune or inflammatory mediators has not been generally effective (Table 3.6). These cytokine treatments are discussed in Chapter 6. Expansion of autologous lymphokine-activated killer (LAK) cells *in vitro*, by using IL-2, followed by reinfusion of the expanded and activated cell population has been extensively investigated. The aim is to divert a large number of activated non-specific cytotoxic lymphocytes to the tumour. There is little evidence that there is an increase in response over that achieved by the lymphokine (IL-2) alone. Curiously, with most of these immunologically

Table 3.6 Potential uses of monoclonal antibodies in cancer, used alone or linked to cytotoxic agents or isotopes as therapeutic agents.

Classification of tumours in tissue sections
Identification of 'undifferentiated' tumours in tissue sections
Diagnosis and classification of leukaemias
Diagnosis of metastatic tumour cells in low frequency, e.g. in bone marrow
Elimination of unwanted cells from bone marrow, e.g. metastatic tumour cells, residual leukaemic cells
Tumour localization by isotopically labelled antibody
Measurement of tumour products and 'markers', e.g. α-fetoprotein, carcinoembryonic antigen, peptide hormones

non-specific approaches to cancer treatment (BCG, IL-2, interferon, LAK cells) responses are confined to the same tumour types, namely, melanoma and renal cell carcinoma. It is clear that there is something exceptional about these two tumours, which renders them occasionally responsive to mediators of inflammation.

Monoclonal antibodies

The development of monoclonal antibody technology has allowed serological definition of the tumour cell surface with a hitherto unattainable precision. Some of the potential uses of monoclonal antibodies are listed in Table 3.6.

So far, monoclonal antibodies to human tumours have not been shown to define an antigen exclusively associated with malignant proliferation. Other antigens may be expressed as a result of rapid cell division, and while they may be demonstrable in some cancers, using monoclonal reagents, they may also be present on some normal tissues. The 'anticancer' monoclonals thus far produced appear to be identifying antigens that are expressed at a particular stage of differentiation of the cell type.

Monoclonal reagents are extremely useful in both the classification of cancer and the diagnosis of undifferentiated tumours (Figure 3.13). Additionally they are of therapeutic value in clearing sites such as the bone marrow of tumour cells in autologous or allogeneic bone marrow transplants. Coupling radioisotopes to these antibodies may be of value in tumour localization and treatment, while coupling of a cytotoxic agent to the monoclonal may provide a means of specific therapy if the antibody can be shown not to 'wrongly' identify vital host cells such as gut or marrow stem cells.

Recent years have seen remarkable progress and the introduction of a new range of therapeutic monoclonal antibodies, several of which now have an established place in cancer treatment. These are discussed further in clinical chapters in relation to the treatment of specific cancers. For example, Ipilimumab is a humanised monoclonal antibody targeting cytotoxic T-lymphocyte antigen-4 (CTLA-4), thereby augmenting antitumour immune responses. Long-term follow-up of patients who received ipilimumab in a phase III trial showed that 24% survived at least two years, and in phase II studies, a proportion of patients survived at least five years. These

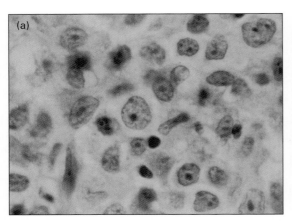
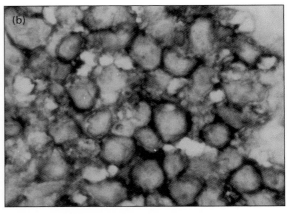

Figure 3.13 Use of monoclonal antibodies for immunocytochemical diagnosis. (a) Undifferentiated nasopharyngeal tumour. Differential diagnosis would include anaplastic carcinoma, lymphoma and melanoma. (b) Same tumour as in (a) stained for common leucocyte antigen using a monoclonal antibody. The tumour cells show dark membrane staining, indicating that the tumour is a lymphoma.

results are unprecedented in metastatic melanoma and studies are underway for other solid tumours.

References

1 Hanahan D, Weinberg RA. The hallmarks of cancer. *Cell* 2000; 100: 57–70.

2 Hanahan D, Weinberg RA. Hallmarks of cancer: the next generation. *Cell* 2011; 144(5): 646–74.

3 Weinberg R. *The Biology of Cancer*. Garland Science, 2013.

4 Shuen AY, Foulkes WD. Inherited mutations in breast cancer genes – risk and response. *J Mammary Gland Biol Neoplasia* 2011; 16(1): 3–15.

5 Bonnet F, Chêne G. Evolving epidemiology of malignancies in HIV. *Curr Opin Oncol.* 2008; 20: 534–40.

6 Arzumanyan A, Reis HM, Feitelson MA. Pathogenic mechanisms in HBV- and HCV-associated hepatocellular carcinoma. *Nat Rev Cancer* 2013; 13: 123–35.

7 Lynch TJ, Bell DW, Sordella R *et al.* Activating mutations in the epidermal growth factor receptor underlying responsiveness of non-small-cell lung cancer to gefitinib. *N Engl J Med* 2004; 350: 2129–39.

8 Burkhart DL, Sage J. Cellular mechanisms of tumour suppression by the retinoblastoma gene. *Nat Rev Cancer* 2008; 8: 671–82.

9 Muller PA, Vousden KH. p53 mutations in cancer. *Nat Cell Biol* 2013; 15: 2–8.

10 Bodmer W, Tomlinson I. Rare genetic variants and the risk of cancer. *Curr Opin Genet Dev* 2010; 20: 262–7.

11 Walther A, Houlston R, Tomlinson I. Association between chromosomal instability and prognosis in colorectal cancer: a meta-analysis. *Gut* 2008; 57: 941–50.

12 Burrell RA, McGranahan N, Bartek J, Swanton C. The causes and consequences of genetic heterogeneity in cancer evolution. *Nature* 2013; 501: 338–45.

13 Gerlinger M, Rowan AJ, Horswell S, *et al.* Intratumor heterogeneity and branched evolution revealed by multiregion sequencing. *N Engl J Med* 2012; 366: 883–92.

14 Bridges EM, Harris AL. The angiogenic process as a therapeutic target in cancer. *Biochem Pharmacol* 2011; 81: 1183–91.

Further reading

Chandel NS, Tuveson DA. The promise and perils of antioxidants for cancer patients. *New Engl J Med* 2014; 371: 177–8.

Pezzella F, Harris AL. When cancer co-opts the vasculature. *New Engl J Med* 2014; 370: 2146–7.

4 Staging of tumours

Although the overall prognosis of malignant tumours is often summarized by stating the proportion of patients alive at 5 or 10 years, such figures usually conceal a wide variation in survival, ranging from cure to death within a few months of diagnosis. The search for indicators of prognosis has occupied the attention of oncologists for many years. The object is to identify those patients for whom a treatment strategy (e.g. surgery alone) is likely to be successful and, conversely, those in whom it is bound to fail, generally because of tumour extension beyond the obvious or visible primary site. For these patients, a different approach must be adopted.

Staging the extent of the disease at presentation is one aspect of the identification of factors that will influence prognosis in any individual patient. The purposes of careful staging of tumour spread are as follows.

To impose discipline in the accurate documentation of the initial tumour.

To assist our understanding of tumour biology.

To give appropriately planned treatment to the patient.

To be able to give the best estimate of prognosis.

To compare similar cases in assessing and designing trials of treatment (see Chapter 2).

Staging notation

For many tumours a useful staging notation is the TNM system developed by the American Joint Committee on Cancer Staging and End Result Reporting [1], which has been widely accepted and used worldwide for many decades, undergoing regular revision as new staging strategies become available. The system has the virtue of simplicity, drawing attention to the prognostic relevance of the size or local invasiveness of the primary tumour (T), lymph node spread (N) and the presence of distant metastases (M). It is widely used for solid tumours including cancers of the breast, head and neck, non-small-cell lung cancer and genitourinary cancers. It has obvious limitations, for example, in disorders such as diffuse lymphoma where the disease is often generalized, and is clearly inappropriate for leukaemias. Even in some solid tumours, such as small-cell carcinoma of the bronchus and ovarian cancer, the practicality and usefulness of the system is limited. In these diseases, different approaches must be used for staging, which are described in the appropriate chapters. For many gynaecological tumours, the FIGO system (International Federation of Gynaecology and Obstetrics) is often preferred (see, e.g., page 313).

Cancer and its Management, Seventh Edition. Jeffrey Tobias and Daniel Hochhauser.
© 2015 John Wiley & Sons, Ltd. Published 2015 by John Wiley & Sons, Ltd.

The primary tumour (T)

In some cancers, the size of the primary tumour relates to prognosis. This is well illustrated by many cancers of the head and neck, for example, in the oropharynx and oral cavity (see Chapter 10). In other tumours, the T stage relates not to size but to depth of invasion, for example, in melanoma and colon and bladder cancer (Figure 4.1a). In squamous lung cancer, the size and site of the primary tumour are both factors of prognostic importance (Figure 4.1b). In some diseases, the mode of spread makes T status largely irrelevant. Examples include ovarian cancer, soft-tissue sarcoma and small-cell carcinoma of the lung. In such tumours, 'stages' or stage groupings are used which are often composites of tumour size and local or distant invasion. In melanoma, the depth of involvement in millimetres is the best predictor of prognosis of the primary tumour. In squamous lung cancer, local invasiveness and tumour site are as important as tumour size (pages 204–206).

Lymph node involvement (N)

Nodal involvement has profoundly important prognostic influence in many solid tumours (Figure 4.2). In head and neck, bladder and large bowel cancers, for example, it is probably the most important determinant of survival. In most types of cancer, fixed (N3) lymph nodes, which are surgically inaccessible, carry a far worse prognosis than mobile ipsilateral (N1) nodes. Nodal involvement often reflects a high probability of haematogenous metastases, as for example in breast carcinoma. In other diseases, particularly cancers of the head and neck, it has considerable prognostic importance because of the higher local failure rate, often with fatal results.

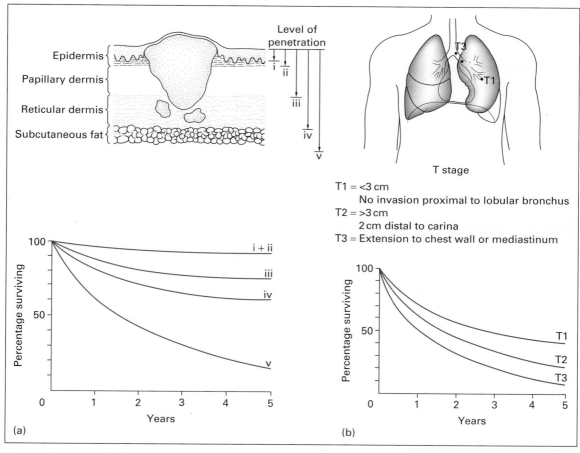

Figure 4.1 Prognosis related to local extent of primary tumour: (a) melanoma; (b) squamous carcinoma of the lung.

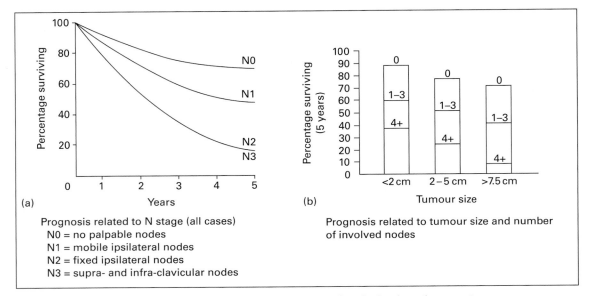

Figure 4.2 Breast cancer: prognosis related to (a) N stage and (b) number of involved nodes and tumour size.

Presence of metastases (M)

This clearly defines a group of patients who are surgically incurable. With few exceptions (notably testicular tumours) the presence of distant metastatic disease has grave prognostic implications, usually proving fatal within months or a few years of diagnosis. Metastases may have been detected by clinical examination alone, or may have been found by investigation using specialized techniques.

Staging techniques

Many techniques are available for determining the extent of spread of a tumour at the time when a patient first presents. Much information can be obtained by investigations such as chest radiography, full blood count and liver enzyme tests. These investigations are performed routinely in a patient who has been diagnosed as having cancer or where the diagnosis is suspected.

A chest radiograph may show metastases in the lungs or the bones or extension of a bronchogenic carcinoma into the pleura or overlying ribs. Hilar or paratracheal lymph node enlargement may also be present. These findings indicate that the tumour has spread beyond its site of origin, and will considerably alter the approach to management.

A full blood count may show anaemia of an iron-deficient type, or normochromic anaemia typical of the anaemia of chronic diseases. Occasionally, the blood film may show leucoerythroblastic anaemia with immature white and red cell precursors present. This is typical of widespread bone marrow infiltration and is most frequently caused by adenocarcinomas, particularly adenocarcinoma of the breast. Bone marrow examination may be performed if infiltration is suspected. In some tumours, for example, small-cell carcinoma of the bronchus, marrow examination is sometimes part of the routine staging and when localized treatment with radiotherapy is considered in addition to chemotherapy. Occult marrow involvement is detected in 5–10% of cases but in 20–30% with immunostaining. Bone marrow examination is usually performed in patients with newly diagnosed non-Hodgkin's lymphoma, where the probability of marrow involvement is higher.

In recent years, diagnostic imaging has been revolutionized by technical advances and has led to a previously unattainable degree of precision in staging the extent of the primary tumour and in assessing whether there has been metastatic spread [2]. Many of these investigations are time-consuming, expensive and very much dependent on the skill and enthusiasm of the radiologist. It is important to maintain a degree of scepticism about equivocal findings, especially if these are not in accordance with the clinical circumstances.

Ultrasound

Diagnostic ultrasound has been greatly refined in the last 15 years. It was first introduced into clinical practice in the 1950s and relies on the differing echo patterns that tissues create when bombarded by sound from an ultrasonic transducer. These echoes are generated at interfaces of tissues whose density differs, then recorded, interpreted and presented as a two-dimensional display. The orientation of the slice or 'cut' is determined by the operator, who places the probe in the position most appropriate for demonstrating the organ and abnormality suspected (Figure 4.3). This flexibility allows images to be obtained in many planes. Ultrasound echoes cannot be obtained if

the organ is shielded by an area of bone or gas since these reflect all the sound from the beam and no echoes can be obtained from beyond these structures. For this reason ultrasound has its main diagnostic use in the abdomen and soft tissues. A great advantage of ultrasound is that it is cheap, quick and non-invasive (though invasive techniques have also been developed, see below). It can therefore be used to monitor responses to treatment, with measurements being made between chemotherapy cycles. Other techniques, such as computed tomography (CT), are more accurate but are too expensive to be used in this way and the dose of radiation is too high.

Ultrasound is particularly useful for diagnosis of liver metastases (Figure 4.3). The type of echo obtained varies depending on the kind of metastases present. Thus, echo-poor areas are often associated with lymphomas

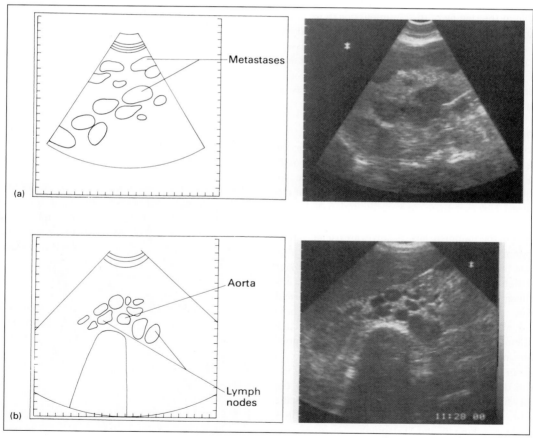

Figure 4.3 Diagnosis of hepatic metastases and lymph node enlargement by ultrasound. (a) Hepatic metastases. Several large metastases are shown in this transverse scan of the liver. (b) Para-aortic lymph nodes. These are demonstrated lying in front of and behind the aorta.

and sarcomas, while gastrointestinal metastases produce a more echo-dense appearance. In colorectal cancer the accuracy of ultrasound approaches that of CT scanning. It is also of value for assessment of obstructive jaundice and is often used in conjunction with CT scanning.

In the kidney, ultrasound examination is frequently able to detect a renal carcinoma and to distinguish this from cysts. The accuracy in this differential diagnosis is of the order of 90%, and the resolving power is approximately 2–3 cm. Ultrasound of the thyroid is useful in making the distinction between solid and cystic lesions, and in the testis it can sometimes demonstrate an occult or doubtfully palpable tumour. It is also often used in distinguishing solid and cystic masses within the breast. Endoscopic ultrasound is increasingly used, for example, by the transrectal route, particularly valuable for the assessment of prostatic carcinomas. Endoscopic ultrasound of the oesophagus is proving valuable in the staging of distal tumours or those at the gastro-oesophageal junction since these may be potentially operable. These are otherwise difficult to assess prior to attempting a hazardous surgical procedure. For pelvic tumours, transvaginal ultrasonography has also proven valuable, for example to assess the thickness or extent of a vulval or vaginal carcinoma.

Computed tomography

Modern CT scanners are able to demonstrate normal anatomy in detail that would have been thought impossible in the early 1970s. The accuracy of the technique has been greatly improved and its use in staging continues to be defined. However, there are many limitations to its use, with both false-positive and false-negative results. For example, in the abdomen, false positives are usually due to confusion with non-specified bowel loops and false negatives to the inability of CT scanning to detect malignant infiltration of normal-sized nodes. Clarity of the CT scanning image depends partly on the presence of the normal fat planes that surround anatomical structures. If these are lost, alteration of the anatomy is less easily detected. The tomographic technique can demonstrate a tumour by showing distortion or enlargement of an organ, or a change in its density. In cancer, the CT scanning is of use both in demonstrating the extent of infiltration of the primary tumour (T staging) and in delineating metastatic spread to adjacent lymph nodes and to other structures such as liver or lung (N and M staging).

CT scanning is of great importance in the definition of the spread of tumours within the chest [3]. Several studies have shown that chest radiography and conventional

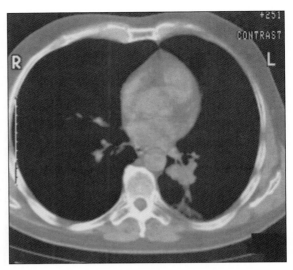

Figure 4.4 CT scanning of thorax. Left-sided bronchogenic carcinoma behind the heart. The tumour extends to the pleura. The chest radiograph was normal.

tomography greatly underestimate the extent of infiltration of lung cancer within the chest, particularly in the mediastinum (Figure 4.4). The CT scanning has also been valuable in demonstrating the true extent of infiltration of tumours arising in the head and neck, particularly in the paranasal sinuses (Figure 4.5). For retroperitoneal structures, CT scanning remains the most

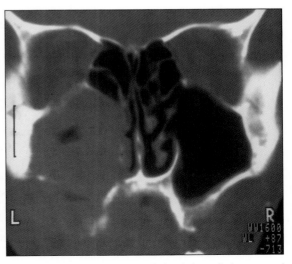

Figure 4.5 CT scanning (coronal plane) through the nose and maxillary antrum. A large tumour fills the left maxillary antrum, destroying its walls and extending medially into the nasal fossa.

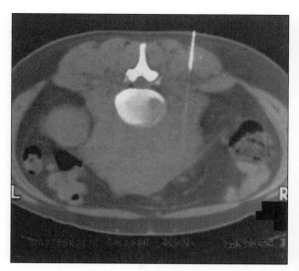

Figure 4.6 CT scanning of the abdomen showing a large para-aortic mass. The track of a CT scanning-guided biopsy needle is visible.

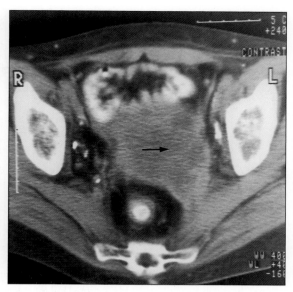

Figure 4.7 CT scanning of the pelvis showing a large central mass (arrow) anterior to the rectum. This was an advanced carcinoma of the cervix.

reliable preoperative investigation and is particularly useful in demonstrating both lymph node enlargement and abnormalities of the adrenal and pancreas. Using fine flexible needles, CT scanning-guided aspiration may help in the distinction between a benign and malignant neoplasm (Figure 4.6), or between an inflammatory mass and a carcinoma, for example, in the pancreas. The extent of retroperitoneal tumours such as sarcomas and lymphomas can be assessed with CT scanning, as can the size of malignant tumours of the kidney. In the pelvis, CT scanning frequently demonstrates the extent of advanced carcinomas of the cervix, bladder, prostate and rectum (Figure 4.7).

However, interpretation requires considerable expertise. CT scanning is also used to determine the degree of lymph node involvement. In the chest, the CT scanning is much more reliable than chest radiography or lung tomography in demonstrating mediastinal and hilar node involvement. In the abdomen, CT scanning delineates pelvic and abdominal lymph nodes, though with lesser clarity than in the chest. Lymph nodes must usually be enlarged to more than twice their normal size before they can be confidently assessed as pathological.

Of the widely available methods, CT scanning remains the most sensitive for assessing pulmonary metastases. It is used for this purpose in testicular germ-cell tumours and osteosarcomas, where occult pulmonary metastases are frequently demonstrated in patients whose chest

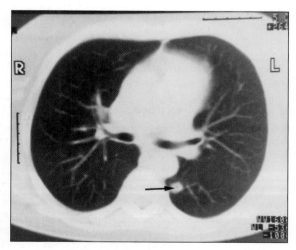

Figure 4.8 CT scanning of thorax showing a solitary metastasis (arrow) behind the heart. In this patient with osteosarcoma, the chest radiograph was normal.

radiograph is normal (Figure 4.8). The technique is particularly valuable in demonstrating metastases that lie in front of and behind the heart or subpleurally, which are not visible on plain radiography. In the liver, CT scanning is now more sensitive than ultrasound examination, though more expensive. The technique is made more

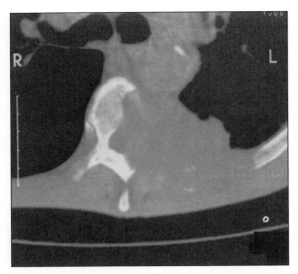

Figure 4.9 CT scanning of a thoracic vertebra at the level of the carina. The vertebra and rib are largely destroyed by local extension of a bronchogenic carcinoma.

accurate by using intravenous contrast, which may also clearly distinguish benign from malignant hepatic lesions. CT scanning is also excellent for demonstrating details of local tumour invasion in the chest (Figure 4.9).

Magnetic resonance imaging

Magnetic resonance imaging (MRI) has provided important additional detail in imaging many body sites, especially the brain and spinal cord, and in sarcomas [4]. In this technique the patient lies within an intense

magnetic field that produces magnetization of atomic nuclei in the patient, in the direction of the field. Electromagnetic pulses are then applied to the patient to change the direction of this nuclear magnetization. Following cessation of the pulse, the nuclei return to their orientation within the static field. This recovery time, which is measured by the scanner, depends on exchange of energy between protons and surrounding atoms and molecules. The recovery time is different in tumours compared with normal tissues. The technique has proved particularly valuable in the brain, where deep-seated primary tumours can be visualized (Figure 4.10). MRI has been able to detect tumours in the brainstem, cerebellum and deep midline structures when CT scanning has been inconclusive. The use of gadolinium contrast techniques has refined the role of MRI still further.

In the spine, MRI has largely replaced myelography since it often demonstrates secondary deposits without the need for lumbar puncture. Use of gadolinium contrast further increases the diagnostic range. In bone and soft-tissue sarcomas, MRI provides unsurpassed detail of the extent of the primary site, which greatly assists the surgeon and radiotherapist in operative and planning technique (Figure 4.11a). Abdominopelvic MRI is also superior to CT scanning, at least in definition of cervical anatomy and pelvic node assessment (Figure 4.11b). Recent results from a large study of MRI for rectal cancer have confirmed that high-resolution MRI accurately predicts whether the surgical resection margins following curative procedures for rectal carcinoma will be clear, with the technique proving reliable even at multiple centres, thus enabling more accurate selection of patients

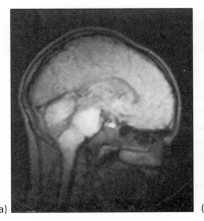

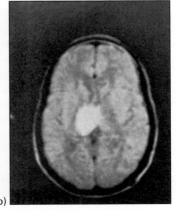

(a)   (b)

Figure 4.10 (a) MRI scan (sagittal view) showing large brainstem tumour. The CT scanning was normal. (b) MRI scan of the brain showing a deep-seated thalamic tumour which was not clearly shown on the CT scanning.

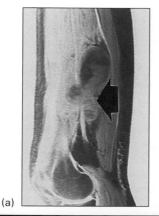

(a)

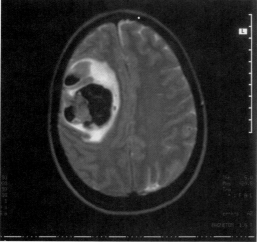

(b)

Figure 4.11 (a) MRI scan of soft-tissue sarcoma in the lower half of the femur. The tumour mass (arrow) is seen to be closely applied to the femur, and the femoral artery is clearly seen passing through the substance of the tumour. (b) MRI scan of the brain showing a very large metastasis. An area of haemorrhage is shown as a dense, black, central opacity. The midline structures are displaced from right to left.

for preoperative treatment with radiotherapy [5]. In prostate cancer, the use of novel contrast agents, including lymphotropic superparamagnetic nanoparticles, has increased the sensitivity and specificity of staging [6].

For imaging of tumours of the pancreatico-biliary tree, magnetic resonance cholangiopancreatography (MRCP) is now increasingly used as an alternative to the more invasive endoscopic retrograde cholangiopancreatography (ERCP). It was originally described in 1991 and has the advantage of avoiding the need for administration of exogenous contrast materials [7], making it ideal for patients with allergy to iodine-containing compounds. Its accuracy is generally considered to be as good as ERCP in many clinical situations, and it is less expensive.

Isotope scanning

Scanning with radioactive isotopes is a simple and widely available technique for assessing metastatic spread. In certain sites it has rather poor accuracy, that is, a low percentage of correct results. This is due to both poor sensitivity of detection (the percentage of positive tests in abnormal tissues) and poor specificity (percentage of negative tests in normal tissues). However, the dose of radiation is small, the technique is safe and reproducible and it is relatively inexpensive.

Skeletal metastases are best demonstrated by isotope scanning, and bone scans are now the most frequent test requested in most service departments. Technetium (Tc)-labelled phosphate compounds are usually used. The isotope is rapidly taken up into bone, rate of uptake being related to both blood flow through the bone and the amount of new bone formation. Metastases cause increase in blood flow and an increase in osteoblastic activity, usually sufficient to be demonstrable as areas of increased uptake of isotope (Figure 4.12). An exception to this is in multiple myeloma where osteoblastic activity is minimal.

Because of the non-specific nature of the uptake, a variety of other conditions will cause increased uptake. Rib fractures, arthritis and vertebral collapse from osteoporosis may all give rise to increased uptake and be misinterpreted as due to metastases in a patient with a malignancy. Single areas of increased uptake in an otherwise fit patient should therefore be interpreted with extreme caution. Radiographs of the affected region should be taken and, if necessary, a CT scanning should be obtained if the presence of a metastasis would materially alter the therapeutic decision. This is especially important if the single site is in the vertebral column, since degenerative disease is common at this site. Despite these problems, an area of increased uptake in a patient with cancer is likely to be due to a secondary deposit and should be carefully evaluated. Multiple areas of increased uptake are almost certainly due to disseminated tumour. An isotope bone scan is generally regarded as an important staging investigation in all patients with newly diagnosed carcinoma of the breast.

In the liver, scanning is performed with ^{99m}Tc-labelled sulphur colloid. Metastases appear as areas of diminished uptake. Isotope liver scanning is less accurate than

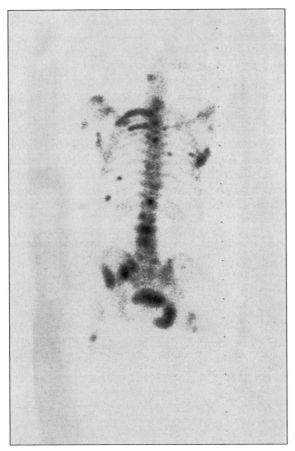

Figure 4.12 Isotope bone scan showing multiple bone metastases. This patient had a carcinoma of the prostate.

ultrasound or CT scanning, and hepatic isotope scanning has now been largely eclipsed.

New techniques of scintigraphy employ tracer doses of labelled monoclonal antibodies to detect metastases from colorectal cancer. In breast cancer and malignant melanoma, the technique of sentinel node staging is becoming established as a likely competitor to formal regional lymphadenectomy. Sentinel node surgery has the potential to eliminate the need for axillary lymph node clearance, for example in many breast cancer patients, since it provides excellent predictive power of the order of 95%, without axillary disturbance [8]. The technique relies on lymphoscintigraphy for localization of the node and minimally invasive surgery to remove it. Unexpected patterns of drainage may be revealed, of considerable value in surgery.

Drugs such as octreotide (a somatostatin analogue) can be labelled and will bind to neuroendocrine tumours bearing somatostatin receptors, and can be used to detect metastases.

Positron emission tomography

In recent years, positron emission tomography (PET) scanners have become widely available, and the image quality has improved dramatically. Its great advantage is to provide reliable information on tumour activity to a far more accurate degree than previously possible with CT scanning or MRI imaging, which gave excellent anatomic visualization but no indication of whether the tumour had remained active, for example after radical treatment by chemo- or radiotherapy. PET imaging relies on computer-assisted image reconstruction using signal-emitting tracers such as radiolabelled sugars. Fluorodeoxyglucose is the most commonly used. The tracer is injected intravenously, with preferential uptake in sites of tumour activity. PET is able to give information on the location, size and nature of tumour deposits, to a level sometimes unobtainable by other techniques. Most malignant tumours show an increase in glucose metabolism, allowing differentiation from benign lesions with PET using ^{18}F-labelled fluorodeoxyglucose. The technique can also distinguish between tumour recurrence and radiation necrosis, another distinct advantage, at least in some situations, over CT scanning or MRI (Table 4.1).

Table 4.1 Indications for fluorodeoxyglucose positron emission tomography in oncology.

Main indications
Preoperative staging of non-small-cell lung cancer [9]
Staging of recurrent disease in lymphoma and colorectal cancer
Assessment of melanoma greater than stage II
Investigation of a solitary pulmonary nodule

Secondary indications
Preoperative staging of head and neck cancer
Staging of recurrent breast cancer
Distinction between scar or recurrence or tissue necrosis or recurrence
Brain tumour grading

Emerging indications
Assessment of tumour response to therapy
In vivo imaging of drug action

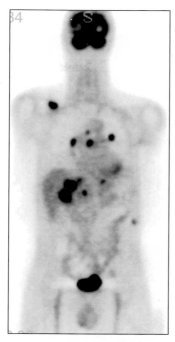

Figure 4.13 PET scan using ^{18}F-fluorodeoxyglucose in non-small-cell lung cancer showing widespread metastases (clinically undetectable) including both hilae, right supraclavicular fossa and porta hepatis.

Detection and localization of metastases may also be more readily accomplished (Figure 4.13); indeed the detection of secondary deposits as part of preoperative or other potentially radical treatment has become one of the major indications for this investigation. Because of the quality of high-resolution MRI or CT scanning for cancer diagnosis, but a lesser power of discrimination of residual activity following treatment, PET scanning may find its most valuable role in the future in tumour monitoring post treatment [10,11]. Indeed, in chemosensitive tumours such as lymphoma, PET appears to have the capability of predicting outcome accurately after as little as one cycle of chemotherapy, clearly an extremely valuable tool in the recognition of early chemoresistance and allowing the appropriate tailoring of treatment. In due course, this could lead routinely to early cessation of chemotherapy, and the use of more appropriate second-line agents in patients whose initial chemoresponse is unsatisfactory. In addition, as techniques for fusing images from PET and CT scanning become better refined and more widely available, the PET/CT fusion scan is increasingly seen as the most

ideal tool for preoperative staging at many tumour sites (Figure 4.14), and is now very widely used. The past few years have seen very rapid advances in this technology, which is widely used and clearly set to expand still further – see, for example, Ref. [12] for a good overview.

More recently still, the advent of PET-MRI scanning has provided better precision and insight into the essential details of tumour location and potential resectability, as well as monitoring of response to treatment with chemotherapy. The first clinically useful whole-body PET–MRI scanners were made available in 2011, and techniques are now advancing rapidly, including the use of gadolinium contrast-enhancement and relatively short acquisition times around 20 min per scan. The work currently being undertaken at our own centre chiefly involves imaging of lymphoma, prostate, colorectal and head-and-neck cancer, particularly in patients where the need for repeated scanning makes the reduction of radiation dose highly desirable, and therefore the avoidance wherever possible of too many CT scanning.

Diagnosis of specific metastatic sites

Pulmonary metastases
A chest radiograph is the most widely used method of screening. CT scanning greatly increases diagnostic accuracy, with overall sensitivity up to 60–65%. Doubtful lesions such as subpleural deposits and isolated opacities can be examined by percutaneous needle aspiration. Small pleural effusions, not apparent on chest radiography, may also be demonstrated.

Bone metastases
Bone scanning is the most accurate and rapid means of screening for bone metastases. Skeletal radiographs are used to demonstrate the degree of bone erosion at a site of metastasis if an alternative explanation for increased isotope uptake, such as trauma or infection, is possible. Percutaneous needle aspiration of bone can be undertaken safely at many sites and is helpful when the diagnosis is uncertain. MRI is useful for demonstrating intramedullary metastasis.

Hepatic metastases
Biochemical tests of liver function are the most widely used screening procedure. For imaging the liver, ultrasound and CT scanning are useful for diagnosis of not only hepatic metastases but also adrenal, mesenteric and other sites of abdominal disease [13]. These investigations

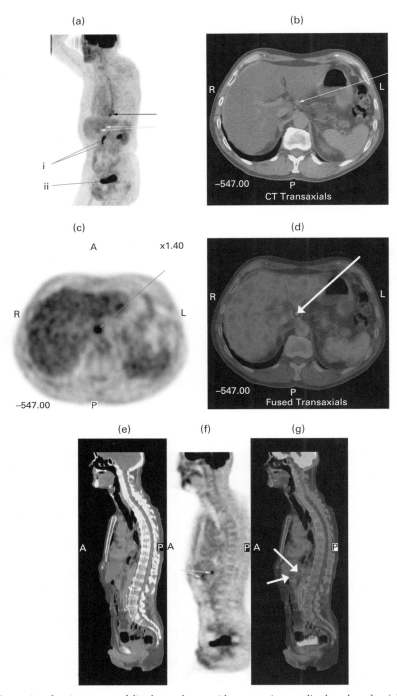

Figure 4.14 CT/PET scanning showing cancer of distal oesophagus with metastasis to coeliac lymph nodes. (a) Maximum intensity projection of a PET study using ^{18}F-fluorodeoxyglucose (FDG). The scan demonstrates the primary oesophageal tumour (black arrow) and metastasis in coeliac lymph nodes (white arrows). Urinary excretion of the isotope is shown by (i) the kidneys and (ii) bladder. (b–d) Corresponding transaxial images through coeliac lymph node as shown by CT scanning (b) and PET (c). Fused coregistered data of CT scanning and PET (d) show intense focal accumulation of FDG in a lymph node (white arrow). (e–g) Additional localization information provided by the sagittal view. CT scanning (e) and PET (f, nodes shown by white arrows) are fused (g), highlighting the lymph nodes (white arrows). (Courtesy of Dr J. Bomanji, Department of Nuclear Medicine, UCL Hospitals.)

may confirm metastatic liver disease even if the liver function tests are normal. In lymphomas (particularly Hodgkin's disease), abdominal CT scanning is now the most widely performed staging procedure, useful both for hepatic deposits and also (more commonly) to demonstrate intra-abdominal lymph node involvement.

Brain metastases

CT scanning is widely available and is the usual preliminary investigation, although it is seldom positive in neurologically normal patients. MRI is more sensitive and can show leptomeningeal spread when CT scanning is normal.

The role of surgery in diagnosis and staging

With the increasing precision of simpler diagnostic techniques, such as aspiration cytology, percutaneous needle biopsy and CT scanning-guided fine-needle biopsy, major surgical procedures are sometimes unnecessary simply to establish the diagnosis. In carcinoma of the pancreas, for example, it has previously been difficult to obtain histological confirmation without laparotomy. The increasing use of non-surgical techniques (or fine-needle aspiration biopsy) often leads to a preoperative tissue diagnosis. This may allow new therapeutic approaches to be considered in the future, in which planned surgery might be undertaken following preoperative radiotherapy or chemotherapy. With the emphasis on tailoring of treatment to the extent of the disease, the cancer surgeon sometimes performs staging procedures that are not in themselves therapeutic but which are intended to assist radiotherapists and medical oncologists in deciding their therapeutic strategy.

Based on these findings, it may sometimes be appropriate to proceed to laparotomy and resection of residual tumour deposits (Table 4.2). However, laparoscopic methods of surgical staging are increasingly used, for instance in upper gastrointestinal cancer to exclude or confirm small-volume peritoneal or nodal disease prior to any attempt at definitive resection [14]. Increasingly sophisticated methods of staging may lead to a spurious improvement in outcome, simply because of the 'stage-shift' effect. Accurate staging is not itself directly therapeutic.

Tumour markers

Some malignant tumours produce proteins that can be detected in the blood and which may serve as a marker both of the presence of the tumour and sometimes of its size. Specific tumour markers are generally fusion protein products associated with the malignancy, in which an oncogene is translocated and fused to an active promoter of a separate gene [15]. Measurement of these tumour markers has become an important part of the management of testicular and ovarian germ-cell tumours, choriocarcinoma and hepatoma. The ideal requirements for a tumour marker are as follows.

The markers should always be produced by the tumour type. This is not the case for the great majority of markers (Table 4.3). In teratoma, α-fetoprotein (AFP) and human chorionic gonadotrophin (HCG) are present in serum in 75% of cases and HCG is present in almost all choriocarcinomas. Apart from carcinoembryonic antigen (CEA) and acid phosphatase, most other markers are of little value in diagnosis or staging.

Table 4.2 Effects of staging on survival ('stage-shift' effect).

	Tumour diagnosed in the 1950s, but with only clinical staging and carefully treated with surgery for stages I and II		Same tumour diagnosed in the 1980s and treated with surgery for stages I and II as in the 1950s	
	All cases (%)	5-year survival (%)	All cases (%)	5-year survival (%)
Stage I: local disease	40	50	10	80
Stage II: local nodules involved	40	20	40	40
Stage III: distant metastasis	20	2	50	10
Overall 5-year survival (%)		28.5		29

The marker should give an accurate and sensitive indication of tumour mass. This is the case with the α-subunit of HCG and AFP in germ-cell tumours and prostate-specific antigen (PSA) (to a lesser extent) in prostate cancer. CEA-producing colorectal cancer and CA-125-producing ovarian cancer can also be monitored by serum levels. In many other tumours the marker is inconsistently produced or is too insensitive to be a useful guide to treatment.

The marker should be produced by recurrent and metastatic disease. One of the major uses of markers is to diagnose recurrence early. Occasionally, in teratomas, recurrent disease is associated with a rise in either HCG or AFP, even though the original tumour produced both. Marker-negative recurrences (from a previously positive tumour) are rare. Similarly, a rise in CEA, PSA or CA-125 may precede clinical evidence of recurrence in bowel, prostate or ovarian cancer, respectively.

The tumour should be amenable to therapy. There is little value in detecting recurrence early if no treatment is available or should be withheld until symptoms develop. For example, recurrence of pancreatic cancer is seldom curable and early diagnosis of metastasis may serve only to alarm the patient. Conversely, in teratoma, a rise in AFP or HCG is a firm indication for full investigation since curative treatment is available.

The marker should be specific for the disease and easy to measure. Some markers, for example, AFP and HCG (α-subunit), are seldom present unless there is a tumour. However, AFP may be raised in pregnancy and with liver disease. CEA can be produced in inflammatory bowel disease as well as in colorectal and pancreatic cancer, and raised levels are found in smokers. The advent of sensitive radioimmunoassay techniques has led to the measurement of AFP and HCG as a routine in germ-cell tumours and hepatoma. Some peptide hormones, for example, antidiuretic hormone (ADH), are extremely difficult to measure accurately.

The marker should ideally be inexpensive and sensitive enough for population screening. In ovarian cancer, for example, most cases are diagnosed at an advanced and incurable stage so the mortality from this condition is now greater than for cancer of the cervix and uterus combined. Use of CA-125 is one of the more promising techniques for population screening for this condition.

Examples of tumour markers are given in Table 4.3. Some of these are in daily clinical use and justify more detailed consideration. Excellent reviews of the overall role together with some of the pitfalls of tumour marker analysis, are given at the end of the chapter (Sturgeon et al. [16]; Kilpatrick and Lind [17]).

Human chorionic gonadotrophin

The β-subunit of HCG is measured to avoid cross-reactivity with luteinizing hormone. HCG is measured by radioimmunoassay. It is used to detect and monitor therapy in choriocarcinoma and testicular and other germ-cell tumours. The half-life $(t_{1/2})$ is 24–36 hours and it is measurable in both blood and urine (where it gives a positive pregnancy test). In addition to its value in monitoring response and relapse, it has been shown that values over 10,000 IU/L are indicative of a poor prognosis in germ-cell tumours [15]. A β-core fragment has recently been described which is of low molecular weight and is found in the urine. It seems to be produced by a wide variety of non-trophoblastic tumours. Its role as a marker is not yet defined.

α-Fetoprotein

This protein is similar in size to albumin and is a major serum component before birth. It may cross the placenta and be detected in maternal blood. It is produced during liver regeneration and is elevated in viral hepatitis and cirrhosis. AFP is produced by malignant yolk-sac elements in germ-cell tumours (see Chapter 19) and by the malignant hepatocytes in hepatomas. Occasionally, after successful treatment with chemotherapy, a persistent rise in AFP occurs, presumed to be a drug effect on the liver. This can be a source of confusion in assessing response. It is also present in small amounts in some patients with pancreatic carcinoma and occasionally in gastric carcinoma. The plasma half-life is 5–7 days.

Placental alkaline phosphatase

This is an isoenzyme of alkaline phosphatase which is found in the serum in patients with seminoma. It is associated with bulky disease and disappears quickly on treatment and is thus of marginal value in monitoring response.

Carcinoembryonic antigen

CEA is one of a family of glycoproteins produced by many epithelial tumours, the molecule usually being demonstrable at the cell surface rather than in the cytoplasm. It is produced by normal colonic epithelium but is not usually present in the blood unless there is inflammation or neoplasia involving the epithelium. It is present in 25% of cases of Dukes B colonic cancer, 45% of Dukes C and 70% of metastatic cases. Its low incidence in early

Table 4.3 Tumour markers in malignant disease: serum markers, and molecular markers for diagnosis.

| Disease | Marker | Marker in use | | | | Marker still at experimental stage |
		Screening	Detection and diagnosis	Staging and prognosis	Follow-up	
Serum markers						
Colon cancer	CEA			(X)	X	
Breast cancer	CA-15-3			X	X	X
	CA-27-29					X
Prostate cancer	PSA	(X)			X	
Ovarian cancer	CA-125		X		X	
	CA-19-9					X
Thyroid cancer	Thyroglobulin		X		X	
(medullary carcinoma)	Calcitonin		X		X	
Testicular cancer	HCG			X	X	
	α-Fetoprotein		X		X	
Molecular markers						
Sarcoma						
Synovial sarcoma	t(X;18)				X	
Ewing's sarcoma	t(11;22)					
Alveolar rhabdomyosarcoma	t(2;13)					
Granulocytic sarcoma	t(9;11)					
Myxoid liposarcoma	t(12;16)					
Round cell liposarcoma	t(12;16)					
Clear cell sarcoma	t(12;22)					
Dermatofibrosarcoma protuberans	t(17;22)					
Melanoma	Tyrosinase					
Adrenal cortical carcinoma	Steroids					
Adrenal medullary carcinoma	Catecholamines					
Lymphoma	t(8;14), t(11;14)					
	t(2;5), t(3;14)					
	CD25, CD44					

(X), use in screening remains controversial (PSA) or possible future use (CEA).
CEA, carcinoembryonic antigen; HCG, human chorionic gonadotrophin; PSA, prostate-specific antigen.

stages makes it of no value in screening. It is also found in plasma in pancreatitis, heavy smokers, ulcerative colitis and gastritis, thus limiting its usefulness in diagnosis. Its value in early diagnosis of recurrent disease is limited by the lack of successful therapy in the majority of patients. Conversely, early surgical exploration of potential local anastomotic recurrences is increasingly undertaken in patients in whom CT scanning coupled with a rise in CEA level has aided the diagnosis while the patient is still asymptomatic. The increasing use of surgical resection, radiation and chemotherapy in patients with advanced colorectal cancer has led to an increased use of this tumour marker. CEA is elevated in approximately 60% of cases of advanced ovarian cancer and 40–70% of advanced breast cancers. It is therefore of little value in diagnosis of metastasis from an unknown primary site.

CA-125

This complex antigen is a glycoprotein of high molecular weight produced in coelomic epithelium and re-expressed in epithelial ovarian, pancreatic and breast cancer. Four-fifths of ovarian cancers are associated with antigenaemia and rising or falling levels correlate with disease in 93%. Levels above the upper limit of normal (35 U/mL) are not specific for ovarian cancer (being found in endometriosis, hepatitis and benign ovarian lesions) and are thus of limited value for screening. During treatment, CA-125 levels fall, but persistent disease is often found even when plasma levels are normal. However, elevated or rising levels can be used to detect early relapse after treatment. A rising level during chemotherapy indicates treatment failure.

CA-19-9

This mucin-like antigen is a polysialylated Lewis blood group antigen. Elevated levels are found in 80% of cases of pancreatic cancer and 75% of cases of advanced colorectal cancer. However, it may also be present in serum in benign hepatic and biliary tract disease [18]. Its value is limited by non-specificity and the lack of effective treatment of pancreatic cancer.

Molecular staging of cancer

Occult locoregional spread of cancer is a common cause of local recurrence, and an early indicator of subclinical dissemination [19]. Since malignancies develop from the progressive accumulation of mutations in genes of somatic cells, these mutations can be used as powerful molecular markers. Useful examples would include the detection of mutations in the urine of patients with bladder cancer and in the stools of patients with colorectal cancer – identical to those present in the primary tumour [20]. Genetic changes can be detected in metastatic tumour cells by fluorescent *in situ* hybridization [21]. Molecular assays can detect small clusters of cancer cells that would otherwise have been missed in routine histopathological staining. Molecular staging of cancer may soon have improved clinical implications. In node-negative breast cancer, for instance, molecular staging might demonstrate a small number of cancer cells, thereby identifying cases in which systemic therapy is clearly indicated. It is becoming increasingly clear that molecular staging of cancer will gain acceptance over the next few years as an important additional tool not only from the classification standpoint, but also to assist with case-selection [22].

References

1 Sobin LH, Wittekind CH, eds. *TNM Atlas: Classification of Malignant Tumours*, 7th edn. Hoboken, NJ: John Wiley & Sons, 2009.

2 Koh D-M, Cook GJR, Husband JE. New horizons in oncologic imaging. *N Engl J Med* 2003; 348: 2487–88.

3 Epstein DM, Stephenson LW, Gefter WB *et al.* The value of CT in the preoperative assessment of lung cancer. *Radiology* 1986; 161: 423–7.

4 Eustace SJ, Nelson E. Whole body magnetic resonance imaging: a valuable adjunct to clinical examination. *Br Med J* 2004; 328: 1387–88.

5 MERCURY Study Group. Diagnostic accuracy of pre-operative magnetic resonance imaging in predicting curative resection of rectal cancer: a prospective observational study. *Br Med J* 2006; 333: 779–82.

6 Harisinghani MG, Barentsz J, Hahn PF *et al.* Noninvasive detection of clinically occult lymph-node metastases in prostate cancer. *N Engl J Med* 2003; 348: 2491–99.

7 Barish MA, Yucel EK, Ferrucci JT. Magnetic resonance cholangiopancreatography. *N Engl J Med* 1999; 341: 258–64.

8 Krag D, Moffat F. Nuclear medicine and the surgeon. *Lancet* 1999; 354: 1019–22.

9 van Tinteren H, Hoekstra OS, Smit EF *et al.* Effectiveness of positron-emission tomography in the preoperative assessment of patients with suspected non-small-cell lung cancer. *Lancet* 2002; 359: 1388–92.

10 Juweid ME, Chaeson BD. Positron-emission tomography and assessment of cancer therapy. *N Engl J Med* 2006; 354: 496–507.

11 Kostakoglu L, Coleman M, Leonard JP *et al.* PET predicts prognosis after one cycle of chemotherapy in aggressive lymphoma and Hodgkin's disease. *J Nucl Med* 2002; 43: 1018–27.

12 Face K, Bradbury I, Laking G and Payne E. Overview of the clinical effectiveness of positron emission tomography imaging in selected cancers. *Health Technology Assessment* 2007; 11: 44

13 Zeman RK, Paushter DM, Schiebler ML *et al.* Hepatic imaging: current status. *Radiol Clin North Am* 1985; 23: 473–87.

14 Conlon KC. Value of laparoscopic staging for upper gastrointestinal malignancies. *J Surg Oncol* 1999; 71: 71–73.

15 Lindblom A, Liljegren A. Tumour markers in malignancies. *Br Med J* 2000; 320: 424–27.

16 Sturgeon C M, Lai L C and Duffy M J. Serum tumour markers: how to order and interpret them. *Brit Med J* 2009;339: 852–58.

17 Kilpatrick ES and Lind MJ. Appropriate requesting of serum tumour markers. *Brit Med J* 2009; 339: 859–70.

18 Begent RHJ, Rustin GJR. Tumour markers: from carcinoembryonic antigen to products of hybridoma technology. *Cancer Surv* 1989; 8: 108–21.

19 Caldas C. Molecular staging of cancer: is it time? *Lancet* 1997; 350: 231.

20 Sidransky D, Tokino T, Hamilton SR *et al.* Identification of *ras* oncogene mutations in the stool of patients with curable colorectal cancer. *Science* 1992; 256: 102–5.

21 Pack S, Vortmeyer AO, Pak E, Liotta LA, Zhuang Z. Detection of gene deletion in single metastatic tumour cells in lymph node tissue by fluorescent in-situ hybridization. *Lancet* 1997; 350: 264–65.

22 Mejia A, Schulz S, Hyslop T, Weinberg DS, Waldman SA. Molecular staging individualizing cancer management. *J Surg Oncol* 2012 ;105 : 468–74.

Further reading

Bomanji JB, Costa DC, Ell PJ. Clinical role of positron emission tomography in oncology. *Lancet Oncol* 2001; 2: 157–64.

Brenner D. Medical imaging in the 21st Century – getting the best bang for the rad. *New Eng J Med* 2010; 362: 943–47.

Gupte C, Padhani AR. New imaging techniques in cancer management. *Br J Cancer Management* 2004; 1: 4–7.

Husband JE, Reznek RH, eds. *Imaging in Oncology*, 3rd edn London: Taylor & Francis, 2009.

Royal College of Radiologists. *Imaging for Oncology: Collaboration Between Clinical Radiologists and Clinical Oncologists in Diagnosis, Staging and Radiotherapy Planning*. London: Royal College of Radiologists, 2004.

Royal College of Radiologists. *Recommendations for Cross-sectional Imaging in Cancer Management*. London: Royal College of Radiologists, 2006.

Shaw A, Dixon A. Cost–benefit analysis in cancer imaging. *Br J Cancer Management* 2005; 1: 8–10.

Wittekind C, Greene FL, Hutter RVP *et al.*, eds. *TNM Atlas: Illustrated Guide to the TNM Classification of Malignant Tumours*, 5th edn. Hoboken, NJ: John Wiley & Sons, 2005.

Wood KA, Hoskin PJ, Saunders MI. Positron emission tomography in oncology: a review. *Clin Oncol* 2007; 19: 237–55.

Zafra M, Ayala F, Gonzalez-Billalabeitia E *et al.* Impact of whole-body ^{18}F-FDG PET on diagnostic and therapeutic management of medical oncology patients. *Eur J Cancer* 2008; 44: 1678–83.

5 Radiotherapy

The Royal College of Radiologists (UK) estimates that, taking cancer patients as a whole and assessing the contributions of differing modalities to cure rates, 'of those cured, 49% are cured by surgery, 40% by radiotherapy and 11% by chemotherapy' [1].

Ever since the discovery of X-rays by Roentgen in 1895, attempts have been made not only to understand their physical nature but also to use them both in the biological sciences and in a variety of human illnesses. The development of the X-ray tube rapidly led to clinical applications, first as a diagnostic tool and later for therapy in patients with malignant disease. The discovery of radium by Marie and Pierre Curie in 1898 also resulted in the use of radioactive materials for the approach to cancer, since surgery was the only alternative available at that time. Over the past 80 years our understanding of the physical characteristics, biological effects and clinical roles of ionizing radiation has greatly increased. Important articles and papers are listed under Further reading.

To understand the nature of radioactivity and radioactive decay, it is important to grasp the concept of a natural spectrum of electromagnetic waves whose energy varies widely, in inverse proportion to the length of the wave itself. This spectrum (Figure 5.1) includes X-rays (very high energy and very short wavelength), visible light rays (of intermediate wavelength and energy) and also radio waves (of generally longer wavelength and lower energy) that are responsible for modern telecommunications and include the transmission signals for radio and television. Of these various types of electromagnetic wave, only X-rays and γ-rays (the terms are almost interchangeable) are of sufficiently high energy to produce the ionization of atoms that occurs when a beam of radiation passes through biological tissue.

In the process of ionization, the essential event is the displacement of an electron from its orbital path around the nucleus of the atom. This creates an unstable or ionized atom, and a free electron which is normally 'captured' by a neighbouring atom, which then becomes equally unstable because of its possession of an extra negative electric charge. When radiation beams pass through living tissue, the intensity, duration and site of these ionization events can be controlled by varying the characteristics of the radiation source. This permits deliberate and controlled cellular destruction in the case of therapeutic radiation (radiotherapy), whereas, with

Cancer and its Management, Seventh Edition. Jeffrey Tobias and Daniel Hochhauser.
© 2015 John Wiley & Sons, Ltd. Published 2015 by John Wiley & Sons, Ltd.

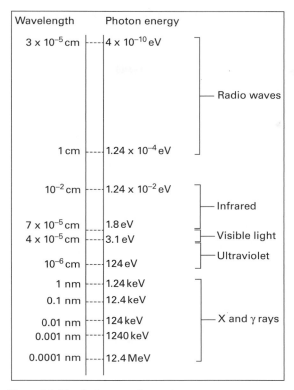

Figure 5.1 The electromagnetic spectrum.

diagnostic radiation, trivial and short-lived alterations occur that usually have no permanent biological effect. The creation of the radiographic image is due to the differential alteration of the X-ray beam by biological tissues containing atoms of differing atomic weights.

Sources and production of ionizing radiation

Radioactive isotopes

Radioactivity is an unalterable property of many naturally occurring atoms that exist in a relatively unstable state. Although the identity of any given atom is defined by the number of protons and electrons it possesses, the atoms of any one element may contain differing numbers of nuclear neutrons, so that their atomic weights (as determined by the proton and neutron component) differ. Such atoms or *isotopes* occur naturally in fixed proportions, and most pure substances (particularly metals such as iron, manganese and cobalt) consist of mixtures of these isotopes. Emission of radioactivity is one of the consequences of

physical decay of unstable atoms, resulting in a final and more stable state. The rate and intensity of these emissions varies with each element.

There is a wide variety of naturally occurring radioactive materials, whose chief characteristic is the emission of electromagnetic waves of a frequency that can produce ionization within biological materials. Historically, these emissions have been divided into α, β and γ waves, depending on the characteristics of the emission. The α particles are no more than helium nuclei, emitted from unstable or decaying radionuclides. It is worth remembering that although many of the properties of radioactive emission are better understood in terms of their characteristic waveforms, the 'wave' also has features of a particle. Thus α and β emissions are best understood in terms of these features since α particles are positively charged helium nuclei, with a substantial mass, and β particles are no more than electrons, with a negative charge but almost no mass; γ rays, on the other hand, carry no charge.

Although α, β and γ rays can all produce ionization in tissues, it is the γ rays which have the greatest application in radiation therapy. For example, in a reaction of great clinical importance, the unstable isotope of cobalt, with an atomic number of 60, disintegrates to a more stable isotope (atomic number 59) by discharging one of its nuclear neutrons, together with γ rays. The characteristics of the emitted γ radiation are constant for this particular reaction, and the rate of nuclear disintegration is unalterable, such that after 5.33 years exactly half of the original radioactive material still remains, thus defining the radioactive half-life of ^{60}Co. The half-life is an important concept in theoretical and clinical work, and varies between a fraction of a second and hundreds or thousands of years (Table 5.1). Radium, widely used before the introduction of more suitable radioactive materials, has a half-life of 1620 years, which meant that radioactive sources for therapeutic use never needed replacing. However, β particles, or electrons, are now increasingly used as their characteristics are generally more suitable. Other atomic fragments are being studied since they have theoretical advantages as a result of their different biological effects. These include neutrons, protons and pi-mesons.

Although the early radioactive substances discovered by the Curies and others were all naturally occurring, modern high-energy physics has provided ready access to many new materials, or artificially manufactured isotopes. These substances, *radionuclides*, are generally manufactured in nuclear reactors by heavy particle

Table 5.1 Therapeutically useful isotopes.

Isotope	Type of radiation	Energy (MeV)	Half-life
^{60}Co	β, γ	0.31 (β), 1.17 and 1.33 (γ)	5.3 years
^{137}Cs	β, γ	0.51 (β) and 0.66 (γ)	30 years
^{131}I	β, γ	0.61 (β) and 0.36 (γ)	8 days
^{198}Au	β, γ	0.96 (β) and 0.41 (γ)	2.7 days
^{32}P	β	1.71 (β)	14 days
^{192}Ir	Γ	0.36–0.6 (γ)	74 days
^{226}Ra (decays to radon, then Ra A,B,C)	α then β, γ	1.0 (γ)	1620 years for radium but 3–27 min for Ra A,B,C

bombardment of natural materials. The chief advantage is that their properties more closely resemble the theoretical ideal for radioactive half-life, γ-ray characteristics and intensity than any natural substance. The changing demands of both diagnosis, for example, in radioisotope imaging, and therapy have led to ever-increasing attempts at producing new radioactive isotopes with differing radiation characteristics. For therapeutic work, this includes the production of both sealed and unsealed sources. For sealed sources, the radioactive material is physically enclosed by an impenetrable barrier such as the platinum casing of a typical radium or caesium needle, so that the radioactive material can be inserted into the tissue to be irradiated and then removed at some predetermined time. With unsealed sources, such as iodine-131 (^{131}I), the isotope is physically ingested by mouth or by injection, passing via the bloodstream to the end organ and taken up (in this case, by the thyroid), where the effects of the radioactive emission cause local damage to both the normal thyroid gland and the cancer within it. The isotope cannot then be recovered.

Unsealed sources are widely used in diagnostic work such as the radioactive technetium bone or brain scan. In therapeutic work, the most specific and ideal application is for carcinoma of the thyroid, where radioactive isotopes of iodine (usually ^{131}I) are given by mouth and selectively taken up by the thyroid gland and thyroid cancer cells, providing 'internal' irradiation to a high intensity without compromising other organs by the delivery of an unacceptable dose of radiation at an unwanted site. Use of injectable radioactive phosphorus (^{32}P) for bone marrow irradiation in polycythaemia rubra vera is another well-known example. Radionuclide therapy provides specificity, efficiency and low toxicity, together with excellent palliation and the prospect of repeated treatment. However, limitations include the unavoidable patient isolation, storage of radioactive waste and the high cost, particularly of some of the newer forms of treatment. Nonetheless, the current therapeutic indications of unsealed radionuclide treatment for malignant disease have expanded in recent years.

For use in clinical work, the choice of either naturally occurring or artificially produced radioactive isotopes will depend on the clinical requirement. For example, in interstitial implantation work, where radioactive needles are directly placed adjacent to or even within the malignant tissue, caesium needles have increasingly been employed in preference to radium because of the more suitable characteristics of the emitted radiation from this material. This is because the specific activity (number of radioactive disintegrations per second) is so high with radium that protection for doctors, radiographers, nurses and other staff has always been a major problem. With caesium, however, the specific activity is substantially lower, making protection easier.

Radioactive isotopes are also used as a source of external radiation (teletherapy). All clinical departments place a heavy clinical reliance on their external therapy techniques since the majority of tumours are deeply situated and inaccessible to irradiation by direct implantation (brachytherapy). Nowadays, when γ irradiation from a major radioactive source is employed, the most common choice of material is ^{60}Co, a material that emits a high-energy γ ray (mean energy 1.2 MeV) of sufficient penetration to allow treatment of deeply situated tumours. Cobalt-60 has a reasonably satisfactory half-life of 5.3 years, so that major source replacement will not be required more than every 3–4 years.

A traditional cobalt unit is in essence no more than a cylindrical source of ^{60}Co produced artificially within a nuclear fission pile, placed in a protective shell made of lead, and supplied with a simple mechanism for moving the source into the treatment position when required. This type of equipment, though largely rendered obsolete because of replacement by linear accelerators (see below), has advantages of reliability and longevity, as well as being relatively inexpensive to purchase and maintain. Its disadvantages are that there is a substantial 'penumbra' of scattered radiation, which forms a significant part of the edge of the beam, and that treatment times can be lengthy, particularly when the source has started to age, since radioactive decay results in a loss of residual radioactive material and treatment time increases proportionately.

Artificial production of X-rays and particles

Shortly before the discovery of radium by the Curies, Roentgen constructed the first X-ray apparatus, consisting of a sealed glass vacuum tube containing an electrode at one end and a target at the other. Heating the electrode resulted in a discharge of electrons, which travelled relatively easily through the vacuum to bombard the target at the other end of the tube. This produced characteristic rays which, like those of radium, could create an image on a photographic plate. The nature of these rays was uncertain; *X-rays*, therefore, seemed the most suitable title. It gradually became clear that X-rays and γ rays were fundamentally similar although their method of production is quite different. Unlike the γ irradiation from radioactive materials, whose characteristics cannot be changed other than by altering either the choice or the purity of the material, X-rays of quite different properties can be produced simply by varying the voltage input to the cathode of the X-ray tube.

X-rays used for diagnostic radiology are generated in a low-voltage machine (e.g. 50 kV) and have a longer wavelength and less penetrating power. By contrast, therapeutic X-rays are much more powerful, varying from 50 kV up to 30 MeV, a 600-fold increase. As voltage is increased, X-rays of shorter wavelength are produced, which have far greater penetration within human tissue.

For therapeutic use, one of the chief criteria for successful treatment is the availability of X-rays of sufficient penetrating power, or depth dose, to deal effectively with deep-seated tumours. For this reason, departments of radiotherapy need a range of equipment with a wide spectrum of clinically useful X-ray beams to deal with both superficial tumours such as skin cancers and those more deeply situated, such as tumours of the mediastinum or pelvis. With conventional or *orthovoltage* X-ray equipment, the maximum deposition of radiation energy is in the superficial tissues, with a steep fall-off (Figure 5.2), such that the dosage received by a deep tumour, which may be 10 cm or more below the skin surface, is low and limited by the skin reaction that this treatment will inevitably cause. The physical and electromagnetic problems of safely applying a very high tension (voltage) input had to be overcome before further progress could be made.

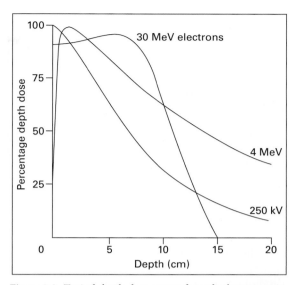

Figure 5.2 Typical depth-dose curves for radiotherapy equipment (kilovoltage, megavoltage and 30 MeV electron beam). There is skin 'build-up' over the first centimetre for megavoltage therapy but not for kilovoltage or electron treatment. Depth dose for both megavoltage and electron beam therapy is much superior to kilovoltage treatment and the 'skin-sparing' effect has great clinical benefit.

Fortunately, most of these technical difficulties were solved in the 1960s with the advent of an entirely fresh approach to the generation of high-energy megavoltage beams and the development of the modern linear accelerator. The principal feature is the acceleration of electrons down a cylindrical 'waveguide' terminating in the deliberate bombardment of a fixed target by electrons travelling almost at the speed of light, thus producing a beam of much higher intensity (Figure 5.3). As well as possessing much greater depth dose, these beams typically have far less in the way of scattered radiation, leading to a much cleaner, higher quality and more precise beam with a narrower penumbra than with traditional cobalt apparatus. In addition, the output (or dose rate) is considerably greater, leading to shorter treatment times. The linear accelerator has now become the standard workhorse of modern radiotherapy departments in the developed world. A further important advantage of this equipment is that the target can be moved out of position, yielding a beam of high-velocity electrons (instead of X-rays) of 30 MeV or more, which can be useful therapeutically in certain clinical situations (see next page).

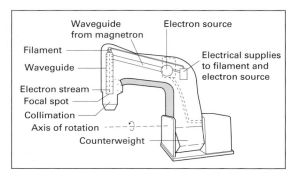

Figure 5.3 Schematic representation of an isocentrically mounted 4–8 MeV linear accelerator. (Source: Meredith and Massey [2])

To the clinician, the fundamental difference between X-ray and electron therapy lies in their entirely different depth-dose characteristics (Figure 5.2). With X-ray or γ-ray therapy, the amount of radiation energy deposited at any given depth of tissue (the depth dose) falls off exponentially, which means that, however, powerful the source and whatever the distance, unwanted areas of tissue will be irradiated, both superficial to the tumour area and also beyond it. The entrance and exit dose will irradiate a substantial volume of normal host tissue, and this unavoidable characteristic is usually the limiting factor in a course of treatment. With electron therapy this disadvantage is at least partly overcome, since the beam decays completely at a depth entirely dependent on the energy of the electron beam.

With low- and medium-voltage X-rays, the energy deposited in the tissues is critically dependent on the mean atomic number of the tissue in which this deposition is occurring. With high-voltage X-rays, γ rays and electrons, the energy absorbed by the tissue is much less dependent on the atomic number, so that the drawbacks of very high bone absorption (with its twin problems of dosage inhomogeneity and radionecrosis) are largely avoided. Radiotherapists are therefore very careful when irradiating superficial lesions situated over bone or cartilage, which require treatment with low-voltage (superficial) beams. For this reason, electron therapy is often preferred in these cases, particularly for skin tumours that overlie an area of cartilage. Common examples include basal cell carcinomas on the nose or pinna of the ear.

A further intriguing possibility under active clinical trial at present is the use of heavy charged and uncharged particles, including neutrons, protons and pi-mesons.

All these beams have theoretical advantages, although the capital expenditure required for the development and building of neutron and charged particle generators is substantially greater than the cost of more conventional equipment. However, trials of neutron therapy have proved disappointing so far. Only a few centres throughout the world have these resources available at present.

Biological properties of ionizing radiation

Tumour sensitivity

Since the beginning of the twentieth century, clinical scientists have been fascinated (and puzzled) by the extraordinary cellular events that occur when living tissue is exposed to a beam of ionizing radiation. It is now clear that radiation-induced damage may be lethal, resulting in cell death, or sublethal, in which case the cellular damage can be partially or completely repaired. In general, the degree of radiosensitivity of any given tumour type will depend not only on the immediate damage sustained by the cell (a measure of its true 'intrinsic' sensitivity) but also on its ability to repair the sublethal damage that has been caused. Although a high degree of radiosensitivity is generally required if there is to be any hope of a radiation cure, other factors may prevent the realization of this aim; radiosensitivity is not in itself sufficient. Acute lymphoblastic leukaemia (ALL), for instance, is highly radiosensitive, since small malignant lymphoblasts are permanently damaged by a relatively low dose of radiation. However, the widespread nature of this disease, which by definition affects the whole of the bone marrow and therefore every organ supplied by the peripheral bloodstream, made it impossible until recently to deliver curative radiotherapy without fatal over-irradiation. The modern technique of allogeneic bone marrow transplantation (BMT) has resulted in safe delivery of total-body irradiation to a sufficiently high dosage for total irreversible ablation of the malignant marrow elements. It is not the bone marrow transplant itself which is the therapeutic event, but the lethal radiation damage inflicted on the leukaemic cell population.

The physicochemical events which take place within radiation-damaged cells are far from understood. Although there is little doubt that the important target site is the nuclear DNA, it is less common for the damage to be inflicted as a result of a 'direct hit', although this mechanism will certainly produce irreversible cleavage of the DNA strands. More commonly the effects are indirect, resulting in the production of unstable, highly reactive and short-lived free radicals that in turn produce destruction of the normal DNA molecule with which they rapidly react. The probability of a lethal cell injury varies not only with the quantity of radiation energy deposited in the tissues (a function of the output of the radiation beam) but also with the intensity of the beam and with its 'type', that is, whether the radiation is produced by γ rays, electrons, neutrons or other particles. These differences give rise to the concept of linear energy transfer (LET), which refers to the amount of radiation energy transferred to the tissue per unit track length by the particular beam. In general, kilovoltage beams of X-rays have a higher LET than megavoltage beams, and neutron beams have a very much higher LET than X-rays or γ rays. Thus, appropriate adjustments in total doses will have to be made if neutron therapy, for example, is offered as an alternative to conventional treatment. Another important principle is that the relatively protective effect of hypoxia (on tumour cells) is particularly apparent with beams of relatively low LET. This is one of the reasons why neutron therapy was long thought to be more effective, regardless of the state of oxygenation of the malignant tissues.

Experimental studies have shown that human tumour cells have markedly different intrinsic radiosensitivities that closely parallel clinical experience. Our present understanding of this correlation postulates two components to cell kill: the α-component which is log-linear (exponential) and, therefore, appears as a straight line in dose–survival curves (Figure 5.4); and a bending or β-component which occurs over a shorter dose range and at low dose levels. Intrinsic differences in sensitivity are most marked in the low-dose region (clinically of greatest importance) below 2 Gy (200 rad) per treatment fraction, and low-dose-rate irradiation is likely to exaggerate these differences. Indeed, at low dose rates, less sensitive cells become relatively more resistant. This is often forwarded as an argument for larger fractions in less sensitive tumours. In the linear quadratic mathematical model, using an α-component that is the linear dose function and β the square of the dose, cell survival is the common end-point. Fractionation tends to spare late-responding tissues more than early-responding tissues and tumours.

In other clinical circumstances, failure of radiation therapy may occur because of the recurrence of disease after apparently successful radiation treatment. This is a frequent event, for example, in squamous cell carcinoma of the bronchus, where careful assessment by chest radiography and even bronchoscopy may well demonstrate

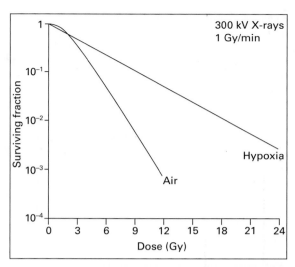

Figure 5.4 Fractionation: the effect of repeated doses of radiation. Fractionation increases the differential cytotoxic effect on normal and malignant tissue.

an apparently satisfactory response to treatment. When relapse occurs, often 1–2 years after primary treatment, what can we suggest by way of explanation? One widely held view, for which there is a good deal of experimental evidence, is that at the time of the initial treatment there is a spectrum of cellular sensitivity to the radiation, and that the degree of oxygenation of each cell is the key determining factor. A great deal of radiobiological work has gone into defining and characterizing this phenomenon, and almost all studies (both with experimental animals and *in vitro* tissue culture systems) have shown that well-oxygenated cells are substantially more radiosensitive than those which are anoxic.

This difference in sensitivity may be reflected in a two- or three-fold increase in the dosage required for tumour eradication in an anoxic environment (Figure 5.4), and the clinical importance of this observation is thought by many to be critical, since cells far removed from a good arterial supply will inevitably be relatively anoxic. In large tumours with a relatively rapid growth rate and in areas of necrosis where vascularization is poor, anoxia may be a major cause of radioresistance, and experiments using microelectrodes for measurement of oxygen tension have confirmed these theoretical predictions.

Quite apart from the oxygen effect, the progenitor cells will not be equally radiosensitive, so that recurrence after apparently successful treatment may be due to repopulation through regeneration of the radioresistant stem cells within the tumour. This can take place either after a complete course of radiotherapy, or rapidly, even between fractions given, say, on a daily basis. There is at least some evidence that regrowth through repopulation may be more delayed with malignant tissues than with normal host cells, and that this may be an important basis for the difference between the relatively adequate regenerative capability of many normal tissues in contrast to the more permanent destructive effects on malignant tumours. This is analogous to the effects of chemotherapy on normal and malignant tissue (see Chapter 6). Recognition of the importance of tumour cell repopulation and cellular hypoxia has led to many experiments using accelerated hyperfractionated radiotherapy and attempts to improve tumour oxygenation, in order to improve local control rates with external beam radiation therapy.

Fractionation and cell death

Fractionation, the use of repeated dosage of radiation within a course of treatment, has long been the subject of considerable interest. Early radiation workers rapidly realized that repeated use of modest radiation doses seemed to be the best method of safely delivering a higher total dose of radiation than would be possible with a single large treatment, and that this generally led to a greater likelihood of cure. Interest in fractionation has developed because of a natural desire not only to understand the mechanisms of radiation-induced cell damage, but also to learn how best to exploit this phenomenon and to advise the clinician as to the optimal choice of fraction size and overall treatment time. These are important details which might make the difference between success and failure. In most single-dose experiments, the degree of damage to the malignant cell (usually measured by inhibition of cell division) is directly proportional, in a log-linear fashion, to the radiation dose (Figure 5.4). The important additional feature is that, at low dosage, the steep curve is flattened to form a characteristic 'shoulder'. With relatively more radioresistant cells (such as malignant melanoma) the shoulder will be broader, and the rest of the curve less steep.

Most theorists agree that the shoulder region represents an area of sublethal damage, from which repair is possible. With repeated or fractionated treatment, further radiation damage can be inflicted before completion of this repair, although naturally the degree of cell recovery between fractions will depend on the interval and intensity of each fraction of treatment (Figure 5.5).

In addition, fractionation of treatment encourages early improvement in tissue oxygenation which, by reduction

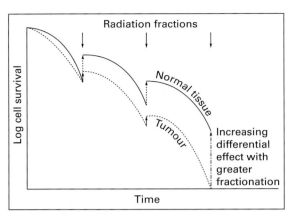

Figure 5.5 Effect of oxygen concentration on cytotoxicity of X-rays. This experiment used Hela cell cultures *in vitro*.

of the tumour bulk, leads to relief of vascular obstruction, a more effective blood supply and greater sensitivity to subsequent doses of irradiation, again due to the oxygen effect. In addition to these theoretical advantages, fractionated treatment has other practical benefits since the earlier fractions often produce a significant improvement in clinical well-being, allowing better tolerance of the total course. This allows much greater flexibility from a course rather than a single treatment, permitting, for example, a change in radiation volume and/or dose rate, which may well be called for as the tumour begins to resolve.

Conversely, lengthy periods of fractionated treatment (often up to 6 weeks in current practice) carry the potential disadvantage of tumour cell repopulation during the course of therapy, with acceleration of repopulating clonogenic cells as little as 1 week after initiation of treatment. For this and other reasons there is increasing interest in the concept of continuous hyperfractionated treatment, using two or three treatment fractions in a single day and treating the patient within a much shorter period of time, even including weekends, for (say) 2–3 weeks rather than the conventional 6-week period.

Despite these general comments, there have been few satisfactory studies comparing different fractionation regimens. Most radiotherapists rely on approaches which have been empirically tested and found acceptable in terms of both effectiveness and toxicity. For example, lengthy fractionation regimens of 6 weeks of daily treatment are often used for squamous carcinomas, while other radiotherapists offer treatment which takes no more than 3 or 4 weeks. Very careful estimates of dose equivalence have to be employed when comparing treatment regimens since all radiotherapists know that, for example, the radiobiological effect of a single dose of 10 Gy is greatly in excess of the effect produced by 10 daily doses of 1 Gy. A yardstick for measurement of dose equivalence is therefore essential, not only for prospective trials of fractionation regimens but also for the radiotherapist, who may sometimes need to deviate from the standard regimen for a whole host of reasons. Unexpected machine breakdown, pressures on equipment and staff shortages can all occur unpredictably from time to time.

Response of biological tissues to radiation

Normal tissues

In clinical practice, successful eradication of malignant cells depends on the difference between the sensitivity (and/or repair capacity) of these cells compared with those of normal surrounding tissues also subjected to radiation therapy. However precise our tumour imaging with isotope scanning, computed tomography (CT) or magnetic resonance imaging, this will always remain a limiting factor. Figure 5.6 demonstrates the relatively narrow gap between tumour and host tissues within which the radiotherapist has to operate. The more radiosensitive the tumour, the wider this therapeutic 'window' and the lower the dose required, allowing a greater chance of

cure with few, if any, side-effects. Since the adverse effects of radiation limit the clinician in choice of dosage, an understanding of the radiation tolerance of normal host tissues is an important facet of the radiotherapist's training and practice. Very wide discrepancies in the radiation tolerance of different organs have been demonstrated (Table 5.2); in general, the most radiosensitive (and easily damaged) tissues are those with rapid cell division – the bone marrow, the stem cells of the gonads and the epithelial lining of the alimentary tract.

A particularly tragic and clear-cut illustration of the critical importance of radiation dose for long-term damage was provided by the unintended over-irradiation of over 200 cancer patients treated in the UK at a single centre in 1988 [4]. Due to the miscalibration of a radiocobalt source, most of these patients received doses of 25% above the recommended prescribed level, with varying effects dependent upon the site. Many patients treated for breast carcinoma suffered profound local effects in the breast itself, together with local chest wall damage (including rib

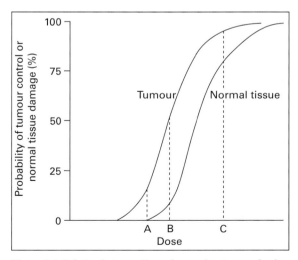

Figure 5.6 Relation between X-ray dose and outcome of radiotherapy. A, low safe dose; B, increasing dose, more normal tissue damage; C, higher chance of a cure but with a greater level of host tissue side-effects, some of which might be long term. (Source: Withers [3]. Reproduced with permission from Elsevier.)

Table 5.2 Radiosensitivity of normal and malignant tissue.

Radio-sensitivity	Normal	Malignant
Highly sensitive	Marrow	Lymphoma
	Gonad	Leukaemia
	Gut (mucosa)	Seminoma
	Lymphatic tissue	Ewing's sarcoma
	Eye (lens)	Many embryonal tumours
Moderately sensitive	Liver	Small-cell lung cancer
	Kidney	Breast cancer
	Lung	Squamous carcinomas (including gynaecological, head and neck, and skin tumours)
	Skin	Adenocarcinomas of the bowel
	Breast	Glioma
	Gut wall	
	Nervous tissue	
Relatively insensitive	Bone	Sarcoma of bone and connective tissue
	Connective tissue	Melanoma
	Muscle	

fracture) and in some cases a brachial plexus radioneuropathy. It seems clear that relatively small dose excesses ('small' at least in comparison with current drug therapy) can, for the radiotherapist, lead to disastrous and in many cases irreversible consequences. Reducing the potential harm from radiotherapy (especially of course when given at radical dose, with intent to cure) has become an even more important issue over recent years. As pointed out by Sir Liam Donaldson, previously Chief Medical Officer for England, highly publicized cases of radiation overdose, though extremely rare, corrode public trust and confidence (see Further reading).

Clinically, there is an important distinction to be drawn between early, *acute*, effects and later, *chronic*, damage. It is not necessarily the intensity of the acute reaction which determines the probability and duration of the long-term effects. Even where recovery from acute irradiation appears complete, the 'reserve' of stem cells in these organs is often permanently depleted, so that further treatment with either radiation therapy or cytotoxic drugs may well produce a surprising degree of tissue damage including, for example, marrow suppression. Understanding this long-term but latent (invisible) damage is of great importance since increasing numbers of cancer patients are likely to be offered both these forms of therapy.

Highly radiosensitive tissues
Haemopoietic tissues
The bone marrow is exceedingly sensitive to irradiation. In humans, a single total-body dose of 4 Gy would prove lethal to about half of all patients, the majority of these deaths due to early myelosuppression producing anaemia, neutropenia and thrombocytopenia. With localized treatment at high dose (a much more common clinical situation), long-lasting inhibition of myelopoiesis occurs, but usually without appreciable effect on the blood count. Lymphopenia is a well-recognized complication of localized radiotherapy at any site, resulting from irradiation of the blood as it passes through the beam, a consequence of the extreme radiosensitivity of the small lymphocyte. Allogeneic BMT has permitted whole-body irradiation to a higher dose (often up to 10 Gy) as part of the therapy for acute leukaemia and other diseases, including non-Hodgkin's lymphoma and myeloma. In addition, large areas of the body can now be treated with therapeutic irradiation for widespread and painful bony metastases (e.g. from myeloma or carcinoma of the prostate) without recourse to marrow transplantation techniques, since the unirradiated marrow is able to

compensate by increased production. This is the basis of so-called hemibody irradiation, an increasingly used method of simple palliation for patients with widespread metastatic disease, which can be repeated to the opposite half of the body, providing a suitable gap of 6–8 weeks is allowed between the two fractions of treatment.

The gonads
In the testes and ovary, small single doses of radiotherapy can permanently damage reproductive function, although the testis is undoubtedly more sensitive. It is likely that some of the primitive spermatogonia (the precursors of the spermatocytes) may be sensitive to a dose of as little as 1 Gy, although a dose as low as this would be unlikely to reduce the human sperm count to zero. The radiation sensitivity of the hormone-producing testicular Leydig cell is very much less, so that large doses of radiotherapy to the human testis do not result in loss of secondary sexual characteristics. In the female, single doses of 4–5 Gy have been used to induce artificial menopause, although some 30% of women appear to continue regular menstruation following this single fraction of radiation. Fractionated treatment to 10–12 Gy results in complete cessation of menses in virtually every patient.

Moderately radiosensitive tissues
This group is characterized by relatively low cell turnover rates which are paralleled by a relative, but by no means complete, insensitivity to radiation; these include nerve cells, including the brain itself, as well as the spinal cord and peripheral nervous system, skin, kidney, gut and other sites (Table 5.2).

Nervous tissue
The nervous system is of great concern partly because the sequelae of damage to the central nervous system can be both profound and irreversible, and also because, for the large majority of malignant brain tumours, radiation therapy is much the most valuable non-surgical modality available (see Chapter 11). During the early acute phase of radiation response, the blood vessels, nerve cells and supporting glial structures are all injured directly; sufficiently large doses may result in acute cerebral oedema and a sudden rise in intracranial pressure. These changes will gradually subside, but chronic effects include demyelination, vascular damage with proliferation of subendothelial fibrous tissue and, eventually, brain necrosis if the dose is sufficiently high. It is generally accepted that the hypothalamus, brainstem and upper cervical spine are rather more sensitive to radiation than other

parts of the brain, and it is also thought that concurrent administration of chemotherapy (chiefly methotrexate and vincristine) may also reduce radiation tolerance.

Irradiation of the spinal cord may pose even more problems, particularly since this may be unavoidable in, for example, the palliation of painful bony metastases of the spine. The radiation tolerance of the spinal cord is governed by a variety of important details such as the length of cord irradiated, the fractionation employed and the total dose given. It is widely held that for a 10-cm length of cord, a total dose of 40 Gy in 4 weeks is safe, although many clinicians err on the side of great caution since radiation myelitis, leading to irreversible paraparesis, is such an appalling complication. Recent work with total-body irradiation has shown that a single dose of about 10 Gy delivered to the whole length of the spinal cord very rarely produces significant neurological sequelae, although the mildest (reversible) late complication, that of Lhermitte's syndrome of paraesthesiae in the extremities on flexion of the neck, is often encountered. Moreover, with prophylactic spinal cord irradiation in children with medulloblastoma, the risk of clinically significant neurological sequelae, after doses as high as 30 Gy applied over 5–6 weeks to the whole of the spinal cord, seems acceptably low. In general, careful fractionation should be employed wherever a significant length of cord is likely to be irradiated in a patient whose survival may be prolonged. For palliative radiation treatment it seems prudent to recommend the lowest effective dose which is compatible with durable pain relief, particularly since further treatment may well be required, inevitably adding to the possibility of cord damage.

The skin

A portion of skin will be irradiated in all patients treated by external methods of X-ray therapy. Historically, the skin reaction was the chief guide in determining the total radiation dose. With modern high-energy (megavoltage) equipment, far fewer severe skin reactions are seen, since the scattered radiation component of these beams is almost exclusively in the forward direction so that maximum energy deposition takes place well beneath the skin surface (see Figure 5.2). Nonetheless, clinically important skin reactions can still pose major problems with orthovoltage and even with megavoltage beams (Table 5.3). Typically, the changes consist of an erythema of increasing severity, leading to dry and then moist desquamation, followed (if the radiation therapy is discontinued) by a repair process associated with progressive fibrosis, hyperplasia of vascular elements

Table 5.3 Skin reactions to radiotherapy.

Early changes	Later changes
Erythema	Fibrosis
Dry and moist desquamation	Loss of pigment
Pigmentation	Telangiectasia
Epilation	Loss of skin appendages
Loss of sweat gland function	Loss of connective tissue
Tissue oedema	

(sometimes resulting in telangiectasia much later on) and also by excessive pigmentation which may be permanent, although depigmentation can also occur. If the skin is further irradiated at a time when moist desquamation is evident, then extensive skin and subcutaneous necrosis may occur; this takes place when the treatment is separated by months or even years. It is, therefore, unwise to attempt re-irradiation of recurrent skin carcinomas, since the risk of necrosis is ever present and such cases are usually better treated by surgery. Skin 'appendages' such as sweat glands, sebaceous glands and hair follicles are also damaged directly by radiation. Radiation-induced epilation of the scalp is an inevitable drawback of whole-brain irradiation for cerebral metastases, which is in other respects an effective technique with few side-effects. Hair regrowth will usually occur, given time, even when a radical dose has been used as, for example, in children with medulloblastoma.

The eye

The eye is frequently irradiated, particularly during the treatment of carcinomas of the maxillary antrum and paranasal sinuses and in the definitive radiation therapy of orbital lymphomas, rhabdomyosarcomas, retinoblastomas and other orbital tumours. It is often not appreciated that, for the most part, the eye is relatively radioresistant, particularly its more posterior structures. Careful attention to detail can result in a healthy eye with very adequate vision even after whole orbital irradiation. However, there are two important points to remember. First, the greatest danger to the eye is posed by dryness of the cornea, leading to keratoconjunctivitis sicca. This generally results from lack of tear formation following irradiation of the lacrimal gland, which can be avoided in most instances by the use of a small lead shield. Second, the most radiosensitive structure of the eye is the lens, which is particularly sensitive to large single fractions of irradiation. Cataract formation can often be prevented by the use of a pencil-shaped corneal shield, although there is always the danger of under-irradiation of important structures deep to the protected cornea and lens.

The kidney

The kidney is frequently irradiated during treatment of abdominal or retroperitoneal tumours, and is a relatively radiosensitive structure. Glomerular filtration rate and renal plasma flow are both reduced after modest radiation doses, and it is often a year or more before recovery begins. Acute radiation nephritis can occur when the dose to both kidneys is no greater than about 25 Gy in 5 weeks. The acute clinical syndrome includes proteinuria, uraemia and hypertension which can be irreversible and even fatal. More chronic changes include persistent albuminuria and poor glomerular and tubular function, which may be lifelong even in patients who recover from the acute syndrome. These complications are particularly likely to occur after whole abdominal irradiation.

The gut

Although both small and large bowel tissues are sensitive to radiation, the rectum deserves special mention since this is frequently the organ of limiting tolerance when treating carcinomas of the cervix and other pelvic tumours. Acute radiation reactions, accompanied by diarrhoea, tenesmus and occasional rectal haemorrhage, are encountered both with external irradiation of the pelvis and with intracavitary treatment. The later radiation effects are of even greater importance, and include oedema and fibrosis of the bowel, which once again may be responsible for diarrhoea, painful proctitis and rectal bleeding, sometimes progressing to stricture, abscess or fistula formation. Occasionally these complications are severe enough to warrant temporary or even permanent colostomy or may cause difficult diagnostic problems by mimicking symptoms of recurrence of the cancer. Radiation damage to the small bowel is pathologically similar to that of the rectum and may limit treatment of intra-abdominal tumours. Late sequelae include stricture formation, which may cause intestinal obstruction.

The heart

Although often overlooked as a moderately radiosensitive tissue, the heart is frequently included within radiation volumes, particularly in treatment of patients with lung and oesophageal cancer, and of course most particularly in the classical 'mantle' supradiaphragmatic treatment of Hodgkin's disease. Radiation-induced cardiac damage is relatively common, affecting the pericardium, myocardium, conducting mechanism or coronary vessels. For the most part, the injury appears chiefly to consist of fibrotic or small vessel damage, and occurs particularly with irradiation of large volumes of the heart [5]. Clinical complications can include pericarditis, arrhythmia, angina and myocardial infarction. The incidence of ischaemic heart disease does not appear to increase rapidly until 10 years after treatment. For this reason, cardiac complications are probably under-reported, particularly as more patients are now being discharged from follow-up following significant irradiation to the chest that might result in long-term survival (e.g. in Hodgkin's disease), especially as cardiotoxic agents such as doxorubicin may have been part of the patient's successful treatment. This issue has become more important in recent years in relation to treatment of breast cancer, first because so many patients are now treated by wide local surgical excision with breast preservation followed by whole-breast radiotherapy, and second because so many patients survive many decades – and many indeed are cured – that late cardiac damage is potentially a hazard to long-term health.

Less radiosensitive tissues
Bone

Therapeutic radiation of bone is a particular problem in children since normal growth may be interrupted, especially when the epiphyseal plate is included in volumes taken to radical dosage, as this area is responsible for the increase in length of any growing long bone. Direct irradiation of the epiphysis interferes with the high mitotic rate of the cartilaginous cells adjacent to the shaft. Radiation damage to the metaphysis may also be severe, though apparently fully reversible provided that the radiation dose is moderate.

The severity of radiation-induced deformity and/or growth disturbance is much greater with high dosage, most particularly with large radiation volumes. The advent of megavoltage irradiation has been particularly helpful in this respect. Nevertheless, in children treated for medulloblastoma, where the whole spine is irradiated to a minimum dose of 30 Gy in 5–6 weeks, the majority of survivors have some deficit in the sitting height. As many as one-third remain persistently below the third centile for height. Younger children are at particular risk but this has to be accepted when radiotherapy is essential for cure, as in medulloblastoma. The late sequelae of radiotherapy and chemotherapy following treatment of childhood cancer are discussed in Chapter 24. Modern treatment with growth hormone replacement has greatly reduced the severity of these problems.

Other connective tissues

Muscle, tendon and connective tissues are all relatively insensitive to radiation and do not usually limit dosage. Fibrosis may occur when high or repeated doses are used, sometimes leading to loss of joint mobility and contractures.

Late sequelae of radiation

In addition to the specific effects on the various organs described above, there are a number of important long-term hazards following the use of radiotherapy. These include carcinogenicity, mutagenicity and teratogenicity, and are all attributable to a fundamental property of ionizing radiation, namely, its biological effect on nuclear DNA with consequent permanent damage to genetic material.

Carcinogenesis

This is a well-documented phenomenon. Survivors from Hiroshima have an increased incidence of neoplasia, particularly leukaemia. An increased incidence of breast cancer was reported almost 40 years after the acute radiation damage was inflicted. Analysis of a large series of patients with ankylosing spondylitis treated by low doses of radiotherapy has demonstrated a 10-fold increase in the incidence of leukaemia. Occasionally, malignant change develops at the site of previous localized irradiation, for example, osteosarcoma of the scapula following radiation for carcinoma of the breast. In children treated for retinoblastoma, late orbital neoplasms may occur (see Chapter 24).

These studies illustrate the general points that neoplasia tends to occur within an organ directly affected by the radiation beam, that there is usually a latent period of at least 10 years before neoplasia develops, and that even moderate doses of irradiation, such as those that used to be employed for benign disease during childhood or young adult life, may lead to a radiation-induced malignancy later on. Much higher doses of radiation are usually given to patients with cancer, but the patients are usually older and have a far smaller likelihood of long survival, so that the true risk of late radiation carcinogenesis is much less amenable to study. Patients with cancer also have a higher probability of developing a second neoplasm. This is sometimes due to common

risk factors, for example, patients cured of early laryngeal carcinomas who continue to smoke and then succumb to carcinoma of the bronchus. Patients with cancer also have an inherent increased probability of developing a second malignancy for reasons that are currently unclear. Increasingly, patients are treated with radiation and cytotoxic chemotherapy, the latter adding to the risk of carcinogenesis. This is well demonstrated by the higher risk of acute leukaemia and breast cancer following treatment of Hodgkin's disease (see Chapters 6 and 25). As more patients are treated with, and cured by, the combination of radiation and chemotherapy, we must expect the incidence of second neoplasms to rise. Although the risk of radiation carcinogenesis is low, it should deter radiotherapists from treating benign skin and other disorders, particularly in children, which could be more safely dealt with by other means. Equally if not more important, the carcinogenic risks of 'routine' diagnostic investigations such as CT scanning are becoming more clearly understood and delineated. This is well described by Sodickson in a recent review, highlighting the apparent 24% increase in the risk of cancer in a large Australian series (Mathews *et al.* [6]) in those exposed to CT scanning during childhood – though the overall risk for children is of course very low, so an increase of 24% while potentially important, is to be kept in sharp perspective: one excess cancer per 1800 head CT's – see both Refs. [6] and [7].

Teratogenicity

Minimal exposure, even to 'soft' X-rays, in pregnant women is extremely hazardous because of the risk of growth retardation and serious malformation in the developing embryo. Irradiation during the last trimester, well after organogenesis is complete, is safer although growth retardation may still occur. Radiation treatment of pregnant women must be avoided wherever possible. This may well lead to difficult clinical decisions, especially when the diagnosis of malignancy is made early in the pregnancy. For example, in patients with pelvic tumours there is general agreement that during the first trimester of pregnancy, treatment should be given as if the patient were not pregnant (unless it can be safely delayed). Spontaneous abortion will always occur but few would feel justified in delaying therapy for perhaps 6 months until the pregnancy is over.

Mutagenicity

This refers to genetic alteration in somatic or germ cells resulting from their direct irradiation. In somatic cells these mutations may be the basis of radiation-induced carcinogenesis. In germ cells, mutation may lead to fetal death or abnormality, although in humans most germ-cell mutations are thought to be non-viable. For these reasons abnormal births following scattered irradiation to the testis are very uncommon.

Technical aspects of radiotherapy

In order to deal adequately with both surface and deep-seated tumours, departments of radiotherapy must possess a suitable range of equipment, comprising superficial (low-energy), orthovoltage (medium-energy) and supervoltage (high-energy) machines. In general, a department will need to draw on a population of at least half a million in order to have a sufficient throughput of new cases. At least 45% of cancer patients require treatment with radiotherapy at some point – the figure seems to be on the rise. Important additional features of the modern department include computer-assisted facilities for planning the radiation treatment, closely liaising with departments of medical physics. For many patients, multifield techniques are essential for best treatment and the physics staff, in conjunction with the radiotherapist, will decide on the most appropriate field arrangement. Modern computing techniques aid us in the generation of isodose curves (similar to contour lines on an Ordnance Survey map) defining points of equal radiation depth dose and making suitable corrections for tissues of unusual density such as lung or bone (Figure 5.7). With the advent of conformal, image-guided and intensity-modulated techniques (see below) we are no longer restricted to geometrically regular radiation volumes: indeed in the majority of modern radiotherapy for radical treatment, with doses often close to normal tissue tolerance, the best compromise between adequate coverage of the tumour and avoidance of unnecessary radiotherapy to surrounding normal structures demands highly individualized radiotherapy volumes.

A treatment simulator is essential in order to reproduce the characteristics of the radiation therapy apparatus in its geometry, capability and limitations, without delivering any treatment. This allows accurate pretreatment appraisal of both the tumour volume to be irradiated and the best alternative techniques. In addition, a mould room will be necessary to produce treatment immobilization devices such as individually manufactured thermoplastic or Perspex head shells for use in head and neck or brain tumour work. Templates

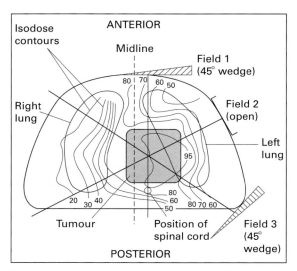

Figure 5.7 Typical plan for multifield irradiation of carcinoma of the left main bronchus showing site of tumour, position of lungs and isodose contours.

for superficial irradiation of irregularly shaped skin cancers, or for individualized shaped fields (such as the 'mantle' or 'inverted-Y' fields for irradiation of patients with Hodgkin's disease) are also produced in the mould room.

As pointed out several years ago by Horwich [8],

> since the birth of radiotherapy at the beginning of this century it has been apparent that the radiotherapist must be fully conversant with the physics of ionizing radiation and with technical aspects of radiation delivery systems, including machine design, dosimetry, treatment planning and simulation, fixation and beam alignment.

Clearly, it is the radiation oncologist's responsibility not only to judge whether radiotherapeutic treatment is indicated but also to decide upon the best technique, field arrangement, choice of therapy unit, total dose and fractionation. Although these technical aspects of radiotherapy are often thought to be synonymous with the total workload of the radiotherapist, they in fact form a limited part of the task. Perhaps even more important is his or her continuing and ever-present role as the clinician responsible for diagnosis, management and follow-up of patients with cancer. In the UK, where the division of radiotherapy from diagnostic radiology occurred early, departments of radiotherapy (now usually termed 'clinical oncology') have been entirely clinical (i.e. non-diagnostic) for well over 30 years.

Radiotherapy planning and treatment techniques

There have been enormous developments in this highly technical part of practical radiation oncology over the past 10 years, some of which are briefly described below. Non-radiotherapists are often puzzled by the technical vocabulary, which radiation oncologists use, making it difficult for the therapists to understand the intentions, achievements and limitations of the techniques employed. Much of the progress in radiotherapy has followed the striking advances in medical imaging which have been so fundamental to recent technical progress in the delivery of an accurate and precisely aimed radiation beam. A short glossary follows.

Treatment prescription

The total dose and treatment time are normally prescribed at the outset of treatment, though in certain circumstances the radiotherapist may prefer to prescribe, say, the first week's treatment and then make a further decision as to whether or not to continue. The units for total absorbed dose are rad (the cgs unit) or grae (Gy, the increasingly preferred SI unit); note that 1 rad = 100 erg/g and 1 Gy = 1 J/kg of absorber, and that 1 Gy = 100 rad. Some radiotherapists (clinical oncologists) prefer the centigray to the grey, since the centigray and the rad are identical. For most treatments, the total dose is split into a number of equal fractions given either on a daily basis or intermittently. The number of fractions of treatment is also prescribed by the radiotherapist. The treatment volume, namely, the volume of tissue to be covered by the prescribed radiation dose, is determined by the radiotherapist using whatever radiological and imaging aids he or she feels to be necessary. With the increasing precision and sophistication of modern radiological imaging, it is now possible to define the treatment or target volume with much greater confidence. The gross tumour volume (GTV) is effectively the volume of tissue defined by the imaging modalities as clearly malignant (Figure 5.8). However, the clinical target volume (CTV) will inevitably cover a larger area, required to ensure that microscopic tumour spread is properly recognized and taken into account, particularly bearing in mind that cell division is often more active at the outer edges of a tumour, presumably due to increased vascularity. The planning target volume (PTV) will be the final target volume selected to be covered by a homogeneous tumour dose; the PTV is often regarded as an 'envelope' within which the CTV (and of course the GTV) would be fully treated

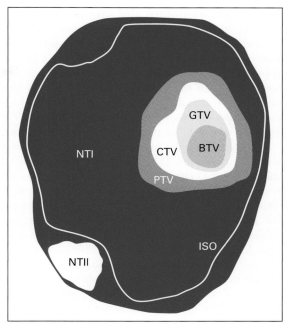

Figure 5.8 Theoretical image of radiotherapy planning volumes in a case of high-grade glioma, incorporating a positron emission tomography-defined biological target volume (BTV) for radiation boost dose. The gross tumour volume (GTV) is defined using high-resolution CT or MRI. The clinical target volume (CTV) is defined by the radiation oncologist to take account of microscopic tumour spread. The planning target volume (PTV) is defined by the oncologist, radiographer and physicist working as a team, to incorporate additional margins of safety, allowing for tumour motion and set-up errors. Careful planning of the 40% isodose (ISO) line to exclude normal tissue at increased risk of radiation damage defined by molecular imaging (NTII) should enable the safe delivery of a reduced dose to the high-risk area. NTI, normal tissue. (Source: West and Charnley [9]. Copyright © British Institute of Radiology 2014)

by the radiation beams chosen, with 100% certainty. With the advent of positron emission tomography as an adjunct to radiotherapy planning, we now also have the so-called biological target volume (BTV) to take account of this important new information. Although the aim is always to produce a homogeneous dose for coverage of the tumour volume, 'hot' and 'cold' spots may occur, although with modern multifield radiation techniques they are usually minimal. Inevitably, the margin between CTV and PTV will include normal as well as malignant tissue, an inescapable everyday problem in radiation oncology, even with the best possible imaging facilities.

Maximum, minimum and modal dose

Since it is impossible to achieve homogeneous irradiation of the desired volume without irradiation of surrounding normal tissue, the radiotherapist must decide on the appropriate compromise. One traditional approach was to prescribe to a *maximum* dose, namely, a dose which would not be exceeded, even if this particular dose level was reached only in a small part of the tumour. The opposite approach, to prescribe to a *minimum* dose, which represented the lowest possible dose level, was also commonly used. The problem with prescriptions of this kind is that neither maximum nor minimum dosage is necessarily representative as a reference dose. A more satisfactory recommendation is the *modal* dose, namely, the particular dose level occurring with the greatest frequency in the prescribed volume, by definition a more representative dose level. The *applied* dose is used where the radiotherapist wishes to prescribe the dose at the surface of the skin. If he or she wishes to state more precisely what the dose at a certain depth should be (e.g. when treating spinal metastases where the dosage at a certain depth is of greater interest than the surface dose) a *depth-dose* prescription may be preferable. The radiotherapist may specify a certain dose at, say, 4 cm depth for metastases in the upper spine, but at 7 cm depth for those in the lower spine, following the expected normal anatomy.

Open (direct) and wedged fields

An open or direct field is usually applied perpendicular to the patient's skin surface and the beam emerging from the treatment machine is not modified in any way. In treatments using several fields (multifield techniques), a number of fields, usually two to four, are used and, by inserting wedges of various dimensions into the beam and using radiation fields applied obliquely, the tumour volume can be irradiated to a more homogeneous level (Figure 5.7). The use of multi-field arrangements, often employing wedged fields, has permitted safer megavoltage irradiation of deep-seated tumours to a high dose level.

Parallel opposed fields

The simplest type of multifield technique is provided by a two-field arrangement where the fields are applied in opposite directions, usually to the anterior and posterior skin surface (Figure 5.9), and the block of tissue in between irradiated. This technique is widely used and, if necessary, the fields can be shaped so that important structures are avoided, for example, the use of the 'mantle'

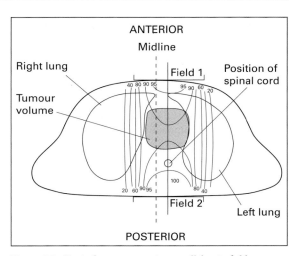

Figure 5.9 Typical anteroposterior parallel pair field arrangement. This is often used for treating thoracic or pelvic tumours. In this instance the patient had an inoperable carcinoma of the bronchus, and the tumour position and size were determined by CT scanning. The spinal cord is also shown since irradiation of this structure is often dose-limiting with this set-up.

irradiation technique for patients with supradiaphragmatic Hodgkin's disease where the lungs are protected from over-irradiation (see pages 506–507). For parallel opposed pairs of fields, the dose normally prescribed is the *midplane* dose since this will define the dose achieved at a point midway between the two fields and indeed midway between the anterior and posterior skin surface of the patient.

Shrinking field technique

During a course of treatment it is sometimes desirable to reduce the treatment volume so that part of the initial treatment volume is treated to a certain dose level and a smaller area then taken to a higher dose. This is often done, for example, in pelvic tumours such as carcinomas of the bladder or prostate, where the original treatment volume might include pelvic lymph nodes with the intention to treat these to a 'prophylactic' dose of irradiation to deal with microscopic disease, while the primary site requires a higher dosage. A further good example is the irradiation technique often employed in a primary bone sarcoma such as Ewing's tumour, where the whole of the long bone might be irradiated to a moderate dose, the field being reduced during treatment so that the primary tumour site receives the full total dose.

Systemic irradiation

This refers to radiotherapy not as traditionally used for specific local sites but throughout the whole body or substantial parts of it. Whole-body irradiation is well established as a means of eradicating leukaemia or lymphoma cells prior to allogeneic or autologous BMT (it is this irradiation which kills the tumour cells, not the transplant itself). Hemibody irradiation, usually to the upper or lower half of the body, is increasingly used as an excellent palliative technique for multiple painful bone metastases and in multiple myeloma (see Chapter 27).

A new form of targeted systemic radioimmunotherapy has recently been reported, using ^{131}I-labelled tositumomab, a monoclonal IgG antibody that selectively binds to CD20 on the surface of normal and malignant B cells [10]. Patients with follicular lymphoma (of whom 90% present with disseminated disease) appear to have a high response rate, even when pretreated with extensive chemotherapy or rituximab (see also Chapter 26, pages 524–525).

Immobilization devices

For precision work, particularly treatment of head and neck cancers, it is essential that the patient be absolutely still and in a reproducible position throughout the whole of the lengthy treatment period. The best means of achieving this is to use an immobilization device such as a Perspex or thermoplastic headcast (Figure 5.10), individually made for each patient, traditionally by

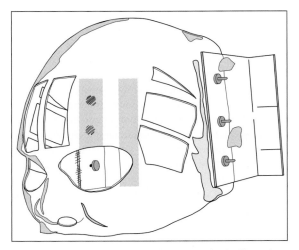

Figure 5.10 Perspex head shell. Shells are individually made to ensure accurate positioning. These are widely used in treatment of tumours of the head and neck, and for pituitary tumours.

obtaining a plaster-of-Paris impression that is then used to produce a Perspex shell which fits the patient snugly and can be screwed to the treatment couch. Newer techniques employing thermoplastic are much easier to use and quicker to prepare. These devices or 'treatment shells' also carry the advantage that field markings can be made on the cast rather than the patient, thereby avoiding unsightly ink marks or tattoos, and ensuring accurate reproduction for each day's treatment.

There have been numerous attempts to enhance the local and regional control of cancer by means of novel approaches using particle beams (see above), stereotactic external beam radiation therapy, radiosensitizing drugs, photodynamic therapy (PDT) and other techniques. Few of these approaches are yet established as standard therapy; indeed most, after promising theoretical preclinical data, have failed to withstand the rigours of the prospectively randomized clinical trial – nitroimidazole radiosensitizers are perhaps the best example. Hyperfractionation, already referred to, and hypofractionation are also areas of major research efforts at present. PDT has been increasingly used in oral and gastrointestinal tumours, and is a form of treatment dependent on the excitation of a number of photoactive compounds by laser-generated light of the appropriate wavelength. Haematoporphyrin derivatives are synthetic haemoglobin compounds which, when administered systemically, may localize in human tumour tissue. When exposed to laser light of the correct wavelength, dose derivatives react with oxygen to form a highly reactive fragment that appears to be locally cytotoxic.

Conformal and intensity-modulated radiation therapy

These are exciting departures in treatment technique, in which the high-dose volume is designed to conform more closely with the target volume. Recently introduced, these approaches are now widely employed in a variety of clinical settings, especially where a complex radiation volume is required.

With *conformal therapy*, the prime intention is to use external beam irradiation to better effect by excluding more normal tissue than was previously possible, thereby increasing the dose that can safely be applied to the tumour volume. Evaluation of these approaches is under active study at present, using customized field shaping designed from three-dimensional 'beam's-eye view' planning. Clear-cut, disease-free survival benefits are increasingly being reported, particularly for irradiation of high-grade prostatic cancers. A further important technique recently developed, with the intention of providing more effective irradiation of the tumour without danger of over-treatment of surrounding tissues, is *intensity-modulated radiation therapy* (IMRT), which provides a unique degree of individualized irradiation and the potential of a further increase in tumour dose. The goal of this treatment is to create a dose distribution closely conforming to the target volume while maximally sparing organs at risk. For example in head and neck cancer, one prime aim is to preserve salivary function by sparing at least one of the parotid glands, normally impossible with the conventional lateral radiation fields so frequently employed, for example, in cancers of the oral cavity or oropharynx.

IMRT is an advanced mode of high-precision radiotherapy that utilizes computer-controlled photon beam modelling or 'shaping' to deliver the radiation dose. The treatment is designed to conform to the three-dimensional outline of the tumour by modulating, or controlling, the intensity of the radiation beam to focus a higher radiation dose to the tumour while minimizing radiation exposure to surrounding normal tissues. Treatment is carefully planned using three-dimensional CT images of the patient in conjunction with computerized dose calculations in order to determine the dose intensity pattern that will best conform to the tumour shape. Typically, combinations of several intensity-modulated fields coming from different beam directions are employed to produce a custom tailored radiation volume. Perhaps 10 or more radiation fields will be necessary to achieve this, with a considerable extra requirement in departmental resources and radiation planning time per patient. The complex planning and radiation delivery may require the use of dynamic multileaf collimation, in which the treated volume actually alters during the exposure, creating a close to ideal, irregularly shaped radiation volume. These newer techniques allow both better shielding of normal surrounding tissues and of course the potential for a higher radiation dose to the tumour itself. With such close attention to detail, many departments regard it as essential to apply 'on-board' imaging technology, which allows frequent verification that the intended target volume is genuinely being treated on each occasion. Repeated imaging at the time of treatment should help to reduce inaccuracies due to a variety of potential problems: organ motion, patient movement, set-up errors and so on. 'Cone beam' CT imaging can also be used for verification of treatment volume at the outset and also as therapy progresses, employing a remarkable new technology. Using a cone-shaped beam enables the scanner to illuminate, image and resolve volumes of tissue rather than simply slices, allowing three-dimensional reconstruction of the volume of interest, with improved precision for both set-up and treatment.

These highly sophisticated and resource-intensive approaches are increasingly used for cancers of lung, head and neck, prostate, pancreas, bladder and deep-seated sarcomas. They may offer a particular advantage in previously irradiated patients by permitting additional treatment with relative avoidance of normal tissue toxicity. These and other novel aspects of radiotherapy are well reviewed by Nutting *et al.* [11] and more recently by Ahmad *et al.* [12].

Integration of radiotherapy and chemotherapy

Remarkable changes in the multimodal therapy of cancer have occurred over the past 25 years. Although it was once unusual for patients to be treated with both radiotherapy and cytotoxic chemotherapy, it has now become commonplace, particularly for squamous cell carcinomas [5]. This exciting trend is certain to continue for at least two reasons. First, radiation therapy is now increasingly used as an alternative to surgery for treatment of the primary tumour, particularly with carcinoma of the larynx and other head and neck sites, carcinoma of the cervix and anus and, over the past few years, with many carcinomas of the breast, bladder and prostate. Second, there is increasing use of chemotherapy both for palliation and, in some tumours, as adjuvant therapy immediately preceding or succeeding the initial local treatment.

There are, however, a number of important risks in the simultaneous use of both treatments. Some cytotoxic agents act as radiation sensitizers, increasing the local reactions from radiotherapy and occasionally producing 'recall' of previous skin reactions. This has even been reported in relation to other non-cytotoxic agents, well after completion of the radiotherapy, including, for example, antibiotic therapy, presumably through the mechanism of enhanced photosensitivity. With respect to cytotoxic agents, the most important example is probably actinomycin D, although there is evidence that other drugs such as doxorubicin may also interact with radiotherapy in this way. For example, oesophageal stricture has been documented in patients undergoing mediastinal irradiation and concurrent treatment with this agent. The danger of doxorubicin-induced cardiomyopathy occurs at a lower dosage in patients who have undergone mediastinal or chest wall radiation, if a significant volume of cardiac muscle has been included. For patients undergoing wide-field irradiation, particularly if a substantial volume of bone marrow is involved (such as in children with medulloblastoma), the use of adjuvant chemotherapy may lead to more troublesome myelosuppression than with radiation alone. In general, it is true that the synchronous use of chemotherapy and radiotherapy (particularly with radiation-sensitizing drugs) leads to greater toxicity. The combination should be avoided particularly when treatment is palliative or large areas of mucosa are being irradiated. However, there is increasing interest in the use of concurrent chemoradiation regimens in order to improve local control (in tumours such as Ewing's sarcoma or small-cell lung cancer), and at the same time to treat micrometastatic disease.

Despite the theoretical drawback of increased toxicity, there are many advantages to combined use of radiotherapy and chemotherapy as initial treatment, especially when administered synchronously. Radiotherapy, as a powerful local tool, is often able to produce tumour control with minimal physiological disturbance, though without effect on occult metastases. It may not be possible to ensure satisfactory irradiation of the primary tumour and its lymph node drainage area if nodal metastases are known to be present, for example, in gynaecological, testicular or bladder tumours with known para-aortic involvement. Conversely, chemotherapy can seldom be relied upon to deal adequately with the primary tumour, though it does at least offer hope in dealing with occult metastatic disease. Combined therapy should then represent a logical approach; indeed it is clear that in a number of major squamous cell primary sites, synchronous chemoradiotherapy now represents the gold standard of treatment with radical intent (cervix, anus, vulva, oesophagus, head and neck; see specific chapters). Use of chemotherapy with curative intent after radiation failure represents a different form of combined therapy, since the treatments are separated in time. This approach is only likely to be successful in highly chemosensitive tumours such as Hodgkin's disease, in which chemotherapy for radiation failure is probably as successful as it is for primary therapy. A more recent concept, still relatively unexplored, is the use of 'adjuvant' radiotherapy in patients treated primarily by chemotherapy. In small-cell carcinoma of the bronchus, for example, chemotherapy is now widely employed as the mainstay of treatment, with mediastinal irradiation, formerly the most widely used method of treatment, now increasingly used as consolidation post chemotherapy

(see Chapter 12). Radiotherapy may also be valuable in a slightly different adjuvant fashion as, for example, in the use of cranial irradiation as prophylaxis for children with ALL in whom meningeal relapse is substantially reduced by routine irradiation, since the cerebrospinal fluid is poorly penetrated by the drugs used for systemic control.

Proton therapy

This exciting approach, a type of particle therapy which uses a beam of protons rather than photons, has attracted great interest in recent years (13, and see Ref. [14]). Its main advantage is the ability to more precisely localize the radiation dosage as a result of the totally different physics of energy deposition within the irradiated tissue. A typical treatment plan for proton therapy is shown in Figure 5.11 which demonstrates the 'dead stop' characteristic of the beam, fundamentally unlike with photons where the unwanted but ever-present exit beam always represents a theoretical hazard. This sometimes causes real clinical harm and distress – the painful pharyngitis

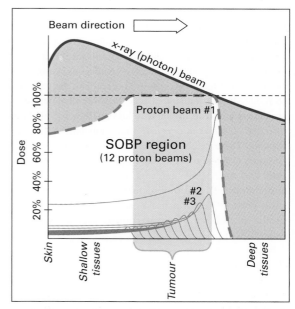

Figure 5.11 Typical dose-distribution curves of proton therapy as compared to photon (Megavoltage X-ray beam) therapy. See text for further explanation. Source: http://commons.wikimedia. org/wiki/File: Comparison of dose profiles for proton vs photon radiotherapy. Created by Mark Filipak and licensed under the Creative Commons Attribution-Share Alike scheme.

seen with irradiation of the cervical spine is a well-known example. The dashed line shows the spread out Bragg peak (SOBP) in the therapeutic radiation distribution. The SOBP is the sum of several 'pure' Bragg peaks (blue lines) at staggered depths. The depth-dose plot of a 10 MV X-ray (photon) beam (red line) is provided for comparison.

To treat tumours situated deeply in the body, the proton accelerator must produce a beam with high energy, given in eV or electron volts. The accelerators used for proton therapy typically produce protons with energies in the range of 70–250 MeV. By adjusting the energy of the protons during application of treatment, the cell damage due to the proton beam is maximized within the tumour itself. Tissues closer to the surface of the body receive reduced radiation and therefore reduced damage. Tissues deeper within the body also receive very little energy deposition so that the dosage becomes immeasurably small.

In most treatments, protons of different energies with Bragg peaks at different depths are applied, in order to treat the entire tumour. These Bragg peaks are shown as blue lines in the figure to the right.

Which types of solid tumour are best treated with protons? This thorny question remains under constant review. Those for which protons are often now used can be separated into two broad categories, firstly those in anatomic disease sites requiring safe delivery of high doses but close to critically placed and easily damaged normal tissues. And secondly, treatments where the increased precision of proton therapy can be expected to reduce unwanted side effects. In some instances dose escalation has been shown to achieve a higher probability of 'cure' (i.e. local control) than conventional radiotherapy. These might include, in the first category, such tumours as uveal melanoma (and other ocular tumours), skull base and paraspinal tumours (e.g. chondrosarcoma and chordoma), and unresectable sarcomas. In all these cases proton therapy achieves significant improvements in the probability of local control over conventional radiotherapy.

In the second major class are clinical situations where the increased precision of proton therapy is used to reduce unwanted side effects, by limiting the dose to normal tissue. In these cases the tumour dose is the same as that used in conventional therapy, and the emphasis is on the reduction of the unwanted dose to normal tissues, and thus a reduction of unwanted effects [13]. Important examples include several (though not necessarily all) tumours in children, where in certain situations there is now convincing data showing the advantage of using protons, resulting in a reduction of long-term damage to the surviving child. Adult head and neck tumours are increasingly being referred for treatment with proton therapy, for similar reasons.

This is an exciting and rapidly moving field of research. As of June 2012, there were a total of 41 proton therapy centres worldwide, and almost 100 000 patients had been treated. However, these are of course extremely expensive treatment units to build, and only two have so far been planned for development in the UK, one in London at University College Hospital and the other in Manchester at the Christie Hospital.

References

1 Royal College of Radiologists. *Equipment, Workload and Staffing for Radiotherapy in the UK 1997–2002*. London: Royal College of Radiologists, 2003.

2 Meredith WJ, Massey JB. *Fundamental Physics of Radiology*. 3rd edn. Bristol: J Wright & Son., 1977.

3 Withers HR. Biological basis of radiation therapy for cancer. *Lancet* 1992; 339: 156–9.

4 Tobias JS. Risk management and radiotherapy for cancer. *Clin Risk* 2000; 6: 13–16.

5 Gaya AM, Ashford RU. Cardiac complications of radiation therapy. *Clin Oncol* 2005; 17: 153–9.

6 Mathews JD, Forsythe AV, Brady Z *et al.* Cancer risk in 680 000 people exposed to computed tomography scans in childhood or adolescence: data linkage study of 11 million Australians. *Brit Med J* 2013; 346: f2360.

7 Sodickson A. CT risks coming into clearer focus. *Brit Med J* 2013; 346: f3102.

8 Horwich A. The future of radiotherapy. *Radiother Oncol* 1990; 19: 353–6.

9 West CML, Charnley N. The potential of PET to increase understanding of the biological basis of tumour and normal tissue response to radiotherapy. *Br J Radiol* 2005; Suppl. 28: 50–4.

10 Kaminski MS, Tuck M, Estes J *et al.* ^{131}I-Tositumomab therapy as initial treatment for follicular lymphoma. *N Engl J Med* 2005; 352: 441–9.

11 Nutting C, Dearnaley D, Webb S. Intensity modulated radiation therapy: a clinical review. *Br J Radiol* 2000; 73: 459–69.

12 Ahmad SS, Duke S, Jena R, Williams MV, Burnet NG. Advances in radiotherapy. *Brit Med J* 2012; 345: e7765.

13 Swanson EL, Indelicato DJ, Louis D *et al.* Comparison of three-dimensional (3D) conformal proton radiotherapy (RT), 3D conformal photon RT, and intensity-modulated RT for retroperitoneal and intra-abdominal sarcomas. *Int J Radiat Oncol Biol Phys* 2012; 83: 1549–57.

14 Gornall J. Proton beam therapy more than a leap of faith? *Brit Med J* 2012; 345: 19–22.

Further reading

Adams GE. The clinical relevance of tumour hypoxia. *Eur J Cancer* 1990; 26: 420–1.

Baumann M. Radiotherapy in the age of molecular oncology. *Lancet Oncol* 2006; 7: 786–7.

Benson RJ, Burnet NG. Altered radiotherapy fractionation: an opportunity not to be missed. *Clin Oncol* 1998; 10: 150–4.

Bentzen SM. High-tech in radiation oncology: should there be a ceiling? *Int J Radiat Biol Phys* 2004; 58: 320–30.

Bernier J, Hall EJ, Giaccia A. Radiation oncology: a century of achievements. *Nat Rev Cancer* 2004; 4: 737–47.

Brown SB, Brown EA, Walker I. The present and future role of photodynamic therapy in cancer treatment. *Lancet Oncol* 2004; 5: 497–508.

Chao KSC, Perez CA, Brady LW. *Radiation Oncology Management Decisions*, 3rd edn. Philadelphia: Lippincott Williams & Wilkins, 2011.

Chatal J-F, Hoefnagel CA. Radionuclide therapy. *Lancet* 1999; 354: 931–5.

Cox JD and Ang KK. *Radiation Oncology: Rationale, Technique, Results, 9e*. St Louis, MO: Mosby, Elsevier Science, 2010.

Dawson LA, Sharpe MB. Image-guided radiotherapy: rationale, benefits and limitations. *Lancet Oncol* 2006; 7: 848–58.

DeLaney TF. Proton therapy in the clinic. *Front Radiat Ther Oncol* 2011; 43: 465–485.

Department of Health. *NHS Cancer Plan: A Plan for Investment, a Plan for Reform*. London: The Stationery Office, 2000.

Dobbs J, Barrett A, Morris SL, Roques T. *Practical Radiotherapy Planning*, 4th edn. London: Edward Arnold, 2009.

Donaldson L. Reducing harm from radiotherapy. *Br Med J* 2007; 334: 272.

Fowler J. The linear quadratic formula and progress in fractionated radiotherapy. *Br J Radiother* 1989; 62: 679–94.

Gilbert HA, Kagan AR. *Modern Radiation Oncology: Classic Literature and Current Management*, Vol. 1 1978; Vol. 2 1984. New York: Harper & Row.

Greco C, Wolden S. Current status of radiotherapy with proton and light ion beams. *Cancer* 2007; 109: 1227–38.

Hall EJ. Cancer caused by X-rays: a random event? *Lancet Oncol* 2007; 8: 369–70.

Hall P, Adami H, Trichopoulos D *et al*. Effect of low doses of ionizing radiation in infancy on cognitive function in adulthood: Swedish population based cohort study. *Br Med J* 2004; 328: 19–21.

Halperin EC. The promise of innovation in radiation oncology. *Lancet Oncol* 2013; 14: 802–804.

Harrington K, Jankowska P, Hingorani M. Molecular biology for the radiation oncologist: the 5 Rs of radiobiology meet the hallmarks of cancer. *Clin Oncol* 2007; 19: 561–71.

Haustermans K, Withers HR. The biological basis of fractionation. *Rays* 2004; 29(3): 231–6.

Herzog P, Rieger CT. Risk of cancer from diagnostic X-rays. *Lancet* 2004; 363: 340–1.

Hopper C. Oncological applications of photodynamic therapy. In: Tobias JS, Thomas PRM, eds. *Current Radiation Oncology*, Vol. II. London: Edward Arnold, 1996: 107–20.

Horsman MR, Overgaard J. Hyperthermia: a potent enhancer of radiotherapy. *Clin Oncol* 2007; 19: 418–26.

International Commission on Radiological Protection. *Release of Patients after Therapy with Unsealed Radionuclides*. ICRP Publication 94. Amsterdam: Elsevier, 2005.

International Commission on Radiological Protection. *Prevention of High-Dose-Rate Brachytherapy Accidents*. ICRP Publication 97. Amsterdam: Elsevier, 2005.

Jones B, Price P. Proton therapy: expanding clinical indications. *Clin Oncol* 2004; 16: 324–5.

Kaanders JH, Bussink J, van der Kogel A. ARCON: a novel biology-based approach in radiotherapy. *Lancet Oncol* 2002; 3: 728–37.

Kang SK. Radiation recall reaction after antimicrobial therapy. *N Engl J Med* 2006; 354: 622.

Kirsch DG, Tarbell NJ. Conformal radiotherapy therapy for childhood CNS tumors. *Oncologist* 2004; 9: 442–50.

Martinez-Monge R, Cambeiro M, San-Julian M *et al*. Use of brachytherapy in children with cancer: the search for an uncomplicated cure. *Lancet Oncol* 2006; 7: 157–66.

Moran JM, Elshaik MA, Lawrence TS. Radiotherapy: what can be achieved by technical improvements in dose delivery? *Lancet Oncol* 2005; 6: 51–8.

Moysich KB, Menezes RJ, Michalek AM. Chernobyl-related ionising radiation exposure and cancer risk: an epidemiological review. *Lancet Oncol* 2002; 3: 269–79.

Nielsen OS, Bentzen SM, Sandburgh E *et al*. Randomised trial of single dose versus fractionated palliative radiotherapy of bone metastases. *Radiother Oncol* 1998; 47: 223–40.

Price P. Advancing radiotherapy: international networking might be the way forward. *Lancet Oncol* 2007; 8: 364–5.

Rosenzweig KE, Amols H, Ling CC. New radiotherapy technologies. *Semin Surg Oncol* 2003; 21: 190–5.

Royal College of Radiologists. *Good Practice Guide for Clinical Oncologists*, 2nd edn. London: Royal College of Radiologists, 2003.

Royal College of Radiologists. *Radiotherapy Dose-Fractionation*. London: Royal College of Radiologists, 2006.

Royal College of Radiologists. *Towards Safer Radiotherapy*. London: Royal College of Radiologists, 2008.

Saunders M, Dische S, Barrett A *et al*. Continuous hyperfractionated accelerated radiotherapy (CHART) versus conventional radiotherapy in non-small cell lung cancer: a randomised multicentre trial. *Lancet* 1997; 350: 161–5.

Scuibba JJ, Goldenberg D. Oral complications of radiotherapy. *Lancet Oncol* 2006; 7: 175–83.

Seiwert TY, Solama JK, Vokes EE. The concurrent chemoradiation paradigm: general principles. *Nat Clin Pract Oncol* 2007; 4: 86–100.

Shatal JF, Hoefangel CA. Radionuclide therapy. *Lancet* 1999; 354: 931–5.

Sidhu K, Ford EC, Spirou S *et al.* Optimisation of conformal radiation therapy using cone-beam CT imaging for treatment verification. *Int J Radiat Oncol Biol Phys* 2003; 55: 757–67.

Symonds RP. Recent advances: radiotherapy. *Br Med J* 2001; 323: 1107–10.

Tobias JS, Ball D. Synchronous chemoradiation for squamous carcinomas. *Br Med J* 2001; 322: 876–8.

Tobias JS, Thomas PRM, eds. *Current Radiation Oncology*, Vols 1–3. London: Edward Arnold, 1994, 1995, 1998.

Turai I, Veress K, Gunalp B, Souchkevitch G. Medical response to radiation incidents and radionuclear threats. *Br Med J* 2004; 328: 568–72.

West CML, Elliott RM, Burnet NG. The genomics revolution and radiotherapy. *Clin Oncol* 2007; 19: 470–80.

Williams MV. Radiotherapy near misses, incidents and errors: radiotherapy incident at Glasgow. *Clin Oncol* 2007; 19: 1–3.

Williams MV, James ND, Summers ET *et al.* National survey or radiotherapy fractionation practice in 2003. *Clin Oncol* 2006; 18: 3–14.

Withers HR. Biological aspects of conformal therapy. *Acta Oncol* 2000; 39: 569–77.

6 Systemic treatment for cancer

The systemic treatment of cancer is the major focus of cancer management. In treatment of some tumours such as childhood cancers, lymphomas and testicular cancers, great progress has been made with the use of cytotoxic drugs. In other more common cancers, the results have been less impressive, although improvements in survival have been obtained with chemotherapy and endocrine therapy in several malignancies including breast and colorectal cancer.

Since such treatments may be both toxic and expensive, a detailed knowledge of the uses and limitations of chemotherapy and other forms of medical treatment is essential for those treating patients with cancer. If there is a reasonable chance of cure, toxicity and expense can usually be accepted. If there is not, then the potential benefits of palliative treatment with anticancer agents must be carefully weighed against unwanted effects. Despite the fundamental advances in understanding of the molecular basis of cancer and the consequent development of targeted therapies, chemotherapy remains the major modality of treatment for most solid tumours. However future improvements in therapy of cancer will come from strategies to inhibit specific molecular pathways implicated in the development of specific cancer types.

Chemotherapy

Nitrogen mustard was introduced into clinical practice in 1946. The effectiveness of this class of compound in producing regression in lymphomas was rapidly established, as was the gastrointestinal and haematological toxicity they produced. In 1947, Farber showed that aminopterin could produce remissions in acute leukaemia. This was followed by the production of the closely related drug methotrexate in 1949. Development of other drugs followed swiftly: 6-mercaptopurine (6-MP) in 1952, and the antitumour antibiotic actinomycin D in 1954. Since 1965, numerous new antimetabolites, alkylating agents and antibiotics with significant activity have been developed, many of which are related to the parent molecules [1]. Examples of important drugs introduced into clinical practice in the last 25 years are epipodophyllotoxins (etoposide), platinum analogues (cisplatin, carboplatin

Cancer and its Management, Seventh Edition. Jeffrey Tobias and Daniel Hochhauser.
© 2015 John Wiley & Sons, Ltd. Published 2015 by John Wiley & Sons, Ltd.

and oxaliplatin) and taxoids (paclitaxel and docetaxel). The process of discovery, preclinical testing and clinical evaluation is slow. The final realization of the value of a new drug may take 10 years or more following its original discovery.

The cellular targets for anticancer drugs

Most anticancer agents in current use produce their effects by reducing the rate of cancer cell proliferation and division, and there is currently a major focus on development of agents that affect invasion, vascularization and metastatic spread. Cell growth and division may be perturbed in several ways:
• by drugs that prevent effective DNA replication by direct binding to DNA bases or by impairing DNA synthesis;
• by damaging the mechanisms of cell division such as formation of the mitotic spindle;
• by blocking the pathways involved in cell growth that are activated by signals such as growth factors or hormones.

Most of the drugs in common use fall into the first two categories, but there has been rapid development of agents designed to block growth pathways. These latter drugs are sometimes referred to as targeted therapies, because they are aimed at defined structures specific for cancer cells such as receptors or enzymes. However, the drugs that fall into the first two categories are also targeted in the sense that they have defined chemical sites of action. The consequent effects of the drug, after binding to DNA or the mitotic spindle proteins, are often complex, involving the activation of cellular responses such as DNA repair or apoptosis. These agents act in a less specific manner than, for example, the action of a hormone binding to its receptor. Nevertheless, alkylating agents that bind to the same base structure in DNA differ widely in their effect on different tumours, and in their relative antitumour efficacies within the same tumour type. Agents with the same DNA target also sometimes show great differences in patterns of normal tissue toxicity. These clinically important differences imply considerable, unexplained, specificity of action, even when the primary cellular target is the same. The effect of these agents is not so much 'non-specific' as imperfectly understood.

The development of an anticancer drug

Before an agent is introduced into practice it undergoes evaluation on human tumour cells in culture, on animals and then in early clinical trials. Preclinical screening is performed using panels of human tumour cell lines.

Evidence is sought for efficacy and efficiency of killing against particular tumour types.

Animal toxicological studies are then performed, together with assessment of responsiveness of human cancers grown as xenografts in nude mice. Data on pharmacokinetics, optimum schedule and toxicity are obtained in animals, including dose, absorption, tissue distribution, plasma half-life and pathways of metabolism and excretion. Drugs showing activity are then taken forward to early (phase I) clinical studies. The patients selected have advanced cancer that is usually resistant to a wide variety of cytotoxic agents. The aims are to determine optimum dosage, schedule, pharmacokinetics and metabolism. Any tumour response or toxicity is noted. Previously treated patients have a much lower tumour response rate than patients whose tumours have not previously been treated. Phase I studies are, therefore, not optimal for determining efficacy. In the next phase (phase II) a more detailed study is made on patients with tumours of defined categories, both previously treated and untreated. Here an assessment of responsiveness is made.

In subsequent studies the drug will be assessed alone or in combination with other agents active in a particular disease. The simplest assessment is in a non-randomized, single-agent study in which a more precise definition of response and toxicity is made in a single tumour type. Such studies are sometimes a randomized comparison against another single, well-established agent.

When evidence of activity has been confirmed, the new agent is combined with other established drugs and again used in a chosen tumour type and stage. Here the aim is to assess efficacy and tolerability of the combination regimen. Such phase III studies carry more weight if a randomized comparison is made with a standard regimen of generally accepted value. The combination may then be assessed in very large-scale studies in which the value of chemotherapy in improving survival in patients with a given tumour is assessed as precisely as possible.

Principles of cancer chemotherapy

The cell cycle

After cell division, cells may enter a growth phase, G_1, in preparation for a subsequent division. This lasts for a variable period of time in different tissues. Alternatively, cells may exit the cell cycle in G_0 phase. After G_1 the cells move into the phase of DNA synthesis, S phase, in which the amount of chromosomal material is doubled. Cell cycle progression into S phase is determined by the presence of exogenous nutrients and growth factors. Until the restriction point of G_1 is reached, withdrawal of these extracellular factors results in entry to G_0 phase. Once the restriction point is passed, the cell is irreversibly committed to continuation of the cell cycle. The cell then passes through a premitotic phase, G_2, and then into mitosis, M, in which the pairs of chromosomes separate and the cell divides.

As with other tissues, tumours are heterogeneous with respect to cell division – some cells are proliferating while others are dying or dormant. The tumours probably contain progenitor or 'stem' cells that are capable of cell division, continuously renewing and increasing the tumour mass (see Chapter 3). The tumour growth rate also depends on the proportion of cells dividing at any given time, called the *growth fraction*. In experimental tumours, the growth fraction falls as the tumour becomes larger; however, in humans, direct proof that small tumours have a higher growth fraction is lacking. Increase in the size of a cancer is a balance between cell division and cell loss. It appears that self-renewal in cancers is often slower than that achievable in the normal tissue counterpart. Vascularization of large tumour masses is often defective and hypoxic cell death is likely to occur in those areas of tumour more than $150\,\mu m$ from a capillary. This defective vascularization presents a problem in drug delivery and is an obstacle to the potential benefits of drugs designed to damage tumour vasculature if these agents are to be used in conjunction with other drugs.

Most cytotoxic drugs produce their effect either by causing direct damage to DNA or by blocking the synthesis of DNA. The more rapidly growing tumours with a high growth fraction are more likely to respond to drug treatment with these agents. However, this generalization that does not explain why some types of cancer (lymphoma, testicular cancer, leukaemia) are sensitive to cytotoxic drugs and other types (pancreatic, colonic cancer) are not is almost certainly not solely a matter of cell kinetics. It may also be related to mechanisms that invoke the cell death (apoptotic) response, and on the relative efficiency of repair of damaged DNA in different tumours.

Most cytotoxic regimens have been derived empirically, not on the basis of cell kinetics. Some drugs (e.g. methotrexate) are only effective within a particular phase of the cell cycle such as during DNA synthesis, while others (e.g. alkylating agents) exhibit some action even against non-cycling cells. Table 6.1 shows the phase specificity of some anticancer drugs.

Table 6.1 Phase specificity of anticancer drugs.

Phase of cell cycle	Effective agents
S phase	Cytosine arabinoside, methotrexate, 6-mercaptopurine, hydroxycarbamide
Mitosis	Vinca alkaloids, taxoids
Phase non-specific	Alkylating agents, nitrosoureas, antibiotics, procarbazine, cisplatin

Attempts have been made to time drug administration in such a way that the cells are synchronized into a phase of the cell cycle that renders them especially sensitive to the cytotoxic agent. For example, in experimental systems, vinblastine can be used to arrest cells in mitosis. These 'synchronized' cells enter cycle together and can be killed by a cycle-active S-phase-specific agent, such as cytosine arabinoside. Other mechanisms of synergy between drugs may be important; for example, cyclophosphamide depletes intracellular glutathione, which may lead to increased sensitivity to agents normally detoxified by glutathione such as other alkylating agents. However, most drug schedules are not devised on the basis of cell kinetics or synergy but on the knowledge of toxicity and practicability. Infusional drug regimens may allow targeting of cells in specific phases (e.g. S phase), as prolonged administration allows those cells in other phases to enter S phase. For example, continuous infusion of the antimetabolite 5-fluorouracil (5-FU) increases response rate in colon cancer compared with bolus administration.

Kinetics of cell killing by cytotoxic drugs

In experimental systems, a given dose of a cytotoxic drug kills a given proportion of cells rather than a given number. This *fractional cell kill hypothesis* is shown diagrammatically in Figure 6.1. A single dose of a drug might, for example, kill 99% of cells and will do so whether 10^{12} cells are treated (leaving 10^{10} cells) or 10^4 cells (leaving 10^2 cells). If true for solid human cancers, the implications are that a small tumour will be killed by fewer chemotherapy cycles than a large one. Because fewer exposures to drugs will be needed, there will be less chance of resistance emerging. Drugs should then be scheduled in such a way as to produce maximum killing. This will depend on the rate of regrowth of the tumour and on the rate of recovery of the normal tissues that have been most damaged by the drug. In humans these tissues are usually the gut and marrow, which regenerate quickly in comparison with most cancer tissue (Figure 6.1). For this reason pulsed intermittent therapy, with time for normal tissues to recover, is the usual method of drug administration. However, this approach has both theoretical and practical limitations.

• The fractional cell kill hypothesis was validated in homogeneous, rapidly growing experimental tumours. Extrapolation of data to slowly growing human cancers may not be valid.

• Experimental tumours grown as ascites or in body fluids (such as leukaemias) can be assumed to have uniform exposure to a drug. This is not the case for poorly vascularized solid cancers, so that the kinetics of killing will be a much more complex function than the first-order kinetics of experimental systems.

• The proportion of inherently insensitive tumour cells may be a function of size of the tumour, being greater with large tumours.

• The rate of regrowth of the tumour may change with repeated chemotherapy. Although this does not appear to occur with experimental ascitic tumours, the situation may be different for solid tumours.

• The rate of recovery of normal tissues, particularly the bone marrow, may be rapidly completed after the first few cycles, but recovery may become prolonged as treatment proceeds (Figure 6.1), which may limit dosage in successive cycles.

• There are few clinical data on the dose–response relationship for a given cytotoxic drug in a particular tumour. The clinical pharmacology of cytotoxic drugs is extremely complex and varies from drug to drug. There is clinical evidence that an antitumour effect of a drug will be seen only if a maximum dose is given, and in practice the range from ineffective to maximum tolerated dose may be quite small.

These considerations notwithstanding, pulsed intermittent therapy is the schedule of drug administration most widely employed in cancer chemotherapy, and this has been derived from both experimental and clinical findings.

The use of drugs in combination

Even in sensitive tumours, such as Hodgkin's disease, single-agent chemotherapy is rarely curative. This led to the critical development of combination chemotherapy pioneered for Hodgkin's and non-Hodgkin's lymphoma by Vincent DeVita in the 1980s. The intention behind combination therapy is to circumvent multiple-resistance mechanisms. This approach soon proved effective in

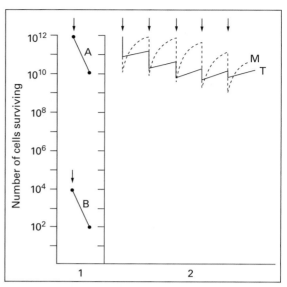

Figure 6.1 Fractional cell kill. In part 1 of the figure, a given dose of a drug is shown killing 99% of cells in both case A and case B. In case A the tumour is reduced from 10^{12} cells to 10^{10} cells and in case B from 10^4 to 10^2 cells. In part 2 of the figure, T shows the effect of repeated drug administration (arrows) on tumour growth. With repeated doses there is less killing of tumour, indicating the emergence of drug resistance. M shows the effect of drug administration on marrow progenitor cells. The marrow recovers quickly, but with repeated doses this is less complete and myelosuppression becomes clinically evident.

childhood leukaemia and adult lymphomas and has been adopted for a wide variety of other tumours.

The development of a combination chemotherapy schedule should follow a number of general principles.

• Only those drugs which are known to be effective as single agents should be used.

• Wherever possible, it is preferable to use drugs of non-overlapping toxicity.

• Pulsed intermittent treatment should be used to allow gut and marrow recovery.

• Ideally, each drug should be used in its optimal dose and schedule.

• Where possible, drugs with synergistic killing effects should be used (normally not known in practice).

• Drugs that work at different phases of the cell cycle are used if practicable.

• Most schedules are derived from an informed empiricism.

The improved efficacy of these combination regimens has several possible explanations.

• The tumour is exposed to a wider variety of agents, and the chances of complete resistance are smaller.

• A maximal killing effect is achieved without undue toxicity.

• There may be less opportunity for the early emergence of a resistant cell population.

Resistance to cancer chemotherapy

The rate of conversion of a drug to its active form and its rate of elimination greatly influence its efficacy. Variations in these enzymic processes are in part *constitutional*, the result of the genetic make-up of the individual. Within the tumour there are, in addition to the constitutional susceptibility, *tumour-related* mechanisms. The latter include over- or under-expression of mechanisms of metabolism within the tumour that have arisen as a result of somatic mutation, and the efficiency of delivery of the drug to the tumour as determined by the properties of the tumour vasculature.

Some of the mechanisms of tumour resistance will therefore be an expression of host metabolism and resistance, while others will be tumour related.

Drug metabolism

The degree of response to a drug in an individual depends on constitutional factors that control absorption, distribution and metabolism of the drug before it reaches the tumour. The efficiency of these processes is affected by genetic differences in individuals, which lead to changes in structure of proteins that are responsible for these functions. Pharmacogenomics is the study of the role of inherited and acquired genetic variation in drug response [2]. For some anticancer drugs the molecular basis for variation is understood and genetic differences in drug metabolism have been linked to important outcomes such as tumour response or, conversely, toxicity. Various genetic changes may be responsible.

Mutations may modify or eliminate the activity of enzymes responsible for metabolism of the drug to an active form or that lead to degradation of the agent. An example is variation in the metabolism of tamoxifen where polymorphisms in the cytochrome P450 enzyme CYP2D6 in the liver change the likelihood of side-effects and drug interactions.

Polymorphisms of genetic structure such as single nucleotide alterations or minor amino acid changes are common; they usually cause minor changes in function but some are of great clinical importance.

Examples

1 *Mercaptopurine* is converted by the enzyme thiopurine methyltransferase to an inactive form. Of the general population, 10% are heterozygous for a mutant allele and 0.3% are homozygous. The mutant allele confers an inability to degrade the drug (severe in the case of homozygotes), with resulting drug toxicity but increased antitumour effect.

2 *Irinotecan* is a topoisomerase I inhibitor. It is converted by CYP3A (a hepatic cytochrome) to an inactive form, and by an enzyme (carboxylesterase) to an active form called SN38. SN38 is inactivated in the liver by glucuronyltransferase (UGT1). Polymorphisms in the promoter region of UGT1 lead to less drug metabolism and more toxicity. Diminished activity of CYP3A has a similar effect.

These examples show the potential of this approach in cancer treatment. With the advent of simple genotyping techniques it will become possible to determine polymorphisms that relate to outcome of cytotoxic treatment in terms of cure rate, susceptibility to acute toxicity, or long-term drug complications such as second malignancy. The aim will be to individualize treatment for patients to a greater extent than what it is currently.

Tumour-related resistance

The cells in a solid tumour are not uniformly sensitive to a cytotoxic drug before treatment starts. Genetic instability develops as cancers grow and somatic mutation causes heterogeneity with respect to resistance to drugs. This provides a partial explanation for greater drug resistance in large tumours where this process has progressed further.

As the tumour grows, the frequency of development of resistant cells increases so that large tumours have a greater number of intrinsically resistant cells. This resistance is produced by one or more of the mechanisms shown in Table 6.2 and discussed below. Its cause is genetic instability, leading to cellular variation in concentration and function of enzyme or transport proteins. Host defence mechanisms and the use of cytotoxic drugs exert a selection pressure, encouraging the survival of the resistant cells, which grow and multiply.

In addition to this type of cellular resistance, at least two other mechanisms are important. The first is diminished vascularity of parts of the tumour as it becomes larger, resulting in hypoxia and decreased drug penetration [3]. There is also evidence to suggest that, as with radiotherapy (see Chapter 5), cellular hypoxia may be a determinant of

Table 6.2 Cellular mechanisms of resistance to anticancer drugs.

Mechanism	Drug (examples)
Efficient repair to damaged DNA	Alkylating agents
Decreased uptake by cell	Methotrexate, doxorubicin
Increased drug efflux (*p*-glycoprotein)	Epipodophyllotoxin, vinca alkaloids, anthracyclines
Decreased intracellular activation	6-Mercaptopurine, 5-fluorouracil
Increased intracellular breakdown	Cytosine arabinoside
Bypass biochemical pathways	Methotrexate, 6-mercaptopurine, asparaginase
Gene amplification or over-production of blocked enzyme	Methotrexate, nitrosoureas

resistance to cytotoxic agents. The second is that only a small proportion of cells may be in cycle, allowing time for repair from cytotoxic damage before cell division.

Cellular mechanisms of resistance to cytotoxic drugs

Somatic mutation and the survival advantage of resistant cells mean that a distinction between 'intrinsic' and 'acquired' cannot be made. The cellular mechanisms are a combination of genetic alteration and selection of cells that express the resistance mechanisms found in normal cells. These resistance mechanisms may be found singly in some cells, or more than one mechanism may coexist in a cell. In the entire tumour we can therefore expect that numerous mechanisms will be operating, unevenly distributed in the cellular population.

One of the unexplained phenomena of cancer chemotherapy is that some tumours are generally sensitive to drugs, while others are resistant. This inherent sensitivity or resistance extends to drugs of many different classes and mechanisms of action. Thus, lymphomas and germ-cell tumours show extreme sensitivity (and curability), while pancreatic cancer and melanoma are highly resistant. This general susceptibility is not easily explained by any of the individual resistance mechanisms detailed below, but might be due to the induction of cell death (apoptosis) more easily in some cell types in response to DNA damage.

Some of the mechanisms of resistance are summarized in Table 6.2 and are outlined briefly below. It must be

emphasized that these mechanisms are the properties of normal as well as malignant cells.

Multidrug resistance

This is related to expression of a membrane glycoprotein (*p*-glycoprotein, PGP, gp170), of molecular weight 170 kDa, that acts as a drug efflux pump to reduce the intracellular concentration of some, but not all, cytotoxic agents [4]. This protein has homology with a bacterial cell wall transport protein and is widely distributed in nature. In normal tissues it is found in the endothelium of the upper gastrointestinal tract, in the adrenal and in the kidney. Its presence confers relative resistance to a series of cytotoxic agents such as vinca alkaloids, anthracyclines and etoposide but not to alkylating agents. Multidrug resistance (MDR) arises when cells exposed to a specific drug develop resistance not only to that drug but to structurally unrelated agents. The *MDR* genes are part of a family of genes that code for drug efflux proteins, the ATP-binding cassette (ABC) family. It is apparent that expression of ABC genes varies widely between cancers. There is some clinical evidence that PGP expression in tumours correlates with worse prognosis (e.g. in childhood soft-tissue sarcoma) but it is not clear whether this is directly due to an adverse response to cytotoxic agents. The effect of PGP can be reversed *in vitro* by calcium channel-blocking drugs (such as verapamil), but with this drug it is difficult to attain appropriate plasma concentrations clinically and, thus far, there has been little clinical success in reversing the MDR mechanism. Other drugs are being evaluated [4].

Glutathione

This small tripeptide is an SH-containing reducing agent that also acts as a general intracellular detoxifying agent. In the cytosol it is kept in the highly reduced SH form by gluthathione reductase and serves to prevent unwanted S–S linkages in proteins that might result in incorrect folding. These are a series of transferases which facilitate the reaction of GSH with a toxin. The transferase specificity of many cytotoxic agents is not yet clear. Polymorphism in the transferases relates to outcome in childhood acute myeloid leukaemia (AML). For alkylating agents and specifically platinum agents, r, the GSH concentration and glutathione transferase activity appear to be important determinants of cellular sensitivity [5]. Concentrations vary widely in different normal tissues and in tumours and do not, in general, correlate with drug sensitivity. It may be possible to alter cellular sensitivity by agents which deplete intracellular

GSH or by agents which inhibit transferases, such as ethacrynic acid. In cells made resistant to nitrogen mustard the increase in transferase activity is due to gene amplification (see below), but it is not clear if this mechanism is important in spontaneous tumours.

Gene amplification

In tumour cell cultures, cells showing resistance to some cytotoxic agents exhibit amplification of genes responsible for mediating resistance. An example is amplification of the dihydrofolate reductase (DHFR) gene, leading to increased intracellular levels of this enzyme, which confers relative resistance to methotrexate. Other examples include amplification of glutathione *S*-transferase isozymes (important in resistance to alkylating agents) and O^6 alkyltransferase (which confers resistance to nitrosoureas). Although amplification occurs frequently in laboratory models where cells are exposed to chemotherapy, the significance clinically is less clear. It is interesting that the amplification which results in increased expression of ErbB2/HER2/neu in breast cancer and hence sensitivity to the antibody Herceptin (Trastuzumab) also frequently amplifies the topoisomerase IIα locus. As increased expression of topoisomerase II contributes to anthracycline sensitivity, these patients may have resultant increased sensitivity to drugs such as doxorubicin [6].

Increase in DNA repair (see also Chapter 3)

Covalent adducts between alkylating agents (and other drugs) and DNA bases are excised by enzymes. The reactions involve DNA glycosylases and polymerases; alterations of DNA repair pathways in cancer are highly complex [7]. Repair mechanisms include *base excision repair*, where glycosylases excise the damaged base from the sugar, and *nucleotide excision repair*, where larger portions of the DNA strand are excised and re-ligated. We know very little about variability and efficiency of DNA repair in cancer cells compared with normal cells, and whether clinical drug resistance is related to increased efficiency of repair of cytotoxic drug-induced DNA damage. The repair mechanisms differ with lesions at chemically distinct sites on the bases, and may vary in efficiency at different sites in the gene and depending on whether the gene is being transcribed.

Decreased drug activation

Agents such as cytosine arabinoside and 5-FU are converted in the cell to an active form before exerting antitumour effect. Low levels of converting enzymes or competing enzyme pathways may decrease intracellular concentrations of the active drug.

Drugs such as cyclophosphamide are converted to the active form in normal tissues (in this case the liver). Heritable differences in efficiency of activation will lead to variation in the amount, and rate of formation, of active drug. These are not intracellular mechanisms in the tumour but may account for diminished drug efficacy. The cellular concentration of a reducing enzyme such as DT-diaphorase may be critical in conversion of bioreductive drugs, such as quinones, to their active form.

Other mechanisms

Increased intracellular drug breakdown is one of the numerous biochemical pathways subverting drug effect; for example, deamination of cytosine arabinoside, inefficient membrane transport (methotrexate), and competing enzyme pathways such as asparagine production by asparagine synthetase, decreasing the efficacy of asparaginase. Many of these are discussed in relation to individual drugs (see below).

Remission induction and maintenance

Clinical complete 'remission' or 'complete response' of a tumour is a clinical description which is compatible with up to 10^{10} cells still being present in the patient. If treatment stops, the relapse-free interval is dependent on the size of the residual tumour and the growth rate of the surviving cells. These two variables adequately account for the shape of the curves of remission duration. The aim of initial chemotherapy is to induce clinical complete response, if possible.

'Maintenance' therapy was a term introduced in treatment of acute leukaemia where, following the induction of a remission, chemotherapy of a less intensive type is used to maintain remission. In acute lymphoblastic leukaemia (ALL), this has been shown to contribute to survival. The improvement is due to continued cytotoxic effect on the tumour when the induction therapy has not completely eradicated the disease.

In most tumours, maintenance therapy has not been shown to improve the results of cyclical combination chemotherapy given over a period of several months. In Hodgkin's disease, for example, survival is not improved by continuing to treat the patient after six cycles have been given. A similar lack of effect has been found in small-cell lung cancer (SCLC) and testicular tumours. In these diseases the patient is cured (or not) during the early phase of treatment. There are strong arguments (discussed above) for a strategy of administering initial treatment as intensely as possible.

Adjuvant chemotherapy

Following resection of an operable cancer (e.g. of the breast or colon) patients may develop local or distant recurrence. Chemotherapy can be used as an adjuvant to surgery to eradicate micrometastases at this early stage. Chemotherapy may be more effective on small tumours than when they have become clinically detectable. There is little doubt that this approach has been very effective in sensitive paediatric tumours such as Wilms' tumour, Ewing's sarcoma and rhabdomyosarcoma. It is now apparent that modest benefits may be obtained, but that the degree of benefit can only be determined in trials of considerable size to exclude moderate biases that influence results of smaller trials (discussed in Chapter 2). Adjuvant chemotherapy is of proven value in many situations including breast cancer, gastrointestinal (gastric, pancreatic and colorectal) cancer, non-small-cell lung cancer (NSCLC), and testicular and bladder cancers. The indications for these important uses of chemotherapy (and hormone and biological therapy) will be better defined, and the regimens improved upon, over the next decade as the necessary studies are completed. Current decisions are made on the basis of the biology and stage of the cancer.

Predicting sensitivity to anticancer drugs

Several techniques have been used to attempt to assess the activity of a drug against the patient's own tumour. These have included measurement of inhibition of cell growth or metabolism in cell suspension or short-term culture, inhibition of the formation of clones of cells grown in soft agar, and growth inhibition in longer-term cell cultures.

The problems, both technical and in interpretation, are formidable: cell suspensions may not be representative of the whole tumour; not all tumours will form clones in soft agar; longer-term cultures often cannot be established; and the pharmacology and exposure of the drug are different in culture than *in vivo*. These difficulties are increased by the methodological problems of proving that there is a benefit in selecting drugs for an individual patient rather than using a standard combination. Drug combinations usually contain many or most of the active drugs so that selection in the assay may be only to predict which drugs to leave out. It will be difficult to show survival benefit by this means, although toxicity may be reduced. It seems probable that the current *in vitro* tests can predict clinical resistance fairly reliably. They

are less accurate in predicting sensitivity. At present they do not have a place as a routine procedure in cancer chemotherapy.

However, there are more recent indications that assessment of the initial cancer can have some value in prediction of chemosensitivity. Examples include the resistance of mismatch-repair deficient colorectal cancers to oxaliplatin and increased sensitivity of HER2-amplified breast cancers to doxorubicin (see above). It is likely that a major focus of research will be molecular profiling of cancers to produce genomic signatures that will predict response not only to chemotherapy but also to the novel targeted therapies.

What cancer chemotherapy has achieved

The majority of curable cancers are uncommon tumours such as childhood cancers, leukaemias, lymphomas and testicular tumours. Other cancers are partially responsive but the impact of chemotherapy on survival in advanced solid tumours is less (although important). These include cancer of the breast, SCLC, ovarian cancer and cancer of the colon. Figure 6.2 shows that the overall contribution of chemotherapy to *cure* is relatively small. However, in advanced cancer, even if cure is not improved, patients may gain significant prolongation of survival and symptomatic relief.

Classes of cytotoxic drugs, mode of action and toxicity

Alkylating agents and nitrosoureas

Alkylating agents and nitrosoureas are very reactive compounds that produce their effect by covalently linking an alkyl group ($R-CH_2$) to chemical moieties in nucleic acids and proteins. The principles are shown in Figure 6.3. Nitrogen mustard, for example, has two chloroethyl side-chains and one of these binds to the 7-nitrogen group of guanine. After forming this bond, for drugs with another side-chain, another link can be formed which results in DNA strands being cross-linked, either within a strand or between strands. The cross-link is the most important lesion determining cellular cytotoxicity. The commonly used alkylating agents bind in the major groove of DNA. There is selectivity in the nucleotide sequence where the drug forms the guanine N_7 bond. The cross-link is dependent on the chemical structure of the drug, which determines the length of DNA over which it can span, the nature of the chemical reaction on the opposite strand and the sequence of bases that is most favourable for binding. Alkylating agent

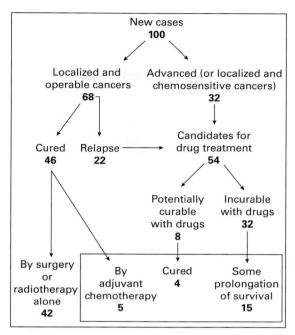

Figure 6.2 The impact of cancer chemotherapy. The flow diagram gives the proportion of new cancer cases which might be expected to benefit from drug treatment (skin and *in situ* cervical cancer are excluded). One in four patients with cancer benefits from chemotherapy.

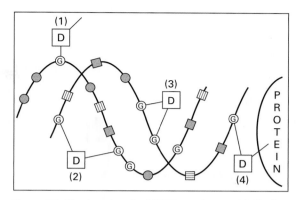

Figure 6.3 The two strands of DNA are shown with the four bases represented by symbols (⬤◎⬛▤). Most alkylating agents react at the N_7 position of guanine (◎). The drug (Ⓓ) forms a mono-adduct (1), an inter-strand cross-link (2), an intra-strand cross-link (3) or a DNA–protein cross-link (4). The strands of DNA are shown with the major (wide) groove and the minor (narrow) groove. Most commonly used alkylating agents bind to guanine in the major groove, but minor groove agents are under development. The toxic lesions are inter- and intra-strand cross-links. The formation of cross-links between guanine is not random but depends on the base sequence, which determines the 'fit' of the agent into the major groove. Mono-adducts are more frequent but more easily repaired than cross-links. The toxicity of DNA–protein cross-links is not known.

damage is therefore chemically selective. This may account for some of the observed differences in the way different tumour types respond, since genes that are essential for maintaining growth in one tumour type, but less important in another, may contain regulatory sequences more vulnerable to alkylation than others or can be repaired more efficiently.

Impairment of DNA replication is the major mechanism of cytotoxicity of alkylating agents. Alkylating agents that are bifunctional (with two alkylation products) are more cytotoxic than monofunctional compounds by virtue of the cross-linking they produce. The cell can repair itself against this damage by excision of the damaged segment of DNA, with the formation of a new segment of DNA, which is then linked to the strand. Although DNA alkylation occurs at any stage in the cell cycle, it seems to have more lethal consequences if it occurs during S phase, possibly because cellular checkpoints (such as *p53*) can initiate apoptosis if repair of damage has not occurred before mitosis is due to begin.

Cyclophosphamide

This is a stable inactive compound that is well absorbed when given orally. It is activated in the liver by the cytochrome P450 system to 4-hydroxycyclophosphamide and thence to phosphoramide mustard and acrolein (Figure 6.4). The latter is responsible for the haemorrhagic cystitis that is a complication of prolonged or high-dose administration. 2-Mercaptoethane sulphonate (mesna), which binds acrolein in the urine, prevents this complication. After oral administration maximal plasma concentrations are reached in 1 hour and the plasma half-life of the drug is 5–6 hours. Little unchanged drug is excreted. The drug is effective in many types of cancer and it is the most versatile alkylating agent in terms of activity and method of administration.

Because the drug must be converted to an active form in the liver, it is not suitable for local use. Haematological toxicity is common, but thrombocytopenia is less marked than with other alkylating agents. Nausea and vomiting accompany intravenous administration, and nausea may also occur when it is given orally. The drug is not vesicant if extravasation occurs. Haemorrhagic cystitis and bladder fibrosis commonly occur, and alopecia is

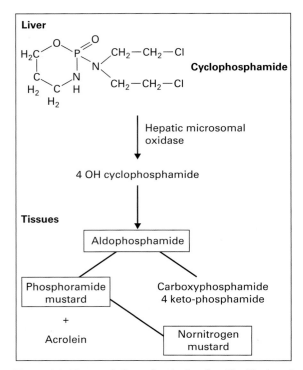

Figure 6.4 The metabolism of cyclophosphamide. The boxed compounds are alkylating agents. Acrolein is the major cause of haemorrhagic cystitis.

frequent with higher doses. Pulmonary fibrosis occurs, as it does with other alkylating agents. High doses may be complicated by inappropriate secretion of antidiuretic hormone (ADH), leading to hyponatraemia. As with most alkylating agents, male infertility is usual. Haemorrhagic carditis has been reported with very high doses. High-dose cyclophosphamide has been used in solid tumour chemotherapy and in allogeneic marrow transplantation for leukaemia and aplastic anaemia.

Ifosfamide

This compound is structurally closely related to cyclophosphamide but one of the two chloroethyl groups is sited on the nitrogen atom and the other on the oxazophosphorine ring nitrogen. Like cyclophosphamide, it is activated by hepatic P450 oxidases. Acrolein, liberated during its metabolism, causes haemorrhagic cystitis, but this is prevented by mesna. Toxicity also includes a neurological syndrome with somnolence, confusion and fits, especially in children and if there is impaired renal function. Toxicity is more frequent when

given in high dose and if there is impaired liver function. The cause is unknown. The half-life is about 6 hours. It is given by short or long infusion and schedules vary greatly. Hydration is necessary. Renal tubular and glomerular toxicity are frequent and are especially severe in children. The drug is moderately myelosuppressive. It may be more active than cyclophosphamide in squamous carcinomas and sarcomas. The schedules of administration are varied, ranging from 1 hour to continuous infusions. There appears to be no pharmacological reason for preferring one over another. Very high-dose administration may increase response in sarcomas.

Melphalan (Alkeran)

Melphalan is a stable alkylating agent in which the two chloroethyl groups are linked to phenylalanine (Figure 6.5). It was originally hoped that this would result in selective activity against melanoma, but this has not proved to be the case. It is usually given orally. It is well absorbed and not vesicant. Delayed leucopenia and thrombocytopenia occur, but nausea, vomiting and alopecia are infrequent. The drug is used in myeloma, less frequently in ovarian and breast cancer, and has a similar activity to cyclophosphamide in these tumours. With prolonged continuous use there is an appreciable risk of the development of myeloid dysplastic states, leading to acute leukaemia. It is used intravenously as part of high-dose chemotherapy regimens in solid tumours using peripheral blood stem cell transplantation.

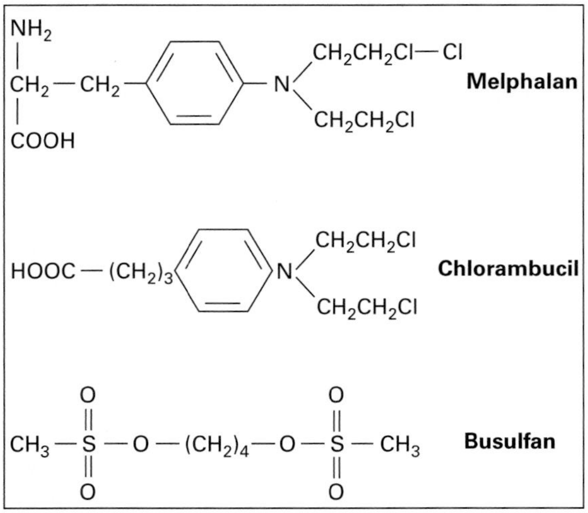

Figure 6.5 The structures of other commonly used alkylating agents.

Chlorambucil (Leukeran)

In this compound, the two chloroethyl groups are linked to a phenyl group (see Figure 6.5). It is a stable compound, well absorbed orally, and is usually given in low continuous dose or as a higher intermittent dose. It produces antitumour effects slowly, and myelosuppressive effects are gradual in onset but persistent. Thrombocytopenia is frequent but haemorrhagic cystitis rarely occurs. It is generally well tolerated and has been widely used in the treatment of low-grade lymphomas, particularly in the elderly, and as part of combination chemotherapy regimens in Hodgkin's disease.

Busulfan (Myleran)

This compound differs in structure from other alkylating agents, being an alkyl sulphonate (see Figure 6.5). Thrombocytopenia is frequent, and pancytopenia develops, which may be irreversible. Pulmonary fibrosis is a complication of long-term administration, which occurs with other alkylating agents but is especially frequent with this drug. Other side-effects include skin pigmentation, glossitis, gynaecomastia and anhidrosis. It is used in the treatment of chronic granulocytic leukaemia and in some very high-dose regimens in childhood cancers.

cis-Diamine dichloroplatinum (cisplatin)

The drug is only active in the *cis* form. It acts as an alkylating agent. It diffuses into cells, and the chloride ions are then lost from the molecule. The compound then binds to DNA, producing inter- and intra-strand cross-links. The binding appears to be mainly to guanine groups. The drug is administered intravenously. The early half-life is about 40 min and the later phase of clearance is slow (half-life 60 hours). It is 90% bound to plasma protein, and is taken up in the kidney, gut, liver, ovary and testis but not the central nervous system (CNS).

The drug is nephrotoxic, and when administered in high dose, a high urine flow is essential, with intravenous fluids being administered before and for 24 hours after the drug. Renal function may worsen during repeated cycles and the plasma creatinine level and clearance should be checked regularly. With some high-dose regimens, mannitol is used to maintain urine flow. Loss of K^+ and Mg^{2+}/Ca^{2+} in the urine may require electrolyte supplementation in both the short and long term. Nausea and vomiting are severe with higher doses, and ototoxicity may be irreversible so that pretreatment audiometry may be carried out. Myelosuppression is not severe, but peripheral neuropathy is frequent and often subclinical. Hypersensitivity is frequent (see below).

Cisplatin is very effective in the treatment of testicular tumours and, in combination with etoposide and bleomycin, has revolutionized the outlook in advanced disease (see Chapter 19). It is also effective in cancer of the ovary and bladder as well as in lymphomas and small-cell carcinoma of the bronchus. It is active in osteosarcoma, oesophagogastric cancer and squamous cancer of the head and neck.

Carboplatin

This analogue of cisplatin has a different spectrum of toxicity from cisplatin and has replaced it in treatment of ovarian cancer and NSCLC. It is given intravenously and the area under the concentration–time curve (AUC) is given by the formula $AUC = [GFR (mL/min) + 25]n$, where n is the desired multiple. Thus the dose required for AUC 5 in a patient with a glomerular filtration rate (GFR) of 120 is $(120 + 25) \times 5 = 725$. Some drug regimens are given according to this formula, others on a conventional dose per square metre basis. The main toxicity is myelosuppression, which may be profound. Typically its onset is at 14–21 days and for this reason intervals between treatments may need to be 28 days. Carboplatin causes less nausea and vomiting than cisplatin and is not as nephrotoxic or neurotoxic. The drug is given by intravenous injection in saline or dextrose/saline. Pre- and post-hydration are not necessary unless there is vomiting. In testicular cancer the drug is less effective than cisplatin since dose reduction is necessary due to myelosuppression. It is active in SCLC and ovarian cancer. In the latter its ease of administration makes it valuable for palliative treatment.

Oxaliplatin

This analogue is active in colorectal cancer in both the adjuvant and advanced settings. It is also active in other gastrointestinal malignancies including pancreatic and oesophagogastric cancers. Oxaliplatin has minimal activity when administered as monotherapy and is combined with fluoropyrimidines (5-FU, capecitabine) for maximal benefit. It is less emetogenic than cisplatin and is not nephrotoxic. The major toxicity is sensory neuropathy which occurs in a substantial proportion of patients and can be debilitating in a minority of patients.

Nitrosoureas

Bis-chloroethyl nitrosourea (carmustine)

Bis-chloroethyl nitrosourea (BCNU) was the first nitrosourea to be used clinically. It has a wide spectrum of activity similar to the alkylating agents. It is lipid-soluble and penetrates the blood–brain barrier that is assumed to exist for primary brain tumours. However, the response rates are low in primary brain tumours and the effect usually transient.

It is usually given intravenously and the half-life is very short, less than 5 min. The major toxic effect is bone marrow depression, which is characteristically delayed for 5–6 weeks. Nausea and vomiting are frequent and renal and hepatic drainage may occur, as do oesophagitis and flushing. It is not vesicant. Long-term follow-up of children treated for brain tumours reveals a high incidence of asymptomatic pulmonary fibrosis, which may become symptomatic at any time.

BCNU and cis-chloroethyl nitrosourea (CCNU) bind to the O^6 position of guanine and the cross-link is formed with the opposite cytosine. Adducts formed by BCNU and CCNU with the O^6 position of guanine are repaired by the enzyme O^6 alkyltransferase. High levels of this enzyme are associated with resistance to nitrosoureas. The enzyme removes the adduct and is itself then inactivated.

cis-Chloroethyl nitrosourea (lomustine)
CCNU is rapidly absorbed and metabolites can be detected in the cerebrospinal fluid (CSF). As with BCNU, the major toxic effects are nausea, vomiting and delayed bone marrow depression. For this reason, the drug is given at 6-week intervals. Nausea and vomiting can be reduced by spreading the dose over 2 or 3 days.

Dimethyltriazenoimidazole carboxamide (dacarbazine)
Dacarbazine probably produces its cytotoxic effect by functioning as an alkylating agent. It is converted to its active form in the liver. It is administered intravenously and is vesicant if extravasated. It was initially introduced as a treatment for melanoma. It is included in some regimens for Hodgkin's disease. It causes severe nausea and vomiting, and myelosuppression is frequent. Damage to liver and peripheral nerves occurs, as do flushing and myalgia.

Temozolomide
This is a nitrosourea that liberates the active species directly without hepatic conversion. Its primary cytotoxic effect is attributable to alkylation at the O^6 position of guanine, where it primarily forms O^6-methylguanine-DNA adducts. The main indication is for treatment of high-grade glioma, melanoma and there is recent evidence of efficacy in neuroendocrine cancers (see Chapter 11). Molecular studies, primarily in patients with

gliomas, suggest that the benefit of temozolomide is greatest in patients whose tumours have a methylated *MGMT* gene promoter with consequently reduced expression and are unable to repair chemotherapy-induced DNA damage [8]. The measurement of MGMT in gliomas is thus one of the few validated biomarkers to inform treatment decisions regarding choice of a chemotherapeutic agent.

Antimetabolites: drugs blocking formation or action of pyrimidines
Methotrexate
Methotrexate (Figures 6.6 and 6.7) is an inhibitor of the enzyme DHFR. This enzyme is essential for reducing dihydrofolate (FH$_2$) to tetrahydrofolate (FH$_4$), which in turn is converted to a variety of coenzymes that are essential in reactions where one carbon atom is transferred in the synthesis of thymidylate, purines, methionine

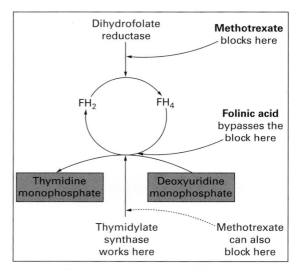

Figure 6.6 The action of methotrexate and folinic acid.

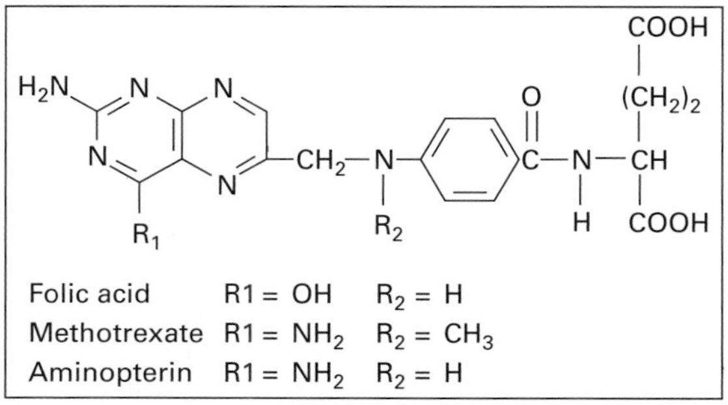

Figure 6.7 Folic acid analogues.

and glycine. Methotrexate and other antifolates are polyglutamated inside the cell. This process increases the efficiency of binding to DHFR. The critical effect in preventing cell replication appears to be the blocking of synthesis of thymidine monophosphate as shown in Figure 6.6. This block results in inhibition of DNA and RNA synthesis and the drug is, therefore, S-phase specific. The block in activity of DHFR can be bypassed by supplying an alternative intermediary metabolite. This is N_5-formyl-FH$_4$, variously termed leucovorin, citrovorum factor or, more commonly, folinic acid. It is converted to the FH$_4$ coenzymes, needed for thymidylate synthase (TS) to function.

The most important mechanism of methotrexate resistance appears to be increased expression of DHFR. In methotrexate-resistant cells there may be an increased copy number of the DHFR gene. This may appear as dense homogeneous staining regions on chromosomes or in small chromosome fragments called double minute chromosomes. These regions appear stable and may be responsible for the continuation of methotrexate resistance in subsequent cell divisions. Other resistance mechanisms are the production of enzyme with decreased affinity for methotrexate, and impaired transport into cells.

The mechanisms of excretion, distribution and metabolism make it one of the most difficult anti-cancer drugs to manage in routine practice. The drug is completely absorbed from the gut at low dosages, but incompletely at higher doses. After intravenous injection there is an initial rapid distribution phase (half-life 45 min), then a slower phase of renal excretion (half-life 2–3 hours) followed by a very slow phase when the drug concentration is low. It is this latter, prolonged, phase of clearance that is responsible for toxicity to marrow, gut and mucous membranes. If there is ascites or a pleural effusion, the drug may accumulate in these sites and then be slowly released from the 'reservoir' (or third space), causing unexpected toxicity even from a low dose. The drug is 50% bound to albumin, from which it can be displaced by drugs such as salicylates, sulphonamides, tetracycline and phenytoin. It is not metabolized significantly but is mainly excreted unchanged in the urine, especially in the first 8 hours by both glomerular filtration and tubular secretion. Drugs which compete for tubular secretion, or the presence of renal failure, may greatly delay excretion of the drug and thereby increase toxicity.

When given at high doses, the CSF concentrations can achieve cytotoxic levels of up to 10% of the plasma concentration. The drug can also be administered intrathecally, usually at a dose of 10 mg/m^2, and high CSF levels are thereby achieved, especially in the spinal CSF.

The toxicity is mainly haematological and on epithelial surfaces. Pancytopenia develops rapidly after a large dose. After 4–6 days, oral ulceration, diarrhoea (which may be bloody) and erythematous skin rashes can occur. Other toxic effects include alopecia, renal failure with high doses, hepatic toxicity (occasionally leading to cirrhosis), pneumonitis, and osteoporosis after long-term therapy.

Methotrexate is part of the established treatment of ALL. It is also used in non-Hodgkin's lymphomas, breast cancer, osteosarcoma and choriocarcinoma. To overcome methotrexate resistance, the drug is often used in high dose followed by folinic acid rescue. Doses of methotrexate can be increased over 100-fold provided the effect of the drug is reversed at 24 hours. Meticulous attention to hydration is essential. Urinary alkalinization is needed to prevent methotrexate deposition in the renal tubule. This is accomplished by using sodium bicarbonate or acetazolamide. Plasma levels of methotrexate must be measured at 24 and 48 hours. If correctly monitored there is little toxicity, but the approach is potentially very dangerous. It is expensive and the value of the procedure uncertain, although improved response rates have been claimed in osteosarcoma (see Chapter 23).

Thymidylate synthase inhibitors

TS is also an attractive target for selective inhibition of thymidine monophosphate formation from deoxyuridine monophosphate (see Figure 6.6).

5-Fluorouracil

A fluorine atom is substituted for hydrogen on the uracil molecule. The 5-FU molecule (Figure 6.8) can enter into many reactions where uracil would be the normal participant. 5-FU has to be activated to 5-fluoro-2-deoxyuridine monophosphate (FdUMP). The conversion of 5-FU to FdUMP can proceed through a variety of pathways, and resistance to the drug is associated with decreased activity of the enzymes necessary for this conversion. FdUMP interferes with DNA synthesis by binding to the enzyme TS and inactivating it. The effect of the block can to some extent be overcome if thymidine is given (similar to the effect of folinic acid rescue for methotrexate). Conversely, folinic acid enhances 5-FU activity by stabilizing the binding of FdUMP to TS. Folinic acid is used as a means of increasing the effectiveness of 5-FU. Response rates of colorectal cancer metastases are increased with the combination. 5-FU is also incorporated into RNA, but the importance of this for its antineoplastic effect is not

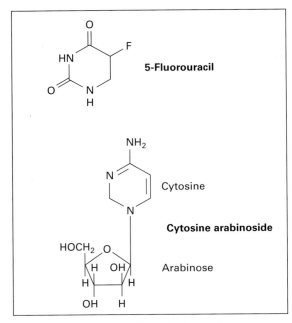

Figure 6.8 The structure of the pyrimidine analogues.

certain. 5-FU is more toxic to proliferating cells (i.e. it is cell-cycle specific) and this may account for efficacy of infusional regimens.

The intestinal absorption of 5-FU is erratic, so the drug is usually given intravenously. Plasma clearance is rapid (half-life 15 min). Much higher plasma concentrations are achieved by rapid intravenous injection than by continuous infusion, and the toxicity of the drug is greater when given by bolus injection. The drug penetrates the CSF well. There are many schedules of administration using 5-FU alone, or with folinic acid, in intermediate dose or in very high dose. Myelosuppression is commonest between 10 and 15 days. Care is necessary in the presence of hepatic dysfunction. Hepatic arterial or portal vein infusion of 5-FU has been used to treat hepatic metastases from colon cancer. The drug has activity against adenocarcinoma of the gastrointestinal tract, breast and ovary. 5-FU is used as adjuvant therapy in colorectal cancer. In this situation, it has been given alone, or with folinic acid. Recent studies indicate that infusional 5-FU is tolerated better than bolus, with increased efficacy. The major disadvantage is the need for indwelling venous access.

The drug is generally well tolerated but toxic effects include nausea, diarrhoea, stomatitis, alopecia, myelosuppression, cardiac disturbances and a cerebellar syndrome. In a small proportion of patients there is a mutation in the dihydropyrimidine dehydrogenase (DPD) gene resulting in impaired metabolism of drug. This may result in severe and life-threatening mucositis and myelosuppression. Prospective identification of patients with DPD deficiency has not been feasible in clinical practice.

Oral fluoropyrimidines (capecitabine, S-1)
Recent advances in oral fluoropyrimidines have allowed more convenient administration of this class of agents. For example, capecitabine is an orally administered prodrug, which is selectively activated by tumour cells to 5-FU. Capecitabine has shown equivalence to 5-FU in randomized trials in the adjuvant treatment of colorectal cancer and has been used in combination with oxaliplatin in both adjuvant and advanced settings. It is also used for treatment of metastatic breast cancer. S-1 is another oral fluoropyrimidine with a favourable toxicity profile which has been shown to be effective in the adjuvant setting for gastrointestinal malignancies including gastric and pancreatic cancers.

Cytosine arabinoside (cytarabine, Ara-C)
In this analogue of cytidine (see Figure 6.8) the pyrimidine base is unchanged but the sugar moiety differs by an alteration in the position of a hydroxyl group. The drug is converted by a series of enzymic steps to its active form known as ara-CTP. This is an inhibitor of DNA polymerase but it is not clear if this is the mechanism of its cytotoxic action. It would explain why the drug is markedly cell cycle (S-phase) specific. Resistance to the effect of the drug could either be due to low levels of one of the converting enzymes (deoxycytidine kinase) or to increased rates of deamination, which is the principal mechanism of inactivation. The former seems to be the major mechanism.

The drug is poorly absorbed from the intestine. After intravenous injection there is a fast phase of clearance (half-life 20 min) followed by a slower phase (half-life 2 hours) and the clearance is largely determined by the speed of deamination in the liver and other tissues. The drug penetrates well into the CSF and deamination occurs slowly at this site. Because it is S-phase specific, it is usually given as multiple intravenous injections or as a continuous intravenous or subcutaneous infusion.

The agent is mainly of use against AML but is also used in ALL and poor-prognosis lymphomas. It is of little value in solid tumours, which usually have a low growth fraction.

The toxic effects include hypersensitivity (see below), marrow suppression, oral ulceration, diarrhoea, nausea and vomiting and, uncommonly, CNS toxicity. It is particularly toxic in the presence of hepatic dysfunction since the liver is the chief site of deamination.

Gemcitabine

This is a fluorinated derivative of deoxycytidine nucleotide. It has multiple intracellular targets, but its chief action is as a substrate for deoxycytidine kinase, which converts the drug to a triphosphate and allows its incorporation into DNA in place of cytosine. The synthesis of DNA is blocked after the next base pair is incorporated in the chain. The drug has linear pharmacokinetics and is excreted in urine in the form of its chief metabolite. It is usually administered as a 30-min infusion once a week. Its dose-limiting toxicity is myelosuppression (especially thrombocytopenia). Fever, rash, abnormal liver function tests and fatigue are other toxicities which depend on schedule of administration. The drug has significant single-agent activity against NSCLC, where it now has an accepted role in combination with other drugs. It also has activity in breast and ovarian cancer. Although responses are uncommon, it has been shown to prolong survival and improve quality of life in pancreatic cancer. Additionally, gemcitabine has been shown to improve survival when used as adjuvant therapy following resection of pancreatic cancer.

Antimetabolites: drugs blocking formation or action of purines

There are several cytotoxic agents that are analogues of the natural purine bases and nucleotides. They are in wide use as cytotoxic and immunosuppressive agents. 6-MP and thioguanine are derivatives of hypoxanthine and guanine, respectively, but with the keto group on C-6 replaced by a sulphur atom. Drugs of this class usually undergo enzymatic conversion to the active form.

6-Mercaptopurine

6-MP (Figure 6.9) must be converted to the nucleotide to become active. This is done by the enzyme hypoxanthine-guanine phosphoribosyltransferase (HGPRT). The resultant nucleotide is 6-MP ribose phosphate (6-MPRP). This accumulates in the cell and inhibits several important metabolic reactions in the formation of normal nucleotides. The cytotoxicity of the drug cannot be ascribed to disruption of a single metabolic pathway and cell death probably results from multiple biochemical abnormalities. However, inhibition of purine nucleotide

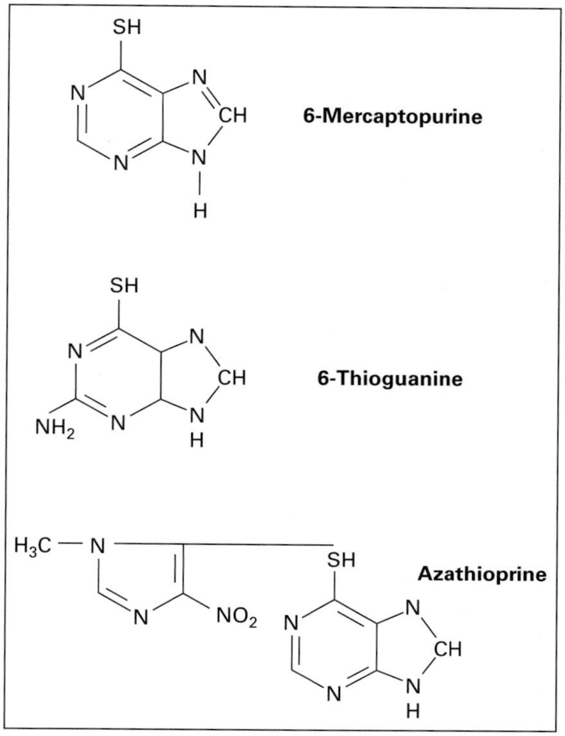

Figure 6.9 The structures of commonly used purine analogues.

biosynthesis is a major action of the drug. 6-MP is also incorporated into DNA as 6-thioguanine (6-TG) but the contribution of this reaction to cytotoxicity is not clear. Resistance to the action of 6-MP is often due to low levels of the converting enzyme HGPRT, and such cells also show resistance to 6-TG and azaguanine. Increased rates of drug breakdown may also be important. Dephosphorylation may also be a mechanism of resistance to 6-thiopurines generally.

6-MP is readily absorbed from the gut, and about half of an oral dose is excreted as antimetabolites in 24 hours. After intravenous injection the drug is rapidly cleared from the plasma (half-life 90 min) due to distribution and metabolism. A major site of metabolism is the liver, where xanthine oxidase rapidly converts the drug to an inactive form. The xanthine oxidase inhibitor allopurinol blocks this conversion, but this increases toxicity as well as effectiveness and the therapeutic ratio is unchanged. If allopurinol is used in the early stages to prevent hyperuricaemia, it will increase the toxicity of 6-MP. 6-MP is widely used in remission maintenance in ALL. Its use as an immunosuppressive agent has largely been superseded by azathioprine. The frequent occurrence of cholestatic jaundice with 6-MP has made it less satisfactory for long-term administration. Its other toxicities are nausea and vomiting with gradual and reversible bone marrow suppression. The usual maintenance dose in ALL is 50–100 mg/day.

Azathioprine (Imuran)

Azathioprine (Figure 6.9) was developed in an attempt to decrease the rate of inactivation of 6-MP. The drug acts as a prodrug, and 6-MP is slowly formed in the tissues. It is degraded in the liver by xanthine oxidase, and allopurinol increases its toxicity. The drug is well absorbed orally and is partly excreted by the kidneys, so that its toxicity is greater if renal failure is present. Reversible bone marrow depression is the major toxicity. It is most widely used as an immunosuppressive agent in connective tissue diseases and renal allograft recipients.

6-Thioguanine

This purine analogue (Figure 6.9) has a mode of action similar to that of 6-MP. It is well absorbed orally and peak concentrations are achieved in 6–8 hours. About half the dose is excreted in the urine as metabolites within 24 hours. Degradation by xanthine oxidase does not appear to be an important aspect of detoxification and the drug can be used safely with allopurinol. The drug is widely used as part of remission induction and maintenance in AML. It has also been used as an immunosuppressive. Reversible bone marrow depression is the major toxicity, but nausea and diarrhoea may also occur.

Fludarabine

This drug is closely related to cytosine arabinoside. The purine is fluorinated and competes for incorporation into DNA, inhibiting cell replication by acting as a chain terminator when incorporated into the newly synthesized DNA. It also inhibits RNA synthesis. It is active in low-grade lymphomas and chronic lymphocytic leukaemia, even in tumours resistant to conventional agents. Its toxic effects include myelosuppression and immunosuppression. It is widely used in the treatment of low-grade lymphomas and chronic lymphatic leukaemia.

Vinca alkaloids and taxanes

Vinca alkaloids are extracted from the periwinkle, *Catharanthus roseus*, and were observed to cause granulocytopenia in animals. Subsequently, they were shown to be mitotic spindle poisons.

The stages of mitosis are described in Chapter 3. The vinca alkaloids and other mitotic inhibitors act by binding to tubulin, which is the constituent protein of the microtubules. The assembly and function of the microtubules during metaphase is shown in Figure 6.10. Exposure of the cell to vinca alkaloids leads to rapid disappearance of the microtubules because no further assembly can take place (Figure 6.10). Conversely, the taxane drugs promote assembly of microtubules and inhibit their disassembly.

In cell lines vinca resistance is associated with the appearance of the 180-kDa membrane glycoprotein and resistance to many other agents (MDR). There is often cross-resistance from one vinca alkaloid to another and between vinca alkaloids and podophyllotoxins. Taxane resistance may also be mediated by decreased binding to tubulin.

Vincristine

Vincristine is administered intravenously and is poorly and unpredictably absorbed from the gut. It is vesicant if it escapes from the vein into the tissues. The pharmacokinetics are similar to those of vinblastine (see below).

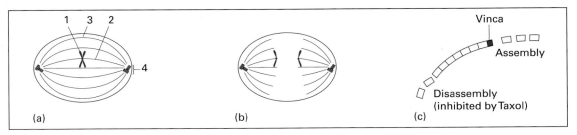

Figure 6.10 The assembly and function of microtubules during metaphase. (a) The chromosome pair (1) is attached to a microtubule (2) which is assembled at the equatorial region (3) and disassembled at the centriole (4). (b) In anaphase the chromosome pair is divided and pulled to opposite ends of the cell. (c) A microtubule is a polymer of the protein tubulin which is made up of α and β subunits. Vinca alkaloids bind to tubulin, blocking further assembly, but disassembly continues. Paclitaxel prevents disassembly.

The drug is useful in treatment of lymphatic malignancies such as Hodgkin's disease, non-Hodgkin's lymphoma and ALL. In these diseases it is usually used in combination with other drugs such as steroids and alkylating agents. It also has a place in the treatment of other cancers such as breast cancers, small-cell carcinoma of the bronchus and brain tumours.

The toxicity of the drug is mainly neurological, and peripheral neuropathy is an almost invariable sequel to long-term administration. It is especially likely to occur in the elderly and those with liver disease, and may be severe and incapacitating. Loss of reflexes and paraesthesiae occur early and are not usually regarded as indications for cessation of treatment, although cautious supervision of further doses is necessary. However, severe myalgic and neuritic pain and motor weakness and/or peripheral sensory loss are signs that treatment should be stopped. Nerve conduction is usually preserved even with severe neuropathy, but electromyography shows a pattern of denervation. Cranial nerve palsies occasionally occur. It is probable that vincristine blocks the passage of tubulin from proximal to distal axonal sites. Autonomic neuropathy often occurs, with constipation and ileus. These symptoms can be partially alleviated with bulk laxatives. Myelosuppression is mild, increasing the usefulness of the drug when used in combination. The drug sometimes causes thrombocytosis and the syndrome of inappropriate secretion of ADH.

Vinblastine

After intravenous injection the drug disappears from the plasma in three phases, with half-lives of 4 min, 1 hour and 16 hours. Much of the drug remains tissue-bound for many days. In the blood it binds to platelets, red cells and plasma proteins. The clinical differences in toxicity cannot be explained on pharmacokinetic grounds. Indications for the use of vinblastine are similar to those for vincristine. In addition, vinblastine is often used in high dose for the treatment of testicular teratoma in combination with cisplatin and bleomycin (see below and Chapter 19). In these high doses, neutropenia and ileus are common. Vinblastine causes more myelosuppression but less neurotoxicity than vincristine. Extravasation leads to cellulitis. Alopecia and mucositis are infrequent side-effects.

Vindesine

This semisynthetic addition to the vinca alkaloids has a similar spectrum of activity but appears to have additional activity in NSCLC. The toxicity of the drug is intermediate between that of vinblastine and vincristine. Myelosuppression and neurotoxicity both occur.

Vinorelbine

This is a vinca alkaloid that has shown significant activity in advanced NSCLC and breast cancer, with a response rate of about 25%. Its toxicity is myelosuppression, but peripheral retinopathy is less marked.

Paclitaxel (Taxol) [9]

This drug is an extract from the bark of the Pacific yew, *Taxus brevifolia*. It promotes assembly of microtubules and inhibits their disassembly. It is poorly water-soluble and is formulated in cremophor oil. When infused, the dose-limiting toxicity is neutropenia. Other side-effects are neuropathy, alopecia and myalgia. It is active in advanced ovarian cancer, with a response rate of 30%, and is also effective for breast cancer; responses have been reported in NSCLC and melanoma. When combined with anthracyclines, mucositis has been dose-limiting. It is often given as a 3-hour infusion three-weekly but there is evidence that lower doses administered weekly may lessen toxicity without compromising efficacy.

Docetaxel (Taxotere)

Docetaxel is a novel semisynthetic taxoid. It has significant activity against breast cancer and NSCLC, and some activity in a number of other tumours, including cancers of the head and neck, ovary and pancreas. The dose-limiting toxicity is neutropenia, but other side-effects are hypersensitivity, skin reactions, fluid retention, neuropathy and alopecia. The current treatment schedule is usually a 1-hour infusion every 3 weeks.

Topoisomerase inhibitors

Topoisomerases are nuclear enzymes that alter the three-dimensional structure of DNA within the nucleus.

They cause protein-associated strand breaks relieving torsional stress within DNA by passing the DNA strand through the break and religating breaks. Two broad classes of enzyme are described: topoisomerase I and topoisomerase II. Topoisomerase I is an essential enzyme involved in DNA replication and transcription; the enzyme forms single-strand DNA breaks. Topoisomerase II (of which there are two isoforms in humans) is involved in DNA replication and chromosomal segregation; interaction with DNA results in double-strand DNA breaks.

Although these drugs are referred to as being topoisomerase inhibitors, they act as cellular poisons by converting the normal protein–DNA complex intermediate (the cleavable complex) into irreversible DNA strand breaks that are toxic to cells. Thus increased cellular expression of topoisomerases results in *increased* sensitivity to these drugs.

Topoisomerase I inhibitors (camptothecin, irinotecan, topotecan)

The prototype drug is camptothecin, derived from *Camptotheca acuminata* (a Chinese tree). It binds to the enzyme–DNA complex, stabilizing it, preventing DNA replication and provoking breaks of the DNA double strand.

Irinotecan has been extensively evaluated. It is active in several cancers, especially of the gut and lung. However, its major use is in the treatment of colorectal cancer. The main toxicities are myelosuppression and diarrhoea. The drug is excreted in bile and urine and has a long half-life. It is a prodrug, which is converted to an active metabolite. Topotecan is a similar agent whose major toxicity is bone marrow suppression.

Drug resistance depends on altered topoisomerase I function, *p*-glycoprotein and poor conversion of irinotecan to its active metabolite.

Topoisomerase II inhibitors

The epipodophyllotoxin derivative etoposide (VP16) is a semisynthetic derivative of extracts of *Podophyllum peltatum*, the American mandrake. Topoisomerase II is an enzyme involved in reversibly cleaving DNA so that it can unwind during cell division. Etoposide has an early rapid phase of clearance followed by a slower phase (half-life 2–13 hours). Etoposide is absorbed erratically from the gut, with plasma availability of about 50% of the intravenous dose. The drug can be infused at high dose, but mucositis then becomes dose-limiting. At conventional doses bone marrow suppression and hair loss are the major toxicities. Etoposide is highly protein-bound and about half the drug is excreted in the urine in 72 hours. After dilution it is stable for about 24 hours, depending on the concentration. Etoposide activity is highly schedule-dependent. In SCLC the response rate is greatly increased by repeated daily administration compared with the same total dose as a single infusion. Hypersensitivity reactions occur (see below).

Antitumour antibiotics

Many antitumour antibiotics have now been produced from bacterial and fungal cultures. They produce their effect by binding to DNA, intercalating between base pairs.

Actinomycin D (dactinomycin)

This antibiotic was first isolated from *Streptomyces* in 1940. At low concentrations it blocks DNA-directed RNA synthesis and at higher concentration also blocks DNA synthesis. The molecule intercalates between guanine/cytosine base pairs and the transcription of DNA is blocked. The drug inhibits the division of all rapidly dividing cells. Resistance appears to be associated with both impaired drug entry and increased drug efflux.

It is given intravenously and is cleared within a few minutes. Its main use has been in the treatment of childhood cancers, such as rhabdomyosarcoma, Wilms' tumour and Ewing's sarcoma. It is of less value in adult tumours. The toxicities are nausea and vomiting, myelosuppression, mucositis and diarrhoea. It sensitizes tissue to radiation.

Bleomycin

This antibiotic was derived from a mixture of glycopeptides isolated from *Streptomyces verticillus* but is now chemically synthesized. The drug inhibits DNA synthesis and causes breaks in the DNA chain. It arrests cells in G_2.

The drug can be given parenterally by any route. It disappears from the plasma with an initial half-life of 1 hour and then more slowly (half-life 9 hours). It is excreted in the urine, and caution is needed with impaired renal function. The drug concentration is very low in the brain and CSF, and it appears to be concentrated mainly in skin and lung. Many tissues contain an inactivating enzyme that hydrolyses the drug, and the levels of this enzyme appear to correlate with resistance. It is active in squamous carcinomas of the head and neck, skin and cervix and against lymphomas and testicular tumours.

The drug is valuable in combination with other agents because it causes little bone marrow toxicity. Acute hypersensitivity reactions are common and are discussed below. Skin toxicity is characterized by pigmentation, erythema and vesiculation. It also causes mucosal ulceration, pulmonary infiltrates and fibrosis. These toxic effects are serious, sometimes disabling, and are related to total dose, with high risk when the dose exceeds $300 \, \text{mg/m}^2$.

Doxorubicin and daunorubicin

These are anthracycline antibiotics produced from a species of *Streptomyces* fungus. Doxorubicin is a highly active agent with a wide spectrum of activity against many tumours, and differs from daunorubicin by the substitution of an OH group for a hydrogen atom.

These intercalating drugs act primarily as topoisomerase II inhibitors. They also produce highly reactive intracellular free radicals, which may be important in producing some of the toxic effects, for example, cardiac toxicity. Drug resistance is mediated, at least in part, through the MDR drug-efflux protein. There appears to be complete cross-resistance between the two drugs as well as some degree of cross-resistance with vinca alkaloids and actinomycin, probably due to the MDR mechanism. The drugs are effective mainly against cells in S phase.

Both drugs are injected intravenously into a fast-running drip, and are highly vesicant. They are cleared rapidly from the plasma, but there is slow terminal clearance of doxorubicin. There is rapid uptake into spleen, kidney, lungs, liver and heart, but not into the brain. The drugs are metabolized in the liver, and severe toxicity may result if they are given to patients with impaired liver function. With doxorubicin, 40% is excreted in the bile as free drug, adriamycinol and other metabolites. With both drugs the major and acute side-effects are bone marrow depression, nausea and vomiting, mucositis, alopecia and gastrointestinal disturbance. Alopecia can be lessened by cooling the scalp before and after drug administration. The most important chronic and dose-limiting side-effect is cardiac toxicity, which can result in arrhythmias and heart failure. It is related to the total dose administered and is a major risk above a total dose of $500 \, \text{mg/m}^2$. However, cardiac damage may occasionally occur with total dose of $300 \, \text{mg/m}^2$. In addition to total dose, the drug schedule may be important. High peak plasma concentrations may be associated with more toxicity. Subclinical cardiac toxicity may be more frequent than suspected previously, which may be of great importance in the treatment of childhood tumours. Cardioprotective agents are currently under evaluation. Mucositis is a troublesome side-effect. It is dose and schedule related. L-Glutamine may confer some protection. Doxorubicin has a wide spectrum of activity in childhood and adult tumours including lymphomas, small-cell bronchogenic carcinoma, adenocarcinomas of ovary, breast and stomach, bone and soft-tissue sarcomas, liver and bladder cancer. Daunorubicin is of value in the treatment of ALL and AML.

Mitoxantrone (mitozantrone)

This is an anthraquinone related to doxorubicin that binds to DNA. When injected intravenously it has a terminal half-life of 36 hours. It is vesicant and has a spectrum of activity similar to that of doxorubicin, with useful effects in metastatic breast cancer, lymphoma and leukaemia. The main toxicity is myelosuppression. It causes less alopecia than doxorubicin and possibly less cardiotoxicity.

Miscellaneous agents

L-Asparaginase (Crasnitin, Elspar)

The enzyme is produced by *Escherichia coli* and *Erwinia carotovora*. Most normal tissues synthesize asparagine but some tumour cells need an exogenous source which the enzyme removes. Resistance may be related to the appearance of asparagine synthetase in the tumour cells.

The drug is initially eliminated rapidly from the circulation, but the later half-life is 6–30 hours. It does not penetrate into the CSF. There is no marrow, gut or hair follicle toxicity, but hypersensitivity including anaphylaxis is very frequent (see below); pancreatitis, hyperglycaemia, raised liver enzymes with fatty change in the liver, confusion, somnolence, coma and hypofibrinogenaemia all occur and the drug is extremely nauseating.

The main use of the drug is in remission induction in ALL. The dosage schedules vary considerably with different combinations of drugs.

Procarbazine (Natulan)

This drug is the most useful of the hydrazine derivatives, which were originally synthesized as monoamine oxidase inhibitors but found to have antitumour activity. The mode of action is unclear. Metabolic activation is needed and the active product may be a methyldiazonium ion, which acts as an alkylating agent. Interphase is prolonged and mitosis is suppressed with breakage of chromatin strands.

The drug is well absorbed from the gut, and rapidly equilibrates with blood and CSF. After intravenous injection the half-life is 7 min and the drug is rapidly metabolized. The toxic effects are hypersensitivity, nausea and vomiting, leucopenia, CNS disturbances (especially psychological upsets), flushing with alcohol, and hypertensive reactions to foods rich in tyramine. It is useful in Hodgkin's disease and in brain tumours.

Hydroxycarbamide/hydroxyurea (Hydrea)

This drug blocks the action of ribonucleoside diphosphate reductase and thereby interferes with DNA synthesis. It causes leucopenia and megaloblastic changes in the bone marrow. It is S-phase specific. The drug is well absorbed orally and enters the CSF. It is excreted in the urine. Toxic effects are mainly marrow suppression and gut disturbances. Its main use is in chronic granulocytic leukaemia.

Targeted therapy for cancer

Strictly speaking, targeted therapy for human cancer is not a new concept. The effects of endocrine manipulation on breast cancer have been known since the late nineteenth century. The discovery that that breast cancers which express the oestrogen receptor (ER) respond to antagonists of the pathway has revolutionized therapy in both the adjuvant and advanced settings. However, increased understanding of the genetics of human cancer has allowed a deeper understanding of the molecular basis of individual cancers. This process has greatly accelerated with the advent of whole exome and deep sequencing technologies which allow the comprehensive molecular anatomy of individual cancers to be characterized. The major focus of therapeutic drug development in cancer is, therefore, personalized therapy in which specific targeted drugs are used to treat specific genetic abnormalities in different cancers.

The discovery of oncogenes implicated in carcinogenesis and the findings that specific mutations occurred in some cancers allowed novel therapeutic approaches to be developed and a better understanding of the use of currently available anticancer drugs [9]. Some tumours express mutated oncogenes to which they are 'addicted' and for which inhibition is an effective treatment. In other cancers for which no 'driver' mutations have been found, targeted therapies may still be of value although the response rates to these agents may be low and of short duration. The section below summarizes the classes of targeted agents currently in use.

Given the sensitivity of cancers to specific pathways the molecular characterization of tumours prior to therapy has become part of standard clinical practice. Thus, genotyping of NSCLC is mandatory to determine the presence of EGFR or ALK mutations which will guide choice of therapies (erlotinib/gefitinib and crizotinib respectively). Similarly, K-RAS mutational status will inform decisions on use of anti-EGFR antibody therapy in colorectal cancer [10]. With the identification of increasing number of such 'actionable' mutations in the coming years the panel of genes to be analysed will increase. Although the technology to obtain whole exome sequencing of cancers is available and likely to become cheaper and more accessible in the coming years there is no indication at present that such information can be used to improve clinical outcomes. Below are included examples of such targeted therapies with more detail in specific chapters. This is a rapidly developing field with novel therapies emerging frequently.

Drugs acting on signalling pathways

The pathways that transmit external signals into the cell have formed targets for new drug development. The aim is to block the subsequent processes of protein production and cell division. These processes are essential for normal cells. There may be many alternative pathways for each signalling event. The therapeutic action in cancer will, therefore, depend on the degree to which the tumour relies on the pathway concerned.

Growth factors, their receptors and receptor tyrosine kinases

The action of receptor tyrosine kinases is shown in a very simplified form in Figure 6.11. Ligands activating the EGFR pathway include epidermal growth factor (EGF), amphiregulin and transforming growth factor (TGF)-α. Members of the EGFR family are denoted as HER1 (EGFR, erbB1), HER2 (erbB2), which has no known ligand, HER3 (erbB3) and HER4 (erbB4). There have been two general approaches to the development of therapeutic agents:

• monoclonal antibodies have been developed that bind to the growth factors or to the cellular receptor, thereby blocking the stimulus
• drugs that bind to the kinase domain

One of the best examples of the use of a monoclonal antibody is *trastuzumab* (Herceptin). Overexpression of HER2 is present in 30% of breast cancers. Trastuzumab is a humanized monoclonal antibody that blocks HER2 but also induces antibody-dependent cell-mediated cytotoxicity. It has been shown to increase response and prolong survival in advanced disease and has significantly improved outcome when used in the adjuvant setting for patients with HER2 amplification. Cardiac complications including myopathy are well described and monitoring of cardiac function is mandatory. Hypersensitivity reactions may also occur.

Cetuximab (chimeric murine/human monoclonal antibody) and *Panitumumab* (a fully human monoclonal antibody) bind to the EGF receptor, thereby blocking activation of the receptor tyrosine kinase by ligands including EGF and TGF-α [11]. Both antibodies have activity in metastatic colorectal cancer given alone and also when combined with chemotherapy. Fatigue and allergic reactions occur. Treatment with cetuximab has also resulted in significant improvement in outcome when given in combination with radiation therapy in squamous cancer of the head and neck [12].

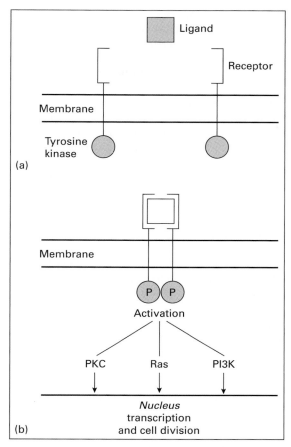

Figure 6.11 Receptor tyrosine kinase action. (a) The receptor is external and tyrosine kinase internal to the cell membrane. (b) The ligand causes dimerization and the kinase is activated by phosphorylation (P). This results in activation of protein kinase C (PKC), Ras and phosphatidylinositol 3-kinase (PI3K) to produce transcription and DNA synthesis.

Several small-molecule inhibitors of tyrosine kinases have now been introduced. *C-abl* is a cytoplasmic tyrosine kinase that forms a fusion protein with *bcr* as a result of the t9;22 translocation in chronic myeloid leukaemia (see Chapter 28). The action of the *bcr/abl* protein appears critical for growth of chronic myeloblastic leukaemia (CML). *Imatinib* is a drug that blocks this action and which produces a high and prolonged response rate in CML. It also has activity against the c-KIT tyrosine kinase overexpressed in gastrointestinal stromal tumours and has major clinical activity in this disease.

Gefitinib and Erlotinib are EGFR inhibitors, active orally. They have moderate activity in NSCLC but major responses are seen in the cohort of patients with mutations in the kinase domain of EGFR [13]. Treatment with gefitinib has revolutionized treatment of mutation-positive cancers with response rates, progression-free and overall survival superior when compared with conventional chemotherapy. Toxicities include corneal damage, rash and diarrhoea.

Crizotinib is an orally available inhibitor of the receptor tyrosine kinase anaplastic lymphoma kinase (ALK) and the c-Met/hepatocyte growth factor receptor (HGFR) with antineoplastic activity. Crizotinib, in an ATP-competitive manner, binds to and inhibits ALK kinase and ALK fusion proteins. In around 5% of NSCLCs which have translocations affecting the ALK locus and consequent overexpression, there are major responses (approximately 90% of patients) to treatment with crizotinib with an almost 5 month improvement in progression-free survival [14]. Toxicities include nausea, vomiting and diarrhoea.

Vemurafenib and *Dabrafenib* are oral tyrosine kinase inhibitors of the oncogenic BRAF V600 protein kinase which is expressed in around half of malignant melanomas. Dramatic responses are seen in a high proportion of patients although the duration of response is between 5 and 7 months when these are used as monotherapies [15]. The use of this agent illustrates the dramatic therapeutic effect of targeting oncogenic 'driver' mutations in cancer. A unique toxicity of these agents is the growth of cutaneous squamous-cell carcinomas induced by activation of the MAPK pathway in cells with RAS mutations.

Synthetic lethality

The development of drugs targeting DNA repair used in combination with DNA-interactive drugs has often been ineffective because of increased toxicities necessitating drastic dose reduction of the chemotherapeutic agent. The Poly ADP Ribose Polymerase (PARP) pathway is a mechanism for repair of single-strand DNA breaks. However, these lesions are usually repaired by the homologous recombination pathway including the BRCA1 and BRCA2 proteins. Clinical studies using PARP inhibitors, such as olaparib, demonstrated that in cancers with defects in the BRCA1 or BRCA2 tumour suppressor proteins, there is increased sensitivity to these agents [16]. This illustrates the principle of synthetic lethality in which molecular alterations within the cancer cell results in dependence on specific survival pathways which can be used to selectively target tumours. There are likely to be wider applications for synthetic lethality in determining therapeutic approaches in several cancer types [17].

Cyclin-dependent kinase inhibitors

Cyclin-dependent kinases are essential components of the cell cycle regulatory mechanism. Various inhibitors have now entered phase I studies. The best studied of these is flavopiridol, which has shown activity against a variety of tumours. Diarrhoea and myalgia are the main toxicities. Other compounds are in development.

Angiotoxic agents and inhibitors of angiogenesis

Damaging tumour vasculature, or inhibiting the growth of new blood vessels, is a new approach to cancer treatment and has led to the introduction of new agents.

Vascular endothelial growth factor

Bevacizumab is an antibody to VEGF that prevents its interaction with its receptors on endothelial cells (Flt-1 and KDR). This interaction normally leads to endothelial proliferation and new vessel formation. It has shown single-agent activity in advanced colorectal cancer and was shown to increase response rate and duration when combined with irinotecan and 5-FU/folinic acid. There is also evidence of activity in other malignancies including ovarian cancer.

Angiotoxins

Another approach to the inhibition of angiogenesis has been to target the tumour endothelium by toxins which disrupt vascular architecture. Combrestatin is the most promising drug of this class at present.

Other targets
CD33

Gemtuzumab is a monoclonal antibody to CD33, a molecule that is overexpressed on blast cells of AML. It has been demonstrated to increase the complete remission rate in patients with AML below the age of 60. Toxicity was minimal but there was a possible increase in risk of veno-occlusive disease.

CD20

Rituximab is a human/mouse chimeric antibody that binds to CD20 on the surface of neoplastic B cells. It is widely used in the treatment of low-grade non-Hodgkin's lymphomas (see Chapter 26).

Proteosome inhibitors

Bortezomib is an agent that interrupts the function of proteosomes, the protein destruction machinery of the cell. It has been used in refractory myeloma and shows significant clinical activity.

Hypersensitivity reactions

Many chemotherapeutic agents are associated with hypersensitivity reactions that may be life-threatening and which, for some drugs, are quite frequent. All those responsible for administration of chemotherapy must be aware of these effects, which cannot be easily predicted. There must be facilities at hand for the urgent treatment of these reactions if they occur. Most acute reactions are typical of type 1 hypersensitivity, with urticaria, angio-oedema, chills, fever and variable degrees of bronchospasm. Treatment is with immediate use of parenteral dexamethasone, diphenhydramine and a bronchodilator. Most patients who have had a reaction will do so again if rechallenged.

Agents producing reactions very frequently
Monoclonal antibodies (e.g. trastuzumab, rituximab, gemtuzumab)

Most of these reactions are fever, chills, urticaria, skin rash and angio-oedema, typical of a type 1 hypersensitivity reaction. Less commonly, the reaction can be life-threatening, with severe bronchospasm and hypotension. Type 3 reactions with pulmonary infiltrates are less common.

Bleomycin

Acute pyrexial reactions commonly occur, and can be relieved or prevented by hydrocortisone. This reaction diminishes with further doses. Other type 1 symptoms are less common. In rare cases, cardiorespiratory collapse occurs. A small subcutaneous test dose at the start of treatment is recommended.

Cisplatin and carboplatin

Both these drugs are associated with type 1 reactions in about 10% of patients. Typically the reactions appear after three or more cycles of treatment. Skin testing can predict those patients who are likely to have a reaction but it is not usual practice to do this. Patients who have had a reaction will do so again if rechallenged. Desensitization is possible in some patients where there is no alternative to the use of the drugs.

L-Asparaginase

About 30% of patients will experience a type 1 reaction by the third dose. The frequency is higher with continued dosage, where there is a history of atopic reactions, when the drug is given intravenously, and when the drug is given as a single agent rather than with steroid and vincristine as part of treatment. A test dose is recommended. Desensitization is possible if the drug is considered essential for treatment.

Agents producing reactions infrequently

Taxanes

When taxanes were first introduced the incidence of acute hypersensitivity was about 30%. Now that appropriate premedication, with steroids and antihistamines, is used as routine, and the infusion time has been prolonged, these reactions occur in about 5% of patients and are less severe. Type 3 reactions with pulmonary infiltrates occur but are much less common. These acute reactions have been attributed to the cromophor in which the drug is dissolved, but it is probable that the drugs themselves are also implicated. Dexamethasone (usually given as 8 mg every 8 hours for 3 days starting the day before the dose) greatly reduces the incidence. Skin tests are of doubtful predictive value. Desensitization and rechallenge are possible.

The administration of cytotoxic agents

Chemotherapeutic drugs are highly toxic and should be prescribed and administered by specialists. This involves a team approach involving oncologists, specialized chemotherapy nurses and pharmacists. The introduction of computerized prescription systems has significantly reduced the incidence of prescribing errors.

Patients on outpatient regimens

Virtually all patients can receive their drugs in this way, especially if the person giving them is the same each time and learns the best antiemetic or sedative regimen for that patient. Some patients are not sick at all, others vomit several hours later and prefer to go home quickly and take a 5-hydroxytryptamine (5-HT)$_3$ antagonist, others vomit at the sight of the needle and require premedication with diazepam or prochlorperazine. There is little doubt that trained nurses are the best people to give the drugs. They become very expert in setting up intravenous infusions and noting side-effects from previous drug treatment, and there are seldom difficulties with extravasation.

Newly qualified house staff are not nearly as capable or as accessible to the patient during the day. Patients undergoing cytotoxic chemotherapy should be aware of the nature of the treatment and its possible hazards. It is easier to make sure that patients receive adequate information if the treatment is the responsibility of a single department. The patient should be told of the nature of the drugs, what the possible side-effects might be and which of these effects should lead the patient to contact the hospital. For example, he or she should be told to report fever or sore throat so that a blood count can be taken. It is worthwhile providing explanatory leaflets about chemotherapy, and drug cards giving the names, dosage and purposes of the drugs are very useful.

Patients on lengthy regimens

These patients, many of whom are on treatments where there is a serious possibility of prolonged myelosuppression, are admitted to hospital. They are under the care of a single team, experienced in the use of intensive cytotoxic regimens and in mitigating the side-effects of the drugs, and familiar with the supportive techniques required (see Chapter 7).

Chemotherapy-induced vomiting

The mechanisms by which chemotherapy induces vomiting [15] are not well understood. Both peripheral (gastric and intestinal) and central stimuli may be important. A schematic representation is shown in Figure 6.12. Blockage of 5-HT$_3$ receptors is part of the action of metoclopramide and led to the introduction of 5-HT$_3$ antagonists as a class of antiemetic.

Intravenous alkylating agents, doxorubicin and cisplatin typically produce nausea and vomiting 2–8 hours after injection, and the symptoms persist for 8–36 hours. Other drugs do not cause vomiting so frequently. After one or two cycles of chemotherapy some patients suffer from anticipatory nausea and vomiting at the sight of the nurse, doctor, intravenous infusion or hospital or even on setting out on the journey to hospital. In these patients prophylactic antiemetic therapy must be given a considerable time before chemotherapy.

Several different types of drug can be used to prevent or treat vomiting (Table 6.3). None is satisfactory in all patients and most are only partially effective. Antiemetic therapy should be started prophylactically, and often a satisfactory regimen can be established in each individual patient by trial and error.

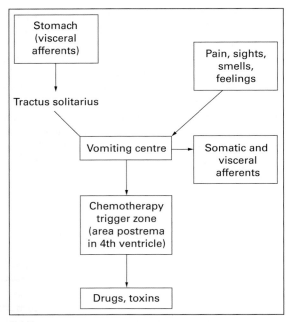

Figure 6.12 A simplified scheme of events in chemotherapy-induced vomiting. The site of action of antiemetics is not shown since the details are not clearly established. 5-Hydroxytryptamine (5-HT)$_3$ receptors are assumed to play a role in the central and peripheral mechanisms. Chemotherapy may damage cells of the intestinal lumen, liberating 5-HT from enterochromaffin cells.

5-HT$_3$ antagonists

This class of compound represented a major step forward in the control of vomiting. Control of cisplatin-induced emesis is achieved in 60% of patients, similar to optimum results obtained with combinations of metoclopramide and dexamethasone. Ondansetron, tropisetron and granisetron are selective 5-HT3 antagonists. The main site of action (central or peripheral) is still unclear. Ondansetron has good oral bioavailability. All are safe and well tolerated. The terminal plasma half-life of ondansetron is approximately 3 hours. Side-effects include headache, flushing and constipation. Hepatic dysfunction decreases metabolism.

Piperazine phenothiazines

These include prochlorperazine and perphenazine. They are effective antiemetics in some patients but must be used near the maximum dose, at which point extrapyramidal reactions are common, particularly with intravenous administration.

Aliphatic phenothiazines

The most commonly used agents are chlorpromazine and promazine. They have more sedative and less antiemetic properties and are more liable to produce hypotension.

Metoclopramide

This drug appears to act on the trigger area, possibly through blocking dopamine receptors. It increases gastric emptying. The drug can be given intramuscularly or intravenously and may cause extrapyramidal side-effects, restlessness and diarrhoea.

Metoclopramide is often used in high dose in the prevention of vomiting. It is probable that it is more effective at high dose, and some studies have shown that it is more effective than phenothiazines and may act as a 5-HT$_3$ receptor antagonist. The incidence of extrapyramidal side-effects does not appear to be greater in high dose. Randomized trials have shown high-dose metoclopramide to be superior to phenothiazines.

Benzodiazepines

Although these drugs have no antiemetic properties, they may make the vomiting more tolerable by inducing a somnolent state in which the patient cannot remember the period of nausea clearly. Intravenous lorazepam is useful for this purpose.

Butyrophenone derivatives

These drugs are dopamine receptor blocking agents that work centrally. Haloperidol is the most widely used and is partially effective against cisplatin-induced vomiting.

Aprepitant

Antagonists of substance P neurokinin (NK)1 receptors in the CNS have marked antiemetic properties. Aprepitant is the first of these antagonists to be introduced into clinical practice. It has good oral bioavailability, with a peak plasma concentration at 4 hours. It is metabolized in the liver but dose adjustment is not needed for mild hepatic dysfunction. In randomized trials it has been shown to add to the control of nausea and vomiting when given with a standard regimen of dexamethasone and ondansetron. An important feature is that the antiemetic effect is exerted for 4 days, resulting in better control of both acute and delayed nausea and vomiting. Aprepitant has important interactions with other drugs that are detoxified by the hepatic cytochrome system, such as anticonvulsants, many antibiotics and antifungal agents. The metabolism of warfarin is accelerated.

Table 6.3 Antiemetic agents.

Agent	Dose	Action	Toxicity
Ondansetron	0.15 mg/kg every 4 hours	5-HT$_3$ antagonist	Constipation, headache
Granisetron	3 mg i.v. over 5–10 min	5-HT$_3$ antagonist	Constipation, headache
Metoclopramide	10 mg p.o. or i.v. or 1–2 mg/kg i.v. repeated every 3 hours	Dopamine and 5-HT$_3$ antagonist (central and peripheral)	Extrapyramidal symptoms, diarrhoea
Dexamethasone	8–16 mg i.v. before treatment	Unclear	Restlessness, mood changes
Benzodiazepines (e.g. lorazepam)	1–2 mg p.o. or i.v. every 4–6 hours	Cerebral cortex, ?histamine receptor blocking agent	Sedation, hypotension, hallucinations, dysphoria, dizziness, ataxia
Phenothiazines (e.g. prochlorperazine)	12.5 mg i.m. or 25 mg suppository	Dopamine antagonist	Extrapyramidal symptoms, drowsiness
Butyrophenones (e.g. haloperidol)	0.5–1 mg p.o. or i.v. repeated every 4–8 hours	Dopamine antagonist	Extrapyramidal symptoms, akathisia
Aprepitant		Neurokinin antagonist	Drug interactions

i.m., intramuscularly; i.v., intravenously; p.o., by mouth.

Long-term complications of cancer chemotherapy

More children and young adults are now surviving diseases such as acute leukaemia, lymphoma and testicular cancer that were formerly incurable. Survival has been achieved by intensive combination chemotherapy. It has become apparent that chemotherapy of this type is associated with long-term complications in some patients. The recognition of these sequelae has emphasized that treatment of great intensity must be justified by a clear benefit in survival and that such drug and radiation therapies must be restricted to those categories of patient in which they are essential for survival. Long-term follow-up of patients is essential since some of the complications may develop many years after treatment is discontinued.

Impaired gonadal function

The prevention of infertility in cancer patient and its management are critical [18]. Suppression of spermatogenesis occurs in the majority of men being treated with combination chemotherapy. Procarbazine and alkylating agents seem to have the greatest adverse effect, methotrexate and doxorubicin less so. The degree of infertility and its permanence vary with different regimens. With MOPP therapy (mustine, vincristine, prednisone and procarbazine) for Hodgkin's disease (see Chapter 25), 95% of men will have long-lasting infertility. This is less with the regimen containing doxorubicin, bleomycin, vinblastine and dacarbazine, and with the cisplatin, vinblastine and bleomycin regimen for teratoma

there is frequent recovery of fertility. Damage to the germinal epithelium is associated with a rise in serum follicle-stimulating hormone (FSH), which normally stimulates spermatogenesis. While prepubertal boys do not appear to experience long-lasting endocrine changes from chemotherapy, intensive chemotherapy during puberty damages Leydig cells and is accompanied by a rise in both FSH and luteinizing hormone (LH), low testosterone levels and gynaecomastia.

The likely effects of chemotherapy must be discussed with all peripubertal and postpubertal males. Sperm-storage facilities must be available for all such patients. Three semen samples should be collected over a week before treatment. This can be reduced to two if treatment is urgent. It is essential that the likely outcome of the storage procedure is discussed in full. The samples should be kept, with the documentation, for at least 10 years together with instructions about destruction of the samples in the event of death. Successful pregnancy by artificial insemination is still infrequent using stored samples. When the quality and number are low, the technique of intracytoplasmic sperm injection is increasingly being used with success.

Ovarian failure is often produced by combination chemotherapy and is more frequent the nearer the patient is to her natural menopause [19]. Even if menstruation does not cease, subfertility is common and the duration of the reproductive years of life is shortened, with earlier menopause. Temporary oligomenorrhoea is common with the onset of chemotherapy. The onset

Table 6.4 Pulmonary and hepatic toxicity of cytotoxic drugs.

Drug	Effect
Pulmonary	
Busulfan and nitrosoureas (and other alkylating agents)	Fibrosis
Bleomycin	Pulmonary infiltrates and fibrosis
Mitomycin C	
Hepatic	
Methotrexate	Fibrosis
6-Mercaptopurine and azathioprine	Cholestatic jaundice and necrosis
Asparaginase	Fatty infiltration

of the true menopause can be determined by a rise in FSH that is not suppressed by hormone-replacement therapy (HRT). HRT should be offered to all women with a premature menopause induced by chemotherapy. Effective methods of cryopreserving oocytes are under investigation.

Pulmonary fibrosis

Pulmonary damage is produced by several cytotoxic drugs (Table 6.4). Most alkylating agents will produce pulmonary fibrosis with long-term impairment of diffusing capacity. However, busulfan is more likely to do so than other drugs. Bleomycin causes pulmonary infiltrates, a phenomenon related to total dose and which is very common over 300 mg/m². These infiltrates may diminish when the drug is stopped but permanent fibrosis often follows.

Liver disease

Many drugs cause a transient rise in plasma enzymes (nitrosoureas, methotrexate, cytosine arabinoside) but permanent hepatic dysfunction is rare. Permanent liver damage can occasionally occur with antimetabolites (Table 6.4). Prolonged administration of cytotoxic drugs may result in steatosis (fatty liver) and this can impact on planned surgical procedures such as liver resection following neo-adjuvant treatment with oxaliplatin and 5-FU.

Second cancers after chemotherapy

Second malignancies have been noted after long-term administration of alkylating agents, particularly melphalan and chlorambucil, typically given to patients with ovarian cancer and myeloma. In both cases there is an increased risk of AML. Almost all alkylating agents are leukaemogenic, and a specific form of AML associated with an 11q23 translocation has been described with etoposide.

Studies have clearly demonstrated the increased risk of leukaemia in Hodgkin's disease and ovarian cancer. In Hodgkin's disease the relative risk is higher in young patients but is greatly outweighed by the survival advantage of treatment. In ovarian cancer the survival benefit of chemotherapy is less marked. Chemotherapy-induced leukaemia is associated with non-random chromosomal deletions (e.g. on chromosomes 5 and 7), and the leukaemia tends to be refractory to treatment. Bladder cancer is a reported complication of cyclophosphamide therapy but the risk appears to be very small.

Long-term immunosuppressive therapy in renal allograft recipients (and the immune suppression in AIDS) also predisposes to the development of cancer. Lymphomas are the commonest malignancy, particularly large-cell lymphoma of the brain. The average time of onset is 2 years but the risk persists indefinitely.

Postulated mechanisms are a direct carcinogenic effect of the drugs, diminished immune surveillance, and activation of oncogenic viruses in immunosuppressed individuals. In radiation-induced cancers of bone there appears to be an added risk if chemotherapy has been used as well.

Principles of hormone therapy

The demonstration by Beatson in 1896 that inoperable breast cancer sometimes regressed after oophorectomy was one of the most remarkable discoveries in the history of cancer treatment. Many years later, Huggins demonstrated that metastatic prostatic cancer would regress with orchidectomy or the administration of oestrogens. In recent years, there has been a transformation in our understanding. In at least one tumour, breast cancer, knowledge of the hormone receptor status of the tumour has become important in guiding treatment decisions.

Steroid hormone receptors

There are receptor proteins for steroid hormones in the cytoplasm, the nucleus and the cell membrane. Interaction between the hormone and its receptor modifies DNA activity and hence cell growth and replication. These events are depicted diagrammatically in Figure 6.13.

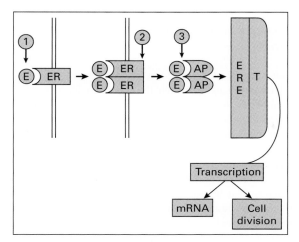

Figure 6.13 Oestrogen (E) binds to the oestrogen receptor (ER) which dimerizes. The complex becomes active (AP) and binds to oestrogen-response elements (ERE) in the nucleus. Other proteins (T) involved in transcription, such as RNA polymerase II, are activated leading to protein synthesis and cell division. Goserelin lowers plasma oestrogen (1); fulvestrant prevents receptor dimerization and activation (2); tamoxifen binds to the active complex, inactivating its role in initiating transcription (3).

The steroid hormone, unbound to plasma protein, crosses the cell membrane by a mechanism which is not well understood. The hormone then links to the cytoplasmic receptor protein and the complex undergoes a conformational change in either the cytoplasm or the nucleus. This hormone–receptor complex binds to a nuclear protein which in turn exerts a controlling activity on DNA. There then follows an increase in RNA polymerase activity that results in the synthesis, first of mRNA, and then of cytoplasmic protein. After 24 hours DNA synthesis occurs, followed by cell division.

This model appears to be generally applicable to a variety of steroid hormones. The synthesis of the receptor proteins is promoted by the hormone to which they bind. Other hormones can reduce the synthesis of receptor proteins, for example, progesterone inhibits the synthesis of ER.

Using these concepts of hormone action, several strategies for modifying tumour growth can be developed.
• The plasma concentration of the stimulating hormone might be lowered by ablative therapy, either surgical, radiotherapeutic or chemical.
• Once the hormone has entered the cell it may be prevented from binding to the receptor by either competitive inhibitors or reduction of receptor synthesis.

• It might also be possible to block the binding of the complex to the nuclear 'acceptor' protein.

In practice it is often difficult to determine the site of action of agents used in hormone therapy. Tamoxifen, for example, appears to bind to the ER but may also affect its synthesis, and the tamoxifen–receptor complex may also block the acceptor site in the nucleus.

Hormone receptor assays

Attempts to use the presence of a hormone receptor to predict the responsiveness of an individual tumour to hormone manipulation have been partially successful. The usual assay is a measure of uptake of isotopically labelled hormone by homogenized tumour cells. The degree of binding varies, and an arbitrary cut-off point is made in what is in fact a gradation from negative to positive. In studies on tissue sections it can be shown that in breast cancer some cells are ER-positive and others ER-negative. The overall expression of ER status is thus an oversimplification of the position. Furthermore, the presence of hormone receptors does not prove that they are functionally active. Oestrogen promotes the synthesis of progesterone receptor (PR) in breast cancer cells, and measurement of PR may thus provide a better measure of functionally active ER than measurement of ER itself. At present it is clear that in breast cancer, for example, the absence (or very low values) of ER strongly predicts a lack of response to hormone manipulation, and that high levels of receptor are indicative of probable response. Intermediate values are associated with a variable response rate.

The role of hormone therapy in individual tumours is discussed in detail in the appropriate chapters.

Approaches to hormone therapy
Lowering the plasma hormone concentration
This may be done by medical or surgical means.

Medical
In premenopausal women, the main source of oestrogens is the ovary, but some oestrogens are formed as a result of the peripheral conversion of androgens, formed in the adrenal. This conversion takes place in muscle, liver and fat, and is mediated by aromatase enzymes. After the menopause the adrenal becomes the main source of oestrogens by production of androgen (Δ^4-androstenedione), which is converted in the peripheral tissues. However, the adrenal is not the only source of oestrogen precursors, and breast tissue itself can synthesize oestrogens. Aromatase inhibitors

block the action of aromatase enzymes and also depress synthesis of androgens and cortisol in the adrenal itself. In premenopausal women the major source of oestrogen synthesis is the ovary, which is not dependent on aromatase enzymes. Inhibition of aromatase prevents the conversion of androgens to oestrogen, the only source of the hormone in postmenopausal women. The new aromatase inhibitors have greatly increased effectiveness and tolerability than the precursors such as aminoglutethimide. Anastrozole (Arimidex) suppresses plasma oestrogen to almost undetectable levels, without affecting the cortisol response to adrenocorticotrophic hormone (ACTH). Eventually it may replace tamoxifen as the hormone treatment of choice in postmenopausal women with breast cancer (see Chapter 13).

Luteinizing hormone releasing hormone (LHRH) is a decapeptide released from the hypothalamus to act on the pituitary (Figure 6.14). Analogues of LHRH such as goserelin and leuprorelin cause initial pituitary stimulation, followed by inhibition of gonadotrophin release that causes a profound fall in plasma testosterone in men and in circulating oestradiol in women. Goserelin (Zoladex) may prove to be the treatment of choice in producing ovarian ablation in premenopausal women with breast cancer. Goserelin is given by subcutaneous injection once a month. If combined with an antiandrogen such

as flutamide (see below), more profound suppression of androgen effect is achieved, which may have some extra benefit in prostate cancer.

Blocking the action of circulating hormones
Antioestrogens, of which the most notable example is tamoxifen, have been a major advance in the treatment of metastatic breast cancer. The action of tamoxifen is not fully understood. The drug appears to exert its effect by binding with the cytoplasmic ER, but its affinity for the ER is much less than that of oestrogen itself. Possibly the drug–receptor complex undergoes a conformational change that blocks its entry to nuclear sites of activity. Other receptor sites which bind tamoxifen but not oestrogen have also been described; however, the balance of evidence at present suggests that tamoxifen exerts its effect by competitively binding with ER, thus displacing oestradiol. Tamoxifen does not increase plasma oestradiol levels in postmenopausal women but does do so in premenopausal women. Tamoxifen has a prolonged terminal half-life in plasma and after 1 month of treatment the plasma concentration exceeds that of oestradiol by as much as 1000-fold. It is for this reason that a dose–response effect is not usually observed clinically. Toxic effects are uncommon, the most frequent being mild nausea and hot flushes. Occasionally, a flare-up of the breast cancer may be seen which is then sometimes followed by a response. The long-term use of tamoxifen is associated with a small increase in uterine cancer, and a possibly beneficial alteration in plasma lipid concentrations.

The mechanism of acquired resistance to tamoxifen is unclear since the cancer cells still contain ER. It is possible that the cell's dependence on oestrogen is bypassed by other mechanisms such as growth factor stimulation.

A new class of antioestrogens binds to the ER and inactivates it. The lead molecule in this class of drugs is fulvestrant. The drug binds to the receptor but impairs the dimerization necessary for the active form of the receptor to be formed (see Figure 6.13). The drug–receptor complex is degraded and ER-mediated gene transcription is prevented.

Megestrol acetate is a synthetic antiandrogen. It blocks the synthesis of testosterone, reducing plasma testosterone levels. Adrenal androgens (androstenedione) are also reduced. The drug also blocks the action of testosterone on prostatic carcinoma cells, and this is a further mechanism for its action in the disease. Cyproterone acetate and flutamide have an antiandrogenic effect that may be valuable in prostatic cancer. Flutamide does not inhibit pituitary LH release and blocks the negative

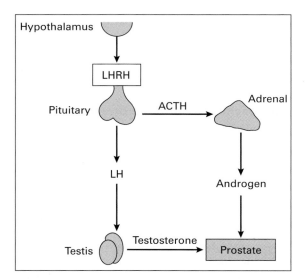

Figure 6.14 Luteinizing hormone releasing hormone (LHRH) analogues at first stimulate and then suppress luteinizing hormone (LH) release, resulting in a fall in testosterone release from the testis. This results in regression in hormone-dependent prostate cancer. ACTH, adrenocorticotrophic hormone.

feedback which testosterone produces, resulting in a rise in serum testosterone. Flutamide has no progestogen activity.

Recent studies indicate the therapeutic potential for increased blockade of the androgen axis in producing improved responses in advanced prostate cancer. Ablation of gonadal androgen production does not interfere with the remaining 20% produced intratumorally and in peripheral tissues. Abiraterone acetate, a specific inhibitor of CYP17 that is key to androgen and oestrogen synthesis, improves progression-free survival and decline of symptoms in metastatic castration-resistant prostate cancer indicating the importance of maximal inhibition of this pathway [20].

Surgical

Oophorectomy (surgical or radiotherapeutic) will abolish oestrogen secretion by the ovary in premenopausal women and was widely used as a first step in hormone treatment of advanced breast cancer. Knowledge of the ER status is useful because the likelihood of response in ER-positive tumours is 50% compared with only 5% in ER-negative tumours, in which the procedure may not be worthwhile.

Adrenalectomy sometimes produces further responses in premenopausal patients with advanced breast cancer responding to oophorectomy. This is probably due to residual sex hormone synthesis by the adrenal. Tumour response occurs despite adequate glucocorticoid replacement. Hypophysectomy produces a similar effect. Both of these operations have been rendered almost obsolete since the advent of aromatase inhibitors (see below). Orchidectomy is effective in reducing plasma testosterone levels and has been widely used as treatment for metastatic prostatic carcinoma.

Additive hormone therapies

In breast cancer these include oestrogens, androgens, glucocorticoids and progestogens. ER-positive breast cancers will sometimes regress with exogenous oestrogen, which indicates that we still have gaps in our knowledge of the mechanism of action of hormone therapies. Medroxyprogesterone acetate and megestrol acetate produce responses in about 20% of patients. They possibly do this by lowering the cytoplasmic ER content and responses are usually only seen in ER-positive tumours but appear independent of PR status. Progesterone derivatives produce responses in about 30% of uterine carcinomas, usually in cases which are ER-positive or PR-positive.

Cytokines in cancer treatment

Cytokines are a group of proteins, some of which regulate the growth of cells while others modulate the immune response and inflammation. They are usually glycosylated and of low molecular weight. They are produced by cells of various types and usually act over short distances (as autocrine or paracrine stimuli). In cancer therapy they may regulate tumour cell growth, be directly cytotoxic, excite an inflammatory or immune response in the tumour, or speed normal tissue recovery from the effect of cytotoxic drugs. Cytokine treatment has an established role in only one or two, rather uncommon, tumours.

Interferons

Three classes of interferon (IFN) have been assessed in cancer therapy, IFN-α, IFN-β and IFN-γ. Their antitumour activity is complex. They may have a direct antiproliferative effect on normal and neoplastic cells, they induce differentiation in some leukaemic cell lines, and they enhance the cytotoxicity of T, natural killer and lymphokine-activated killer (LAK) cells (see below). Expression of major histocompatibility class I and II is increased on tumour cells.

The clinical activity of IFNs is summarized. Side-effects include an influenza-like illness with rigours, headache, muscle pains and fever; leucopenia may occur. These symptoms are dose-related. Neutralizing antibodies may develop.

Interleukins

Interleukins are a family of peptides that act as modulators of immune and inflammatory responses. Interleukin (IL)-2 has received most clinical attention.

Interleukin-2

This is a glycoprotein (molecular weight 15) produced by activated T cells. It binds to a cell-surface receptor on T cells. This receptor has two subunits, each of which can bind IL-2 with low affinity but together bind with high affinity. IL-2 stimulates production of IFN-Iγ, and tumour necrosis factor (see below) and activates cytotoxic lymphocytes. These kill cells without the need for antigen recognition or histocompatibility specificity.

As a single agent, IL-2 produces responses in 15–30% of patients with metastatic renal carcinoma and melanoma. Some of these responses are very durable. Continuous infusion may have some advantages over bolus injection (continuous activation, fewer side-effects). The combination of LAK cells (where the patient's own lymphocytes are activated and expanded *in vitro* and then returned to the patient) and IL-2 may produce more complete responses, but overall response rates are similar. The side-effects of IL-2 are considerable: fever, lethargy, hypotension, adult respiratory distress syndrome, nausea, vomiting, anaemia, neutropenia, disorientation and somnolence. These effects are dose-related.

Interleukin-6

This cytokine is produced in the bone marrow and by human osteoblasts. It appears to act as a paracrine growth factor in myeloma and is overproduced in this disease. The reason for the overproduction is unclear. Its production is dependent on IL-1. IL-6 stimulates osteoclast activity and appears to stimulate platelet production.

Monoclonal antibodies in cancer therapy

After many years of development, monoclonal antibodies now have an established place in cancer treatment. The technical advances that have made this possible include:

• humanization of mouse antibodies, avoiding formation of anti-antibodies;
• development of high-affinity antibodies by techniques using bacterial phages;
• production of antibodies of varying size and affinity with different degrees of tissue penetration.

Antibodies may be altered to produce an antitumour effect by many means. The most commonly employed techniques are shown in Figure 6.15 and are described in the accompanying legend. For each of these approaches there are limitations and possibilities.

1 Direct killing by complement or by antibody-dependent cell cytotoxicity. In this approach the Fc portion of the antibody must bind to the Fc receptor (FcRI and FcRII) on the effector cell and avoid binding to FcRIII which is inhibitory. This mechanism of cell killing is the mode of action of trastuzumab, which binds to the ErbB2 receptor in breast cancer, and rituximab, an anti-CD20 monoclonal antibody used to treat B-cell lymphoma.

2 Monoclonal antibody carrying a toxin or radioactivity or an activating enzyme. One example is gemtuzumab, which comprises humanized anti-CD33 conjugated to the DNA minor-groove binding agent calicheamicin. CD33 is expressed on AML blasts. Gemtuzumab induces remission in drug-resistant relapse. The approach using toxins such as ricin coupled to monoclonal antibodies

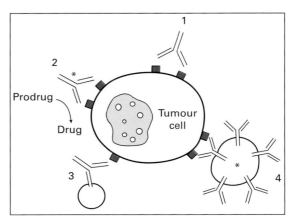

Figure 6.15 Methods of tumour killing by monoclonal antibodies. 1 The monoclonal antibody binds to the tumour antigen and results in cell killing by direct complement-mediated cell killing or via antibody-dependent cell killing by macrophages. 2 The monoclonal antibody carries radioactivity, or a toxin or a cytokine that mediates the tumour cell killing, or the monoclonal antibody may carry an enzyme that converts a prodrug to an active drug. 3 The monoclonal antibody is bispecific: one binding site attaches to tumour, the other to an antitumour effector cell. 4 The monoclonal antibody may be attached to a liposome that contains drugs or toxins.

has not proved practicable due to unacceptable vascular toxicity. Coupled radioisotopes such as yttrium-90 (^{90}Y) or iodine-131 (^{131}I) are attractive strategies because of the possibility of bystander killing. ^{90}Y-labelled anti-CD20 and ^{131}I-labelled anti-CEA (carcinoembryonic antigen) are in clinical trial. The HER2-directed antibody-drug conjugate Trastuzumab emtansine (T-DM1) consisting of the anti-microtubule agent DM1, linked to the HER2-specific monoclonal antibody trastuzumab has shown efficacy (T-DM1) in advanced breast cancer [21]. This is a novel strategy for breast cancer which combines delivery of chemotherapy to tumour, blockade of HER2 pathway and activation of antibody-dependent cellular cytotoxicity (ADCC). The role of this agent in earlier stages of the disease and in the neoadjuvant setting is under investigation.

3 The approach using bispecific antibodies is still in the early phase of development. Attachment to effector T cells has led to extensive toxic cytokine release, limiting the use.

4 Immunoliposomes are an effective means of increasing delivery of a toxin or radioactivity, but are difficult to produce. They have considerable promise in approaches where the target is the tumour vasculature.

Gene therapy

The possibility of changing the genetic structure of cancer cells to kill the tumour, or change its growth rate, has become more of a reality now that so much is known about the genetic changes that accompany malignant transformation. To exert its effect, the gene must gain access to the cell. The delivery is via a *vector*. This may be a virus that is defective in replication and into which the gene has been inserted, usually with a promoter that becomes active in the cell. An alternative strategy is to package the gene in a liposome. It is possible to use viruses that replicate selectively in cancer cells. Such selectivity may be based on the necessity for cell division for the gene to be active, or on the absence of an active *p53* or *RB* (retinoblastoma) gene. A related approach is to use a replication-deficient virus that will divide only if a normal tissue gene promoter is expressed, for example, the promoter for prostate-specific antigen in prostate cancer.

Gene therapy for cancer may have one of several aims.
1 To restore function of a defective tumour-suppressor gene. The restoration of function of a defective suppressor gene such as *p53* or *APC* (adenomatous polyposis coli) has been shown to inhibit tumour cell growth in model systems. This is perhaps a surprising result in view of the multiplicity of genetic defects in cancer cells.
2 To block the action of a mutated or overexpressed oncogene. Viral gene vectors have been used to insert factors (oligonucleotides or ribozymes) that block the action of dominant oncogenes and thereby inhibit tumour growth. However, the most successful method has been the use of small molecules (i.e. drugs) that block oncogene action (e.g. imatinib).
3 To insert a gene that can activate a prodrug or produce other cell-killing effects. The advantage of the approach using genes that convert an inert prodrug into an active drug is that the active agent can kill cancer cells near the cell into which the gene has penetrated, the so-called *bystander effect*. A bystander effect on the vascular system occurs when antiangiogenesis genes are inserted into tumour cells.
4 To modify susceptibility to immune attack. Vectors may be used that increase the expression of antigens that increase susceptibility to cellular cytotoxicity.

Immunotherapy

There has been a revolution in the field of immunotherapy over the past few years [22]. This has now become a major area of development in oncology with novel and effective therapies in melanoma and NSCLC as well as other malignancies. There are several excellent recent reviews on this rapidly changing field. Specifically progress has been dramatic in the area of immunological checkpoint inhibition [22]. Checkpoint inhibitors modulate T cell regulation, which may act to inhibit the immune response to cancer. The antibody Ipilimumab binds and blocks inhibitory signalling mediated by the T cell surface co-inhibitory molecule cytotoxic T lymphocyte antigen 4 (CTLA-4). When the function of CTLA-4 is inhibited, there is activation of the immune antitumour response. A pivotal study in 2010 demonstrated improved survival for Ipilimumab in advanced melanoma and this was the first drug of this class to be approved by the FDA.

Second generation antibodies under development target programmed cell death protein 1 (PD-1) and programmed cell death 1 ligand 1 (PD-L1), which regulate T cell activation in peripheral tissues and allow escape from immune surveillance. The first antibody of this class nivolumab, a fully human IgG4 blocking monoclonal antibody against PD-1 showed objective responses in 16–30% of diverse tumour types, many of which were of long duration (over one year). In contrast to conventional agents, responses to these agents are often delayed pending the development of an anticancer immune response.

References

1 DeVita VT Jr., Chu E. A history of cancer chemotherapy. *Cancer Res* 2008; 68: 8643–53.
2 Wang L, McLeod HL, Weinshilboum RM. Genomics and drug response. *N Engl J Med* 2011; 364(12): 1144–53.
3 Rohwer N, Cramer T. Hypoxia-mediated drug resistance: novel insights on the functional interaction of HIFs and cell death pathways. *Drug Resist Updat* 2011; 14(3): 191–201.
4 Pluchino KM, Hall MD, Goldsborough AS, Callaghan R, Gottesman MM. Collateral sensitivity as a strategy against cancer multidrug resistance. *Drug Resist Updat* 2012; 15: 98–105.
5 Rabik CA, Dolan ME. Molecular mechanisms of resistance and toxicity associated with platinating agents. *Cancer Treat Rev* 2007; 33(1): 9–23.
6 Press MF, Sauter G, Buyse M *et al.* Alteration of topoisomerase II-alpha gene in human breast cancer: association with responsiveness to anthracycline-based chemotherapy. *J Clin Oncol* 2011; 29:859–67.
7 Lord CJ, Ashworth A. The DNA damage response and cancer therapy. *Nature* 2012; 481(7381): 287–94.
8 Hegi ME, Diserens AC, Gorlia T *et al.* MGMT gene silencing and benefit from temozolomide in glioblastoma. *N Engl J Med* 2005; 352(10): 997–1003.

9 Lønning PE, Knappskog S. Mapping genetic alterations causing chemoresistance in cancer: identifying the roads by tracking the drivers. *Oncogene* 2013; 32: 5315–30.

10 Ong FS, Das K, Wang J *et al.* Personalized medicine and pharmacogenetic biomarkers: progress in molecular oncology testing. *Expert Rev Mol Diagn* 2012; 12: 593–602.

11 Heinemann V, Douillard JY, Ducreux M, Peeters M. Targeted therapy in metastatic colorectal cancer – an example of personalized medicine in action. *Cancer Treat Rev* 2013; 39: 592–601.

12 Bonner JA, Harari PM, Giralt J *et al.* Radiotherapy plus cetuximab for squamous-cell carcinoma of the head and neck. *N Engl J Med* 2006; 354: 567–78.

13 Lynch TJ, Bell DW, Sordella R *et al.* Activating mutations in the epidermal growth factor receptor underlying responsiveness of non-small-cell lung cancer to gefitinib. *N Engl J Med* 2004; 350: 2129–39.

14 Shaw AT, Kim DW, Nakagawa K *et al.*Crizotinib versus chemotherapy in advanced ALK-positive lung cancer. *N Engl J Med* 2013; 368: 2385–94.

15 Sosman JA, Kim KB, Schuchter L *et al.* Survival in BRAF V600-mutant advanced melanoma treated with vemurafenib. *N Engl J Med* 2012; 366: 707–14.

16 Farmer H, McCabe N, Lord CJ *et al.* Targeting the DNA repair defect in BRCA mutant cells as a therapeutic strategy. *Nature* 2005; 434: 917–21.

17 Brough R, Frankum JR, Costa-Cabral S, Lord CJ, Ashworth A. Searching for synthetic lethality in cancer. *Curr Opin Genet Dev* 2011; 21: 34–41.

18 Loren AW, Mangu PB, Beck LN *et al.* Fertility preservation for patients with cancer: American Society of Clinical Oncology clinical practice guideline update. *J Clin Oncol* 2013; 31: 2500–10.

19 Blumenfeld Z. Chemotherapy and fertility. *Best Pract Res Clin Obstet Gynaecol* 2012; 26: 379–90.

20 Ryan CJ, Smith MR, de Bono JS *et al.* Abiraterone in metastatic prostate cancer without previous chemotherapy. *N Engl J Med* 2013; 368: 138–48.

21 Verma S, Miles D, Gianni L *et al.* Trastuzumab emtansine for HER2-positive advanced breast cancer. *N Engl J Med* 2012; 367: 1783–91.

22 Page DB, Postow MA, Callahan MK, Allison JP, Wolchok JD. Immune modulation in cancer with antibodies. *Annu Rev Med* 2014; 65: 185–202.

7 Supportive care and symptom relief

Talking about the diagnosis and treatment

Major disease brings anxiety and worry, but few diseases are associated with such dread as cancer, with its imagined inevitable sequel of certain death, pain, lingering and suffering. One of the most difficult and rewarding tasks for the physician is to set the disease in its right context, to explain the treatment, to give enough information at the correct rate and time, to sustain hope, and to be accessible, supportive, competent, open-minded and, above all, kind.

The patient has a life outside the consulting room. He or she will interpret what is said in the light of his or her own experience and apprehensions. Cancer is commonest in the elderly. In the course of a long life, many patients will have had friends or relatives who have died of the disease. They may perhaps have cared for a member of the family with cancer. These experiences will have an important influence on a patient's expectations. Cancer and its treatment are widely discussed in the media. Although patients are better informed now, their knowledge is often fragmentary and disorganized. Some patients may have recognized the seriousness of a symptom – haemoptysis, unexplained weight loss, a lump or backache – but be too anxious (or too afraid of surgery) to voice their suspicions. Other patients may have no idea of the possible diagnosis.

As with patients, the attitude of physicians is influenced by their experience and training. Frequently, the first diagnosis of cancer is made by a specialist in another area such as general surgery, gynaecology or chest medicine. Some of these doctors may themselves have a very pessimistic view of cancer and what can be achieved by treatment. Furthermore, the specialist has often had little opportunity to get to know the patient before the diagnosis has been made. A lack of familiarity, both with what can be achieved by treatment and with the patient, combined sometimes with fear of the disease, may lead the physician or surgeon into euphemisms and half-truths. Words such as 'growth' or 'ulcer' may be used to soften or obscure the diagnosis, while the doctor often betrays his or her real meaning by appearing evasive or unclear.

This attitude means that unless the patient is bold and asks for a more frank statement of the diagnosis, the doctor may be unable to assess what impact his or her words have had. Because the meaning of the diagnosis is being avoided, it becomes difficult to allow the patient to

Cancer and its Management, Seventh Edition. Jeffrey Tobias and Daniel Hochhauser.
© 2015 John Wiley & Sons, Ltd. Published 2015 by John Wiley & Sons, Ltd.

express his or her fears or ask the appropriate questions. The patient may in fact be under the impression that the diagnosis is worse than it actually is: that he or she has only a short time to live or that treatment will be to no avail. The doctor's evasions may then strengthen this opinion. An ill-informed patient may learn of the diagnosis by other means – from a pathology request form, a hospital porter, a well-meaning friend or an overheard remark. If the diagnosis is discovered accidentally, the patient may realize that the intention behind concealment was to spare him or her anxiety, but may feel let down by the doctor and be cautious in accepting any further reassurance.

The attitude of cancer specialists has now moved towards a fuller discussion of the diagnosis and treatment. However, what is said to the patient must be well judged and carefully delivered. All physicians make errors of judgement which shake their confidence with the next patient they see, but it is essential not to retreat from these discussions when difficulties have occurred. It is important to learn from one's mistakes.

If possible, it is useful to assess the attitude of the patient before the diagnosis is made. Questions such as 'What do you feel is wrong with you?' or 'Have you any particular anxieties about what might be wrong?' are often very revealing since the patient will sometimes admit, for example, to a fear of malignancy. Such information allows the physician to ask the patient whether, if this proves to be the diagnosis, he or she would want to know the details of what is found.

Nowadays it is usual to make the diagnosis before major surgery is undertaken: by bronchoscopy for lung cancer, needle biopsy in breast cancer or endoscopy for gastrointestinal disease. When the diagnosis has been established preoperatively and treatment by surgery is necessary, it is hardly possible, still less desirable, that the diagnosis is not discussed and the probable operative procedure described. Sometimes the diagnosis only becomes apparent after an operation and the patient will be waiting to hear what has been found. In either case, when talking to patients about their diagnosis, doctors need to have a clear idea of what they are going to say and the words they will use, although they must be prepared to modify their approach if the situation demands it.

In explaining the diagnosis, the word 'cancer' is the only word that unequivocally conveys the nature of the complaint. Many physicians use the words 'malignancy', 'tumour' or 'growth' with the best of intentions, but this carries the risk that the patient will fail to realize the true nature of the disease (indeed, this is often what is

intended). It is true that in an elderly or very anxious patient, the word 'cancer' may be very frightening and there are some patients for whom other terms may be necessary. Many patients have only a vague idea of what cancer means and are surprised that the disease is nearly always treatable and often curable. The explanation of the diagnosis must be combined with a realistic but hopeful account of what can be done. Few patients can exist without hope of any kind. This does not mean that a cure is promised but patients must feel confident that every attempt will be made to cure them and know that there is a possibility of success, if that is the case. If a cure is likely, this must be stressed and a much more optimistic account of the disease can be given. Even when the prognosis is poor, the doctor must show how treatment may help to achieve a reasonable period of healthy and enjoyable life.

The manner in which the explanation is given is all-important. The doctor should be unhurried, speak clearly and not technically, look at the patient's face while speaking, show that he or she is not frightened or discomfited by the diagnosis, and indicate by look and gesture that he or she is competent and prepared to discuss the problem calmly. There is a limit to the number of facts which a patient can assimilate during one conversation, particularly under stressful circumstances. Too much information may progressively extinguish the understanding which a short account would achieve. Frequently, the patient may seem to understand, but in fact be too anxious to take in anything of what is being said. This failure of understanding is not 'denial' but is due to confusion and anxiety. It is a good policy to stop frequently and enquire if what is being said is clear or if there are questions that the patient wants to ask. When the patient is able to ask questions it implies that he or she has understood at least part of the explanation. Simple drawings often clarify the site of the illness or what radiotherapy or surgery is attempting to achieve. The doctor should make it quite clear that members of the team will always be pleased to answer questions and that there will be an opportunity to talk again in a day or two. One discussion is seldom enough. It may take a few days for the patient to start to understand and to take a realistic view of the situation, and at that stage want to know more. It is usually advisable, therefore, to impart the details of the diagnosis and treatment over a period of time. The facts of the diagnosis are given first with a brief outline of treatment, gradually giving more information as the patient begins to come to terms with his or her position.

Some physicians ask relatives for advice on how much to tell the patient, particularly when they are in doubt about the correct approach. This can be helpful, but there is a risk that the relatives may misjudge the patient and, out of love and sympathy, suggest that the truth be withheld or modified, when the patient would have wished otherwise. It is, of course, essential that relatives have a clear understanding of what has been said, and why, and that the medical team do not give contradictory accounts. For this reason, the doctor should explain to the rest of the medical and nursing team exactly what has been said, with an idea of the words that have been used and what the reaction has been. The same information should be conveyed to the relatives, but the discussion about prognosis may sometimes have to be more pessimistic with relatives than with the patient. It is unwise to give patients a prognosis measured in a finite time because they tend to remember the stated number of months or years, however, many qualifications are made. Such predictions are often incorrect.

The patient's reaction may be a mixture of acceptance, anxiety, anger and grief. It is essential to be understanding and not to be irritated by unjustified hostility if it occurs. This demands a lot from the doctor, who must have enough self-confidence and maturity to realize that, in the end, the patient will come to trust his or her honesty and support.

At a later stage the physician, while discussing the details of investigation and treatment, may wish to explain that an illness such as cancer will alter the patient's self-perception. That is, the patient will tend for a while to view himself or herself as 'ill', and minor aches and pains that would previously have been ignored may be magnified in the patient's mind and be interpreted as symptoms of relapse. In explaining that this is an understandable but usually temporary phase, the physician should make it clear that he or she will be seeing the patient regularly and, if symptoms occur which cause anxiety, the patient should get in touch. The best cancer departments operate an 'open-door' policy of this type, eliminating a lot of bureaucratic difficulty for the patient who may otherwise be given an appointment weeks ahead for a problem that is immediate. The ideal arrangement is where the hospital specialist works in close collaboration with the family doctor in providing support and reassurance. The family practitioner may have long and invaluable experience of the patient and his or her family.

Whenever a patient visits, either for a regular review or because of a symptom, the physician should give as much time to discussion as to the technical aspects of examination and investigation. It is greatly to be regretted that some doctors and most health administrators regard heavily booked clinics as a sign of efficiency. A five-minute consultation with a cancer patient is nearly always bad medicine.

Many cancer treatments have a bad reputation. Fear of being burned or scarred by radiotherapy is very common and a careful explanation of modern advances is sometimes needed. Alopecia, nausea and vomiting are unpleasant side-effects of chemotherapy. Patients have heard of these and, understandably, fear them. If chemotherapy is judged necessary, then the reasons should be explained. Patients will easily grasp the idea that cancer may not be localized and that a systemic treatment is being given to prevent or treat any recurrence from cancer cells which may have spread to other sites. Indeed, they often find the idea of a systemic as well as a local treatment reassuring. The ways in which the side-effects can be mitigated should be clearly explained.

Although patients will usually accept the need for radiotherapy or chemotherapy, they may find reality worse than they had imagined. This is particularly true for chemotherapy, which often goes on for many months. There can be few things more miserable than repeated, predictable episodes of severe nausea and vomiting. Patients may begin to feel that they cannot go through with treatment and then find themselves in a frightening dilemma. On the one hand, they are fearful of jeopardizing their chance of cure and of disappointing the doctor; but on the other, the side-effects may produce progressive demoralization. In the case of a potentially curative treatment, for example: Hodgkin's disease, testicular tumours or acute lymphoblastic leukaemia, the doctor must try to sustain the patient through the treatment and do all he or she can to see it completed. However, for many cancers of adult life the benefits of chemotherapy are much less clear. In these cases, the worst outcome is that a patient is made to feel wretched by the treatment and guilty at stopping treatment and is then frightened at the prospect that he or she has jeopardized the chance of survival. If relapse occurs there may be self-blame and depression. The responsibility for this situation is as much the doctor's as the patient's. When chemotherapy is being given without a reasonable prospect of cure and the patient cannot continue, the physician should be sympathetic and reassuring, and explain that he or she does not feel let down by the patient and that the prognosis has not been materially worsened.

There are few other branches of medicine that demand simultaneously such technical expertise and kindly understanding as cancer medicine. The strains on doctors are considerable, especially if they take the human aspect of their work seriously. It is a great failing in doctors if they talk to patients only about the physical and technical aspects of their illness, rely heavily on investigation in making treatment decisions, and find it difficult to give up intensive measures and accept that patients cannot be cured. Technical prowess has then replaced a thoughtful analysis of patients' feelings and what is in their best interests.

Sustaining and counselling a patient and his or her relatives is a matter of teamwork, and the psychological aspects of the disease are as important as the physical aspects. Patients' increasing use of the Internet has brought many benefits but at the same time can make medical consultations more difficult, sometimes undermining well-judged advice given by the physician, based on many years of clinical experience [1]. The special problems of dealing with children with cancer are discussed in Chapter 24. Treating patients with cancer demands great resources of emotional energy on the part of doctors and others in the medical team. In some units, part of the work of talking to patients is taken over by psychiatrists, psychologists, social workers or other counsellors. Invaluable though this help may be, we do not think it desirable that some members of the medical team should see themselves as technical experts and that patients should be sent to talk to someone else about their problems when human feelings are expressed.

Guidance from the NHS National Institute for Clinical Excellence has recently been issued in the form of an invaluable manual for improving supporting and palliative care [2]; this is highly recommended.

Support, counselling and rehabilitation

With any disease it is important to put oneself in the patient's position and try to anticipate the problems which are likely to arise. For example, it may seem obvious that mastectomy is a mutilating operation and that some preoperative and postoperative psychological support will be necessary. Nevertheless, some women do not receive adequate advice. What may be less obvious (until one thinks of it) is that partners of women with mastectomy may be in need of explanation too. Indeed, the reaction of a partner to the operation may be of prime importance in helping the patient to recover from her illness. Such advice is seldom offered.

In addition, many patients with cancer face specific problems of rehabilitation as a result of surgical and other treatments. Rehabilitation and counselling are an essential part of the general care of cancer patients. In recent years specialized support services have developed to help patients overcome the effects of the illness and its treatment, and to return as soon as possible to normal life.

Stoma care

Successful treatment of cancer of the bowel or bladder will sometimes require permanent colostomy or ileostomy. Similarly, in the treatment of gynaecological cancers, there will be a few patients in whom a permanent colostomy, resulting from radiation damage to the large bowel, is the price of a radiotherapy cure (see Chapter 17). Although some patients manage their stoma without difficulty, others require a great deal of education and help, and the role of the stoma therapist has now become established. Patients must learn not only how to keep the stoma clean and healthy but also how to recognize the complications that might demand further surgical review, such as prolapse or stricture. Although a left-sided colostomy is relatively easy to manage, there are considerable difficulties with an ileostomy because of the daily fluid loss of 400–500 mL, which can lead to electrolyte disturbance, dehydration (especially if gastrointestinal infection occurs) and greater aesthetic difficulties. Advances in surgery may lead to continent ileostomies, but at present most patients need to wear an appliance. The British Colostomy Association and Ileostomy and Internal Pouch Support Group offer support and practical help.

Breast prostheses

Most large hospitals should now have some form of mastectomy counselling service, not only to provide psychological support for patients who have undergone mastectomy but also to offer expert advice regarding external prostheses. Almost all patients, including those with very radical operations, can now, when clothed, disguise their defects since a wide variety of prostheses, brassieres and swimsuits are available. A nurse or counsellor specializing in the problems of mastectomy is of great help and many patients will benefit from the advice available from the Mastectomy Association. Nevertheless, a rapidly increasing number of women are unhappy with any form of external prosthesis and request reconstructive, oncoplastic or prosthetic implantation surgery to give a more normal contour, greater confidence and sense of personal control, and the opportunity for more adventurous dressing. Part of the mastectomy counsellor's job is to advise such patients that, contrary to their expectation, following surgery, they cannot always expect to look completely normal, though surgical techniques are improving all the time and the oncoplastic breast surgeon is obviously a key member of any busy breast surgical service.

Laryngectomy rehabilitation

Following total laryngectomy, the patient has to be taught how to create an oesophageal voice, using techniques of air swallowing and careful phonation that can only be acquired with the help of an experienced speech therapist. Although some patients find this straightforward, the majority requires careful tuition, and some never achieve a satisfactory voice. For these patients, a vibrating device or 'artificial larynx' should be available. The vibrating device is held against the neck, and permits a vibrating column of air to be produced which, with careful phonation by the patient, gives monotonous, barely acceptable but comprehensible speech. In a few centres, permanent valves are now being implanted which increase the power and durability of speech. Although these experimental techniques may well have a place in the future rehabilitation of laryngectomy patients, it should be stressed that well-taught oesophageal speech can be very acceptable indeed. The National Association of Laryngectomy Clubs may provide further helpful advice.

Limb prostheses

The regional limb-fitting centres are responsible for providing both temporary and permanent external prostheses for those who have lost limbs, whether through trauma or surgery. Traditionally, amputation has been the mainstay of treatment for bone and soft-tissue sarcoma. Most patients, including children, adapt remarkably well to the loss of a limb, and many are able to drive a car, participate in sport and lead a full and active life. In children, the limb must be replaced as the child grows and care must be taken with the details of weight, length, construction and fitting in order to avoid unequal pressure on the spine, which might lead to scoliosis.

Other prostheses

Other sophisticated prostheses may also be necessary, particularly for patients with facial defects following radical surgery of the head and neck region. In particular, radical surgery for tumours of the maxillary antrum, orbit and nasal fossa, though curative, may result in substantial disfigurement that can only be covered by external prostheses. Remarkable results can be obtained, but the work is highly specialized.

Home support

Learning how to use a colostomy bag or walk with an artificial limb is the start of a much more complex process of rehabilitation, in which the development of self-reliance and self-esteem needs encouragement. While many patients achieve this with the help of their family, some are more isolated and require more professional help. The importance, for example, of a modified bathroom with supporting rails and wheelchair access may well be underestimated compared with the surgical and oncological challenge that the patient represented, but may help to make possible an independent existence at home. Community nursing help may allow patients to leave the hospital relatively early after major operations, improve morale and reduce both the cost of the operation and its morbidity from postoperative complications.

National counselling organizations

In a general hospital the work of counselling patients and their families is made easier if much of the inpatient treatment is in a specialized unit. In such a unit, the nursing staff become very skilled in anticipating the problems of the disease and its treatment. When frequent admissions are necessary, for example, for chemotherapy, it is of great help to the patient to see familiar faces. There is also considerable benefit to be gained by having medical social workers who are especially skilled and interested in the problems of cancer. They not only provide another source of advice and reassurance but will also be knowledgeable about the local availability of counselling groups, nursing support, bereavement organizations and facilities for the care of the dying.

Self-help groups have arisen in many counties, organizing themselves nationally. Such groups have an enormous amount to offer, provided that they take care to give well-balanced and sensible advice. Many patients find it very helpful to talk about their problems with fellow sufferers, and much detailed practical advice may be given which few doctors are in a position to match.

Cancer treatment and the quality of life

Most cancer treatments are unpleasant, producing short- and long-term side-effects that interfere with the patient's quality of life. Assessment of this quality of life is not straightforward. Important criteria include the length of time spent in hospital, the ability to return to work, or at least to an independent life after treatment, and the degree of relief from troublesome symptoms, particularly pain.

Other aspects of morbidity, such as nausea, fatigue, depression and anorexia, are more difficult to measure.

The distinction between *radical* and *palliative* treatment intent should be kept in mind. For example, patients with widely metastatic breast cancer are often treated with combination chemotherapy, and remissions, often lasting several months, are frequently seen. However, since cure is never achieved, such treatment is palliative and offered to patients with symptomatic disease that is likely to respond. Frequently this approach is not followed and patients with metastatic cancer (including far less sensitive tumours than carcinoma of the breast) are treated routinely with combination chemotherapy without mature consideration being given to the objectives of treatment.

Where two types of treatment appear to give similar results, one should choose the less toxic. For example, chemotherapy for Hodgkin's disease has been made much more acceptable by the substitution of other alkylating agents for mustine (see Chapter 25). In certain situations, where there is a slight possible advantage to a more toxic treatment, the greater toxicity might outweigh the slight improvement in results. For example, in infiltrating carcinoma of the urinary bladder, there may be a slight survival advantage in a combination of irradiation and radical cystectomy, compared with treatment by radiotherapy alone. However, the extra few months of median survival are obtained at the cost of both a permanent ileostomy and a high risk of impotence. Given a choice, many of us might opt for radiotherapy alone, despite the slightly greater risk, particularly since surgery is still possible if there is local recurrence. As with the example of asymptomatic non-small-cell carcinoma of the bronchus noted below, in recent years this type of decision has become more difficult, with the advent of more effective chemotherapy that is capable of down staging the tumour to a significant degree.

For a number of malignancies, radical treatment by radiation, or more often nowadays chemoradiation, therapy (see specific chapters) can give local control rates that are the equal of surgery. This is reflected by the increasing use of such treatment for carcinoma of the cervix, head and neck, bladder, prostate, oesophagus and breast.

In each of these sites, there are important physiological and psychological advantages to treatment with radiotherapy, either alone or with chemotherapy. Radical surgery can usually be performed if relapse occurs. Finally, one should remember that there are some patients with malignant disease in whom treatment may not be immediately necessary. For many patients with follicular lymphoma, the course is so indolent that treatment is unnecessary, often for several years. In patients with asymptomatic but inoperable squamous carcinoma of the bronchus, there is often little advantage to early treatment with radiotherapy or chemotherapy, since such treatment does not prolong life and may cause side-effects (see Chapter 12), although the advent of increasingly effective and well-tolerated chemotherapy has made this type of decision more difficult, particularly in frail or unfit patients. Treatment may be better withheld until a troublesome symptom such as haemoptysis, dyspnoea or pain from a secondary deposit becomes apparent.

For these reasons, when trials of cancer treatments are undertaken it may be important to include some assessment of quality of life, especially if there is unlikely to be a substantial difference in cure rate. In this way, any advantage in terms of survival or local control can be set against the morbidity which the treatment has induced.

Symptom control [3,4]

Pain

Relief of pain is a particularly important aspect of the management of cancer. Cancer pain may arise from viscera, when it is often poorly localized and variable; from the bones and limbs (e.g. bone metastasis), when it is persistent and localized; and is often worse at night or 'shooting' when neuropathic. Patients often have more than one cause of pain.

The first step in management is to make an accurate clinical assessment of the pain that the patient is experiencing, and its site, severity and duration. The use of a pain assessment chart is helpful in defining the main problem and in monitoring progress with time.

Analgesics

There is no such thing as a single and ideal analgesic, and most patients will require drugs of different strength and dosage during the course of their illness. It is convenient to group analgesics into three classes according to their strength, as shown in Table 7.1.

Mild analgesics

This group includes aspirin, paracetamol and non-steroidal anti-inflammatory agents. These can be valuable for considerable periods of time. Aspirin and the non-steroidal anti-inflammatory agents (e.g. indometacin, ibuprofen) are particularly helpful in bone

Table 7.1 Analgesics for pain relief in cancer.

Drug	Duration of action (hours)	Toxicity
Mild analgesics		
Aspirin	4–6	Gastrointestinal bleeding and abdominal pain
Paracetamol	2–4	Skin rash; hepatic damage with overdose
Propionic acid derivatives (e.g. ibuprofen)	2–6	As aspirin
Indole derivatives (e.g. indometacin)	8	As aspirin
Moderate analgesics		
Codeine and dihydrocodeine	4–6	Constipation, excitement
Oxycodone	8–10	Constipation, hypotension, nausea, dysphasia
Pentazocine	3–4	Nausea, dizziness, palpitations, hypertension, dysphasia
Dipipanone	6	Constipation, mental confusion, respiratory depression
Tramadol	6	Nausea, vomiting, sweating, constipation
Paracetamol with codeine (longer with sustained-release preparations)		
Powerful analgesics		
Morphine sulphate	4–6 (longer with sustained-release preparations	Constipation, hypotension, nausea, dysphasia
Diamorphine	4–6	As morphine sulphate
Methadone	15–30	As morphine sulphate, more nausea, cumulative
Hydromorphone	4–6	Useful in patients with morphine intolerance
Dextromoramide	6	Dizziness, sweating, constipation, respiratory depression
Pethidine	3	Nausea, dry mouth, respiratory depression

pain. Side-effects include dyspepsia and gastrointestinal bleeding. They can be combined with agents from a more powerful class (e.g. combined aspirin and papaveretum tablets). Intravenous preparations of paracetamol have recently become available, resulting in a much higher peak plasma concentration than with the oral preparation, and an improved analgesic effect, claimed to be comparable to a 10-mg intramuscular dose of morphine.

Moderate analgesics

This group includes codeine, oxycodone, pentazocine and dipipanone. These agents are more effective than those in the mild analgesic group but at the cost of greater side-effects, particularly constipation. Dextropropoxyphene is sometimes combined with paracetamol, but this preparation (co-proxamol) has recently been withdrawn in the UK. Oxycodone is particularly valuable as it is available in the form of suppositories. Pentazocine should be avoided because it commonly produces hallucinations. It has a partial antagonist action to morphine and should not be used in combination with opiates. Tramadol, a synthetic opioid phenylpiperidine analogue

of codeine, was initially synthesized in Germany. It is increasingly used as an alternative to other agents in the moderate analgesic group, and in many countries is not regarded as a 'controlled substance', making it convenient for extended use. However, this situation is likely to change as its unique dual action clearly increases the risks of adverse effects, particularly in overdose. Deaths attributed to this agent have increased in recent years. The drug has weak agonist activity at opiate receptors in the brain, which may cause euphoria and respiratory depression. It also enhances serotoninergic and noradrenergic systems in the brain (by inhibiting their reuptake mechanisms). The potential harm comes from the fact that the opioid effects of tramadol are reversible only with naloxone. Doses range from 50–400 mg daily, and the drug can be given by mouth (every 4–6 hours) or parenterally.

Powerful analgesics

These drugs, which include morphine and related compounds (synthetic and semisynthetic derivatives), are powerful in their pain-relieving effects and are the mainstay of analgesic therapy for patients with unremitting pain – see Ref. [5] for a fuller account of this important topic, with recommendations from the European Association for Palliative Care (EAPC). These agents mimic the actions of the endogenous brain mediators known as opioid peptides. Almost all patients with severe cancer pain require regular medication with analgesics of this type. Useful agents include morphine analogues such as diamorphine, morphine and codeine; phenylpiperidine derivatives such as methadone, pethidine, fentanyl and dextropropoxyphene; thebaine derivatives such as buprenorphine; and benzomorphans such as pentazocine. Agents such as fentanyl and oxycodone are metabolized via the cytochrome P450 pathway. Ordinary morphine and diamorphine are active for only 4 hours and should therefore be given 4-hourly, but long-acting oral tablets of morphine sulphate are now available. Morphine is metabolized via a different biochemical pathway, chiefly through glucuronidation.

The choice of opiate analgesic and dosages should be determined by the patient's need [6]. For example, many patients are comfortable and pain-free with small, regular doses (10–20 mg every 4 hours) of morphine or diamorphine, while others require 20 times this dose. There are few other drugs with as wide a dose range as a result of variable degrees of pharmacological tolerance, which develops rapidly. In most patients, oral medication is appropriate and effective although absorption is slow and variable. In patients with, for example, complete obstruction from pharyngeal or oesophageal cancer, an alternative route will have to be found. Sublingual buprenorphine can be a useful alternative but it antagonizes the effect of morphine and should therefore be neither abruptly substituted for morphine nor given with it concurrently. Treatment using rectal suppositories of oxycodone or morphine can be extremely effective. In very occasional cases, where both the oral and rectal routes are unavailable, suppositories can be given vaginally.

Regular intravenous treatment with opiates is necessary only rarely but subcutaneous infusions of diamorphine can be valuable if treatment by other routes proves unsatisfactory. Diamorphine is preferable because of its very high solubility, allowing volumes for injection to be small. 'On-demand' use may allow the patient to be more in control of the pain relief. Very rarely, regular administration of epidural morphine may be necessary for relief of severe localized pain, but this should never be considered as a long-term solution unless other methods of regular opiate administration have been tried.

Long-acting morphine, available in tablets, is a very important addition to the family of opiates. Since both morphine and diamorphine must be given frequently throughout the day, the availability of long-acting morphine is of real value, particularly to the active patient. When changing the treatment from diamorphine to long-acting morphine, the dose ratio of diamorphine to morphine is 2:3, so that a patient on, say, diamorphine 20 mg 4-hourly (total daily dosage 120 mg) will require 180 mg of morphine daily, or long-acting morphine 90 mg twice daily. Hydromorphone HCl, a semisynthetic opioid derivative, can be useful in morphine-intolerant patients and is available in sustained-release preparations (given 12-hourly). Transdermal patches of fentanyl (a semisynthetic opioid) at an initial dose of 25 mg/hour (in patients not previously exposed to opioids) or by appropriate dose transfer in patients taking morphine may offer excellent pain control with less constipation, nausea and daytime drowsiness and is often especially useful for nauseated patients. Fentanyl is sometimes given in the form of an oral 'lollipop', a type of approach favoured by a surprisingly high number of adults as well as children!

All patients taking regular opiate medication will require advice regarding constipation. Regular laxatives are usually (but not always) necessary, and may need to be given in above-normal doses. Regular dantron–poloxamer mixture (or capsules) is effective. The standard daily dose of 10–15 mL (or one to three capsules) in divided daily doses may be insufficient for patients on large doses of morphine and a stronger suspension is available. Nausea, vomiting and sedation are the other important side-effects of opiate analgesics but are less consistent. Although sedation usually disappears with time, nausea may persist and require treatment. Haloperidol is effective as is cyclizine, although phenothiazines are more sedating (see Table 7.2).

In recent years other useful potentiating agents have been increasingly employed, for example, the anticonvulsant group that includes gabapentin, pregabalin, carbamazepine and sodium valproate. The advantages include their good interaction profiles with more conventional analgesics, together with favourable pharmacokinetic handling. Generally speaking, they are not metabolized by the liver and are excreted via the kidney. These agents are widely used for patients with neuropathic pain. In addition, the modern tricyclic antidepressants are also capable of potentiating major opioid or non-opioid analgesia, which is likely to remain the most important part of the patient's pain management.

Table 7.2 Classification of drugs used to control nausea and vomiting.

Putative site of action	Class	Example
Central nervous system		
Vomiting centre	Antimuscarinic*	Hyoscine hydrobromide, prochlorperazine
	H_1 receptor antagonist*	Cyclizine, dimenhydrinate
	5-HT_2 receptor antagonist	Levomepromazine
	D_2 receptor antagonist	Metoclopramide, domperidone
	5-HT_3 receptor antagonist	Granisetron, ondansetron, tropisetron
Cerebral cortex	Benzodiazepine	Lorazepam
	Cannabinoid	Nabilone
	Corticosteroid	Dexamethasone
Gastrointestinal tract		
Prokinetic	5-HT_4 receptor antagonist	Metoclopramide, cisapride
	D_2 receptor antagonist	Metoclopramide, domperidone
Antisecretory	Antimuscarinic	Hyoscine, glycopyrrolate
	Somatostatin analogue	Octreotide, vapreotide
	Vagal 5-HT_3 receptor antagonist	Granisetron, ondansetron, tropisetron
Anti-inflammatory	Corticosteroid	Dexamethasone

*Antihistamines and phenothiazines both have H_1 receptor antagonistic and antimuscarinic properties.
Source: Twycross [7].

Guidelines for pain control in terminal cancer patients

The guidelines are summarized in Figure 7.1.

1 *Use enough analgesia to be effective.* Regular aspirin, or compound paracetamol–codeine tablets can be effective for many weeks especially in musculoskeletal pain. A change to dihydrocodeine will then usually give further pain relief. Use of morphine or related agents should be considered when drugs of lesser effect are inadequate for the patient's pain. At this stage, less powerful agents such as dipipanone, aspirin or non-steroidal anti-inflammatory agents may be useful to supplement the regular morphine dose. A common useful starting dose of diamorphine elixir is 10 or 20 mg every 4 hours but some patients need more than 1 g of diamorphine daily for adequate pain relief. Addiction is not a problem and opiates should not be withheld for fear of producing it. Dysphoria and loss of lucidity may occur and can be distressing. In such cases, a lower dose may have to be accepted, even if pain relief is incomplete, and additional analgesia attempted by other means (see below) [9] (Figure 7.2).

2 *Give analgesics regularly rather than on a 'when required' basis.* Patients should not have to 'earn' their analgesia. Morphine and diamorphine need to be given every 4 hours to be effective, but most patients can manage on slow-release morphine tablets (see above).

3 *Warn patients about side-effects.* This particularly applies to constipation. High-fibre diet and regular laxatives are sufficient to deal with this important and painful problem in most cases. Metoclopramide, prochlorperazine or cyclizine can be useful if nausea is a persistent problem.

4 *Keep drug prescriptions as simple as possible.* Some opiates antagonize each other and should never be given together (e.g. sublingual buprenorphine and oral diamorphine).

5 Consider *alternative methods of pain control.*

(a) Alternative routes of analgesic administration: oral, sublingual, rectal, vaginal or even (rarely) via colostomy; subcutaneous, intramuscular, intravenous, transcutaneous using fentanyl. The past 5 years have seen an increase in familiarity with subcutaneously administered morphine infusions, using a simple, constant-rate syringe driver that the patient can usually manage very effectively at home, with a boost facility for additional flexibility.

(b) Alternative approaches: consider radiotherapy for painful bone metastases, surgical internal fixation for pathological fractures and other procedures such as nerve block and neurosurgical approaches.

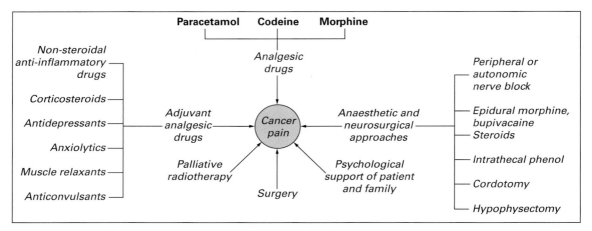

Figure 7.1 Treatment of cancer pain. (Source: Baines [8]. Reproduced with permission from BMJ Publishing Group Limited.)

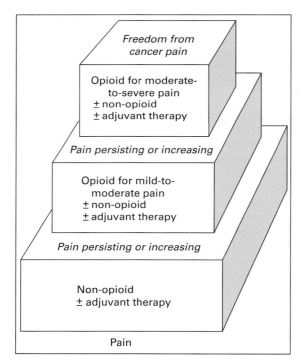

Figure 7.2 WHO's cancer pain ladder for adults. (Source: http://www.who.int/cancer/palliative/painladder/en/ (accessed March 2014). Reproduced with permission from the World Health Organization.)

Nerve blocks, surgical procedures and other approaches

Some patients with cancer have intractable pain at a particular site, which responds poorly even to high doses of opiates. Radiation is often a highly effective treatment for localized pain, particularly when it arises in bone. If this is ineffective, an alternative technique is a nerve block, which destroys pain and other sensations in the affected part of the body. The technique requires great skill and is usually performed by an anaesthetist with special training. Local dorsal root block using fine-needle insertions of phenol or absolute alcohol is the commonest method (Figure 7.3). A similar technique can be used to produce coeliac or brachial plexus block.

Surgical destructive procedures are rarely necessary but may have to be considered if all else fails. Spinothalamic tractotomy is an operation performed on the spinal cord in which the fibres carrying pain are divided. Anatomical specificity is often possible since the pain fibres are arranged in the lateral spinothalamic tract in an orderly fashion. However, pain relief may not be complete since other spinal pathways may also subserve pain sensation. Operations can also be considered at higher levels (e.g. thalamotomy) if tractotomy is ineffective.

Epidural infusions

Epidural infusions of local anaesthetic or opiates can sometimes be used to control pain when the oral route proves difficult due to nausea. The infusions are intermittent or continuous and use an infusion pump (such as that used for subcutaneous infusion), connected to a catheter in the epidural space. Tolerance to local anaesthetics occurs quickly so that the effect lasts only a few weeks. Infection may occur. Pain relief may be obtained without paralysis or autonomic disturbance.

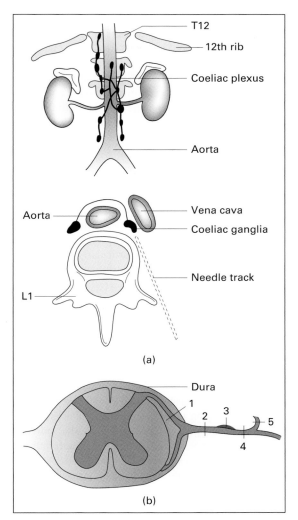

(a)

(b)

Figure 7.3 Coeliac plexus and dorsal root blocks to relieve pain. (a) Anatomical relations of coeliac plexus. The plexus comprises a number of ganglia situated in front of T12 and L1. The injection is made in front of the anterior border of the body of L1. The needle is inserted below the 12th rib. (b) Dorsal root block and section: 1, block of root inside dura; 2, block of dorsal root outside dura; 3, excision of dorsal root ganglion; 4, coagulation of nerve trunk; 5, coagulation of medial branch of primary ramus.

Other procedures

These include transcutaneous nerve stimulation and acupuncture analgesia, both of which can be valuable even in patients taking large doses of opiates. The mechanisms of these methods may involve stimulation of endogenous endorphins at a central level.

Anorexia and nausea [10]

Anorexia is a very common accompaniment of terminal cancer and there is, of course, no long-lasting remedy. There is, however, much that can be done to relieve the anxiety which the patient feels about the continued wasting [11]. Small meals should be offered, particularly the patient's favourite dishes, and a glass of wine or sherry may stimulate appetite. One of the great ironies of faddish 'alternative' diets, advocated as natural ways for the patient to build resistance to cancer, is that they may detract from the simple pleasure of eating and drinking in the final weeks of a patient's life. Steroids may be valuable to help stimulate appetite in this situation. Steroid side-effects will not be a problem if the prognosis is a matter of weeks. The drug of choice is probably dexamethasone, 2 mg given three or four times daily, although lower doses may be adequate. Other helpful drugs are progestogens (especially megestrol), anabolic steroids and phenothiazines.

Treatment of nausea (and vomiting) may be difficult and depends on the cause (Table 7.2). Drug-induced nausea (due to morphine) may require treatment with metoclopramide, haloperidol or phenothiazines. Nausea due to intestinal obstruction or other causes of gut stress is often difficult to treat. Metoclopramide may help, as may domperidone. Rectal administration is often effective. 5-Hydroxytryptamine (5-HT)$_3$ antagonists can also be valuable in treatment of nausea in advanced cancer. If there is a mechanical cause, such as intestinal obstruction from an intra-abdominal mass, a fine-bore nasogastric tube may have to be passed for aspiration of stomach contents. In most cases symptomatic treatment with prochlorperazine, chlorpromazine or metoclopramide, given regularly before meals, may help. Rectal administration may occasionally be necessary. Chemotherapy-induced nausea and vomiting are dealt with separately in Chapter 6.

Oral mucositis

This distressing and under-recognized symptom frequently accompanies chronic ill-health or the administration of chemotherapy [12], particularly with methotrexate, fluorouracil, bleomycin or doxorubicin. Principles of management include both prevention (oral hygiene and use of a regular mouthwash), and treatment with ice chips during chemotherapy, to decrease oral mucosal blood flow.

Constipation

There are many causes of constipation in patients with cancer. One of the most common is anorexia and low bulk intake. This can sometimes be helped by dietary fibre supplements if tolerated. Lack of fluid intake leads to hard stools and can be helped by increasing fluid intake and by a stool-softening agent such as docusate or a lubricant (liquid paraffin). Drugs (morphine, codeine and derivatives) are a very frequent cause of constipation and require a combined stimulant and stool softener such as a co-danthramer or senna, as well as a review of analgesic dosage.

Intestinal obstruction

Intestinal obstruction [13], a common complication of advanced intra-abdominal malignancy, is often a cause of great distress and is difficult to treat. The tumour is usually diffusely scattered on the bowel surface, infiltrating the wall and the mesentery. A stiff immobile bowel results in areas which are encircled and compressed. If a localized obstruction cannot be relieved by laparotomy, then pain control must be achieved by opioids and antispasmodics; antiemetics will be needed for nausea, and a stool-softening agent (without stimulating laxatives) for constipation. Octreotide may help control vomiting and a nasogastric tube may be needed if vomiting is intractable and cannot be relieved by other means. Most patients can be made more comfortable for a time, but this is often a miserable complication of cancer.

Depression and anxiety

Most patients will have episodes of depression and anxiety, and sympathetic conversation with family, friends, doctors and nurses will usually help the patient through bad days. Persistent, disturbing or suicidal depression (fortunately very uncommon) may require additional treatment with tricyclic or tetracyclic antidepressants, and occasionally skilled psychiatric help is needed. Some authorities find amphetamines are helpful in special circumstances. Benzodiazepines are useful for acute or persistent anxiety. In the long term, recent studies have suggested that anxiety is a more frequent problem than persistent depression and that more support for families and care takers is urgently needed – see, for example, Ref. [14].

The care of the dying

In England and Wales alone, over 135 000 people die each year from cancer, accounting for some 20% of all deaths. Of these about 60% die in non-specialist hospitals, 30% at home and the remainder in hospices, nursing homes and private hospitals. About half of all cancer patients present with incurable conditions at the time of diagnosis, and in the more fortunate half with potentially curable cancers, the majority develop recurrent disease and require palliative symptomatic care. The World Health Organization has estimated that over 3.5 million people are suffering worldwide from cancer-induced pains each day, a sad reflection on the quality of care available to the majority of cancer patients.

It has become increasingly apparent that patients dying from cancer have particular needs which are often poorly served by traditional means of support. Even the most well-meaning doctors frequently find themselves out of their depth either through inadequate training in the use of the appropriate drugs (particularly analgesics) or because of the difficulties of exploring patients' needs. It is against this background that interest and expertise in the management of terminally ill patients has developed and, as so often happens, it is the determined work of a few individuals that has identified the problem and developed principles which are now widely adopted. In recent years, the Liverpool Care Pathway, which sets out to encourage the best possible care of the dying patient and provide an evidence-based protocol of support and medication, has been increasingly used to assist in this challenging task. Despite many attacks on it as potentially damaging or 'insensitive' to the individual need of a patient or the family, it found great favour with most practitioners experienced in this work – see, for example, Ref. [15] – although public pressure forced it to be abandoned in the UK during July 2013 as it was being implemented in a less than thoughtful manner, with insufficient attention to specific patient needs. Sadly this illustrated all too clearly the gap between good intentions and clinical practice in busy general hospital wards with so many competing priorities.

First and foremost, it is always wrong for a doctor to say, or feel, that there is nothing more that he or she can do. The enthusiastic oncologist may feel that his or her work is over when the specific anticancer treatment is at an end. The patient will, in general, make a much less clear distinction between active and supportive treatment so that, from the patient's point of view, careful treatment with analgesics, concern about appetite, constipation, mobility and so on, may be equally important. Second, it is largely through the work of hospice staff that we are beginning to learn the critical importance of adequate symptom control. The symptoms most commonly causing distress are pain, anorexia, nausea and vomiting, constipation, weakness and lassitude.

Terminal care: home, hospice and support teams

Many patients like to remain at home for as long as they can and to die there if possible. Familiar surroundings and family life offer great comfort. The care of a dying patient is, however, extremely demanding and a great deal of support is always required if home care is to be achieved successfully. Women generally look after dying men much better than men care for dying women. There are many factors which determine the feasibility of home care. These include whether the patient lives alone; the continued presence of family or friends to provide support (the spouse or partner may have to go to work); whether there are young children at home to be cared for; the availability of adequate local support services such as nursing, laundry, home helps and meals on wheels; and the degree and nature of the patient's disability and symptoms. It may be necessary to provide specialized aids to nursing and mobility, such as handrails in the bathroom, commodes, a ripple or water bed, a hoist or a wheelchair.

A flexible approach is essential – see, for example, Ref. [16], for an excellent, contemporary and level-headed brief review. Even if the intention is to care for the patient at home, the circumstances may change and the situation more difficult, making hospital or hospice care necessary. This may lead to feelings of guilt or of defeat in the family; the doctor should realize this and explain that continuous care of the dying patient is a highly skilled task, that professional help is often needed and that a change in plan is not a sign of failure.

There has been considerable expansion of palliative care teams and inpatient hospices such that palliative care has now emerged as a new medical specialty. Hospices for terminally ill cancer patients have taught us the importance of careful pain control, attention to patients' physical and spiritual needs, and the important ways in which medical, nursing and other staff can make enormous contributions by spending a little more time with patients, often just by listening or simply being there. Nevertheless, the hospice movement is itself aware of the disadvantages of hospice care. Hospices are expensive to set up and maintain, and demand a high staff to patient ratio. Some patients find the concept of moving to a 'terminal home' difficult to accept even though the majority is content once they arrive. Psychologically, many patients find it difficult to accept that the doctor

who has been treating them, in whom they have had trust and confidence, no longer has any treatment to offer. Doctors with a genuine interest in the management of terminally ill cancer patients often find it upsetting if they are made to feel that they have no further role, as sometimes happens when a hospice support team takes the view that it should be entirely responsible for a patient. For the general practitioner who will have to look after the family after the death of the patient with cancer, this sudden role change can create real difficulty.

The traditional alternative, and the place where many cancer patients die, has been the general hospital ward. Undoubtedly there are advantages, particularly the continuity of care afforded by familiar staff and surroundings. Some patients might gain comfort from the fact that many of the patients on the ward will be suffering from non-malignant conditions, and that the general atmosphere is likely to be brisk and active. However, most of us would agree that for patients in the final stages of their illness, the ideal environment would be more tranquil and the staff rather less busy, so that there is more time for reflective discussion. It is well known that on many general medical or surgical wards, the cancer patient is all too often hurriedly passed by, particularly by the medical staff, who perhaps feel pressured and unable to help, and embarrassed or discomfited by this inadequacy. Furthermore, as expressed by Sleeman and Collis [17], 'doctors are notoriously poor at prognosticating, and recognizing that a person is dying is a skill that develops over time. In the patient who is close to death, clinical signs such as reduced consciousness level, respiratory changes (for example, Cheyne–Stokes breathing) and cardiovascular changes (for example, peripheral vasoconstriction) are common. For the patient and his or her family to have time to express their preferences for end-of-life care, however, recognition must occur earlier'.

A solution is the setting up of community- or hospital-based supportive care teams, which consist of medical and nursing staff, usually with a social worker. Such teams exist to help both hospital specialists and local general practitioners, by providing expertise, assistance and time for terminally ill cancer patients, maintaining continuity of support whether the patient has been admitted to a hospital bed or is at home under the care of the local practitioner. From our own experience of working with such a team it is apparent that there are benefits both for the patient and for his or her family. Supportive care teams can assist by providing an expert service regarding, for example, choice of analgesic or antiemetic, as well as arranging for essential facilities such as commodes, home oxygen, rapid installation of telephone services and so on. Although all these roles could be undertaken by general practitioners, district nurses or social workers, there is no doubt that the presence of a team entirely committed to the improvement of standards in terminal care enormously improves the efficiency of the service. Many teams also take on a bereavement counselling role and remain closely in touch with bereaved relatives, particularly if problems have been perceived before the death of the patient. Although there is no ideal time to refer patients to such a team, we feel that early referral is to be encouraged so that possible problems can be rapidly identified, and a close relationship quickly established. Moreover, the increased recognition of our limitations in respect of effective further treatment for end-of-life patients with cancer, has stimulated 'Death with Dignity' programmes of support, even including bold and controversial 'physician-assisted' approaches to dying. This has already led to legislation in Washington State and Oregon despite religious and ethical concerns – see Ref. [18]. This movement, clearly popular with many patients close to the end of their lives, looks certain to become more powerful and widespread.

Cancer quackery

Quackery: the pretensions or practice of a quack
Quack: shortened form of quacksalver – a charlatan
Quacksalver: one who quacks about his salves

(derived from Dutch)

Patients with cancer may decide to abandon medical treatment and opt for false or unproven remedies such as dietary manipulation, 'natural' or herbal medicines, homeopathy, faith healing, visualization therapy, immunizations, multivitamin supplements and enemas. They may be urged to do so by relatives or other cancer patients, and they sometimes try these treatments in addition to conventional methods.

Patients who do this are usually frightened and anxious; some may see doctors as members of a conspiratorial establishment who have closed minds to any alternative approach. They may have strong ideas about the way their body works or what causes cancer, believing, for example, that the disease is the result of lifestyle, diet, psychological stress or pollution. However, even if dietary factors are important in aetiology it is illogical to expect that the cancer can therefore be cured by alterations in diet or

emotional attitude, or by taking natural products such as herbal remedies. Sadly, giving up smoking does not cure lung cancer. Many august personages are prepared to lend their support to these notions, their names often being more impressive than their intellectual credentials. There is also no shortage of doctors, naturopaths or homeopaths to support the public in these beliefs, as well as some more tough-minded charlatans out to make money [19]. There are many damaging aspects to their activities.

First, there is no evidence that these remedies work. No evidence for antitumour activity is presented, no evaluation of results and no independent or critical assessment of data. Instead, cases are quoted, anecdotes offered and spurious facts and figures produced. In one of the few controlled studies of alternative cancer treatments, Laetrile (amygdalin), a 'harmless yet effective' remedy approved by most alternative cancer 'authorities', was found to be entirely without benefit and with significant side-effects when assessed in over 500 cancer patients [20]. High levels of oral vitamin A, sometimes offered as part of a dietary supplement, are known to be teratogenic [21]. Both mistletoe and Chinese herbs, increasingly used for cancer patients in the UK and USA, can be dangerously nephrotoxic [22–24]. Randomized trials of the 'holistic' approach against conventional treatment have not been undertaken, partly due to reluctance by the practitioners of alternative medicine to put their beliefs to the test, and partly due to the ethical difficulties. Two case–control studies have been carried out in advanced cancer, neither of which has shown any benefit for survival in the 'alternative' approach, and one of which showed no improvement in quality of life either [25]. Vitamin C was shown in a randomized trial to be of no value in advanced cancer. Objective but uncontrolled studies of macrobiotic diets and immuno-augmentative therapy have found no evidence of efficacy. Furthermore, even homeopathic remedies with high dilution may represent a potential hazard to the patient [26], although generally the risk is admittedly low. A recent well-researched (and much publicized) large-scale meta-analysis from a Danish group, working as part of the Cochrane Library, has suggested that using large doses of vitamins and/or mineral supplements adds nothing to a standard healthy diet, and may even do harm [27]. In particular, the so-called antioxidants such as β-carotene, vitamin A and vitamin E 'given singly or combined with other antioxidant supplements significantly increase mortality'. As one of the journalists commenting on this report pointed out:

Every vitamin devotee in the country will be outraged. Anyone who has ever pondered the life-enhancing claims on the seductive tubs of supplements lining the shelves of Boots [a well-known chain-store of chemists/drugstores in the UK] must be doing a double-take.

Second, the proponents may say that they do not pretend to offer a cure-all, but some patients believe that they will be cured or the disease arrested. The process of mental adjustment to the diagnosis may be badly shaken by false optimism followed by despair at failure. The terms *alternative medicine* and *alternative therapy* are themselves lies when they are used to imply that proven methods of treatment are being offered. Third, the patient may delay conventional treatment, occasionally with tragic consequences in the case of a potentially curable tumour. Fourth, the treatment is often expensive and patients may waste a lot of money. Finally, these 'remedies' may create a great deal of conflict within the family. Patients with advanced cancer can be cajoled or even bullied by their well-meaning relatives into taking an entirely 'natural' diet; then find it intolerable and lose what remaining interest they may have in nutrition. They may even feel that they have to continue in order not to let their children down.

However, it must be admitted that one reason why patients seek these remedies is a dissatisfaction with conventional medicine or with their doctor, which may in part be well founded [28,29]. Patients will often say that they tried these treatments because they were given no hope or emotional support, because they found the prospect of radiotherapy or chemotherapy unnatural, because there was inadequate explanation and reassurance or because treatment was being unreasonably and thoughtlessly prolonged or aggressive without any hint of benefit. The first question doctors should ask themselves when faced with a patient who has decided to undergo a quack treatment is whether they have given enough explanation and reassurance. Furthermore, there is no doubt that many patients feel a great deal better if offered additional support beyond what has traditionally been available – so complementary therapies are here to stay, regardless of what the medical profession think is useful or not! Treatments such as aromatherapy, massage, reflexology and acupuncture are good examples of the type of supportive care which many patients value.

If a patient or relative decides to discontinue treatment it is, of course, essential to say what the consequences might be, but cruel to overstate the case in order to browbeat the patient into continuing [30]. Some cancer treatment is palliative and no great harm may be done by stopping it. It is kind to make it clear that although the proposed alternative is of unproven value, the patient will be welcome to come back at any time.

References

1 Ziebland S, Chapple A, Dumelow C *et al.* How the internet affects patients' experience of cancer: a qualitative study. *Br Med J* 2004; 328: 564–7.

2 National Institute for Clinical Excellence. *Guidance on Cancer Services: Improving Supportive and Palliative Care for Adults with Cancer – The Manual.* London: NICE, 2004.

3 Levy MH. Pharmacologic treatment of cancer pain. *N Engl J Med* 1996; 335: 1124–32.

4 Saunders CM, Sykes N. *The Management of Terminal Malignant Disease.* London: Edward Arnold, 1993.

5 Caraceni A, Hanks G, Kaasa S *et al.* Use of opioid analgesics in the treatment of cancer pain: evidence-based recommendations from the EAPC. *Lancet Oncol.* 2012; 13: e58–68. doi: 10.1016/S1470-2045(12)70040-2.

6 Hanks GW, Hoskin PJ. Opioid analgesics in the management of pain in patients with cancer. A review. *Palliative Med* 1987; 1: 1–25.

7 Twycross R. Guidelines for the management of nausea and vomiting. *Palliative Care Today* 1999; 32.

8 Baines M. Pain relief in active patients with cancer: analgesic drugs are the foundation of management. *Br Med J* 1989; 298: 36–8.

9 Jadad AR, Bowman GP. The WHO analgesic ladder for cancer pain management: stepping up the quality of its evaluation. *JAMA* 1995; 274: 1870–3.

10 Bruera E, Higginson I, eds. *Cachexia–Anorexia in Cancer Patients.* Oxford: Oxford University Press, 1996.

11 Rimmer T. Treating the anorexia of cancer. *Eur J Palliative Care* 1998; 5: 179–81.

12 Mead GM. Management of oral mucositis associated with cancer chemotherapy. *Lancet* 2002; 359: 815–16.

13 Ripamonti C, Mercadante S. Pathophysiology and management of malignant bowel obstruction. In: Doyle D, Hanks GW, Cherny N, Calman K, eds. *Oxford Textbook of Palliative Medicine*, 3rd edn. Oxford: Oxford University Press, 2005: 496–507.

14 Addington-Hall J. The legacy of cancer on depression and anxiety. *Lancet Oncol* 2013; 14: 675–6.

15 Chinthapalli K. The Liverpool Care Pathway: what do specialists think? *Brit Med J* 2013; 346; f1184.

16 Collis E, Al-Qurainy R. Care of the dying patient in the community. *Brit Med J* 2013; 347: 27–30.

17 Sleeman KE, Collis E. Caring for a dying patient in hospital. *Brit Med J* 2013; 346: f2174.

18 Loggers ET, Starks H, Shannon-Dudley M *et al.* Implementing a death with dignity program at a comprehensive cancer centre. *New Engl J Med* 2013; 368:1417–24.

19 Willams AN, Birmingham L. The art of making ineffective treatments effective. *Lancet* 2002; 359: 1937–9.

20 Moertel CG, Fleming TR, Rubin J *et al.* A clinical trial of amygdalin (Laetrile) in the treatment of human cancer. *N Engl J Med* 1991; 306: 201–6.

21 Rothman KJ, Moore LL, Singer MR *et al.* Teratogenicity of high vitamin A intake. *N Engl J Med* 1995; 333: 1369–73.

22 Lord GM, Cook T, Arit VM, *et al.* Urothelial malignant disease and Chinese herbal nephropathy. *Lancet* 2001; 368: 1515–16.

23 Lord GM, Tagore R, Cook T *et al.* Nephropathy caused by Chinese herbs in the UK. *Lancet* 1999; 354: 481–2.

24 Steuer-Vogt MK, Bonkowsky V, Ambrosch P *et al.* The effect of an adjuvant mistletoe treatment programme in resected head and neck cancer patients: a randomised controlled clinical trial. *Eur J Cancer* 2001; 37: 23–31.

25 Cassileth BR, Lusk EJ, Guerry P *et al.* Survival and quality of life among patients receiving unproven as compared with conventional cancer therapy. *N Engl J Med* 1991; 324: 1180–5.

26 Kirby BJ. Safety of homeopathic products. *J R Soc Med* 2002; 95: 474–5.

27 Bjelakovic G, Nikolova D, Gluud LL *et al.* Mortality in randomized trials of antioxidant supplements for primary and secondary prevention: systematic review and meta-analysis. *JAMA* 2007; 297: 842–57.

28 Cassileth B, Lush EJ, Strouse TB *et al.* Contemporary unorthodox treatment in cancer medicine: a study of patients, treatments and practitioners. *Ann Intern Med* 1984; 101: 105–12.

29 Downer SM, Cody MM, McCluskey P *et al.* Pursuit and practice of complementary therapies by cancer patients receiving conventional treatment. *Br Med J* 1994; 309: 86–9.

30 Fried TR, Bradley EH, Towle VR, Allore H. Understanding the treatment preferences of seriously ill patients. *N Engl J Med* 2002; 346: 1061–6.

Further reading

Agarawal JP, Swangsilpa T, van der Linden Y *et al.* The role of external beam radiotherapy in the management of bone metastases. *Clin Oncol* 2006; 18: 747–60.

Anon. Cancer survivors. Living longer, and now, better. *Lancet* 2004; 364: 2153–4.

Anon. Opioid analgesics for cancer pain in primary care. *Drug Ther Bull* 2005; 43: 9–12.

Bardia A, Barton DL, Prokop LJ *et al.* Efficacy of complementary and alternative medicine therapies in relieving cancer pain: a systematic review. *J Clin Oncol* 2006; 24: 5457–64.

Bosely S. Hard to swallow, *The Guardian.* 14 April 2008. (http://www.theguardian.com/society/2008/apr/17/health .healthandwellbeing)

Brydoy M, Fossa SD, Klepp O *et al.* Paternity following treatment for testicular cancer. *J Natl Cancer Inst* 2005; 97: 1580–8.

Cherny N, Ripamonti C, Pereira J *et al.* Strategies to manage the adverse effects of oral morphine: an evidence based report. *J Clin Oncol* 2001; 19: 2542–54.

Doyle D, Hanks G, Cherny N, Calman K, eds. *Oxford Textbook of Palliative Medicine*, 3rd edn. Oxford: Oxford University Press, 2005.

Ellershaw J, Ward C. Care of the dying patient: the last hours or days of life. *Br Med J* 2003; 326: 30–4.

Fallon M, guest ed. Palliative medicine: the art and the science. *Eur J Cancer* 2008; 44: 1069–179.

Gilron I, Bailey JM, Tu D *et al.* Morphine, gabapentin, or their combination for neuropathic pain. *N Engl J Med* 2005; 352: 1324–34.

Goldacre B. Benefits and risks of homoeopathy. *Lancet* 2007; 370: 1672–4.

Jager A, Sleijfer S, van der Rijt CC. The pathogenesis of cancer-related fatigue: could increased activity of pro-inflammatory cytokines be the common denominator? *Eur J Cancer* 2008; 44: 175–81.

Jones LW, Demark-Wahnefried W. Diet, exercise, and complementary therapies after primary treatment for cancer. *Lancet Oncol* 2006; 7: 1017–26.

Kalso E, Aldington DJ, Moore RA *et al.* Drugs for neuropathic pain. *Brit Med J* 2013; 347: f7339.

Katz, N. *Opioid Prescribing Toolkit*. Oxford University Press, 2011. ISBN 978-0-19-978236-9.

Laird MA, Gidal BE. Use of gabapentin in the treatment of neuropathic pain. *Ann Pharmacother* 2000; 34: 802–7.

Laviano A, Mequid MM, Rossi-Fanelli F *et al.* Cancer anorexia: clinical implications, pathogenesis, and therapeutic strategies. *Lancet Oncol* 2003; 4: 686–94.

Laviano A, Meguid MM, Inui A *et al.* Therapy insight: cancer anorexia–cachexia syndrome. *Nat Clin Pract Oncol* 2005; 2: 158–65.

Lee H, Schmidt K, Ernst E. Acupuncture for the relief of cancer-related pain: a systematic review. *Eur J Pain* 2005; 9: 437–44.

Lieb J. The multifaceted value of antidepressants in cancer therapeutics. *Eur J Cancer* 2008; 44: 172–4.

Mannix K. Palliation of cancer-related nausea and vomiting. *Br J Cancer Management* 2006; 2: 20–3.

Patrick DL, Ferketich SL, Frame PS *et al.* National Institutes of Health State-of-the-Science Conference Statement: Symptom Management in Cancer: Pain, Depression and Fatigue, 15–17 July 2002. *J Natl Cancer Inst* 2003; 95: 1110–17.

Pittrof R, Rubenstein I. The thinking doctor's guide to placebos. *Br Med J* 2008; 336: 1020.

Raja SN, Haythornthwaite JA. Combination therapy for neuropathic pain: which drugs, which combination, which patients? *N Engl J Med* 2005; 352: 1373–5.

Roos DR, Fisher RJ. Radiotherapy for painful bone metastases: an overview of the overviews. *Clin Oncol* 2003; 15: 342–4.

Saarto T, Wiffen PJ. Antidepressants for neuropathic pain. *Cochrane Database Syst Rev* 2005; 3: CD005454.

Wallace WHB, Anderson RA, Irvine DS. Fertility preservation for young patients with cancer: who is at risk and what can be offered? *Lancet Oncol* 2005; 6: 209–18.

Werneke U, Earl J, Seydel C *et al*. Potential health risks of complementary alternative medicines in cancer patients. *Br J Cancer* 2004; 90: 408–13.

Wong GY, Schroeder DR, Carns PE *et al*. Effects of neurolytic coeliac plexus block on pain relief, quality of life, and survival in patients with unresectable pancreatic cancer: a randomised controlled trial. *JAMA* 2004; 291: 1092–9.

World Health Organization. *Cancer Pain Relief, With a Guide to Opioid Availability*, 2nd edn. Geneva: WHO, 1996.

8 Medical problems and radiotherapy emergencies

Acute and often life-threatening medical problems may arise as a result of cancer and its treatment. Iatrogenic deaths occur because many treatments, particularly intensive chemotherapy, are inherently very dangerous. Nevertheless, the majority of deaths are avoidable. The risks are minimized if patients are managed in specialized cancer units with staff skilled in anticipating, avoiding and managing these problems.

Bone marrow failure and its consequences

Cytotoxic drugs damage the reproductive integrity of cells. Bone marrow haemopoietic cells are among the most rapidly dividing cells in the body and are extremely sensitive to the action of most antineoplastic agents.

Some drugs, for example, vincristine and bleomycin, produce only slight bone marrow depression, while the majority of cytotoxic agents impair haemopoiesis. With drugs such as doxorubicin, myelosuppression is one of the major toxicities. Cytotoxic agents affect different proliferative compartments within the marrow. This leads to nonuniform patterns of toxicity even within the same class of cytotoxic agent. For example, cyclophosphamide, administered as a single intravenous injection, causes predictable granulocytopenia 4–7 days later, with a less marked effect on platelet count. In contrast, melphalan and busulfan produce slower marrow suppression with onset at 7–8 days and maximum depression of white cell count at about 2–3 weeks. Nitrosoureas such as cis-chloroethyl nitrosourea (CCNU) characteristically exert a delayed effect on the blood count at about 4–5 weeks. The reason for these differences is unknown and

Cancer and its Management, Seventh Edition. Jeffrey Tobias and Daniel Hochhauser.
© 2015 John Wiley & Sons, Ltd. Published 2015 by John Wiley & Sons, Ltd.

is not explained by the known chemical reactivity of the drugs. For example, carboplatin regularly causes bone marrow suppression, while cisplatin does not do so to the same degree. These differential patterns of action exphasize how oversimplified is the view that the action of, for example, alkylating agents is in some sense non-specific in the cellular damage they cause.

The speed of onset and the severity with which the marrow is affected also depends on dose and timing of drug administration. Although the platelet count does not fall significantly with cyclophosphamide given in conventional doses, it will do so at much higher doses. Similarly, although neutropenia and thrombocytopenia usually occur at 4–5 weeks after CCNU administration in conventional doses, at very high doses, such as those which have been used experimentally in the treatment of brain tumours, an earlier onset of neutropenia and thrombocytopenia may occur, occasionally as early as 4–5 days after the drug has been given.

Although some agents (melphalan, busulfan, CCNU) may cause prolonged marrow suppression even when given on the first occasion, in a patient receiving intermittent cytotoxic chemotherapy for the first time the marrow depression is usually transient and the blood count normal in 2–3 weeks, when the next cycle can be given. With increasing duration of chemotherapy, however, the proliferative compartments in the marrow may become progressively more depleted and the nadir of the white cell count then becomes lower and recovery less rapid, so that chemotherapy cycles may have to be delayed or the dose reduced. In order to avoid life-threatening marrow suppression a familiarity with the cytotoxic regimen is essential, and the physician must be aware of the likelihood of increasing marrow depression with time.

However, experienced the clinician may be, marrow depression sometimes occurs unexpectedly. With some treatment regimens – for example, during the induction of remission in acute myeloblastic leukaemia, or with the use of very high-dose chemotherapy in some solid tumours – pancytopenia is an inevitable consequence of treatment.

Granulocytopenia is symptomatic only when infection supervenes. There is usually fever, malaise, shaking and chills, sometimes accompanied by oral ulceration. If the platelet count is severely depressed, the patient may develop epistaxis or purpura. It is unusual for symptoms of anaemia to occur acutely even if erythropoiesis ceases altogether, because the half-life of red cells (25 days) is such that the haemoglobin does not usually fall appreciably after a single treatment before recovery has occurred.

The management of marrow depression by blood component therapy
Blood transfusion

Many patients undergoing combination intermittent chemotherapy for solid tumours gradually develop moderate anaemia, with a haemoglobin level of 10–12 g/dL. The blood count will recover when treatment is discontinued, and transfusion [1] is not usually required unless the haemoglobin falls below 9 g/dL. In deciding whether to transfuse a patient, the symptoms of anaemia (fatigue, malaise and breathlessness) must be balanced against the risks of transfusion, in particular volume overload in elderly patients. In the presence of thrombocytopenia, a transfusion can precipitate episodes of bleeding, particularly intracerebral haemorrhage. For this reason, many physicians prefer to use a platelet transfusion before giving blood or packed cells in severely thrombocytopenic patients.

Many patients with advanced malignant disease become anaemic due to an effect of the tumour itself or to marrow infiltration (e.g. in myeloma, leukaemia or widespread bone secondaries). This occurs even when patients are not having treatment with chemotherapy or radiotherapy. Even if no active treatment for the tumour is planned, a patient may gain symptomatic relief from blood transfusion. Precise guidelines cannot be drawn, but in general, transfusion should be considered only if the haemoglobin falls below 9 g/dL or if, above that level, there are symptoms that can be attributed to the anaemia.

Platelet transfusion

The risk of bleeding is related to the platelet count and rises sharply below 20×10^9/L. Ecchymosis and purpura are then characteristically found in pressure areas and on the shins. Major bleeding is life-threatening and intracerebral haemorrhage is often fatal.

Transfused platelets have a half-life of only a few days. Platelets have a variety of surface antigens, including human leucocyte antigens. Repeated transfusion may be accompanied by immunization against these antigens, with the result that further platelet transfusions lead to rapid platelet destruction and a failure to elevate the platelet count. Nevertheless, platelet transfusion has been a major factor in decreasing the morbidity of intensive chemotherapy regimens and most patients can be protected during periods of hypoplasia without serious haemorrhage [2].

There is no single level of platelet count at which transfusion should be given. Platelet transfusion is rarely required at counts above 30×10^9/L. Indications for platelet transfusion are as follows.

1 A rapidly falling platelet count following the start of intensive chemotherapy in which it can be predicted that circulating platelets will fall below 20×10^9/L within a 24-hour period. This is particularly important when making arrangements for the care of patients at weekends. The trend of the platelet count will help in deciding if a further transfusion will soon be necessary.

2 If there is evidence of bleeding (such as widespread ecchymoses, epistaxis or gastrointestinal bleeding), platelet transfusion is essential, even at levels higher than 30×10^9/L.

3 Platelet transfusions are sometimes necessary at higher levels of platelet count ($>30 \times 10^9$/L) if there are other complicating factors such as anaemia, peptic ulceration or infection which predispose to bleeding.

Occasionally, patients will become refractory to platelet transfusions, with little or no rise in platelet count. Fever, infection and splenomegaly may all contribute to this, but the usual cause is immunization to platelet antigens. This can be avoided by using HLA-matched donors, generally obtained from the patient's family. In immunized patients a rise in platelet count can sometimes be produced by the use of corticosteroids.

Haemopoietic growth factors [3]

Short-term cultures of human bone marrow cells have allowed identification of progenitor cells that form colonies and whose growth is dependent on colony-stimulating factors. The progenitor cells may form cells of several lineages but they are not the self-renewing stem cells (detected in mouse spleen colony-forming assays). Cloning of the genes of these colony-stimulating factors has led to the characterization of many of these molecules, many of which are interleukins. Colony-stimulating factors are glycoproteins, are active at extremely low concentrations, and may stimulate a variety of functions in marrow precursor and mature cells. The chromosomal location and source of the factors are shown in Table 8.1.

The colony-stimulating factors bind to specific high-affinity receptors on the target cell. Granulocyte colony-stimulating factor (G-CSF) and macrophage colony-stimulating factor (M-CSF) stimulate the late stages of division and the differentiation of the granulocyte and macrophage lineage, respectively, and affect the function of mature cells. Other factors such as granulocyte/macrophage colony-stimulating

Table 8.1 Haemopoietic growth factors: chromosomal location and cellular source.

Factor	Molecular weight (kDa)	Chromosome	Source
Glycoprotein			
G-CSF	18	17q11.2–21	Monocytes, endothelium
M-CSF	40–50	5q23–31	Monocytes, T cells, endothelium
GM-CSF	14–35	5q23–31	Monocytes, T cells
Endothelium			
Erythropoietin	36	7q11–22	Renal peritubular cells, macrophages
IL-3	14–28	5q23–31	T cells

factor (GM-CSF) stimulate several cell lineages earlier in differentiation. GM-CSF also increases neutrophil phagocytosis of bacteria and yeasts. Interleukin (IL)-1 and IL-6 act on early progenitor cells, stimulating cell division and making cells more sensitive to GM-CSF, G-CSF and M-CSF by increasing the number of surface receptors. The earlier return of the white cell count may allow increased intensity of chemotherapy and possibly improve results of treatment. This has not yet been shown to occur in any chemocurable cancer. This important area is comprehensively discussed in a recent report by Bennett *et al.* [4].

Clinical use of haemopoietic growth factors
Granulocyte colony-stimulating factor

G-CSF has been shown to hasten the return of the neutrophil count with conventional myelosuppressive chemotherapy [5] and after autologous bone marrow transplantation (BMT). The platelet count is unaffected. G-CSF has become widely and rather uncritically used in cancer therapy. Before using G-CSF the physician should decide whether it is wise or necessary to use chemotherapy at a dose that will dangerously depress the white cell count. This is clearly not the case for palliative treatment. Using drugs intensively can only be justified if the cure rate is thereby increased. G-CSF may then have a role in improving treatment. There is no place for its routine use, the more so since it is very expensive and inconvenient. G-CSF is used when severe neutropenia has occurred, especially if accompanied by infection. It is used prophylactically when previous cycles have caused severe neutropenia.

Granulocyte/macrophage colony-stimulating factor

GM-CSF causes a rise in granulocyte and platelet count in patients not receiving chemotherapy. It accelerates recovery following conventional chemotherapy and after autologous BMT. Fever and thrombophlebitis are side-effects. Despite the more rapid recovery of the blood count, length of hospital stay and mortality do not appear to be reduced during autologous BMT. In patients undergoing combined radiotherapy and chemotherapy for small-cell lung cancer (SCLC) the use of GM-CSF was associated with more severe thrombocytopenia [6].

Erythropoietin

Anaemia due to malignant disease will improve with recombinant human erythropoietin, resulting in amelioration of quality of life. Erythropoietin has been shown to diminish the degree of anaemia and transfusion requirements in patients undergoing intensive chemotherapy for SCLC, and to decrease the period of transfusion dependence after allogeneic marrow transplantation [7]. A new form with more sialic acid side-chains has a much longer half-life, allowing once weekly administration. Erythropoietin is expensive and its routine use in mild anaemia is not justified. There are also emerging concerns about potential negative impact on survival in solid tumours.

Infections in the immunocompromised patient

Infections are a major cause of death in cancer. They not only occur frequently but also are often more severe than in other patients, less responsive to therapy and sometimes produced by organisms which are not pathogens in healthy people. This susceptibility results from depression of host defence mechanisms produced by the tumour and its treatment.

The skin and mucosal surfaces are a barrier to infection. Tumour infiltration and local radiotherapy may lead to damage to lymphatic or venous drainage, with resulting susceptibility to local infection. The turnover of gastrointestinal epithelial cells is depressed by chemotherapy, leading to mucosal damage and ulceration, which allows gut organisms to escape into the portal system. The skin is breached by intravenous needles and cannulae, especially tunnelled subcutaneous lines. These are frequently sources of infection with skin organisms such as *Staphylococcus epidermidis*. Nasogastric tubes act as a focus for infection with *Candida albicans*.

Advanced cancer is sometimes associated with reduced function of both neutrophils and monocytes. Depressions of chemotactic, phagocytic and bactericidal activity have all been described.

Impaired delayed hypersensitivity is common in advanced untreated Hodgkin's disease but less common in other malignancies. Lymphopenia is an invariable accompaniment of treatment with alkylating agents and extensive radiotherapy. Cell-mediated immunity is particularly important in host defence against fungi, viruses, tuberculosis and protozoa. Intensive cytotoxic chemotherapy leads to impaired production of antibody to bacterial and viral antigens.

Circulating bacteria are cleared by the phagocytic cells lining the sinuses of the reticuloendothelial system, especially in the liver and spleen. Antibody and complement are important for this clearance. Splenectomy increases the risk of severe bacterial infection, especially pneumococcal septicaemia in young children and to a lesser extent in adults [8].

Bacteraemia and septicaemia

Bloodstream infections are particularly frequent in granulocytopenic patients [9]. Gram-negative bacteria (*Escherichia coli*, *Pseudomonas aeruginosa*), staphylococci and streptococci are frequent pathogens. Infections with Gram-positive bacteria have increased in frequency, especially *Staphylococcus epidermidis*. Patients with tunnelled subcutaneous lines are prone to infection with this organism. Fever in a neutropenic cancer patient is an indication for blood cultures, and cultures through the subcutaneous line. If there is an obvious source of infection such as infected infusion sites, cultures should be taken and the cannula removed. Treatment should not be delayed in the neutropenic patient. These patients should be admitted to hospital. Recent trials have indicated that oral amoxicillin–clavulanate combined with oral ciprofloxacin is as effective as intravenous chemotherapy in this group (70% of all patients). The high-risk patients (with uncontrolled cancer or inpatients on intensive therapy) are treated with intravenous antibiotics that include a β-lactam and an aminoglycoside, or ceftazidime.

Table 8.2 Causes of fever and pulmonary infiltration in immunocompromised patients.

Bacteria: *Streptococcus pneumoniae*
Gram-negative organisms: mycobacteria, *Legionella*
Fungi: *Aspergillus, Candida, Cryptococcus*
Viruses: cytomegalovirus, herpes simplex, measles
Protozoa: *Pneumocystis*
Treatment: cytotoxic drugs, radiation pneumonitis

Respiratory infection

Fever with pulmonary infiltration is a common occurrence in the severely immunocompromised patient. The major causes are given in Table 8.2. The difficulties in making a diagnosis can be considerable because sputum and blood cultures may be negative, and more invasive procedures such as transbronchial biopsy may be impossible because of thrombocytopenia or the general condition of the patient.

There are some clinical features that are helpful in diagnosis. Cavitation is more common with anaerobic bacteria, staphylococci and mycobacteria. *Pneumocystis* infection causes marked dyspnoea, and the chest radiograph shows bilateral infiltrates typically radiating from the hilum. However, the disease may be indolent, and can cause lobar consolidation. Cytomegalovirus (CMV) infection mainly occurs in severely immunodepressed patients, particularly during allogeneic BMT. The disease may also cause myocarditis, neuropathy and ophthalmitis. The pulmonary infiltrate is usually bilateral. *Candida* infection can cause a wide variety of radiographic changes. There is often *Candida* infection elsewhere. Panophthalmitis may occur and the organism can sometimes be isolated from the blood. *Aspergillus* infection is usually rapidly progressive in these patients. Blood cultures are usually negative and the infiltrate can be in one or both lungs. Faced with this diagnostic uncertainty, the following scheme can be adopted.

In patients without neutropenia or thrombocytopenia, investigate with blood cultures, sputum culture, bronchoscopic washings and transbronchial biopsy, where possible. If blood and sputum cultures are negative, treat with broad-spectrum bactericidal antibiotics (usually with an aminoglycoside, penicillin and metronidazole or an equivalent combination). If *Pneumocystis* is a possible cause, high-dose co-trimoxazole should be given. If there is no response, consider aciclovir for herpes simplex infection and antifungal therapy with amphotericin or ketoconazole. Aciclovir is not effective against CMV.

If blood or sputum cultures are positive treat as appropriate, but if there is no response, consider a mixed infection.

In patients with neutropenia or thrombocytopenia, bronchoscopy can be carried out, but biopsy may not be possible and treatment may have to proceed along the lines indicated above without further diagnostic investigation. Before and after bronchoscopy, antibiotics and platelet transfusion may be necessary.

Urinary tract infections

Infection is common in patients with obstruction to outflow, particularly from the bladder. Obstruction may be by tumour or due to an atonic bladder in a patient with cord compression. Diagnosis is made by urine culture, and treatment is with antibiotics and relief of obstruction if possible.

Gastrointestinal infections

Oral thrush (infection with *Candida albicans*) is a frequent complication of chemotherapy. It is particularly likely to occur in immunosuppressed patients, in patients on steroids and in those treated with broad-spectrum antibiotics. The mouth and pharynx become very sore and white plaques of fungus are visible on an erythematous base. The infection may penetrate more deeply in some malnourished patients and extend down into the oesophagus, stomach and bowel. Oral nystatin, amphotericin or miconazole are usually effective.

Herpes simplex cold sores are often troublesome in leucopenic patients, and the lesions may become very widespread. Treatment is with aciclovir, given topically for minor infections in immunosuppressed patients and systemically for more serious infections.

Candida infection in the oesophagus requires treatment with oral nystatin suspension, but if this is ineffective treat with ketoconazole or a short course of amphotericin. *Candida* infections of the bowel should be treated with amphotericin.

Perianal infections are common in neutropenic patients. Preventive measures should always be employed, with scrupulous perineal hygiene and stool softeners to prevent constipation and anal fissures. Spreading perineal infection can be a life-threatening event, and urgent treatment with intravenous antibiotics active against Gram-negative and anaerobic bacilli is required.

Meningitis

Central nervous system (CNS) infections are rare, but patients with lymphoma or leukaemia occasionally develop meningitis due to *Cryptococcus neoformans*. The onset is insidious with headache. The organism can be detected by India ink staining of the cerebrospinal fluid (CSF). Detection of *Cryptococcus* antigen in blood and CSF is possible in most patients. Many patients will improve with amphotericin and some will be cured.

Skin infections

Apart from infection introduced at infusion sites the most common skin infection is shingles (varicella zoster). This infection, which is due to reactivation of varicella zoster virus in dorsal root ganglia, is a dermatomal vesicular eruption that is particularly severe in immunocompromised hosts and which may disseminate as chickenpox and cause fatal pneumonia. Patients should be treated with aciclovir as early as possible.

Prevention of infection in the leucopenic patient

When a patient is leucopenic, reverse barrier nursing procedures are usually used. For most episodes of granulocytopenia, disposable aprons, face masks and careful washing of hands is probably satisfactory. For a more persistent type of leucopenia (e.g. with allogeneic BMT) a protected environment has much to commend it. Here the air is filtered free of bacteria and a laminar airflow is established from one end of the room to the other. The patients are 'decontaminated' before entry with oral antibiotics, to kill intestinal bacteria, and cutaneous antiseptic cleansing. Protected environments can lower the infection rate but their contribution to overall reduction in mortality is small since the hazards of the disease and other effects of treatment are greater. The psychological stress and cost of isolation are other major disadvantages. Other important preventive measures are scrupulous hygiene in the placing of intravenous drugs, perineal hygiene and high standards of staff training.

Antibiotic prophylaxis has been studied extensively [10]. Several randomized trials have shown that ciprofloxacin is effective in preventing infection with Gram-negative organisms in neutropenic patients. The combination of ciprofloxacin and rifampicin with vancomycin has been shown to be effective prophylaxis in stem cell transplantation. However, bacterial strains resistant to ciprofloxacin are now beginning to occur in the community.

Prophylactic use of antibiotics has been shown to reduce the incidence of fungal infections in patients undergoing BMT. Fluconazole has been widely used; it reduces the frequency of *Candida* infection and is as effective as amphotericin in leukaemia induction treatment.

Aciclovir is effective in preventing varicella zoster in patients undergoing BMT and stem cell transplantation or those who are in the recovery period. High-dose aciclovir and ganciclovir are also effective prophylactics for CMV. In patients undergoing very intensive therapy, prophylaxis with co-trimoxazole (trimethoprim/sulfamethoxazole) helps prevent *Pneumocystis carinii* infection. Recent work has underscored still further the recurring problem of CMV infection in patients who have undergone allogeneic bone marrow transplants for leukaemia, lymphoma or other disorders. The use of antiviral agents has been limited by frequent toxic effects and also the emergence of resistance, but an important US-based study has outlined the value of oral CMX001, a lipid acyclic nucleoside phosphonate. It was given at the generally tolerable dose of 100 mgm twice weekly, in a group of 230 patients randomized to receive CMX001 or placebo, with patients stratified by the presence or absence of graft-versus-host disease and CMV DNA in plasma – see Ref. [11]. Treated patients had a significantly reduced incidence of CMV-related events, when the agent was given from about 3 – 12 weeks after transplantation, an important step forward in a difficult and challenging clinical situation.

Cancer cachexia and the nutritional support of the cancer patient

Cachexis is a condition associated with a variety of illnesses including cancer, AIDS and congestive heart failure [12]. Clinical symptoms include weight loss (both adipose tissue and skeletal muscle), wasting and progressive weakness. Weight loss is of course a common symptom of cancer, but profound and rapid weight loss usually indicates disseminated tumour. When cancer recurs and is widespread, loss of weight is an almost invariable accompaniment. This leads finally to the cachectic state in which the patient becomes wasted, weak and lethargic [13].

Molecular pathways resulting in cachexia are beginning to be understood. Various factors are released by both tumour cells and immune effector cells responding to the tumour, and current research suggests that inflammatory

Table 8.3 Weight loss in cancer.

Reduced intake
Anorexia/cachexia syndrome
Treatment-induced effects: anorexia, nausea, oral ulceration
Depression and anxiety

Nutrient malabsorption
Gut surgery
Gut toxicity from radiation or drugs
Bowel obstruction
Malabsorption syndrome: obstructive jaundice, pancreatic
  carcinoma

Loss of protein and nutrients
Diarrhoea
Ulceration of the gut mucosa by tumours
Gut mucositis (drugs and X-rays)

Metabolic changes induced by tumour
Increased protein and fat metabolism
Altered glucose metabolism induced by tumour
Tumour consumption of carbohydrate and protein

cytokines such as tumour necrosis factor (TNF)-α, IL-1β and interferon (IFN)-γ may all be important [14].

Pathogenesis of malnutrition in cancer

Anorexia is a major factor in reducing food intake (Table 8.3). The nausea and vomiting of chemotherapy are evident causes, as is depression and anxiety. However, the mechanism of tumour-induced anorexia and cachexia is poorly understood. It frequently accompanies widespread disease, in particular, the presence of hepatic metastases. Typically the patient loses all interest in food and has an altered perception of taste and smell such that the thought of eating can become repugnant.

Nutrient malabsorption may be due to mechanical causes such as surgical resection (partial gastrectomy or major gut resection) or gut obstruction, or be due to mucosal damage by drugs or radiation. Tumours ulcerating the gut and mucosal damage by treatment cause loss of blood and protein. Metabolic abnormalities have been found in advanced cancer but there is no uniform abnormality that is always present in cachectic individuals.

Maintaining nutrition

In considering nutritional support for an individual cancer patient, the objectives of treatment must be clear.

If a potentially curative treatment is being considered, with surgery, chemotherapy or radiotherapy, effective nutritional support will usually improve the tolerance of treatment. Well-nourished cancer patients frequently lose weight as a result of cancer treatment, whether with surgery, chemotherapy or radiotherapy. If the effects of radical treatment are likely to persist over a week or more, and considerable weight loss can be anticipated, it is probable that nutritional supplements will decrease morbidity. If there is no prospect of cure, then nutritional support is a palliative procedure. Aggressive and uncomfortable means of maintaining nutrition are then completely inappropriate. There is no evidence at present that the progressive malnutrition and wasting which accompany advanced and incurable cancer can be reversed by any form of feeding. Every cancer patient should have an assessment of weight loss and appetite. If there has been loss of more than 10% body weight it is advisable to have a dietitian's advice in developing a plan for nutritional support.

Enteral nutrition

Attention to diet and to the foods available to the patient is of great importance. This involves discussions with the patient about favourite foods. Dietary advice from a dietitian and the support of the family in providing favourite foods are an essential part of the plan. Small but frequent meals are often helpful. Nutritional supplements can be added to the patient's diet, including high-calorie liquids such as Hycal and more complete protein and carbohydrate mixtures (e.g. Complan or Clinifeed). Protein hydrolysates, providing small peptides and amino acid fragments, are also available (Vivonex). They provide calories in liquid form at a time when the patient finds it difficult to eat solid food. They can cause osmotic disturbances and for many patients they are quite unpalatable. Appetite stimulants such as medroxyprogesterone acetate and dexamethasone may be helpful in the short term.

Occasionally a patient may find it difficult to swallow or eat at all. Enteral support with liquid dietary supplements can be given by using a fine-bore flexible nasogastric feeding tube or by per-endoscopic gastrostomy feeding. The latter has been widely used in cancer of the head and neck, and of the oesophagus. The aim is to provide about 2000–3000 kcal/day. These supplements have a high osmolality. They can cause nausea and diarrhoea and provide a large solute load for renal excretion. Large amounts of fluid are required to excrete this solute load, even in the presence of normal renal function.

Total parenteral nutrition

Adequate calorific support can be given intravenously for patients who cannot take food by mouth or by nasogastric tube, and this approach is now increasingly employed as oncology units have become more aggressive both in the active treatment and support of patients undergoing cancer chemotherapy. Access is through a catheter placed in a deep vein, since parenteral nutritional solutions are an irritant. The incidence of venous thrombosis when catheters are inserted into the subclavian vein is small. With all subcutaneous catheters there is a risk of infection, which is particularly likely to occur in the immunocompromised individual. A variety of synthetic total parenteral nutrition solutions are available commercially, usually consisting of amino acid solutions with dextrose, vitamins, electrolytes and trace elements.

Several of the metabolic defects present in the malnourished patient can be reversed by total parenteral nutrition. Although it is difficult to demonstrate benefit, it is sometimes justifiable to support a patient with parenteral nutrition during intensive but potentially curative treatment. This includes patients undergoing major gastrointestinal surgery, or chemotherapy with marrow ablation. Total parenteral nutrition is complex, expensive and potentially hazardous. It is of no proven value as a routine measure in patients undergoing cancer therapies though as mentioned above, may be extremely valuable in highly selected cases where aggressive chemotherapy is justified in difficult circumstances, in the grossly undernourished patient.

Acute metabolic disturbances

Hypercalcaemia

Raised plasma calcium is a frequent accompaniment of cancer. In a hospital population, carcinomas of the bronchus, breast and kidney are, together with multiple myeloma, the commonest malignant causes of hypercalcaemia. Life-threatening hypercalcaemia is usually due to cancer. Minor elevations of plasma calcium (up to 2.8 mmol/L) are not usually associated with any symptoms. As the plasma calcium rises, patients experience anorexia, nausea, abdominal pain, constipation and fatigue. There may be proximal muscle weakness, polyuria and polydipsia. With increasing hypercalcaemia, severe dehydration, confusion and finally coma may supervene.

Bone metastases are much the commonest cause of hypercalcaemia in cancer. Most patients with severe hypercalcaemia have demonstrable metastases on radiography or on bone scanning. Bone marrow aspiration may show infiltration with tumour. Even if metastases are not detectable at presentation, they usually quickly become apparent. Metastases in bone stimulate osteoclast activity by the local release of parathyroid hormone (PTH)-related protein (PTHrP). The bone resorption liberates factors such as transforming growth factor (TGF)-α, TGF-β, epidermal growth factor, and IL-1 (α and β forms) [15]. These factors may not only act locally to cause bone resorption but may also, in the case of breast cancer, cause further release of PTHrP from tumour cells.

In addition to direct bone lysis by metastases, cancers may produce hypercalcaemia by remote, humoral mechanisms – the syndrome of humoral hypercalcaemia of malignancy. The syndrome is largely due to circulating PTHrP released from the tumour but other cytokines may also play a part, especially in lymphoma and myeloma. The protein has striking homology to PTH in the first 13 amino acids but differs in the remainder. Alternatively spliced forms of mRNA may yield two or more different proteins. Most squamous carcinomas express the protein (whether the patient is hypercalcaemic or not). Its metabolic effect is similar to PTH, with increased bone reabsorption of calcium.

The treatment of hypercalcaemia in cancer may be a medical emergency, particularly in the elderly and in patients with myeloma. Hypokalaemia may also accompany hypercalcaemia, and may in part be due to a renal loss of potassium. Elderly patients, and those with impaired renal function, are unable to withstand the effects of the raised plasma calcium, and life-threatening renal failure may quickly develop. In myeloma, it is particularly likely to occur since other causes of renal failure are present (see Chapter 27).

In severe hypercalcaemia, the first line of treatment is salt and water replacement using isotonic saline. In the first 24 hours, 4–8 L may be required. This may be sufficient to lower the plasma calcium to normal. In the elderly, care must be taken not to overload the patient with fluids. If the plasma calcium does not begin to fall within 24 hours, prednisolone given orally (30–60 mg/day) or hydrocortisone intravenously (50–100 mg 6-hourly) is often helpful in reducing the calcium, but not all patients will respond. Furosemide (frusemide) promotes calciuresis but care must be taken with volume replacement, to avoid further salt and water depletion.

Bisphosphonates reduce serum calcium by inhibiting bone resorption and are effective in hypercalcaemia due to metastases or PTHrP. Pamidronate is effective in

90% of patients. A dose of 60–90 mg given in a 2-hour infusion is the usual procedure. It can be repeated every 2–3 weeks. Mild fever and skin irritation can occur, and it is preferable to use bisphosphonates after rehydration since temporary renal impairment can occur. Etidronate seems rather less effective; it is usually given as three infusions of 7.5 mg/kg. Clodronate in a dose of five daily infusions of 300 mg restores normocalcaemia in 90% of cases. Oral clodronate can be given (1600 mg/day) but causes gastrointestinal upset.

Mithramycin has been largely replaced by the bisphosphonates. A single injection usually causes a fall in plasma calcium after 24–48 hours. Occasionally it may be necessary to use mithramycin on two or three successive days. This carries a risk of thrombocytopenia.

Intravenous or oral phosphate therapy is seldom necessary to control the plasma calcium, but phosphate infusions (usually with serum calcium of 4 mmol/L or more) may be helpful in patients who are gravely ill.

Calcitonin produces a more rapid fall in the plasma calcium but its effect is variable and its use is limited to patients with severe acute hypercalcaemia.

Although it is not usually difficult to diagnose the cause of malignant hypercalcaemia, diagnostic problems can occur when hyperparathyroidism is an alternative diagnosis in cancer patients who do not have evidence of disseminated disease. The steroid suppression test will not reduce the plasma calcium in hyperparathyroidism, but 75% of patients with cancer show a fall after 10 days of hydrocortisone administration. If serious doubt remains, elevation of plasma PTH is found in 80% of patients with primary hyperparathyroidism, but not in patients with cancer.

Tumour lysis syndrome

An acute metabolic disturbance may occur as a result of the rapid dissolution of tumour following chemotherapy. This is particularly likely to occur in children with Burkitt's lymphoma or acute lymphoblastic leukaemia, and in non-Hodgkin's lymphomas in children, adolescents and young adults. The syndrome occurs when there is extreme sensitivity of the tumour to treatment, and is uncommon in adults with non-lymphoid neoplasms. When it occurs, tumour masses may disappear very rapidly, and as the cells are killed they release products of nitrogen metabolism, especially urea, urate and large amounts of phosphate.

The rapid reduction in tumour mass causes hyperuricaemia, hyperphosphataemia, hyperkalaemia and uraemia. Hyperuricaemia may result in acute urate deposition in the renal tubules (urate nephropathy), leading to acute renal failure or, less dramatically, to reduction in glomerular filtration rate that exacerbates the hyperuricaemia. Occasionally, the syndrome can be sufficiently severe to cause an acute and prolonged uraemia. Hyperphosphataemia results in a reciprocal lowering of the plasma calcium and can result in tetany.

The syndrome is more likely to occur in children with Burkitt's lymphoma who have extensive disease, particularly if there are intra-abdominal masses, impaired renal function from tumour infiltration of the kidney or postrenal obstruction due to lymph node enlargement. The syndrome is rare in adults since the tumours are generally less sensitive to chemotherapy, and their dissolution less rapid. It may, however, occur if there is coincidental renal failure due to some other cause, ureteric obstruction or infiltration of the kidney with tumour.

Tumour lysis syndrome is usually preventable. Before beginning chemotherapy in a high-risk patient, allopurinol should be given (usually by mouth) in full dose (50–100 mg 8-hourly in children, twice this dose in adults) for 24 hours. This xanthine oxidase inhibitor partly prevents the formation of uric acid. The precursors, xanthine and hypoxanthine, are, therefore, present in great excess but are much more soluble than uric acid and do not cause nephropathy. Allopurinol should be continued for the first few days of treatment and discontinued when the plasma urate is in the normal range. If 6-mercaptopurine is being given the dose should be reduced since allopurinol inhibits its metabolism. At the same time, the patient should be given adequate fluids, usually in the form of intravenous saline, to establish a good diuresis. These measures should prevent both hyperuricaemia and hyperphosphataemia. In Burkitt's lymphoma, the induction chemotherapy is sometimes given at reduced dose until there has been considerable tumour shrinkage and then the full dose is administered. Allopurinol should be given to adults with high-grade lymphoma starting treatment with intensive chemotherapy; its use should be considered in other cases if there is any possibility of renal impairment.

If hyperuricaemia and acute renal failure develop, these can usually be treated by cessation of chemotherapy, cautious administration of intravenous fluids with alkalinization of the urine to promote urate excretion, and allopurinol. If the blood urea and plasma urate continue to rise, peritoneal dialysis may be needed to tide the patient over the acute renal failure. If preventive measures are taken, this should rarely be necessary.

An excellent recent review by Gemici [16] gives further details of aetiology, prevention and management.

Serous effusions

Many patients with cancer develop a pleural or pericardial effusion or ascites during the course of their illness. These can be difficult to treat and can be a major cause of discomfort and breathlessness. The effusions are exudates caused by the presence of tumour on the serosal surface. It is not clear how the increased permeability occurs. It is possible that it is due to factors produced by the tumour. The protein content is greater than 30 mg/L.

Pleural effusion [17]

Pleural fluid must reach a volume of about 500 mL before it can be detected clinically, although lesser degrees can be radiologically apparent. Typically the effusion is substantial in volume (1–4 L), accumulates rapidly, and may be blood-stained. It often causes dyspnoea with dry cough, sometimes with pleuritic chest pain. In addition to the fluid, there is usually a thick coating of malignant infiltrate on both pleural surfaces. The parietal layer can cause chest wall infiltration, pain and swelling. Although cytological demonstration of cells confirms the nature of the effusion, it is common for a malignant effusion to be repeatedly cytologically negative, in which case pleural biopsy will often be indicated if there is clinical doubt as to the diagnosis. However, pleural biopsy is only diagnostic in 50% of cases. Thoracoscopy increases the accuracy of biopsy, a diagnosis being made in 90% of cases of malignant disease. The malignant diseases causing pleural effusion (in descending frequency) are as follows: lung, breast and genitourinary cancers, lymphoma and gastrointestinal cancer.

Occasionally, patients with cancer develop a pleural effusion from a non-malignant cause, and alternative explanations should always be considered if a patient with apparently controlled cancer unexpectedly develops a pleural effusion.

Management is rarely straightforward. Most patients require therapeutic aspiration (thoracocentesis) to improve symptoms of cough and dyspnoea, and large volumes (1–5 L) may have to be removed for worthwhile benefit. The fluid often forms sealed-off collections (loculations), especially when recurrent after aspiration. These loculated areas may make control of the effusion difficult. In patients with secondary pleural deposits, chemotherapy or endocrine therapy will be given as primary treatment (e.g. in lymphoma or breast cancer). In these patients, this systemic treatment may prove effective in preventing reaccumulation of pleural fluid. In others, where effective systemic therapy is unavailable, the question of whether to instil an intrapleural sclerosant, to prevent or reduce fluid accumulation, will arise.

Pleurodesis using physical, antibiotic or bacterial sclerosants (talc, tetracycline, quinacrine or *Corynebacterium parvum*) and cytotoxic drugs (such as bleomycin) is common. Sclerosants depend on the production of an inflammatory reaction to obliterate the pleural space. Each is effective only in a proportion of case. Tetracycline can cause severe local pain, and bleomycin can cause fever and chills.

There are a few comparisons of one treatment with another. Instillation of talc (hydrated magnesium silicate) appears to provide the highest rate of control and is currently regarded as treatment of choice. One recent large-scale trial (over 550 patients recruited) of talc poudrage together with formal thoracoscopy [18] showed clearly how oxygen requirements after treatment can fall sharply, using this feature as an index of success. Talc can be instilled under local or general anaesthesia after the effusion has been drained to dryness, but it is undoubtedly a procedure requiring both experience and technical expertise. Control rates of 90% are achieved. Simpler but less taxing procedures, such as instillation of bleomycin, tetracycline or *C. parvum* can control up to 70% of effusions, and are indicated for patients whose condition is too poor for thoracoscopy. Occasionally, pleurectomy will be required for adequate control of an effusion due to pleural secondary deposits and should be considered if the patient's general condition warrants.

Pericardial effusion

This is an infrequent clinical problem and, in contrast to pleural effusion, pericardial effusions are less commonly due to malignancy than other causes such as infections, myxoedema, collagen disorders and rheumatoid arthritis. The diagnosis is often a radiological one, with 'globular' enlargement of the heart shadow. The clinical features are dyspnoea, orthopnoea, cough and central chest pain. The commonest signs are pulsus paradoxus, raised jugular venous pressure and hypotension. There may be a pleural rub, faint heart sounds and hepatomegaly. The diagnosis should be suspected in any patient with cancer who develops the rapid onset of unexplained breathlessness.

The commonest causes are carcinomas of breast and bronchus, and lymphoma including Hodgkin's disease.

In patients with widespread metastases, it may occur concurrently with a malignant pleural effusion. The diagnosis can be simply confirmed by echocardiography, which also gives useful quantitative information about the volume of the effusion. Because pericardial aspiration is both more hazardous and technically more difficult than pleural aspiration, it should not be undertaken in asymptomatic patients without expert cardiology advice.

Treatment is mainly with the same chemicals used for pleural effusion including cytotoxic drugs and tetracycline, but not talc. There may in addition be a useful response to systemic chemotherapy or endocrine therapy. The formation of a surgical 'pericardial window' into the mediastinum is often beneficial if the effusion is persistent. The operation can be performed, if necessary, under local anaesthesia and high local control rates are achieved [19].

Ascites

Ascites [20] is a common clinical problem in cancer. The usual cause is widespread peritoneal seedlings which cause exudation of fluid and diminish reabsorption by blocking lymphatic drainage. Liver metastases are often present, and hypoalbuminaemia contributes to the accumulation of fluid by lowering plasma osmotic pressure. Common cancers causing ascites include carcinomas of ovary, breast, bronchus (especially small cell), large bowel, stomach and pancreas, and melanoma.

Patients usually present with abdominal distension, bulging of the flanks and with peripheral oedema if there is associated hypoalbuminaemia and/or inferior vena caval obstruction. The umbilicus may be everted and some patients have a fluid thrill. It is important not to assume a malignant diagnosis, particularly when the tumour was previously thought to be localized or controlled by treatment. Important non-malignant causes include portal hypertension (usually from cirrhosis or portal vein thrombosis), hepatic vein thrombosis (Budd–Chiari syndrome), raised systemic venous pressure as in long-standing cardiac failure and hypoalbuminaemia from other causes.

Diagnosis is by clinical examination, abdominal ultrasound and aspiration cytology. Ultrasound examination is a sensitive technique for demonstrating ascites and associated tumour masses. Malignant cells may be detected cytologically, though this examination is negative in 50% of cases of proven malignancy.

Treatment includes both therapeutic aspiration (paracentesis) and general measures designed to prevent recurrence. Some patients will have control of ascites, at least for a while, using spironolactone (50 mg 8-hourly) with or without furosemide. Slow drainage over several days, via a peritoneal dialysis catheter, may be necessary to give relief of symptoms. Instillation of cytotoxic agents is less frequently practised and less frequently successful than in malignant pleural effusion, but intraperitoneal bleomycin, quinacrine and TNF have all been used. Systemic chemotherapy (or endocrine therapy in breast cancer) may occasionally help to control ascites in appropriately sensitive cancers.

Surgical procedures such as peritoneovenous (LeVeen and Denver) shunts can be helpful if the patient is likely to survive at least 3–6 months and is suffering repeated episodes of ascites. The initial success rate is about 70% but ascites almost always recurs after a few months. The prognosis for patients with malignant ascites is poor, the majority dying within 6 months of diagnosis.

Carcinomatous meningitis

This complication of cancer is increasingly recognized [21]. Its frequency is not known with certainty, but some estimates suggest that as many as 5% of patients with solid tumours will be affected. It is commoner in lymphoma and leukaemia than in solid tumours. It is most frequently found in breast cancer (especially the lobular subtype) and SCLC but may occur in any tumour, including melanomas.

The tumour cells line the meninges in sheets and nodules, and penetrate into the substance of the brain, tracking down blood vessels. A dense fibrotic reaction may occur which may cause additional ischaemic neurological damage. The tumour cells reach the meninges either by direct extension from an underlying intracerebral metastasis, or possibly by direct haematogenous spread.

The presenting features are very varied and the diagnosis should be considered in any unexplained neurological disturbance in a patient with cancer. Central symptoms are altered consciousness, confusion, dysphasia, headache and meningism. Cranial nerve involvement is frequent (50% of cases), the oculomotor and facial nerves being the most frequently affected. Individual spinal nerve roots are very frequently involved, causing weakness and sensory disturbance. More generalized long tract signs occur due to cord involvement.

Investigation should include computed tomography (CT) or preferably magnetic resonance imaging (MRI) with gadolinium enhancement, which is much more sensitive. The scans will also demonstrate hydrocephalus, which indicates that diagnostic lumbar puncture may be hazardous. MRI may show diffuse meningeal enhancement and focal deposits and nodules. In the spinal cord the investigation is less reliable, about 50% of cases showing a normal appearance.

Lumbar puncture will demonstrate tumour cells in most, but not all, cases. The sensitivity is increased by repeating the investigation if the first sample is abnormal but not diagnostic. CSF protein is usually raised and the glucose level is reduced in 50% of cases.

Treatment is essentially palliative and there are no absolute guidelines. Certain drugs are useful. Methotrexate concentrations are much higher when the drug is administered directly into the CSF. The half-life is about 12 hours and CSF drug concentrations have fallen to 0.1 μmol/L by 48 hours, when it is safe to repeat the dose. The drug is usually given two to three times per week. There are difficulties with repeated administration, especially in the presence of malignant infiltration, and the distribution of the drug is less certain than when it is given prophylactically. Side-effects include arachnoiditis, transient paralysis, headache and vomiting. The use of intraventricular reservoirs does not appear to improve outcome, although they are reasonably well tolerated and convenient. Cytosine arabinoside can also be given intrathecally, with high concentrations being achieved in normal CSF. It is subject to the same limitations as methotrexate when given in carcinomatous meningitis. The half-life in the CSF is approximately 3.5 hours, with a level of 1 μmol/L at 24 hours, below which the drug is not active. Thiotepa has been used in intrathecal treatment, but it is a prodrug whose intermediary metabolites are unknown. The usual regimens are twice weekly administration for 5 weeks and then weekly for 5 weeks.

Brain irradiation is often given, especially in those patients showing a response to intrathecal treatment. The usual regimen is 30 Gy in 10 fractions. Maintenance intrathecal treatment has not been shown to be of benefit, although, as with most aspects of treatment for this condition, there is a lack of data from randomized trials addressing this and other issues in management.

Patients treated with intrathecal therapy alone will often respond and survival may be improved. Dramatic responses may occur but are uncommon. The prognosis of carcinomatous meningitis remains very poor. The reported median survival is 6–12 weeks, but some patients survive much longer. Survival is worse in SCLC, in patients with widespread disease elsewhere, with poor previous performance status and with widespread neurological signs.

Progressive multifocal leucoencephalopathy

This rare syndrome is not always associated with cancer, but lymphoma is by far the commonest associated disorder. The clinical features are aphasia and dementia leading to coma, visual field loss (which may progress to blindness), fits and focal paralyses. The differential diagnosis includes metastases, lymphomatous meningitis, herpes encephalitis and cerebrovascular disease. The CSF is usually normal.

The brain shows patchy demyelination throughout the white matter with abnormal oligodendroglia, the nuclei of which contain viral inclusions. Papovaviruses (JC and SV40) have been isolated from these brains. Antibodies to these viruses may be present in blood or CSF and may help in diagnosis. The disease is usually fatal in 6–12 months, although some patients live for years. Responses to intrathecal and intravenous cytosine arabinoside have been reported.

Management of hepatic metastases

Many patients with cancer will develop hepatic metastases, and when these are widespread the expectation of life is only 2–3 months. In many cases there will be widespread dissemination and liver involvement will not be a separate medical problem. In some tumours such as small-cell carcinoma of the bronchus, breast cancer or lymphoma there is a reasonable likelihood of a response to chemotherapy, with symptomatic and biochemical improvement. There are, however, many occasions when the liver is involved with metastatic cancer, for which chemotherapy is inappropriate due to primary or acquired drug resistance.

The usual symptoms are fatigue, weight loss, anorexia and right upper quadrant pain. There may be abdominal distension from ascites. Episodes of sudden severe pain may occur when there is haemorrhage into a metastasis. Later, jaundice develops with advancing cachexia. Survival is usually a few months, depending on the extent of involvement and rate of progression. Metastatic carcinoid tumours may be very slow-growing, and in this disease hepatic metastases are compatible with survival of 3–5 years.

Almost all treatment of hepatic metastasis is palliative and the value of each approach depends on the circumstances of each patient. The main symptoms are anorexia, nausea, pain, fever and malaise. Jaundice is a late feature unless there is obstruction to the porta hepatis by a tumour or lymph node mass. Itching and steatorrhoea may then be major symptoms. The following approaches can be taken to relieve symptoms.

Pharmacological

Anorexia, fever and malaise may all be relieved for a time by corticosteroids. Prednisolone 20–30 mg/day is usually adequate, but the symptoms often recur after a few weeks and muscle wasting becomes profound if this dose is continued for long. Phenothiazines or metoclopramide before meals may help a little with the nausea, and aspirin or indometacin may also relieve fever. Pain is treated with analgesics, as described in Chapter 7.

Radiotherapeutic (and radiofrequency) ablation

Although the liver does not tolerate large doses (>35 Gy), radiotherapy has a useful role in palliation of pain and may also improve nausea and vomiting. With a dose of 20–35 Gy to the whole liver, over 70% of patients will experience a degree of improvement, particularly relief of pain. In chemoresistant tumours, the addition of chemotherapy or hypoxic cell sensitizers does not improve these results. Often, a particularly painful metastasis can be treated with a local field using a few large fractions, producing quick relief of pain without adverse effects. Increasingly, radiofrequency ablation in the hands of experts may offer excellent palliation of symptoms, together with a modest improvement in overall survival time. It is particularly valuable for solitary lesions (or where there are only a few) under 4 cm in size, and is sometimes combined with either surgical resection and/or tumour embolization. This modality is increasingly used to treat liver metastases from colorectal cancer, sarcomas and neuroendocrine tumours.

Surgical

Hepatic artery ligation or embolization can produce pain relief and shrinkage of metastases, but they recur rapidly with regeneration of the blood supply. Occasionally a slow-growing solitary metastasis is worth resecting in a fit patient with, for example, a carcinoid tumour. Surgical resection of isolated hepatic metastases has been increasingly performed in patients with colorectal cancer (see Chapter 16).

Radiotherapeutic emergencies

There are two common clinical situations that require urgent consideration by the radiotherapist or clinical oncologist. These are acute spinal cord compression and superior vena caval obstruction (SVCO).

Acute spinal cord or cauda equina compression

Acute spinal cord or cauda equina compression [22, 23] results from pressure on the cord, usually as a result of a tumour extending from a vertebral body to compress the cord from the epidural space (Figure 8.1). Compression may also occur as a result of direct extension from a mediastinal tumour or the cauda equina from a retroperitoneal tumour. If the vertebra is weakened, a crush fracture may precipitate cord compression. Very occasionally, intramedullary metastases will cause acute cord compression from within. Cord compression most commonly occurs in diseases where bony metastases (particularly vertebral metastases) are frequent. Myelomas and carcinomas of the prostate, breast and lung (particularly small-cell carcinomas) are the commonest causes. The thoracic vertebrae are the commonest site of compressive lesions (the cord ends at L1). Compression of the spinal venous drainage quickly leads to oedema and ischaemia of the cord.

The onset may be acute or gradual. Characteristically, the patient complains of back pain often with a root distribution; weakness of the legs; dribbling, hesitancy and incontinence of urine; and sluggish bowel action. In most cases, only one or two of these symptoms will be present. Limb weakness and bladder dysfunction are later signs, but in many patients the symptoms will only have been present 48 hours or so before paraplegia occurs. Higher cord lesions will also be accompanied by symptoms and signs in the upper limb (Table 8.4).

Cauda equina syndrome, where the compression occurs below the lower level of the spinal cord, that is, L1 or L2, is often difficult to diagnose. Features include leg weakness, sacral anaesthesia, retention of urine and erectile failure. Clinical diagnosis is particularly important since in this syndrome radiological studies, including myelography, often fail to demonstrate any definite abnormality. Careful neurological examination

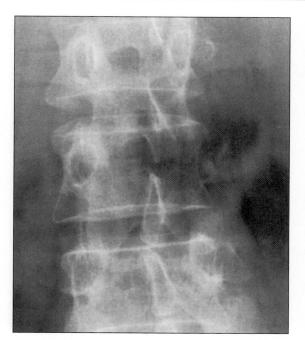

Figure 8.1 Radiograph of lumbar vertebrae showing destruction of the left pedicle L3.

Table 8.4 Syndromes of spinal cord compression.

Complete compression
Sensory loss just below level of lesion
Loss of all modalities of sensation – variable in degree at first
Bilateral upper motor neurone weakness below lesion
Bladder and bowel dysfunction

Anterior compression
Partial loss of pain and temperature below lesion
Bilateral upper motor neurone weakness below lesion
Bladder and bowel dysfunction

Lateral compression (Brown–Séquard)
Contralateral loss of pain and temperature (touch much less affected)
Ipsilateral loss of proprioception and vibration
Ipsilateral upper motor neurone weakness

Posterior compression
Loss of vibration and position below lesion
Pain, temperature and touch relatively spared
Painful segmental paraesthesia at level of lesion

may reveal loss of sacral sensation (saddle anaesthesia), which will only be detected if perianal sensation is tested with a pin, and anal sphincter tone is assessed on rectal examination.

Spinal cord compression may occasionally occur at more than one site, giving rise to neurological signs (e.g. a mixture of upper and lower motor neurone weakness), which would otherwise be difficult to explain on the basis of a single lesion.

Investigation should include plain radiography of the spine, which may show evidence of multiple bone metastases, a paraspinal mass, a crush fracture at the site of pain, or less obvious changes such as erosion of a pedicle (Figure 8.2). A normal radiograph is not uncommon; MRI is the most useful investigation. It demonstrates the site of blockage with great accuracy and usually gives a clear view of its extent (of the tumour inside and outside the spinal canal) and whether multiple lesions are present (Figure 8.3). When MRI is not immediately available, CT often offers a reliable alternative.

Cord compression is a medical emergency in which treatment must begin within hours, not days. Any patient with cancer who develops severe back pain with a root distribution is at very high risk and must be investigated

at once. Treatment of cord compression is by radiation therapy, surgery or a combination of both. For tumours that are radiosensitive (myeloma, lymphoma, SCLC, breast cancer) radiotherapy is usually the initial treatment. A common treatment dose recommendation is 30 Gy given in 10 fractions, with the dose generally prescribed 'at depth'. Dexamethasone is usually given before and during radiation, and is strongly recommended as an initial intervention prior to radiotherapy, which can take many hours to organize and implement. If there is evidence of neurological deterioration at any stage, the need for surgery must be reassessed at once. For tumours insensitive to radiation, surgery may be the preferred initial treatment, especially for solitary lesions. If the tumour is anterior, approaches to decompression are technically more difficult, but anterior approaches are now much more widely used. Posterior lesions are treated by decompressive laminectomy. Postoperative complications are not uncommon and instability of the spine occurs in 10% of cases.

The prognosis for patients with cord compression relates to the degree of neurological damage before treatment and to the underlying cancer. Delayed diagnosis results in a poor outcome. Speedy and efficient treatment is essential. If the patient has progressed to paraplegia before treatment, the chance that he or she will walk after treatment is less than 5%. Early diagnosis is essential

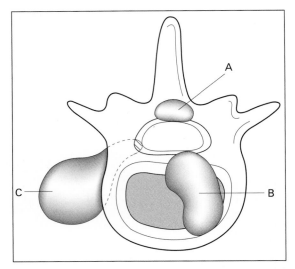

Figure 8.2 Epidural compression of the cord may be caused by metastasis from the vertebral body (A and B) or from paravertebral metastasis penetrating the intervertebral foramen (C). The vertebral body is the commonest site.

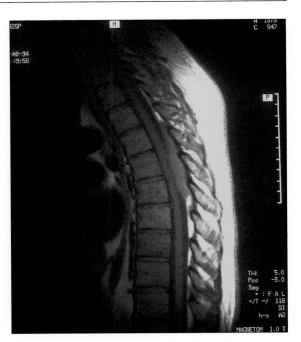

Figure 8.3 MRI scan showing acute spinal cord compression. A large posterior mass, extending over three vertebrae, is compressing the spinal cord.

since, with less severe damage, 50% will be ambulatory. Widespread radioresistant tumour (e.g. melanoma) has a poor prognosis. Chemotherapy plays no part in the initial management of cord compression.

Superior vena caval obstruction

This most commonly results from a right-sided carcinoma of the bronchus (particularly small-cell carcinoma). It also occurs in lymphoma (particularly Hodgkin's disease, in which mediastinal involvement occurs in about one-quarter of all patients), as well as carcinoma of the breast, kidney and other tumours that may metastasize to mediastinal nodes. Occasionally, it may be a presenting feature of a primary mediastinal tumour such as a thymoma, or a germ-cell tumour. It is characterized by swelling of the face, neck and arms, with a typical plethoric cyanotic appearance. There is non-pulsatile engorgement of veins, and large collateral veins may be visible over the surface of the shoulders, scapulae and upper chest. Retinal veins may also be engorged, and there is often conjunctival oedema. The most constant physical sign is the occurrence of leashes of tiny bluish venules over the chest wall, particularly in the precordial, subcostal and infrascapular regions. Patients are almost always dyspnoeic and hypoxic, and the chest radiograph usually shows a substantial right-sided or central mediastinal mass (Figure 8.4).

Urgent treatment with radiotherapy is the mainstay of management and is undoubtedly the treatment of choice for non-small-cell carcinomas of the bronchus and other tumours not amenable to chemotherapy, and where treatment must be started before the diagnosis is known. However, with the advent of effective chemotherapy for lymphoma and small-cell carcinoma of the bronchus, combination chemotherapy should be considered in SVCO due to these conditions and has a number of advantages. First, patients may be several kilometres from a radiotherapy centre; second, many of them will have extensive disease that would be left untreated by local irradiation; third, chemotherapy is given as a single intravenous injection, whereas radiotherapy has to be given daily for several days or weeks; and finally, the response to chemotherapy is often at least as quick as with radiotherapy, which can still be given if chemotherapy fails. Radiation dosage in treatment of SVCO should depend on the primary diagnosis. As with spinal cord compression, dexamethasone is often a valuable addition to treatment. Endovascular stenting is increasingly used for supportive management in SVCO, and can of course be combined with radiotherapy [24].

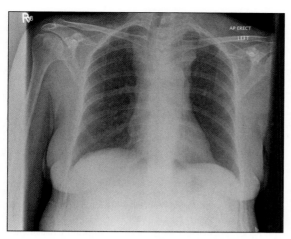

Figure 8.4 Typical radiological findings in superior vena caval obstruction. The tumour is almost always bulky and right-sided. This patient has locally advanced Hodgkin's disease.

Other radiotherapy emergencies

Orbital or intraocular metastases most commonly occur in carcinoma of the breast and in malignant melanoma. They present with proptosis, oculomotor palsy or visual loss, which may be acute if there is bleeding into the eye from a choroidal deposit. These metastases may be bilateral. Early treatment with radiotherapy is important since permanent visual loss or ocular palsy may occur in a patient whose lifespan may be several years. Careful radiation planning is required in order to avoid treatment to the anterior half of the eyes and to the contralateral lens. A single lateral radiation field with a dose of 30 Gy in 10 daily fractions over 2 weeks of treatment is usually adequate. Chemotherapy plays no part in the management of these complications.

Primary or secondary cancers at other critical sites may also lead to the necessity for urgent treatment. Impending collapse of a lung from severe bronchial narrowing may be the cause of an urgent referral from a chest physician who has been following an asymptomatic patient with known carcinoma of the bronchus for months or even years. The development of a unilateral monophonic wheeze, usually heard at its loudest over the main or lobar bronchus, is the most reliable physical sign. The sequence of chest radiographs often shows increasing shadowing and obstruction of part of the lung. Radiotherapy may well reverse this picture and relieve the patient's dyspnoea. The role of radiotherapy in carcinoma of the bronchus is more fully discussed in Chapter 12.

For the severe, localized and unremitting pain of bony metastases, radiotherapy is pre-eminently the treatment of choice. Palliative radiotherapy is often given as a matter of urgency in patients with severe bone pain who have not previously been treated maximally with radiotherapy to the painful site, especially if a single metastatic site is evident on clinical examination, radiography or isotope bone scan. Analgesics (usually opiates) will need to be given during the course of treatment and often afterwards as well (see Chapter 7 for discussion of pain control). If an area of spinal cord is included in the field, the treatment is often fractionated over 2 weeks (30 Gy in 10 daily treatments), although shorter treatment periods are certainly acceptable for patients with a short lifespan and may be perfectly safe. Common regimens for the relief of bone pain include five fractions of 5 Gy calculated at depth, or four fractions of 6 Gy. Single-fraction treatments of 8–14 Gy are becoming more popular and are certainly more convenient [23]. It is becoming increasingly clear that such treatments are probably as effective as more conventional regimens.

Cancer during pregnancy

Cancer is not uncommon in women during the child-bearing years of life [25]. Breast and cervical are the commonest tumours, but leukaemia, lymphoma, melanoma and colorectal cancers frequently affect this age group, especially as more women start families later. The approach to management will depend on the curability of the tumour, the stage of pregnancy and the wishes of the patient with respect to continuation of the pregnancy.

Treatment with cytotoxic drugs is especially hazardous during the first trimester. Pooled data suggest that the risk of fetal malformation if alkylating agents are used at this period is about 15%. For antimetabolites the figure is the same. Methotrexate is particularly likely to cause malformation. There are few data on other drugs. Large doses early in pregnancy will often cause abortion. The deformities are in skeletal and limb formation. There is no evidence of increased risk of malformation if treatment is in the second or third trimester, but it is not known if long-term consequences of drug treatment such as leukaemia will occur.

If the patient refuses termination and the cancer is curable with drug treatment, then this must be given in full dosage (there is no evidence that drug combinations or full dosage carry a greater risk of fetal injury).

Where possible, this treatment should be delayed to the second trimester. Local treatment, for example, surgery for breast cancer, or involved field radiation for lymphoma, can be given safely. Abdominal radiation must be avoided throughout pregnancy, and if given is very likely to lead to abortion. Radiation causes fetal growth retardation, CNS damage (microcephaly) and malformation of the eyes. The degree of microcephaly is related to radiation dose. The malformations can occur with irradiation at any stage in the pregnancy but are more severe earlier. Abdominal surgery for cancer can be performed but clearly presents major difficulties if the pregnancy is advanced. Safe delivery of the fetus can now usually be attained at 30 weeks' gestation. This has made cancer management easier during the third trimester.

References

1 Varlotto J, Stevenson MA. Anemia, tumor-hypoxemia, and the cancer patient. *Int J Radiat Oncol Biol Phys* 2005; 63: 25–36.

2 Kelton JB, Ali AM. Platelet transfusion: a critical appraisal. *Clin Oncol* 1983; 2: 549–85.

3 Vose JM, Armitage JO. Clinical applications of haematopoietic growth factors. *J Clin Oncol* 1995; 13: 1023–35.

4 Bennett CL, Djulbegovic B, Norris LB, Armitage JO. Colony-stimulating factors for febrile neutropenia during cancer therapy. *New Engl J Med* 2013; 368: 1131–1139.

5 Gabrilove JL, Kubowski A, Scher H *et al*. Effect of granulocyte colony stimulating factor on neutropenia and associated morbidity due to chemotherapy for transitional cell carcinoma of the urothelium. *N Engl J Med* 1988; 318: 1414–22.

6 Bunn PA, Crowley J, Kelly K *et al*. Chemoradiotherapy with or without granulocyte-macrophage colony stimulating factor in the treatment of limited stage small cell lung cancer: a prospective phase III randomized study of the South West Oncology Group. *J Clin Oncol* 1995; 13: 1632–41.

7 Henry DH, Abels RI. Benefits of erythropoietin alfa in anemic cancer patients receiving chemotherapy. *J Clin Oncol* 1995; 13: 2473–4.

8 Weitzman S, Aisenberg AC. Fulminant sepsis after the successful treatment of Hodgkin's disease. *Am J Med* 1977; 62: 47–50.

9 Finberg RW, Talcott JA. Fever and neutropenia: how to use a new treatment strategy. *N Engl J Med* 1999; 341: 362–3.

10 Klastersky J, Paesmans M. Risk-adapted strategy for the management of febrile neutropenia in cancer patients. *Support Care Cancer* 2007; 15: 477–82.

11 Marty FM, Winston DJ, Rowley SD *et al*. CMX001 to prevent cytalomegavirus disease in haemopoietic-cell transplantation. *New Engl J Med* 2013; 369: 1227–36.

12 Chamberlain JS. Cachexia in cancer: zeroing in on myosin. *N Engl J Med* 2004; 351: 2124–5.

13 Bozetti F. Nutritional support in patients with cancer. In: Payne-James J, Grimble G, Silk D, eds. *Artificial Nutrition Support in Clinical Practice*. London: Edward Arnold, 1995: 511–33.

14 Rubin H. Cancer cachexia: its correlations and causes. *Proc Natl Acad Sci USA* 2003; 100: 5384–9.

15 Mundy GR, Guise AT. Hypercalcaemia of malignancy. *Am J Med* 1997; 103: 134–45.

16 Gemici C. Tumour lysis syndrome in solid tumours. *Clin Oncol* 2006; 18: 773–80.

17 Rahman NM, Davies RJO, Gleeson FV. Investigating suspected malignant pleural effusion. *Br Med J* 2007; 334: 206–7.

18 Janssen JP, Collier G, Astoul P *et al*. Safety of pleurodesis with talc poudrage in malignant pleural effusion: a prospective cohort study. *Lancet* 2007; 369: 1535–9.

19 Park JS, Rentschler R, Wilbury D. Surgical management of pericardial effusions in patients with malignancies. *Cancer* 1991; 67: 76–80.

20 Cheung DK, Raaf JH. Selection of patients with malignant ascites for a peritoneo-venous shunt. *Cancer* 1982; 50: 1204–9.

21 Jayson GC, Howell A. Carcinomatous meningitis in solid tumours. *Ann Oncol* 1996; 7: 773–86.

22 Rades O, Fehlaur F, Schulte R *et al*. Prognostic factors for local control and survival after radiotherapy of metastatic spinal cord compression. *J Clin Oncol* 2006; 24: 3388–93.

23 Prasad D, Schiff D. Malignant spinal-cord compression. *Lancet Oncol* 2005; 6: 15–24.

24 Watkinson AF, Yeow TN, Fraser C. Endovascular stenting to treat obstruction of the superior vena cava. *Br Med J* 2008; 336: 1434–7.

25 Doll DC, ed. Cancer and pregnancy. *Semin Oncol* 1989; 16(5): 337–455. See reviews by Doll *et al*. (p. 337) for effects of cytotoxic drugs, and Brent (p. 347) for effects of radiation.

Further reading

Agarawal JP, Swangsilpa T, van der Linden Y *et al*. The role of external beam radiotherapy and the management of bone metastases. *Clin Oncol* 2006; 18: 747–60.

Bohlius J, Weingart O, Trelle S, Engert A. Cancer-related anemia and recombinant human erythropoietin: an updated overview. *Nat Clin Pract Oncol* 2006; 3: 152–64.

Gillams AR, Lees WR. Five-year survival following radiofrequency ablation of small, solitary, hepatic colorectal metastases. *J Vasc Intervent Radiol* 2008; 19: 712–17.

National Institute for Clinical Excellence. *Percutaneous Cementoplasty for Palliative Treatment of Bony Malignancies*. Interventional Procedure Guidance 179. London: NICE, 2006.

National Institute for Clinical Excellence. Metastatic spinal cord compression. Available at www.nice.org.uk/guidance/index (Accessed July 2008).

Senior K. Why is progress in treatment of cancer cachexia so slow? *Lancet Oncol* 2007; 8: 671–2.

Smith TJ, Khatcheressin J, Lyman GH *et al.* 2006 update of recommendations for the use of white blood cell growth factors: an evidence-based clinical practice guideline. *J Clin Oncol* 2006; 24: 3187–205.

Wilkinson AN, Raymond V, Brudage MD. Managing skeletal related events resulting from bone metastases. *Br Med J* 2008; 337: 1101–5.

Wilson LD, Detterbeck FC, Yahalom J. Superior vena cava syndrome with malignant causes. *N Engl J Med* 2007; 356: 1862–9.

Working Party of the Royal Colleges of Physicians, Radiologists and Obstetricians and Gynaecologists. *The Effects of Cancer Treatment on Reproductive Functions: Guidance on Management.* London: Royal College of Physicians, 2007.

9 Paraneoplastic syndromes

Fever due to malignant disease, 148
Ectopic hormone production in cancer, 149
  Syndrome of inappropriate antidiuretic
    hormone secretion, 149
  Ectopic adrenocorticotrophic hormone
    production, 150
  Hypoglycaemia, 151
  Gynaecomastia and gonadotrophin
    production, 151
  Other ectopic hormones, 151
Haematological syndromes, 151
  Anaemia, 151
  Erythrocytosis, 152
  Thrombotic disorders, 152
  Disseminated intravascular coagulation, 152
Neurological syndromes, 152
  Encephalomyelitis, 153
  Cerebellar degeneration, 153
  Carcinomatous myelopathy, 153

Peripheral neuropathy, 153
  Lambert–Eaton myasthenic syndrome, 154
Muscle and joint syndromes, 154
  Polymyositis and dermatomyositis, 154
  Hypertrophic pulmonary
    osteoarthropathy, 154
  Polyarthritis, 154
Dermatological syndromes, 155
  Acanthosis nigricans, 155
  Hypertrichosis (lanuginosa acquisita), 155
  Erythroderma, 156
  Vasculitis, 156
  Pyoderma gangrenosum, 156
  Bullous eruptions, 156
  Ichthyosis, 156
  Alopecia, 156
  Generalized pruritus, 156
Nephrotic syndrome, 156

Cancers are frequently associated with constitutional disturbances that are not due to the local effect of the tumour. For example, although cancer of the head of the pancreas will frequently cause obstructive jaundice, leading to steatorrhoea and weight loss, these metabolic upsets are due to the physical presence of the tumour obstructing the common bile and pancreatic ducts. However, the tumour may occasionally give rise to a remote effect such as fever, thrombophlebitis or mood change. The mechanisms whereby these symptoms are caused are poorly understood. Such remote systemic effects of cancer are common and often add to the patient's symptoms. These syndromes, which are termed 'paraneoplastic', may sometimes be the presenting feature of cancer and lead to other diagnoses being made in error, before a cancer is suspected. An awareness of these complications of cancer is therefore essential for correct management because the symptoms can often be controlled even when the primary tumour cannot be removed. Furthermore, the symptoms may be wrongly interpreted as being due to metastases,

and an opportunity for effective treatment of the primary tumour may be lost.

In recent years, the pathogenesis of some of these syndromes has become clearer. The syndromes of ectopic hormone production have been further elucidated, antibody-mediated syndromes have been defined and syndromes due to secretion of colony-stimulating and growth factors have been described. These syndromes may cause significant morbidity in cancer patients especially in the case of associated neurological manifestations [1,2].

Table 9.1 illustrates some metabolic and other paraneoplastic syndromes in non-endocrine neoplasms. The pathogenesis and management of weight loss, cachexia and hypercalcaemia are discussed in Chapter 8.

Fever due to malignant disease

Most patients with cancer who develop a fever do so because of infection. However, fever is a symptom

Cancer and its Management, Seventh Edition. Jeffrey Tobias and Daniel Hochhauser.
© 2015 John Wiley & Sons, Ltd. Published 2015 by John Wiley & Sons, Ltd.

Table 9.1 Metabolic paraneoplastic syndromes in non-endocrine neoplasms.

Syndrome	Tumour
Endocrine and metabolic	
Cushing's syndrome	Small-cell bronchogenic cancer, thymoma, bronchial carcinoid, neuroblastoma, phaeochromocytoma, medullary carcinoma of thyroid
Inappropriate ADH secretion	Small-cell bronchogenic cancer, thymoma, lymphoma, duodenal carcinoma, pancreatic carcinoma
Gynaecomastia	Teratoma, large-cell lung cancer, adenocarcinomas (breast, pancreas and gut, tumours of liver and adrenal)
Hypoglycaemia	Retroperitoneal sarcoma and lymphoma, hepatoma
Hypercalcaemia (see Chapter 8)	All cancers with widespread bone metastases, squamous cancers, renal and ovarian carcinoma
Hyperpigmentation	Small-cell bronchogenic cancer
Cachexia, anorexia, altered taste	All tumours
Haematological	
Multiple thromboses	Pancreatic cancer, other adenocarcinomas
Erythrocytosis	Renal carcinoma, hepatoma, uterine cancer, cerebellar haemangioblastoma
Disseminated intravascular coagulation	Thymomas

of cancer itself and may be the presenting feature. Lymphomas, especially Hodgkin's disease, are often accompanied by fever and in these diseases the pyrexia usually indicates an aggressive and advanced tumour. The typical relapsing Pel–Ebstein fever is present only in a minority of patients with Hodgkin's disease. Non-specific intermittent or remittent fever is more common. The pathogenesis is not well understood. Interleukin (IL)-1, IL-6 and tumour necrosis factor (TNF) are pyrogenic and are produced in cell culture by some tumour cell lines. They probably cause fever by inducing synthesis of prostaglandin $(PG)E_2$ in vascular endothelial cells in the hypothalamus, which affects the function of temperature-regulating neurones.

Hypernephroma is notable for its propensity to cause fever and leucocytosis and thus mimic a pyrogenic infection. Other carcinomas may present with similar features, especially if they are metastatic to the liver and bone marrow. Sarcomas and primary liver cancer are also frequently associated with pyrexia.

When cancer is the cause of the presenting pyrexia it can usually be diagnosed fairly easily. When fever occurs on treatment, the first priority is to exclude infection and then to investigate for tumour recurrence. In the absence of effective treatment for the specific cancer, symptomatic relief can sometimes be obtained by aspirin, non-steroidal anti-inflammatory agents and steroids.

Ectopic hormone production in cancer

Many cancers produce hormone precursors and peptides, some of which have biological activity. In the synthesis of a hormone in an endocrine gland, the precursor hormone (prohormone) is often the major storage form and is biologically inactive but is cleaved to the active hormone at the time of secretion. In the blood and tissues, the hormone is degraded to the inactive carboxyl fragment and the amino fragment, which may retain activity. Tumours may produce both inactive prohormones and the active principle. They may also produce biologically active peptides such as human chorionic gonadotrophin (HCG) or variants of HCG that have reduced carbohydrate content and which have lost activity. Similarly, a biologically active glycopeptide hormone may have two chains, both of which are necessary for biological activity. If only one chain is made by the tumour it will be inactive. The mechanism of ectopic synthesis is not clear, but may be due to abnormal gene activation as a result of malignant transformation.

In this section, 'ectopic' hormone is taken to mean production of a hormone by a non-endocrine tumour. Cancers of endocrine organs such as the adrenal, pancreas or endocrine cells in the gut may cause hormonal disturbances. These are discussed in the appropriate chapters.

Syndrome of inappropriate antidiuretic hormone secretion

This syndrome which should be distinguished from hyponatraemia which is common in cancer patients [3] occurs as a result of two separate mechanisms: (i) formation and release of antidiuretic hormone (ADH) from the tumour, and (ii) release of normal ADH from the pituitary as a stress response in ill patients.

Ectopic production of arginine vasopressin by the tumour, usually small-cell lung cancer (SCLC), may cause profound hyponatraemia. An elevated level of ADH and impaired water handling are present in 30% of patients with SCLC. The syndrome is characterized biochemically by plasma sodium below 130 mmol/L, with low plasma and high urine osmolality. Clinically it usually becomes apparent only when the plasma sodium reaches 120 mmol/L or lower, when the patient becomes tired, then drowsy and confused. The commonest underlying tumour is SCLC, which is usually apparent on chest radiography. Computed tomography (CT) of the brain may be necessary to exclude cerebral metastases as a cause of the neurological picture, since these are common in SCLC. In SCLC, marked hyponatraemia (assumed to be a reflection of ectopic ADH) is associated with a worse prognosis.

Treatment of the tumour with drugs and radiotherapy may improve the metabolic abnormality. While this is being done, demeclocycline may be effective in correcting the plasma sodium. It does this by rendering the distal tubule unresponsive to the ectopic ADH. This drug can impair renal function, and the blood urea should be measured regularly. In severe cases, water restriction may be temporarily required, but this is difficult to sustain and is sometimes ineffective. In an acutely ill patient with life-threatening hyponatraemia, a 3% saline infusion combined with intravenous furosemide (to increase free water clearance) is an effective emergency treatment.

Cyclophosphamide, vincristine and morphine can also cause hyponatraemia, due to either pituitary ADH release or a direct effect on the renal tubule. Low plasma sodium may be found in very ill patients regardless of cause. This is probably due to inappropriate ADH release from the posterior pituitary. This syndrome is occasionally difficult to distinguish from ectopic ADH production.

As demeclocycline is effective in only around 60% of patients, there has been development of antagonists of the vasopressin-2 receptor such as tolvaptan which is indicated for treatment of clinically significant hypervolemic or euvolemic hyponatremia that is symptomatic and has resisted correction with fluid restriction. This requires initial administration in a controlled hospital environment to monitor serum levels of sodium carefully.

Ectopic adrenocorticotrophic hormone production

Excess production of adrenocorticotrophic hormone (ACTH) is an uncommon metabolic complication of cancers that are normally neuroectodermal in origin. The commonest tumour to produce the syndrome is small-cell carcinoma of the bronchus. Small carcinoid tumours in the lung, thymus and pancreas may also cause the syndrome. Raised ACTH levels have been found in half of all patients with SCLC, and immunoreactive ACTH can be extracted from the majority of these tumours. Normal ACTH is derived from pro-ACTH which is, in turn, derived from pro-opiomelanocortin. In SCLC, most of the immunoreactive ACTH is derived from these precursor molecules with little ACTH itself. Nevertheless, pro-ACTH can produce Cushing's syndrome.

In SCLC, clinical manifestations of ectopic ACTH production are very unusual, and when they occur the clinical picture is usually different from classical Cushing's syndrome. There is usually hypokalaemia, glucose intolerance, hypertension, pigmentation and muscle weakness, but without the long-term weight gain of typical Cushing's syndrome. These patients usually have extensive disease with a poor prognosis. Estimates of the frequency of this syndrome in SCLC vary depending on the criteria used to define it.

In indolent or benign tumours such as bronchial or thymic carcinoid, typical Cushing's syndrome occurs. The syndrome also occurs rarely in squamous lung cancer, adenocarcinomas of the lung, gut or kidney, and medullary carcinoma of the thyroid. It also occurs in thymoma and ganglioneuroblastoma in childhood. Some of these tumours contain molecules of a prohormone with a higher molecular weight than normal ACTH which may not be biologically active. Rarely, tumours can produce a corticotrophin-releasing factor that acts on the pituitary to produce Cushing's syndrome by ACTH release.

Clinically, the syndrome caused by SCLC is rarely confused with other forms of Cushing's syndrome. The diagnosis is more difficult when the tumour is a bronchial carcinoid. The urinary free cortisol is increased and plasma cortisol is greatly raised. In SCLC with ectopic ACTH, high-dose dexamethasone does not suppress the plasma cortisol level, in contrast to pituitary-dependent Cushing's syndrome. Some patients with ACTH produced from carcinoid tumours will show suppression of plasma cortisol with dexamethasone. The plasma ACTH will be very low with an autonomous adrenal adenoma or carcinoma. In the latter, the plasma cortisol may also fail to suppress with dexamethasone.

Treatment is to the primary tumour. If this is ineffective, then aminoglutethimide and ketoconazole will block steroid synthesis. If total blockade is produced, a replacement dose of hydrocortisone must be given. Metyrapone will also block 11-hydroxylation of corticosteroids, causing a fall in plasma cortisol. This drug can be useful in seriously ill patients before definitive treatment of the tumour begins, but neither drug will produce lasting benefit in the absence of treatment of the disease.

Hypercalcaemia

This important paraneoplastic manifestation is discussed in Chapter 10.

Hypoglycaemia

Hypoglycaemia is a very uncommon complication of some cancers. It occurs with large thoracic and abdominal sarcomas, especially those situated retroperitoneally, and with hepatomas, mesotheliomas, adrenal carcinomas and lymphomas. It does not seem to be produced by insulin, which cannot be found in plasma or tumour extracts. Elevated plasma levels of somatomedin-like (insulin-like growth factor II) peptides have been demonstrated in some patients. These are peptides normally synthesized in the liver as a result of growth hormone (GH) and which have an action like insulin. The insulin-like growth factor II peptides also inhibit pituitary secretion of GH, thereby impairing the compensatory response to hypoglycaemia.

Hypoglycaemic attacks may be spontaneous or associated with fasting, and can be very severe. Emergency treatment requires glucose infusion. Clinically, the episodes are indistinguishable from those produced by islet cell tumours, but the plasma insulin is not raised. If the tumour cannot be completely removed, the hypoglycaemia may be partially controlled by frequent feeding, diazoxide, glucagon or corticosteroids.

Gynaecomastia and gonadotrophin production

Gynaecomastia is an increase in the glandular and stromal tissue of the male breast as a result of the inappropriate production of oestrogen induced by ectopic HCG. In most instances, when it complicates a non-endocrine malignancy, it is probably caused by tumour-related HCG production. In women, oligomenorrhoea may occur. In children, precocious puberty may occur with hepatoblastoma or hepatoma. Teratoma and seminoma may both be associated with HCG production and so may carcinoma of the bronchus of all histological types. Other HCG-producing tumours include those

of the pancreas (both exocrine and islet cell tumours), liver, adrenal and breast. In most cases of non-germ-cell neoplasms, HCG is produced in amounts too small to be clinically significant, although it may occasionally be useful as a tumour marker. In other cases, the hormone may not be glycosylated by the tumour, and this results in its rapid removal from the blood. Some tumours secrete free subunits which are not associated with biological activity. The increased oestrogen production, which is the cause of the gynaecomastia, is probably due to the action of the ectopic HCG on the testis or within the tumour itself. The correct treatment is removal of the tumour, but if this is not possible, or is incomplete, the HCG inhibitor danazol may be useful if the gynaecomastia is painful. Painful gynaecomastia can also sometimes be relieved by mammoplasty or local irradiation of the breasts. Further details on HCG are given in Chapters 4 and 19.

Other ectopic hormones

Bronchial carcinoids and pancreatic islet cell tumours may, rarely, produce GH-releasing substances over sufficient length of time to cause acromegaly. Galactorrhoea has been reported with cancer, due to hyperprolactinaemia. Hyperthyroidism may occur in trophoblastic tumours producing HCG. This does not appear to be due to thyroid-stimulating hormone (TSH) production, but the HCG may have TSH-like activity. Hypercalcaemia is discussed in Chapter 8.

Haematological syndromes

Anaemia

Anaemia is an almost universal accompaniment of advanced cancer [4]. Many factors contribute, including gastrointestinal bleeding leading to iron deficiency, and poor appetite with resulting iron and folate deficiency. Even if there are no secondary deficiency states, anaemia can still develop and can be regarded as a 'paraneoplastic' syndrome. Characteristically, it is similar to the anaemia of other chronic diseases. It takes a few months to develop and the haemoglobin does not usually fall below 8–9 g/dL. The anaemia is normocytic and normochromic or slightly hypochromic. The serum iron is low but so is total iron-binding capacity (TIBC), in contrast to the anaemia of iron deficiency where TIBC is high. The marrow shows stainable iron in macrophages. The red cell survival is often shortened without an increase in erythropoiesis sufficient to compensate for this. There also appears to be a block in release of iron from macrophages into the plasma. Serum erythropoietin (EPO) levels are low.

Treatment of the anaemia depends on successful treatment of the cancer. If this is impossible, and there are no secondary deficiencies of iron or folate, the anaemia can be corrected, albeit temporarily, by blood transfusion. Response to EPO occurs but is temporary.

An autoimmune haemolytic anaemia, which usually responds to treatment with steroids, may complicate B-cell lymphomas and Hodgkin's disease. It is much less common to find autoimmune haemolytic anaemia associated with non-lymphoid neoplasms, but it has been reported as a rare association with cancers of many types. As anaemia may contribute to the fatigue of patients with cancer, there has been interest in the development of erythropoiesis stimulating agents (ESA) such as erythropoietin and darbepoietin to reduce the need for transfusions and to enhance quality of life. Several studies have suggested that the risk of thromboembolic disease and death may be increased with treatment and that outcome may be worse with ESA. Research is ongoing to define the indications for this treatment which is not in routine clinical use [4,5].

Erythrocytosis

The commonest cancer to produce this syndrome is renal carcinoma. Rarer causes include cerebellar haemangioblastoma, hepatoma, uterine leiomyosarcoma and fibroids. The explanation is the production of EPO. Only 2–5% of cases of renal cancer are associated with polycythaemia, although excess production of EPO occurs in over half of all patients. It is not clear if the hormone itself is inactive or if there is a block to its action.

If the investigation of a high haematocrit confirms a true polycythaemia, a renal carcinoma should be excluded unless the patient is hypoxic. Erythrocytosis usually responds to removal of the primary tumour whether or not it is due to EPO production by the tumour.

Thrombotic disorders

Thrombotic complications of cancer are common and a frequent cause of morbidity and mortality. Although there may be treatment-related causes such as chemotherapy and intravenous catheters, venous thromboembolism may occur especially with mucin-secreting adenocarcinomas of the gastrointestinal tract (especially pancreas). Rarely there may be multiple arterial occlusions. Substances produced by the tumour react with factor VII and provoke coagulation through the extrinsic pathway.

Low molecular weight heparins are the preferred treatment rather than Vitamin K antagonism in view of their short half-life, relative lack of drug interactions and lack of need for monitoring [6]. Detailed internationally agreed guidelines for the management of this important complication of cancer and its treatment are now available [7].

Carcinoma of the pancreas, especially of the body or tail, is occasionally associated with multiple thromboses, often in superficial veins and migratory in nature. Other adenocarcinomas may give rise to the same syndrome of *migratory thrombophlebitis*. The tumours tend to be inoperable. The venous thromboses are sometimes in an unusual site such as the arm, and this may arouse suspicion of the underlying diagnosis. Pulmonary embolism seldom occurs.

Disseminated intravascular coagulation

Disseminated intravascular coagulation (DIC) [8] is a complication of malignancy that has been described in many different types of cancer, of which the commonest are adenocarcinomas (prostate, breast, pancreas, ovary) and other tumours such as metastatic carcinoid, neuroblastoma and rhabdomyosarcoma. It is probably due to the liberation of thromboplastin-like material from cancer cells, but some cancers secrete thrombin-like enzymes. Many patients with cancer have increased levels of fibrin degradation products in the blood, but the degree of intravascular coagulation is usually mild. Problems with haemorrhage are very unusual except in acute promyelocytic leukaemia, where DIC can be severe when treatment is first started. In solid tumours, where the DIC is chronic and low grade, treatment is by removal of the cancer where possible. Occasionally, DIC can be associated with red cell fragmentation (microangiopathic haemolytic anaemia) especially in stomach cancer. This syndrome may also be accompanied by acute renal failure (haemolytic–uraemic syndrome).

Neurological syndromes

Cancers can be associated with neurological syndromes [9] unrelated to direct compression or infiltration. Minor, or subclinical, manifestations are frequent in some cancers such as lung cancer. However, clinically significant, non-metastatic, neurological complications of malignancy are infrequently encountered. Most neurological complications of cancer are due to metastases or compression. The mechanism of damage is immunological, but ill-understood. Both humoral and T-cell-mediated cytotoxicity appear to be involved. The major clinical syndromes are discussed briefly below.

Encephalomyelitis

This is a general term embracing a wide variety of paraneoplastic neurological syndromes affecting the brain and spinal cord. The commonest associated cancer is SCLC. Here the mechanism is immunological. Polyclonal anti-Hu antibodies are often present in the blood but the role of these antibodies in producing the lesions is not understood. The central lesions are sometimes associated with severe sensory neuropathy due to dorsal root ganglia involvement. Treatment is often ineffective even when the primary tumour is removed.

Limbic encephalitis is a rare variant. An underlying small-cell carcinoma is likely to be responsible. It is characterized by the fairly rapid onset of confusion, memory disturbance and agitation. There is temporal lobe degeneration with some perivascular infiltrate. Anti-Hu antibodies are usually present. As with cerebellar degeneration, the main differential diagnosis is from intracranial metastasis.

Cerebellar degeneration

Syndromes of cerebellar degeneration are associated with carcinoma of the bronchus, ovary and uterus, and Hodgkin's disease. They differ from the chronic idiopathic cerebellar degenerations of adult life by being more rapid in evolution, sometimes progressing to severe disability in a few months, even before the primary tumour is apparent. Symptoms include unsteadiness of gait, truncal ataxia, vertigo and diplopia. Long tract signs due to spinal cord degeneration may develop. Pathologically, there are two variants. One is part of the encephalomyelitis spectrum with perivascular inflammatory infiltrate. In other cases, there is Purkinje cell loss without inflammation. Anti-Yo antibodies are polyclonal anti-Purkinje cell antibodies typically present when the cause is breast or ovarian cancer. Anti-Hu antibodies are present when SCLC is the cause. Anti-Hu antibodies are associated with inflammation but anti-Yo is not. Treatment of the primary tumour, although necessary, does not usually help. A CT scan is essential to exclude a cerebellar metastasis as far as possible. The response to treatment of the tumour is very disappointing, most cases showing at best stabilization of the neurological process even when the disease is cured or is in remission.

Carcinomatous myelopathy

This exceedingly rare syndrome can present as a flaccid paraplegia of acute onset with loss of sphincter control. The primary tumour is usually lung cancer. There is necrosis of the cord with little inflammation. The mechanism is unknown and the damage irreversible. A less acute myelopathy can also occur, associated with loss of anterior horn cells and a slowly progressive lower motor neurone weakness. It is usually associated with lymphoma and lung cancer.

The diagnosis of carcinomatous myelopathy is difficult to make. Cord compression must be excluded and the cerebrospinal fluid (CSF) examined for malignant cells. Other diseases such as amyotrophic lateral sclerosis may cause a similar picture. The association with carcinoma may become apparent only late in the evolution of the disease.

Peripheral neuropathy

Paraneoplastic neurological syndromes may frequently precede the appearance of cancer and hence recognition may lead to an earlier diagnosis of the primary cancer. The commonest variety of neuropathy seen in association with cancer is a *sensory neuropathy*. Pathologically there is segmental demyelination of nerves, usually distally, and axonal degeneration. SCLC is the commonest association and anti-Hu antibodies are usually present. The neuropathy varies in its severity. There is a severe form occurring earlier, sometimes before the tumour is manifest and occasionally following an intermittent course. The CSF shows a modest increase in protein (1 – 2 g/L), without excess cells. There is also a slowly progressive sensory neuropathy, associated with pains and paraesthesiae in the limbs, which may spread to the trunk and face. There is degeneration of dorsal root ganglia sometimes associated with a mononuclear cell infiltrate. Later, there is loss of the posterior columns leading to ataxia. The patient may become immobilised before the primary tumour has declared itself. Cancer of the lung (especially SCLC) is the commonest tumour but lymphoma and many other cancers can be associated. Removal of the tumour usually does not produce improvement and the neuropathy is progressive. In view of the infrequent occurrence of cancer-associated neuropathy no randomised controlled studies have been performed to allow definitive recommendations for therapy [10]. There are numerous case studies in the literature with some evidence that intravenous methylprednisone, immunoglobulins and occasionally plasma exchange may provide benefit in selected cases.

A pure motor neuropathy may occur in association with Hodgkin's disease but is rare. An *acute ascending paralysis* of the Guillain–Barré type may also occur, and has been noted in Hodgkin's disease especially.

The diagnosis of carcinomatous neuropathy is often very difficult. Infiltration of the meninges with carcinoma and lymphoma may occasionally cause peripheral sensory and motor damage. The CSF should therefore always be examined for malignant cells. In young patients with lymphoma, where the risk of central nervous system (CNS) involvement is high, it is usually best to treat the patient for CNS relapse if there is doubt about the diagnosis. The presence of anti-Hu antibodies is strongly suggestive of the diagnosis.

Lambert–Eaton myasthenic syndrome

In the rare Lambert–Eaton myasthenic syndrome, which is found almost exclusively with SCLC, the patient complains of weakness, aching and fatigue in the shoulder and pelvic girdle muscles, and sometimes impotence. It resembles myasthenia except that the relationship of fatigue to repeated muscular activity is less clear-cut and the electromyogram shows an increase in muscle action potentials at higher rates of nerve stimulation. The ocular and bulbar muscles are usually spared. The syndrome may appear before the tumour. Unfortunately there is little response to oral anticholinesterases. The syndrome is produced by IgG antibodies that bind in the proximity of voltage-gated calcium channels and which impair calcium influx and acetylcholine release. Treatment of the tumour may help. Plasma exchange and intravenous immunoglobulin may produce improvement as may 3, 4-diaminopyridine, which prolongs calcium channel activation.

Muscle and joint syndromes

Many patients with cancer complain of fatigue and sometimes of aching in the muscles that is occasionally out of proportion to the amount of weight loss. It has often been postulated that some of these patients have a more specific muscle disturbance. Conversely, unequivocal myopathic syndromes are unusual. Rheumatological complications of cancer are well-described [11].

Polymyositis and dermatomyositis

A syndrome typical of polymyositis, and which may be associated with skin changes indistinguishable from dermatomyositis, can rarely accompany cancer. All types of tumours have been reported in association. In a patient presenting with polymyositis, the likelihood of an occult, localized and remediable tumour being discovered is small, only 10–15% of cases are associated with a neoplasm. One therefore has to judge the extent to which investigation should be undertaken in each patient. A cancer is much more likely to be present in men over the age of 50 and when the syndrome is dermatomyositis. In this group, bronchial carcinoma is by far the commonest associated malignancy. A reasonable policy is to carry out a minimum of investigations in middle-aged patients presenting with dermatomyositis. These would include chest radiography, acid phosphatase and abdominal ultrasound in a man and pelvic ultrasound and mammograms additionally in a woman. Clinical indications such as rectal or vaginal bleeding or persistent cough should, of course, be further investigated.

The syndromes are characterized by symmetrical proximal muscle weakness that is slowly progressive. The skin changes consist of facial erythema and oedema, especially over the nose and around the eyes. The chronic contractures and calcification typical of the childhood disease do not usually have time to occur. Steroids produce temporary improvement, and azathioprine may also be of benefit. Where possible, the underlying cancer should be treated.

Hypertrophic pulmonary osteoarthropathy

Nowadays, bronchogenic carcinoma is almost exclusively the cause of the uncommon syndrome of hypertrophic pulmonary osteoarthropathy, although it can occur with lung metastases. The periosteum at the ends of the long bones (tibia, fibula, radius and ulna especially) is raised, thickened and inflamed, and periosteal new bone formation is shown by a typical layer of calcification parallel to, and 2–3 mm above, the periosteal surface of the bone. The bone is tender and the neighbouring joints may be hot and swollen, and clubbing is usually present. The pathogenesis of the syndrome is unknown, but it may regress on treatment or removal of the cancer. A rare form of the syndrome may be associated with features of acromegaly, with raised GH levels in the plasma.

Polyarthritis

An asymmetrical polyarthritis is a rare complication of cancer, particularly lymphoma and lung cancer. The differential diagnosis is from rheumatoid arthritis, but tests for rheumatoid factor are negative and the arthritis is less erosive. The syndrome may subside with removal of the tumour.

Table 9.2 Non-metastatic dermatological manifestations of malignancy.

Tumour	Marker
Disorders of pigmentation	
Hyperpigmentation	MSH-producing carcinoma (usually bronchial)
Vitiligo	Melanoma
Acanthosis nigricans	Adenocarcinomas, lymphomas
Erythema and inflammation	
Dermatomyositis	Most cancers
Thrombophlebitis	Adenocarcinomas
Thrombophlebitis migrans	Adenocarcinomas, especially pancreas and ovary
Erythroderma	Lymphomas
Pyoderma gangrenosum	Myeloproliferative syndromes, leukaemia, myeloma, lymphoma
Erythema	Carcinoid, glucagonoma
Fat necrosis	Pancreatic carcinoma
Bullous eruptions	Lymphoma
Vasculitis	Hairy cell leukaemia, other lymphomas, many solid tumours
Generalized pruritus	Lymphoma, leukaemia, polycythaemia
Acquired ichthyosis and hypertrichosis	
Hodgkin's disease	
Lung cancer	
Breast cancer	

MSH, melanocyte-stimulating hormone.

Table 9.3 Inherited disease (associated with cancer and with non-malignant skin lesions).

Gardner's syndrome: epidermal cysts and dermoids with multiple colonic polyps leading to carcinoma

Neurofibromatosis: neurofibromas, café-au-lait patches and other skin lesions, with sarcomatous change, medullary carcinoma of thyroid and phaeochromocytoma

Tylosis palmaris: hyperkeratosis of palms and soles with oesophageal cancer

Peutz–Jeghers syndrome: buccal, oral and digital pigmentation with multiple intestinal polyps leading uncommonly to gut carcinomas, ovarian tumours

Ataxia telangiectasia: telangiectases on neck, face, behind elbows and knees with cerebellar ataxia, IgA deficiency and increased incidence of lymphoma and leukaemia

Chédiak–Higashi syndrome: defective skin and hair colour, recurrent infections, high incidence of lymphoma and leukaemia

Wiskott–Aldrich syndrome: eczema, purpura, pyoderma, thrombocytopenia, low IgM, leukaemia and lymphoma

Tuberous sclerosis: adenoma sebaceum on cheeks, mental retardation and epilepsy, hamartomas and astrocytoma

Bloom's syndrome: photosensitive light eruptions, facial erythema, dwarfism, leukaemia, squamous cell carcinoma of the skin

Adult progeria (Werner's syndrome): thickened tight skin, soft-tissue calcification, growth retardation, soft-tissue sarcomas

Fanconi's anaemia: patchy hyperpigmentation, skeletal abnormalities, anaemia leading to acute myelomonocytic leukaemia

Dermatological syndromes

The skin manifestations of malignancy are extremely varied [12]. First, the skin may be infiltrated by primary or secondary cancer (Table 9.2). Second, it may be indirectly affected by general metabolic consequences of cancer at other sites (e.g. due to obstructive jaundice or steatorrhoea). Third, some inherited disorders are associated with skin manifestations and an increased likelihood of developing cancer (Table 9.3). Finally, some skin eruptions are non-specific manifestations of internal malignancy. Some of these (such as dermatomyositis and thrombophlebitis) have been described previously in this chapter. The following is a brief account of some dermatological syndromes not discussed elsewhere.

Acanthosis nigricans

This is a brown/black eruption in the armpits, groins and on the trunk that has a velvety surface and multiple papillary outgrowths. A familial form occurs which is not associated with cancer, and the syndrome can develop without any underlying malignancy in middle age. However, when it occurs in adult life, a cancer is often present, usually an adenocarcinoma and often a gastric neoplasm. Lymphomas are also associated. The skin lesion may antedate the cancer and, when it recurs after treatment, may herald a recurrence.

Hypertrichosis (lanuginosa acquisita)

Very rarely an adenocarcinoma of the lung, breast or gut, or a bladder carcinoma, may be associated with lanugo, which is fine downy hair on the face, trunk or limbs. The syndrome may be associated with acanthosis nigricans or ichthyosis. The hair growth does not usually regress after treatment of the primary tumour.

Erythroderma

A generalized, red, maculopapular rash may complicate cancer and the underlying disease is nearly always a lymphoma. The condition may progress to exfoliative dermatitis. Control of the underlying lymphoma is essential in treatment. As the rash fades it becomes slightly scaly and bran-coloured. Relapses of the lymphoma may result in further skin rash.

Sweet's syndrome is a febrile disorder with erythema of the face and trunk associated with leukaemia and lymphoma.

Vasculitis

Many variants of vasculitis (polyarteritis, leucocytoclastic vasculitis) may be associated with underlying cancer. Hairy cell leukaemia is the tumour with the closest association and the skin disorder may precede the clinical appearance of the malignancy.

Pyoderma gangrenosum

This is an infrequent complication of malignancy and can occur with other diseases such as ulcerative colitis. The lesions start as red nodules and then expand rapidly, breaking down in the centre to form necrotic, painful, infected ulcers with a rolled erythematous edge. Although the condition responds to steroids, the dose needed is usually very high. An underlying lymphoma or myeloproliferative syndrome is the most commonly associated malignancy, and the skin lesion may regress with successful treatment of the tumour.

Bullous eruptions

Very uncommonly, typical bullous pemphigoid and dermatitis herpetiformis are associated with underlying cancers, usually lymphomas.

Ichthyosis

Hodgkin's disease, other lymphomas and occasionally cancer of the lung are sometimes associated with thickened and flaking skin, usually affecting the face and trunk. The skin changes appear after the clinical appearance of the disease. Histologically, there may be epidermal atrophy or hyperkeratosis.

Tylosis palmaris is an inherited hyperkeratosis of the palms associated with oesophageal cancer.

Alopecia

Patchy alopecia occasionally accompanies lymphoma (usually Hodgkin's disease). There may be follicular mucinosis. The disorder may be self-limiting.

Generalized pruritus

Occasionally, patients present with generalized itching without any rash. Although cancer is not a frequent cause of this problem, it is an important one and the itching may precede the clinical appearance of the tumour, sometimes by a few years.

Hodgkin's disease is one of the commonest cancers to be associated and the itching can, in this disease, become intolerable. Pruritus is usually worse at night, and in the case of polycythaemia, worse after a hot bath. Lung, colon, breast, stomach and prostate are other primary tumours. Effective treatment of the cancer will often alleviate the condition and will certainly do so in Hodgkin's disease.

Nephrotic syndrome

The kidney may be involved by cancer in many ways but clinically evident non-metastatic manifestations are unusual, apart from amyloidosis complicating myeloma (see Chapter 27). Massive proteinuria leading to nephrotic syndrome may occur as a direct result of glomerular damage. In membranous lesions, it is thought that complexes of tumour products and antibody are deposited in the glomeruli. In the elderly, especially, a small proportion of patients with membranous glomerulonephritis have an underlying cancer, removal of which results in remission of the renal lesion. The cancer is usually an adenocarcinoma (breast, colon, stomach). Hodgkin's disease is also associated, although here there is usually minimal-change glomerulonephritis.

References

1 Pelosof LC, Gerber DE. Paraneoplastic syndromes: an approach to diagnosis and treatment. *Mayo Clin Proc* 2010; 85: 838–54.

2 Graus F, Dalmau J. Paraneoplastic neurological syndromes. *Curr Opin Neurol* 2012; 25: 795–801.

3 Castillo JJ, Vincent M, Justice E. Diagnosis and management of hyponatremia in cancer patients. *Oncologist* 2012; 17: 756–65.

4 Aapro M, Österborg A, Gascón P, Ludwig H, Beguin Y. Prevalence and management of cancer-related anaemia, iron deficiency and the specific role of i.v. iron. *Ann Oncol* 2012; 23: 1954–62.

5 Tonia T, Mettler A, Robert N *et al.* Erythropoietin or darbepoetin for patients with cancer. *Cochrane Database Syst Rev* 2012; 12: CD003407.

6 Lee AY, Peterson EA. Treatment of cancer-associated thrombosis. *Blood* 2013; 122: 2310–7.

7 Farge D, Debourdeau P, Beckers M *et al.* International clinical practice guidelines for the treatment and prophylaxis of venous thromboembolism in patients with cancer. *J Thromb Haemost* 2013; 11: 56–70.

8 Levi M Disseminated intravascular coagulation in cancer patients. *Best Pract Res Clin Haematol* 2009; 22: 129–36.

9 DeAngelis LM, Posner JB. *Neurologic Complications of Cancer*, 2nd edn. New York: Oxford University Press, 2009.

10 Giometto B, Vitaliani R, Lindeck-Pozza E, Grisold W, Vedeler C. Treatment for paraneoplastic neuropathies. *Cochrane Database Syst Rev* 2012; 12: CD007625.

11 Ashouri JF, Daikh DI. Rheumatic manifestations of cancer. *Rheum Dis Clin North Am* 2011; 37: 489–505.

12 Thiers BH, Sahn RE, Callen JP. Cutaneous manifestations of internal malignancy. *CA Cancer J Clin* 2009; 59: 73–98.

10 Cancer of the head and neck

Introduction, aetiology and epidemiology

Carcinomas of the upper air and food passages are a varied and important group of tumours with particular epidemiological features [1]. Worldwide, head and neck cancer is the sixth commonest type of malignancy and its incidence is rising [2]. The global incidence is thought to be over 600 000 new cases annually, that is, around 6% of all cancers worldwide, with approximately 350 000 deaths. These tumours pose exceptionally difficult management problems, and account for approximately 4% of all carcinomas in the UK. In Europe, the 2002 figures give an estimated incidence of around 143 000 total cases and over 68 000 deaths. Figure 10.1 shows age-specific incidence rates for the UK.

Important aetiological factors include excessive intake of tobacco either by smoking or chewing (a common practice in many parts of Asia and India where, as a result, oral cancer is among the commonest of all tumours).

Alcohol, particularly spirit, ingestion is also an important contributing agent [3] and these two factors are clearly synergistic (Figure 10.2). Although tobacco use is declining in many Western countries, alcohol ingestion is not; in the UK, for example, alcohol sales have increased by 7% over the past 20 years. Syphilitic leucoplakia was previously an important predisposing factor in carcinoma of the tongue. Dental and mechanical trauma have also been incriminated, but with improvements in oral and dental hygiene these factors are less important now [2]. The Paterson–Kelly (Plummer–Vinson) syndrome of chronic anaemia, glossitis and oesophageal web is known to predispose to postcricoid carcinoma, particularly in women. More recently, adenocarcinoma of the nasal cavity has been described in hardwood workers in the furniture industry. Several clusters have now been reported.

Important racial differences have also emerged, particularly in relation to carcinoma of the nasopharynx,

Cancer and its Management, Seventh Edition. Jeffrey Tobias and Daniel Hochhauser.
© 2015 John Wiley & Sons, Ltd. Published 2015 by John Wiley & Sons, Ltd.

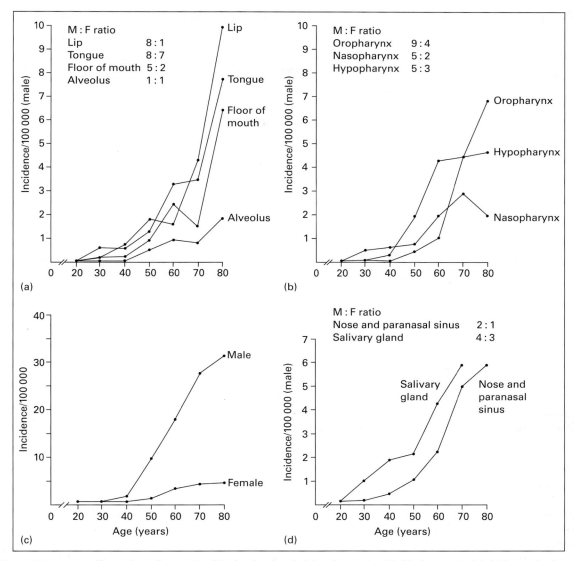

Figure 10.1 Age-specific incidence for cancers of the head and neck: (a) oral cavity (male); (b) pharynx (male); (c) larynx (male and female); (d) nose and paranasal sinuses and salivary gland (male).

commonly seen in the Chinese, particularly those of the Mongolian race. It is especially common in Hong Kong and south China, and in male Taiwanese is by far the commonest cause of death, three times the rate of any other neoplasm. It is also common in the Philippines, Malaysia, Greenland, Malta, North Africa and Saudi Arabia. Curiously, it often develops at a far younger age than other head and neck cancers, with a bimodal age distribution.

Of all cases 20% (in high-prevalence areas) are diagnosed in patients (usually male) under the age of 30.

Alterations of the tumour-suppressor gene *p53* and its protein product have been noted in head and neck cancers. Genetic mutations are also present in both normal oral mucosa and tumour tissues, with evidence of a tumour-associated *p53* mutation [4]. There is increasing evidence that genetic abnormalities within tumour cells

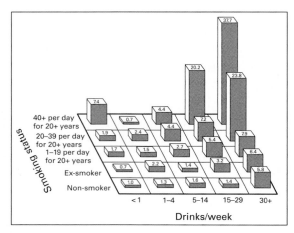

Figure 10.2 Relative risk of oral/pharyngeal cancer in males by alcohol and tobacco consumption. (Source: Cancer Research UK 2006. Reproduced with permission.)

of selected head and neck cancer cases may have a bearing on outcome following treatment. Metastasis is apparently often mediated by a low oxygen tension within the malignant cell, possibly then acting via a mechanism involving the *TWIST* gene, so patients with tumours showing high levels of this gene have a greater likelihood of distant metastasis, and a worse prognosis. Aetiologically, environmental agents have been implicated, including dietary factors such as salted fish and vegetables popular among many Chinese, Inuit (Eskimo) and North Africans. Case–control studies in Chinese patients have suggested a link between salted fish consumption and incidence of nasopharyngeal carcinoma [5].

Apart from possible dietary causes of nasopharyngeal carcinoma, it is also known that patients with this condition generally have evidence of Epstein–Barr virus (EBV) genome in the epithelial tumour cells [6] and a characteristic EBV antibody pattern with a rise in IgA and IgG antiviral capsid antigen and EBV-associated nuclear antigens [7].

A causal role for human papillomavirus (HPV) in head and neck cancer has increasingly been postulated, analogous to the role of HPV in other squamous sites such as the cervix and anus, now so clearly established [8]. It is important to retain perspective, however – even in oral cancer, figures from Cancer Research UK suggest that overall, HPV infection accounted for about 8% of cancers compared with the much larger contributions from tobacco (64%) and alcohol (20%) – 2010 figures. However, in contrast with cervical cancer, high-risk HPVs

are not necessary for the development of all cases of head and neck squamous cell carcinoma. In some of these tumours, HPV DNA (particularly type 16) is present in primary and metastatic tumour-cell nuclei – in high copy-numbers frequently integrated and transcriptionally active. These tumours are characteristically tonsillar in origin, with poorly differentiated histopathology and disproportionate diagnosis in younger patients. The molecular profile of HPV-associated head and neck squamous cell cancers is distinct from that of HPV-negative tumours, indicative of viral oncogene function in the tumours, as in cervical cancer. Recognition that HPV can be causative for some head and neck squamous cell cancers may have important implications for their prognosis, prevention and therapy. For example, an important recent case–control study confirmed that oral HPV infection is strongly associated with oropharyngeal cancer among subjects 'with or without the established risk factors of tobacco and alcohol use' [9]. In this study, serum antibodies against HPV-16 oncoprotein E6, E7, or both, were found in 64% of 'case' patients and only 4% of the control patients. One intriguing diagnostic possibility is the proposal for a cervix-analogous 'oral Pap-smear' for earlier diagnosis and treatment, one recent study identifying such patients as comprising 7% of controls investigated in this way. Australia recently became the first nation in the world to offer HPV vaccination to boys in order to reduce the incidence of this disease (along with penile and anal cancer), and calls have been made for both the UK, USA and other countries to follow this lead. The proposal is for three doses of the quadrivalent Gardasil to be given at ages 12–13 years and with a catch-up programme for 14–15 year-olds until the end of 2014.

In nearly all head and neck cancers there is a male predisposition (except possibly for postcricoid carcinomas), with a male to female ratio of approximately 3:1. For some sites, notably carcinoma of the larynx, the male to female ratio has been reportedly as high as 10:1.

Improvements in dental and oral hygiene led for a period (1960–1980) to a falling incidence of cancers of the head and neck, although the incidence now appears to be rising again. American data provide age-adjusted incidence rates of 17.3 per 100 000 (white males) and 5.6 per 100 000 (white females). Approximately 40% of these tumours prove fatal. In the UK, Scandinavia, Germany, Japan and Israel the figure is somewhat lower, but elsewhere in northwest Europe (France, Switzerland, Italy and Scotland) the death rate is slightly higher. These survival figures probably correlate with alcohol intake.

Pathology

The overwhelming majority (about 90%) of these tumours are squamous cell carcinomas, although frequencies of other histological types and degree of differentiation vary with site. Nasopharyngeal carcinoma is clearly an exception, and differs from other head and neck cancers in a number of ways. For example, in one large series the commonest tumours from this primary site were anaplastic and squamous cell carcinomas, although lymphoepithelioma (undifferentiated squamous cell carcinoma), malignant lymphoma, adenoid cystic carcinoma (cylindroma) and plasmacytoma also occurred, as well as rarer tumours such as melanoma or undifferentiated sarcoma. Together, these constituted a significant group of carcinomas of nonsquamous origin amounting to almost 30% of all cases. In contrast, in a series of over 2000 cases of carcinoma of the larynx, 95% were squamous, showing varying degrees of differentiation and including 97 patients with carcinoma *in situ*. Of patients with head and neck carcinomas, 20% or more develop multiple primary lesions, most notably within the oral cavity.

Malignant lymphoma can arise anywhere within the head and neck but particularly from Waldeyer's ring. In such cases special care should be taken to establish the correct histological diagnosis since prognosis and management of lymphoma is very different from epithelial carcinoma.

Clinical staging

Careful staging is essential, both as a reminder to carry out a full clinical and radiological assessment in each case and in order to develop logical treatment strategies and to document for case comparison [10]. In Europe, the proposals of the Union Internationale Contre le Cancer (UICC) for standard tumour node metastasis (TNM) staging have gained wide acceptance [11]. This has been facilitated by the adoption of the same staging notation for lymph node status regardless of the primary head and neck site (Table 10.1). Unfortunately this uniformity of notation has not been possible for T staging, where some primary sites are still staged according to their spread (see Tables 10.2 and 10.3, for examples). Cancers of the head and neck have always been associated with particular challenges in cancer staging. Not only are these cancers highly variable in terms of primary anatomical site, but unlike most other major cancers they frequently

Table 10.1 Staging of nodes and metastases in head and neck cancers (except thyroid gland).

N	Regional lymph nodes
NX	Regional lymph nodes cannot be assessed
N0	No regional lymph node metastasis
N1	Metastasis in a single ipsilateral lymph node, 3 cm or less in greatest dimension
N2	Metastasis in a single ipsilateral lymph node, more than 3 cm but not more than 6 cm in greatest dimension, or in multiple ipsilateral lymph nodes, none more than 6 cm in greatest dimension, or in bilateral or contralateral lymph nodes, none more than 6 cm in greatest dimension
N2a	Metastasis in a single ipsilateral lymph node, more than 3 cm but not more than 6 cm in greatest dimension
N2b	Metastasis in multiple ipsilateral lymph nodes, not more than 6 cm in greatest dimension
N2c	Metastasis in bilateral or contralateral lymph nodes, none more than 6 cm in greatest dimension
N3	Metastasis in a lymph node more than 6 cm in greatest dimension

Source: Sobin *et al.* [11].

lend themselves to adequate clinical assessment by visual inspection and palpation, facilitating proper documentation by the trained clinician. Furthermore, when the site of the primary cancer involves organ-sparing approaches, full anatomical and histological data for comprehensive pathological staging are often not available. Even so, the processes involved in surgical decision-making and radiotherapy treatment planning require meticulous assessment and documentation of the extent of locoregional disease. Furthermore, many patients who succumb to head and neck cancer do so as a result of locoregional disease.

For all these reasons it is essential to perform reliable and accurate pretreatment clinical staging of head and neck cancers. The current staging system takes into account detailed local anatomical features that influence management, since the degree of involvement of these structures may be as important as distant metastasis, in the overall outcome. For this reason the most recent cancer staging classification (sixth edition) of the UICC and the American Joint Committee on Cancer (AJCC) includes new criteria for the more advanced cases (e.g. T4 categories and stage IV disease). These new features reflect the fact that in heterogeneous populations, as is

Table 10.2 Current UICC staging system in nasopharyngeal carcinoma. (Data from [11].)

Nasopharynx

T1	Nasopharynx, oropharynx, or nasal cavity
T2	Parapharyngeal extension
T3	Bony structures of skull base/paranasal sinuses
T4	Intracranial, cranial nerves, hypopharynx, orbit, infratemporal fossa/masticator space
N1	Unilateral cervical, unilateral or bilateral retropharyngeal lymph nodes, above supraclavicular fossa, ≤ 6 cm
N2	Bilateral cervical above supraclavicular fossa, ≤ 6 cm
N3a	> 6 cm
N3b	Supraclavicular fossa

Stage grouping (Nasopharynx)

Stage 0	Tis	N0	M0
Stage I	T1	N0	M0
Stage II	T1	N1	M0
	T2	N0, N1	M0
Stage III	T1, T2	N2	M0
	T3	N0, N1, N2	M0
Stage IVA	T4	N0, N1, N2	M0
Stage IVB	Any T	N3	M0
Stage IVC	Any T	Any N	M1

Table 10.3 T staging for tumours of the lip and oral cavity.

TX	Primary tumour cannot be assessed
T0	No evidence of primary tumour
Tis	Carcinoma *in situ*
T1	Tumour 2 cm or less in greatest dimension
T2	Tumour more than 2 cm but not more than 4 cm in greatest dimension
T3	Tumour more than 4 cm in greatest dimension
T4a	Lip: tumour invades through cortical bone, inferior alveolar nerve, floor of mouth, or skin of face (i.e. chin or nose)*
	Oral cavity: tumour invades through cortical bone, into deep (extrinsic) muscle of tongue (genioglossus, hyoglossus, palatoglossus, and styloglossus), maxillary sinus, or skin of face
T4b	Tumour involves masticator space, pterygoid plates, or skull base and/or encases internal carotid artery

*Superficial erosion alone of bone/tooth socket by gingival primary is not sufficient to classify as T4.
Source: Edge *et al.* [12]. Reproduced by permission of Springer Science + Business Media.

clearly the case with head and neck cancer, cure may be a realistic possibility in some patients with locally advanced disease, but not in others.

Distant metastasis

The definitions of the M categories for all head and neck sites are:

M   Distant metastasis
MX   Presence of distant metastasis cannot be assessed
M0   No distant metastasis
M1   Distant metastasis

Routine assessment and staging should always include careful inspection of the primary site, with measurement of its dimensions and examination for direct extension into adjacent tissues and local lymph node areas. Although a reasonable attempt at clinical examination and staging can be made with indirect laryngoscopy and nasopharyngoscopy with mirror techniques, most patients require an examination under anaesthesia, with direct endoscopic evaluation, before firm conclusions can be drawn. This is particularly true of nasopharyngeal carcinoma, since mirror examination of the postnasal space can be demanding for the patient, and unreliable even in the hands of an expert. Outpatient fibreoptic nasendoscopy has become standard practice since the mid-1980s. Histological confirmation must ideally be obtained in every case.

Investigation

Plain radiography, computed tomography (CT) and magnetic resonance imaging (MRI) are of great value. In carcinomas of the larynx and hypopharynx, for example, the soft-tissue lateral radiograph of the neck often gives a useful indication of the anatomical extent of the lesion, of particular value in subglottic tumours of the larynx, where extension or origin of the lesion may be difficult to assess. CT and MRI scanning have made a dramatic impact on the accuracy with which deep-seated lesions can now be visualized, particularly those of the nasopharynx, parotid gland, retro-orbital area and paranasal sinuses, and where there is involvement of the skull base or other evidence of bone erosion (Figure 10.3).

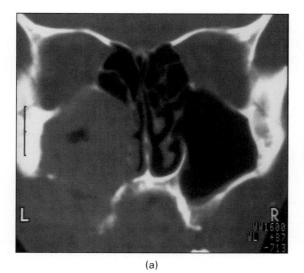

(a)

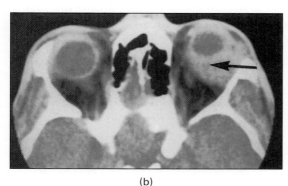

(b)

Figure 10.3 CT in head and neck tumours. (a) Coronal-plane CT scan through the nose and maxillary antrum: a large tumour fills the left maxillary antrum, destroying its walls and extending medially into the nasal fossa. (b) CT scan through orbits showing large left-sided tumour (arrow) displacing the globe forwards and downwards.

Haematogenous spread is uncommon at presentation, but when it does occur the lungs are the most common site of spread. The risk is highest with advanced tumours and in cases of nasopharyngeal carcinoma. A chest radiograph is essential and will also disclose the occasional simultaneous carcinoma of the bronchus. A routine blood count and liver function tests should also be performed.

These tumours are best managed jointly by a surgeon and a radiotherapist with particular interest in this area, since they present technical problems of management unequalled by those at any other site. Additional important members of the team include the medical oncologist, specialized pathologist, dental surgeon, plastic surgeon, specialist nursing and nutritional teams, and rehabilitative physiotherapists and/or occupational therapists. Because of the extreme variation in presentation, natural history and response to treatment, this chapter only gives a brief outline of general principles of management; for those with a particular interest, specialist texts can be recommended [13].

Carcinoma of the larynx

In the Western world, carcinomas of the larynx form the largest numerical group. Historically, the first laryngectomy for carcinoma is generally credited to Billroth in 1873.

The human larynx is an unusually complex organ (Figure 10.4) that combines the role of a protective sphincter for keeping the lower respiratory tract free from foreign bodies with the highly sophisticated function of speech production. This demands extraordinary precision in the tone of the laryngeal musculature and in the approximation of the vocal cords themselves.

Laryngeal cancer accounts for about 2–3% of all malignant disease, but the distress it causes is disproportionately high because of the severe social consequences of loss of speech. Indeed, the quality of voice and speech production is an important factor in choice of treatment. The larynx is sufficiently accessible to be viewed directly with ease, using mirror techniques (indirect laryngoscopy), nasendoscopy or by direct vision under anaesthesia. It contains epithelial and mesodermal tissue components, which lend themselves well to the study of radiation effects on both normal and abnormal tissues. For these reasons, the larynx has always been of particular interest to the radiotherapist.

Cigarette smoking is undoubtedly the most important aetiological factor, accounting for the male predominance. There is a known correlation between premalignant laryngeal mucosal changes and the number of cigarettes smoked. The rise in incidence of laryngeal carcinoma has been shown to parallel the rising incidence of carcinoma of the bronchus, and in patients cured of early laryngeal carcinoma but continuing to smoke, bronchial carcinoma has become the commonest cause of death.

Hoarseness is the principal and often the only symptom, and any patient with hoarseness of more than 3 weeks' duration should be referred for immediate laryngoscopy since early (T1–2N0) carcinomas can almost always be

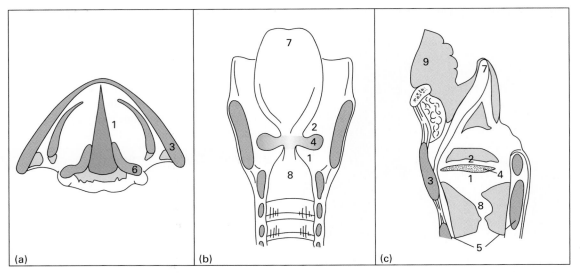

Figure 10.4 Anatomy of the larynx: (a) from above; (b) coronal plane; (c) median sagittal plane. 1, True vocal cord; 2, false vocal cord; 3, thyroid cartilage; 4, laryngeal ventricle; 5, cricoid cartilage; 6, arytenoid; 7, epiglottis; 8, subglottic area; 9, base of tongue.

cured by radiotherapy (see below). Dysphagia is much less common, though important in patients with supraglottic carcinoma, particularly when there is extension to the oropharynx. Dyspnoea, sometimes with stridor, is a feature of subglottic carcinoma where early obstruction is the rule and immediate tracheostomy frequently required before definitive management can be undertaken.

Carcinomas can arise from any of the three anatomical regions of the larynx, although not with equal frequency (Figure 10.5). Lesions of the glottis are much the commonest, followed by supraglottic and finally subglottic cancers. Although early supraglottic cancer is uncommon in the UK, these tumours are commoner than cancer of the glottis in some parts of Europe including Spain, Italy and Finland. In glottic lesions, the commonest site is the anterior third of the cord, often with extension to anterior or (more rarely) the posterior commissure. However, the whole cord can be involved. Direct spread can take place upwards via the laryngeal ventricle to the false cord and then to the remainder of the supraglottic region, or downwards directly to the subglottic area. Lymph node metastases are uncommon in early glottic carcinoma since the lymphatic drainage of the true cord is so sparse, but prognosis is highly dependent on the T stage. Most patients with T1 and T2 tumours are curable, whereas the majority of T3 and T4 lesions are not. Tumours of the epiglottis are usually advanced at presentation because there is little anatomical hindrance to direct tumour

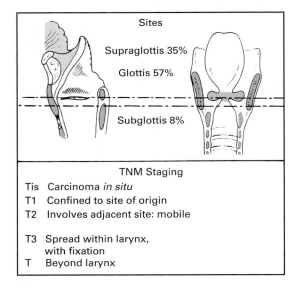

Figure 10.5 Relative frequency and TNM staging system in laryngeal cancer.

extension, particularly into the pre-epiglottic space. They do not cause hoarseness initially, and may elude diagnosis at laryngoscopy, particularly if the tumour arises on the inferior surface.

Management and prognosis
Carcinoma of the glottis

Radiotherapy to a *minimum* radical dose of 66 Gy (daily fractions over 6.5 weeks, or equivalent) will cure the majority of patients where the vocal cord remains mobile (T1, well over 90%; T2, 70%). Many centres now increasingly employ routinely higher doses, around 70 Gy. Where failure occurs with radiotherapy treatment, salvage surgery is curative in over half of all cases. Total laryngectomy is usually necessary but some cases can be treated successfully by partial laryngectomy with preservation of the voice, particularly if the initial tumour was well localized. Although conservative surgery (usually by partial vertical laryngectomy) can deal effectively with most early glottic carcinomas, the resulting voice is inferior to what can be achieved with radiotherapy. There are few drawbacks to radiotherapy, for early cases, since the field of treatment is small (often only 5 × 5 cm) with no need, at least in T1 tumours, to irradiate local lymph node areas.

Treatment of the *advanced* case is more difficult, requiring full discussion between surgeon and radiotherapist. There is an increasing emphasis on laryngeal preservation, which seems fully justified by recent data [14]. Surgery is occasionally required as an emergency procedure, particularly with subglottic extension. Many centres still employ a policy of planned radiotherapy and surgery in combination for the majority of these advanced lesions, especially if there is evidence of cartilage invasion, perichondritis, extralaryngeal spread or nodal metastases where the ultimate prospect for cure is so poor. However, radiotherapy in combination with multiagent chemotherapy has gradually replaced this approach whenever possible (see below), reserving 'salvage' surgery for cases in which non-surgical treatment had been unsuccessful. This has become more widely practised in recent years, and has led to a higher proportion of patients cured of the carcinoma yet with retention of the larynx and satisfactory speech production [15]. Adverse prognostic factors such as fixation of the primary tumour, early local invasion, extrinsic spread and lymph node metastasis are interrelated and often occur together. The potential role of both chemotherapy and biological targeted therapies is discussed below (pages 174–177). Great strides have been made in the management of laryngeal carcinomas with combined concurrent chemoradiation therapy, allowing organ preservation in the majority of patients [15,16]. Most regimens in current use include cisplatin, often with 5-fluorouracil (5-FU). For the majority of these patients, even the most intensive

combinations of surgery, radiotherapy and chemotherapy will fail to cure, and the ultimate 5-year survival rate for T3 lesions is about 25%.

Carcinoma of the supraglottis

These tumours are more difficult to treat. They often present late because early symptoms are few. Dysphagia may not develop until ulceration and local extension take place. Both local invasion and lymph node involvement are more common than with glottic carcinomas, and almost one-quarter of supraglottic lesions extend down to the glottis. By locally invading in other directions, these tumours frequently involve the oropharynx (particularly the posterior third of the tongue) and the hypopharynx (particularly the pyriform fossa). For early lesions, a policy of radical irradiation with salvage surgery (total laryngectomy) where required (as for glottic tumours) is usually recommended, although surgery may be preferable for accessible lesions, such as those at the tip of the epiglottis. Conservative surgery is not normally possible. An important difference in radiotherapy technique between treatment of this region and the true glottis is that the radiation fields should routinely include the local lymph node areas, since clinical and occult lymph node metastases are common. For more advanced supraglottic lesions, the combination of total laryngectomy with preoperative radiotherapy has traditionally been employed, and a 5-year survival rate of around 60% has been achieved. However, histological examination of the specimen may show that the preoperative radiation had already produced a probable cure. For this reason it may be preferable to withhold surgery until there is evidence of recurrence or residual disease after radiation.

Carcinoma of the subglottis

The outlook is much less satisfactory with these difficult tumours. Often there is vocal cord fixation at diagnosis, and invasion of the cricoid cartilage is common. Involvement of the thyroid gland or paratracheal lymph nodes occurs in about half of all cases, and surgical excision, if undertaken, must be radical. Such operations are performed less often nowadays, in favour of a planned combination of radiotherapy and chemotherapy, with surgery reserved for residual or recurrent disease.

Conservative surgery in laryngeal cancer

Although long-term survival in patients with laryngeal cancer has remained almost unchanged for the past 20 years, the quality of life of survivors has improved considerably. Where surgery proves necessary in radiotherapy

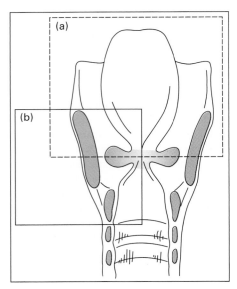

Figure 10.6 Conservative laryngectomy operations in laryngeal cancer: (a) horizontal supraglottic laryngectomy; (b) vertical partial laryngectomy.

failures, it is sometimes possible to offer conservative surgery, offering the patient some chance of reasonable speech production. With *horizontal supraglottic laryngectomy* (Figure 10.6), the upper part of the larynx is removed but the cords preserved. In *vertical partial laryngectomy*, the surgeon removes one vocal cord, the false cord and the vocal process of the arytenoid with part of the adjacent thyroid cartilage, and if necessary up to one-third of the contralateral vocal cord. Success in these procedures lies in accurate evaluation of tumour extent even though preoperative assessment can never be completely reliable.

Rehabilitation

Following laryngectomy, social and vocal rehabilitation is of great importance (see Chapter 7, page 117). With the appropriate training of oesophageal voice technique and stoma care, most patients can look forward to a full life, usually with an adequate voice. Although this is difficult to define, the ability to speak on the telephone is often used as an important criterion.

Permanent vocal prostheses are often now used in patients who find it difficult to develop adequate oesophageal speech. These devices contain valves, which sometimes offer a striking improvement in voice quality. An example is the Blom–Singer valve, which requires a permanent pharyngeal puncture with placement of a small tube which is brought forward to the skin of the anterior neck. By occluding the opening with a finger, many patients can produce adequate speech, although care of the valve can be difficult and a high standard of hygiene is essential.

Carcinoma of the pharynx

Anatomy and patterns of metastasis

The pharynx is best considered a passage with two distal sphincters serving the function of channelling both food and air in the right directions – the digestive and respiratory passages. During deglutition the respiratory tract is effectively closed off by laryngeal constriction, protecting the trachea and bronchi from inhalation of food or foreign bodies. The pharynx has three concentric coats: an internal mucous membrane, a supporting fibrous tunica and a muscular coat with a series of deficiencies for entry of vessels and nerves. These defects are important because they are the principal sites through which malignant tumours of the pharynx spread to adjacent tissues, particularly lymph nodes, in the neck.

Anatomically, the pharynx is usually described in three contiguous parts (Figure 10.7). The *nasopharynx*

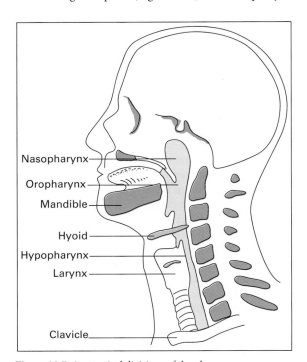

Figure 10.7 Anatomical divisions of the pharynx.

cancers arising from the nasopharynx are typically poorly differentiated or undifferentiated, or even anaplastic. Three-quarters of all nasopharyngeal lesions present with obvious lymphadenopathy, whereas in hypopharyngeal cancer almost half of all cases are clinically free of nodes [17]. Lymphomas are also relatively common in the oropharynx (particularly the tonsil) and nasopharynx.

Carcinoma of the nasopharynx

Although relatively uncommon in the Western world, these tumours are the commonest of all malignant tumours in many parts of China, accounting in some areas for half or more of all cancers. Clinical staging is more difficult than in any other head or neck site because of the inaccessibility of the lesion and its drainage routes. The TNM staging system is now widely used.

Cancers of the nasopharynx often have an insidious onset and present late, often with nodal disease in the neck. Nasal obstruction, usually unilateral, and secretory otitis media are also common. Bone erosion or destruction is common because of the close proximity of the nasopharynx to the base of the skull, many patients presenting with cranial nerve involvement, particularly nerves III–VI, which pass through the cavernous sinus. Cranial nerves IX–XII may also be involved by direct tumour extension where they pass through the parapharyngeal space in proximity to the lateral nasopharyngeal wall. Other extrapharyngeal sites of extension include the paranasal sinuses, nasal cavity, orbit and middle ear. Involvement of these regions causes pain, nasal stuffiness or discharge, unilateral deafness and ophthalmoplegia.

Treatment is by radical radiotherapy (increasingly by means of intensity-modulated radiation therapy; see Chapter 5, pages 73–75), with or without chemotherapy (see below). The irradiation volume must be large in order to encompass likely sites of local extension and nodal involvement. This must be achieved without any concession in total dosage, which should be at least 60 Gy delivered within 6–6.5 weeks. Higher doses may be delivered to the primary site but the many challenging technical difficulties include avoidance of the upper part of the spinal cord and temporal lobe of the brain (both of which have limited radiation tolerance), as well as the minimization of mucosal reaction as far as possible. The classical approach of Lederman (Figure 10.9) is still widely employed and aims at non-uniform high-dose irradiation to the primary and bilateral cervical nodes [18]. Lateral and anterior fields are employed, with appropriate shielding and field changes to avoid dangerous over-treatment of the upper cervical spinal cord

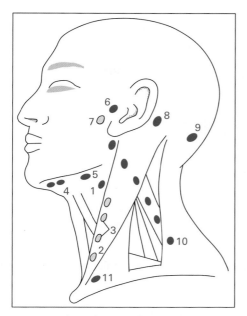

Figure 10.8 Lymphatic drainage of the head and neck: 1, jugulodigastric; 2, jugulo-omohyoid; 3, deep cervical; 4, submental; 5, submandibular; 6, preauricular; 7, parotid; 8, postauricular; 9, occipital; 10, posterior triangle; 11, supraclavicular.

is situated behind the nasal cavity and extends from the base of the skull above to the superior aspect of the soft palate below. It is bounded posteriorly by prevertebral fascia, extending anteriorly to the junction of the hard and soft palate. The *oropharynx* is situated behind the oral cavity, extends inferiorly to the floor of the vallecular sulcus and includes the posterior third of tongue, vallecula, soft palate, uvula, faucial pillars and tonsils. The *laryngopharynx* (or *hypopharynx*) is situated behind the larynx, extending from the floor of the vallecular sulcus above to the level of the lower border of the cricoid cartilage below, where it joins the oesophagus. It includes the pyriform fossae, posterior pharyngeal wall and postcricoid area. The whole pharynx has a rich lymphatic drainage and early nodal involvement is common, with a predictable clinical pattern (Figure 10.8). The important but inaccessible node of Rouvière is situated in the lateral retropharyngeal area, closely related to the jugular foramen and situated over the lateral masses of the atlas. Its importance lies in its critical position, making it an early site of invasion, particularly by nasopharyngeal tumours.

Most pharyngeal carcinomas are squamous in origin (oropharynx 60%, hypopharynx 75%), although primary

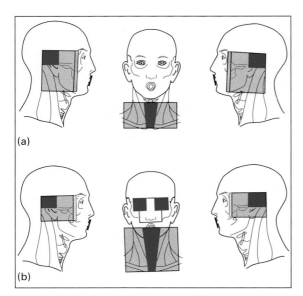

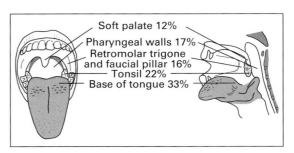

Figure 10.10 Carcinoma of the oropharynx: relative frequency at different sites.

Figure 10.9 Typical radiation for radical treatment of carcinoma of the nasopharynx: (a) first phase of treatment (40 Gy in 4 weeks); (b) second phase of treatment (to 60 Gy total dose in 6 weeks). (Source: Lederman and Mould [18]. Copyright © British Institute of Radiology 2014.)

without compromising the dosage to the lymph nodes. Even with this technique, a small portion (usually about 4 cm) of the spinal cord may inevitably receive a dose of 50 Gy, and treatment complications will be inevitable in some cases. Other complications of treatment such as perichondritis or radionecrosis are uncommon with careful fractionation and avoidance of overdosage. It is important to avoid removal of teeth during or shortly after treatment. Surgery has no place other than biopsy of the primary lesion, and occasionally in removal of residual lymph node disease by block dissection if the primary appears controlled.

Results of treatment are closely related to stage (see Table 10.2); median disease-free 5-year survival, even in patients with early disease, is less than 50%. The largest single group (T2N0–1), with an intermediate prognosis, has a 5-year disease-free survival of about 30%. A significant number of patients alive at 5 years will ultimately die of recurrence, and prolonged control followed by late relapse is common in this tumour. With T3-4N2-3 disease very few patients survive 5 years. Overall 5-year survival is better in younger people and in women. Recent attempts to improve results have included the use of intracavitary radioactive implants (often using caesium) to increase the dose to the primary site. The role

of chemotherapy is discussed below (pages 174–177), but is now regarded by almost all authorities as a standard part of treatment for nasopharyngeal carcinoma.

Carcinoma of the oropharynx

These tumours are somewhat more accessible, and in many ways simpler to treat. The important sites include the soft palate, faucial pillars, tonsil, posterior third of tongue and pharyngeal wall. The relative incidence and TNM staging are shown in Figure 10.10 and Table 10.4. Presenting symptoms include dysphagia with pain as well as aspiration of liquids. There may also be dysarthria with large tumours of the posterior tongue. The tumour is usually visible providing the anterior portion of the tongue is carefully retracted, but cancers arising from the posterior third of the tongue can be notoriously difficult to visualize and cervical lymph nodes may be enlarged [19] and sometimes precede definition of the primary site by more than a year. Radiological assessment can be very useful, using plain lateral views of the neck, tomography, barium contrast studies and CT scanning. There are differences in the presenting stage of tumours at different sites within the oropharynx; lesions of the tonsillar fossa are more often locally advanced (T3 and

Table 10.4 Tumours of the orbit (excluding globe).

Benign	Malignant
Haemangioma	Lymphoma
Lacrimal gland tumours	Rhabdomyosarcoma
Meningioma	Optic nerve glioma
Lymphangioma	Metastases
Neurofibroma	Angiosarcoma and other sarcomas
Dermoid cysts (pseudotumour)	Myeloma

T4) at presentation than tumours of the retromolar trigone or anterior faucial pillar.

Combinations of surgery and radiotherapy are routinely used in managing these lesions, although increasingly the emphasis has been on radical radiotherapy (sometimes in combination with chemotherapy), with surgery reserved for radiotherapy failures. The radiotherapeutic technique is much simpler than with carcinoma of the nasopharynx since direct extension of tumour can usually be dealt with simply by extension of the field in the appropriate direction. An important randomized study from Europe [20] has suggested a real advantage in tumour control following hyperfractionated radiotherapy using two fractions of treatment per day (see also Chapter 5). Difficult problems arise when there is extension into the hard palate, mandible, tongue or larynx, and these are usually best dealt with by high-dose radiation (with or without chemotherapy), or by surgery if treatment by irradiation and chemotherapy is unable to control the primary tumour. This is also true of lymphatic metastases. *En bloc* radical neck dissection may be required and can even be performed bilaterally ifx necessary.

Surgery and radiation are probably equally effective in controlling both the primary and the node metastases though with a far better functional result in patients treated by radiotherapy. Combined surgery and radiation may be valuable in more advanced tumours, particularly those arising in the anterior faucial pillar. For tonsillar tumours, excision biopsy of the whole tonsil is usually advisable for reliable histology, and may be sufficient if the resection margins are unequivocally clear.

For patients with local recurrence, surgical removal offers the only prospect of cure. These operations are complex and require careful consideration, demanding close cooperation between the head and neck surgeon who will undertake the radical excision and the plastic surgeon responsible for the reconstruction. Modern techniques, for example, using jejunal replacement of the pharynx, have improved the functional results, but rehabilitation of oropharyngeal function, especially deglutition, can be exceptionally difficult. Patients may need many months of skilled support and may suffer long-term problems with oral lubrication since the radiation fields frequently cover the parotid glands.

Lymphoma of the pharynx

A significant proportion of nasopharyngeal and tonsillar tumours will prove histologically to be lymphomas rather than epithelial tumours. Invariably these are non-Hodgkin's lymphomas, usually lymphocytic B-cell neoplasms. It is wise to undertake full investigation as for non-Hodgkin's lymphomas at other sites, because distant spread occurs. The stomach is involved in 20% of cases at some stage but spread to the marrow and other extra-nodal sites is unusual at presentation. Nasopharyngeal lymphomas also have a tendency to spread directly to the paranasal sinuses and nasal fossae. Routine treatment of these contiguous areas is often recommended whenever a primary nasopharyngeal lymphoma is encountered. Although this represents an unusually large treatment volume, local control can usually be achieved with a more modest dose than for epithelial tumours. A dose of 40 Gy in 4 weeks has traditionally been considered adequate, though higher doses are increasingly being recommended in order to make use of modern radiation technology (particularly intensity-modulated radiation therapy; see Chapter 5) and apply a higher dose to a smaller volume.

Carcinoma of the laryngopharynx (hypopharynx)

These are at least as common as those of the oropharynx, and as with other sites excessive cigarette and spirit consumption are the chief aetiological factors. Common symptoms include dyspnoea, dysphagia, anorexia, inanition and sometimes stridor. Most are well-differentiated squamous carcinomas and are locally advanced at presentation. Palpable lymph nodes are present in about half, and one-quarter of these are bilateral.

Although the prognosis is generally poor, some sites are prognostically more favourable than others. Carcinomas of the upper part of the laryngopharynx, including the aryepiglottic fold and exophytic lesions of the pharyngo-laryngeal fold, have a better prognosis than those of the more infiltrating or ulcerative variety, arising from the pyriform fossa, cervical oesophagus and posterior pharyngeal wall. They have a poor prognosis despite intensive treatment with radiotherapy, surgery and chemotherapy (in patients whose general condition warrants it). The 5-year survival rates remain no better than 10–15% overall, regardless of the specific hypopharyngeal subsite or method of treatment. A small subgroup has a better prognosis, including a remarkable 5-year survival rate of 50% for early (T1N0) lesions of the pyriform fossa. Although good results with radiotherapy alone have occasionally been claimed for individual patients with advanced disease, it is clear that the chief use of radiotherapy lies in palliation, and the avoidance of mutilating surgery that would in all probability fail to cure. Radical surgery is, however, occasionally indicated in patients with operable lesions and in good general health; these individual decisions are best made by a surgeon and radiotherapist working jointly in a combined clinic. Most patients ultimately die of local or regional recurrence (rarely because of lymph node disease alone), although an increasing proportion have evidence of more widespread dissemination.

Radiation technique is complicated by the large volume frequently required. Delineation of the lower extent of spread in laryngopharyngeal tumours is often very difficult. The technique usually consists of lateral opposed field treatment with either open (direct) or wedged fields (see Chapter 5). A major technical problem arises when the tumour has extended below the thoracic inlet since easy access by lateral fields is limited by the shoulders. These tumours pose some of the greatest technical challenges in clinical radiotherapy, particularly with postcricoid primary tumours. For treatment to be curative, a minimum radical dose of 64 Gy in 6.5 weeks, or equivalent, is always necessary. As with laryngeal cancers, an increasing number of centres routinely advocate a higher dose.

For both this and other head and neck sites, evidence is accumulating that re-irradiation with synchronous chemotherapy may be both feasible and effective for recurrent disease [21].

Tumours of the oral cavity

Tumours of the oral cavity include those arising from the lip, the mobile portion of the tongue (anterior to the circumvallate papillae), buccal mucosa, alveolae (gingiva), floor of mouth, hard palate and retromolar trigone. They are among the commonest tumours seen in many combined head and neck oncology clinics (see Figure 10.1), and are often surprisingly advanced at presentation. The incidence is rising fast, particularly among younger men [22], with a substantial change from 4400 new cases reported in the UK 10 years ago increasing to 5900 in 2008 and over 6200 in 2012. However, there is at least some evidence that use of retinoids in high-risk populations may prevent the development of dysplastic premalignant intraoral lesions into frankly invasive tumours [23].

The commonest symptom is of a non-healing ulcer on the lip, tongue, cheek or floor of mouth. Cancers of the lip can arise on the upper or lower vermillion border, or an adjacent area such as the philtrum, with direct involvement of the lip itself. The primary lesion can be raised, ulcerated, excavated, pigmented, well or poorly demarcated, painful or painless. Many oral cavity lesions are first diagnosed by a dentist and are sometimes hidden by dentures. Leucoplakia is a predisposing cause, although the value of surgical intervention and full resection of these lesions remains uncertain, current policies ranging from watchful waiting at some centres to aggressive surgical intervention in others [24]. On examination the usual findings are of a raised erythematous ulcerated lesion, often with an area of necrosis. Large tumours of the tongue may reduce mobility and interfere with speech.

Clinical examination should include careful bimanual palpation and the lesion should always be measured. Examination of the neck may reveal enlarged lymph nodes.

Investigation should include chest radiography, full blood count and liver function tests. In patients with tumours of the floor of mouth or lower alveolus, investigation should always include radiological examination (orthopantomogram) of the lower jaw since asymptomatic involvement can occur, even when the lesion is not tender. Fine-needle aspiration cytology of neck nodes is easily performed.

The clinical behaviour and probability of metastases varies with the site [19,22]. Carcinomas at the tip of the tongue are far easier to control than tumours of its lateral margins; cancers of the dorsum are most difficult of all (Figure 10.11). In general, tumours of the floor of the mouth, buccal mucosa, hard palate and alveolus show similar and relatively low metastatic rates, whereas

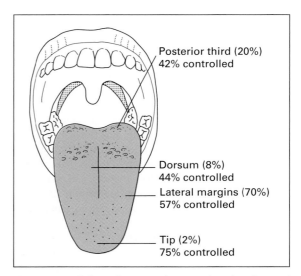

Figure 10.11 Relative frequency (in parentheses) and control rates in carcinoma of the tongue.

tumours of the oral tongue have a higher propensity for nodal spread.

Metastases are more frequent with poorly differentiated tumours. Larger tumours (>4 cm in diameter) are more difficult to control and likely to be accompanied by cervical node metastases. Bilateral node involvement is common with lesions of the floor of the mouth and faucial arch. The anatomical position of the abnormal nodes varies with the primary site. For carcinomas of the oral tongue and floor of mouth, the commonest sites are the jugulodigastric and submaxillary nodes, whereas palatine and retromolar trigone lesions are more frequently accompanied by lymphadenopathy at the angle of the jaw. Second primary cancers are relatively common within the oral cavity.

Management

Optimum management is best achieved in joint consultative clinics staffed by a surgeon, radiotherapist (clinical oncologist) and medical oncologist [25]. Principles of management are similar for the major sites within the oral cavity and are considered together, except for carcinomas of the lip (see page 172). See also Ref. [26], for a fuller account of evidence-based radiotherapy strategies for head and neck cancer. With improved tumour localization and routine use of conformal and IMRT radiation techniques, higher tumour doses can now be given more safely – see also Chapter 5, page 74–75.

Small accessible tumours of the oral cavity (T1)

These have an excellent cure rate with radical radiotherapy, with very good preservation of function. Interstitial implantation techniques are often ideal for intraoral tumours (i.e. excluding those of the lip), since the treatment volume can be kept small and a high dose given safely. Implants of radium, caesium, gold, tantalum and iridium are all satisfactory. Intraoral sites often treated by interstitial irradiation include tongue, buccal mucosa, floor of mouth, palate and lower alveolus. Very small lesions (<1 cm) can be treated with an interstitial implant alone, without external beam irradiation, although most radiotherapists use a combination of interstitial and external irradiation in larger tumours which are still small enough to implant (T1 and small T2 cancers). With an interstitial implant, a tumour dose of 60 Gy is usually given over 4–7 days. Where interstitial and external radiation are used together, many authorities recommend that the volume implant is taken to 50 Gy in 5–7 days, followed by external beam irradiation to 30 Gy in 3 weeks. In some clinics, excisional surgery is

preferred for small tumours of the anterior tip of the tongue, sometimes using the laser excision technique.

Larger tumours of the oral cavity (T2–T4)

In these tumours, external beam irradiation has traditionally been the mainstay of treatment, although a dual modality approach using combined radiation and chemotherapy is increasingly being employed (see below). With external irradiation, doses of 60 Gy over 6 weeks are usually considered essential; tolerance is related to the volume irradiated. Radiation technique involves treatment by lateral open (direct) or wedged fields, to include both the primary tumour and the initial drainage node group. For cancers of the tongue, floor of mouth and lower jaw, the palate can safely be excluded from treatment by means of a mouth gag which depresses the tongue.

The proper management of metastases in neck nodes remains contentious. Many clinics recommend routine radical neck dissection in patients with mobile nodes, and prophylactic node dissection in clinically node-negative patients has revealed a significant incidence of micrometastatic tumour. In patients without evidence of neck node involvement (N0), most radiotherapists give prophylactic treatment to the neck, to a slightly lower dose (50 Gy in 5 weeks or equivalent) than radical dosage, on the grounds that occult nodal spread is common and that nodal recurrence is reduced by such treatment. Most centres employ external beam irradiation, sometimes in combination with surgery, to control metastatic neck nodes, although ultimate survival rates in patients with N2 and N3 nodes are poor whatever the approach.

In patients treated initially by surgical resection, the question arises of which patients routinely require postoperative radiation therapy. Increasingly a 'high-risk' group is recognized, whose features include either extracapsular extension of nodal disease or any two or more of the following risk factors: microscopically positive mucosal margins: nerve involvement invasion; more than two involved neck nodes; node size greater than 3 cm; more than one positive nodal group in the neck. Whilst these points hold true for many head and neck primary sites, they seem particularly relevant for cancers of the oral cavity and oropharynx.

Patterns of recurrence and overall survival are clearly dependent on the size and stage of the tumour. In one large study the cumulative 3-year survival in mobile tongue and floor of mouth lesions without lymphadenopathy was 57%, whereas for patients with palpable lymphadenopathy the survival rate fell to

42% [27]. In general, patients whose oral carcinoma seems most likely from the clinical history (including tobacco/alcohol use) to be related to HPV infection, the overall outcome is better stage for stage, possibly related to the fact that these patients tend to be younger and fitter, with less intensive tobacco consumption and better nutrition. Where lymph node involvement is obvious at presentation, failure at the primary site is common despite intensive radiotherapy. Occasionally it is possible to control a limited relapse (usually the primary site) with an interstitial radioactive implant, although radical surgery is usually required later since durable control is rarely achieved.

In the UK, surgery is usually undertaken if local relapse occurs after primary radiation therapy, though increasingly some centres recommend primary surgical excision instead of radical irradiation because of the long-term problems of radiation damage within the oral cavity. A wide resection is invariably required, with immediate reconstruction.

The advent of free flap grafting with microvascular anastomosis has dramatically improved the cosmetic results. However, complete surgical extirpation of the initial area at risk has to be undertaken, often resulting in substantial local damage with loss of function. A typical operation for a recurrent lesion of the floor of the mouth might include a hemiglossectomy, excision of the floor of the mouth, hemimandibulectomy, and neck dissection (commando procedure) with pedicle and/or microvascular free flap grafting in order to achieve adequate healing, a major undertaking in patients who are often debilitated enough to require hyperalimentation before surgery. Intensive rehabilitation and speech therapy are also critically important. Chapter 7 (page 117) provides a fuller discussion of patient rehabilitation. For persistent radiation-induced dry mouth (xerostomia) the use of oral pilocarpine has been shown to increase salivary production, generally with fairly minor side-effects such as sweating and urinary frequency [28]. A further attempt at modifying the often severe and painful radiation-induced mucositis is currently under investigation, using the human keratinizing growth factor receptor binding-agent palifermin, which has already been shown to reduce radiation-induced mucositis following total body irradiation for leukaemia (see Chapter 28). This agent appears to protect during the painful ulcerative phase of mucositis by mediating cytokine release, without evidence (to date) of tumour cell protection – potentially an important advance.

Chemotherapy may also be valuable in the primary or secondary management of these tumours and is further discussed in the final section of this chapter.

Carcinoma of the lip

These are almost always squamous cell carcinomas, often well differentiated and presenting relatively early since the tumour is usually visible. The incidence has fallen rapidly during the past 25 years, and less than 300 new cases are now seen annually in the UK. Cancers of the lower lip are much commoner than those of the upper lip (20:1) but upper lip cancers are relatively commoner in women.

Metastasis is relatively uncommon, and is to local lymph nodes. About 7% of patients have involvement of local nodes at diagnosis, and the same proportion will develop metastases in local lymph node groups after primary treatment. Nodal invasion is usually directly to the submaxillary or submental nodes and metastases rarely occur elsewhere.

Treatment

Treatment is by surgery or radiotherapy. Most carcinomas of the lip are curable by radiation therapy, particularly where the tumour is small (T1). External beam therapy with photons or electrons, and brachytherapy with radium moulds or interstitial iridium implants, have all been used, all with high cure rates. Surgery also offers excellent local control, although the cosmetic result may be slightly less satisfactory, particularly where excision of a substantial portion of the lip needs to be undertaken. In larger tumours (T2), radiotherapy is generally accepted as a better method of treatment both cosmetically and functionally, since surgical excision often leads to poor closure of the mouth and may interfere with phonation. With large destructive cancers of the lip (T3, T4, now relatively uncommon), it is difficult to achieve an adequate cosmetic and functional result by either method of treatment, and the incidence of local recurrence is higher. Healing may be excellent even following large doses of radiation therapy, but surgical reconstruction is often necessary.

External beam irradiation is most commonly employed, using either electron beam therapy or moderate-energy photons, although the lip is also one of the classic sites for brachytherapy. As with treatment of skin cancer, an individually designed lead cut-out can be used to allow external beam treatment of any size and shape of field. Treatment schedules are varied, though the best cosmetic schedules include 40 Gy applied dose in 10 fractions daily over 2 weeks, 50 Gy applied dose in 20 fractions over 4 weeks, 45 Gy in 10 fractions (given on alternate weekdays over 3.5 weeks) or, in centres preferring lengthy radical dosage, 60 Gy in 30 consecutive daily fractions over 6 weeks. This latter regimen is probably the most suitable for large volumes.

In the rare patient with nodal metastases, radical neck dissection is the treatment of choice, although radiotherapy can also be effective. With radical radiation therapy, surgery or a combination of both techniques, the results in carcinoma of the lip are excellent, and virtually all patients without lymph node involvement should be considered curable. Even with lymph node metastases, the overall survival is 60–70% at 5 years.

Nasal cavity and paranasal sinuses

These uncommon tumours, where presentation is often late and accompanied by early invasion of critical structures, are among the most difficult of all tumours of the head and neck region [29,30]. The exposed nature of these facial cancers demands great skill both in eradicating the tumour and in providing accept-able reconstruction. They tend to be slow-growing, well-differentiated squamous carcinomas, in which local recurrence is the major problem. Melanoma of the nasal cavity accounts for almost 10% of nasal cavity cancer. Tumours of the nasal cavity/paranasal sinuses spread locally and to the nasopharynx (Figure 10.12). Although late presentation is the rule, those originating from within the nasal cavity tend to present earlier, usually with nasal obstruction, stuffiness or offensive discharge.

Olfactory neuroblastoma is a rare but important tumour, accounting for about 3% of all primary intranasal tumours. They are also known as esthesioneuroblastoma or olfactory neuroepithelioma. Although commonest in adult life, about 20% occur in younger patients, below the age of 20. They are generally staged according to the Kadish system (stage A, nasal cavity only; stage B, nasal cavity and one or more paranasal sites; stage C, more widespread disease, for example, to the skull base, neck nodes or more distant dissemination).

Anatomically, the commonest nasal/paranasal sinus sites are the maxillary antrum, followed by nasal cavity and ethmoid sinus. Localized tumours of the maxillary antrum are usually asymptomatic; symptoms such as swelling and erythema of the cheek should raise suspicion of extension beyond the confines of the primary site. Erosion of the floor of the orbit and displacement of

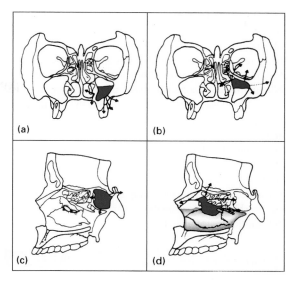

Figure 10.12 Pathways of local spread of tumours of the nasal cavity and paranasal sinuses: (a, b) lower and upper maxillary tumours spreading to orbit, nasal fossa, palate, upper alveolus and soft tissues; (c) sphenoid sinus tumours (lateral view) into nasopharynx, base of brain, ethmoid and nasal cavity; (d) nasal fossa tumours (lateral view) into orbit, base of skull, sphenoid and posterior choana. (From Boone *et al.* [30].)

the globe may occur, leading to diplopia and ophthal-moplegia. Spread downwards (into the oral cavity) or posteriorly (into the pterygoid region) are also common, and other adjacent sites such as nasal cavity and ethmoid and sphenoidal sinuses are often involved (Figure 10.12).

Little is known of the predisposing factors, although excessive alcohol intake, cigarette smoking and oral hygiene are held to be important. Adenocarcinoma of the nasal cavity is an occupational hazard in hardwood furniture makers, presumably due to inhalation of an occupational carcinogen. Staging by TNM or other conventional criteria has been disappointing but CT and MRI give far more practical information (see Figure 10.3).

The concept of combined-modality treatment is well established. In 1933, Ohngren advocated treatment by a combination of surgery and irradiation on the grounds that this gave better results than either treatment alone. In general, this approach has been validated and remains the standard policy in many large centres, particularly for treatment of the maxillary antrum. Surgical healing, even after radical doses of radiotherapy, is not usually a problem at this site, since the head and neck region is so well vascularized. Conversely, there seems little prospect of reducing the extent of surgery for tumours that have usually spread beyond their primary confines at the time of diagnosis. No worthwhile comparative trials have been reported, but several series have demonstrated a 5-year survival of up to 40% with combined treatment. In patients too frail to undergo an operation, a 5-year survival of 20% has been achieved with the use of radiotherapy alone. For olfactory neuroblastoma, the Kadish stage provides useful prognostic information, with a good outcome for localized cases treated by combined surgical and radiotherapeutic techniques, particularly where the tumour is of low histological grade. Modern prosthetics have allowed many of these patients to face the world with a reasonably normal appearance despite substantial anatomical deficiencies.

Tumours of the middle ear

Cancer of the middle ear is extremely unusual, chiefly occurring in middle-aged men with a history of chronic otitis media, often making diagnosis difficult since the symptoms may be little more than an accentuation of the chronic discharge, with the addition of bleeding and pain. Direct local spread to mastoid air cells or external auditory canal is the rule, sometimes producing severe pain, particularly if bone erosion has occurred. The tumours are usually squamous carcinomas, arising as a result of squamous metaplasia of the columnar epithelial cells normally present. Adenocarcinoma is very rare. Complete surgical removal is often impossible, and local control difficult to achieve. Extension beyond the temporal bone makes the prognosis very poor. Local extension to the brain may occur. Since survival rates are similar (about 25% at 5 years) whichever local method of treatment is employed, radical irradiation is usually preferred. Other rare tumours include soft-tissue sarcomas and primary tumours of bone. In these cases, radical surgery is seldom possible and the mainstay of treatment is radiotherapy.

Glomus jugulare tumours arise from neuroendocrine chemoreceptors of the jugular bulb, and should be considered with similar tumours (chemodectoma, paraganglioma) arising at other sites such as the bifurcation of the carotid artery (carotid body tumour) or posterior mediastinum. They are three times commoner in women, and may sometimes be bilateral. Although histologically benign, these tumours invade locally. Surgery is hazardous, since they are highly vascular and usually involve the middle ear and petrous temporal bone. Presentation is with a classical cluster of symptoms including deafness, cranial nerve palsies, local pain and tinnitus. Radiotherapy is often the treatment of choice and modest doses (40–50 Gy in 4–5 weeks) are adequate though regression may be slow.

Carcinoma of the pinna and external auditory canal

Tumours of the external auditory canal are usually squamous cell carcinomas, but on the pinna (much the commoner site) the commonest cell type in the UK is the basal cell carcinoma, although squamous carcinomas are commoner in the USA. Malignant melanoma is occasionally encountered. Usually there is a visible lesion of the pinna; in the case of tumours of the external canal, crusting, discharge or unilateral deafness occur. Pain is unusual. Local extension may occur to preauricular structures, tympanic membrane, middle ear or mastoid.

Although radical surgery can be curative, it is widely accepted that treatment by radical radiotherapy is equally effective and offers a better functional result, even though mucosal oedema, sterile fluid collections in the middle ear and perforation of the eardrum may occur with high-dose radiation.

Chemotherapy in squamous carcinomas of the head and neck

Although both surgery and radiotherapy can be curative for localized squamous cancers of the head and neck [31,32] (even in some cases with lymph node involvement), the prognosis of patients with recurrent or disseminated disease is very poor [33]. The first attempts at using cytotoxic chemotherapy in these patients were made at least 30 years ago, often using intra-arterial perfusion. More recently, interest has shifted from the use of single agents to combination chemotherapy, and from treatment of recurrent disease to the use of adjuvant chemotherapy in the initial management. It is now widely accepted that chemotherapy plays a critically important role in the initial management of locally advanced cancers of the head and neck, reducing the likelihood of recurrence and in several large studies and meta-analyses improving the overall survival rate.

Active drugs include methotrexate, cisplatin, bleomycin, 5-FU, the taxanes and mitomycin C. All these show some degree of activity, and in the past few years there has been a tendency towards combination chemotherapy for recurrent disease, increasingly employing cisplatin/5-FU or methotrexate/bleomycin combinations, although the duration of response tends to be short. There is no definite evidence that multidrug regimens are superior in survival to single-agent therapy [34], although it has become customary to use multiagent chemotherapy, as with so many other adult solid tumours. Other newer agents with activity include paclitaxel, docetaxel (see Chapter 6 for a fuller discussion), vinorelbine, gemcitabine and topoisomerase inhibitors such as topotecan.

A major area of controversy surrounds the use of adjuvant combination chemotherapy immediately following (or in some cases preceding) local treatment with surgery or radiotherapy [35–38]. Large cooperative American and European groups have reported better local control and survival in comparison with historical controls. Indeed, randomized studies using chemoradiotherapy compared with conventional radical irradiation have been reported [38,39], increasingly suggesting a clear-cut benefit for the combined-modality group, especially in terms of freedom from local recurrence. In a large study from the Christie Hospital, Manchester, for example, the addition of just two pulses of single-agent methotrexate proved clearly beneficial in a series of over 300 patients with advanced disease [36]. A large prospective meta-analysis of adjuvant chemotherapy in squamous cell carcinomas of the head and neck [33] has confirmed the following:
- over 10 700 patients were included in analysis, from 76 trials;
- 34% were classified as UICC/TNM stage III, 56% as stage IV;
- there was a small but statistically highly significant improvement in overall and event-free survival in favour of chemotherapy (hazard ratio 0.90, $P < 0.0001$) in risk of death, corresponding to a 4% absolute increase in overall survival at both 2 and 5 years;
- the benefit appeared dependent on timing of chemotherapy – synchronous chemoradiation clearly produced better results;
- there is no evidence of benefit with neoadjuvant or subsequent chemotherapy;
- no obvious advantage for platinum-containing programmes compared with other regimens.

See also Ref. [40] for an account of the largest single chemoradiation study and in addition, a meta-analysis update of this topic from Ref. [41]. This later French-based analysis confirmed their initial findings published in 2000, added several new trials, and showed an increased absolute survival for concomitant chemo-radiotherapy studies of 6.5% (measured at 5 years median post-treatment), that is, somewhat larger than the original estimate.

Several uncontrolled series have investigated cisplatin/5-FU combinations and found them both active and feasible in combination with radical irradiation. Other active agents, apart from the well-established group (cisplatin, bleomycin, methotrexate and 5-FU), include carboplatin, the taxanes and ifosfamide. Despite encouraging data from a number of studies and meta-analyses, it remains difficult to evaluate the role of chemotherapy in primary treatment until larger-scale randomized trials have been completed. The first major meta-analysis [33] suggested a 6.5% increase in overall survival (all trials taken together) but almost double this figure (12.1%) with synchronous chemoradiation therapy. There is no doubt that chemotherapy has now become established as a major component of therapy for most patients with locoregionally advanced disease. Molecular targeted agents such as the epidermal growth factor receptor (EGFR) inhibitor cetuximab are also becoming more widely used (see below).

An important and encouraging study in advanced oropharyngeal carcinomas was reported from the French multicentre head and neck oncology group in 2004 [38]. Concomitant chemoradiotherapy (carboplatin plus 5-FU) was compared with radiotherapy alone in a group of 226 patients. Overall survival was 22% in the combination group compared with 16% with radiotherapy alone; median survival times were 22 months compared with 13 months, although not surprisingly the complication rate was higher in the combined-modality treatment group. Recent work employing the combination of chemoradiation postoperatively (i.e. following attempted curative resection) has again supported the use of this multimodal approach in the adjuvant postoperative setting [39]. In this large clinical trial of 459 patients, those receiving chemoradiation therapy following radical surgical resection had a 2-year locoregional control rate of 82%, compared with only 72% in the radiotherapy group. Clearly, multimodal therapy for locally advanced squamous cell carcinomas of the head and neck has now become increasingly established, and further studies have supported this view, even in the postoperative setting [42].

Patients with nasopharyngeal carcinoma undoubtedly have a higher response rate to chemotherapy. Attention has naturally turned to the use of chemotherapy as an adjuvant to primary treatment by radical irradiation.

Although at least one large study has proven positive [43], results from other study groups have been less successful, with one large trial failing to demonstrate an improvement either in relapse-free survival or in overall survival between two treatment arms [44]; however, in the subgroup of 49 patients with very bulky neck lymph nodes (greater than 6 cm) the results of multimodal treatment were superior, the chemotherapy apparently doubling the survival rate from 37% to 73%. Other recent studies have also been more positive [44], and recent overviews of all the published randomized trials have concluded that synchronous chemotherapy (i.e. given concomitantly with radical irradiation) probably improves survival. The benefits of adding of synchronous chemotherapy to radical irradiation are seen over all the major head and neck tumour sites – see Ref. [45].

It is now widely accepted that synchronous schedules are superior, that radical chemoradiation programmes are well tolerated by the majority of patients and that disease-free survival is improved. Choice of agents remains controversial; the Pignon meta-analysis does not favour platinum-containing regimens over the generally less toxic non-platinum-based combinations. One recent study investigating the novel combination of carboplatin with paclitaxel concluded that it was probably as effective as standard therapy with cisplatin/5-FU but had a better toxicity profile [46]. Mature survival analysis gave a long-term (3-year) survival rate of 70%. On the other hand, cisplatin-based chemoradiation therapy has certainly become the standard of care at most centres, particularly since the publication of the important US-based Intergroup study demonstrating an absolute 3-year survival rate advantage of 14% [46,47]. Interestingly, the magnitude of this improvement was even greater than that observed with radiotherapy plus cetuximab in the widely discussed report by Bonner and colleagues (see immediately below). More recently, studies from both US and European cooperative groups have confirmed an impressive advantage for the combination of cisplatin, 5-FU and docetaxel, in comparison with the current standard of the first two agents alone, in patients with unresectable head and neck cancer [48]. In the European study, for example, the median overall survival was increased from 14.5 months (cisplatin/5-FU) to 18.8 months (cisplatin, 5-FU and docetaxel), and a reduction in the risk of death at the assessment point (32.5 months) of 27%.

Newer systemic approaches for the management of advanced or refractory disease include attempts to target EGFR (which is known to be over-expressed in most patients with head and neck carcinoma), *p53* or H-*ras* gene mutations; use of novel chemotherapy with transforming growth factor and antisense therapy; use of the differentiation agent 13-*cis*-retinoic acid for both treatment and prophylaxis; and intratumoral injection of ONYX-015, a gene-deleted replication adenovirus that both replicates and causes clear-cut cytopathogenicity in a variety of cancer cells. All the above, as well as attempts at re-irradiation, are under current trial [49]. Molecular targeted therapies are rapidly becoming established, at least within the clinical trial setting. Results from one substantial study showed that the IgG1 monoclonal antibody cetuximab (Erbitux) enhances the effects of conventional chemotherapy and also appears to act as a radiosensitizer. In both untreated and recurrent cisplatin-resistant cases, cetuximab has now demonstrated proven activity, improving the therapeutic index without increasing the toxicity of treatment. A recent report from a US-led international group will almost certainly lead to a new standard of care for patients with locally advanced disease [50]. This large-scale study (424 patients) compared intensive radiation therapy alone with the same treatment plus cetuximab, given as a loading dose just before the definitive radiation therapy, and also during the full course, generally a 7–8 week period. The results were extremely impressive, with improvements in local control (from 14.9 to 24.4 months) and, even more importantly, overall survival (from 29.3 months to over 49 months) in the combined-modality group; with the additional benefit that most of the toxicity normally associated with cytotoxic chemotherapy was avoided. The greatest benefit was seen in patients with oropharyngeal tumours, although the current standard of care in this group, namely, chemoradiation therapy, was not used here as the 'control' arm (which employed radiotherapy alone). These data were recently updated, and confirm a substantial 5-yr survival improvement with cetuximab (49 months vs 29 months, for patients with locally advanced disease), particularly in patients developing the treatment-related characteristic rash – see Ref. [51]. An increasing number of EGFR inhibitors have also shown activity against head and neck cancer, including gefitinib, erlotinib, lapatinib, zalutumumab and panitumumab – all of which are the subject of current trials. This important area of current research is well covered in [52,53].

Dual-agent molecular targeting of EGFR may be achieved even more effectively by combining an anti-EGFR antibody with a tyrosine kinase inhibitor [54], which theoretically would augment the potency of both EGFR signalling inhibition and, in consequence, tumour responsiveness. Finally, recent analyses have shown a similar survival benefit either from the routine use of synchronous chemoradiation or by hyperfractionation of radiotherapy [55]. Using six rather than five radiotherapy fractions per week gives a clear advantage, as does strict adherence to a standard daily protocol with avoidance of unplanned treatment gaps or delays in commencing radiotherapy – an important point now taken increasingly seriously by most radiotherapy departments. These newer approaches to the treatment of locally advanced, recurrent or metastatic head and neck cancer represent one of the most exciting areas of oncology at the present time (see Ref. [56]).

Tumours of salivary glands

Although uncommon, accounting for about 2% of all neoplasms, salivary tumours are of great interest since they are of such varied histology and present technical problems in management [57]. The most common primary site is the parotid (almost 80% of all cases), although the other major (submandibular and sublingual) and minor salivary glands can be affected. Occasionally, tumours of minor salivary glands can grow to a large size, mimicking cancers of the nasopharynx or palate.

The parotid gland is an accessible organ, overlying the styloid process, situated between mastoid and mandible, and mostly lying anterior to the pinna. Its deep boundary is close to the parapharyngeal space and lateral pharyngeal wall. Superiorly, it rarely extends beyond the zygomatic arch. The gland is divided by the facial nerve and it branches into a superficial and deep lobe; excision is often limited for fear of surgical damage to this nerve. The submandibular gland lies beneath the horizontal portion of the mandible, and the sublingual gland (the smallest of the three major salivary glands) lies in the floor of the mouth, in contact with the inner surface of the mandible, often extending to the midline where it meets the contralateral gland.

Pathologically, the wide variety of histological types of salivary tumour encompasses both benign and malignant disorders (Table 10.5). Three-quarters are benign, mostly pleomorphic adenomas or 'mixed salivary tumours', which is much the commonest tumour in the parotid gland and less frequently found in other sites (only 40% of tumours in minor salivary glands). About 65% occur in women, mostly in the 50–65 year age group, although pleomorphic adenomas of the parotid have been reported even in children. The tumours are histologically

Table 10.5 Histological types and prognosis in salivary gland tumours.

	Frequency (%)	5-year survival (%)
Pleomorphic adenoma	75	96
Adenocarcinoma	8	50
Mucoepidermoid		
Low grade	3	90
High grade	3	20
Adenoid cystic	4	60
Malignant mixed	2	55
Acinic cell	1	80
Squamous	3	25

varied, often with several populations of cells. However, the overall pattern, though bizarre, pleomorphic and disorganized, is not one of malignancy.

Approximately one-quarter of parotid tumours are malignant. *Malignant mixed tumours*, or pleomorphic adenocarcinomas, often resemble pleomorphic adenomas histologically although foci of malignant change are typically scattered throughout the specimen. These patients usually give a history of slow-growing and painless parotid swelling, often for several years, followed by a sudden change, with increased swelling and pain. This well-recognized development represents one of the best examples of malignant change within an area of benign neoplasia, a most unusual phenomenon at other sites. *Adenoid cystic carcinomas* or cylindromas are rather more common (about 15% of malignant salivary tumours) and arise in major salivary glands but also quite typically in the minor glands, for example, in the palate. Characteristically, these tumours spread by direct extension along perineural spaces, a feature that may lead to unusual clinical presentations. *Mucoepidermoid carcinomas* are well recognized, and consist histologically of two distinct populations of cells, with mucus secretion together with typical epidermoid morphology. These often tend to be less malignant tumours and the lowest grade ones are clinically benign, although at the other end of the spectrum is the high-grade mucoepidermoid carcinoma, which can be difficult to control and may be rapidly fatal. *Acinic cell tumours* are rare, more common in females, with a slow clinical evolution and an unusual histological picture suggesting an origin in acinic epithelial cells. Squamous cell and *anaplastic carcinomas* of the salivary glands must be diagnosed with caution, since there is a problem in distinguishing these from secondary deposits arising from a head and neck tumour site of more typical squamous origin. Histologically, the squamous or anaplastic element may be one component of a mixed malignant or other type of salivary tumour. True anaplastic or squamous tumours of the salivary gland are among the most malignant of tumours, with a very poor prognosis. *Lymphoma* of the parotid is occasionally seen, but it is difficult to be sure if its site of origin is the parotid itself or an adjacent lymph node. *Adenolymphoma* (Warthin's tumour) is an unusual lesion, sometimes misdiagnosed as an abscess, and of doubtful origin. It is never malignant, may even be degenerative, and is characterized by large pink-staining cells surrounded by a lymphoid 'follicle', often with a centrally cystic area.

Clinical features and management

Benign salivary tumours usually present with a slowly growing, painless mass. The onset of pain or a facial palsy is a sinister development suggestive of malignancy. The most rapidly growing tumours are anaplastic and squamous carcinomas, other malignant salivary tumours typically presenting with a more insidious onset. With adenoid cystic carcinomas, pain is a common feature due to the perineural spread. Lymph node involvement is unusual in salivary tumours though reportedly more common in high-grade mucoepidermoid carcinoma. However, haematogenous spread is well recognized, particularly with anaplastic, mixed malignant tumours and cylindromas.

Surgical excision is undoubtedly the most important approach for both benign and malignant salivary tumours. For benign parotid tumours (occurring most commonly in the superficial portion of the gland), superficial parotidectomy with preservation of the facial nerve is the operation of choice, giving excellent results if complete excision is achieved. When excision is incomplete, postoperative radiotherapy will reduce recurrence rates and is mandatory in this situation. Although some surgeons recommend follow-up observation after incomplete excision, this policy carries the disadvantage that a second operation may then be required, with the consequent risk of damage to the facial nerve. It is far safer to offer routine postoperative radiotherapy to patients with incompletely excised parotid tumours. At other sites such as the submandibular and sublingual glands, wider excision may be possible since there is no risk of facial nerve trunk damage.

The indications for routine radiotherapy in malignant tumours include inadequate surgical excision margins; tumours of high grade (particularly squamous, anaplastic and mixed malignant lesions); when surgery has been performed for recurrent disease; and for malignant lymphoma of the parotid, where surgery plays no part in the management, other than for biopsy. There is justification for the suggestion that postoperative radiotherapy should be offered in all cases of malignant salivary tumours. Lymphomas and adenocarcinomas are generally the most radiosensitive types of salivary tumour. Occasionally, surgery is contraindicated, for example, in unfit or elderly patients, or in those with malignant tumours of the minor salivary glands in the nasopharynx or palate. In these circumstances, long-term control can sometimes be achieved with radiotherapy alone.

The radiotherapy technique may be technically demanding since large volumes of tissue need to be uniformly irradiated and care is required to avoid over-treatment to sensitive structures, that is, brainstem, eye and mucous membranes. The usual arrangement is a wedged pair of fields. Particular care must be taken to avoid irradiation of the contralateral eye from the exit beam. A dose of 50–55 Gy in 5–5.5 weeks is adequate treatment for residual benign tumours. Malignant parotid tumours need higher doses. If there is residual disease postoperatively, 60–70 Gy in 6–8 weeks is recommended. Because of the initially large volume, a shrinking field technique may be necessary (see Chapter 5). The whole parotid bed should be treated up to the zygomatic arch and inferiorly to the level of the hyoid, to include both the jugulodigastric and upper cervical nodes. For submandibular and sublingual tumours, large treatment volumes are also required since the whole gland will need to be irradiated. Adenoid cystic lesions must be irradiated generously in view of the perineural invasion; with parotid cylindromas, the mastoid should always be treated.

Should the whole of the cervical node chain be irradiated in patients with malignant parotid tumours? Since the frequency of lymph node involvement varies with the histology, routine cervical node irradiation is only necessary in patients with squamous or anaplastic tumours, adenocarcinomas or mucoepidermoid and malignant mixed tumours of high grade. In some clinics, particularly in the USA, these patients are treated by elective lymph node dissection.

Prognosis

The outcome depends on the histological type [58] as well as operability. Routine use of postoperative radiotherapy increases local control in all the major types, but squamous, anaplastic and high-grade mucoepidermoid carcinomas carry a poor prognosis because of both local recurrence and metastatic spread. Better results are seen with low-grade mucoepidermoid tumours and acinic cell tumours, with adenoid cystic and malignant mixed tumours carrying an intermediate prognosis. Overall, women have a better prognosis than men (10-year survival 75% and 60%, respectively).

Further surgical excision is sometimes possible for localized recurrent disease, while palliative radiotherapy may be useful for distant metastases, particularly with less aggressive slow-growing tumours. Pulmonary and other distant metastases are encountered, particularly with adenoid cystic carcinoma. Treatment with chemotherapy has no established role.

Tumours of the orbit and eye [59,60]

Orbit

Both primary and secondary neoplasms occur in the orbit (see Table 10.4). Lymphoma and rhabdomyosarcoma are the commonest primary tumours. Soft-tissue sarcoma, nerve and nerve sheath tumours (including optic nerve gliomas) and meningiomas are all seen occasionally. Orbital secondary deposits are likely to be due to carcinomas of the breast, bronchus or thyroid.

Clinical features

Because of the orbit's rigid structure, forward displacement of the globe (proptosis) is the cardinal physical sign. Ophthalmoplegia may also occur because of interference with the external ocular muscles or, less commonly, because of a third cranial nerve palsy, particularly with posteriorly placed tumours. Proptosis can be extreme and disfiguring, particularly in children. Chemosis and infection are common and may lead to a misdiagnosis of cellulitis. Panophthalmitis can lead to perforation of the globe and unilateral blindness is common with advanced tumours. The rapid onset of chemosis and lid oedema suggest that the tumour is malignant. Marked proptosis with normal ocular movement usually indicates a slow-growing benign tumour. Tumours within the muscle cone produce less disturbance of ocular movement but more proptosis and greater visual loss; those outside the cone produce eccentric proptosis and affect vision later.

Investigation

Plain radiography and tomography can be extremely helpful and give good views of the orbital margins and optic canals. Greater detail is obtained with CT scanning, which gives information on the site, size and degree of intraorbital and extraorbital spread as well as a clear indication of bony erosion and soft-tissue tumour invasion (see Figure 10.3). Ultrasound examination may be helpful in providing rapid demonstration that a tumour is present. Biopsy confirmation of the diagnosis should be obtained where possible, but there may be formidable difficulties, with a risk of tumour spillage, haemorrhage and blindness. If the tumour is encapsulated it is usually best to excise it entirely.

Lymphoma

Malignant lymphomas of the orbit are almost always of the non-Hodgkin variety and may be isolated or encountered as part of a more generalized lymphoma (see Chapter 26). Full investigation is required as for any other lymphoma, since evidence of systemic disease will sometimes be found. Biopsy is usually straightforward since the lymphomas tend to be anteriorly placed, and treatment with radiotherapy is usually successful. Even where systemic lymphoma is discovered, radiotherapy is used as an addition to systemic treatment in order to prevent local recurrence, and modest doses of the order of 30 Gy over 3 weeks are usually adequate.

Orbital pseudotumour

This condition usually presents as a painful ophthalmoplegia often accompanied by swelling of the eyelids. CT shows a retro-orbital mass, often ill defined and surrounding the optic nerve. Histologically, there is a pleomorphic inflammatory infiltrate but occasionally monotypic B cells can be demonstrated, indicating a low-grade lymphoma.

The disease responds rapidly to steroids, which may prevent visual loss. Relapses occur and the 'tumour' may spread back through the orbital fissure to the base of the brain. Radiotherapy may help but, in rare cases, the disease can be relentlessly progressive.

Rhabdomyosarcoma

This is usually embryonal in type, occurring chiefly in infants, young children and adolescents, slightly more commonly in males. Local spread involves the maxilla, paranasal sinuses, frontal bone or even the brain, via the anterior or middle cranial fossae. Haematological spread is primarily to lung or bone but is less common than with rhabdomyosarcomas from other sites. Lymph node involvement, present in 25% of cases, usually involves upper deep cervical or preauricular nodes. These tumours often advance rapidly, leading to particularly severe proptosis with chemosis and lid oedema. Wherever possible, full pretreatment staging, including bone marrow aspiration, should be performed. Surgery was formerly used for control of the primary lesion, but radiotherapy has become increasingly preferred and has a low local recurrence rate. High doses of the order of 50 Gy over 5–6 weeks are required and a high proportion of these patients preserve useful vision provided that the lacrimal apparatus is shielded to ensure against xerophthalmia (see below).

Adjuvant chemotherapy is now an established part of treatment, with combinations of cyclophosphamide, vincristine and actinomycin D or doxorubicin. At least one course of combination chemotherapy is given before orbital radiation, because of the high probability of extraocular spread and also because rapid resolution occurs that will make the child more comfortable and the radiotherapy technically easier. The chemotherapy should normally be continued for about 1 year. Local irradiation is important as a means of ensuring local control even when metastases are present. Routine use of chemotherapy has improved 5-year survival from 40% using surgery and radiotherapy alone to about 75%, with a particular improvement in tumours of younger children, which were previously notorious for their high probability of dissemination (see Chapter 24).

Lacrimal gland tumours

These are usually considered with orbital tumours, although they are extremely rare. Commonest in young adults, their histological spectrum is reminiscent of that of salivary gland tumours, with pleomorphic adenomas and adenoid cystic carcinomas the most frequently encountered types. There is usually a long history (>1 year) of a slowly expanding, hard, painless mass. With more rapidly growing lesions, a biopsy is imperative and complete surgical removal of the tumour should be carried out if possible. Where total removal of the lacrimal gland cannot be performed (for a patient with either a pleomorphic adenoma or any of the malignant tumours) radiotherapy should also be given. Local recurrence is very common even after a high dose, so every effort should be made to remove these tumours. True carcinomas of the lacrimal gland are rare, and extraorbital spread tends to occur early. Malignant lacrimal gland tumours are a miscellaneous group, difficult to treat and with a poor overall prognosis and a 5-year survival rate of the order of 20%. Mucosa-associated lymphoid tissue (MALT) lymphoma also occurs at this site, often accompanied clinically by Sjögren-like syndrome (see Chapter 26). The prognosis is usually excellent as this variety of non-Hodgkin lymphoma is characteristically indolent.

Optic nerve glioma

These are predominantly low- to medium-grade astrocytes of young people, and are generally treated by surgical excision (if possible) and/or radiotherapy with particular care to preserve vision in the contralateral eye.

Radiation techniques for tumours of the orbit

Although lead shielding of the cornea, lens and lacrimal sac is routinely recommended, it is impossible to arrange for homogeneous irradiation of the whole of the orbital content as well as adequate shielding of sensitive structures. A wedged pair of fields (see Chapter 5) is the usual arrangement. Great care must be taken to avoid irradiation of the contralateral eye, even though useful vision is often retained in the treated one. It is useful to ask the patient to look directly into the beam during treatment in order to fix the gaze and to avoid the inevitable build-up effect of the closed lid. With supervoltage beams, the maximal energy deposition is deep to the cornea and may even partly spare the lens. Partial or complete corneal shielding can usually be achieved with a simple cylindrical shield, and conjunctival damage is uncommon, particularly as low doses of radiation are well tolerated by this part of the eye. Where shielding is impossible, painful keratitis, sometimes with iridocyclitis or even corneal ulceration, may occur. Failure to shield the lacrimal gland will usually pose a greater threat to the integrity of the eye since the lacrimal apparatus has a lower tolerance, and doses of greater than 30 Gy over 3 weeks will cause significant reduction of tear production with consequent dryness of the eye, requiring regular instillation of lubricant drops.

The most radiosensitive structure in the eye is the lens itself (see Chapter 5, pages 69–70) and cataracts can develop after doses of a few grays, although clinically important lens opacity is rarely seen with doses below 15 Gy. With doses above 25 Gy, progressive cataract is almost invariable; fortunately, these cataracts can be removed and an intraocular lens implanted. Other parts of the eye such as the retina and the sclera have a much higher radiation tolerance, closely similar to that of the central nervous system, and clinically important changes are uncommon where doses of less than 60 Gy are given by carefully fractionated external beam therapy.

Tumours of the eyelid and conjunctiva

Tumours of the eyelid are not uncommon and include basal cell and squamous cell carcinomas, mostly occurring in elderly patients. The lower lid and inner canthus of the eye are the commonest sites (see Chapter 22). In the conjunctiva both melanoma and squamous cell carcinoma are occasionally encountered, and it is important to diagnose these early since small lesions can be effectively treated by radiation, with conservation of the eye and preservation of vision. In general, local surgical excision is advisable, followed by radiotherapy using an applicator carrying a radioactive source, often ^{90}Sr. It is important to distinguish true melanomas from precancerous ocular melanosis (a diffuse flat pigmented lesion), which can be clinically diagnosed with confidence and which should be observed without biopsy since malignant change may take years to develop. Overall prognosis of conjunctival melanoma is good (5-year survival about 75%), although patients with bulky lesions have a high risk of early fatal dissemination. Squamous carcinomas have an even better prognosis provided that adequate surgery and/or radiotherapy are expertly given.

Tumours of the globe

The two most common tumours are retinoblastoma and uveal (choroidal) melanoma. Retinoblastoma is discussed in Chapter 24.

Malignant melanoma of the uveal tract is the commonest intraocular tumour of adults (6 per million per year). Blood-borne metastases are common, but may not become clinically apparent for many years. Only 15% arise in the ciliary body and iris, but these present earlier and are more easily visible. Choroidal melanoma (85% of the total) may cause no symptoms at first unless arising from the macula. At other sites a peripheral field defect may go unnoticed. Retinal detachment may occur.

The diagnosis is normally made on inspection. Primary choroidal melanoma must be distinguished from secondary deposits since the choroid is a known site of metastasis of cutaneous melanoma.

In the past, immediate enucleation has been preferred to biopsy in the belief that biopsy was dangerous. A more conservative approach is now adopted, especially in the elderly. Small melanomas can probably be watched and surgery only considered when the tumour enlarges. Treatment is then by photocoagulation, cryotherapy, local irradiation to a high dose or surgery. In small lesions and tumours of the iris, enucleation can sometimes be avoided though it may be necessary for large lesions or where there is macular or optic nerve involvement or retinal detachment. Pain, local extension and secondary glaucoma are also indications for enucleation.

References

1 Forastière A, Koch W, Trotti A, Sidransky D. Medical progress: head and neck cancer. *N Engl J Med* 2001; 345: 1890–900.

2 Shah JP, Lydiatt W. Treatment of cancer of the head and neck. *CA Cancer J Clin* 1995; 45: 352–68.

3 Grønbaek M, Becker U, Johansen D *et al*. Population based cohort study of the association between alcohol intake and cancer of the upper digestive tract. *Br Med J* 1998; 317: 844–8.

4 Cheng Y, Poulos NE, Lung ML *et al*. Functional evidence for a nasopharyngeal carcinoma tumor suppressor gene that maps at chromosome 3p21.3. *Proc Natl Acad Sci USA* 1998; 95: 3042–7.

5 McDermott AL, Dutt SN, Watkinson JC. The aetiology of nasopharyngeal carcinoma. *Clin Otolaryngol* 2001; 26: 82–92.

6 Vokes EE, Liebowitz DN, Weichselbaum R. Naso-pharyngeal carcinoma. *Lancet* 1997; 350: 1087–91.

7 Tsai ST, Jin YT, Mann RB, Ambinder RF. Epstein–Barr virus detection in nasopharyngeal tissues of patients with suspected nasopharyngeal carcinoma. *Cancer* 1998; 82: 1449–53.

8 Gillison ML, Lowy DR. A causal role for human papillomavirus in head and neck cancer. *Lancet* 2004; 363: 1488–9.

9 D'Souza G, Kreimer AR, Viscidi R *et al*. Case–control study of human papillomavirus and oropharyngeal cancer. *N Engl J Med* 2007; 356: 1944–56.

10 Janot F, Klinjanienko J, Russo A *et al*. Prognostic value of clinico-pathological parameters in head-and-neck squamous cell carcinoma: a prospective analysis. *Br J Cancer* 1996; 73: 531–8.

11 Sobin LH, Gospodarowicz MK, Wittekind Ch, eds. *TNM Classification of Malignant Tumours*, 7th edn. Chichester: Wiley-Blackwell, 2009.

12 Edge S, Byrd DR, Compton CC, *et al*., eds. *AJCC Cancer Staging Manual*, 7th edn, Springer, 2010: 29.

13 Shah JP. *Head and Neck Surgery*, 2nd edn. St Louis: Mosby, 1996.

14 Forastiere AA, Goepfert H, Maor M *et al*. Concurrent chemotherapy and radiotherapy for organ preservation in advanced laryngeal cancer. *N Engl J Med* 2003; 349: 2091–8.

15 Vokes EE, Stenson K, Rosen F *et al*. Weekly carboplatin and paclitaxel followed by concomitant paclitaxel, fluorouracil and hydroxyurea chemoradiotherapy. *J Clin Oncol* 2003; 21: 320–6.

16 Lin JC, Jan JS, Hsu CY *et al*. Phase III study of concurrent chemoradiotherapy versus radiotherapy alone for advanced

nasopharyngeal carcinoma: positive effect on overall and progression-free survival. *J Clin Oncol* 2003; 21: 631–7.

17 Don DM, Anzai Y, Lufkin RB *et al.* Evaluation of cervical lymph node metastases in squamous cell carcinoma of the head and neck. *Laryngoscope* 1995; 105: 669–74.

18 Lederman M, Mould RE. Radiation treatment of cancer of the pharynx: with special reference to telecobalt therapy. *Br J Radiol* 1968; 41: 251–74.

19 Martinez-Gimeno C, Rodriguez EM, Vila CN, Varela CL. Squamous cell carcinoma of the oral cavity: a clinicopathologic scoring system for evaluation risk of lymph node metastasis. *Laryngoscope* 1995; 105: 728–33.

20 Horiot JC, Le Fur R, N'Guyen T *et al.* Hyperfractionation vs. conventional fractionation in oropharyngeal carcinoma: final analysis of a randomized trial of the EORTC cooperative group of radiotherapy. *Radiother Oncol* 1992; 25: 229–32.

21 Garofalo MC, Haraf DJ. Re-irradiation: a potentially curative approach to locally or regionally recurrent head and neck cancer. *Curr Opin Oncol* 2002; 14: 330–3.

22 MacFarlane GJ, Boyle P, Scully C. Rising mortality from cancer of the tongue in young Scottish males. *Lancet* 1987; ii: 912.

23 Lippman SM, Batsakis JG, Toth BB *et al.* Comparison of low-dose isotretinoin with beta-carotene to prevent oral carcinogenesis. *N Engl J Med* 1993; 328: 15–20.

24 Sudbø J, Lippman SM, Lee JJ *et al.* The influence of resection and aneuploidy on mortality in oral leukoplakia. *N Engl J Med* 2004; 350: 1405–8.

25 Hutchison I. Complications of radiotherapy in the head and neck: an orofacial surgeon's view. In: Tobias JS, Thomas PRM, eds. *Current Radiation Oncology*, Vol. 2. London: Edward Arnold, 1996: 144–77.

26 Corvo R. Evidence-based radiation oncology in head and neck squamous cell carcinoma. *Radiother Oncol* 2007; 85: 156–170.

27 Montana FS, Hellman S, von Essen CF, Kligerman MM. Carcinoma of the tongue and floor of the mouth: results of radical radiotherapy. *Cancer* 1969; 23: 1284–9.

28 Johnson JT, Ferretti GA, Netuery WJ *et al.* Oral pilocarpine for post-irradiation xerostomia in patients with head and neck cancer. *N Engl J Med* 1993; 329: 390–5.

29 Robin PE, Powell DJ, Stansbie JM. Carcinoma of the nasal cavity and paranasal sinuses: incidence and presentation of different histological types. *Clin Otolaryngol* 1979; 4: 431–56.

30 Boone MLM, Harle TS, Higholt HW, Fletcher GH. Malignant disease of the paranasal sinuses and nasal cavity. Importance of precise localization of extent of disease. *Am J Roentgenol Radium Ther Nucl Med* 1968; 102: 627–36.

31 Lamont EB, Vokes EE. Chemotherapy in the management of squamous-cell carcinoma of head and neck. *Lancet Oncol* 2001; ii: 261–9.

32 Argiris A. Update on chemoradiotherapy for head and neck cancer. *Curr Opin Oncol* 2002; 14: 323–9.

33 Pignon JP, Bourhis J, Domengue C, Designe L. Chemotherapy added to locoregional treatment for head and neck squamous cell carcinoma: three meta-analyses of updated individual data. *Lancet* 2000; 355: 949–55. See also Ref. [41].

34 Tobias JS. Current issues in cancer. Cancer of the head and neck. *Br Med J* 1994; 308: 961–6.

35 Munro AJ. An overview of randomized controlled trials of adjuvant chemotherapy in head and neck cancer. *Br J Cancer* 1995; 71: 83–91.

36 Gupta NL, Swindell R. Concomitant methotrexate and radiotherapy in advanced head and neck cancer: 15 year follow-up of a randomized clinical trial. *Clin Oncol* 2001; 13: 339–44.

37 Merlano M, Vitale V, Rosso R *et al.* Treatment of advanced squamous-cell carcinoma of the head and neck with alternating chemotherapy and radiotherapy. *N Engl J Med* 1992; 327: 1115–21.

38 Denis F, Garaud P, Bardet E *et al.* Final results of the 94-01 French Head and Neck Oncology and Radiotherapy Group randomized trial comparing radiotherapy alone with concomitant radiochemotherapy in advanced-stage oropharynx carcinoma. *J Clin Oncol* 2004; 22: 69–76.

39 Cooper JS, Pajak TF, Forastiere AA *et al.* Postoperative concurrent radiotherapy and chemotherapy for high-risk squamous-cell carcinoma of the head and neck. Radiation Therapy Oncology Group 9501/Intergroup. *N Engl J Med* 2004; 350: 1937–44.

40 Tobias JS, Monson K, Gupta N *et al.*, on behalf of the UK Head and Neck Cancer Trialists' Group. Chemoradiotherapy for locally advanced head and neck cancer: ten-year follow-up of the UK Head and Neck (UKHAN1) trial. *Lancet Oncol* 2010; 11: 66–74.

41 Pignon JP, Maître A, Maillard E, Bourhis J. on behalf of the MACH-NC collaborative group. Meta-analysis of chemotherapy in head and neck cancer (MACH-NC): an update on 93 randomised trials and 17,346 patients. *Radiother Oncol* 2009; 92: 4–14.

42 Zakotnik B, Budihna M, Smid L *et al.* Patterns of failure in patients with locally advanced head and neck cancer treated postoperatively with irradiation or concomitant irradiation with mitomycin C and bleomycin. *Int J Radiat Oncol Biol Phys* 2007; 67: 685–90.

43 Chua DTT, Sham JST, Choy D *et al.* Preliminary report of the Asian-Oceanic Clinical Oncology Association randomised trial comparing cisplatin and epirubicin followed by radiotherapy vs. radiotherapy alone in the treatment of patients with loco-regionally advanced nasopharyngeal carcinoma. *Cancer* 1998; 83: 2270–83.

44 Chan AT, Teo PM, Leung TW, Johnson PJ. The role of chemotherapy in the management of nasopharyngeal carcinoma. *Cancer* 1998; 82: 1003–12.

45 Blanchard P, Baujat B, Holostenco V *et al.* Meta-analysis of chemotherapy in head and neck cancer (MACH-NC):

a comprehensive analysis by tumour site. *Radiother Oncol* 2011; 100(1): 33–40.

46 Al-Sarraf M, LeBlanc M, Shanker Giri PG *et al.* Chemoradiotherapy vs. radiotherapy in patients with advanced nasopharyngeal cancer: phase III randomised intergroup study 0099. *J Clin Oncol* 1998; 16: 1310–17.

47 James N, Hartley A. Improving outcomes in head and neck cancer. *Clin Oncol* 2003; 15: 264–5.

48 Vermorken JB, Remenar E, van Herpen C *et al.* Cisplatin, fluorouracil, and docetaxel in unresectable head and neck cancer. *N Engl J Med* 2007; 357: 1695–704. [Correspondence in *N Engl J Med* 2008; 358: 1075–8.]

49 Kim ES, Kies M, Herbst RS. Novel therapeutics for head and neck cancer. *Curr Opin Oncol* 2002; 14: 334–42.

50 Bonner JA, Harari PM, Giralt J *et al.* Radiotherapy plus cetuximab for squamous-cell carcinoma of the head and neck. *N Engl J Med* 2006; 354: 567–78.

51 Bonner JA, Harari PM, Giralt J *et al.* Radiotherapy plus cetuximab for locoregionally advanced head and neck cancer: 5-year survival data from a phase 3 randomised trial, and relation between cetuximab-induced rash and survival. *Lancet Oncol* 2010; 11: 21–8.

52 Vokes EE, Seiwert TY. EGFR-directed treatments in SCCHN. *Lancet Oncol* 2013; 14: 672–3.

53 Soulieres D, Senzer NN, Vokes EE *et al.* Multicentre phase II study of erlotinib, an oral epidermal growth factor receptor tyrosine kinase inhibitor, in patients with recurrent or metastatic squamous cell cancer of the head and neck. *J Clin Oncol* 2004; 22: 77–85.

54 Huang S, Armstrong EA, Benavente S *et al.* Dual-agent molecular targeting of the epidermal growth factor receptor EGFR: combining anti-EGFR antibodies with tyrosine kinase inhibitor. *Cancer Res* 2004; 64: 5355–62.

55 Adelstein DJ, Li Y, Adams GL *et al.* An Intergroup phase III comparison of standard radiation therapy and two schedules of concurrent chemoradiotherapy in patients with unresectable squamous cell head and neck cancer. *J Clin Oncol* 2003; 21: 92–8.

56 Cripps C, Winquist E, Devries MC *et al.* Epidermal growth factor receptor targeted therapy in stages III and IV head and neck cancer. *Curr Oncol* 2010; 17: 37–48.

57 Jones AV, Craig GT, Speight PM, Franklin CD. The range and demographics of salivary gland tumours diagnosed in a UK population. *Oral Oncol* 2008; 44: 407–17.

58 Hickman R, Cawson RA, Duffy SW. The prognosis of specific types of salivary gland tumours. *Cancer* 1984; 54: 1620–4.

59 Hernandez JG, Brady LW, Shields JA *et al.* Radiotherapy of ocular tumours. In: Tobias JS, Thomas PRM, eds. *Current Radiation Oncology*, Vol. 1. London: Edward Arnold, 1994: 101–25.

60 Darsaut TE, Danzino G, Lopez MB, Newman S. An introductory overview of orbital tumors. *Neurosurg Focus* 2001; 10(5): E1.

Further reading

Dulguerov P, Allal AS, Calcaterra TP. Esthesioneuroblastoma: a meta-analysis and review. *Lancet Oncol* 2001; 2: 683–90.

Haddad RI, Shin DM. Recent advances in head and neck cancer. *N Engl J Med* 2008; 359: 1143–54.

Harari PM, Huang S. Radiation combined with EGFR signal inhibitors: head and neck cancer focus. *Semin Radiat Oncol* 2006; 16: 38–44.

Lefebvre JL. Laryngeal preservation in head and neck cancer: a multi-disciplinary approach. *Lancet Oncol* 2006; 7: 747–55.

Lin A, Kim HM, Terrell JE *et al.* Quality of life after parotidsparing IMRT for head-and-neck cancer: a prospective longitudinal study. *Int J Radiat Oncol Biol Phys* 2003; 57: 61–70.

National Institute for Cinical Excellence. *Guidance on Cancer Services: Improving Outcomes in Head and Neck Cancers – The Manual.* London: NICE, 2004.

O'Sullivan B, Shah J. New TNM staging criteria for head and neck tumors. *Semin Surg Oncol* 2003; 21: 30–42.

Prellop P, Ove R. New approaches to postoperative radiotherapy for cancer of the head and neck. *Curr Cancer Ther Rev* 2005; 1: 63–70.

Rieger JM, Zalmanowitz JG, Wolfaardt JF. Functional outcomes after organ preservation treatment in head and neck cancer: a critical review of the literature. *Int J Oral Maxillofac Surg* 2006; 35: 581–7.

Rosenthal DI, Ang KK, eds. Head and neck cancer. *Semin Radiat Oncol* 2004; 14: 101–95.

Samant S, Kruger E. Cancer of the paranasal sinuses. *Curr Oncol Rep* 2007; 9: 147–51.

Scuibba JJ, Goldenberg D. Oral complications of radiotherapy. *Lancet Oncol* 2006; 7: 175–83.

Shah JP. *Head and Neck Surgery*, 2nd edn. St Louis: Mosby, 1996.

Shah JP, Singh B. Keynote comment: why the lack of progress for oral cancer? *Lancet Oncol* 2006; 7: 356–7.

Syrjänen S. Human papillomaviruses in head and neck carcinomas. *N Engl J Med* 2007; 356: 1993–5.

11 Brain and spinal cord

Brain tumours

Although relatively unusual (<2% of all primary cancers), brain tumours are among the most devastating of all malignant diseases, frequently producing profound and progressive disability leading to death. They are often difficult to diagnose and are invariably challenging to treat. The incidence appears to be rising steadily, at least in the USA; peak incidence is in the first decade of life and at age 50–70 years (Figure 11.1). Brain tumours are one of the most important groups of childhood tumours, second only to the leukaemias and lymphomas in frequency. In the UK, the incidence is just over 7 per 100 000, with 2200 deaths each year. In the USA, almost 22 500 new cases of primary brain tumour are diagnosed each year [1].

Very little is known of the aetiology. Brain tumours are slightly more common in males (1.2:1.0), with the exception of meningiomas, which are commoner in women. In addition, several familial syndromes (all uncommon) are known to be associated with a high incidence of glioma (Table 11.1). An increase in both benign and malignant brain tumours has also been noted following radiation of the scalp for benign conditions in childhood. Cranial radiation (together with antimetabolite therapy) has also been implicated as a cause of brain tumour development in children given central nervous system (CNS) prophylaxis for acute leukaemia. Significant differences exist in the frequency of brain tumours throughout life, suggesting the possibility of different aetiological factors in their causation [3]. Most childhood brain tumours occur at infratentorial sites (especially glial tumours and medullablastoma) or in the midline (especially germ-cell tumours, craniopharyngiomas). In adults, most brain tumours arise from supratentorial sites. Clearly, childhood and adult CNS tumours have different biological behaviour; only haemangioblastoma has an equal incidence in both childhood and adult life. Hormonal influences in pituitary adenoma and meningioma may explain the earlier peak age incidence of these tumours in females, and to some extent account for the apparent sex ratio differences.

Brain metastases are even more common than primary brain tumours and are now attracting more attention in the research arena. The commonest primary sites are lung (both small-cell and non-small-cell), breast and melanoma. They appear to be becoming more frequently encountered, with increasing longevity of cancer patients.

Primary cerebral lymphoma has become far more frequently diagnosed with the advent of the AIDS pandemic over the past two decades (see pages 13, 28–31). The other important recent aetiological factor in cerebral lymphoma is the increase over the past 20 years in successful organ transplantation.

Over the past 25 years, neurosurgical and radiotherapeutic techniques have improved with, in some instances, a positive impact on prognosis or a reduction

Cancer and its Management, Seventh Edition. Jeffrey Tobias and Daniel Hochhauser.
© 2015 John Wiley & Sons, Ltd. Published 2015 by John Wiley & Sons, Ltd.

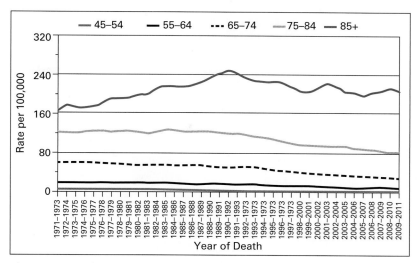

Figure 11.1 Brain, other CNS and intracranial tumours, average number of new cases per year and age-specific incidence rates by sex, UK, 2008–2010. (Source: http://info.cancerresearchuk.org/cancerstats/types/brain/incidence/, accessed February 2014. (© 2014 Cancer Research UK, Reproduced with permission.))

Table 11.1 Main familial tumour syndromes associated with gliomas.

Syndrome	Chromosome	Gene	CNS tumours	Main other tissue tumours
Li–Fraumeni disease	17p13	TP53	Astrocytomas, primitive neuroectodermal tumours	Breast carcinoma, bone and soft-tissue sarcomas, leukaemia, adrenocortical carcinoma
Neurofibromatosis type 1	17q11	NF1	Optic nerve gliomas, astrocytomas (frequently pilocytic), neurofibromas, MPNST	Osseous lesions, phaeochromocytoma, leukaemia, iris hamartomas
Turcot's disease type 1	3p21, 7p22	HMLH1, HPSM2	Astrocytomas	Colorectal polyps, cancer
Tuberous sclerosis	9q34, 16p13	TSC1, TSC2	Subependymal giant-cell astrocytoma	Skin angiofibroma, renal hamartoma, cardiac myxoma

MPNST, malignant peripheral nerve sheath tumour.
Source: Behin *et al.* [2]. Reproduced with permission from Elsevier.

in treatment morbidity. More recently, a possible role for cytotoxic agents has begun to emerge, although their contribution is not yet fully established.

Cellular biology of brain tumours

The growth kinetics of malignant brain tumours have been widely studied in recent years, mostly using incorporation of radiolabelled DNA precursors such as ^{3}H-thymidine or bromodeoxyuridine (BrdU) and quantifying the result by immunological techniques with a specific anti-BrdU-DNA monoclonal antibody. Higher-grade tumours have much higher labelling indices [4], and are more likely on flow cytometry studies to exhibit aneuploidy.

Oncogene analysis has also proven valuable [2]. In over 50% of glioblastoma multiforme, for example, amplification of N-*myc*, c-*myc*, N-*ras* or other oncogenes is present, often with simultaneous over expression of more than one. In addition, the epidermal growth factor receptor (EGFR; see Chapter 3) is usually highly expressed, and encoded by the *erb*-B oncogene [5].

At least six specific and frequently occurring molecular genetic alterations have been identified in the pathogenesis of gliomas (Figure 11.2). In the amplification of

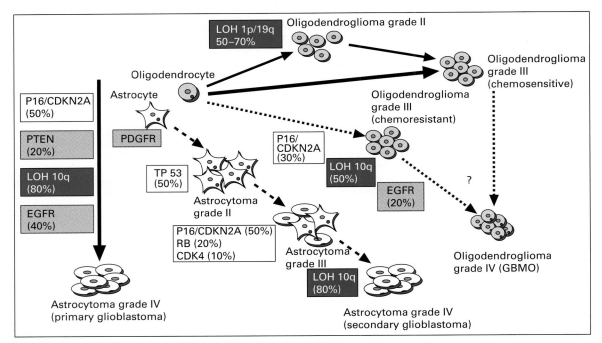

Figure 11.2 Genetic pathways in glioma progression. White squares correspond to genetic alterations of cell cycle control: TP53, mutation; RB, mutation; P16/CDKN2A, homozygous deletion; CDK4, amplification. Light red squares correspond to genetic alterations affecting signal transduction pathways: EGFR, amplification; PDGFR, overexpression; PTEN, mutation. Dark red squares correspond to loss of heterozygosity (LOH) on chromosomes 1p/19q or 10q. GBMO, glioblastoma multiforme with oligodendroglial component; EGFR, epidermal growth factor receptor; PDGFR, platelet-derived growth factor receptor. (Source: Behin *et al.* [2]. Reproduced with permission from Elsevier.)

EGFR, a specific gene appears responsible. In high-grade tumours, hemizygous and homozygous deletion of interferon loci at chromosome 9p has been demonstrated. Major karyotypic alterations also occur: in primitive neuroectodermal tumours including medulloblastoma, deletion of the short arm of chromosome 17 is common. Furthermore, it is now clear that medulloblastoma can be divided by reference to gene expression profiles into at least four groups, each with a distinct pattern of mutational changes, clinical features and behaviour – see Ref. [6]. This new insight provides the opportunity of targeting tumour-stromal interactions in this disease, to block tumour growth. One therapeuetic consequence showing promise in preclinical testing is the targeting of the placental growth factor/neuropilin pathway, raising the prospect of stromal-targeted therapies as well as tumour-targeted treatment – see Ref. [7]. Loss of heterozygosity (LOH) on chromosome 10 is also frequent, with a specific association with glioblastoma [8]. Tumour suppressor gene(s) are present on the distal portion of this chromosome's long arm. Other early changes include loss of tumour-suppressor function (e.g. loss of *p53* as well as the chromosomal mutations). In anaplastic oligodendroglioma, LOH at 1p and 19q is common, and appears to carry prognostic weight, with a longer survival time for patients with this condition in whom LOH was demonstrated. Other cytogenetic abnormalities in this condition include deviations on chromosomes 4, 9p, 15 and 18. In high-grade glioma (glioblastoma), recent work has centred on the demonstration that the enzyme O^6-methylguanine-DNA methyltransferase (MGMT) is abnormally methylated in up to 40% of patients. The importance of this relates to its control by a promoter, whose function is activated by methylation, leading to intracellular gene silencing, with consequent enhancement of sensitivity to alkylating agents such as bis-chloroethyl nitrosourea (BCNU; see below). The significance of this observation has now been demonstrated by recent studies [9,10] showing the prognostic value of identifying the methylation status of the promoter of the MGMT gene see also Ref. [11]).

Further specific aberrations have also been identified, particularly involving chromosomes 1, 3, 7 and 22 [12]. One particularly well-studied tumour is the meningioma, which frequently displays monosomy 22.

Pathological classification of brain tumours

The majority of primary brain tumours are gliomas, thought to arise from malignant change of mature glial elements, usually with differentiation towards one particular type of glial cell [13]. Although it now seems clear that tumour progression can occur, for example, from astrocytoma to glioblastoma, no predisposing premalignant states have been recognized in human glioma, unlike many other human solid tumours.

Taken together, astrocytomas, ependymomas, oligodendrogliomas and medulloblastomas account for over 90% of all primary brain and spinal cord tumours. In cases where the tumour is well differentiated, there is usually no difficulty in recognizing the type of cell from which the tumour has arisen. These tumours are classified according to the cell of origin and a widely accepted working classification is given in Table 11.2. Other more detailed classifications have been proposed by the World Health Organization (WHO).

Gliomas
Astrocytomas

These are much the commonest variety and arise from astrocytes (the supporting cells of the brain). Astrocytomas account for about 70% of all new cases of primary brain tumour. They are divided into four grades (according to Kernohan) on the basis of cytomorphological characteristics. Grade I is the least malignant. Grades II–IV show progressively more malignant characteristics, with the degree of malignancy assessed according to histological features such as invasion, tumour necrosis, cellularity, pleomorphism and mitotic activity. Low-grade gliomas (Figure 11.3a) chiefly occur in the frontal, parietal and temporal lobes and in the brainstem and cerebellum of children. Local destruction is unusual, in contrast to high-grade gliomas, in which degeneration, necrosis, haemorrhage, infarction and local destruction are characteristic.

Biopsy specimens are not always representative of the whole tumour: mixed varieties are common. Descriptive terms are sometimes used where a particular morphological feature predominates and the terms *fibrillary*, *protoplasmic*, *gemistocytic* or *pilocytic* are used to describe relatively well-differentiated types of astrocytoma. These subdivisions may have considerable prognostic

Table 11.2 Simplified classification of brain tumours.

Primary tumours
Gliomas
Astrocytoma
Glioblastoma multiforme
Ependymoma
Oligodendroglioma
Primitive neuroectodermal tumours (including
   medulloblastoma)
Pituitary tumours
Pituitary adenoma
Craniopharyngioma
Pituitary carcinoma
Meningiomas
Benign
Malignant (meningiosarcoma)
Pineal tumours
Pinealoblastoma
Pinealocytoma
Germinoma
Teratoma
Intracranial lymphoma
'Histiocytic' lymphoma
Microglioma
Acoustic
Chordoma
Neuronal tumours
Ganglioneuroma
Ganglioglioma
Colloid cyst

Secondary tumours
Common sites of origin
Lung
Breast
Melanoma
Less common sites of origin
Ovary
Testis
Gut
Bladder
Kidney
Pancreas
Liver
Leukaemia and lymphoma
Miscellaneous
Langerhans' cell histiocytosis

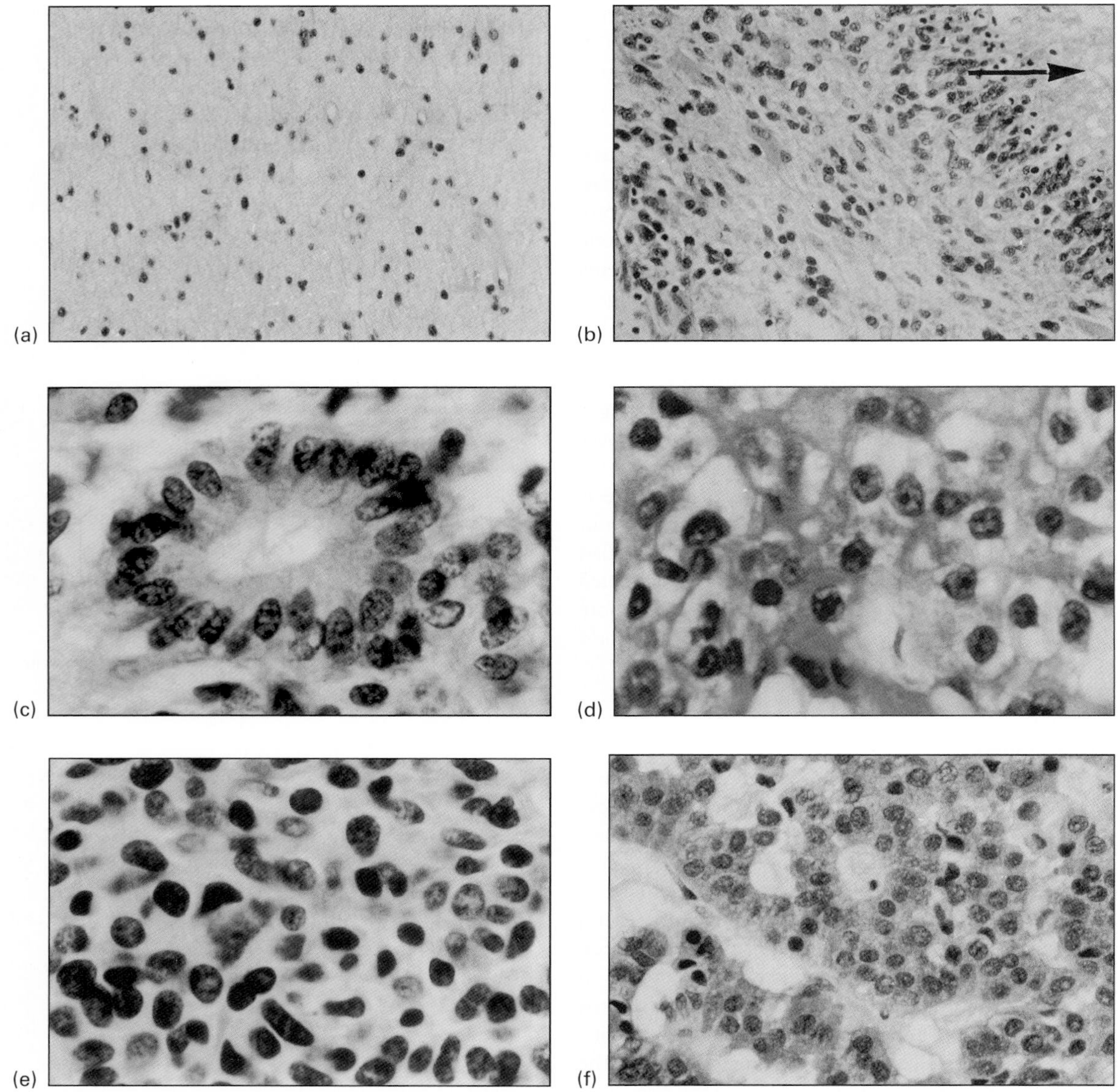

Figure 11.3 Histological appearance of the common brain tumours. (a) Low-grade glioma showing sparse cellularity with no vascular proliferation (original magnification ×200). (b) High-grade glioma showing cellular pleomorphism and necrosis (arrow) (×200). (c) Ependymoma: tumour forms typical rosettes (×400). (d) Oligodendroglioma showing typical 'boxed-in' cell appearance (×400). (e) Medulloblastoma showing small, darkly staining, closely packed cells (×400). (f) Pituitary adenoma: appearance is characteristic of endocrine tumours (×250).

significance (see below). In highly malignant gliomas, it may be impossible to recognize the initial cell of origin since they are among the most bizarre and undifferentiated of all tumours, often termed *glioblastoma multiforme* (Figure 11.3b). Growing rapidly by direct extension, they are always much larger than suggested by imaging studies such as computed tomography (CT) or magnetic resonance imaging (MRI). They are rarely operable, do not as a rule respond impressively to irradiation and are usually fatal within a year. In contrast, low-grade gliomas enlarge much more slowly and can often be excised completely, although local recurrence does sometimes occur. They constitute over 30% of all childhood brain tumours [13]. However, true grade I gliomas are extremely unusual, and most low-grade gliomas are grade II. Gliomas at different sites may behave quite differently despite a similar histological appearance. For this reason, localized gliomas of the optic nerves are often left untreated and may regress spontaneously, while gliomas of the pons or brainstem are much more aggressive and demand urgent attention with wide-field irradiation.

Of particular interest is the recognition of at least two types of glioblastoma. The *de novo* or primary glioblastoma tends to occur in older patients, with no prior history of tumour. It is characterized by oncogene amplification (e.g. EGFR), *p16* deletions and mutations of the tumour-suppressor gene *PTEN* on chromosome 10 and has a particularly poor prognosis. Secondary or progressive glioblastoma arises in younger patients, frequently with preceding astrocytoma and has a slightly better prognosis. Common abnormalities are *p53* mutations and platelet-derived growth factor receptor (PDGFR) amplification. LOH on chromosome 10 is common in both types of glioblastoma. Of special interest is the recognition that the majority of oligodendrogliomas are characterized by LOH 1p,19q and this is associated with very high response to chemotherapy. These tumours must be recognized because, properly treated, they have a relatively good prognosis.

Ependymal tumours

These represent about 5% of all primary brain tumours and are derived from the ciliated lining cells of the CNS cavities. The tumour cells form characteristic rosettes (Figure 11.3c). This most commonly occurs in childhood and early adult life, just over half arising from infratentorial sites. Tumour spread occurs by direct invasion and also by seeding throughout the CNS, particularly with high-grade ependymoma and where the primary tumour is infratentorial. Although tumour grading is perhaps less important with astrocytomas, low-grade ependymomas have a far better prognosis than the higher grades. Most aggressive of all is the ependymoblastoma.

Oligodendrogliomas

These are derived from other supporting cells and are usually very indolent in their growth pattern, with a long history, often calcifying. The cells have a typical appearance (Figure 11.3d) with a clear zone around the nucleus, the cells appearing 'boxed in'. Typical sites are the frontal, parietal and temporal lobes. The commonest age range is 40–60 years. The clinical history is often lengthier than with astrocytomas, and these tumours can be surprisingly radiosensitive.

Medulloblastoma

The term *primitive neuroectodermal tumour* is now increasingly preferred to describe these, and certain other, embryonal tumours (Figure 11.3e). At present, the WHO classifies medulloblastoma as one of five embryonal tumours, all of which share a primitive cellular morphology. Gene-array studies suggest that medulloblastoma represents a distinct tumour type. Cytogenetically, there is a characteristic loss of genetic information, often from chromosome 17. They account for 3% of all brain tumours and are predominantly diagnosed in childhood and young adult life, with few cases occurring after the age of 25 years. It is the commonest brain tumour of childhood, with a peak age incidence of 4–10 years. Over 500 cases are diagnosed in the USA each year, and the tumour chiefly arises in the posterior fossa or from the vermis, cerebellar hemispheres or the fourth ventricle. About 30% of children have evidence of cerebrospinal fluid (CSF) involvement at diagnosis. Patients usually present with raised intracranial pressure (see below). Because of close proximity to the CSF, the tumour metastasizes via the CSF either to the spinal cord or elsewhere in the brain. Occasionally, distant metastases are seen outside the CNS, and bone metastases (mostly osteosclerotic) and marrow involvement are occasionally encountered. Other sites include lung and lymph nodes.

The large-cell anaplastic histological subtype carries a worse prognosis than the classic or desmoplastic pathology. The anaplastic tumours tend to carry other features such as over expression of ErbB2 or c-MYC amplification, which probably explain the aggressive phenotype.

Pituitary tumours

Constituting about 10% of primary intracranial neoplasms, these usually arise from the glandular epithelial cells, producing tumours that are histologically classified according to the staining characteristics of the cytoplasmic granules. Granular staining is mostly absent (chromophobe tumours, Figure 11.3f) but in a minority there is characteristic acidophilic or basophilic staining. Increasingly, however, these tumours are pathologically classified using functional and immunological criteria. Non-epithelial pituitary tumours arise from cell rests

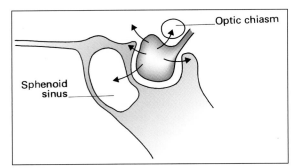

Figure 11.4 Local effects of pituitary tumours. Extension commonly produces pressure on the optic chiasm, base of brain and anterior and posterior clinoid processes. Extension occurs inferiorly and laterally, to sphenoid and cavernous sinuses.

from Rathke's pouch, producing tumours known as *craniopharyngiomas*. This part of the brain is also a common site of secondary cancer, chiefly from breast cancer and small-cell lung cancer (SCLC).

Chromophobe adenomas comprise about three-quarters of all pituitary tumours, and are more common in adult life. They tend to be non-functional (endocrine-inactive), although adrenocorticotrophic hormone (ACTH), growth hormone (GH), prolactin and other hormones are sometimes produced. They frequently attain a large size, particularly if non-functioning, and may extend upwards out of the sella to involve the optic chiasm, leading to the characteristic visual disturbance of bitemporal hemianopia (Figure 11.4). Of the chromophil tumours, the acidophil adenomas are chiefly associated with excessive production of GH, leading either to acromegaly if the tumour arises in adult life, or very rarely to gigantism when the tumour occurs in childhood. Basophilic tumours tend to be smaller, usually secreting ACTH and/or melanocyte-stimulating hormone, leading to Cushing's syndrome sometimes with hyperpigmentation. These tumours are usually small and rarely involve the suprasellar area, so visual signs are unusual.

Meningioma

Meningiomas are much the commonest tumours arising from the meninges, and are the commonest benign intracranial tumour, accounting for 13–26% of all primary intracranial tumours [13,14]. They are twice as common in females as males, with an incidence highest after the fifth decade of life. They sometimes appear to arise as a consequence of previous radiation therapy, usually for a low-grade glioma.

They can be classified according to their dural site of origin, the involvement of adjacent tissues (e.g. venous sinuses, bone, brain and nerves) and their histological grading. There is a predilection for certain sites, particularly the parasagittal region and sphenoid ridge. They often cause cerebral compression but frank invasion is very uncommon except for the rare malignant meningioma, sometimes referred to as meningiosarcoma. Pressure outwards may cause erosion of the inner table of the skull, while inward displacement of the brain may lead to epilepsy as an early feature. Meningiomas may be chiefly fibrous in nature (fibroblastic meningioma) or very vascular (angi-oblastic meningioma), the latter having a more rapid evolution and more frequent malignant transformation.

A specific genetic abnormality, monosomy 22, is present in up to 70% of cases. Mutations of the *NF2* gene, located at chromosome 22q12, often occur and are probably an early event in tumour development. Up to 60% of sporadic meningiomas show a somatic mutation of *NF2*, with a clear association between the histological variant and the frequency of *NF2* mutations; 80% of transitional and fibroblastic meningiomas carry *NF2* mutations, compared with only 25% of meningothelial meningiomas.

Others

Tumours of the pineal gland and third ventricle

This is a highly diverse group of tumours arising from the pineal itself, the third ventricle, or less commonly from ectopic sites of pineal tissue, particularly in the hypothalamus. Common types include the *pinealoblastoma*, which histologically resembles medulloblastoma; the *pinealocytoma*, which is a tumour of mature pineal cells; and *germ-cell tumours*, which can be either pure seminoma (pineal germinoma) or teratoma, often containing highly differentiated mesenchymal structures. These latter tumours may produce α-fetoprotein (AFP) and human chorionic gonadotrophin (HCG), which can be measured in CSF or blood, often critical for diagnosis and management (see Chapter 4). At the anterior end of the third ventricle, the histological types are even more varied and include *pituitary tumours, germinomas, meningiomas, optic nerve glioma, Langerhans' cell histiocytosis* and *non-malignant granulomas*, which can occasionally cause diagnostic difficulty, with tuberculosis and sarcoidosis, for example. In proven pineal and suprasellar germinomas there is a high risk of spinal seeding (20–30%), possibly aggravated by attempts at surgical excision.

Intracerebral lymphomas (see also Chapter 26)

These are unusual, but now far more common as one of the recognized AIDS-related malignancies. The incidence of primary CNS lymphoma is 4–5 per 1000 person-years in AIDS patients but only 0.3 per 100 000 person-years in the fully immunocompetent population [2]. The two main types are the 'histiocytic' lymphoma, which can occur at any site in the brain and appears more frequently in immunosuppressed patients such as renal transplant recipients, and the microglioma, a rare intracranial lymphoma not seen outside the CNS.

Thalamic and brainstem tumours

These are usually gliomas, although surgical biopsy is generally regarded as inadvisable. Thalamic gliomas are seen in children (usually well-differentiated tumours) and in adults (usually glioblastoma multiforme). Brainstem tumours are also chiefly encountered in children and are usually astrocytomas of variable differentiation.

Tumours of cranial nerves and nerve sheaths

Acoustic neuroma is a tumour of adult life, rather more common in females, and arising from the VIII cranial nerve, usually in its vestibular part. These tend to be slow-growing tumours that present with unilateral deafness, vertigo, tinnitus and involvement of other cranial nerves. Although strictly benign, they exert a local space-occupying mass effect. Other less common neuronal tumours include the ganglioneuroma and ganglioglioma, which are also typically benign though dangerous because of local pressure effects.

Chordomas

These uncommon malignant tumours originate from the remnants of the embryonic notochord. Although occasionally encountered in children and young adults, the peak age of incidence is 50–60 years and the characteristic sites are in the extremes of the spinal cord: a spheno-occipitocervical group (40% of all cases) and a sacrococcygeal group (equally frequent). The tumour consists of very characteristic solid cords of polygonal or mucin-containing 'physaliphorous' cells, sometimes with a lobulated pattern. Local pressure symptoms are common, including bulbar, occipital or neck symptoms from tumours at the upper end of the spine, or constipation and low back pain from sacrococcygeal tumours. Extensive bone destruction may occur.

Clinical features

Brain tumours can be difficult to diagnose. The onset of symptoms may be late, particularly in tumours situated in less critical areas of the brain, where they often grow to a substantial size before diagnosis, only producing subtle changes in personality, muscular power or coordination. In more critically sited tumours, obvious symptoms such as convulsions, ataxia or sensorimotor loss lead to much earlier diagnosis.

Symptoms can be divided into the following groups.

1 The tumour can exert a *mass effect* and lead to raised intracranial pressure, with headache, drowsiness, nausea and vomiting as the cardinal symptoms. The headache is often worse in the morning, typically clearing by lunchtime. Vomiting may be sudden, unexpected and not preceded by nausea. Tumours situated around the fourth ventricle, in the cerebellum and around the pons are particularly likely to lead to raised intracranial pressure (Figure 11.5), often with ventricular enlargement.

2 There is a large group of *focal symptoms* caused by damage to local structures. Space-occupying lesions can cause devastating symptoms if sited in the motor cortex, Broca's area or the base of the brain. Accurate siting of tumours is often possible as a result of these specific symptoms: myoclonic seizures, development of late-onset grand mal epilepsy and hemiparesis all point to lesions in the motor cortex, whereas lip-smacking, hallucinations and other psychotic disturbances are typical of a temporal lobe lesion. For tumours situated more deeply, visual disturbances occur due to interruption of the visual pathways. At the base of the brain, the classical features are those of cranial nerve lesions, often multiple. Tumours near the jugular foramen cause a specific pattern of cranial nerve palsies since many of the lower cranial nerves exit at or near this point. Ataxia, nystagmus and diplopia are typical of cerebellar lesions, often coupled with nausea and headache due to raised intracranial pressure.

3 The third group of symptoms results from *remote endocrine effects*, occurring with tumours of the pituitary and hypothalamus. Damage to local structures is of great importance in pituitary tumours, which can extend upwards to the suprasellar area and optic chiasm, inferiorly into the sphenoid sinus or laterally to the cavernous sinus or beyond, sometimes into the middle or posterior fossa (Figure 11.4). Damage to cranial nerves III, IV and VI may occur. Bleeding into a pituitary tumour (pituitary apoplexy) results in sudden deterioration of vision, severe headache and hypopituitarism. Lesser degrees of panhypopituitarism are common in pituitary tumours, although different end organs may be variably affected. The florid syndrome includes hypothyroidism from reduction in thyroid-stimulating hormone (TSH) production, hypocorticism with hypotension from reduction in ACTH, and hypogonadism with loss of secondary sexual characteristics and libido and amenorrhoea with infertility. Sophisticated endocrinological investigations are often required for full assessment, but simple measurements of tri-iodothyronine (T_3), thyroxine (T_4), TSH, cortisol and gonadotrophins (and GH in children) are usually sufficient for demonstration of the basic defects.

4 Tumours of the CNS occasionally *metastasize*. This usually occurs late in the disease. Although very unusual in adults, metastases are well recognized in children with medulloblastomas and poorly differentiated ependymomas. Secondary spread from these tumours is almost always via the CSF, usually presenting as spinal or meningeal deposits. Bone metastasis is also a well-recognized complication of medulloblastoma.

5 Childhood brain tumours may present with other symptoms including weight loss, precocious puberty, growth failure and macrocephaly in addition to the classical symptoms noted in tumours of adults [15]. Trying to diagnose brain tumours in young patients who so frequently present with headache, behavioural problems or even epilepsy of a quite different aetiology, is a recurring challenge for primary care physicians, as pointed out in an excellent recent editorial – see Ref. [16]. Figures from the UK suggest that an average general practice (primary care centre) will only see a new case of a childhood cancer every six years, of which about a quarter will be brain tumours.

The accurate diagnosis of brain tumours has of course been revolutionized by the advent of contrast-enhanced CT and MRI (Figure 11.5). Both carry the advantages of high definition and easy repeatability [17]. However, CT brain scanning does have its limitations, particularly in tumours of the posterior fossa and brainstem. In these sites, MRI is clearly superior. Pituitary tumours require high resolution since they are often small and close to bony structures. Most CT scanning machines can reliably detect lesions greater than 1 cm^3, but low-grade gliomas are sometimes poorly visualized. Angiography is still indicated to exclude arteriovenous malformations, and occasionally to visualize posterior fossa, deep-seated and thalamic lesions, or other sites poorly visualized by CT or MRI. In addition, preoperative angiography may be helpful in defining the tumour's vascular supply. Digital subtraction techniques provide excellent images in these situations.

Management of brain tumours

Surgical removal or biopsy is desirable both for histological diagnosis and sometimes for definitive treatment. However, radical excision can be extremely hazardous and stereotactic CT-guided biopsy is used for histological confirmation in inoperable cases. Where hydrocephalus is present, surgical decompression by ventriculoperitoneal drainage results in dramatic improvement. For deep-seated (e.g. thalamic, pineal and brainstem) tumours even a biopsy may be out of the question. Urgent reversal of acute cerebral oedema may be necessary, which may include the use of intravenous urea or mannitol, or high doses of dexamethasone (see page 201 for management details). Radiotherapy is frequently employed as an adjunct to surgery and sometimes as the

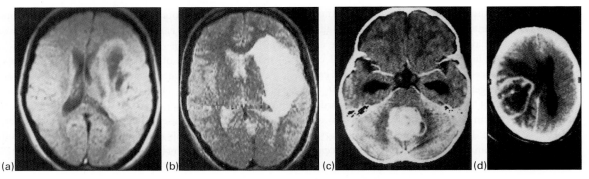

(a)   (b)   (c)   (d)

Figure 11.5 (a) CT scan showing a large mass (glioma) in the left hemisphere. (b) MRI scan from same case as (a). (c) CT brain scan showing large midline tumour of the posterior fossa. This was a medulloblastoma. (d) CT brain scan showing large parieto-occipital glioma. Note the obvious rim of contrast with oedema and ventricular dilatation.

definitive treatment in both adults and children [18,19]. The role of chemotherapy is still debatable, although cytotoxic drugs are increasingly used.

Gliomas

Low-grade (Kernohan grades I and II)

Complete surgical excision is often attempted since these lesions tend to be well localized and can often be removed from adjacent structures without causing too much damage. In many cases, surgery is the sole method of treatment. However, late local recurrences may occur, sometimes at a higher tumour grade. Routine irradiation is now established as an important mode of treatment in incompletely resected tumours, at least in adults. A study (from the Mayo Clinic) of 167 low-grade astrocytomas showed that in the pilocytic group (41 cases) there was a good prognosis regardless of postoperative treatment. In the remainder, radiotherapy clearly prolonged survival, especially if the tumour dose exceeded 53 Gy, in which case the 5-year survival rate was 68% compared with 21% when radiotherapy was not given [18]. Interestingly, complete surgical excision did not appear critically important so radiotherapy may become the dominant therapeutic modality in low-grade gliomas. In childhood brain tumours, the same general principles seem to apply (see also Chapter 24).

Although postoperative irradiation is now increasingly recommended in all cases, a recent large-scale European multicentre study has failed to demonstrate a clear-cut radiation dose-response for low-grade cerebral glioma [20]. A total of 379 patients were randomly assigned to treatment with either low-dose (45 Gy over 5 weeks) or high-dose (59.4 Gy over 6.6 weeks) radiotherapy, with a median follow-up of 74 months; overall survival (58%) and progression-free survival (48%) were similar in both groups. On the other hand, a further study from the same EORTC (European Organization for Research and Treatment of Cancer) group gave support to early radiotherapy, at least on symptomatic grounds and also in lengthening the period between diagnosis, initial surgical resection and recurrence [21]. The current confusing controversy regarding management of low-grade adult glioma has been well reviewed [22].

High-grade (Kernohan grades III and IV)

For these tumours radiotherapy is almost always employed as an adjunct to surgery (Figure 11.6): first, because complete surgical removal is rarely possible; and second, because the results of surgery alone are so poor. Recent studies of postoperative irradiation

for glioblastoma multiforme have demonstrated that although at 1 year there are no survivors with surgery alone, almost one-fifth of patients receiving postoperative radiation are still alive. Large radiation volumes are required, sometimes including the whole of the brain. Doses of 40–50 Gy in 4.5–6 weeks are often used (Figure 11.6), or higher doses if the target volume can be sufficiently focused. However, the ultimate prognosis remains very poor, less than 6% of patients with grade IV disease surviving for 5 years. For patients with grade III tumours, the survival is better, and over half of the surviving patients achieve an independent life (Figure 11.7). An important study from France addressing the question of whether radiotherapy should be offered routinely to elderly patients (aged 70 years or over) with glioblastoma was discontinued early, at the first interim analysis, because the results were so positive [23]. A total of 85 patients (median age 73) were randomly assigned radiotherapy or supportive care alone; at a median follow-up of 21 weeks, the median survival was 29.1 versus 16.9 weeks in favour of active treatment, a hazard ratio of 0.47.

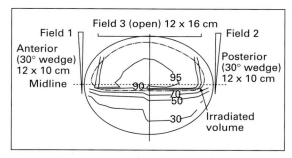

Figure 11.6 External beam radiation for cortical glioma. Typical three-field plan treating whole hemisphere. The irradiated volume is shown.

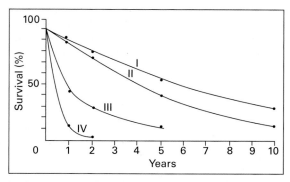

Figure 11.7 Survival related to grade in malignant glioma. Note the small proportion of 10-year survivors even with low-grade tumours.

Attempts to improve these dismal figures have led to the use of wide-field irradiation or treatment to higher dosage, since local recurrence at the initial tumour site is almost always the cause of death. If a safe means of increasing the dose could be found, better local control might be possible and there is increasing interest in at least three novel radiation techniques: interstitial brachytherapy, stereotactic external beam irradiation and hyperfractionated radiotherapy.

Interstitial brachytherapy, often using ^{125}Ir or ^{60}Co sources, permits the delivery of high doses of radiotherapy to the volume without unnecessary treatment of large areas of normal brain, and can be used in conjunction with stereotactic surgery. A large series from San Francisco suggested that this technique might be valuable for both primary treatment and recurrent disease [24], particularly in grade III lesions, although the excellent results from this group probably reflect careful selection of tumours which are limited by size and the performance status of the subject. Indeed, these features, together with age and clinical history, are known to be important prognostic factors. Unfortunately, however, the use of high-dose brachytherapy has failed to prevent a familiar pattern of locoregional failure [25].

External beam stereotactic radiosurgery has been widely tested in recent years [26]. Compared with interstitial irradiation, it has the advantage of non-invasiveness and can also be employed together with more conventional wide-field external beam therapy, even including whole-brain irradiation. Only a limited number of patients are suitable for treatment by radiosurgery but the technique seems promising with small tumours which, due to their precise location, are unsuitable for surgical resection (e.g. brainstem, thalamus, optic tract). The precision of stereotactic radiosurgery offers the hope of higher-dose treatment to a more restricted volume than would be possible by other external beam approaches.

Cytotoxic agents are sometimes used as an adjuvant to surgery and radiotherapy for high-grade gliomas. The nitrosoureas BCNU and *cis*-chloroethyl nitrosourea (CCNU) have received most attention, since they are known to be lipid-soluble and cross the hypothetical blood-brain barrier (see Chapter 6). Assessment of response of brain tumours to chemotherapy is difficult, but there is no doubt that some patients with recurrent disease benefit, though most of these responses are short-lived. In a large prospective multicentre trial, Walker and coworkers showed that routine use of BCNU as an addition to surgery and radiotherapy prolonged the median survival only by a few weeks [27]. Treatment by surgery and chemotherapy (but no irradiation) was much less successful. There is a possible slight superiority for CCNU over BCNU. However, recent studies have suggested a possible benefit of BCNU given as an intraoperative local wafer (Gliadel Wafer), a relatively novel way of employing chemotherapy as a form of local therapy.

Temozolomide is a relatively new cytotoxic drug active against gliomas [28]. It is an alkylating agent, a derivative of mutozolomide but less toxic, with myelosuppression as the main side-effect. It is more active in recurrent glioblastoma than procarbazine. Its precise role in newly diagnosed glioblastoma multiforme is still being evaluated, but it is clearly a genuinely active agent and is the most important of all agents currently available for the common brain tumours in adults. It is now very widely used for malignant tumours and is well tolerated by most patients. It has now been used in a large number of well-conducted randomized trials. A recent analysis of the large EORTC/NCI-Canada study (573 patients treated either with radiotherapy alone or with radiotherapy plus temozolomide) confirmed that the addition of this agent both during and after radiotherapy significantly improved the outcome, with an approximately 16% additional absolute survival benefit without any negative effect on health-related quality of life, which was carefully recorded in this study [29]. Many would now argue that use of concurrent radiation therapy with temozolomide, followed by adjuvant temozolomide, represents the best available means of treatment for these difficult tumours (see, e.g. Khanduri and Gerrard in Further reading), certainly superior to the use of the previously established cytotoxic agents of choice.

Despite many small randomized trials over 30 years, the role of chemotherapy in high-grade malignant glioma is still contentious. A relatively recent meta-analysis (published in 2002, i.e. before the most recent results with temozolomide were available) showed a 6% increase in 2-year survival, a result that will undoubtedly stimulate further study of chemotherapy in these tumours [30]. Intra-arterial drug treatment has proved to be unacceptably toxic.

Other agents with known activity include vincristine and procarbazine. These drugs have the added advantage of being relatively non-toxic. Cisplatin, carboplatin and etoposide (VM26) have also been shown to have a degree of useful activity. One commonly used combination is procarbazine, CCNU and vincristine (PCV), a fairly well-tolerated regimen often used as adjuvant therapy and given on a 6-weekly outpatient basis.

A number of exciting but as yet unproven newer therapies are currently under study, including targeted molecular therapy, focusing chiefly on inhibitors of tyrosine kinase receptors such as EGFR, PDGFR and vascular endothelial growth factor receptor (VEGFR) [1] (see also Chapter 6). Other approaches include signal transduction inhibitors targeting mTOR, farnesyltransferase and phosphatidylinositol 3-kinase. Antiangiogenic agents have also been extensively investigated, but no clear-cut major advances have been secured with these newer types of treatment.

Ependymoma

Ependymoma is far less common than astrocytoma and behaves differently [31]. It arises from cells lining the ventricles and central canal of the spinal cord, and has a tendency to seed throughout the subarachnoid space, giving rise to symptomatic spinal deposits in about 10% of patients, particularly in patients with high-grade lesions, especially if arising from the fourth ventricle. For this reason, routine craniospinal irradiation has traditionally been recommended in all patients with high-grade ependymomas and for ependymomas of the posterior fossa, regardless of grade (see pages 196–198 for details of technique and toxicity). Spinal cord primaries tend to be of lower grade than intracerebral tumours, with a better survival rate. Until recently, the policy has often been to treat the primary site to a high radiation dose (50 Gy or greater in 5–7 weeks) with full craniospinal treatment in patients with high-grade tumours. However, the role of chemotherapy in this tumour has recently been expanded, following a number of reports confirming its value either as a form of induction treatment, prior to radiotherapy, or in some cases (especially in younger children) substituting entirely for the radiation therapy [32,33]. It is increasingly accepted that chemotherapy has an important role in the management of this rare tumour in children and probably also in adult patients.

The overall survival is better than with astrocytomas, over 50% of patients surviving 5 years. In a report by Phillips and coworkers recording the results with postoperative radiotherapy alone (i.e. before the era of chemotherapy) [34], the 5-year survival rate of patients given *intensive* radiotherapy was almost 90%, twice the overall survival rate of 40% (which included those who died postoperatively without treatment as well as patients who received inadequate irradiation dosage).

The exceptionally rare choroid plexus carcinoma is also best treated by surgery with routine postoperative radiotherapy. In the largest series reported to date [35], a thorough review of the medical literature from 1966 to 1998 revealed 566 well-documented choroid plexus tumours. These were analysed to determine prognostic factors and treatment modalities. Most patients with a supratentorial tumour were children, while the most common sites in adults were the fourth ventricle and the cerebellopontine angle. Cerebellopontine angle tumours were more frequently benign. Histology was the most important prognostic factor: 1-, 5- and 10-year projected survival rates were 90, 81 and 77% in choroid plexus papilloma ($N = 353$) compared with only 71%, 41% and 35% in choroid plexus carcinoma, respectively. Radiotherapy was associated with significantly better survival in choroid plexus carcinomas. In addition, when given chemotherapy for relapse, 8 of 22 documented carcinomas responded.

Oligodendroglioma

These uncommon tumours are often relatively well differentiated, slow-growing and amenable to complete surgical removal. Postoperative irradiation is advisable where there has been incomplete surgical excision or where there are histologically aggressive features (sometimes termed *oligodendroblastoma*). In a classic study assessing a group of over 30 patients, Sheline and coworkers reported that the 5-year survival rate with surgery alone was 31%, compared with an 85% survival rate in patients receiving postoperative irradiation [36]. From these and other data, the 10-year survival rate is of the order of 35% with 'traditional' surgery and radiotherapy.

For recurrent oligodendroglioma there has been for many years increasing evidence of chemoresponsiveness, using agents such as either PCV (see above) or cisplatin [37]. As pointed out by the authors of a large recent study from France, 'the optimal therapy of oligodendroglioma remains uncertain. Although chemosensitive, these tumours are not chemocurable' [38]. Although the results were somewhat difficult to interpret, these authors favoured the use of initial or 'neoadjuvant' chemotherapy, which appeared to prolong overall survival in patients with histologically confirmed pure oligodendroglioma. A more recent report from the EORTC gave a more favourable outlook, showing clear evidence that for anaplastic oligodendroglioma, the use of PCV regimens provided long-term benefit in both overall and progression-free survival, especially in patients with 1p/19q codeleted tumours (see Ref. [39]). The results were surprising and impressive – an increase in overall survival from 31 to 42 months with 6 cycles of treatment ($n = 368$, median follow-up 140 months).

Deep-seated gliomas

Gliomas situated deep to the cerebral cortex present particular problems of diagnosis and management. Important sites include the thalamus and hypothalamus, pons, brainstem, pineal region and optic nerves. Histological confirmation is often impossible because surgical intervention could be so hazardous, although gliomas of the pineal area are increasingly considered suitable, particularly since histology at the site is so critical to management. Their clinical behaviour varies greatly. Optic nerve gliomas, which usually present with proptosis or blindness, are often associated with neurofibromatosis (NF) 1 and are frequently thought to be benign and unresponsive to radiotherapy, though this is clearly mistaken (see below). In children with NF1, the disease often develops under the age of 7 years. In some cases, the tumours are bilateral, involve the optic chiasm or extend backwards to the ventricles, sometimes with hydrocephalus. These should be treated with radiotherapy. Although uncomplicated lesions may be self-limiting, radiotherapy may produce complete relief of distressing proptosis, and objective response verified on CT or MRI scanning. Pierce and coworkers [40] reported a series of 24 children with optic nerve glioma with lengthy follow-up (median 6 years) and an overall 6-year survival rate of 100%. Over 90% of patients had improvement or 'stabilization' of vision. In a further more recently reported series, 25 consecutive unselected patients with optic pathway glioma were observed in the first instance, and treated with radiotherapy only if clinical progression was evident [41]. Diagnosis was based on MRI. The natural history was more indolent in patients with NF1 than in the others, and regressions were commonly observed; 13 non-NF1 patients had larger tumours at diagnosis and more rapid progression of disease. There were five intra-orbital optic nerve tumours (one with progression), 19 chiasmatic tumours (12 with progression) and one diffuse tumour. Progressive intra-orbital optic pathway gliomas are best treated by surgical resection, provided that sight can be maintained; if this is unlikely, a trial of radiotherapy seems much preferable. Progressive chiasmatic tumours are also best treated by radiotherapy, and respond well by marked regression. Exceptionally, exophytic chiasmatic tumours may sometimes be better treated by chiasm-preserving surgery.

For thalamic tumours, radiotherapy is almost invariably indicated since surgical excision or even histological confirmation is so dangerous at this site. The prognosis appears to vary with age, although, as expected, histological grade (usually obtained only at autopsy) is also important. The 5-year survival rate in young patients with grade III lesions is about 25%.

Tumours of the pons and brainstem carry a particularly poor prognosis, often presenting with florid symptoms including cranial nerve palsies, ataxia or involvement of the long tracts. These are usually high-grade astrocytomas and infiltrate widely, often attaining a large volume before diagnosis. They are a challenge to the radiotherapist since they are surgically untreatable, but often present with urgent problems in management. The majority showed a symptomatic response to radiotherapy, but the ultimate survival rate (approximately 15%) is poor. A large review of patients with brainstem tumours showed an average survival of 4 years for irradiated patients, compared with only 15 months if untreated. With a documented response to treatment, average survival was over 5 years. Large lateral opposed fields are required since the tumour has usually spread throughout the whole of the pons, brainstem and medulla and often to the upper cervical spine. Doses of 40–55 Gy in 4–5 weeks of daily treatment are usually recommended although some centres employ fewer fractions, for example, a total dose of 45–48 Gy in 15 daily fractions.

Medulloblastoma (and other primitive neuroectodermal tumours)

Surgical treatment alone is unsuccessful, and postoperative radiotherapy has been routinely employed since the 1920s, when the marked radiosensitivity of this tumour was first noted. With increasingly accurate treatment planning, supervoltage equipment, prophylactic irradiation of the whole brain and spinal cord, and the increasing use of chemotherapy, the 10-year survival rate has improved and is now around 60%.

An attempt at surgical removal is generally the first important therapeutic step. Although these tumours are radiosensitive, they do recur at the primary site, and removal of tumour bulk clearly reduces the rate of local recurrence. In general, neurosurgeons always aim to excise as much tumour as is safely possible, and for many years now it has been routine practice to offer postoperative irradiation. The degree of residual postoperative tumour left unresected is an important prognostic factor, highly influential in defining an 'average' or high risk of recurrence, with treatment consequences (see below). In children over the age of 3 years, the whole of the craniospinal axis should be treated as soon as possible after surgery. Increasingly, children over the age of 3 years are classified as 'standard' or 'high' risk, depending on extent of disease beyond the primary tumour, presence of tumour cells in the CSF and/or the demonstration of any frank metastatic sites within the neuraxis [42]. Children with standard risk are treated with a lower dose of radiotherapy to the craniospinal axis (of the order of 23.4 Gy), with a boost to the posterior fossa to a total of 55.8 Gy. For the higher-risk group, the neuraxis is treated to a higher dose, around 35.0 Gy. For both groups, chemotherapy is increasingly employed, indeed in almost every case, unlike say even 10 years ago, when the use of chemotherapy was far more selective. Single-agent concurrent treatment is often employed, followed by multiagent chemotherapy for the standard-risk group, and a more aggressive regimen for the higher-risk group. For younger children, using chemotherapy together with irradiation of the primary site, but avoiding the extensive spinal irradiation which can be so damaging to developing organs, has become more widely practised during the past decade. Treatment planning must be meticulous, taking particular care to treat the base of the brain, retro-orbital area and brainstem (Figure 11.8). These sites can be under-treated if adult surface anatomical boundaries are used without regard to the anatomy of the developing brain. It is important to monitor the blood count during treatment of the spine, but with this technique and dose rate the treatment rarely has to be discontinued, although the white blood cell count frequently falls to about 2×10^9/L by the end of treatment.

Irradiation of the whole neuraxis carries a number of drawbacks including cognitive impairment, psychiatric disorders, endocrine dysfunction and skeletal growth retardation [42]. Fortunately, skull growth is usually almost complete by the time of treatment, so permanent reduction in skull volume is very rare. Nevertheless, some degree of shortness of stature (particularly sitting height) must be expected from irradiation of the whole spine coupled with pituitary irradiation (see Chapter 5). In addition, midline organs such as the thyroid, larynx, oesophagus, thymus and heart are directly in the path of the exit beam, and the kidneys and female gonads are also likely to receive significant scattered irradiation despite the most careful planning. The need for whole-spine irradiation has, therefore, been questioned, especially as only 10% of children will develop spinal cord metastases. Risk-adapted craniospinal irradiation has now been recognized as a legitimate approach, with differing radiation doses increasingly used: 23.4 Gy for average-risk disease and 36.0–39.6 Gy for high-risk disease, as recommended by the St Jude's Children's Cancer Group [43]. In addition, this highly influential group has argued for intensive

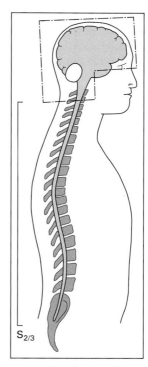

$S_{2/3}$

Figure 11.8 Craniospinal irradiation. Schematic representation of the field arrangement for craniospinal irradiation in medulloblastoma and other tumours which seed through the cerebrospinal fluid.

chemotherapy in selected cases (see below), claiming a cure rate of over 70% for average- and high-risk patients (see also Crawford *et al.* in Further reading).

Increasingly, chemotherapy is now recognized as an important part of treatment for most children, and over the past few years has become an established part of the management of medulloblastoma and other primitive neuroectodermal tumours. One additional advantage of this approach is the reduction in dose of craniospinal radiotherapy required for average-risk cases. High-risk patients include those with residual disease greater than 1.5 cm after surgery, or metastatic disease in the brain, spine or elsewhere. In the St Jude series, treatment included dose intensification with stem-cell rescue, using a cyclophosphamide-based regimen that also included topotecan [43]. Despite these hazards and the possible added problem of cognitive/learning defects, over 75% of surviving children lead independent and active lives and at least one study has shown that intellectual achievement in these children is not impaired. In the context of curative treatment by whole-CNS irradiation, there is little doubt that possible hazards of treatment have to be accepted.

In the past, chemotherapy was mainly used for treatment of recurrent disease and as initial treatment in very young children (<2 years) in whom CNS irradiation carries particular toxicity. Lipid-soluble agents have been used both singly and in combination. With recurrent disease, responses are usually short-lived, and combination chemotherapy may be difficult if relapse follows soon after craniospinal irradiation because of the volume of irradiated bone marrow. Methotrexate, which may be of some value, may be hazardous within 6 months of irradiation as it can cause leucoencephalopathy. Combination chemotherapy is increasingly preferred to single-agent treatment, and response rates up to 75% have been reported. It is clear that both cisplatin and carboplatin are active agents. At the present time, for *Average-risk disease*, the most encouraging results with adjuvant chemotherapy have been reported in children receiving 8 cycles of lomustine (CCNU), vincristine, and cisplatin chemotherapy for approximately 1 year following conventional dose radiotherapy and concomitant vincristine. The latest trials indicate that children aged 3–10 years who received this regimen with reduced-dose craniospinal radiation had a superior survival rate compared to those receiving standard radiation alone, with a current 3-year progression-free survival rate of approximately 80%. For those with *Poor-risk disease*, the most effective agents identified to date include cisplatin, carboplatin, cyclophosphamide and vincristine.

Chemotherapy is also used for recurrent childhood malignant glioma, and a few studies have produced encouraging results using CCNU, vincristine and prednisone [44].

Cytotoxic chemotherapy has also been used as an adjuvant to surgery and radiotherapy. The International Society for Paediatric Oncology undertook a large trial to assess the role of adjuvant chemotherapy with vincristine and CCNU [45]. From a series of over 330 cases, the main beneficiaries appear to be those individuals for whom the tumour was incompletely removed, with brainstem spread and below 3 years of age. Recent reports have suggested that it may be possible, in very young children, to avoid the potential long-term hazards of radiotherapy, and treat with adjuvant postoperative chemotherapy alone. Despite the obvious potential advantages, this approach should still be regarded as 'not fully established'. Many experts feel that it is still important in most cases to use at least the whole-brain and posterior fossa radiation boost in order to secure primary tumpour

control. One real problem here is the issue of 'competing toxicities' – for instance, in the increasing use of platinum-based cytotoxic chemotherapy as an alternative to the traditional spinal component of radiotherapy, we are now seeing more long-term chemo-induced nerve deafness in survivors, a major and life-longer incursion on the quality of life and educational prospects of these children and young adults.

It is often possible to obtain symptomatic improvement in patients with recurrence by further radiotherapy, particularly if the initial treatment was given at least 3 years beforehand.

Pituitary tumours [46]

For small tumours without suprasellar extension, many surgeons now favour resection via the trans-sphenoidal, sublabial or (increasingly) the endonasal route, which avoids the complications of craniotomy, although infection and CSF rhinorrhoea are occasionally encountered. Over 90% of patients with visual field defects have satisfactory postoperative reversal of the visual symptoms, with only a few requiring craniotomy after trans-sphenoidal resection, even with relatively large non-active macroadenomas with suprasellar extension. For larger tumours and those with extension outside the pituitary fossa, craniotomy may still be necessary. In children with craniopharyngioma, surgery can be particularly difficult.

Postoperative irradiation for patients with pituitary tumours decreases the likelihood of local recurrence. Chromophobe adenomas are more radiosensitive than chromophil tumours. In patients with acromegaly (almost always due to a chromophil tumour), arrest or reversal of the syndrome can be achieved with surgery and postoperative irradiation in 75% of cases. Pituitary irradiation is clearly the treatment of choice after unsuccessful surgery for patients with Cushing's disease [47]. Craniopharyngioma requires a high local dose for eradication (50–60 Gy in 5–7 weeks), although wide variation was confirmed in a recent national audit [48].

Multifield planning and attention to localization detail are essential for successful radiation treatment. A three-field plan is normally employed, with particular care to avoid over-treatment of the eyes and optic chiasm. For most tumours the field size can be limited, although chromophobe pituitary adenomas can reach a very large size. In some centres a rotational plan is used. The radiation technique is the same regardless of whether the patient is treated postoperatively as an adjuvant to surgery, or later for recurrence, although in the latter instance the treatment volume may have to be larger. Complications of radiotherapy are relatively unusual but include visual impairment, hypopituitarism and radiation carcinogenesis.

Alternatives to the use of conventional external beam irradiation include interstitial yttrium-seed irradiation, gamma-knife or 'cyberknife' radiosurgery, and heavy-particle (proton or α-particle) irradiation. Fractionated stereotactic radiotherapy is also increasingly used, and probably represents the most ideal form of radiation delivery technology at the present time, coupling the precision and dose focusing of stereotactic radiosurgery with the biological advantages of fractionation [49].

The use of bromocriptine has been advocated in recent years as an alternative to surgery and/or radiotherapy. This agent is particularly useful for small tumours producing prolactin only (prolactinomas). Although widely used, patients on bromocriptine do sometimes develop frank recurrence; it is also uncertain how long the drug needs to be continued. If bromocriptine fails, prolactinomas may have to be removed surgically.

Meningioma

Meningiomas should be surgically excised. If inaccessible and difficult to remove, radiotherapy should be given to reduce the rate of local recurrence. As these tumours are not very sensitive, high doses are usually required (50–60 Gy over 5–7 weeks). For patients with 'malignant' meningioma, radiotherapy is always required, although the overall prognosis in these cases is very poor. Occasionally they metastasize to distant sites. Sporadic small series have suggested a possible benefit from chemotherapy with oral hydroxycarbamide or other chemotherapy agents [50].

Pineal tumours

These present particular problems of management since they are often not biopsied by the surgeon for fear of causing irreparable damage. Many pineal tumours are curable by radiotherapy (particularly the 'pure' non-teratomatous pineal germinomas), and in patients without histological verification of the type of pineal tumour a brief trial of radiotherapy is often justified unless there is strong evidence of a teratomatous tumour such as raised markers (AFP or β-HCG, see below) or clear-cut radiological heterogeneity within the primary tumour. Germinoma and pinealoblastoma are the most radiosensitive of pineal tumours, and repeat CT or MRI scanning after as little as 2 weeks' treatment often

shows dramatic reduction in size. In this case, it can reasonably be assumed that the diagnosis is either germinoma or pinealoblastoma since other pineal tumours (generally glioma or pineal teratoma, pinealocytoma) are far less radiosensitive. Radiotherapy technique varies with the type of tumour, and in most patients with germinoma there is an increasing tendency to treat with platinum-containing chemotherapy in the first instance [51] (for chemotherapy details see Chapter 19). With the radiosensitive group, there is a tendency for involvement by tumour seeding throughout the CNS, and full craniospinal irradiation should be employed. This is not required with other pineal tumours, though if radiotherapy is selected as the treatment of choice, they do require a high local dose to the primary itself. Biopsy or even total removal of pineal tumours may be possible, providing accurate histological diagnosis. For the less radiosensitive group, total surgical removal offers the best result. Pineal teratomas, like teratomas at other sites, can produce AFP and HCG both in CSF and in the blood.

Overall survival is close to 80% in patients under the age of 30 with pineal tumours (including unbiopsied cases), reflecting the high incidence of radiocurable or chemocurable germinomas in this group. For older patients the prognosis is much worse, of the order of 25% survival, due no doubt to the higher incidence of gliomas and other less radiosensitive tumours.

Intracranial lymphoma

Microgliomas and histiocytic lymphomas are also radiosensitive. The surgical approach depends on the site of the lesion and surgery is sometimes complete. Nevertheless, radiotherapy should be offered in all high-grade cases and a remarkable degree of radiosensitivity is sometimes encountered, although durability of response is often disappointing (see Chapter 26). In general, the best results have been obtained with high dosage, and full craniospinal irradiation is often advocated since these tumours can spread throughout the nervous system.

Chordoma

Surgical removal is essential though often difficult because of the anatomy of the tumour. These tumours often have a 'dumb-bell' appearance with an intraspinal component, making total removal impossible. Postoperative radiotherapy is therefore usually necessary, although these lesions are rather insensitive. High radiation dose is particularly difficult to achieve in the cervical spine, although sacral chordomas can be treated to a higher dose since there is no danger of damage to the spinal cord. Despite the marginal radiosensitivity of chordomas, long survival has occasionally been documented in patients treated by subtotal surgical removal and radical postoperative radiotherapy. The advent of modern techniques in radiotherapy has been especially beneficial in this rare group of tumours, allowing high doses to be offered with far greater safety despite the close proximity of these tumours to the spinal cord – see, for example, Ref. [52].

Other tumours

Acoustic neuromas, and other neuronal tumours, are best treated surgically or by fractionated sterotactic radiosurgery [53]. Conventional postoperative radiotherapy should certainly be considered where surgery has been incomplete. The surgical approach depends both on the site of the tumour and on the degree of hearing loss. The prospect for preservation of functional hearing is much better with tumours under 2 cm and where auditory brainstem responses and other audiological assessments are only minimally abnormal. With elderly patients or poor operative risk candidates, sequential MRI may allow a conservative non-intervention policy without significant danger. A large study of radiosurgery (162 patients) from the USA has claimed a 98% control rate with low toxicity [53].

Treatment on relapse

For recurrent brain tumours, the question of retreatment radiotherapy often arises. When the disease-free interval has been short, as with high-grade gliomas, there is little value in retreatment since only a modest radiation dose can be safely achieved – of doubtful benefit where more intensive radiotherapy has already failed. However, in patients with low-grade glioma of any type, or those with medulloblastoma, late recurrences are common. Feasibility of retreatment increases with time from initial treatment, and if a sufficient time has passed (10 years or more), a complete retreatment dose can be contemplated. Chemotherapy is increasingly used as the first type of relapse treatment, and sometimes has the virtue of delaying for as long as possible a second course of radiotherapy. With medulloblastoma particularly, widespread late primary, cerebral and spinal metastases can develop, with continued responsiveness to repeated courses of radiotherapy. Dexamethasone often provides valuable symptomatic relief. Chemotherapy may produce transient responses and is discussed above.

Prognosis of brain tumours

For malignant gliomas, the prognosis is heavily dependent on tumour grade and on other well-established prognostic factors (see Figure 11.7). Patients with malignant glioma fall chiefly into two prognostic groups (see page 193–195 et seq) since those with grade I and II tumours have a relatively good prognosis and 5- and 10-year survival rates of approximately 65 and 35%, whereas those with grade III and IV tumours have a 5-year survival rate of under 10% (Figure 11.7), with a much worse prognosis in the grade IV category. The median survival for patients with glioblastoma remains very poor, about 11 months [54]. In all grades, incomplete removal is associated with a worse prognosis. Recent studies have suggested that patients with tumours that have hemizygous loss of 1p and 19q have a survival advantage, which might reflect a more durable response to radiotherapy or chemotherapy. Methylation of MGMT also seems to predict a better than average prognosis.

In medulloblastoma, a variety of factors contribute to prognosis. Age at diagnosis and completeness of excision are both important; children over 15 years of age have a better prognosis. Children with spinal metastases at presentation are not usually cured. The adequacy of the irradiation, with regard to both technique and dose, is crucial and 5-year survival rates of over 40% should now be achieved with modern techniques.

In ependymoma, prognosis depends on tumour grade. The median survival following surgery in low-grade ependymoma is approximately 10 years. Recurrences are frequently of a higher histological grade, and median overall survival in high-grade ependymoma is no better than 2–3 years.

Both pituitary tumours and meningiomas have an excellent prognosis following surgical removal and, where appropriate, postoperative radiotherapy. Few large series of pineal tumours have been reported. Survival is very variable (see above). In chordoma, the prognosis is poor since these tumours are not usually entirely resectable or fully radiosensitive. In children with high-grade glioma, Pollack and coworkers have suggested that overexpression of p53 protein is strongly associated with an adverse outcome, independently of clinical or pathological features [55]. Overall, there were 3400 deaths from brain and CNS tumours in the UK in 2001, representing 2% of all cancer deaths. Over the last two decades, the European standardized mortality rates have risen slightly in the UK, from 5.5 to 6.3 (per 100 000 men) and from 3.6 to 3.9 (per 100 000 women).

Secondary deposits in the brain

Cerebral metastases are common and account for about one-third of all brain tumours. Common primary sites include carcinoma of the bronchus (about 35% of all cases of brain metastases), breast cancer (about 15%) and melanoma (about 8%), with renal cell cancers, colorectal cancer and 'unknown primary site' accounting for most of the remainder. In each of these tumours, autopsy series confirm that the probability of dissemination to the brain is very much greater than the frequency of premortem diagnosis. About 60% of all patients with SCLC have demonstrable brain metastases at autopsy, and in melanoma about three-quarters of patients who die from disseminated disease have brain metastases. Many other tumours can metastasize to the brain, though at a much lower frequency (see Table 11.2).

Metastases may be either single or multiple and diagnostically (particularly when solitary) may be difficult to distinguish from primary brain tumours, or when, as occasionally occurs, there is no known primary.

Cortical, cerebellar, thalamic and pituitary deposits are all encountered. As with primary brain tumours, the characteristic symptoms are those of raised intracranial pressure, focal neurological damage and convulsions. The diagnosis is usually suggested by contrast-enhanced MRI or CT. Although local oedema is often present, this is usually less than that seen with high-grade primary brain tumours. In patients with known cancer, particularly lung, breast or melanoma, further investigation is not usually indicated, especially where the primary diagnosis has been made within the previous 5 years, although alternative diagnoses should always be considered. With apparently solid metastases, the most important differential is from a benign brain tumour, particularly meningioma (especially, of course, if the tumour is anatomically located at a common meningioma site). In cases of multiple metastases, the presumed diagnosis is almost always correct, although occasional confusion with intracerebral abscesses may occur.

Treatment
Reversal of oedema

Treatment with dexamethasone, often at high oral dosage (6 mg every 6 hours, or if necessary by intramuscular or intravenous administration) can provide rapid, even dramatic relief from symptoms of raised intracranial pressure. Response to this powerful agent is a useful indicator that an intracerebral tumour is present, and a helpful pointer to the likelihood of response to radiotherapy. Its effect is rapid, and can often be reduced in dosage within a week or two. It is a great mistake to allow patients to remain on dexamethasone for too long because of the inevitability of steroid complications, particularly proximal myopathy and facial swelling. In general, we usually recommend gradual discontinuation of dexamethasone over 3–6 weeks, although this policy occasionally results in patients redeveloping symptoms and signs of raised intracranial pressure because of excessively rapid reduction, in which case the dose can easily be increased again. There is considerable variation in the rapidity with which patients can be weaned off dexamethasone. In those where dexamethasone is ill-advised or dangerous (e.g. where there is a history of bleeding peptic ulcer, severe hypertension or diabetes) it is sometimes possible to achieve the desired reduction in cerebral oedema by the use of intravenous urea (1 g/kg, in dextrose solution), mannitol (2 g/kg as a 20% solution) or oral glycerine which can be made palatable by making up a 50% mixture with lemonade. Most patients dislike this latter treatment because it rapidly induces diarrhoea, but it can be highly effective in improving symptoms of raised intracranial pressure. Occasionally, the dexamethasone dose may need to be elevated still further, with benefit, over a very short period, up to a dose of 24 mg/day.

Radiotherapy

Radiotherapy is indicated in a high proportion of patients with secondary brain deposits, though the decision to treat requires careful thought [56], and it has become clearer in recent years that some patients, particularly those with a poor performance status and poor prognosis, may be better untreated. It is certainly unhelpful to treat those with a likely survival that can be measured only in just few weeks. Patients likely to benefit include those with known radiosensitive tumours (particularly SCLC of the bronchus and to a lesser extent carcinoma of the breast), those in whom there has been a good response to dexamethasone, those whose general condition is good (particularly if there is no other evidence of distant metastases), and those with multiple intracerebral deposits in whom there can be no question of surgery. Patients with brain metastases from a primary breast carcinoma have a better prognosis than those in the other large group of primary lung cancers (both SCLS and NSCLC).

The choice of fractionation and dosage remains contentious. Recent large multicentre studies have shown no advantage for prolonged fractionation, and a total dose of 12 Gy in two consecutive daily fractions may be as effective as much more prolonged regimens, is more convenient for patients, requires less transportation (as these patients are often too unwell to attend independently), and frees up valuable resources. Patients with less radiosensitive tumours (adenocarcinomas, melanoma and others) may require higher doses, particularly in the case of surgically unsuitable single metastatic deposits where the relatively limited volume can be treated to a higher dose. Other commonly used radiotherapy fractionations include 20 Gy given over 1 week (the most commonly employed regimen in our own department) or 30 Gy given as 10 fractions over 2 weeks. In certain patients with good prognosis (i.e. with a limited number of brain metastases, the so-called oligo-metastatic group), a combination of whole-brain irradiation with stereotactic radiosurgery boosting can apparently deliver an enhanced result, including improved quality of life and neurological function [57]. This approach is now commonly used though still in a relative minority of cases. The use of recursive partitioning analysis (RPA) has helped define patients in different risk groups, who are best treated by differing combinations of surgery, whole-brain radiotherapy and stereotactic irradiation [52, and see also Ref. [58]]. In the large landmark study from Gaspar and colleagues [59], the RPA decision tree was based on characteristics such as age, number of brain metastases and Karnofsky performance status. Three groups were defined, with survival outcomes from over 7 months (best group) to 2.3 months (worst group). Several trials are presently underway, for example, to assess the role of consolidation whole-brain irradiation after surgical resection of up to three brain metastases and the potential of supportive care with dexamethasone (without whole-brain irradiation) in the treatment of patients with inoperable brain metastases from non-small-cell lung cancer. The role of both whole-brain external beam radiotherapy and stereotactic radiosurgery for less radiosensitive tumour deposits (typically melanoma, sarcoma or renal-cell carcinoma) has become clearer over recent years, particularly since the publication of an important study from the ECOG group (2005), especially at the role of stereotactic radiosurgery – see Refs. [60] and [61].

Surgery

Neurosurgical removal of metastases is occasionally performed in the mistaken supposition that the surgeon is dealing with a primary brain tumour. In these cases, where there has been complete macroscopic removal, treatment with postoperative radiotherapy is usually given as well, in case of unrecognized deposits elsewhere in the brain. Surgical removal of metastases is unquestionably of value in a small proportion of patients, and an important randomized study demonstrated that postoperative whole-brain irradiation should then be routinely offered [59]. Recurrence of tumour anywhere in the brain was less frequent in patients in the radiotherapy group compared with those in the surgery-only group: 9 of 49 (18%) versus 32 of 46 (70%) during the observation period. Relative indications for surgical resection include young patients with a solitary brain metastasis without evidence of disease elsewhere, particularly where they have maintained a high performance status; where there has been a long treatment-free interval (often the case in patients with breast cancer); and where the single metastasis is unlikely to be radiosensitive (e.g. in adenocarcinoma of the bronchus or thyroid). In this selected group, surgical removal with whole-brain radiotherapy is probably the treatment of choice [59,62].

Chemotherapy

In chemosensitive tumours such as small-cell carcinoma of the bronchus or testicular germ-cell tumours, intravenous chemotherapy is effective in producing tumour response [63]. The role of chemotherapy requires further definition, and a recent study of temozolomide in addition to whole-brain radiotherapy certainly suggested a benefit in terms of local control (from 54% to 72% at 3 months) and a (non-significant) improvement in survival (4.5 months in the combined modality arm vs 3.1 months with whole-brain radiotherapy alone) [64]. The long-held concept of a blood–brain barrier may be erroneous, because the changes in vasculature following establishment of a secondary deposit result in a breach of the physiological boundary. Intrathecal chemotherapy is of no value for intracerebral metastases.

Overall survival is poor, particularly where the primary diagnosis is SCLC or melanoma. In other cases, such as breast cancer and adenocarcinoma from other primary sites, survival may be more prolonged, particularly where neurosurgical removal of a solitary metastasis is possible, and in patients where the cranial involvement represents a late solitary site of recurrence.

Lymphomatous and carcinomatous meningitis are discussed in Chapters 8 and 26, respectively.

Tumours of the spinal cord [65,66]

Primary tumours of the spinal cord are very uncommon, comprising about 10% of all CNS tumours, although secondary deposits involving the cord are frequently

Table 11.3 Classification of tumours of spinal cord (with percentage frequency).

Intradural (55%)
Extramedullary
Meningioma (15%)
Neurofibroma (10%)
Congenital and others (7%)
Intramedullary
Ependymoma (5%)
Astrocytoma (5%)
Angiomas (6%)
Others (7%)

Extradural (45%)
Metastases (25%)
Myeloma (6%)
Lymphoma (5%)
Sarcomas (5%)
Others (5%)

encountered. They are often classified into three groups, based on location within the spine, namely, extradural, intradural extramedullary, and intramedullary spinal tumours. Table 11.3 shows the main types of spinal cord tumour. Ependymoma is the commonest, particularly in children and young adults, whereas astrocytoma is much less frequently seen. Schwannomas, vascular tumours and meningiomas are the other relatively common types. The dorsal spine is the commonest primary site, with lumbosacral and cervical primary sites less common. Secondary deposits may be intramedullary but are more often extramedullary (usually extradural), frequently resulting from direct spread from an adjacent involved vertebral body. Management of acute cord compression is also dealt with in Chapter 8.

Symptoms

Pain and tenderness may be presenting symptoms (especially with metastasis) and is generally felt directly over the cord lesion, although the site of pain can be misleading. More laterally situated tumours (often involving the nerve roots as well) may cause more specific and focally sited pain than centrally placed tumours, for example, fusiform intramedullary lesions which can extend in a clinically silent way throughout several segments. Sensorimotor loss is frequently present, with defects of both power and sensation at and below the level of involvement. There may be obvious sensory loss (especially evident in lesions of the dorsal and

lumbar spine involving loss of sensation over the trunk). Muscular weakness in the upper limbs is a feature of lesions of the cervical spine. Below the affected area of an incomplete cord compression there may be partial preservation of function with less obvious neurological abnormalities and only patchy sensory loss, but complete cord compression or major interruption of the vascular supply leads to paraplegia or severe paraparesis. Loss of sphincter function is a late sign with a poor prognosis (see Chapter 8), but lesser degrees occur earlier and their significance is often missed.

Tumours situated below the lower end of the spinal cord (L1 or L2) may produce a typical *cauda equina syndrome* with sacral anaesthesia, sciatic pain (often bilateral), gluteal weakness, wasting, impotence, and bladder dysfunction with retention and overflow incontinence. Most cases are less symptomatically clear-cut and in practice the diagnosis is often very difficult, although MRI has made such cases easier. A myelogram is likely to be normal and cannot reliably exclude the diagnosis. Ependymomas constitute the largest single group of primary tumours at the lower end of the cord (conus medullaris and filum terminale). Lateral compression of the spinal cord may cause a complete or partial Brown–Séquard syndrome, with ipsilateral spastic weakness, reduced vibration sense and proprioception, together with contralateral insensitivity to pain and temperature change. Tumour progression causes an increasingly florid clinical picture with weakness, sensory loss, hyperreflexia and autonomic dysfunction (see Table 8.4). Acute spinal cord compression is discussed in Chapter 8.

Destructive secondary deposits, which more often involve the vertebral column than the spinal cord, produce more local pain and tenderness than some of the less common primary cord lesions. Common primary sites of vertebral or cord metastases include carcinoma of the bronchus (particularly small-cell), carcinoma of the breast and myeloma. Less common primary sites include thyroid, large bowel malignancies, kidney and cutaneous melanoma.

Differential diagnosis

Although the clinical syndrome of spinal cord compression usually implies a malignant aetiology, a few non-malignant lesions can produce a similar clinical picture. These include inflammatory cord lesions (particularly transverse myelitis, infectious polyneuropathy or Guillain–Barré syndrome), anterior spinal arterial occlusion, abscess of the cord, syringomyelia and haemorrhage into the cord (haematomyelia). Very occasionally an

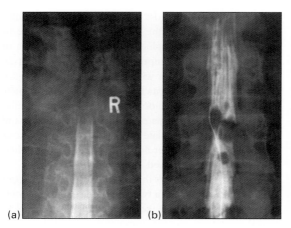

(a)   (b)

Figure 11.9 Radiological changes in spinal cord compression: (a) complete cord compression; (b) partial cord compression due to multiple deposits from an ependymoma.

acutely prolapsed intervertebral disc may produce symptoms of cord compression.

Investigation

Radiological investigation is essential. Plain radiographs of the spine may show an obvious lytic deposit in the vertebrae at the level of compression, but radiographic changes may be very subtle, with loss of the pedicle of the spine but no other significant features. Myelography used to be widely employed, gives good anatomical demonstration of the spinal cord lesion and will show whether the block is partial or complete (Figure 11.9) but has now been almost completely replaced by MRI (see Figure 8.3). With a complete block, it is difficult to be certain of the upper extent of the abnormality, and very occasionally a cisternal myelogram will need to be performed if full anatomical definition is considered important for therapy. Metrizamide gives good definition of root pathology but, being water-soluble, is rapidly cleared so that re-examinations require a further lumbar puncture. In tumours with doubtful or difficult physical signs, CT scanning can be invaluable. This investigation can be even more informative when combined with metrizamide myelography. In general, however, MRI has rapidly become the imaging modality of choice with spinal tumours. Myelography is now largely outmoded.

Management

For primary tumours of the spinal cord, surgical removal is the treatment of choice if it can be safely attempted without permanent neurological deficit. However,

major technical difficulties are often encountered, and intramedullary tumours are almost always unresectable. Surgical decompression is invaluable even where the tumour cannot be removed, and this is generally achieved by laminectomy, often encompassing several segments. Biopsy will be diagnostically valuable even if little more can be surgically achieved. Spinal neoplasms often extend over a considerable length of the cord. These are typically low-grade gliomas and can sometimes be fully excised. Many benign or extramedullary and intradural tumours of borderline malignancy can be removed without need for further treatment. This group includes meningiomas, low-grade gliomas, neurofibromas and tumours of the coverings of the cord (angiomas, fibromas and lipomas).

For more malignant tumours and in patients with secondary deposits involving the spinal cord, surgical decompression followed by postoperative radiotherapy is usually the treatment of choice. If rapid transfer to a neurosurgical centre is difficult or if the patient is unfit or unsuitable for surgery (perhaps because of widespread malignant disease), intensive radiotherapy can often provide excellent palliation, particularly if the cord lesion is a secondary deposit of a radiosensitive tumour. In malignant primary cord tumours such as high-grade glioma, total surgical removal is usually impossible and postoperative radiotherapy is mandatory. A high radiation dose will be required since these tumours are not usually very radiosensitive, generally to the tolerance dose (see below). Very careful judgement of anatomical details, field length, fractionation and total dose is always required.

High doses of dexamethasone are invaluable in reducing cord oedema, making intensive radiotherapy safer. The role of chemotherapy is not established and it has no routine place in the management of spinal cord tumours.

Tumours of the peripheral nerves

These are rare tumours, more often benign than malignant. Multiple neurofibromatosis (von Recklinghausen's disease), the commonest peripheral nerve tumour, is most frequently encountered. In 5–10% of cases, sarcomatous change takes places (neurofibrosarcoma). Tumours of the nerve sheath (schwannomas) can occur in both cranial and peripheral nerves, particularly the acoustic nerve, spinal nerve roots, peripheral nerves and occasionally cranial nerves V, IX or X. These may occasionally undergo malignant change. *Neuroepithelioma* is an exceedingly rare malignant tumour of peripheral nerve, sometimes occurring in conjunction with von Recklinghausen's disease. The histological appearance suggests a neural crest origin, and metastases are frequent.

Treatment of peripheral nerve tumours is by surgical excision if the tumour is producing troublesome pressure symptoms or where there is any suspicion of malignant change. Routine surgical excision of neurofibromas in patients with von Recklinghausen's disease should be discouraged unless there is a sudden increase in size of one of the peripheral lesions. Management of sarcomatous tumours is discussed in Chapter 23.

Radiation damage in the brain and spinal cord

With radical radiotherapy, particularly of midline tumours, the treatment volume may include the spinal cord. For example, in lung cancer a portion of the cord is usually irradiated. Radiation tolerance of the brain, pituitary and spinal cord are of great clinical importance since this frequently sets the dose limit [67,68]. Particularly difficult questions arise when a further dose of radiation to the spinal cord is inevitable, for example, following the need for additional radiotherapy to a new intrathoracic primary cancer which proves unresectable [69]. Both acute and late damage may occur, the latter being of much greater importance. In the brain, early effects include headache, nausea, vomiting and lassitude from raised intracranial pressure, both as a result of the tumour itself and from acute cerebral oedema produced by the radiotherapy. Drowsiness and irritability have been described as side-effects of whole-brain irradiation in children (somnolence syndrome) but are transient and self-limiting. An early syndrome of demyelination may develop but is extremely rare. Late changes include haemorrhage, gliosis, demyelination and necrosis of the brain. The clinical features are those of progressive focal or generalized neurological damage, occurring months or even years after radiation. Damage to the optic chiasm is well recognized in patients treated for pituitary tumours and is clearly dose-related, with minimal risk when daily fraction size is kept between 1.8 and 2.0 Gy.

At least one recent report of drug therapy for improvement of cognitive function and quality of life after radiotherapy for brain tumours has suggested a possible benefit from drugs generally used to treat the symptoms of Alzheimer's disease [70]. Patients treated with donepezil for 6 months showed significant improvements in mood, memory, function and fatigue. The study may represent a new approach to the treatment of long-term cognitive dysfunction in brain tumour survivors, although many would question the American view that 90% of patients receiving brain irradiation (for a primary brain tumour or metastasis) develop cognitive problems that significantly contribute to poor quality of life, even if the tumour has been eradicated. Nonetheless, considerable improvements occurred in memory scores, measures of confusion and fatigue, and a brain-specific quality-of-life scale, possibly resulting from donepezil's documented augmentation of cerebral acetylcholine levels.

Early radiation damage to the spinal cord is more frequently encountered and usually transient. The commonest feature is Lhermitte's syndrome, characterized by 'electric shock' sensations in the extremities (usually the feet), particularly marked on flexion of the neck. It usually occurs a few weeks after the treatment, and is usually self-limiting and without long-term effects.

With late radiation damage, myelopathy can cause progressive motor and sensory changes at the irradiated site, leading to paraparesis, anaesthesia and, in exceptionally severe cases, paraplegia with physiological transection of the cord. If less than the total width of the cord has been irradiated, Brown–Séquard syndrome may result. These changes are due to direct damage to neurological tissue with loss of anterior horn cells, other neurones and oligodendroglia as well as direct vascular damage leading to infarction of the cord. Progressive and chronic radiation myelopathy is usually irreversible and leads to spastic paraplegia with sphincter disturbance. This is fatal in over 50% of cases, particularly where the lesion is in the cervical or upper dorsal cord.

Radiation tolerance of the cord is inversely related to the length of cord irradiated. It is generally accepted that for a 10-cm length of cord, a dose of 40 Gy in daily fractions over 4 weeks is safe, although this dose may have to be exceeded in patients with relatively insensitive lesions that cannot be completely excised, for example, a chordoma. Fraction size is clearly important since treatment to 50 Gy in daily fractions over 5 weeks is usually safe, whereas many cases of cord damage have been documented following treatment to a dose of 40 Gy in daily fractions over 3 weeks [67].

References

1 Wen PY, Kesari S. Malignant gliomas in adults. *N Engl J Med* 2008; 359: 492–507.
2 Behin A, Huong-Xuan K, Carpentier AF, Delatto J-Y. Primary brain tumours in adults. *Lancet* 2003; 361: 323–31.

3 Relling MV, Rubnitz JE, Rivera GK *et al.* High incidence of secondary brain tumours after radiotherapy and
antimetabolites. *Lancet* 1999; 354: 34–9.

4 Hoshino T, Nagashima T, Cho KG *et al.* Variability in the
proliferative potential of human gliomas. *J Neurooncol* 1989;
7: 137–43.

5 Nishikawa R, Ji XD, Harmon RC *et al.* A mutant epidermal
growth factor receptor common in human glioma confers
enhanced tumorigenicity. *Proc Natl Acad Sci USA* 1994; 91:
7727–31.

6 Kool M, Korchunov A, Remke M *et al.* Molecular subgroups
of medulloblastoma: an international meta-analysis of
transcriptome, genetic aberrations, and clinical data of
WNT, SHH, Group 3 and Group 4 medulloblastomas. *Acta
Neuropathol* 2012; 123: 473–484.

7 Pollack IF. Tumor-stromal interactions in medulloblastoma.
New Engl J Med 2013; 368: 1942–43.

8 James CD, Olson JJ. Molecular genetics and molecular biology advances in brain tumours. *Curr Opin Oncol* 1996; 8:
188–95.

9 Stupp R, Mason WP, van den Bent M *et al.* Radiotherapy plus
concomitant and adjuvan temozolomide for glioblastoma. *N
Engl J Med* 2005; 352: 987–96.

10 Hegi ME, Diserens A-C, Gorlia T *et al.* MTMG gene silencing and benefit from temozolamide in glioblastoma. *N Engl
J Med* 2005; 352: 997–1003.

11 Bady P, Sciuscio D, Diserens AC *et al.* MGMT methylation
analysis of glioblastoma on the Infinium methylation
BeadChip identifies two distinct CpG regions associated
with gene silencing and outcome, yielding a prediction
model for comparisons across datasets, tumor grades, and
CIMP-status. *Acta Neuropathol* 2012; 124: 547–60.

12 Bigner SH, Mark J, Burger PC *et al.* Specific chromosomal
abnormalities in malignant gliomas. *Cancer Res* 1988; 48:
405–11.

13 Russell DS, Rubenstein LJ. *Pathology of Tumors of the Nervous System*, 4th edn. Baltimore: Williams & Wilkins, 1982.

14 Whittle IR, Smith C, Navoo P, Collie D. Meningiomas.
Lancet 2004; 363: 1535–43.

15 Wilne S, Collier J, Kennedy C *et al.* Presentation of childhood
CNS tumours: a systematic review and meta-analysis. *Lancet
Oncol* 2007; 8: 685–95.

16 Wilne SH, Dineen RA, Dommett RM and Walker DA. Identifying brain tumours in children and young adults. *Brit Med
J* 2013; 347: f5844.

17 Gilman S. Medical progress: imaging the brain. *N Engl J Med*
1998; 338: 812–20 and 889–98.

18 Shaw EG, Daumas-Duport C, Scheithauer BW *et al.* Radiation therapy in the management of low-grade supratentorial
astrocytomas. *J Neurosurg* 1989; 70: 853–61.

19 Freeman CR, Farmer JP, Montes J. Low-grade astrocytoma
in children: evolving management strategies. *Int J Radiat
Oncol Biol Phys* 1998; 41: 979–87.

20 Karim ABMF, Maat B, Hatlevoll MD *et al.* A randomised
trial on dose–response in radiation therapy of low-grade

cerebral glioma: EORTC study 22844. *Int J Radiat Oncol
Biol Phys* 1996; 36: 549–56.

21 van den Bent MJ, Afra D, deWitte O *et al.* EORTC radiotherapy in Brain Tumour Groups and the UK Medical Research
Council. Long-term efficacy of early versus delayed radiotherapy for low-grade astrocytoma and oligodendroglioma
in adults: the EORTC 22845 randomised trial. *Lancet* 2005;
366: 985–90.

22 Shaw EG, Tatter SB, Lesser GJ, Ellis TL, Stanton CA,
Stieber VW. Current controversies in the radiotherapeutic
management of adult low-grade glioma. *Semin Oncol* 2004;
31: 653–8.

23 Keime-Guibert F, Chinot O, Taillandier L *et al.* Radiotherapy for glioblastoma in the elderly. *N Engl J Med* 2007; 356:
1527–35.

24 Larson D, Gutin P, Leibel S *et al.* Stereotaxic irradiation of
brain tumors. *Cancer* 1990; 65: 792–9.

25 Schupak K, Malkin M, Anderson L *et al.* The relationship
between the technical accuracy of stereotactic interstitial
implantations for high-grade gliomas and the pattern of
tumor recurrence. *Int J Radiol Biol Phys* 1995; 32:
1167–76.

26 Brada M, Graham JD. Stereotactic external beam radiotherapy in the treatment of glioma and other intracranial lesions.
In: Tobias JS, Thomas PRM, eds. *Current Radiation Oncology*, Vol. 1. London: Edward Arnold, 1994: 85–100.

27 Walker MD, Green SB, Byar DP *et al.* Randomized comparisons of radiotherapy and nitrosoureas for the treatment
of malignant glioma after surgery. *N Engl J Med* 1980; 303:
1323.

28 National Institute for Clinical Excellence. Guidance on
the use of temozolomide for the treatment of recurrent malignant glioma (brain cancer). Available at
www.nice.org.uk/pdf/temozolomideguidance.pdf

29 Taphoorn MJ, Stupp R, Coens C *et al.* Health-related quality
of life in patients with glioblastoma: a randomized controlled
trial. *Lancet Oncol* 2005; 6: 937–44.

30 Glioma Meta-analysis Trialists Group. A systematic review
and meta-analysis of individual patient data from 12 randomised trials. *Lancet* 2002; 359: 1011–18.

31 Agaoglu FY, Ayan I, Dizdar Y, Kebudi R, Gorgun O,
Darendeliler E. Ependymal tumors in childhood. *Pediatr
Blood Cancer* 2005; 45: 298–303.

32 Reni M, Brandes AA, Vavassori V *et al.* A multicenter study
of the prognosis and treatment of adult brain ependymal
tumors. *Cancer* 2004; 100: 1221–9.

33 Grundy RG, Wilne SA, Weston CL *et al.* for the Children's
Cancer and Leukaemia Group (formerly UKCCSG) Brain
Tumour Committee. Primary postoperative chemotherapy
without radiotherapy for intracranial ependymoma in
children: the UKCCSG/SIOP prospective study. *Lancet
Oncol* 2007; 8: 696–705.

34 Phillips TL, Sheline GE, Boldrey E. Therapeutic considerations in tumours affecting the central nervous system:
ependymomas. *Radiology* 1964; 83: 98–105.

35 Wolff JE, Sajedi M, Brant R et al. Choroid plexus tumours. *Br J Cancer* 2002; 87: 1086–91.

36 Sheline GE, Boldrey EB, Karlsberg P, Phillips TL. Therapeutic considerations in tumours affecting the central nervous system: oligodendrogliomas. *Radiology* 1964; 82: 84–9.

37 Bouffet E, Jouvet A, Thiesse P et al. Chemotherapy for aggressive or anaplastic high grade oligodendrogliomas and oligoastrocytomas: better than a salvage treatment. *Br J Neurosurg* 1998; 12: 217–22.

38 Sunyach MP, Jouvet A, Perol D et al. Role of exclusive chemotherapy as first line treatment in oligodendroglioma. *J Neurooncol* 2007; 85: 319–28.

39 van den Bent MJ, Brandes AA, Taphoorn MJ, et al. Adjuvant procarbazine, lomustine, and vincristine chemotherapy in newly diagnosed anaplastic oligodendroglioma: Long-term follow-up of EORTC Brain Tumor Group Study 26951. *J Clin Oncol* 2013; 31: 344–50.

40 Pierce SM, Barnes PD, Loeffler JS et al. Definitive radiation therapy in the management of symptomatic patients with optic glioma. *Cancer* 1990; 65: 45–52.

41 Astrup J. Natural history and clinical management of optic pathway glioma. *Br J Neurosurg* 2003; 17: 327–35.

42 Polkinghorn WR, Tarbell NJ. Medulloblastoma: tumorigenesis, current clinical paradigm, and efforts to improve risk stratification. *Nat Clin Pract Oncol* 2007; 4: 295–304.

43 Gajjar A, Chintagumpala M, Ashley D et al. Risk-adapted cranio-spinal radiotherapy followed by high-dose chemotherapy and stem-cell rescue in children with newly diagnosed medulloblastoma (St Jude Medulloblastoma-96): long-term results from a prospective, multicentre trial. *Lancet Oncol* 2006; 7: 813–20.

44 Sposto R, Ertel IJ, Jenkin RDT et al. The effectiveness of chemotherapy for treatment of high-grade astrocytoma in children: results of a randomised trial. *J Neurooncol* 1989; 7: 165–77.

45 Tait D, Thornton-Jones H, Bloom HJG et al. Adjuvant chemotherapy for medulloblastoma: the first multicentre controlled trial of the International Society for Paediatric Oncology. *Eur J Cancer* 1990; 26: 464–9.

46 Powell MF, Lightman SL, eds. *Management of Pituitary Tumours: a Handbook.* Edinburgh: Churchill Livingstone, 1995.

47 Estrada J, Boronat M, Mielgo M et al. The long-term outcome of pituitary irradiation after unsuccessful trans-sphenoidal surgery in Cushing's disease. *N Engl J Med* 1997; 336: 172–7.

48 Jephcott CR, Sugden EM, Foord T. Radiotherapy for cranio-pharyngioma in children: a national audit. *Clin Oncol* 2003; 15: 10–13.

49 Colin P, Jovenin N, Delemer B et al. Treatment of pituitary adenomas by fractionated stereotactic radiotherapy: a prospective study of 110 patients. *Int J Radiat Oncol Biol Phys* 2005; 62: 333–41.

50 Schrell UMH, Rittig MG, Anders M et al. Hydroxyurea for treatment of unresectable and recurrent meningiomas. II.

Decrease in the size of meningiomas in patients treated with hydroxyurea. *J Neurosurg* 1997; 86: 840–4.

51 Balmaceda C, Heller G, Rosenblum M et al. Chemotherapy without irradiation: a novel approach for newly diagnosed CNS germ cell tumors: results of an international cooperative trial. *J Clin Oncol* 1996; 14: 2908–15.

52 Foweraker KL, Burton KE, Maynard SE et al. High-dose radiotherapy in the management of chordoma and chondrosarcoma of the skull base and cervical spine: Part 1--Clinical outcomes. *Clin Oncol (R Coll Radiol)* 2007; 19: 509–16.

53 Kondziolka D, Lunsford LD, McLaughlin MR et al. Long-term outcomes after radiosurgery for acoustic neuromas. *N Engl J Med* 1998; 339: 1426–33.

54 Rampling R. *CancerStats: Brain and Other Central Nervous System Tumours – UK.* London: Cancer Research UK, 2003. Available at www.cancerresearchuk.org

55 Pollack IF, Finkelstein SD, Woods J et al. Expression of p53 and prognosis in children with malignant gliomas. *N Engl J Med* 2002; 346: 420–7.

56 Lock M, Chow E, Pond GR et al. Prognostic factors in brain metastases: can we determine patients who do not benefit from whole-brain radiotherapy? *Clin Oncol* 2004; 16: 332–8.

57 Andrews DW, Scott CB, Sperduto PW et al. Whole brain radiation therapy with or without stereotactic radiosurgery boost for patients with one to three brain metastases: phase III results of the RTOG 9508 randomised trial. *Lancet* 2004; 363: 1665–72.

58 Patil CG, Pricola K, Sarmiento JM. Whole brain radiation therapy (WBRT) alone versus WBRT and radiosurgery for the treatment of brain metastases. *Cochrane Database Syst Rev.* 2012; 9: CD 006121.

59 Gaspar L, Scott C, Rotman M et al. Recursive partitioning analysis (RPA) in three Radiation Therapy Oncology Group (RTOG) trials. *Int J Radiat Oncol Biol Phys* 1997; 37: 745–51.

60 Manon R, O'Neill A, Knisely J et al. Phase II trial of radio-surgery for one to three newly diagnosed brain metastases from renal cell carcinoma, melanoma, and sarcoma: an Eastern Cooperative Oncology Group study (E 6397). *J Clin Oncol* 2005; 23: 8870–76.

61 Hanson PW, Elaimy AL, Lamoreaux WT et al. A concise review of the efficacy of stereotactic radiosurgery in the management of melanoma and renal cell carcinoma brain metastases. *World J Surg Oncol* 2012; 10: 176. doi: 10.1186/1477-7819-10-176.

62 Patchell RA, Tibbs PA, Regine WF et al. Postoperative radio-therapy in the treatment of single metastases to the brain: a randomized trial. *JAMA* 1998; 280: 1485–9.

63 Twelves CJ, Souhami RL, Harper PG et al. The response of cerebral metastases in small cell lung cancer to systemic chemotherapy. *Br J Cancer* 1990; 61: 147–50.

64 Verger E, Gil M, Yaya R et al. Temozolomide and concomitant whole brain radiotherapy in patients with brain metastases: a phase II randomised trial. *Int J Radiat Oncol Biol Phys* 2005; 61: 185–91.

65 Rossi A, Gandolfo C, Morana G, Tortori-Donati, P. Tumors of the spine in children. *Neuroimaging Clin North Am* 2007; 17: 17–35.

66 Gelabert-González M. Primary spinal cord tumors. An analysis of a series of 168 patients. *Rev Neurol* 2007; 44: 269–74.

67 Wara WM, Phillips TL, Sheline GE *et al.* Radiation tolerance of the spinal cord. *Cancer* 1975; 35: 1558–62.

68 Nieder C, Grosu AL, Andratschke NH, Molls M. Update of human spinal cord reirradiation tolerance based on additional data from 38 patients. *Int J Radiat Oncol Biol Phys* 2006; 66: 1446–9.

69 Constine LS, Woolf PD, Cann D *et al.* Hypothalamic–pituitary dysfunction after radiation for brain tumors. *N Engl J Med* 1993; 328: 87–94.

70 Shaw EG, Rosdhal R, D'Agostino RB *et al.* Phase II study of donepezil in irradiated brain tumor patients: effect on cognitive function, mood and quality of life. *J Clin Oncol* 2006; 24: 1415–20.

Further reading

Barker FG, Chang SM. Improving resection of malignant glioma. *Lancet Oncol* 2006; 7: 359–60.

Benson VS, Pirie K, Green J, Casabonne D, Beral F. Lifestyle factors and primary glioma and meningioma tumours in the Million Women Study cohort. *Br J Cancer* 2008; 99: 185–90.

Bezjak A, Adams J, Barton R *et al.* Symptom response after palliative radiotherapy for patients with brain metastases. *Eur J Cancer* 2002; 38: 487–96.

Cancer Genome Atlas Research Network. Comprehensive genomic characterization defines human glioblastoma genes and core pathways. *Nature* 2008; 455: 1061–8.

Collins VP. Mechanisms of disease: genetic predictors of response to treatment in brain tumors. *Nat Clin Pract Oncol* 2007; 4: 362–74.

Crawford JR, MacDonald TJ, Packer RJ. Medulloblastoma in childhood: new biological advances. *Lancet Neurol* 2007; 6: 1073–85.

Deangelis LM. Chemotherapy for brain tumors: a new beginning. *N Engl J Med* 2005; 352: 1036–8.

Henson JW, Gaviani P, Gonzalez RG. MRI in treatment of adult gliomas. *Lancet Oncol* 2005; 6: 167–75.

Jenkins PJ, Bates P, Carson MN, Stewart PM, Wass JA. Conventional pituitary irradiation is effective in lowering serum growth hormone and insulin-like growth factor-I in patients with acromegaly. *J Clin Endocrinol Metab* 2006; 91; 1239–45.

Kaal EC, Niel CG, Vecht CJ. Therapeutic management of brain metastasis. *Lancet Neurol* 2005; 4: 289–98.

Khanduri S, Gerrard G. Defining the standard of care for high-grade glioma: a NICE deal for UK patients? *Clin Oncol* 2007; 19: 507–8.

Khanduri S, Gerrard G, Barton R *et al.* Clinical trials assessing the optimal management of brain metastases: the state of play. *Clin Oncol* 2006; 18: 744–6.

Lavy C, James A, Wilson-MacDonald J *et al.* Cauda equina syndrome. *Br Med J* 2009; 338: 881–4.

Macbeth FR, Wheldon TE, Girling DJ *et al.* for the Medical Research Council Lung Cancer Working Party. Radiation myelopathy: estimates of risk in 1048 patients in three randomized trials of palliative radiotherapy for non-small cell lung cancer. *Clin Oncol* 1996; 8: 176–81.

Mellinghoff IK, Wang MY, Vivanko I *et al.* Molecular determinants of the responsive glioblastomas to EGFR kinase inhibitors. *N Engl J Med* 2005; 253: 2012–24.

Melmed S. Medical progress: acromegaly. *N Engl J Med* 2006; 355: 2558–73.

Omuro AM, Leite CC, Mokhtari K, Delattre JY. Pitfalls in the diagnosis of brain tumours. *Lancet Neurol* 2006; 5: 937–48.

Omuro AM, DeAngelis LM, Yahalom J, Abery LE. Chemoradiotherapy for primary CNS lymphoma: an intent-to-treat analysis with complete follow up. *Neurology* 2005; 64: 69–74.

Papagikos MA, Shaw EG, Stieber VW. Lessons learned from randomised clinical trials in adult low-grade glioma. *Lancet Oncol* 2005; 6: 240–4.

Parsons DW, Jones S, Zhang X *et al.* An integrated genomic analysis of human glioblastoma multiforme. *Science* 2008; 321: 1807–12.

Shaw EG, Robbins ME. The management of radiation-induced brain injury. *Cancer Treat Res* 2006; 128: 7–22.

Tsao MN, Mehta MP, Whelan TJ *et al.* The American Society for Therapeutic Radiology evidence-based review of the role of radiosurgery for malignant glioma. *Int J Radiat Oncol Biol Phys* 2005; 63: 47–55.

12 Tumours of the lung and mediastinum

Carcinoma of the bronchus

Introduction, aetiology and epidemiology

Carcinoma of the bronchus is the commonest cancer in the Western world, having increased steadily in incidence since the 1930s. The overall incidence in the United Kingdom is currently 82 per 100 000 (male) and 50 per 100 000 (female), with the highest incidence in Scotland, with an annual incidence of over 41 000 cases in the United Kingdom (see Ref. [1]). Mortality from lung cancer accounts for over 450 000 deaths annually in China, 342 000 in Europe and 162 000 in the United States – globally, about 1 million deaths each year. These figures are strongly related to age (Figure 12.1). As a result of the increasing prevalence of cigarette smoking after the First World War, carcinoma of the bronchus had become the leading cause of cancer death in males during and beyond the latter half of the twentieth century. In recent years, more women have become cigarette smokers, with the result that lung cancer has become increasingly common in women. Moreover, there is increasing evidence that women who smoke are more likely than men to develop lung cancer [2]. Indeed, in British women there are now more deaths each year from lung cancer than from breast cancer. Perhaps surprisingly, women with lung cancer appear to have a better survival than men, an effect unrelated to either stage or histological subtype at diagnosis.

Although several aetiological factors have been implicated, including exposure to radioactivity and possible environmental hazards, these are insignificant compared with the highly carcinogenic effect of prolonged exposure to cigarette smoke. Cigarette smoke contains a variety of harmful substances and chemicals, including nicotine (the drug which makes cigarettes so addictive), carbon monoxide, tar, benzene, formaldehyde, nitrosamines and benzopyrene, to name but a few. Recent studies have shown that non-smokers married to lifelong smokers are at double the expected risk for developing lung cancer. Case–control studies have also suggested an increased incidence of lung cancer in non-smokers who lived in a household of heavy smokers during childhood and adolescence. About 15–20% of cases of lung cancer develop in non-smokers [3], and a proportion of these appear to be clearly related to passive smoking; indeed, it is the risk of passive smoking in employees of various organizations that has so powerfully driven the recent widespread

Cancer and its Management, Seventh Edition. Jeffrey Tobias and Daniel Hochhauser.
© 2015 John Wiley & Sons, Ltd. Published 2015 by John Wiley & Sons, Ltd.

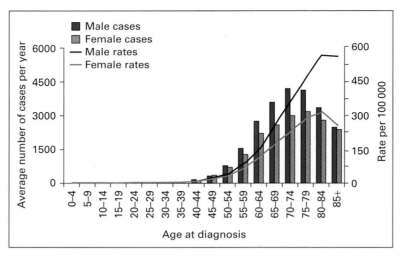

Figure 12.1 Lung Cancer: Average Number of New Cases per Year and Age-Specific Incidence Rates by sex, UK, 2008–2010. (http://info.cancerresearchuk.org/cancerstats/types/lung/incidence/?a=5441, accessed February 2014. © Cancer Research UK. Reproduced with permission.)

legislation restricting cigarette smoking in public places over the past few years (see below). It has been estimated that in the United Kingdom about 600 people die each year because of exposure to passive (or 'second-hand') smoking, particularly those working in the hospitality industry including bar workers and waiters, to say nothing of a much higher estimate of deaths (over 10 000 in all) annually from second-hand smoke in the home.

A great deal of political debate has followed the demonstration of an incontrovertible link between cigarette smoking and lung cancer, in which health education, cost of treatment, possible loss of tax revenue, reduction in productivity resulting from ill-health, and freedom of choice have been the principal points for discussion. In the United Kingdom, approximately one-quarter of adults are smokers (down from half just 30 years ago). Sadly there is a clear age and class prevalence trend: almost one-third of girls aged 15–16 smoke cigarettes regularly, and people in the 20–24 year age group smoke the most (38% of men and 34% of women of this age). Every year, about 100 000 people die as a result of smoking – one-third of these deaths are due to lung cancer alone and life expectancy in long-term smokers has been reduced by about a decade. Despite these gloomy figures, British adults are about half as likely to smoke as was the case four decades ago. In 1974, 45% of adults smoked (51% of men, 41% of women). The figures for 2011 are 20% (total) – 21% of men, 19% of women (see Ref. [4]).

At an international level, there has been a wide variety of approaches towards the restriction of smoking, stemming from the differing philosophies of different countries. It is estimated that tobacco use, chiefly smoking-related, is associated with about 5 million deaths annually worldwide. This figure is expected to rise to about 10 million per year by 2025 (see Ref. [5]). Of the 1.2 billion smokers in the world, about half will die of smoking-related causes. In China, smoking rates are rising sharply; smoking was responsible for only 12% of deaths in middle-age during the 1990s; by 2030 this figure will have risen to about one-third. Smoking in public places has been banned in Scotland, Wales, Ireland, Malta, Italy, Norway, Sweden and New Zealand. Just before the free vote in the British Parliament in February 2006, which resulted in a clear mandate for a total ban on smoking in all public places in England (with the exception of prisons and long-stay mental homes), a large survey found that over 70% of the British population were indeed in favour of a total smoking ban. In many Scandinavian countries, it is now socially unacceptable to smoke in public places, and cigarettes have become extremely expensive, with the result that smoking-related illnesses are beginning to decline. In the United Kingdom, tobacco accounted for about half of all premature deaths during the 1970s, whereas the figure is now (2012) about 20% of deaths in middle-aged men, less than half the 47% in the same group 40 years earlier (see Ref. [6]). In the United States, smoking rates have steadily declined from a high of 57% of adult men in 1955 and 34% of women in 1965, to a new level of 19% in recent years (see Ref. [7]). There is a clear inverse relationship between the cost of cigarettes and the amount smoked. In the United Kingdom, restriction of smoking in public areas has been a protracted and uphill battle. There is a clear inverse relationship in both the United Kingdom and the United States between socioeconomic status and incidence of lung cancer. The death rate from this disease is disproportionately high in comparison to incidence because of the low cure rates currently achieved (<10% at 5 years overall). So far, attempts at screening, even in high-risk groups, have met with very little success even though considerable resources – and resourcefulness – have been deployed; see, for example, Ref. [8]. In developing countries, cigarette consumption is rapidly rising and high-tar brands, which are no longer popular in this country, are widely advertised. Despite overwhelming evidence of the dangers of cigarette smoking, major tobacco companies are urging farmers in developing countries to change from production of staple arable crops to growing tobacco. At present, three of the world's five biggest tobacco firms are British, and each year make about £2.9 billion in pretax profits. It has been estimated that smoking costs the NHS almost £2 billion a year.

Fortunately, the carcinogenic effects of cigarette smoke are to a considerable extent reversible. In their classic study of the smoking habits of British doctors, Doll and Hill were able to demonstrate a gradual reduction in mortality of British doctors who gave up smoking. Lung cancer declines in incidence when smokers give up the habit. After 12 years of total abstinence from cigarette smoking, the risk of developing lung cancer is almost as low as in non-smokers, except for heavy smokers (more than 20 per day), in whom the risk never falls to that of the non-smoker (Figure 12.2). In the lower age groups (30–45 years), there is evidence for a fall in death rate over the past 15 years (Figure 12.3). These findings were updated in a powerful landmark study published 50 years later [9], and see also an update from the United States by Jha *et al.* [10]. It is doubtful that this reduction is due to the introduction of low-tar brands; it is more likely attributable to smoking cessation. In the US-based study, after quitting smoking, adults who had stopped at ages 25–34, 35–44 or 45–54 years of age gained 10, 9, and 6 years of life respectively, as compared with those who continued to smoke. Attempts to prevent the development of lung cancer by the administration of retinoids to high-risk individuals have been unsuccessful; indeed, lung cancer deaths were increased [11]. On the other hand, we do at least have increasing evidence for the effectiveness of nicotine patches to aid quitters, with a 'stop rate' among those receiving nicotine replacement therapy of around 20% [12]. In this large study of over

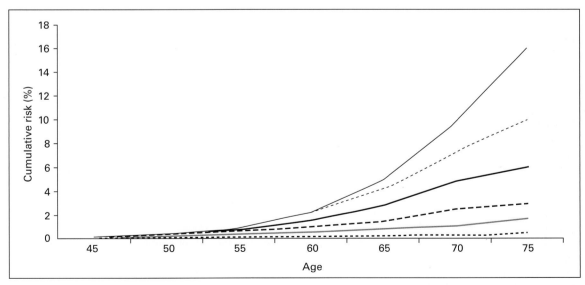

Figure 12.2 Effects of stopping smoking at various ages on the cumulative risk (%) of death from lung cancer by age 75 for men. ____Current cigarette smoker; ____stopped aged 60; ____stopped aged 50; _ _ _stopped aged 40; ____stopped aged 30; ....lifelong non-smoker.

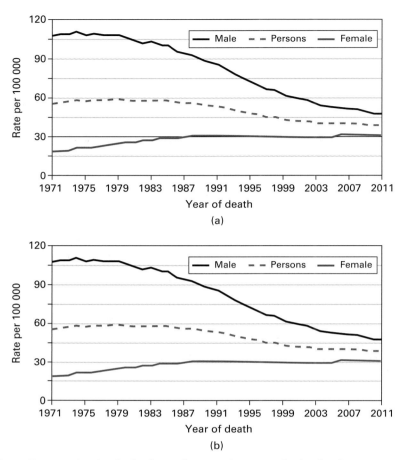

Figure 12.3 Lung Cancer European Age-Standardized Mortality Rates, By Age, England and Wales, 1950–2011. (a) for men (b) for women. (http://info.cancerresearchuk.org/cancerstats/types/lung/mortality/?a=5441, accessed February 2014. © Cancer Research UK. Reproduced with permission.)

34 000 eligible smokers who phoned a toll-free quitline, over 6000 successful quits were attributable to receipt of nicotine replacement therapy, at a cost of only about £300 per quitter, far better value than any other form of intervention or, of course, treatment of the established disease. See also Ref. [13].

Other aetiological factors thought or known to have a role include asbestos exposure, industrial pollution, ionizing radiation and occupational hazards (see also Chapter 2). The potential importance of air pollution as an aetiological factor has been underscored by a recent report from nine European countries with a mean follow-up of almost 13 years, showing a clear association for development of an adenocarcinoma of the lung with increasing levels of particulate matter

of less than 10 μm in diameter – see Ref. [14]. Some of the potential carcinogens accessed occupationally include inorganic arsenicals, tin, nickel, cadmium, sulphuric acid or zinc vapour, strontium chromate, beryllium and haematite, plus many others. Of these, asbestos exposure is probably the most critical, for both lung cancer and mesothelioma (see page 217). This is particularly important when combined with cigarette smoking: in smokers with occupational exposure to asbestos, the risk of lung cancer is 45 times above that of the normal population. This remarkable statistic has led to several attempts at screening for lung cancer in the appropriate population, usually by radiological methods that increasingly have included spiral computed tomography (CT) [15].

Perhaps it is worth mentioning here that even now, over 50 years since Doll's classic paper, smoking is still being linked with new diseases, including non-malignant disorders [16]. For example, we now know that smoking in pregnancy appears to be linked with a variety of congenital disorders in the child, including, for example, polydactyly or other abnormalities of the hand. A second recent example is the uncovering of a link between smoking and early rheumatoid arthritis, to say nothing of the known pulmonary, cardiac, dermatological and other disorders.

Screening for lung cancer is clearly still in its infancy. In a large, recently reported study of over 31 500 asymptomatic people at risk for lung cancer, screening was undertaken with low-dose CT scans (1993–2005), with repeated screening for the majority. Lung cancer was diagnosed in 484 of these people, of whom 85% had clinical stage 1 (i.e. potentially surgically curable), with an estimated 10-year survival in this subgroup of 88% [17]. More recently, results were presented from the US-based National Lung Screening Trial Research Team [18]. 55 439 participants were randomized to either low-dose CT-scanning or chest radiography. 27% and 9% respectively had a positive screening result, ultimately leading to a diagnosis of lung cancer in 292 participants −1.1% of the CT-scanned group and 0.7% in those undergoing chest radiography. Of these, stage 1 cases likely to be surgically curable were diagnosed in 158 versus 70 patients; stages IIB-IV in 120 versus 112. The authors suggested that a reduction in mortality is potentially achievable but clearly, this approach is likely to remain both prohibitively expensive and inefficient on a national scale especially outside the United States, a far less attractive alternative to persuading smokers to stop, and using current techniques to help them to do so.

The molecular pathology of lung cancer

The carcinogens in cigarette smoke cause mutations in genes, some of which result in further genomic instability. By the time the cancer is clinically apparent numerous mutations in dominant or recessive growth-regulatory genes are apparent. Many types of abnormality occur, including deletions, rearrangements, point mutations, splicing errors and amplification. Figure 12.4 shows diagrammatically some of the abnormalities which are consistently observed at the various stages of tumour growth during the progression from hyperplasia/dysplasia to invasive cancer in non-small-cell lung cancer (NSCLC). The genes deleted at chromosomes 3p and 9p21 are not yet defined, but will be of great

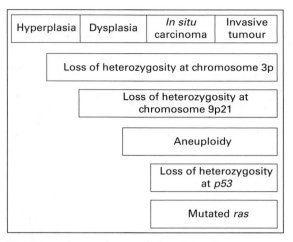

Figure 12.4 Genetic changes which accompany progression to invasive lung cancer.

interest in understanding lung cancer growth. Over the past few years, molecular markers have become integrated into decisions about treatment for lung cancer, largely through the discovery of mutations in the epidermal growth factor receptor (EGFR) that are predictive of responses to agents such as gefitinib or erlotinib. For example, *RRM1*, the gene that encodes the regulatory subunit of ribonucleotide reductase, is important in NSCLC. Low levels of expression of this gene are associated with poor survival, a feature used in the study by Zheng and colleagues [19] to give useful prognostic information following surgical treatment of apparently localized disease. Overall survival was over 10 years for patients whose tumours had high expression of *RRM1*, compared with 5 years for those with low expression.

Pathology of lung cancer
Histological types

Lung cancer is only rarely a tumour of the true lung parenchyma, arising far more frequently in large and medium-sized bronchi. There are many histological types of lung cancer. However, it is convenient to consider the commonest varieties in four major groups, although there is substantial histological variation within each of these (Table 12.1). There has been considerable debate as to whether the cell of origin is different in the differing histological types. There is, however, evidence to suggest that the cancers arise from a common precursor cell, which has the capacity to differentiate into a variety of histological types.

Table 12.1 Histological classification of lung cancer.*

	Frequency (%)
Squamous carcinoma	35–45
Small-cell carcinoma	20
Adenocarcinoma (bronchogenic, acinar bronchioalveolar)	15–50[†]
Large-cell carcinoma (with or without mucin, giant and clear-cell variants)	10
Mixed forms	10–20
Other tumours (carcinoid, cylindroma, sarcoma and mixed histological types)	2

*Data from the World Health Organization classification.
[†]Geographical variation.

Primary tracheal tumours are extremely unusual. Histologically they are generally non-small-cell carcinomas, indistinguishable from their far more common bronchogenic counterpart. For many reasons, notably their extremely proximal anatomical situation and early tendency to obstruct, they do of course pose exceptional problems in management [20].

Squamous cell carcinoma

This is the commonest histological type and is characterized by the presence of keratinization and intercellular bridging, and is often subdivided on the basis of differentiation. Most of these tumours arise proximally in large bronchi (though they may also arise peripherally), and tend to be polypoid or infiltrating, often with distinct borders. Since the bronchi at this level are not normally lined by squamous epithelium, it is likely that neoplastic change at this site is preceded by squamous metaplasia, although studies of carcinoma *in situ* have suggested that this may not always occur. Mutations and loss of heterozygosity of the *p53* gene have been found in many tumours.

Small-cell lung cancer

Small-cell lung cancer (SCLC) is characterized by a diffused growth of small cells with fine granular nuclei, inconspicuous nucleoli and scanty cytoplasm. SCLC accounts for about 12% of all newly diagnosed lung cancers and morphologically the cells tend to be tightly packed or moulded, with little evidence of supportive tissue. Occasionally, combinations of small-cell and squamous cell carcinomas are seen, although many pathologists think that such tumours should be classified

as poorly differentiated squamous cell carcinoma. Neurosecretory granules are often present on electron microscopy (Figure 12.5). These may be the site of origin of hormones such as adrenocorticotrophic hormone (ACTH), antidiuretic hormone (ADH) and calcitonin that are sometimes produced and which give rise to ectopic hormone syndromes that may be clinically significant (see Chapter 9). Small-cell carcinomas express other markers of neural differentiation. Chief among these is the presence on the cell surface of the neural-cell adhesion molecule (NCAM). The cells secrete autocrine growth factors such as gastrin-releasing peptide which, after secretion, binds to receptors on the tumour cell surface and causes a mitotic stimulus. Numerous other peptide hormones also bind to receptors on the SCLC cell surface and there has been considerable interest in the possible therapeutic effects of blocking such autocrine growth mechanisms. The tumours also show overexpression or amplification of one or more *myc* family oncogenes. Karyotypically, there is an almost invariable deletion of part of the short arm of chromosome 3 (bands 14–23), and loss of heterozygosity at the site of the *p53* gene (17p). As in NSCLC, *p53* mutations occur frequently. Small-cell carcinomas typically develop in proximal large bronchi and are characterized by extensive local invasion associated with early blood-borne and lymphatic metastases, making them almost invariably unsuitable for surgery as a definitive treatment. Some tumours are diagnosed by biopsy of enlarged supraclavicular or cervical lymph nodes.

Adenocarcinomas

These show the typical features of neoplastic cells derived from glandular epithelium, with formation of acini, papillae and mucus. Many adenocarcinomas are peripheral in site of origin, frequently invading the pleura. These cancers sometimes arise in scar tissue, and may occur in fibrotic lung disease. Adenocarcinoma is less clearly related to cigarette smoking than either squamous cell or small-cell carcinoma, and was the predominant cell type before the advent of cigarette smoking. Unlike other forms of lung cancer, it is slightly commoner in females. In some countries it is increasing in frequency. In large series from the United States, adenocarcinoma now accounts for 50% of all NSCLC.

The uncommon bronchioalveolar carcinoma sometimes presents as a multicentric tumour with alveoli lined by neoplastic columnar cells. Like the more typical adenocarcinoma it is commoner in women and less frequently associated with smoking.

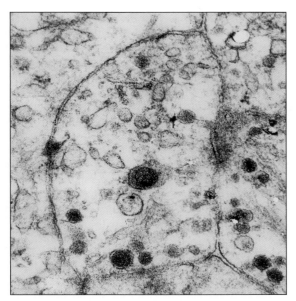

Figure 12.5 Electron microscopy appearances in small-cell carcinoma. Dense neurosecretory granules are shown in cell processes (×52 250).

Large-cell carcinoma

Large-cell carcinoma refers to undifferentiated tumours with a variety of appearances. The cells are large, often with featureless cytoplasm and show little tendency towards keratinization or acinar formation. In a proportion of these tumours, there is evidence of mucus production, and there may also be other ultrastructural characteristics which are reminiscent of adenocarcinoma. The tumour borders are generally well defined, and the tumour itself may arise from a subsegmental or more distal bronchus.

Mixed histologies

Approximately 20% of tumours show a mixed histological appearance (small/large-cell, adeno/squamous, squamous/small-cell). Of interest is the finding that 10–20% of typical adenocarcinomas have some cellular features of neuroendocrine cells such as expression of chromogranin (found in dense core granules), NCAM and neurone-specific enolase. There have been some studies that purport to show that these tumours may, like SCLC, show sensitivity to chemotherapy, but the issue is not settled.

Pathological diagnosis

In over 80% of patients with lung cancer, malignant cells are found in the sputum, using exfoliative cytology. The likelihood of a positive sputum diagnosis increases from 60% with a single specimen to 80% when four specimens are obtained. This proportion is also increased when specimens are obtained at bronchoscopy from trap, brush or lavage specimens. The four major categories can be distinguished with an accuracy of 80% by either cytological or histological methods. Occasionally, a mixture of cell types is seen, for example, mixed small-cell and large-cell carcinoma or adenosquamous tumours. About one-quarter of autopsy cases show mixed histologies, although this high proportion may be related to a treatment-induced change in the histology. Cases with mixed histology represent one line of evidence suggesting that these carcinomas do not arise from different cells, but that the cancer-inducing event results in cells which can differentiate along more than one pathway.

The clinical distinction between primary adenocarcinoma of the bronchus and secondary pulmonary deposits from primary adenocarcinomas at other sites may be a difficult one, especially if no endobronchial lesion is seen at bronchoscopy. Similarly, the clear-cell carcinoma variant of large-cell carcinoma can be mistaken for metastatic hypernephroma. One important clinical feature of squamous cell carcinomas is that they may cavitate and can therefore be confused with a lung abscess.

Patterns of local invasion and metastasis

Carcinoma of the bronchus spreads by local invasion and by lymphatic and haematogenous routes (Figure 12.6). Locally, the tumour may spread into the mediastinum or through the bronchial wall and lung parenchyma to the pleural space and chest wall. There may be erosion of overlying ribs. Apical tumours typically spread from the apex of the lung to involve the brachial plexus, with erosion of upper thoracic ribs and local nerves such as the thoracocervical sympathetic chain (Pancoast syndrome). At the hilum of the lung the tumour may damage the phrenic or left recurrent laryngeal nerve. It may also erode posteriorly into the oesophagus or vertebrae.

Lymphatic spread within the chest is chiefly to hilar and mediastinal, subcarinal, tracheobronchial and paratracheal nodes. Beyond the chest, involvement of supraclavicular, cervical and axillary nodes may occur. Lymphatic involvement below the diaphragm is frequent in small-cell carcinoma, especially to upper para-aortic nodes.

Blood-borne spread is especially frequent in small-cell carcinoma and typically occurs earlier than with other lung cancers. The skeleton is frequently involved, particularly vertebrae, ribs and pelvis, and widespread infiltration into bone marrow occurs, especially in

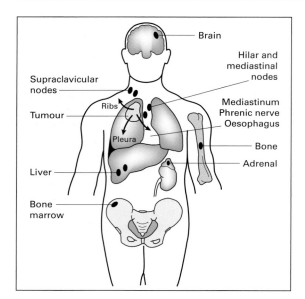

Figure 12.6 Local and metastatic spread in lung cancer.

small-cell carcinoma where estimates of frequency vary from 5–30%, depending on the number of marrow aspirations, the extent of the tumour and the sensitivity of the methods used to detect the infiltrating cells. Other common sites include the brain (65% of autopsies in small-cell carcinoma), liver and adrenals, but secondary deposits can be found in any organ. Early and rapid dissemination is particularly characteristic of small-cell carcinoma, which also has the most rapid volume doubling time.

Clinical features

Most patients with lung cancer present with symptoms directly related to the tumour such as haemoptysis, cough, dyspnoea or chest pain. Since many are smokers, some of these symptoms (particularly a cough) will already be present as a result of chronic bronchitis and emphysema. This may delay them in seeking advice, although a substantial number are sufficiently aware of the increased intensity of their symptoms to give up smoking, often after a lifetime of being unable to do so. The cough is often persistent, nocturnal and may be productive. Sputum may be blood-streaked or persistently discoloured as a result of infection that cannot resolve due to atelectasis beyond an obstructing endobronchial tumour. Haemoptyses, though intermittent, usually become increasingly severe. Pain, usually aching, is present in over 50% of patients. It seems to be commoner

in patients with mediastinal involvement or atelectasis, and is much commoner than the typical, sharper, pain of bone metastases. At present, the National Institute for Health and Clinical Excellence (NICE) recommendations for obtaining an urgent referral from a family practitioner for chest radiography are clear-cut: haemoptysis and/or unexplained cough, chest or shoulder pain, weight loss, dyspnoea, hoarseness or finger clubbing, with any of the above lasting for more than 3 weeks. In addition, any features suggestive of a metastasis (e.g. to skin, liver, bone or brain) should also prompt an urgent referral. These are important practical points for the general practitioner.

More peripheral tumours often present rather late, when already of significant size. They may cause pain in the chest wall by direct extension to the pleura or periosteum of the ribs, often trapping or invading intercostal nerves. Direct tumour invasion of the left recurrent laryngeal nerve may result in hoarseness of the voice, which is a frequent presenting symptom. Pleural effusion, phrenic nerve palsy and lobar or total lung collapse may all contribute to increasing dyspnoea. Pneumonias that fail to resolve completely after antibiotics raise the suspicion of underlying cancer. Dysphagia may result from enlarged mediastinal lymph nodes that compress the oesophagus, usually at its mid or lower third, or by direct invasion. Wheeze and stridor are important signs of obstruction of large airways, generally due to proximal tumours.

Tumours at specific sites may produce typical syndromes. A Pancoast tumour, situated at the apex of the lung, causes severe pain in the shoulder, chest wall and arm as a result of relentless local invasion which destroys ribs and infiltrates the brachial plexus. Weakness of the small muscles of the hand may occur, with paraesthesiae on the inner aspect of the arm, due to C5/6 infiltration and T1 motor loss. Tumours of the right main or right upper lobe bronchus (often with associated right paratracheal node enlargement) may compress the great veins leading to superior vena caval obstruction (SVCO), producing a typical clinical syndrome consisting of swelling of the face, neck and upper arms, plethora or cyanosis and rapid development of a visible collateral circulation over the scapula and upper chest wall. In severe cases, conjunctival oedema (chemosis) occurs. The majority of cases of SVCO are caused by small-cell carcinomas and prompt treatment may produce a gratifying resolution of these symptoms (see Chapter 8).

Some patients notice a 'mass' in the neck due to lymph node enlargement. In other patients, the presenting symptoms are caused by secondary deposits, especially in small-cell cancer. Pain in the back may be due to vertebral collapse, and is particularly important since cord compression with paraplegia may develop with great rapidity unless the diagnosis is made and treatment started promptly. Other typical metastatic presentations include neurological symptoms and signs (focal lesions, raised intracranial pressure, cerebellar syndromes) and weight loss and nausea from hepatic involvement.

Constitutional symptoms are also common and most patients with lung cancer complain of anorexia, weight loss, weakness and fatigue. Although many patients do not notice clubbing of the fingers, this is a common manifestation particularly associated with squamous cell carcinoma and rare in small-cell carcinoma. Pain in the limbs may result from the much less common hypertrophic pulmonary osteoarthropathy, which can be severe.

A wide variety of paraneoplastic non-metastatic syndromes has been described in association with lung cancer. These are discussed in Chapter 9. Many of these syndromes are uncommon. Hypercalcaemia (without obvious bone metastases) is most frequently found in squamous cell cancer, and the syndromes of inappropriate ADH secretion and ectopic ACTH production are both commoner in small-cell carcinoma. The symptoms and management of hypercalcaemia are discussed in Chapter 8 and of ectopic hormone production in Chapter 9.

Staging notation

Although complex, the tumour node metastasis (TNM) staging system and stage grouping are widely used in NSCLC (Table 12.2) and has been shown to be useful prognostically. It has little value in small-cell carcinomas, in which local and distant dissemination is so common and the role of surgery so limited that staging systems have little relevance.

Investigation and staging
Non-small-cell lung cancer

Most patients with suspected lung cancer are first seen by a chest physician and the diagnosis made by fibreoptic bronchoscope. This instrument has the advantage of permitting good access to lobar and segmental bronchi and is especially helpful in evaluating upper lobe tumours out of biopsy range of the rigid bronchoscope. However, the rigid instrument is sometimes useful since it may give a better view of proximal bronchi and allows a larger biopsy in doubtful cases.

Staging of NSCLC is important since a crucial distinction between operable and inoperable tumours has to be made. To the surgeon, the most important criteria are the tumour site, absence of metastases and the general

Table 12.2 TNM staging system for non-small-cell lung cancer.

T	**Primary tumour**			
T0	Primary tumour not demonstrable			
TX	Positive cytology but tumour not demonstrable			
Tis	Carcinoma *in situ*			
T1	Tumour <3 cm in diameter, no proximal invasion			
T2	Tumour >3 cm in diameter, or invading pleura or with atelectasis, >2 cm from carina			
T3	Tumour of any size with extension into the chest wall, diaphragm, mediastinal pleura or within 2 cm of carina			
T4	Tumour of any size with invasion of mediastinal organs or vertebral body			
N	**Regional lymph nodes**			
N0	Nodes negative			
N1	Ipsilateral hilar nodes			
N2	Ipsilateral mediastinal and subcarinal nodes			
N3	Contralateral mediastinal or hilar nodes, scalene or supraclavicular nodes			

Stage grouping				*5-year survival**
Stage IA	T1	N0	M0	61
Stage IB	T2	N0	M0	38
Stage IIA	T1	N1	M0	34
Stage IIB	T2	N1	M0	24
	T3	N0	M0	
Stage IIIA	T1–3	N2	M0	13
Stage IIIB	T4	Any N	M0	5
	Any T	N3	M0	
Stage IV	Any T	Any N	M1	1

*Data from International Early Lung Cancer Action Programme Investigators [17].

fitness of the patient. Before any consideration of surgery, the maximum amount of information must therefore be obtained. Chest radiographs may indicate that the tumour is inoperable. Findings indicating inoperability include large central primary tumours particularly extending across the midline; widening of the superior mediastinum due to enlargement of paratracheal nodes; intrapulmonary, rib or other bony metastases; pleural effusion; and bilateral tumours. Further assessment is often needed; bronchoscopic evaluation is usually required to make the diagnosis and is essential to assess operability.

At bronchoscopy, some tumours can be shown to be inoperable. Features indicating inoperability include endobronchial tumour within 2 cm of the main carina;

extrinsic compression and widening of the angle of the main carina indicating mediastinal spread; and paralysis of the left vocal cord resulting from recurrent laryngeal nerve palsy.

With very few exceptions, mediastinal involvement is a strong contraindication to surgery. Assessment of the mediastinum is therefore essential in any patient being considered for operation. Clinical evidence of involvement includes a hoarse voice with a typical 'bovine' cough, resulting from recurrent laryngeal palsy, Horner's syndrome from involvement of the cervical sympathetic chain, pain in the shoulder, SVCO, cardiac dysrhythmia and dysphagia. Further assessment can be made by tomographic views of the mediastinum, and by barium swallow, which may show enlarged mediastinal nodes causing extrinsic oesophageal compression. CT scanning is essential in the preoperative assessment of tumour extent, sometimes demonstrating unexpected lymph node involvement or direct invasion of other structures (Figure 12.7). Chest wall involvement, for example, usually indicates inoperability. However, it is important not to rule out surgery on the basis of an equivocal CT scan since not all lymph node enlargement will prove to be neoplastic at thoracotomy.

The mediastinum can be directly visualized by mediastinoscopy (Figure 12.8). In this procedure, the surgeon makes a small incision in the suprasternal notch and the mediastinum is inspected through a mediastinoscope. Biopsies of the nodes are taken where possible. For

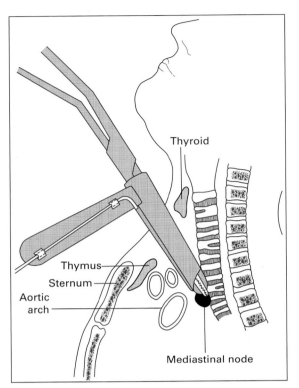

Figure 12.8 The technique of mediastinoscopy. (Cancer Research UK 2006. Reproduced with permission.)

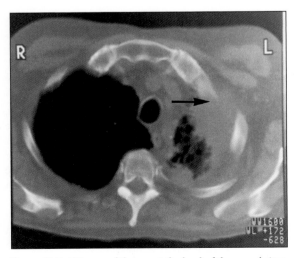

Figure 12.7 CT scan of thorax, at the level of the manubrium, in a patient with squamous carcinoma of the lung. The tumour is shown extending through the pleural space into the chest wall, eroding the ribs (arrow).

left-sided tumours an additional mediastinotomy may be necessary, and it is generally performed through the bed of the second intercostal cartilage. In patients whose mediastinoscopy is negative the resectability rate is at least 85%, and in over 50% of cases the nodes will not be involved at thoracotomy. In a further 30% the stage will be N1 only (Table 12.2). Clearly, if the diagnosis has been made from supraclavicular node biopsy or biopsy of metastatic lesions, these patients are unsuitable for surgery. Other signs of obvious distant spread, such as abnormal liver function tests combined with an abnormal liver scan or hepatic ultrasound, are also obvious contraindications to operation. If the liver function tests are normal and there are no neurological symptoms or signs, ultrasound scan of the liver or CT brain scan will seldom be positive and are therefore not routinely indicated. A bone scan may, however, show unsuspected metastases.

Finally, the surgeon needs to know whether his or her patient is likely to withstand a surgical operation. Routine exercise testing, spirometry and other lung function tests such as ventilation–perfusion scanning can all be valuable. Patients with poor pulmonary reserve may have to be excluded from surgery even though their tumours are operable by other criteria. As a rough guide, patients with forced expiratory volume less than 1.2 L/s do not withstand pneumonectomy, although this also depends on age, sex, size and especially height. Patients over 70 years of age also tolerate pneumonectomy poorly (particularly right-sided).

In the past few years, several attempts have been made to use genetic profiling by means of microarrays and reverse-transcriptase polymerase chain reaction (RT-PCR). The aim is to provide useful prognostic information, recognizing the inadequacy of current staging methods. One impressive result has come from work in Taiwan, in which 16 genes were identified by analysing microarray data and correlating with survival [21]. The technique was further refined such that five genes provided a genetic signature, behaving as an independent predictor for both relapse-free and overall survival. As the authors pointed out, the identification of five genes that can predict clinical outcome might reveal targets for therapeutic development, particularly since the five chosen genes are each associated with a specific task; for example, *STAT1* causes arrested growth and apoptosis in many types of cancer cells, while *DUSP6* inactivates extracellular signal-regulated kinase II resulting in tumour suppression.

Small-cell lung cancer

For patients with SCLC, the rationale for staging is altogether different. The characteristic early and widespread dissemination of this tumour makes surgical intervention inappropriate in the large majority of cases, although the occasional instance of 'surgically resectable' SCLC is encountered.

In some patients, determination of the degree of spread in SCLC is both logical and necessary. For example, although radiotherapy alone is no longer considered the best treatment for this disease (see below), it is sometimes used in patients considered unsuitable for chemotherapy. More commonly, in patients undergoing treatment with chemotherapy, radiotherapy is often given to those with 'limited' disease in whom no metastases can be demonstrated and disease is confined to one hemithorax. If the proposed treatment is only with cytotoxic drugs, irrespective of extent of disease, routine staging is unnecessary, although investigation of specific symptoms is sometimes indicated on clinical grounds.

If staging in SCLC is to be undertaken, the most useful investigations include liver function tests (including

measurement of serum albumin), plasma electrolytes and calcium determination, full blood count, isotope bone scanning and ultrasound liver scanning in patients with abnormal liver function tests. CT scanning of the brain in asymptomatic patients is seldom abnormal and not performed as routine. Bone marrow examination is positive (using conventional stains) in only 5% of patients with limited disease and normal blood counts. The proportion rises if staining with monoclonal antibodies is used. Marrow examination is therefore not always used in staging, and contributes nothing if the disease is already known to be disseminated.

Treatment

The principles of treatment of NSCLC and SCLC are very different. SCLC is seldom surgically resectable, is usually widespread at presentation and is both more chemosensitive and more radiosensitive. For these reasons its management is considered separately.

Non-small-cell lung cancer
Surgery

For NSCLC, which accounts for about 85–90% of all lung cancer, surgical resection, wherever possible, offers the best hope of cure. The percentage of operable cases varies with the philosophy of the surgeon, but the criteria for operability are not usually met in more than about 30% of cases. Approximately 50% of tumours are obviously unresectable by chest radiographic or bronchoscopic criteria. Physiological evaluation, biochemical testing and mediastinoscopy raises the unresectability rate still further (see above).

For patients in whom surgery is possible, the choice of operation depends on the location of the tumour and the patient's respiratory capacity. If the tumour is peripheral with no evidence of local extension, a wedge or segmental resection may occasionally be sufficient, particularly in patients whose pulmonary reserve is poor. In patients with more centrally located tumours contained within a single lobe, lobectomy is the usual procedure, provided the hilar nodes are clear. An adequate margin of normal-looking lung should be removed where possible. Pneumonectomy is necessary for tumours originating within the main-stem bronchus, where the primary tumour involves more than one lobe, or where the hilum is involved. Clearly, these patients should undergo careful measurement of respiratory function before such an operation can be contemplated.

Although patients with evidence of local spread are usually considered to have inoperable lesions, many surgeons are prepared to undertake an operation in Pancoast tumour since cancers at this site (superior sulcus) may be biologically more favourable. Despite local invasion of pleura and ribs, they can sometimes be removed surgically, and regional lymphatic metastases appear to be unusual. Several encouraging new surgical techniques have recently been described [22].

The mortality (5%) and morbidity associated with pneumonectomy are greater than with a lesser operation such as a lobectomy (2% mortality); many surgeons do not operate in patients over the age of 70, since mortality rises steeply with advancing age.

There is considerable controversy over the role of surgery when mediastinal nodes are involved (N2). Many surgeons are now prepared to operate on some of these patients, especially after previous (neoadjuvant) chemotherapy (discussed below). The results of randomized trials comparing this approach with radical radiotherapy are awaited.

Postoperative treatment with adjuvant platinum-based chemotherapy is now established as standard practice for patients with resected Stage IB, IIA, IIB or IIIA disease, with a survival benefit of almost 5% at 5 years (see Ref. [23]).

Results of surgical treatment

The results of surgical treatment depend largely on the degree of patient selection; surgeons using the most stringent criteria for operability will have the best results. Histological type and stage of the tumour are important prognostic criteria. Patients with squamous cell carcinoma have the best survival rates – 37% of all patients surviving 5 years. Those with adenocarcinoma or large-cell carcinoma do less well, the overall 5-year survival being 27%. The importance of tumour stage is shown in Table 12.2. For patients with stage I disease, the 5-year survival rate is over 60% for all histologies (but approaching 80% for T1 squamous carcinomas), suggesting that in NSCLC tumour stage is more important than histology in determining survival. In patients with squamous cell carcinoma, the presence of local nodal involvement does not always imply early death from metastases. In these patients, radical surgery may be possible if mediastinal node involvement was limited. Early mediastinal nodal involvement should not be regarded as an absolute contraindication to surgery. Nevertheless, despite modern operative techniques and more careful case selection, current overall survival outcomes are not dramatically better than those obtained in the 1950s.

Several attempts have been made to provide useful prognostic data, giving weight to a variety of clinico-pathological features. In a recent study from France, prospectively enrolling 4669 patients from 137 centres, a number of independent variables were identified and given due prognostic weighting. These included age (with older patients doing worse), gender (male patients doing worse), performance status (the more active the better), histological type (large-cell NSCLC patients doing worse than the others) and TNM stage (as expected, far worse for the more advanced stages) [24].

Radiotherapy

Although patients with NSCLC have always formed a large part of the clinical oncologist's work, there is continued debate regarding the indications for the use of this treatment. In judging which patients are suitable for treatment, the radiotherapist has to decide whether the intention is radical or palliative. In the majority of cases, palliation is the only realistic expectation, though long-term survival is occasionally seen in patients irradiated only with palliative intent.

Palliative radiotherapy

The majority of patients with NSCLC have inoperable disease. Palliative radiotherapy is often recommended for locoregional disease considered unsuitable for surgery but without evidence of distant metastases. Such patients include those with tumours of the main-stem bronchus within 1 cm of the carina, those with invasion of important mediastinal structures such as the recurrent laryngeal or phrenic nerves, and those with troublesome symptoms including haemoptysis, obstruction of a major bronchus, severe cough and pain. Finally, in patients in whom obstruction to a bronchus is imminent or where SVCO is present, radiotherapy is indicated, whether the patient is symptomatic or not.

Relative contraindications to radiotherapy include metastases beyond the locoregional nodes, multiple lesions, bronchial fistula, supraclavicular node involvement or a large tumour mass. Even under these adverse circumstances, palliative treatment may still offer benefit, if the patient's symptoms demand it. If the patient is symptomatic, treatment should be given as soon as possible.

When should treatment be used in asymptomatic patients with inoperable disease? In an early study, treatment with radiotherapy, chemotherapy or both was compared with no initial treatment. Survival was the same in all groups (approximately 8.5 months), with no advantage for active treatment unless specific symptoms were present. Delaying radiotherapy until the onset of a specific symptom frequently allowed a patient 4–5 months before treatment proved necessary, and this group had the best palliation of all. Some radiotherapists in the United Kingdom therefore delay palliative treatment, but this is not the practice in many large centres, especially in North America and other European countries. Increasingly, palliative radiotherapy schedules have become shortened and simplified without apparent loss of benefit.

Photodynamic therapy is becoming recognized as potentially valuable for non-small-cell bronchial carcinoma [25]. This minimally invasive treatment involves intravenous injection of a photosensitizing agent, followed a few days later by photoradiation of the affected area through a bronchoscope. The intention is to reduce the bulk of the tumour, therefore reducing symptoms caused, for example, by bronchial obstruction. The recent NICE guidelines (see Refs [72,73]) have supported the use of this technique though recognizing that data are still relatively sparse.

Radical radiotherapy
Occasionally, patients with operable lung cancer are referred for radiotherapy either because they decline the offer of surgery or because of coexistent medical conditions that would make surgery hazardous. In these operable cases and other inoperable localized tumours where the tumour can be encompassed by the radiation fields, radical irradiation may be justifiable, though even in these selected patients the 5-year survival following radiotherapy alone is only about 10%.

It seems likely therefore that radiotherapy can occasionally cure patients with carcinoma of the bronchus, particularly those with small, technically operable tumours. In these patients, a radical approach should be employed, requiring treatment to a higher dose than generally employed for palliation of symptoms, in the region of 50–60 Gy over 5–6 weeks in daily fractions or equivalent (see Chapter 5, Figure 5.7). Such treatments may be accompanied by side-effects including dysphagia, pericarditis and skin reactions. In addition, irradiation of a portion of spinal cord is unavoidable even with the most sophisticated planning techniques. With careful tumour imaging and the use of multifield techniques this problem can be minimized. Radiation damage to the spinal cord is discussed on pages 192–193.

There have been several new approaches to radical radiation treatment. Over 10 years ago, a much discussed trial of continuous hyperfractionated accelerated radiotherapy (CHART) reported improved survival for this technique compared with conventional radiotherapy [26]. In another approach, a European trial used cisplatin as a radiation sensitizer during radiotherapy and, in a randomized trial [27], it provided some evidence of improved survival. Neither technique has become part of widely accepted standard practice, but both results emphasize that effective local treatment may have an impact on survival. One extremely important new technology is the increasing use of conformal and/or intensity-modulated radiation therapy, described in more detail in Chapter 5, in an attempt to increase the delivery of high doses in a part of the body containing many highly radiosensitive structures – the lungs, spinal cord, oesophageal mucosa and so on. Although the case for such sophisticated, resource-consuming treatment has not yet been fully established, there seems little doubt that it offers the potential for building up the dose to levels that were previously impractical [28,29]. Still more important has been the increasing recognition that, as with so many other sold tumours, particularly squamous-cell carcinomas at many sites, the use of concurrent chemo-radiation therapy has brought a real improvement in overall response and even survival rates – see, for example, Ref. [30]. This may even be true for carefully selected older patients who previously would not have been thought suitable for this approach. As with squamous-cell cancer of the head and neck, it is the concurrent rather than sequential approach with chemotherapy that is the key here – see Ref. [31].

There is no place for routine preoperative radiotherapy in operable lung cancer. Occasionally, a patient with stage III disease, with mediastinal involvement, may achieve a useful clinical regression with radiotherapy. However, even in such cases, it is exceptional for surgery to become a practical proposition. Combined treatment with surgery and preoperative radiotherapy is often recommended for Pancoast tumour (see above), but overall the results do not appear better than those of surgery alone. A large and widely quoted patient-data-based meta-analysis of randomized trials of postoperative radiotherapy following surgical resection of stage I tumours suggested a higher mortality in the treated group, with 2-year survival reduced from 55–48% [32].

Chemotherapy
Several drugs have been shown to have some activity in NSCLC (Table 12.3). The response rates for single agents are relatively low but are greater when drugs are

Table 12.3 Chemotherapy in non-small-cell lung cancer.

Agent	Response rate (%)
Single agents	
Ifosfamide	15
Mitomycin	15
Vinorelbine	20
Cisplatin	12–15
Gemcitabine	20
Paclitaxel/docetaxel	20–30
Doxorubicin	12
Etoposide	10–12
Combination therapy in advanced disease	
Mitomycin, ifosfamide and cisplatin	45
Mitomycin, vinblastine and cisplatin	40
Cisplatin, vindesine or vinorelbine	25–35

used in combination. Typical combinations are shown in Table 12.3.

Most of the active regimens (whether given as adjuvant therapy, as is increasingly the case, or for recurrent disease) include cisplatin, with its concomitant nausea, vomiting and other side-effects. Newer active regimens include carboplatin and gemcitabine (now very widely used), and carboplatin with etoposide or paclitaxel. The combination of carboplatin and gemcitabine has relatively low toxicity, and has become the standard regimen in our hospital and in many others in the United Kingdom. Among the vinca alkaloids, vinorelbine is a useful agent, with a reasonable toxicity profile. It is also now available in oral form, a distinct advantage, with effectiveness apparently equal to the intravenous preparation. One large European study which assessed the use of adjuvant vinorelbine plus cisplatin versus observation in patients with completely resected NSCLC confirmed the benefit of such chemotherapy [33]. Over 800 patients were randomly assigned to chemotherapy or not, and at follow-up of over 6 years the median survival was 66 months in the chemotherapy group compared with 44 months in the observation group. The overall 5-year survival with chemotherapy was improved by 8.6%, maintained at 7 years. This was one of the studies included in the comprehensive NSCLC meta-analysis published in 2010 referred to above. The precise details of chemotherapy regimens vary across international centres but ESMO guideline recommendations are well laid out and were currently up to date at the time of writing – see Ref. [34].

The most powerful meta-analysis data show an increase in overall survival from cisplatin-based chemotherapy of the order of 64–67% for stage IB, from 39% up to 49% for stage II and from 26% up to 39% for stage III NSCLC at a median follow-up of 5.1 years, though the meta-analysis confirmed a potential *detrimental* effect of chemotherapy in stage IA cases. More recent work has suggested that patients with tumours which express the excision repair cross-complementation group 1 (ERCC1) protein will not benefit from adjuvant cisplatin-based chemotherapy, whereas ERCC1-negative tumours have a substantial advantage, with significantly prolonged survival [35] – though this claim remains highly controversial (see Ref. [36]). For patients with metastatic NSCLC, platinum-based chemotherapy can prolong life and improve quality of life in carefully selected patients, but careful risk assessment is essential in each case as many of these patients are far from enjoying the ideal performance status which would be preferred.

For non-squamous carcinomas, pemetrexed has emerged as the agent of choice; other useful cytotoxics in this setting include gemcitabine and taxanes – see Ref. [37], for the ESMO guideline group. Further, small improvements in survival and quality-of-life measures have also been claimed with the use of maintenance therapy, at least in non-squamous non-small cell cancer – for example, in the recently reported PARAMOUNT study of over 1000 patients, maintenance treatment with pemetrexate resulted in a gain from 2.8 months to 4.1 months in progression-free survival, with acceptable treatment-related complications – see Ref. [38].

Recent additions to drug treatment have focused on the use of targeted therapy using agents which block the function of the EGFR [39–41] (also see Chapter 6). It is now clear that the signalling pathway of the EGFR is activated in over half of all patients with NSCLC, often resulting from protein over-expression, increased gene copy number or genetic mutation(s) – see Ref. [42]. This opens up a potential new strategy for effective treatment with targeted agents such as the monoclonal antibody cetuximab (Erbitux) and the selective tyrosine kinase inhibitors gefitinib (Iressa), erlotinib (Tarceva), nintedanib (Vargatef) and crizotinib (Xalcori). An important recently reported study from the Harvard group showed impressive activity for this agent when compared with either docetaxol or pemetrexed in a relatively rare group of previously treated patients (only comprising about 3–5% of all NSCLC but nonetheless a fairly large number overall, because of the continued high frequency of this disease) with ALK (anaplastic lymphoma kinase)-positive disease (Shaw *et al.* [43]). ALK is a tyrosine kinase target in several types of cancer and in NSCLC is activated by chromosomal rearrangement: the cancer cell seems to require ALK-activation to survive. This new agent doubled progression-free survival from 3 to 7.7 months, making this agent now 'standard of care' in this particular clinical setting, though the drug is not yet as widely available as it would have to be, to address the unmet need – Cataldo *et al.* [42], provide a useful clinically based discussion.

Recent studies have identified gene mutations targeting the kinase domain of the EGFR that are related to the response to these inhibitors; in general, they appear to act by inhibiting the tyrosine kinase activity of the EGFR by competition with ATP for the ATP-binding site. These drugs produce objective responses in 10–15% of patients even when pretreated with conventional cytotoxic agents. The responses appear more frequent in women (especially Japanese), and in patients with adenocarcinoma, for reasons which are unexplained. Indeed the molecular requirements for response are not yet understood: increased EGFR expression, common in NSCLC, does not itself reliably predict response. Recent studies have begun to suggest a probable overall survival benefit for erlotinib as second-line therapy following failure of chemotherapy, at least in the short term (6- and 12-month survival rates). Nintedanib in combination with docetaxel has also given promising results in an important European study LUME Lung-1, a double-blind placebo-controlled trial. The investigators reported a prolongation of survival in patients with adenocarcinoma refractory to their initial chemotherapy regimen, as well as an improvement in progression-free survival in other histologies – see Ref. [44]. In addition, it is also clear that agents such as cetuximab, gefitinib and bevacizumab, as well as the increasingly used erlotinib, are effective in a proportion of patients for relieving symptoms, maintaining stable disease and improving quality of life without the adverse events that may be associated with cytotoxic drug treatment. Anecdotal reports suggest continuing value when given as maintenance following palliative treatment for, for example, suitably fit patients with brain metastases. Patients developing the typical erlotinib-associated rash clearly seem to do better than those who do not, probably relating to a greater uptake of the drug. Similar findings have been noted in other tumour populations, for example, those with pancreatic, colorectal and head-and-neck cancer. For an individual patient with advanced metastatic disease, the use of chemotherapy is a matter of clinical

judgement, particularly in elderly or infirm patients (see, e.g., Refs [45] and [30]). The survival benefit is small (but unquestionable) compared with best supportive care [27] but this oversimplifies the issue. The toxicity of chemotherapy (which is reduced in the more recent regimens) must be balanced against the improvement in symptoms that accompanies response. Responses are more frequent, long-lasting and complete in patients who are fit, and many patients have a strong wish for active treatment. Nonetheless there is increasing clinical evidence to support the more widespread use of chemotherapy in relapsed NSCLC. NICE recommend that docetaxel monotherapy should be considered as second-line treatment, often providing both symptomatic benefit and also a modest extension in overall survival in this difficult group.

There has been considerable interest in the combination of chemotherapy before surgery in localized, initially inoperable, tumours and of chemotherapy before radical radiotherapy for localized tumours. There is no doubt that preoperative chemotherapy is associated with a higher response rate (up to 60%) than in metastatic disease, that some tumours are rendered operable and that there may even be no viable tumour at resection. A few trials of this approach have suggested benefit, but others have not. Chemotherapy before or after radical radiation has been assessed in several randomized trials, but these were too small for a convincing survival difference to be shown (see, e.g., Ref. 46). The meta-analysis of all data from these trials [47] indicates a potential benefit of 2–7%. A similar benefit of chemotherapy is present in all stages of localized NSCLC treated with surgery or radiotherapy [48]. Such small differences are nevertheless very important in such a common disease. The value of *concomitant* chemoradiation is still undecided and awaits the results of definitive large-scale randomized trials.

However, it is clear that both cetuximab and gefitinib, as well as the increasingly used erlotinib, are effective in a proportion of patients for relieving symptoms, maintaining stable disease and improving quality of life, without the unpleasant side-effects often associated with cytotoxic drug treatment (see Ref. [49]). One recent study from the Eastern Cooperative Oncology Group compared the use of paclitaxel/carboplatin alone or with the addition of bevacizumab (878 patients), confirming a small additional overall survival advantage for the bevacizumab group (about 7% at 1 and 2 years). This prompted approval of bevacizumab for use in selected patients with NSCLC by the Food and Drug Administration in the United States, even though there was a modest increase in treatment-related death [40]. An important study criterion was the exclusion of cases of squamous cell carcinoma; most of the patients had adenocarcinoma. Further studies are in progress.

Small-cell lung cancer

The majority (two-thirds) of patients present with extensive disease, namely, thoracic disease involving more than one hemithorax or with metastatic spread. In these patients, radiotherapy has a palliative role only and even with modern chemotherapy the prognosis is very poor. In patients with limited disease (confined to one hemithorax) chemotherapy is the mainstay of treatment.

Chemotherapy

It has long been apparent that SCLC is a rapidly dividing tumour, usually metastatic at the time of presentation. For this reason, a systemic approach to treatment is essential. SCLC is relatively sensitive, at least at first, to cytotoxic agents and chemotherapy has become the mainstay of treatment. An early randomized study comparing radiation alone with radiation and combination chemotherapy showed a clear short-term survival advantage for the patients treated with both chemotherapy and radiation compared with radiation alone.

Numerous single agents have since been shown to have activity. Cyclophosphamide and ifosfamide are among the most useful alkylating agents. Many other drugs such as etoposide, taxanes, irinotecan, vinca alkaloids, cisplatin, and anthracyclines also have activity (Table 12.4). Single-agent chemotherapy has largely been discarded except under special circumstances (discussed below). Numerous trials of combination chemotherapy, using a wide variety of regimens and schedules, have shown a high rate of complete (25–50%) and partial (30–50%) responses (Table 12.5).

The duration of conventional chemotherapy has been assessed in several large studies. The balance of evidence suggests six cycles of conventional chemotherapy to be adequate. Neutropenia is a major dose-limiting toxicity that can be partially overcome by the use of haemopoietic growth factors, which are now used almost routinely in this setting, to support the intensive chemotherapy regimen offered to the majority of patients as their initial treatment. Our own practice is to recommend a combination of carboplatin and etoposide with G-CSF, as first choice of treatment from the outset. Randomized trials have assessed survival is improved by increasing dose intensity. This has been approached either by acceleration of cycles or by dose increase with the use

Table 12.4 Single-agent chemotherapy in small-cell lung cancer (response data are approximate and depend on case selection).

Agent	Response rate (%)
Carboplatin	60
Etoposide	40–70
Irinotecan	45
Paclitaxel	35
Cyclophosphamide	35
Ifosfamide	35
Cisplatin	35
Doxorubicin	30
Docetaxel	25
Gemcitabine	20
Methotrexate	20
Vincristine	15
CCNU	10

Table 12.5 Combination chemotherapy in small-cell lung cancer.

Regimen	Approximate response rate (%)
Cisplatin and etoposide	80
Ifosfamide, cisplatin and etoposide	75
Vincristine, doxorubicin and cyclophosphamide	70
Cisplatin, doxorubicin and etoposide	85
Doxorubicin, cylophosphamide and etoposide	80

of haemopoietic growth factors. In general these trials have not shown a clinically worthwhile survival benefit when judged against the increased toxicity and expense. Attempts to increase the intensity of chemotherapy by giving drugs weekly have not improved survival. Similarly, the use of very high-dose chemotherapy with autologous peripheral blood stem-cell support as initial treatment has not been shown to be of value, although the overall response rates with these approaches are high. A commonly used regimen at present is the combination of cisplatin (or carboplatin for more vulnerable or frail patients), together with etoposide, which is generally well tolerated and has an objective response rate of over 75% following treatment with six courses. Other authorities advocate the use of ifosfamide in addition to the above combination, and even the possible use of high-dose stem-cell supported chemotherapy in selected good-prognosis cases [50]. Second-line treatment is usually worth considering after failure of the initial chemotherapy, and modern drug choices often include topotecan and paclitaxel. The ESMO guidelines working group keep current chemotherapy recommendations up to date and this important topic is well covered in their recent publication (See Ref. [51]).

The toxicity of chemotherapy is considerable, and despite the high initial response rate the gains in survival are, as yet, modest. It is clear that adding radiotherapy to the primary tumour volume is of great importance for limited-disease patients, increasing their likelihood of cure from about 8% to about 14% (limited disease cases). An analysis of survival in SCLC from 20 years ago [52] showed that only 8% of limited disease patients and less than 3% of extensive disease patients were alive at 2 years and that relapse of SCLC continues for at least 6 years after treatment; even though there is a chance of long survival, and possibly cure, with chemotherapy, the morbidity of treatment is sufficient to justify more palliative approaches, especially in elderly or frail patients. Such approaches must be judged critically since symptoms relating to treatment can be a major component of poor quality of life. Oral etoposide, for example, was widely promoted as a simple palliative treatment, yet two randomized trials showed it produced worse response and survival, worse toxicity and worse quality of life.

A number of factors are known to be associated with poor prognosis in SCLC (Table 12.6). Of these, the most important are extensive disease, poor performance status, low plasma albumin and sodium and abnormal liver function tests (Figure 12.9). In elderly patients, in whom these poor prognostic factors are often present, it is unwise to persist with chemotherapy beyond the first

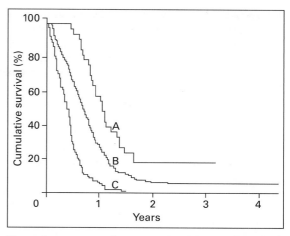

Figure 12.9 Prognostic factors in small-cell lung cancer. In A all patients had good performance status and normal biochemistry (see Table 12.6). In C patients had poor performance status and more than two biochemical abnormalities. Group B is by exclusion. (Cancer Research UK 2006. Reproduced with permission.)

two or three cycles unless there is a clear improvement in the tumour and in the patient's well-being. For younger patients with limited disease and in whom there are no adverse prognostic features, intensive combination chemotherapy offers the best chance of long-term survival. There will be many patients who fall between these two extremes, and here the oncologist must make a judgement on a case-by-case basis.

SCLC is radiosensitive, with complete radiological response of the primary tumour in over 80% of cases. Even large primary lesions associated with massive hilar and mediastinal lymphadenopathy may regress completely following moderate doses of radiotherapy (40–50 Gy over 4–5 weeks). There has been interest in the use of twice-daily (hyperfractionated) radiotherapy but without proof of benefit in randomized studies.

Although the initial response to radiotherapy is usually gratifying, recurrence within the irradiated area is frequent and long-term local control of the disease is not always achieved. As might be expected, there is evidence that more durable local control may be obtained by higher radiation dosage though at the cost of greater toxicity, particularly if chemotherapy is also used.

The combination of chemotherapy and radiotherapy for the primary tumour has been investigated in several randomized trials in which patients treated with chemotherapy were assigned to receive thoracic irradiation or not. The studies were too small to detect

Table 12.6 Adverse prognostic factors in small-cell lung cancer.

Poor performance status
Extensive disease
Low plasma albumin and sodium
Raised alkaline phosphatase or lactate dehydrogenase
Brain metastases
Marrow infiltration or anaemia
Radiotherapy

a moderate difference reliably, but an overview [53] in which individual data have been reanalysed has shown a 5% benefit in survival at 3 years (from 7–12%), a 60% relative improvement. The morbidity of thoracic irradiation may be considerable in combination with chemotherapy. Nevertheless, thoracic irradiation now has an established role in patients with limited disease who are fit enough to receive it and who are responding to chemotherapy. An improvement in response rate has been reported with concomitant radiotherapy and chemotherapy, but no substantial improvement in survival was evident in the first randomized trial to have been published. The optimum timing of irradiation is also unclear. Although a Canadian study [54] suggested a benefit for early treatment, other studies have not, and the meta-analysis [55] showed no difference in survival with respect to timing. Furthermore, a large study from our own London-based group [56] showed no obvious survival advantage for early thoracic consolidation radiotherapy, unlike the NCI Canada study.

In summary, thoracic irradiation should be considered under the following circumstances:

in patients with limited disease, where there is a partial or complete response to chemotherapy;
for local recurrence;
for SVCO unresponsive to chemotherapy.

Radiotherapy is often of considerable palliative value in SCLC, and is the treatment of choice for painful bone metastases and for brain metastases. Clinical evidence of brain metastases occurs in 25% of patients with SCLC and is demonstrable in about two-thirds of patients at autopsy. Treatment with radiotherapy to the whole brain to a total dose of 20 Gy in five fractions in a week is often effective and well tolerated; there seems to be no advantage for more prolonged regimens. Similar fractionation is usually satisfactory for painful bony deposits.

The frequent occurrence of brain metastases in SCLC, and the morbidity which they cause, has led to the assessment of prophylactic cranial irradiation (PCI). A number of large-scale randomized trials and a meta-analysis have shown that routine use of PCI has decreased the clinical frequency of brain metastases from 40% to less than 10%, with a real benefit for survival. In a recent large study from the European Organization for Research and Treatment of Cancer that addressed the question in the context of patients with extensive disease, the 1-year survival rate improved from 13.3% (control group) to 27.1% in the treated group [57]. PCI therefore reduces the undoubted morbidity of brain metastasis. Conversely, PCI is itself associated with short-term toxicity (confusion, unsteadiness, memory loss) and possible long-term neurological morbidity, although this seems very uncommon. The usual policy is to offer PCI to patients who have had a good response to chemotherapy, thereby avoiding unnecessary cerebral irradiation in non-responding patients whose survival time will be short.

In summary, a number of important questions remain with respect to the use of thoracic radiation in limited-stage SCLC, including the volume of irradiation, choice of technique, optimal total dose (fractionation, timing and sequencing of radiation), and so on. It is becoming clear, for example, that the relative chemosensitivity of SCLC does not mean that a modest radiation dose is all that is required, and the most appropriate timing of radiation therapy in relation to chemotherapy remains controversial. An additional modality, percutaneous radiofrequency ablation, for both primary and secondary lung cancers is increasingly being used, and has now received approval from NICE (see Refs [72,73]).

Surgery

Very uncommonly SCLC presents as a small peripheral tumour without mediastinal node involvement. Such tumours can be resected and it is usual to give postoperative chemotherapy. Clinical trials have shown that there is no benefit in surgery after chemotherapy as a 'debulking' procedure. The role of surgical intervention is therefore small in SCLC generally.

Prognosis of lung cancer: geographical variation of lung cancer mortality rates

Within the United Kingdom, variations in lung cancer mortality rates clearly reflect regional smoking patterns. As with incidence, the highest male mortality rates are in Scotland. Within England and Wales there is also a north–south differential, with lung cancer mortality rates higher in the north, again a reflection of regional smoking patterns. European lung cancer mortality rates also vary markedly. For example, age-standardized rates for Hungarian men are over three times higher than those for Swedish men. Countries are at different stages in their lung cancer epidemic as a result of different histories of tobacco consumption and the long latent period between smoking and lung cancer development. Male lung cancer mortality rates in the United Kingdom and many other European countries have decreased quite rapidly, together with falls in tobacco consumption. While female lung cancer mortality rates began to decline in the United Kingdom, especially in younger women during the 1990s and subsequent decade, it looks as though it may be on the rise again, and elsewhere in Europe rates continue to climb, with effective antismoking policies urgently needed to control the epidemic of lung cancer in women. In the United Kingdom, deaths in women have increased by 7% since 2009 (now running at 21 per 100 000 women) – expert opinion is that by 2015 it will be responsible for more deaths than breast cancer, a gloomy prospect in a tumour almost entirely preventable and whose aetiology, unlike that for breast cancer, we almost fully understand. The predicted mortality estimates for 2013 are worth presenting: 88 886 European women (breast) and 82 640 (lung), with the breast statistic set to fall and that for lung cancer to rise. It may still be possible in some countries, for example, Spain and Portugal, to prevent widespread smoking in disadvantaged women whose smoking prevalences are currently low. It is estimated that there are around 243 100 lung cancer deaths each year in the European Union (around 188 000 in men and 55 000 in women). Overall, smoking is estimated to cause over half-a-million deaths each year in the European Union and 1 million in Europe.

Sadly, both lung cancer incidence and mortality rates have a clear positive association with deprivation, particularly for men. For example, for men aged 15–64 in England and Wales who died between 1999 and 2003, the lung cancer mortality rates were 3.7 times higher in the most deprived category compared with the least deprived category, when deprivation was divided into twentieths (Figure 12.10). This type of association is strongly related to the smoking behaviour in different deprivation groups.

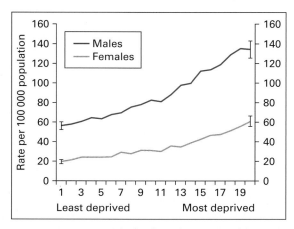

Figure 12.10 Age-standardized incidence rates of lung cancer by deprivation category, England and Wales, 1993. (Cancer Research UK 2006. Reproduced with permission.)

Tumours of the mediastinum

The mediastinum lies at the centre of the chest and is bordered by the thoracic inlet superiorly, the diaphragm inferiorly, the vertebral column posteriorly, the sternum anteriorly and the pleural reflections laterally (Figure 12.11). A great variety of tumours can arise in the mediastinum [58] and tend to occur at different sites within it.

The *anterosuperior compartment* of the mediastinum is bounded inferiorly by the diaphragm, anteriorly by the sternum and posteriorly by the vertebral column down to the fourth thoracic vertebra, and then by the anterior pericardium. It contains the upper trachea and oesophagus, the aortic arch and the thymus and may also include a retrosternal portion of a normal thyroid gland, with parathyroid structures and embryonic cell rests. The *middle compartment* of the mediastinum is bounded anteriorly by the anterior pericardium and

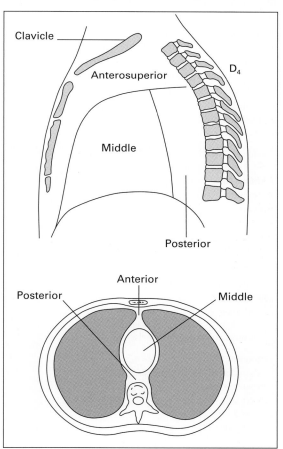

Figure 12.11 Simplified anatomy of the mediastinum.

posteriorly by the oesophagus, and extends downwards to the diaphragm. It contains the heart, ascending aorta, main bronchi, hila and carina, and the subcarinal and other closely related tracheobronchial lymph nodes. The *posterior mediastinum* lies between the vertebral column and posterior pericardium and contains the oesophagus, the descending thoracic aorta and the sympathetic nerve chains. The pattern of tumours arising in the mediastinum reflects these anatomical divisions (Table 12.7).

Anterosuperior mediastinum

The commonest malignant tumours of the anterosuperior mediastinum are thymomas and germ-cell tumours, including teratomas of various types and seminomas. In addition, thyroid and parathyroid adenomas occur at this site and can cause diagnostic difficulties, and carcinomas of the thyroid may occasionally arise from the retrosternal portion of the gland. Symptoms from superior mediastinal tumours are usually caused by pressure on local structures such as the oesophagus, trachea and laryngeal or phrenic nerves. Dysphagia, dyspnoea, stridor, cough and SVCO are relatively common, and vocal cord palsy and/or diaphragmatic paralysis are sometimes seen. These symptoms occur less frequently with slow-growing tumours (such as retrosternal goitre and some thymomas).

Table 12.7 Tumours of the mediastinum.

Anterosuperior
Thymoma
Teratoma
Thyroid and parathyroid tumours
Sarcoma (haemangiosarcoma, haemangiopericytoma)
Mesothelioma
Lipoma

Middle
Malignant lymphoma
Tumours of the heart
Secondary lymph node involvement
Pericardial tumours

Posterior
Neurofibroma, neurilemmoma, schwannoma
Neuroblastoma
Neurofibrosarcoma
Phaeochromocytoma
Chordoma
Paraganglioma

Thymoma

Thymic tumours form a mixed histological picture often including more than one population of cells. Lymphocytes, epithelial cells and spindle cells tend to predominate, and 'typical' thymomas may contain lymphocytic and epithelial components as apparently distinct populations. Unfortunately, thymic tumour histology is a poor predictor of the behaviour of the tumour, although the macroscopic appearance is more valuable. Some thymic tumours grow very slowly over many years, others more rapidly.

The criteria for malignancy are difficult to define in thymomas, and the tumours have traditionally been described (using a system known as Masaoka staging) as invasive or non-invasive. However, a World Health Organization (WHO) classification system is now increasingly used [59]. An impressively large study of over 1300 patients was recently reported from Japan, with information on resectability, recurrence rates and 20-year prognosis [60]. Distant metastases are relatively unusual, although thymomas are often locally invasive, for example, to pericardium, pleural surfaces and other intrathoracic sites. Occasionally, Hodgkin's disease can arise from thymic tissue, without evidence of lymphadenopathy elsewhere. In these cases, surgical excision is clearly less important than with other types of thymic tumour. *Thymic carcinomas* are rare tumours which show clear histological features of malignancy. Many variants have been described (squamous, clear cell, spindle cell, small cell, mucoepidermoid, adenocystic).

A variety of clinical syndromes are associated with thymomas. Much the commonest is *myasthenia gravis*, which occurs in 44% of patients. Myasthenia is often the presenting feature of an otherwise asymptomatic tumour, either benign or malignant. Myasthenia gravis is associated with antibodies to acetylcholine receptors, but its relationship to the tumour is only poorly understood. Removal of the thymoma (thymectomy) results in remission of the myasthenia in approximately 30% of cases. *Red cell aplasia* occurs in 4%, and may be associated with leucopenia and/or thrombocytopenia; in these cases, a spindle cell thymic tumour is the commonest pathology. Occasionally the aplasia recovers after removal of the tumour. Other syndromes include hypogammaglobulinaemia, connective tissue diseases, pernicious anaemia and autoimmune thyroiditis. Together, one or other of the associated diseases occur in 80–90% of thymomas, with myasthenia gravis and cytopenias as the commonest.

Diagnosis may be difficult, and a core biopsy is usually necessary. Investigation includes chest radiography

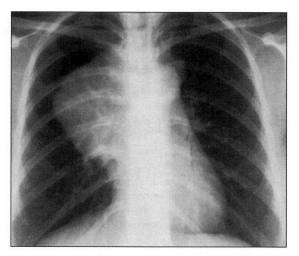

Figure 12.12 Typical posteroanterior chest radiographic appearance in a patient with a thymic tumour. There is a well-demarcated tumour mass and the lung fields are clear.

(Figure 12.12) and CT, which may demonstrate pleural metastases (again, often only mildly symptomatic with cough or shortness of breath). Treatment is by surgical removal of the primary whenever possible. Complete removal is usually achieved if the tumour is encapsulated, and in such cases local recurrence is unusual – see, for example, Ref. [61]). Capsular invasion, direct extension to the pleura or pericardium and incomplete resection are all indications for postoperative radiotherapy, which reduces the local recurrence rate [60,62] and is often recommended for stage III cases. An alternative strategy, employing preoperative chemotherapy, radiation therapy, or synchronous use of both modalities, has increasingly been advocated for unresectable cases, though some authorities advocate chemotherapy alone for patients with locally advanced disease, reserving radiotherapy as a postoperative strategy in selected cases. Chemotherapy regimens are usually cisplatin/anthracycline-based, for example, the PAC combination of cisplatin, doxorubicin and cyclophosphamide, with reported response rates of up to 75% when used pre-operatively. Radiation doses of 40–50 Gy in 3–5 weeks are often used. More distant spread of recurrence after radiotherapy is treated by chemotherapy, although experience is limited and the results are often poor. The most active agents appear to be doxorubicin, ifosfamide, cisplatin and etoposide. Cisplatin/etoposide regimens are now often used, and responses occur in 70% of cases, 40% being complete. Responses usually last 2–3 years.

Encapsulated thymomas have an excellent prognosis and 60% of patients are alive 20 years later. Invasive thymomas have a much worse prognosis, and only 50% of patients are alive after 5 years.

Carcinoid of the thymus

This tumour is uncommon and probably develops from neuroendocrine cells within the thymus (see Chapter 15). These rare tumours may give rise to Cushing's syndrome by producing ACTH and causing adrenal hyperplasia. They are occasionally malignant and are much more common in men. Although they may be completely resected, they often recur locally and metastasize. They do not cause carcinoid syndrome. The prognosis is not good, with 5-year survival as low as 15% in some series.

Germ-cell tumours

Primary germ-cell tumours of the mediastinum are uncommon but are potentially curable. Although teratomas and mixed tumours are the commonest, pure seminoma is also described. The tumours may produce β-human chorionic gonadotrophin (β-HCG) and α-fetoprotein (AFP) as do testicular tumours (see Chapter 19). As with thymomas, the usual clinical presentation is with local pressure symptoms, chiefly dyspnoea, cough and dysphagia. Occasionally, gynaecomastia is the presenting feature. Haematogenous metastasis is unusual, lung and brain being the commonest sites. Local lymphatic invasion may occur. Any young male with an unexplained superior mediastinal tumour of uncertain origin should have plasma tumour markers (AFP and β-HCG) measured since histological interpretation can be difficult even in experienced hands and these tumours can be misdiagnosed as adenocarcinoma. There is an association between Klinefelter's syndrome (XXY) and mediastinal germ-cell tumours.

Plain chest radiography and CT are essential for delineating the tumour and for following progress after treatment. CT lung scanning will occasionally reveal unsuspected metastases. The principles of management are essential as for testicular germ-cell tumours (see Chapter 19). Primary treatment is with combination chemotherapy (currently using combinations including cisplatin, bleomycin, vinblastine and etoposide). As with the commoner primary gonadal seminoma, these tumours are highly radiosensitive and in some cases curable by local radiotherapy (40 Gy in 20 daily fractions over 4 weeks is a commonly recommended dose, though some authorities prefer a higher dose, up to 50 Gy); however, chemotherapy is now considered an essential component of treatment and radiotherapy less frequently used.

In mediastinal teratomas, the role of radiation for residual disease is uncertain. Surgical removal of suspicious residual masses should always be considered, ideally when tumour markers have returned to normal. Previous treatment with large doses of bleomycin may lead to pulmonary toxicity with stiff lungs and poor lung compliance, which may make the post-thoracotomy period particularly hazardous. Recent reports of high-dose chemotherapy and surgical treatment have been encouraging [63], with several long-term survivors (probable cures), in contrast to earlier reports in which cure was rare.

Middle mediastinum

In the middle compartment of the mediastinum, lymphomas are the commonest malignant tumours, and both Hodgkin's disease and non-Hodgkin's lymphomas occur. The differential diagnosis includes an important group of non-malignant conditions: pericardial and bronchogenic cysts, mediastinal lipoma, tuberculosis, sarcoidosis and infectious or malignant causes of hilar and/or mediastinal lymphadenopathy. In the absence of palpable lymphadenopathy in an accessible site, the diagnosis is usually made by mediastinoscopy or limited thoracotomy. Tissue diagnosis is essential and examination of fresh (unfixed) tissue is valuable for the histopathologist since the use of immunocytochemical stains can help distinguish difficult lymphomas from each other and from anaplastic carcinomas (see Chapter 3).

Staging and management of mediastinal lymphomas follow similar principles to those at other sites (see Chapter 26). Surgical excision has no place in the routine management of these tumours, which are sensitive to both chemotherapy and radiotherapy. Occasionally, mediastinal lymphoma causes severe SVCO that requires emergency treatment (see Chapter 8).

Two particular characteristic non-Hodgkin's mediastinal lymphomas occur. The first is T-cell convoluted, lymphoblastic, diffuse lymphoma, seen predominantly in adolescent males. The second is a sclerosing B-cell lymphoma, occurring most frequently in young women (see Chapter 26). Hodgkin's disease of the mediastinum, usually in association with obvious lymphadenopathy in the neck and/or axilla, occurs in about 30% of all supradiaphragmatic cases, but the mediastinum may occasionally be the sole site of involvement.

Posterior mediastinum

Tumours of the posterior mediastinum are chiefly neurogenic in origin, and usually arise from the thoracic sympathetic chain or intercostal nerves (Table 12.7). They are frequently asymptomatic but may cause back pain, dysphagia or ptosis due to Horner's syndrome. Neurofibromas are the commonest, and can usually be removed surgically. They can arise sporadically or in patients with von Recklinghausen's disease. Other neurogenic tumours include schwannomas (both benign and malignant) and neurofibrosarcoma. These neurogenic tumours may extend through the intervertebral foramina (dumb-bell tumours) and cause cord compression. This is suggested by vertebral erosion on the lateral chest radiograph. Ganglioneuromas are probably the commonest of the sympathetic nerve tumours and are generally well differentiated, encapsulated and surgically resectable. In some cases, urinary vanillylmandelic acid may be raised and can be useful for monitoring progress. A less well-differentiated form (ganglioneuroblastoma) is also encountered, and has a worse prognosis because of local recurrence and metastases. Phaeochromocytoma, another hormonally active tumour, frequently presents with symptoms of catecholamine excess, such as paroxysmal hypertension, headache, palpitation, chest pain and excessive sweating, rather than with pressure symptoms. It should be surgically excised where possible. In children, neuroblastoma is a common cause of posterior mediastinal tumour, accounting for about one-fifth of all childhood neuroblastomas. The management of neuroblastoma is discussed in Chapter 24.

Of the rare tumours, chordoma occasionally presents as a posterior mediastinal tumour, and its management is discussed in Chapter 11. Paraganglioma (chemodectoma) is rare and may be locally invasive, usually involving the great vessels.

Diagnosis of posterior mediastinal tumours requires careful radiological assessment (sometimes with contrast studies such as aortography or contrast CT scanning) as well as precise tissue diagnosis, which usually requires thoracotomy. Management is by surgical removal of the tumour wherever possible. For incompletely excised malignant tumours, postoperative radiotherapy is usually recommended.

Mesothelioma

This relentlessly progressive malignant tumour arises from the surface of the pleura, occasionally remaining well localized at the primary site but more often spreading diffusely and involving a substantial area of the pleura including the inner surface of the visceral pleura, thereby encroaching on the pericardium. Pleural effusion is common, and the disease is occasionally bilateral. Primary peritoneal mesothelioma, without pleural involvement, may also occur, and peritoneal disease occasionally develops in patients in whom the pleura is the main or primary site of disease. Most patients with mesothelioma give a history of asbestos exposure, which is documented in about 75% of cases, although there is characteristically a delay of 20 years or so before the disease becomes apparent. The incidence of mesothelioma is rising, presumably because of the widespread use of asbestos products. In the United Kingdom, it is estimated that the number of deaths from this condition is likely to rise from about 1500 in 2000 to a peak of probably double this number by 2020. Although the past 10 years have seen increasingly stringent constraints on the use of asbestos, the full impact has not yet been felt [64] and the incidence is likely to increase, at least until 2020. Having climbed the 'league table' of male cancers over the past 30 years, mesothelioma is now approximately as common as cancers of the liver, bone and bladder, particularly in Europe and Australia [65]. Crocidolite is thought to be the most carcinogenic fibre. Simian virus (SV)40 has frequently been found in mesotheliomas but the role of the virus as a cofactor in carcinogenesis is not established. The polyomaviruses are a group of small double-stranded DNA viruses, and SV40, which blocks tumour-suppressor genes, is a potent cancer-causing virus for human and rodent cells. Up to 60% of human mesotheliomas apparently contain SV40 DNA. With little active or effective treatment available, the mortality rate has risen sharply over the past 30 years.

Pathology

Pathologically the tumours may appear sarcomatous, often with both fibrous and epithelial elements, and may be so anaplastic as to be almost indistinguishable from a poorly differentiated carcinoma. The degree of anaplastic change correlates poorly with clinical behaviour. In other cases the distinction from adenocarcinoma may be very difficult. Direct extension is characteristic, and mesotheliomas typically invade ribs and chest wall. Early and widespread involvement of intercostal bundles probably accounts for the severe pain so typical of this tumour. In addition, extension through the diaphragm, invasion of local lymph nodes and distant blood-borne metastases are all commonly found. It is now known that both

Table 12.8 Current staging for mesothelioma.

T1	Ipsilateral parietal pleura
T2	Parietal and visceral pleura (including mediastinal and diaphragmatic pleura)
T3	Locally advanced but potentially resectable tumour. Both pleural surfaces, extends into mediastinal fat
T4	More extensive unresectable tumour
N0	No regional nodes
N1	Ipsilateral bronchopulmonary nodes
N2	Mediastinal nodes (ipsilateral)
N3	Contralateral nodes

Stage grouping

Stage I	T1	N0	M0
Stage II	T2	N0	M0
Stage III	Any T3	M0	
	Any N1–2	M0	
Stage IV	Any T4, N3 or M1		

Source: From Sobin & Wittekind [67]. Reproduced by permission of John Wiley and Sons.

vascular endothelial growth factor and platelet-derived growth factor are important autocrine growth factors in this condition; EGFR is also significantly overexpressed. Cytotoxic drugs and biological agents that target these factors have real potential, such as thalidomide, bevacuzimab and gefitinib. The subject is well reviewed by Stahel *et al.* [66].

A staging system has been introduced that allows more precise prognosis and trial design [67] (Table 12.8).

The cytogenetics of mesothelioma are now increasingly understood, with loss of chromosome 22 as the most common gross change, although structural rearrangement of 1p, 3p, 9p and 6q are often noted. Most mesotheliomas have an abnormal karyotype, often with extensive aneuploidy and structural rearrangements [65].

Clinical features

Patients typically complain of increasing chest pain, which can be very severe, coupled with shortness of breath on exertion. The dyspnoea tends to be progressive and unremitting, often leading to severe incapacity even at rest. On examination there are signs of diminished chest movement and pleural effusion. Radiologically, the most typical feature of asbestos exposure is the pleural plaque, often multiple, and usually associated with pleural effusion (Figure 12.13). In mesothelioma there is extensive pleural infiltration extending into the mediastinum

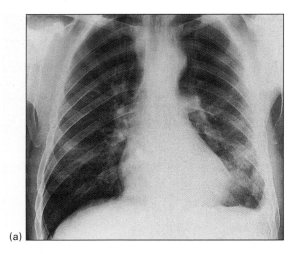

(a)

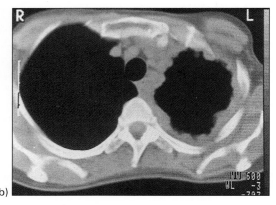

(b)

Figure 12.13 Mesothelioma. (a) Typical radiographic findings, including pleural shadowing with nodulation behind the heart, in the costophrenic angle and along the lateral chest wall, together with partial destruction of ribs. (b) Typical CT appearance, with involvement of the whole of the pleura of the left lung and complete sparing on the right. (Courtesy of Professor M.E. Hodson.)

and causing 'crowding' of the ribs on the affected side because of contracture caused by the tumour.

Diagnosis

The diagnosis can usually be confirmed by pleural biopsy. In cases with such widespread involvement that surgical resection is impossible, diagnostic thoracotomy should be avoided, particularly since tumour seeding of thoracotomy scars is common and can produce additional severe pain. CT scanning is essential for definition of the extent of the tumour, particularly with respect to the

juxtapericardial reflection of the pleura and the adjacent pericardium.

Treatment

Treatment of mesothelioma is tragically unsatisfactory and symptom control unusually difficult, with severe chest pain being a constant concern. Surgery is possible only in the small proportion of cases with localized involvement, although surgical cures can be obtained. Local recurrence is common, and most surgeons favour wide excision where possible, including sacrifice of part of the chest wall, diaphragm, pericardium and adjacent lobe of lung where necessary – often formally termed extra-pleural pneumonectomy, and often requiring resection of the hemi-diaphragm and pericardium *en bloc*.

Radiotherapy is of limited value, though pain relief and apparent reduction in the rate of tumour growth occasionally occur. Adequate irradiation of the whole pleural surface is technically difficult because of the proximity of the lung, but new methods of tangential arc irradiation may allow this technique to be explored further. However, the most useful role for radiotherapy so far has been in the prevention of tumour cell seeding in the wound site, following surgery or even insertion of a chest drain. Presumably this implies, frustratingly, that provided the tumour cell burden is sufficiently small, radiotherapy can be of real benefit in an otherwise therapeutically bleak situation.

A wide variety of chemotherapeutic agents has been used in mesothelioma but with no long-term success until recently [68,69]. The most active agents (with approximate percentage response rates) are methotrexate (30%), vinorelbine (20%), mitomycin (20%), cisplatin (15%), doxorubicin (15%), docetaxel (10%) and gemcitabine (10%). The new antifolates pemetrexed and raltitrexed have shown even higher response rates (40–50%) in relatively small studies and these may well be the most active drugs in the disease. Pemetrexed, a multitargeted antifolate that inhibits at least three enzymes in the nucleic acid synthesis pathways, has recently been approved for use (in combination with cisplatin) in advanced malignant pleural mesothelioma, following demonstration of response rates over 40% in a recent phase III study [70]. This is a remarkable result in such an intractable tumour, and this new agent may be the most effective yet identified. This combination is, at present, the preferred choice for routine treatment. In highly selected suitable cases, radical surgical resection is combined with neoadjuvant or postoperative adjuvant chemotherapy, with platinum-based regimens or pemetrexed as the preferred options. The combination of gemcitabine and cisplatin produces responses in about 35% of cases, but was not superior to cisplatin in a randomized comparison. Responses to α-interferon have also been reported. Combinations of cisplatin and interferon produce responses in about 20% of patients, and some responses last for many months. More studies are needed to determine the survival benefit of other combinations. However, the role of chemotherapy is now becoming established in this intractable disease. Intrapleural chemotherapy is occasionally attempted for control of the malignant pleural effusion, but the results are discouraging. Overall median survival is little over 1 year [71]; negative prognostic factors include sarcomatous histology, male gender, poor performance status and a raised white cell count at diagnosis.

Gene therapy has also been used. This approach, involving administration of engineered viruses into which a gene of interest has been inserted with the aim of inducing prolonged expression in the tissues of the protein product of the inserted gene, is of theoretical interest at present. Suicide gene therapy involves transfer to tumour cells of DNA encoding an enzyme which, after administration of the antiviral agent ganciclovir, is capable of converting this drug into a toxic metabolite that can destroy both tumour cells and their malignant neighbouring cells. Immunomodulatory gene therapy involves the local delivery of a vector producing a cytokine that would mimic the inflammatory or immune processes occurring in organs undergoing autoimmune destruction.

Fewer than 15% of patients survive for 5 years. Patients unsuitable for surgery, treated with 'best supportive care', have a median survival of around 6 months. These very poor results argue strongly for rigid control of the use of asbestos products, and patients with mesothelioma and a clear history of industrial asbestos exposure are usually considered by independent tribunals to be strong candidates for compensation. British law has recently altered in this area: successful claims are increasingly being brought, for example, in patients who developed pleural plaques from washing work clothes contaminated by asbestos, or even following a single exposure to asbestos in the workplace.

Primary tracheal tumours

These are extremely unusual, but when encountered pose enormous challenges in management [20]. Often misdiagnosed as asthma or chronic lung disease as a result

of their presentation with noisy stertorous breathing, they may later present with haemoptysis or obstructive breathing. A conservative approach to surgery, with organ preservation and postoperative radiotherapy, often represents the best approach to treatment, which should ideally be undertaken at a specialist centre. Although generally benign in children, these tumours are normally malignant when encountered in adult life. Squamous cell carcinoma is the commonest histological variety, generally associated with long-term cigarette smoking, and is at least twice as common in men than women. If the tumour is surgically inoperable, an endobronchial stent may give useful palliative relief. Chemotherapy has also been employed, as for NSCLC, although no worthwhile studies are available since the disease is so uncommon.

References

1 Ferlay J, Shin HR, Bray F *et al*. Estimates of worldwide burden of cancer in 2008: GLOBOCAN 2008. *Int J Cancer* 2010; 127 : 2893–17.

2 Henschke CI, Yip R, Mietinnen OS. Women's susceptibility to tobacco carcinogens and survival after diagnosis of lung cancer. International Early Lung Cancer Action Program Investigators. *JAMA* 2006; 296: 180–84.

3 Jamrozik K Estimate of deaths attributable to passive smoking among UK adults: database analysis. *Br Med J* 2005; 330: 812–15.

4 Torjesen I Britons are making healthier lifestyle choices than 40 years ago. *Brit Med J* 2013;346: f1583.

5 Hatsukami DK, Stead LF, Gupta PC. Tobacco addiction. *Lancet* 2008; 371: 2027–38.

6 Ferriman, A Finding the smoking gun. *Brit Med J* 2012; 345: 31 (27 Oct 2012).

7 Schroeder S. Stranded in the periphery: the increasing marginalization of smokers. *N Engl J Med* 2008; 358: 2284–86.

8 Tammemagi MC, Katki HA, Hocking W G *et al*. Selection criteria for lung-cancer screening. *New Engl J Med* 2013; 368: 728–36.

9 Doll R, Peto R, Boreham J, Sutherland I. Mortality in relation to smoking: 50 years' observations on male British doctors. *Br Med J* 2004; 328: 1519.

10 Jha P, Ramasundarahettige C, Landsman V *et al*. 21st-century hazards of smoking and benefits of cessation in the United States. *New Engl J Med* 2013; 368: 341–50.

11 Omenn GS, Goodman GE, Thornquist MD *et al*. Effects of a combination of beta carotene and vitamin A on lung cancer and cardiovascular disease. *N Engl J Med* 1996; 334: 1150–55.

12 Miller N, Frieden TR, Liu SY *et al*. Effectiveness of a large-scale distribution programme of free nicotine

patches: a prospective evaluation. *Lancet* 2005; 365: 1849–54.

13 West R, May S, West M *et al.* Performance of English stop smoking services in first 10 years: analysis of service monitoring data. *Brit Med J* 2013; 347: f4921.

14 Raaschou-Nielsen O, Andersen ZJ, Beelen R, *et al.* Air pollution and lung cancer incidence in 17 European cohorts: prospective analyses from the European Study of Cohorts for Air Pollution Effects (ESCAPE). *Lancet Oncol* 2013; 14: 813–22.

15 Gohagan J, Marcus P, Fagerstrom R *et al.* Baseline findings of a randomized feasibility trial of lung cancer screening with spiral CT scan versus chest radiograph: the Lung Cancer Screening Study of the National Cancer Institute. *Chest* 2004; 126: 114–17.

16 Vineis P, Alavanja M, Buffler P *et al.* Tobacco and cancer: recent epidemiological evidence. *J Natl Cancer Inst* 2004; 96: 99–106.

17 International Early Lung Cancer Action Programme Investigators. Survival of patients with stage I lung cancer detected on CT screening. *N Engl J Med* 2006; 355: 1763–71.

18 National Lung Screening Trial Research Team. Results of initial low-dose computed tomographic screening for lung cancer. *New Engl J Med* 2013; 368: 1980–91.

19 Zheng Z, Chen T, Li X *et al.* DNA synthesis and repair genes *RRM1* and *ERCC1* in lung cancer. *N Engl J Med* 2007; 356: 800–8.

20 Macchiarini P Primary tracheal tumours. *Lancet Oncol* 2006; 7: 83–91.

21 Chen H-U, Uyu S-L, Chen CH *et al.* A 5-gene signature and clinical outcome in non-small-cell lung cancer. *N Engl J Med* 2007; 356: 11–20.

22 Rusch VW. Management of Pancoast tumours. *Lancet Oncol* 2006; 7: 997–1005.

23 NSCLC Meta-analyses Collaborative Group. Adjuvant chemotherapy, with or without postoperative radiotherapy, in operable non-small-cell lung cancer: two meta-analyses of individual patient data. *Lancet* 2010; 375: 1267–77.

24 Blanchon F, Grivaux M, Asselaine B *et al.* Four year mortality in patients with non-small-cell cancer: development and validation of a prognostic index. *Lancet Oncol* 2006; 7: 829–36.

25 National Institute for Clinical Excellence. Interventional Procedure Guidelines. Photodynamic Therapy for Advanced Bronchial Carcinoma. Available at www.nice.org.uk/ip100overview.

26 Saunders M, Dische S, Barrett A *et al.* Continuous hyperfractionated accelerated radiotherapy (CHART) versus conventional radiotherapy in non-small-cell lung cancer: a randomised multicentre trial. *Lancet* 1997; 350: 161–65.

27 Schaake-Koning C, van den Bogaert W, Dalesio O *et al.* Effects of concomitant cisplatin and radiotherapy on inoperable non-small-cell lung cancer. *N Engl J Med* 1992; 326: 524–30.

28 Rosenzweig KE, Amols H, Ling CC. New radiotherapy technologies. *Semin Surg Oncol* 2003; 21: 190–95.

29 Sidhu K, Ford EC, Spirou S *et al.* Optimisation of conformal radiation therapy using cone-beam CT imaging for treatment verification. *Int J Radiat Oncol Biol Phys* 2003; 55: 757–67.

30 Wisnievsky JP and Strauss GM. Treating elderly patients with stage III NSCLC. *Lancet Oncol* 2012; 13: 650–51.

31 Curran WJ, Paulus R, Langer C J *et al.* Sequential vs concurrent chemoradiation for stage III non-small cell lung cancer: randomized phase III trial RTOG 9410. *J Natl Cancer Inst* 2011; 103: 1452–60.

32 PORT Meta-analysis Trials Group. Postoperative radiotherapy in non small-cell lung cancer: systematic review and meta-analysis of individual patient data from nine randomized clinical trials. *Lancet* 1998; 352: 257.

33 Doullard J-Y, Rosell R, De Lena M *et al.* Adjuvant vinorelbine plus cisplatin versus observation inpatients with completely resected stage IB–IIIA non-small-cell lung cancer (ANITA trial). *Lancet Oncol* 2006: 7; 719–27.

34 Crino L, Weder W, van Meerbeeck J, *et al.* Early stage and locally advanced (non-metastatic) non-small-cell lung cancer: ESMO clinical practice guidelines for diagnosis, treatment and follow-up. *Ann Oncol* 2012; 21 (Supplement 5): v103–v105.

35 Olaussen KA, Dunant A, Furet P *et al.* DNA repair by ERCC1 in non-small-cell lung cancer and cisplatin-based adjuvant chemotherapy. *N Engl J Med* 2006: 355; 983–91.

36 Friboulet L, Olaussen KA, Pignon J-P, *et al.* ERCC1 isoform expression and DNA repair in non-small-cell lung cancer. *New Engl J Med* 2013; 368: 1101–10.

37 Peters S, Adjei AA, Gridelli C *et al.* Metastatic non-small-cell lung cancer (NSCLC) :ESMO clinical practice guidelines for diagnosis, treatment and follow-up. *Ann Oncol* 2012; 23 (Supplement 7): vii56–vii64.

38 Paz-Ares L, de Marinis F, Dediu M *et al.* Maintenance therapy with pemetrexed plus best supportive care after induction therapy with pemetrexed plus cisplatin for advanced non-squamous non-small-cell lung cancer (PARAMOUNT): a double-blind, phase 3, randomized controlled trial. *Lancet Oncol* 2012; 13: 247–55.

39 Silvestri G, Rivera MP. Targeted therapy for the treatment of advanced non small cell lung cancer: a review of the epidermal growth factor receptor antagonists. *Chest* 2005; 128: 3975–84.

40 Sandler A, Gray R, Perry MC *et al.* Paclitaxel–carboplatin alone or with bevacizumab for non-small-cell lung cancer. *N Engl J Med* 2006; 355: 2542–50. [Correspondence *N Engl J Med* 2007; 356: 1373–75.]

41 Blackhall F, Ranson M, Thatcher N. Where next for gefitinib in patients with lung cancer? *Lancet Oncol* 2006; 7: 499–507.

42 Cataldo VD, Gibbons DL, Perez-Soler R and Quintas-Cardama A. Treatment of non-small-cell lung cancer with erlotinib or gefitinib. *New Engl J Med* 2011; 364: 947–55.

43 Shaw AT, Kim D-W, Nakagawa K, *et al*. Crizotinib versus chemotherapy in advanced ALK-positive lung cancer. *New Engl J Med* 2013;368: 2385 – 94.

44 Reck M, Kaiser R, Mellemgaard A, *et al*. Nintedanib (BIBF 1120) plus docetaxel in NSCLC patients progressing after first-line chemotherapy: LUME Lung 1, a randomized, double-blind phase III trial. *J Clin Oncol* 2013; 31 (suppl; abstr LBA8011).

45 Davidoff AJ, Tang M, Seal B, *et al*. Chemotherapy and survival benefit in elderly patients with advanced non-small-cell lung cancer. *J Clin Oncol* 2010; 28: 2191 – 97.

46 Dillman RO, Seagreen SL, Propert KJ *et al*. A randomized trial of induction chemotherapy plus high-dose radiation vs. radiation alone in stage III non-small-cell lung cancer. *N Engl J Med* 1990; 322: 940 – 45.

47 Non-Small-Cell Lung Cancer Collaborative Group. Chemotherapy in non-small cell lung cancer: a meta-analysis using updated data on individual patients from 52 randomized trials. *Br Med J* 1995; 311: 899 – 909.

48 Arriagada R, Bergman B, Dunant A *et al*. Cisplatin-based adjuvant chemotherapy in patients with completely resected non-small-cell lung cancer. *N Engl J Med* 2004; 350: 351 – 63.

49 Lee SM, Khan I, Upadhyay S, *et al*. First-line erlotinib in patients with advanced non-small-cell lung cancer unsuitable for chemotherapy (TOPICAL): a double-blind, placebo-controlled, phase 3 trial. *Lancet Oncol* 2012; 13: 1161 – 70.

50 Buchholz E, Manegold C, Pilz L *et al*. Standard versus dose-intensified chemotherapy with sequential reinfusion of hemopoietic progenitor cells in small-cell lung cancer patients with favorable prognosis. *J Thorac Oncol* 2007; 2: 51 – 58.

51 Sorensen M, Pijls-Johannesma M and Felip E. Small-cell lung cancer: ESMO clinical practice guidelines for diagnosis, treatment and follow-up. *Ann Oncol* 2010; 21 (Supplement 5): v120 – v125.

52 Souhami RL, Law K. Longevity in small-cell lung cancer. *Br J Cancer* 1990; 61: 584 – 89.

53 Pignon J-P, Arriagada R, Ihde DC *et al*. A meta-analysis of thoracic radiotherapy for small-cell lung cancer. *N Engl J Med* 1992; 327: 1618 – 24.

54 Murray N, Coy P, Pater JL *et al*. Importance of timing for thoracic irradiation in the combined modality treatment of limited-stage small-cell lung cancer. *J Clin Oncol* 1993; 11: 3363.

55 Faivre-Finn C, Lee LW, Lorigan P *et al*. Thoracic radiotherapy for limited-stage small-cell lung cancer: controversies and future developments. *Clin Oncol* 2005; 17: 591 – 98.

56 Spiro SG, James LE, Rudd RM *et al*. Early compared with late radiotherapy in combined modality treatment for limited disease small-cell lung cancer: a London Lung Cancer Group multi-centre randomized clinical trial and meta-analysis. *J Clin Oncol* 2006; 24: 3823 – 30.

57 Slotman B, Faivre-Finn C, Kramer G *et al*. Prophylactic cranial irradiation in extensive small-cell lung cancer. *N Engl J Med* 2007; 357: 664 – 72.

58 Harper PG, Addis B. Unusual tumours of the mediastinum. In: Williams CJ, Krickorian JC, Green MR, Raghavan D, eds. *Textbook of Uncommon Cancer*. Chichester: Wiley, 1988: 411 – 49.

59 Müller-Hermelink HK, Marx A. Thymoma. *Curr Opin Oncol* 2000; 12: 426 – 33.

60 Kondo K, Monden Y. Therapy for thymic epithelial tumors: a clinical study of 1,320 patients from Japan. *Ann Thorac Surg* 2003; 76: 878 – 85.

61 Okereke IC, Kesler KA, Freeman RK *et al*. Thymic carcinoma: outcomes after surgical resection. *Ann Thoracic Surg* 2012; 93: 1668 – 72.

62 Kim ES, Putnam JB, Komaki R *et al*. Phase II study of a multidisciplinary approach with induction chemotherapy, followed by surgical resection, radiation therapy, and consolidation chemotherapy for unresectable malignant thymomas: final report. *Lung Cancer* 2004; 44: 369 – 79.

63 de Georgi U, Rosti G, Slavin S *et al*. Salvage high-dose chemotherapy for children with extragonadal germ-cell tumors. *Br J Cancer* 2005; 93: 412 – 17.

64 Peto J, Hodgson JT, Matthews FE, Jones JR. Continuing increase in mesothelioma mortality in Britain. *Lancet* 1995; 345: 535 – 39.

65 Robinson BW, Musk AW, Lake RA. Malignant mesothelioma. *Lancet* 2005; 366: 397 – 408.

66 Stahel RA, Weder W, Lievens Y and Felip E. Malignant pleural mesothelioma: ESMO clinical practice guidelines for diagnosis, treatment and follow-up. *Ann Oncol* 2010; (Supplement 5): v126 – v128.

67 Sobin LH, Wittekind Ch, eds. *TNM Classification of Malignant Tumours*, 6th edn. New York: Wiley-Liss, 2002.

68 Andreopoulou E, Ross PJ, O'Brien ME *et al*. The palliative benefits of MVP (mitomycin C, vinblastine and cisplatin) chemotherapy in patients with malignant mesothelioma. *Ann Oncol* 2004; 15: 1406 – 12.

69 Tomek S, Manegold C. Chemotherapy for malignant pleural mesothelioma: past results and recent developments. *Lung Cancer* 2004; 45: 103 – 19.

70 Vogelzang JN, Rusthoven JJ, Symanowski J *et al*. Phase III study of pemetrexed in combination with cisplatin versus cisplatin alone in patients with malignant pleural mesothelioma. *J Clin Oncol* 2003; 21: 2636 – 44.

71 Curran D, Sahmoud T, Therasse P *et al*. Prognostic factors in patients with pleural mesothelioma: the European Organisation for Research and Treatment of Cancer experience. *J Clin Oncol* 1998; 16: 145 – 52.

72 National Institute for Clinical Excellence. Interventional Procedure Guidance 185. Percutaneous Radio-frequency Ablation for Primary and Secondary Lung Cancers. Available at www.nice.org.uk/IPG185distribution list.

73 National Institute for Clinical Excellence. Lung Cancer: Diagnosis And Treatment. Clinical Guideline 24.

Developed by the National Collaborating Centre for Acute Care. Available at www.nice.org.uk, ref. NO825-IP-80K.

Further reading

Advice for stopping smoking is available at an excellent website: www.givingupsmoking.co.uk. A Freephone line is available on 0800 002200 or 0800 1690169 (UK subscribers); alternatively try www.reducetherisk.org.uk.

Analysis of the Science and Policy for European Control of Tobacco (ASPECT). *Tobacco or Health in the European Union: Past, Present and Future.* Luxembourg: Office for Official Publications of the European Union, ASPECT Consortium, 2004.

Brandt AM. *The Cigarette Century: The Rise, Fall, and Deadly Persistence of the Product that Defined America.* New York: Basic Books, 2007.

Brandt AM. FDA regulation of tobacco: pitfalls and possibilities. *N Engl J Med* 2008; 359: 445–48.

Christakis NA, Fowler JH. The collective dynamics of smoking in a large social network. *N Engl J Med* 2008; 358: 2249–58.

Clark S Personal account on giving up smoking. *Lancet* 2005; 365: 1855.

Curfman GD, Morrissey S, Drazen JM. The FDA and tobacco regulation. *N Engl J Med* 2008; 359: 1056–67.

Currie GP, Watt SJ, Maskell NA. An overview of how asbestos exposure affects the lung. *Br Med J* 2009; 339: 506–10.

Eberhardt W, Pöttgen C, Stuschke M. Chemoradiation paradigm for the treatment of lung cancer. *Nature Clin Pract Oncol* 2006; 3: 188–99.

Einhorn LH. First-line chemotherapy for non-small-cell lung cancer: is there a superior regimen based on histology? *J Clin Oncol* 2008; 26: 3485–86.

Erridge SC, Møller H, Price A, Brewster D. International comparisons of survival from lung cancer: pitfalls and warnings. *Nat Clin Pract Oncol* 2007; 4: 578–90.

Gruer L, Hart CL, Gordon DS *et al.* Effect of tobacco smoking on survival or men and women by social position: a 28 year cohort study. *Br Med J* 2009; 338: 643.

Gu D, Kelly TN, Wu X *et al.* Mortality attributable to smoking in China. *N Engl J Med* 2009; 360: 150–59.

Hajek P, Stead LF, West R *et al.* Relapse prevention interventions for smoking cessation. *Cochrane Database Syst Rev* 2009; 1: CD003999.

Herbst RS, Heymach JV, Lippman SM. Lung cancer. *N Engl J Med* 2008; 359: 1367–80.

Jha P, Peto R, Zatonski W *et al.* Social inequalities in male mortality, and in male mortality from smoking: indirect estimation from national death rates in England and Wales, Poland and North America. *Lancet* 2006; 268: 367–70.

Kris MG, Natale RB, Herbst RS *et al.* Efficacy of gefitinib, an inhibitor of the epidermal growth factor receptor tyrosine kinase, in symptomatic patients with non-small-cell lung cancer. *JAMA* 2003; 290: 2149–58.

Kurfman GD, Morrissey S, Drazen JM. Tobacco, public health, and the FDA. *N Engl J Med* 2009; 361: 402–3.

Le Chevalier T, Arriagada R, Pignon J-P, Scagliotti GV. Should adjuvant chemotherapy become standard treatment in all patients with resected non-small-cell lung cancer? *Lancet Oncol* 2005; 6: 182–84.

McMahon PM, Christiani DC. Computed tomography screening for lung cancer: results of randomized trials are needed before recommending its adoption. *Br Med J* 2007; 334: 271.

Massarelli E, Herbst RS. Use of novel second-line targeted therapies in non-small-cell lung cancer. *Semin Oncol* 2006; 33 (1 Supplement 1): S9–S16.

Potti A, Mukherjee S, Petersen R *et al.* A genomic strategy to refine prognosis in early-stage non-small-cell lung cancer. *N Engl J Med* 2006; 355: 570–80.

Rasmussen SR, Prescott E, Sørensen TI, Søgaard J. The total lifetime health cost savings of smoking cessation to society. *Eur J Public Health* 2005; 15: 601–6.

Seffrin JR. We can eradicate the global scourge of tobacco. *Nat Clin Pract Oncol* 2005; 2: 378–79.

Shepherd FA, Pereira JR, Ciuleanu T *et al.* For the National Cancer Institute of Canada Clinical Trials Group. Erlotinib in previously treated non-small-cell lung cancer. *N Engl J Med* 2005; 353: 123–32.

Spira A, Ettinger DS. Multidisciplinary management of lung cancer. *N Engl J Med* 2004; 350: 379–92.

Sweeney K, Toy L, Cornwell J. A patient's journey: mesothelioma. *Br Med J* 2009; 339: 511–12.

Warner KE, Longstaff Mackay J. Smoking cessation treatment in a public-health context. *Lancet* 2008; 371: 1976–78.

Watkinson AF, Yeow TN, Fraser C. Endovascular stenting to treat obstruction of the superior vena cava. *Br Med J* 2008; 336: 1434–37.

Wilson LD, Detterbeck FC, Yahalom J. Superior vena cava syndrome with malignant causes. *N Engl J Med* 2007; 356: 1862–69.

PROQUEST LLC:

ISBN	Qty	Sales Order
9781118468739	1	F 21913122 1

Customer P/O No
MEDWC9726/1

Cust P/O List
70.99 GBP

Title: Cancer and its management.

Author: Tobias, Jeffrey S.,

Publisher: Wiley Blackwell,

Fund: MEDWC

Location: WHITECHAPL

Loan Type: 5 x owls

Coutts CN: 28629340

Format: P (Paperback)

Order Specific Instructions

Ship To: UK 21036007 F
BARTS & THE LONDON SCHOOL OF
MEDICINE & DENTISTRY
WHITECHAPEL LIBRARY
TURNER STREET
LONDON
E1 2AD

Volume:
Edition: Seventh ed
Year: 2015.,
Pagination: 1 online resour
Size: 25 x 20 cm

Routing *5

Catalog
Sorting Y12L09X
Inpro
RFID
Covering – BXXXX
Despatch

BARTS & THE LONDON SCHOOL OF

P20SJRSH2

37   257

260498888 ukrwls10 RC2

13 Breast cancer

Incidence, aetiology and epidemiology

Breast cancer is the commonest of all malignant diseases in women, with an annual incidence of over 40 000 new cases in the UK and 145 000 new cases in the USA. The incidence has risen steadily over the past 50 years, with a striking geographical variation across the world. Incidence figures in the developed Western world are much higher than in poorer developing countries (Figure 13.1), although rates are clearly rising in the developing world, probably due to both increasing longevity and changes in lifestyle and diet, leading to increasing body weight. In China, for example, a change in eating habits, with increased likelihood of the adoption of the typical Western 'meat/sweet' diet, seems to be an important predictor of risk. Globally, an estimated 1 million cases are now diagnosed annually, and the age-related incidence is shown in Figure 13.2. One woman in nine will develop breast cancer during her lifetime, making it the leading cause of death from malignant disease in Western women. In the UK, the prevalence of breast cancer is so high that approximately half of all live female cancer patients are suffering from this single disease. In the USA, over $8 billion annually is spent in diagnosis and treatment of this single disease, and most are diagnosed at an early and highly treatable stage. In contrast, in South Africa, for example, this would apply to only 5–10% of cases; in India, about half of all patients diagnosed with breast cancer effectively receive no treatment at all.

There are a number of known aetiological factors [1,2]. Age is important, over 75% of cases occur in women of 50 years or greater. Women with a first-degree relative with breast cancer have a threefold increase in risk. In particular, a history of breast cancer diagnosed premenopausally confers on the patient's daughters an additional risk of 3–11 times the normal rate. It is estimated that familial breast cancer susceptibility accounts for just under 25% of all cases, and the BRCA1 and BRCA2 genes are now known to be high-penetrance predisposition genes identified by genome-wide linkage analysis and positional cloning – see Balmana et al. [3]. Women bearing their first child when over the age of 30 are three times more likely to develop breast cancer than those who do so when under 20 years, and there is an increased risk in

Cancer and its Management, Seventh Edition. Jeffrey Tobias and Daniel Hochhauser.
© 2015 John Wiley & Sons, Ltd. Published 2015 by John Wiley & Sons, Ltd.

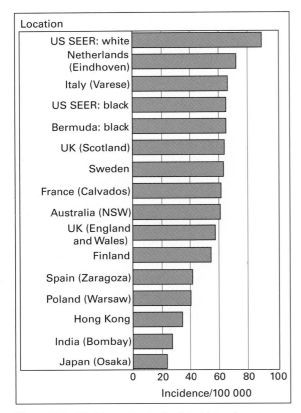

Figure 13.1 World age-standardized incidence breast cancer rates, females, world regions, 2008 estimates. Source: http://www.cancerresearchuk.org/cancer-info/cancerstats/types/breast/incidence/#world, accessed March 2014. © 2014 Cancer Research UK, Reproduced with permission.

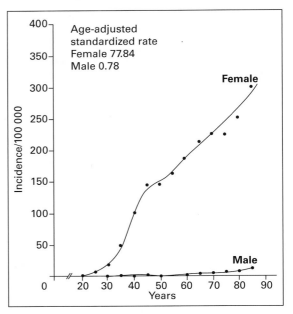

Figure 13.2 Age-specific incidence of breast cancer.

patients who have a history of benign breast disease, particularly epitheliosis and benign cellular atypia. Early menarche and late menopause predispose to a higher incidence, whereas oophorectomy, carried out early in life, offers some degree of protection. It is also clear that prophylactic oophorectomy in women with a *BRCA1* or *BRCA2* mutation considerably reduces the risk of their developing breast cancer [2]. Mutation testing of at-risk families is now commonly performed and many women from families with hereditary breast or ovarian cancer will consider bilateral prophylactic mastectomy and/or salpingo-oophorectomy as a strategy to reduce their risk of developing cancer [4]. Decisions about early detection and prophylactic options for high-risk women are particularly difficult because of the uncertain effectiveness of cancer screening and the complexity of these issues (Table 13.1).

In the UK, the National Institute for Health and Clinical Excellence (NICE) has recently issued guidelines for the identification and care of women at risk of familial breast cancer in the primary, secondary and tertiary care settings [5]. Although the evidence relating to use of oral contraceptives has been contentious, it seems likely that breast cancer is not more common in patients who have used these, and there is of course a substantial benefit from these agents in respect of protection from the risk of ovarian cancer (see Chapter 17). With widespread use of hormone-replacement therapy (HRT), great attention has been paid to the potential risk of breast cancer. A recent large-scale study from the Women's Health Initiative in the USA confirmed an additional risk of 26% after 5.2 years of use of a combination oestrogen/progestin medication, as well as additional risks of stroke and heart disease [6]. An increased risk in women taking HRT has been repeatedly documented either with oestrogens alone or in combination with progestins [7]. The small additional risk may be offset, at least partly, by other clinical advantages (including a clear reduction in the risk of osteoporosis) and has virtually disappeared after 5 years' cessation of HRT. The HRT risk may be particularly important in the pathogenesis of lobular breast cancer, according to recent data from the USA. A large international study has clarified the important protective role of breast-feeding [8]. There was a clear relationship between the duration of breast-feeding and the subsequent risk of breast cancer, with a relative reduction decreasing 4.3% for every 12 months of breast-feeding, and a decrease of 12% for each birth. The authors estimated that the cumulative incidence of breast cancer in developed countries could be reduced by more than half, from 6.3 to 2.7 per 100 women by age 70 years, if women had the average number of births and lifetime duration of breast-feeding that had been prevalent in developing countries until recently.

Follow-up of victims of Hiroshima have shown a late increase in incidence of breast cancer due to the carcinogenic effect of low- or moderate-level radiation fallout. Demographic differences are also marked, and are probably due more to dietary, cultural or geographic variability than to racial characteristics since Japanese and Hawaiian women who settle in the USA have daughters and grand-daughters whose breast cancer prevalence follows the American pattern after as little as two generations. On the other hand, recent studies have suggested that black British women may be at an increased risk of developing breast cancer compared with white women, at a lower age, and with more adverse prognostic factors. As far as diet is concerned, the possible importance of a high-fat diet as a causal agent has been strongly queried by a negative cohort analysis from international studies, although a link has clearly emerged between breast cancer incidence and alcohol intake. Other possible important protective dietary links include organosulphur compounds (e.g. S-llylcysteine, which is present in garlic and cruciferous vegetables such as Brussels sprouts), indole-3-carbinol (also present in cruciferous vegetables), carotenoids (e.g. β-carotene, which occurs in green and yellow vegetables), vitamin E, selenium, tea and polyphenolic oxidants, and flavonoids [9].

Several cohort studies have now suggested a reduced risk of breast cancer in women who are physically active and exercising regularly. Even minimal exercise (as little as 30 min per week) seems, perhaps surprisingly, to have a measurable protective effect. It may even prolong the life of women already diagnosed. Circulating oestrogens are directly linked to breast cancer incidence, and since body fat produces oestrogen (particularly in the post-menopausal years), weight gain might be linked as a risk factor for breast cancer, a suggestion strongly supported by the very large Nurses' Health Study from the USA [10] and now widely accepted as a genuine aetiological factor. Almost 90 000 people were followed for 30 years, and the research has recently estimated that 15% of postmenopausal cancers were directly attributable

Table 13.1 Genetic counselling issues in women considering prophylactic surgery.

Bilateral prophylactic mastectomy
Effectiveness in reducing risk of breast cancer including residual risk
Timing of prophylactic mastectomy (e.g. when risk increases)
Surgical considerations
  Total vs. skin-sparing vs. subcutaneous mastectomy
  Plans for breast reconstruction, including nipple reconstruction
  Type of breast reconstruction (implants or tissue transfer)
  Surgical complications
  Cost of surgery
Psychosocial motivations
  Discussion of motivating factors (perceived risk, family experiences, cancer worry)
  Psychological impact
  Psychosexual impact (body image and sexuality)
  Plans for breast-feeding

Bilateral prophylactic salpingo-oophorectomy
Effectiveness of reducing risk of ovarian and breast cancer, including residual risk
Timing of prophylactic oophorectomy (e.g. when risk increases, after child-bearing)
Surgical considerations
  Laparotomy vs. laparoscopy
  Consideration of hysterectomy (to eliminate need for progesterone and risk of endometrial cancer if taking tamoxifen)
  Surgical complications
  Cost of surgery
Hormonal considerations in premenopausal women
  Loss of fertility
  Onset of menopause
  Increased risk for coronary artery disease and osteoporosis
  Role of hormone replacement therapy in reducing symptoms
  Effect of hormone replacement therapy on risk of breast cancer
Psychosocial considerations
  Plans for child-bearing
  Psychosexual impact (libido)
  Family experiences of ovarian cancer
  Familial obligations

Source: Lobb and Meiser [4]. Reprinted with permission from Elsevier.

to becoming fatter since the teenage years. This link was particularly clear-cut in women who had never taken HRT. The more weight they gained, the greater the risk. The relationship between obesity and breast cancer is probably mediated by excess oestrogens produced by adipocytes. It seems increasingly likely that breast-cancer incidence is more closely related to weight gain *per se,* rather than due to a particular dietary component such as ingested fats – see, for example, Khaw [11]. Alcohol consumption has also emerged as an independent aetiological factor, particularly for hormone receptor-positive disease. Overall, there is strong evidence of a recent fall in breast cancer mortality, probably from earlier diagnosis and better treatment, and predating the application of the UK national screening programme. Recent studies have suggested that the use of daily aspirin may reduce this risk still further, with a reduction in the incidence of breast cancer by 28% from daily use. One important point to have emerged more recently is that with the increasing choice by women to undergo breast-augmentation using cosmetic implants, they may face a risk of being diagnosed, if they later develop breast cancer, with a disease that is less likely to present at a fully localized stage – see Lavigne *et al.* [12]. These Canadian authors conducted a meta-analysis of 12 studies published after 1993, chiefly in the USA, Canada and northern Europe. The hypothesis was that although breast implants do not cause breast cancer they do seem to make early diagnosis more difficult – and with a suggestion from the five studies that actually addressed outcome, that the risk of death from breast cancer was 38% higher than in those without. A worrying result indeed, though the authors rightly urged caution in the interpretation of the data.

Identification and cloning of *BRCA1* and *BRCA2* has led to a rapid increase in understanding molecular events in hereditary breast cancer. Possession of *BRCA1* or *BRCA2* implies a 50–85% probability of the disease developing at some point during a patient's life, usually during the postmenopausal period (and also an ovarian cancer risk of 15–45%). However, the overwhelming majority of sporadic breast cancer cases are not related to *BRCA1* or *BRCA2* and there are other genes such as *p53* that also confer a predisposition to the disease – these also include *PTEN* and *STK 11*, which are more often associated with the rarer forms of cancer syndrome such as Li-Fraumeni, Cowden and Peutz-Jeghers. Heterozygotes for mutations in the ataxia telangiectasia gene may also be at increased risk. *BRCA1* itself is a large gene, encoded by 5592 nucleotides distributed over a genomic region of approximately 100 kb. Furthermore, recent work from Cambridge University [13] has suggested that there are at least seven more recognizable variants ('susceptibility alleles'), in addition to the well-studied *BRCA* genes, which are now known to increase a woman's chances of developing breast cancer, particularly if present, in particular, combinations. These include *CASP8, FGFR2, TNRC9, MAP3K1, LSP1* and others. In the case of *CASP8,* for example, about three-quarters of women carry two copies of the version of this gene that is associated with an increased risk of breast cancer. For *FGFR2,* the figure is one in six women, and for *MAP3K1,* about one in thirteen. *RAD51C* has also been discovered as a potentially high-risk cancer predisposition gene in breast/ovarian cancer families. Testing more women in this way, perhaps at around the age of 30 years, could open up a dramatic new area of breast screening, even on a national scale. This is clearly a landmark study, which has attracted considerable media interest and has major ethical, medical and economic implications, though it has to be admitted that despite all this recent work in genetic testing and mapping, no obvious predisposing factor is discovered in well over half – probably about 75% – of all patients presenting with breast cancer.

Pathology and mode of spread

Almost all breast cancers arise from the glandular epithelium lining the lactiferous ducts and ductules, and are therefore typical adenocarcinomas. True intraduct carcinomas (or ductus carcinoma *in situ*, DCIS) do occur, particularly in screen-detected cases (see below), but most primary breast cancers have invaded into the stroma of the breast by the time of diagnosis (invasive carcinoma). The great majority of these present as breast lumps, although a very small number have eroded through the skin of the breast by the time they are first seen, presenting as fungating tumours. Lesser degrees of skin involvement lead to skin dimpling or tethering and *peau d'orange* in which skin infiltration leads to local lymphatic obstruction. The wide variability in histological appearance has led to classifications of these tumours according to microscopic characteristics (recently with the help of histochemical stains). Tumour grade, essentially the degree of differentiation, is of great prognostic importance.

Intraduct carcinomas of the breast (DCIS and lobular carcinoma *in situ*), without evidence of true invasiveness, are undoubtedly premalignant in a proportion of cases, often with widespread abnormalities within the breast. With the advent of mass screening, DCIS is now encountered far more frequently; indeed, pure intraduct carcinoma is rightly regarded as a 'new disease'. It accounts for about 20% of all newly diagnosed cases of breast cancer in the USA each year (i.e., about 60 000 cases), mostly oestrogen-receptor-positive – see Smith [14] for a useful brief review. There is still considerable uncertainty about its natural history, but both radiotherapy and tamoxifen appear to reduce the risk of development towards invasive disease [15,16].

Much of our recent understanding of the prognostic importance of these observations comes from studies of genomic and proteomic analysis, which has permitted a 'molecular portrait' to be obtained for individual tumours. The terminal duct-lobular unit of the breast, the structure from which the majority of breast cancers arise, is composed of two types of epithelial cell [17]. The inner or luminal cells, which are potential milk-secreting cells, are surrounded by an outer basal layer of contractile myoepithelial cells. Most breast carcinomas (in some series, as high as 95%) express phenotypic markers that are consistent with an origin from luminal cells. The biology of normal luminal cells is the key to understanding breast cancer initiation, with the genetic alterations in normal cells and epithelial hyperplastic lesions driving the earliest stages of progression. Despite the luminal origin of breast tumours, some invasive ductal carcinomas in the breast also express markers specific for myoepithelial cells. Recent studies using cDNA microarray analysis of primary human breast tumours have also identified a basal-like subset of invasive ductal carcinomas, based on their patterns of gene expression. These tumours, i.e. those exhibiting a basal phenotype, have a generally more aggressive phenotype and correspondingly poorer prognosis.

Triple-negative breast cancer (TNBC), in which the cellular staining pattern is negative for ER (oestrogen receptor), PR (progesterone receptor) and human epidermal growth factor receptor (HER)-2, accounts for 15–20% of breast cancers. This is now known to be a group of widely heterogeneous diseases, not only on the molecular level, but also on the pathologic and clinical levels – see Metzger-Filho *et al.* [18] for an excellent review. TNBC is associated with a significantly higher probability of relapse and poorer overall survival in the first few years after diagnosis when compared with other breast cancer subtypes, despite relatively high sensitivity to chemotherapy. In the advanced setting, responses observed with chemotherapy tend to lack durability. The molecular complexity of TNBC has led to proposed

subclassifications which will be of real value for the development of targeted therapies – see below.

Modes of spread in breast cancer (Figure 13.3) have been the subject of great controversy. The main focus of dispute previously was whether breast cancer always spread 'centrifugally' or by direct lymphatic dissemination, before more widespread involvement in the bloodstream; or whether the latter route was possible even in the absence of local nodal involvement. It is now clear that blood-borne metastases do occur independently, although axillary node involvement is highly predictive of the probability of haematogenous spread. Local dissemination may occur to the underlying chest wall and related structures (ribs, pleura and brachial plexus), or to overlying skin. Lymphatic spread is to axillary lymph nodes and the supraclavicular, internal mammary or contralateral groups. Blood-borne metastasis occurs particularly to bone (especially the axial skeleton), liver, lung, skin and central nervous system

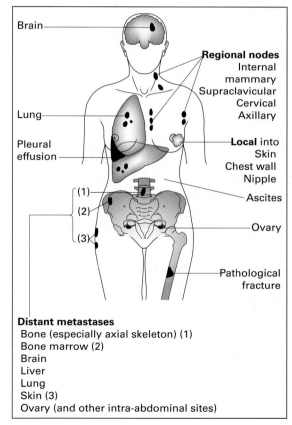

Figure 13.3 Local, nodal and distant spread in breast cancer.

(both brain and spinal cord). Intra-abdominal and pelvic metastases, including ovarian and adrenal deposits, are common. Many patients manifest particular patterns of spread, for example, widespread bone involvement without evidence of soft-tissue disease. Some patients develop relentless local recurrence of disease, cancer *en cuirasse*, without distant metastasis but with a deep fungating ulcer affecting much of the chest wall. The reasons behind these patterns are unclear and apparently unrelated to histological characteristics or pathological grade.

Haematogenous spread is of crucial importance, since patients die from distant metastases rather than from uncontrolled local disease. The likelihood of axillary lymph node metastases correlates closely with the size of the primary tumour. There is a quantitative relationship between the number of metastatic lymph nodes and survival (see also Figures 4.2 and 13.7). Internal mammary node involvement is an important early site of spread of medially placed tumours, which have a reputation for higher risk of relapse and death than tumours located elsewhere in the breast. The finding of supraclavicular lymphadenopathy at diagnosis is a particularly adverse clinical sign. Recent evidence suggests that detection of tumour cells in the bone marrow carries considerable prognostic weight [19]. Such cells presumably disseminate via the haematogenous route and recent studies have suggested that the number of identifiable circulating tumour cells prior to treatment may be an independent prognostic factor, even for overall survival. Observations relating to the natural history of breast cancer using evidence from screening programmes have suggested that breast cancer does indeed behave as a progressive disease, that time of diagnosis is important in determining outcome, and that local treatment can sometimes be totally effective for small tumours. Assessment of individual risk has also become increasingly precise.

Over the past few years, the results of clinical studies evaluating the prognostic and predictive value of genetic signatures identified through the use of gene microarray technology have become increasingly established. An important study from Holland investigated the value of a 70-gene signature in 295 early breast cancer patients, which clearly divided them into two prognostic groups. The first group consisted of 180 patients with poor prognosis (10-year survival of 55%) and the second of 115 patients with an excellent prognosis (10-year overall survival of 95%) [20]. The 70-gene signature appears to be a more powerful predictor of disease outcome than standard systems based on traditional clinical or pathological criteria, offering, for example, a better

opportunity to tailor the appropriate chemotherapy as a reflection of individual risk.

Clinical features

Most women with breast cancer present to their family doctor with a lump in the breast, although screen-detected cases are increasingly frequently encountered since the widespread adoption of mass population screening (see below). In a recent study of almost 3500 UK and European patients treated within the large TARGIT-A trial for early breast cancer (see below), over 60% of patients presented with a screen-detected cancer. (M Baum, personal communication). Most breast lumps are benign and the commonest causes are cysts, fibroadenomas or areas of fibroadenosis. Although a skilled surgeon often gives the correct clinical diagnosis, all breast lumps should be regarded as potentially malignant and firm histological diagnosis is nearly always necessary. Not all women with breast cancer present with a lump; pain in the breast, discharge or bleeding from the nipple, and pain or swelling in the axilla are also occasionally encountered.

Signs suggesting malignancy include an asymptomatic impalpable but radiologically typical lesion, with microcalcification and an opacity with radiating fibrous strands; a change within the breast noticed by the patient herself; or signs of locally advanced disease, including a large mass, tethering to skin and/or chest wall, axillary or supraclavicular lymph node enlargement, *peau d'orange*, nipple inversion and skin infiltration. Although cancers are typically firm or indurated, this may also be true of a simple cyst. Although women now present more often with relatively early disease, the lump is sometimes deliberately ignored, and can even be present for years before it becomes a fungating mass, although this now fortunately has become less common. Patients may present with symptoms from a secondary deposit, for example, in the spine or brain. These may include pain in the back due to vertebral metastasis leading to vertebral collapse and/or spinal cord compression (see pages 134–135). General symptoms such as lassitude and anorexia may reflect advanced and widespread disease, particularly liver involvement.

Confirming the diagnosis

There are several methods of confirming the diagnosis. Aspiration of cysts is easy and frequently performed.

The finding of a cyst with typical greenish fluid and disappearance of the lump after aspiration makes the diagnosis of cancer extremely unlikely. Aspiration cytology from solid lesions is fully established as a reliable diagnostic technique and it is even possible to provide prognostically useful cytological grading. If there is real diagnostic uncertainty, a much larger piece of tissue can be obtained by core biopsy with a 'Tru-cut' or other percutaneous biopsy needle, which usually yields an adequate core of tissue for histology. If the diagnosis cannot be obtained in this way, excision biopsy will be necessary. It is unjustifiable to proceed to mastectomy without giving the patient an opportunity to consider both the implications of the diagnosis and the alternative approaches for primary control of the tumour.

Mammography is widely used. On the whole, carcinomas have a characteristic mammographic appearance, with fine calcification and areas of obvious radiological irregularity; fixation of deep lesions to either chest wall or skin can sometimes be seen. The permissible radiation dose for a mammogram has now been reduced to around 7 mSv (maximum), the equivalent of 10 standard chest radiographs or an individual's average radiation exposure over a period of 3 months. There is no longer any need to compromise exposure time for fear of radiation exposure. Mammography is particularly valuable for excluding synchronous primary cancers within the breast, a finding which would have considerable bearing on the choice of operation. Additional imaging techniques include ultrasonography (often particularly valuable in the younger patient where a high breast density may make mammography unreliable) and, increasingly, magnetic resonance imaging (MRI). Although sometimes difficult to interpret with confidence, there is no doubt that an MRI can demonstrate small lesions which may be unidentifiable by other means. These imaging techniques are described more fully in Chapter 4.

Preoperative investigation

A good deal of controversy has surrounded the question of preoperative investigations that are helpful in influencing management. In some centres, patients are extensively investigated with isotope bone, liver and brain scans, together with skeletal radiography, tumour marker analyses and estimations of urinary hydroxyproline. However, the general view at present is that the most valuable tests are a chest radiograph, full blood count, simple assessment of liver function and abdominal (hepatic) ultrasonography. In short, staging is only important if it defines 'early' breast cancer, distinguishing it clearly from more advanced cases unlikely to be surgically curable. Increased scepticism regarding the role of routine (and expensive) staging investigations has led to a reduction in their use.

Staging notation

There have been several attempts to devise a simple staging system; most of the classifications depend on tumour size, the presence or absence of axillary node metastases, and the confirmation of distant metastases. The tumour node metastasis (TNM) staging system proposed by the Union Internationale Contre le Cancer (UICC) has become widely accepted (Table 13.2). Future modifications are likely to take account of more detailed information regarding the pathological grade of the tumour, and its endocrine receptor status.

Hormone receptors in breast cancer

A proportion of breast cancers carry cellular receptors for oestrogen and other steroid hormones (including progestogen) in the cell nuclei and also the cytoplasm. These receptors are present in 65% of cancers in postmenopausal women but in far fewer cancers, about 30%, in premenopausal women. *BRCA1*-associated tumours are generally negative for both oestrogen and PRs whereas *BRCA2* tumours are characteristically positive [13]. Hormone dependence of some breast cancers can be demonstrated clinically by alteration of the hormonal

Table 13.2 Simplified staging notation for breast cancer based on current UICC/TNM classification (Sobin *et al.* [111])

Stage	Description
T1*	Tumour less than 2 cm in diameter
T2*	Tumour 2–5 cm in diameter
T3*	Tumour more than 5 cm
T4	Tumour of any size with direct extension to chest wall or skin
N0	No palpable node involvement
N1	Mobile ipsilateral nodes
N2	Fixed ipsilateral nodes
N3	Supraclavicular or infraclavicular nodes or oedema of arm
M0	No distant metastases
M1	Distant metastases

*T1, T2 and T3 tumours further divide into (a) no fixation and (b) with fixation to underlying pectoral fascia or muscle.

environment (see pages 234–236). It is now established that the presence of ER in a breast cancer cell correlates with the probability of hormone dependence in an individual tumour, making it possible to predict response to hormonal treatments. This has considerable clinical implications. Oophorectomy, for example, can be avoided in patients who are known to have an ER-negative tumour. It is not entirely clear whether ER status is the reflection of a genuine and fundamental difference between 'negative' and 'positive' breast cancers or whether there is a continuum from ER-rich tumours to those with no detectable ERs whatever. The evidence at present favours the latter view, and ER 'positivity' is normally used to describe tumours in which the level of ERs is greater than a certain defined figure, usually 5 fmol/mg cytoplasmic protein, or 25 fmol/mg nuclear DNA (see Chapter 6).

ER positivity is associated with well-differentiated tumours (particularly tubular, lobular or papillary types) and with microscopic elastosis in the tumour. Clinically, it is apparent that slow-growing tumours tend to be ER-positive. Both primary tumours and metastases show similar ER content, although ER-negative metastases are sometimes encountered from an ER-positive primary tumour. The reverse is rarely true. This may relate to the fact that both ER and PR are ligand-activated transcription factors, and possibly to the complex issue of functionally distinct subtypes of ER, namely ERα and ERβ. At present, only ERα is used clinically, to help with treatment decisions [21]. How successful have ER measurements been in the prediction of hormone responsiveness? At most, only 5–7% of ER-negative tumours respond to hormone manipulation. Conversely, 55% of ER-positive tumours will respond, so ER positivity, though useful, is not entirely reliable. However, there is a detectable semi-quantitative response: tumours very rich in ERs are clinically hormone-dependent in 90% of cases. Tumours rich in PRs are usually clinically hormone-responsive (>80% of cases).

Screening for breast cancer

The general principles of cancer screening have been discussed in Chapter 2. At first sight, breast cancer would appear to be an ideal tumour for a screening programme: relatively common (1–2 cases per 1000 women per year) and relatively accessible to clinical examination by doctors, nurses, paramedical staff and by the patient herself. In addition, mammography often demonstrates a breast cancer before it is clinically evident. Furthermore, there are known groups of patients at relatively high risk: those

with a strong family history of breast cancer, those with late first pregnancies and those with a history of benign breast disease.

However, many authorities feel that unselected mass clinical and mammographic screening has still not yet been unequivocally justified by the results [22], even after massive financial input, decades of studies and exhaustive analysis of many end-points – in fact the debate has undoubtedly intensified over the past few years (and since the last edition of this text). Apart from the considerable cost, it is not entirely clear whether the true cure rate would be appreciably higher as a result of earlier detection [23], although several studies have suggested a reduction in mortality in patients over 50 years old, presumably from detection of the cancer at an earlier stage. It is often forgotten that the key point – the sole purpose and justification – of cancer screening is *not* earlier diagnosis but a proven benefit in terms of overall survival. Without a reduction in the death rate, the whole of the expensive and resource-consuming programme is pointless. These points are well discussed in the much-quoted Independent Panel Report from the UK chaired by Sir Michael Marmot and published in 2012 (See Independent UK Panel on Breast Screening report [24]). A major population-based study from Oxford, analyzing deaths over a thirty-year period, clearly failed to demonstrate any advantage for the screened cohort, attracting a great deal of national interest. In particular, a reduction in mortality was more clearly identified in the younger (unscreened) age group – see Mukhtar *et al.* [25]. However, screening of selected high-risk patients is likely to be more worthwhile. In the UK, the Forrest Report which kicked off the screening programme recommended regular screening of all women between the ages of 50 and 64 (the highest-risk age group), in line with results published in the 1980s. Taking all age groups together, the overall results so far are not entirely encouraging, which may well reflect the great advancements in treatment seen over the past 20 years – the greater the efficacy of therapy, the less is the value of the screening process. The value of screening appears particularly dubious in young women who, in more than one report, have had an overall worse survival than the unscreened group, perhaps due to a more rapid cancer growth rate in the younger patient, coupled with a sense of false security between routine scanning appointments. Breast self-examination, though widely practised, cheap and easily repeated, does not appear beneficial. Regrettably, international evidence remains substantially inconsistent – and even fundamental questions regarding, for example, the most appropriate yardstick by which to measure success, remain highly contentious: see, for instance, Penston *et al.* [26].

Several studies have now confirmed an increased rate of mammographic detection of early cancers [27] with a probable survival advantage over unscreened cases, although the false-positive rate is considerable, the cost high and the anxiety produced distressing – a point increasingly emphasized over the past few years. To give an idea of the benefit, a recent Cochrane systematic review [28] examined all the past available data and published the results in 2006. The authors concluded that screening is associated with, at best, a 20% *relative* reduction in breast cancer mortality (with higher-quality programmes and reports giving a lesser figure of about 15%). In absolute terms, this translates into one life saved by repeatedly screening 2000 women over a 10-year period. And against this small benefit is a 30% 'over-diagnosis' rate, and over-treatment, of lesions (including some cases of low-grade DCIS) that would never at any point have threatened the patient's life. This small degree of survival benefit was echoed by a further study in younger women [29], which calculated a 17% relative reduction in this group in breast cancer-specific mortality (statistically non-significant). In the UK, about 1.3 million women are now screened with mammography every year, and about 10 000 new cancers (including pure DCIS as well as cases of invasive disease) are detected annually. On the positive side, for every 1000 women aged 50–70 years who are regularly screened over a 10-year period, 10 will develop a cancer that will require mastectomy compared with 12 non-attenders who would require mastectomy. A recent estimate from the chair of the independent advisory committee of the UK's national breast screening programme (possibly the best in the world) suggested that in the UK about 1400 lives are saved annually [30]. When a screening programme begins, about 20 (prevalent) cases are detected per 1000 women. When these 'screened' women are followed up, the new (incident) cases are about 2 per 1000 per year; the cost of incident screen-detected cases is therefore between £10 000 and £25 000, and the cost of each life saved as a result of screening perhaps two to five times greater, though admittedly some authors quote a lower figure [31]. These are particularly important considerations in the context of expensive but appropriate newer targeted treatments for breast cancer, as discussed below. The effectiveness of screening depends heavily on the population uptake, and is more clear-cut in a compliant well-motivated group than, for instance, an inner-city population that might be harder to reach because of their greater social or demographic mobility. Moreover, increasing attention is now (at last) being paid to the possible disadvantages of screening, which of course must include the costs – financial, psychological and even potentially surgical – of false-positive screening tests [32]. In April 2007, the American College of Physicians issued new guidelines for younger women (40–49 years), recommending that women make an informed decision 'after learning about the benefits and harms of mammography'. One important problem only recently identified is that the effectiveness of screening mammography seems to be compromised in women taking HRT [33], presumably because of the 'high proportion of their mammograms occupied by radiologically dense tissue'.

Important questions relating to screening techniques, interval and management of intraduct non-invasive lesions have yet to be answered – see, for example, Bleyer and Welch [34]. If a screening policy is to be logically pursued, the 3-yearly interval recommended in the UK is probably too long, since a large number of 'interval' cancers still develop. In Scotland, a 'two-view' screening approach has now been adopted, despite the additional cost, in order to increase detection rate. Despite all these pitfalls, breast cancer screening is here to stay and possibly even set to expand in England to include women aged 47–73 years by 2012. Figures issued by the UK NHS Breast Screening Programme for the 12-month period between April 2006 and March 2007, are worth reproducing (see Cancer Research UK, under "Further Reading"). During this period, 1 955 825 women were screened by mammography in the UK; 15 856 cancers were detected, a rate of 8.1 per 1000 women screened. Of these, 79% were invasive cancers, 20% were non-invasive and 1% was microinvasive. Of the 12 491 patients with invasive cancers (detection rate 6.4 per 1000), 26% underwent mastectomy and 72% underwent a breast-conserving procedure. These important details have been transmitted more clearly to patients in recent years, with the recognition that the possible harms of screening – particularly in relation to over-diagnosis and possible over-treatment – have been insufficiently explained to patients in the past. The pros and cons have now been more clearly balanced in the current written advice, at least within the UK national screening programme, and many of us would see this as a most welcome step and somewhat overdue.

Attention has also increasingly turned to the possibility of chemoprevention in susceptible (but otherwise entirely normal) women – usually identified by a positive family history. Recent data from the SERM Chemoprevention group – a meta-analysis of four large randomized trials – have been much discussed (see Cuzick *et al.* [35]), largely because of the implications for possible preventative treatment using selective oestrogen-receptor modulators ("SERMs") which though highly bio-active are of course accompanied in some cases by important side-effects. The background to this work was the clear evidence over many decades of tamoxifen (and also raloxifene and others) reducing the risk of breast cancer in women at an elevated risk of disease, though with unknown effects in respect of duration of benefit. They assessed the effectiveness of selective ER modulators on breast cancer incidence, performing a meta-analysis with individual participant data from nine prevention trials which compared four selective ER modulators (SERMs; tamoxifen, raloxifene, arzoxifene, and lasofoxifene) with placebo, or in one study with tamoxifen. The primary endpoint was the incidence of all breast cancer (including ductal carcinoma *in-situ*) during a 10 year follow-up period. The Cuzick study analysed data for 83 399 women with 306 617 women-years of follow-up with a median follow-up of 65 months. Overall, they noted a 38% reduction (hazard ratio 0·62) in breast cancer incidence, with 42 women needing to be treated to prevent one breast cancer event in the first 10 years of follow-up. The reduction was larger in the first 5 years of follow-up than in years 5–10, but they noted no heterogeneity between these time periods. Perhaps not surprisingly, thromboembolic events were significantly increased with all SERMs (odds ratio [OR] 1·73), but there was a significant reduction of 34% in vertebral fractures (OR 0·66), and a smaller effect for non-vertebral fractures (OR 0·93). As a result of these observations the UK-based NICE has for the first time recommended intervention, namely that women whose family history puts them at moderate or high risk should be offered tamoxifen to be taken for 5 years. This might apply, for example, to women who have first-degree relatives developing breast cancer under the age of 40 years; two first-degree, or one first and one second-degree who developed it at any age; close relatives with ovarian cancer also carry a risk 'score'. If the computer-assisted programme following a careful family history comes out at greater than 17% overall risk, and the woman (not 'patient!' – please note) is over the age of 35 years, then treatment with tamoxifen is probably justified, unless of course there is a major complication such as a personal history of deep vein thrombosis, pulmonary embolus or other thrombotic tendency. Sensibly the NICE guideline also

stresses weight control, breastfeeding and no smoking as important additional measures to reduce the risk still further. More recently a further study from the collaborative group led by Cuzick and colleagues has demonstrated the remarkable effectiveness of anastrozole in disease prevention – this is the long-waited IBIS – II study recently published, showing a halving of reported cases of breast cancer in patients taking this agent daily for 5 years, matched against placebo control – see Cuzick *et al.* [36]. The authors randomized almost 4000 high-risk post-menopausal women; at a median follow-up of 5 years, they recorded 40 cases in the treatment group and 85 cases in the controls, though no survival difference has yet emerged. Endocrine-based prevention seems here to stay, but the risks and benefits will need careful assessment in view of the side-effects most particularly osteopenia and osteoporosis that these agents frequently produce: the key advantage of improvement in overall survival has not yet been demonstrated.

Management of the primary tumour in 'early' breast cancer

Surgical operations for breast cancer

A good deal of controversy has previously surrounded the choice of operation in patients with 'early' breast cancer, as it does, to some extent, even now. It is worth remembering that the principle of surgery in breast cancer is 'adequate control of locoregional disease' and there is no doubt that very good results, in terms of freedom from local recurrence, are achieved by mastectomy. In patients with axillary node involvement the additional use of postoperative radiotherapy will reduce the local recurrence rate still further but at the cost of an increased risk of arm swelling (lymphoedema).

With increased understanding that patients with breast cancer die not from uncontrolled local disease but from distant blood-borne metastases, there is now a much greater readiness to offer less mutilating procedures than mastectomy, wherever possible. In the USA and western Europe, conservative breast-preserving procedures are routinely employed and regarded as the treatment of choice (see below), though simple mastectomy with axillary dissection is still required in about 20% of cases, a dramatic difference from even 10 years ago. Patients requiring mastectomy include those with large or retroareolar tumours (especially in a small breast), widespread intraduct carcinoma, and multiple lesions within the same breast. Surgical reconstruction of the breast has advanced considerably over the past 10 years and there is a variety of techniques now available. The most commonly used are silicone prostheses and myocutaneous flap reconstruction. The improved contour is valuable and helps both confidence and self-image. However, the cosmetic result can be mediocre by comparison with the best results from radiotherapy, and reconstruction of the nipple is not generally performed, which is a further drawback. Myocutaneous flap reconstruction is cosmetically the most successful surgical method, but it is a far lengthier procedure than simple insertion of silicone prosthesis.

An important surgical advance, now fully established, is the recognition that the sentinel node, namely those nodes (sometimes a single one) first receiving drainage from a tumour, can be removed by very limited surgery, usually directed by radioactive-tracer scintigraphy [37]. The pathological findings correlate closely with the results of a more formal axillary dissection, offering an opportunity in the majority of patients for avoiding axillary dissection altogether, although in some parts of even the developed world, the technique is still not sufficiently widely available outside of specialist centres. Advantages of sentinel node biopsy include the avoidance of a more substantial axillary surgical procedure, with a corresponding reduction in both short- and long-term surgical morbidity, and length and cost of hospital stay. Recent interest has centred on the use of OSNA ('One-step nucleic acid amplification'), a powerful new molecular technique which assesses the axillary sample for CK-19 protein and permits almost instant and reliable analysis – see, for example, Osako *et al.* [38]. This new and less invasive approach to diagnosis has already been approved for use by the NHS in the UK and seems set to make a real impact in refining diagnosis in patients with early breast cancer.

Combinations of surgery and radiotherapy [39–41]

Following treatment by surgery alone, local recurrence of disease in the chest wall, ipsilateral lymph nodes or residual breast occurs with a frequency of 7–30% (see Table 13.3). It is more common with large tumours (above 5 cm) and with axillary node involvement. Postoperative radiotherapy greatly reduces the frequency of local recurrence, particularly in patients with axillary node-positive disease. However, most studies have shown no *survival* benefit from the routine use of radiotherapy in axillary node-positive cases, although an extremely important randomized study of postoperative radiotherapy in

Table 13.3 The 5-year survival rates in operable breast cancer.

Operation	5-year survival rate (%)
Extended mastectomy (Urban)	67
Radical mastectomy (Halsted)	69
Total mastectomy (Patey)	67
Simple mastectomy and radiotherapy (McWhirter)	66
Radical radiotherapy with local excision of tumour (Calle)	74

high-risk premenopausal women suggested a genuine survival advantage [41]. All patients (a total of 1708) received adjuvant chemotherapy following mastectomy with axillary dissection. At 10 years post mastectomy, local recurrence (9% vs 32%), overall survival (54% vs 45%) and disease-free survival (48% vs 34%) were significantly better in the irradiated group. This and similar studies will stimulate a fresh look at our current understanding of the biology of breast cancer since localized treatments are not generally held to contribute greatly to freedom from distant recurrence and overall survival. From the point of view of local recurrence, it is clear that local irradiation plays a crucially important role, an observation well documented by the large Cancer Research Campaign King's/Cambridge study (published in 1980) which compared simple mastectomy with simple mastectomy plus local irradiation [42].

Techniques of postoperative irradiation vary widely. For example, some authorities omit regional node irradiation entirely (unless there is histological evidence of axillary disease), treating only the chest wall in patients who have undergone mastectomy. Axillary irradiation should usually be avoided in patients who have undergone axillary node dissection, unless there is major involvement or extranodal disease. An example of a field arrangement with dose distribution is shown in Figure 13.4. Recent years have seen an important shift away from lengthy 6-week treatment programmes in favour of regimens using a higher dose per fraction in order to allow the overall treatment period to be halved. An important British study (the "START trial") has now confirmed that this policy is both safe and effective (see Haviland *et al.* [43]).

The initial impetus towards minimal surgical excision with breast preservation came from Geoffrey Keynes in London and, later, Baclesse in Paris and Crile in

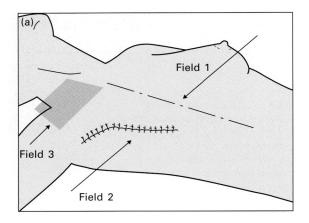

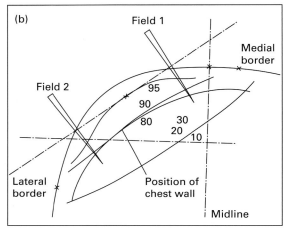

Figure 13.4 Postoperative irradiation following mastectomy. (a) Use of two wedged fields tangentially applied to irradiate chest wall, axilla and internal mammary nodes. Field 3 irradiates the supraclavicular and lower cervical nodes using a directly applied radiation beam. Many other field arrangements are in common use. (b) Transverse view showing isodose distribution from the two tangential fields (1 and 2) in relation to the breast and the chest wall.

the USA. Subsequently, large series from Calle (Institut Curie, Paris) and others have lent strong support to the safety and effectiveness of these approaches. In Calle's classic account of over 1000 cases, the results at 5 and 10 years are certainly within the range achieved by more traditional surgical approaches, and only the minority of patients in this series later required surgical resection for local recurrence [44]. About half requiring 'salvage' mastectomy subsequently proved to be long survivors, suggesting that local recurrence following 'adequate'

initial treatment may not necessarily be accompanied by widespread metastases.

An important American study from the National Surgical Adjuvant Breast Project (NSABP) on the role of breast-conserving primary treatment was initially reported in 1985 and later updated [45]. These data give strong support for the concept of breast preservation. Over 1800 patients were randomized to undergo treatment with either simple mastectomy alone, or local excision ('lumpectomy') with or without postoperative radiotherapy. After full axillary node dissection, patients with node-positive disease were given adjuvant chemotherapy. The 5-year disease-free survival rate after local excision plus radiotherapy was better than with simple mastectomy alone. Furthermore, overall survival with local excision was, if anything, also slightly better. A total of 98% of node-positive patients treated by local excision, axillary dissection, radiotherapy and adjuvant chemotherapy remained free of local recurrence, compared with 64% without radiotherapy. More recently, interest has centred on the use of partial breast irradiation techniques, including the intriguing possibility that a single dose of intraoperative irradiation may be all that is necessary in selected low-risk cases [46]. A large-scale international prospective randomized study is in progress to assess its potential, the comparison treatment being conventional external beam irradiation.

The conventional approach for early breast cancer has sharply altered over the past decade in favour of these more conservative treatments. In general, the cosmetic result of radical irradiation is highly satisfactory in the majority of cases, unlikely to be equalled by surgical reconstruction techniques. The psychological and sexual implications of mastectomy are beginning to be understood, and it is likely that the demand for radiotherapy as an alternative to mastectomy will increase even further. The question of local excision versus mastectomy has largely been answered, both by the changing preferences of surgeons and by the patients themselves. An important recent study from the USA (Eastern Cooperative Oncology Group) has strongly suggested that in women with small (T1N0M0) primary cancers who were over the age of 70 years, had undergone total surgical excision by lumpectomy and also had ER-positive tumours, radiotherapy is entirely unnecessary, provided that they receive treatment for 5 years with tamoxifen [47] (see below).

Long-term follow-up is essential, especially since features have already emerged which might, in the individual case, argue against local excision with breast preservation rather than mastectomy. These include large primary size, inadequate excision with positive margins, high *in situ* component and high tumour grade. Moreover, potential late side-effects of radiotherapy are increasingly recognized, including breast discomfort, chest wall tenderness, cardiac risks and the small but significantly increased risk of radiation-induced lung cancer [48], although fortunately the doses used nowadays are smaller than those on which these observations were initially made. For these and other reasons, including patient convenience and the heavy resource requirement of standard postoperative radiotherapy regimens, the use of partial breast irradiation (including 'single-fraction' intraoperative radiotherapy) is currently the subject of intense study, with encouraging results now published from the large international TARGIT-A randomized trial [49]. In this large UK-led international trial initially pioneered at University College London, UK, over 3400 patients were randomized between conventional external beam radiotherapy and 'single-shot' intra-operative radiotherapy given at the time of surgery, or a few weeks later when the final pathology review had confirmed that the patient was suitable for randomization. Perhaps surprisingly, the real benefit as seen in the group of patients treated with *immediate* intra-operative radiotherapy (i.e., under the same anaesthesia as the surgical resection) even though in some cases, the final pathology review later revealed unexpected adverse features, in which case the study protocol allowed for additional external beam radiotherapy. It seems likely that for patients with relatively good prognosis disease, this treatment will become more widely applied; it is certainly preferable for the many patients who live a considerable distance from a radiotherapy centre and who cannot easily remain close to the hospital for a prolonged period of weeks for treatment. A further benefit is the strong hint that the overall survival may be better than with conventional radiotherapy because of avoidance of radiotherapy-related damage to the heart and also the carcinogenic effect of external-beam radiotherapy. The 2013 update of the TARGIT trial confirmed a rate of fatal cardiovascular complications of 11 cases in the external-beam group compared with 2 in the TARGIT group, and 16 versus 8 cases of fatal new or second cancers (all deaths coded for cause-of-death by a senior clinician unconnected with the study and blinded to initial treatment). Breast cancer-related mortality was the same in both groups. An alternative approach to intra-operative radiotherapy pioneered by the Veronesi group in Milan – the ELIOT trial (Electron Intra-operative radiotherapy Trial) - has yielded less satisfactory results in terms of local control of the primary tumour – see Veronesi *et al.* [50].

Adjuvant hormone and cytotoxic therapy are discussed on pages 234–240.

Management of the primary tumour in advanced breast cancer

For patients with locally advanced disease (T3, T4 and the majority of patients with N1B or N2 disease) the results of mastectomy have been disappointing. Surgery is contraindicated apart from debulking operations (often referred to as 'toilet' mastectomy), which can be extremely valuable together with radiotherapy, chemotherapy and hormone treatment to give the best possible chance of local control. Such surgical procedures are particularly helpful with fungating, bulky, exophytic cancers.

Radiotherapy is generally preferred; given cautiously, a high dose can often be achieved, with a local control rate as high as 90% at 5 years, although the overall survival in such patients is only 20–25%. The probability of local control is inversely related to the size of the primary tumour [51,52], and features such as fixation to the chest wall, fixed axillary lymphadenopathy or involvement of supraclavicular lymph nodes contribute both to inoperability and to a higher probability of local recurrence. A high local dose is essential.

In some cases, particularly elderly patients with hormone receptor-positive disease, radiotherapy can initially be withheld and the patient treated with an aromatase inhibitor such as letrozole or anastrozole. These agents can produce remarkable responses even in patients with advanced fungating local disease, and it is usually clear by 6 weeks after starting treatment whether or not there has been a worthwhile response. In younger women, treatment with chemotherapy may be more rapidly effective; this is usually regarded as the treatment of choice (see below). Where appropriate, even elderly patients should be considered for chemotherapy since tolerance in this age group can be surprisingly good, with appropriate antiemetics and other supportive measures.

Complications of local treatment
Lymphoedema
This is due to lymphatic and venous obstruction and is a frequent (about 10%) and troublesome sequel to treatment for breast cancer, particularly when both radical surgery and radiotherapy have been used. Other factors contributing to its development include infection

and recurrent or persistent disease. If lymphoedema appears years after primary treatment, axillary recurrence of tumour is the likely explanation. Apart from the disfigurement, the swelling can be very uncomfortable, and can also be a focus for spreading subcutaneous infection (cellulitis).

Management of the swollen arm is difficult and often unsuccessful. The patient should be instructed in isometric exercises with the arm elevated, in an attempt to improve the muscle pump. Avoidance of infection is essential; the patient must take care not to damage the skin of the affected arm, and wear gloves for tasks such as gardening. Cellulitis must be treated promptly with antibiotics. If local recurrence of tumour is confirmed, it is usually better treated with systemic therapy rather than further radiotherapy, in order to avoid additional radiation damage. Compression sleeves are sometimes helpful in massaging fluid out of the limb but they often need to be used for several hours to be effective. Nocturnal elevation of the arm (e.g. by a roller towel arrangement or by resting on pillows) is often recommended if the patient can tolerate it. Nurse-led lymphoedema clinics skilled in management of this complication are an important part of the oncology department – an effective but labour-intensive aspect of care.

Stiff or frozen shoulder

Patients undergoing mastectomy should be given a programme of graded exercises postoperatively in order to increase shoulder mobility, prevent stiffness and help prevent lymphoedema. The aim is to develop normal elevation and rotation in the shoulder joint. Abduction and elevation of the arm are most important. If a frozen shoulder has developed, physiotherapy and short-wave diathermy are helpful.

Restoring a normal breast contour

Many women adapt well to an external prosthesis, but breast reconstruction – either performed by a skilled surgeon or wherever available an oncoplastic surgeon with a special interest in breast reconstruction – should in general be considered for those women who wish to pursue it. Not all women will wish to proceed, and it can be an exhausting though often very rewarding part of "aftercare" for patients who inevitably have already been through a great deal of anxiety and discomfort. It is often helpful to reassure patients who are about to undergo mastectomy that early breast reconstruction is feasible, and regarded by the surgeon as part of the primary treatment, if the patient so wishes. Of the various alternative techniques, simple silicone or saline implant (with a tissue expander if necessary) is the most straightforward, but more complex surgery including the latissimus dorsi or transverse rectus abdominis muscle flap, though more demanding for the patient, do provide a better final result. Nipple reconstruction is best achieved by use of pigmented skin transfer (from upper thigh) but remains a difficult surgical challenge. These and other details of breast reconstruction are well covered in a recent review – see Thiruchelvam et al. [53]. One cautionary note is that it is imperative to consider the oncological needs of the patient first and the reconstructive or cosmetic aspects of care as an important but secondary consideration; no point in proceeding to an aesthetically beautiful reconstruction in an inadequately treated patient.

Psychological disturbance

Any form of mastectomy is mutilating, especially radical mastectomy. The incidence of depression and psychosexual disorders is about 25% during the first year and these are more severe in women who place particular emphasis on their body image. Preoperative and postoperative counselling is certainly helpful and the role of patient support and counselling groups is discussed in Chapter 7. Although patients undergoing treatment without loss of the breast clearly suffer a range of psychological disturbances, these seem to be different from those encountered in patients who have required mastectomy. The most difficult period is generally the initial 6 months after primary treatment.

Adjuvant hormone therapy, chemotherapy and targeted therapy

Since patients with breast cancer often develop disseminated disease from undetectable micrometastases present at the diagnosis, attention has increasingly been paid to the concept of adjuvant systemic therapy following primary local treatment. The aim is to eradicate these deposits before they become clinically apparent, an approach supported by animal data suggesting that small metastases are more chemosensitive. Although most of the initial trials were far too small to detect the difference with certainty, more recent studies and large powerful meta-analyses have clarified the degree of benefit and long-term outcome from adjuvant systemic treatment [51,52,54].

Adjuvant hormone therapy

Following the demonstration that oophorectomy caused regression of advanced breast cancer, many studies of ovarian ablation following primary surgery have been performed, and its effect in randomized comparisons of patients with ER-positive disease has been repeatedly and convincingly demonstrated. In the early 1970s, the increasing use of tamoxifen, essentially an agent with antioestrogenic properties but also a weak oestrogen agonist, revolutionized breast cancer treatment. The large Oxford-based 2005 overview of all prospectively randomized studies of tamoxifen (and adjuvant chemotherapy as well) showed unequivocally that there is a real, worthwhile and long-term survival benefit in patients given tamoxifen for at least 2 years after initial treatment [52] (Figure 13.5). The benefits of adjuvant tamoxifen therapy for patients who are ER-positive, in terms of reduction in overall mortality from breast cancer, applies to both node-negative and node-positive cases, and clearly persist for at least 15 years following therapy; this remarkable biological observation following a treatment which was discontinued years previously was accurately described as 'a long-term gain from a short-term treatment'. Perhaps unexpectedly, the benefit is even greater at 15 years despite discontinuation of treatment at 5 years, and it

now seems clear from at least two studies that treatment beyond 5 years is required for maximum effect. These are the UK-based aTTom (Adjuvant Tamoxifen: Offer More?) and ATLAS (Adjuvant Tamoxifen, Longer against Shorter) trials.

The large multicentre aTTom trial randomized 6952 patients between 1991 and 2005 to 5 versus 10 years treatment, and was recently presented (Gray et al. [55]), demonstrating a clear-cut benefit of longer exposure to tamoxifen, as follows: overall recurrence rates were 16.7% (10 year group) and 19.3% (5 year group). Compared with 5 years of treatment, 10 years of tamoxifen was associated both with a significant 15% reduction in risk of recurrence and also a 25% reduction in risk of breast cancer mortality starting at year 10. These findings aligned closely with those from the multicentre ATLAS Trial (C. Davies and R. Peto, ATLAS preliminary results, San Antonio Breast Cancer Conference, 2012). Pooled analysis of the 17 477 patients enrolled in these two trials showed an impressive 9% reduction in the risk of death for patients receiving 10 versus 5 years of tamoxifen for the entire follow-up period. Furthermore, the relative risk reduction increased to 16% starting at year 10. In the ATLAS trial, the largest breast cancer study yet reported, the preliminary results are broadly similar. Over 11 500 patients from 38 countries were randomized at 5 years if still disease-free and either ER-positive or unknown. At 5–9 years from randomization, there was a statistically significant reduction in recurrence rate, with a hazard ratio (HR) of 0.88 – a 12% benefit ($P = 0.005$).

Taken together, these two studies will certainly prove to be highly influential in future management. There may also be additional benefits from the cholesterol-lowering effect of tamoxifen (with reduction in frequency of death from myocardial infarction) and from the significant protection it appears to offer against postmenopausal bone loss. On the other hand, there is no doubt that tamoxifen is associated with an increased incidence of both endometrial carcinoma and, much more rarely, uterine sarcoma [56,57]. As pointed out by Fisher and colleagues in a recent landmark article [54], the benefits of tamoxifen are sustained for at least 15 years following treatment; they also pointed out that 'the notion that use of tamoxifen or chemotherapy should be based only on age is too restrictive'. Recent work from a community-based study from Scotland also underscored the key importance of adhering to the full course of tamoxifen. McCowan and colleagues calculated that the lives of more than 400 women from the UK annually could be saved each year if patients took a full 5-year

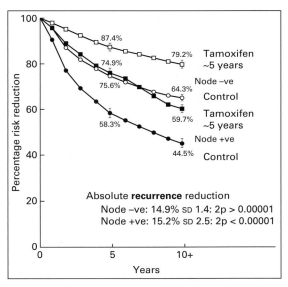

Figure 13.5 Absolute reduction in risk of recurrence of breast cancer following tamoxifen. Open symbols, node-negative cases; closed symbols, node-positive cases. (Source: Early Breast Cancer Trialists' Collaborative Group [52]. Reproduced with permission from Elsevier.)

course despite the sometimes severe side-effects – see McCowan et al. [58]. They analysed prescription records for 1263 women diagnosed with breast cancer between 1993 and 2000, to see how often they took tamoxifen, and for how long. Women who collected fewer than 80% of their prescriptions were classed as having low adherence to treatment and the findings showed 434 lives a year could be saved alongside millions of GBP pounds if women took the full course. About 13 000 women a year are prescribed a five-year course of tamoxifen but sadly, too many are clearly not completing this, complaining of hot flushes, joint pain, fatigue, weight gain and sweats. The Glasgow group found that low-adherence patients had a higher chance of their cancer recurring, with earlier death and on average, loss of reasonable quality of life of about 13 months. Difficult decisions often need to be made in respect of 'best choice' adjuvant therapy in each individual case, balancing against side-effects which some (a small but sizeable minority) find barely acceptable (see also below). This problem becomes more urgent still, when considering that many more patients now will be advised to continue for ten years, bearing in mind the recent aTTom and ATLAS study results.

Several large-scale studies have now been reported in which aromatase inhibitors have been compared with standard tamoxifen therapy for postmenopausal patients. The largest of these, the ATAC trial, showed that anastrozole (1 mg orally per day) was both more effective and less toxic than tamoxifen given at the standard 20-mg daily dose, with benefits clearly persisting well beyond discontinuation of the 5 years of adjuvant treatment [59]. The major end-points of disease-free survival, time to recurrence and time to distant recurrence were all significantly improved in the anastrozole group, with the outcome curves still separating at over 8 years. The absolute benefit in terms of disease-free recurrence rose from 2.8% at 5 years to 4.8% at 9 years, and the long-term relative benefit was approximately 15% (HR for all recurrences 0.85). Moreover, the newer agent was better tolerated, with a dramatic reduction in the risk of serious thromboembolic complications and gynaecological symptoms such as vaginal bleeding and discharge. In the group of 3116 patients treated with tamoxifen, 24 patients developed endometrial carcinoma, compared with only five in the similar-sized anastrozole group. Another important study suggested that offering the aromatase inhibitor letrozole for an additional 5 years beyond the standard 5-year tamoxifen regimen also gives additional benefit in reducing the risk of recurrence [60], although the recent ATLAS results suggesting at

least some continued benefit for tamoxifen given beyond 5 years clearly blunts the potential benefit seen in the letrozole study, as the tamoxifen comparator group consisted only of 5 years' treatment in all cases. In addition, in an important 'switching' study, exemestane, an oral steroidal aromatase inhibitor, has been shown to benefit patients when substituted for tamoxifen in a 5-year programme, approximately halfway through the treatment [61]. In this large and influential study of over 4700 patients, Coombes and colleagues showed that this 'switch' approach led to an impressive improvement in disease-free survival with an absolute benefit of 3.3% and, for the first time in any study involving the use of an adjuvant aromatase inhibitor, 'a modest improvement in overall survival'. Likewise, a switch from tamoxifen to anastrozole after 2–3 years has also shown an impressive improvement [62], strongly suggesting that for postmenopausal patients whose initial adjuvant treatment has been with tamoxifen, there are clear-cut advantages of switching to an aromatase inhibitor after 2–3 years, regardless of which of the available agents is chosen. One interesting new departure is the opportunity for offering neoadjuvant endocrine therapy, that is, prior to the conventional 'surgery first' approach. In postmenopausal hormone receptor-positive patients, the use of an aromatase inhibitor (anastrozole or letrozole) given preoperatively for just 2 weeks is currently being trialled (Pre-Operative Endocrine Therapy Individualising Care or POETIC). Surrogate end-points will include a dynamic assessment of Ki67 activity before and after treatment, which is already known to give a reliable indicator of long-term benefit.

In ER-positive premenopausal patients, ovarian ablation with luteinizing hormone releasing hormone (LHRH) agonists such as goserelin (Zoladex) has been claimed to be as effective as CMF (cyclophosphamide, methotrexate and 5-fluorouracil) chemotherapy [63], and for selected patients international breast cancer guidelines now recommend this form of treatment as an alternative or addition to chemotherapy [64]. LHRH agonists provide the first reliably reversible form of oestrogen suppression, leading to a temporary postmenopausal state. The benefits appear to be enhanced by simultaneously delivering tamoxifen, in contrast to the situation in postmenopausal patients where we now know that the anastrozole–tamoxifen combination is no more effective than tamoxifen alone. A recent meta-analysis of almost 12 000 premenopausal women with early breast cancer, randomized within 16 prospectively controlled trials using an LHRH agonist alone or together with tamoxifen and/or chemotherapy, showed how effective this form of treatment could be [65]. In combination with tamoxifen, LHRH agonists reduced the recurrence rate by 12.7% and death after recurrence by over 15%, a similar level of efficacy to results obtained with chemotherapy, but with a far better degree of tolerability.

Adjuvant chemotherapy

Chemotherapy in breast cancer is firmly established as one of the major therapeutic modalities. Although introduced much more recently than other treatments, chemotherapy has assumed increasing importance, both in primary management (as adjuvant therapy) and for patients with metastatic disease. Responses have been documented to many classes of drug, including alkylating agents, antimetabolites, spindle poisons, antitumour antibiotics, taxanes and several others. The observation of objective tumour response, coupled with frequent improvement in subjective well-being, makes these agents well worth considering in the management of metastatic disease. In general, skin, lymph node and soft-tissue metastases respond more readily than deposits in the liver or lung, which in turn are more likely to respond than bone metastases. Previous responsiveness to hormone therapy does not appear to predict the probability of response to chemotherapy. Over the past few years, it has become clear that taxanes such as docetaxel and paclitaxel have marked activity in breast cancer and may be particularly useful in treating recurrent or metastatic tumours that are no longer responsive to traditional agents.

It is usual to employ cytotoxic drugs in combination in breast cancer, rather than as single agents. Early work using a five-drug regimen comprising vincristine, methotrexate, cyclophosphamide, prednisolone and 5-fluorouracil suggested that very high response rates could be obtained, but greater experience showed that the response rate was nearer 50%. Since that time a variety of different combination regimens have been used (Table 13.4), although the most effective combination of drugs is uncertain. Many include doxorubicin or epirubicin, clearly amongst the most active single agents for breast cancer, both at relapse and as part of adjuvant regimens (see below). Treatment with intermittent combination chemotherapy has now replaced low-dose continuous administration, and toxicity is largely predictable but usually no worse than would be expected from the additive use of the single agents chosen. For CMF, for example, the major problems are nausea, stomatitis and cystitis; for VAP (vincristine, doxorubicin and

prednisone) the commonest side-effects are neuropathy and alopecia. Treatment regimens change and progress rapidly in breast cancer, and neither CMF nor VAP are now in such widespread use. The taxane group has emerged as an important additional class of agents in patients resistant to doxorubicin, and is now increasingly used in adjuvant regimens (see pages 237–240). Use of weekly adjuvant paclitaxel programmes is becoming more widespread, particularly since the publication of an important study comparing this regimen with more standard 3-weekly treatment (see Sparano *et al.* in Further reading). The advent and widespread use of adjuvant chemotherapy has revolutionized breast cancer care over the past 30 years. The very first study, that of Nissen-Meyer and coworkers at the Oslo Cancer Institute [66], suggested that cyclophosphamide given immediately after surgery could improve survival at 10 years.

The unpredictable nature of breast cancer and the need for lengthy follow-up (Figure 13.6) make interpretation of more recent studies extremely difficult, but it is clear (again from worldwide data generated by the Early Breast Cancer Trialists Collaborative Group) that adjuvant chemotherapy had a substantial impact on both disease-free and overall survival in node-positive premenopausal patients, particularly in women aged 30–40 years. As Peto has pointed out, small improvements in survival may be translated into thousands of lives saved in a condition such as breast cancer where the incidence is so high. Recent work has also focussed on the serious detriment to overall survival relating to poor patient compliance with tamoxifen in patients unable to complete at least five years of adjuvant treatment. Subgroups of node-negative patients with adverse features such as large or high-grade primary tumour also benefit from adjuvant chemotherapy. Adverse prognostic features include tumour size greater than 3 cm, poorly differentiated tumours, nuclear pleomorphism, hormone receptor negativity, high proliferation rate and expression of ErbB2 protein. Young patients, diagnosed under the age of 35 years, should also be treated with adjuvant chemotherapy regardless of node status or other features, since they have much to gain from chemotherapy. More recently, neoadjuvant therapy has been tested for breast cancer in a number of randomized controlled trials. In this approach, the chemotherapy is given as primary treatment, prior to surgery or radiotherapy. Although an interesting concept in breast cancer, it is too early to know whether such preoperative treatment will prove in the long run more effective than the conventional sequence of treatment. In patients with smaller, operable tumours,

Table 13.4 Examples of combination chemotherapy regimens for advanced breast cancer.

Regimens	Dose and route
CMF	
Cyclophosphamide	100 mg/m^2 p.o. days 1 – 14
Methotrexate	40 mg/m^2 i.v. days 1 + 8
5-Fluorouracil	600 mg/m^2 i.v. days 1 + 8 (repeated every 28 days) (many variants)
VAP	
Vincristine	2 mg i.v. days 1 + 8
Doxorubicin	40 – 50 mg/m^2 day 1
Prednisolone	30 mg/day for 7 days (repeated every 21 days)
AC	
Cyclophosphamide	1 g/m^2 i.v. day 1
Doxorubicin M-M-M	40 mg/m^2 i.v. day 1 (repeated every 21 days)
Melphalan	10 mg p.o. per day for 3 days
Methotrexate	50 mg i.v. bolus day 1 (every 21 days)
Mitomycin C	15 mg i.v. bolus (given every alternate course, i.e. every 6th week)

Standard chemotherapy regimens

Anthracycline-containing chemotherapy should be considered the norm. There is no objective evidence to distinguish between the various 'second-generation' anthracycline regimens. However, there is evidence for a dose-response effect for epirubicin, with doses of 90 – 100 mg/m^2 being more effective than lower doses; FEC100 and E-CMF are preferred for fitter patients.

FEC100: 5-fluorouracil 500 mg/m^2, epirubicin 100 mg/m^2 and cyclophosphamide 500 mg/m^2 every 3 weeks for six cycles

E-CMF: epirubicin 100 mg/m^2 every 3 weeks for four cycles *then* cyclophosphamide 600 mg/m^2, methotrexate 40 mg/m^2 and 5-fluorouracil 600 mg/m^2 on days 1 and 8 every 4 weeks for four cycles

For higher-risk patients

The NICE Technology Assessment recommends that docetaxel be considered as an option for women with node-positive disease. A taxane regimen is advised for all fit patients who can expect a 3% or greater marginal benefit, equating to a benefit of about 12% or greater from an anthracycline regimen (see above). FEC – docetaxel (the PACS 01 regimen) is preferred over TAC on the grounds of (probably at least) equivalent efficacy, reduced toxicity with no automatic requirement for primary granulocyte colony-stimulating factor, and cost.

FEC100 – docetaxel: FEC every 3 weeks for three cycles *then* docetaxel 100 mg/m^2 every 3 weeks for three cycles

Other regimens

FEC75 is probably of intermediate efficacy between FEC100 and CMF-type chemotherapy and may be considered for patients who are unlikely to withstand FEC100. Patients who are fit enough to be treated with docetaxel should not be given FEC75 in place of FEC100. AC (×4) and CMF have equivalent efficacy, which is approximately two-thirds of that of FEC or E-CMF. Their use should be reserved for patients for whom anthracyclines are contraindicated (CMF) or for elderly or unfit patients or where longer or more intensive treatment is unlikely to be tolerated (AC).

FEC75: 5-fluorouracil 600 mg/m^2, epirubicin 75 mg/m^2 and cyclophosphamide 600 mg/m^2 every 3 weeks for six cycles

AC: doxorubicin 60 mg/m^2 and cyclophosphamide 600 mg/m^2 every 3 weeks for four cycles

CMF: cyclophosphamide 600 mg/m^2, methotrexate 40 mg/m^2 and 5-fluorouracil 600 mg/m^2 on days 1 and 8 every 4 weeks for six cycles

Cardiac assessment and anthracyclines

Routine pre-anthracycline assessment of left ventricular function is advised for all patients who:

- have a cardiac history
- are treated for a cardiovascular condition including hypertension
- have an obviously abnormal ECG
- are 65 or older.

Anthracyclines should be avoided in patients with a baseline left ventricular ejection fraction (LVEF) of <50%. LVEF should be rechecked after a cumulative epirubicin dose of not more than 400 mg/m^2 for patients with a baseline LVEF of <60%; treatment should only be continued in exceptional cases.

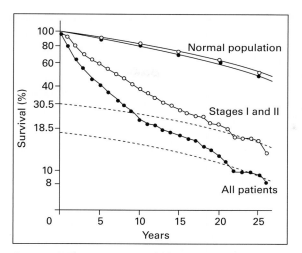

Figure 13.6 The 25-year survival of patients with breast cancer. Dashed lines are an extrapolation parallel to the indicated proportion 'cured' at 25 years. (Source: Brinkley and Haybittle [88]. Reproduced with permission from Elsevier.)

however, it now seems clear that administering adjuvant chemotherapy should take precedence over postoperative radiation therapy [67]. This means that for a large proportion of premenopausal women (including virtually all node-positive cases), the current sequence of therapy should be, first, local surgical excision plus axillary dissection or sentinel-node biopsy wherever available; second, adjuvant systemic combination chemotherapy; and, finally, radiation therapy – a dramatic change even from 15 years ago. Patients should also receive systemic adjuvant hormone therapy (generally with either tamoxifen or an aromatase inhibitor) if they are ER-positive. In addition, the use of trastuzumab (Herceptin) has also become fully established in selected cases (see below).

The difficulty in assessment of early results of adjuvant therapy is discussed more fully in Chapter 2. These problems are particularly acute in breast cancer in view of the lengthy follow-up required. It is not a simple matter to give an unqualified answer to the question whether adjuvant chemotherapy is of benefit to *all* patients with early breast cancer. The advantage is probably confined to subgroups of patients, and may not be substantially greater than with adjuvant hormone therapy, generally a far less toxic form of treatment. The toxicity of combination chemotherapy can be considerable (although many patients have little difficulty), so this is clearly an area where a possible benefit must be weighed against the quality of the patient's life (see Chapter 7), particularly

bearing in mind that hormone therapy in ER-positive premenopausal patients clearly has a major role, possibly as great as chemotherapy [52,59–62].

Adjuvant chemotherapy is now widely used in postmenopausal and, more particularly, premenopausal patients. It is almost always offered to patients with premenopausal node-positive tumours and, in addition, to many patients with high-grade tumours even if node-negative. The initial CMF programme has now been almost completely superseded by anthracycline-containing regimens such as AC (doxorubicin plus cyclophosphamide) or FEC (using the less toxic anthracycline epirubicin). Sequential use of anthracyclines as well as CMF has become widely practised, following presentation of results from the NEAT trial [68]. In this large prospective randomized study, four cycles of epirubicin (E) followed by four cycles of CMF were compared with six to eight cycles of CMF alone (2391 women in total). At a median follow-up of 4 years, the relapse-free and overall survival rates were significantly higher in the E-CMF groups. The 5-year overall survival was increased from 75% with CMF alone to 82% with E-CMF.

In addition, the taxanes are increasingly used in the adjuvant setting, particularly for patients with high-risk disease [69]. Mature data from four large randomized studies using either paclitaxel or docetaxel have now been presented, notably the CALGB 244 study [70], in which patients with node-positive disease were randomly assigned to receive either four cycles of AC or the same regimen followed by further cycles of paclitaxel. The latter group had a consistently lower rate of relapse, which became apparent at an early follow-up (21 months, sustained at 5 years). This benefit was disproportionately seen in patients with hormone receptor-negative disease. However, recent studies have strongly suggested that the benefit of adding a taxane to the adjuvant chemotherapy protocol for node-positive patients is strongly linked to overexpression of HER2 [71]. In this large trial (data from 1322 patients), for HER2-negative cases there was no appreciable advantage in ER-positive patients, whereas the outcome in ER-negative patients was indeed improved by adding paclitaxel. Moreover, a recent large UK-based study investigating the incorporation of docetaxel to standard therapy for high-risk patients has failed to support the initial finding of additional benefit for this taxane agent (see Ellis *et al.* in Further reading). In light of the increasing use of newer therapies such as the taxanes and targeted therapy, particularly trastuzumab and lapatinib (see below), some authorities are beginning to challenge the long-held view that hazardous treatment with doxorubicin, previously a mainstay of adjuvant chemotherapy, is unavoidable for best outcomes (see Pegram *et al.* in Further reading). The question is of course particularly acute when considering the potential long-term cardiotoxicity that complicates treatment with both doxorubicin (irreversible) and trastuzumab (partly, if not fully reversible). Recent work suggests that the real value of using doxorubicin, with its many side-effects, may well be confined to patients who are HER2-positive. Another suggestion rapidly gaining ground is that amplification of the topoisomerase IIα gene may be even more important than HER2 amplification in the prediction of response to anthracycline agents such as doxorubicin and epirubicin. These recent observations are set to have a profound effect on the tailoring of breast cancer adjuvant therapy over the next few years.

Treatment with dose-dense chemotherapy programmes has also become increasingly widely used over the past few years. The most influential demonstration of chemotherapy 'acceleration' comes from a study by Citron and colleagues, who demonstrated a statistically superior survival for the dose-dense schedules [72].

Decisions regarding the potential benefit from offering adjuvant chemotherapy for both premenopausal and postmenopausal patients have become easier since the widespread introduction of computer-aided risk-benefit assessment tools, for example, Adjuvant! (www.adjuvantonline.com). These are based on simple criteria such as age, nodal status, size and pathological grade of the primary tumour, receptor characteristics and so on, and are now widely available as hand-held PC programs.

The current guidelines for use of adjuvant chemotherapy in our department at University College Hospital are shown below.

Guidelines for adjuvant chemotherapy
General principles

- Patients should be considered for and offered adjuvant therapy clinical trials whenever available.
- Adjuvant systemic therapy with endocrine treatment and/or cytotoxic chemotherapy improves relapse-free and overall survival in all age groups.
- The absolute reduction in risk is greatest in those women at greatest risk of relapse.
- The risk–benefit ratio of adjuvant systemic therapy must be considered for each patient individually.

- Assessment of the trade-off between potential benefits and toxicity from adjuvant systemic therapy is subjective; women should be supported in making an informed choice.
- The benefits of endocrine therapy and chemotherapy are independent and should not be considered as alternatives.

Patient selection

Recent studies have in general supported the emerging view that, at least in principle, there is no group of women with primary breast cancer who will not derive some benefit from adjuvant chemotherapy. However, decisions regarding specifically which patients should be offered this demanding treatment should be based on their individually estimated risk of breast cancer death and/or reduction of risk of recurrence offered by chemotherapy, together with the toxicity of treatment and the other co-morbidities from which the patient might be suffering. Four of the main factors that determine the likely benefit from treatment are discussed below. In addition, the past few years have seen an important additional advance in the ER-positive group, namely the use of genetic Recurrence Score testing ('Oncotype DX') which relies on a panel of 21 genes for analysis – the purpose being to assess the potential value of adjuvant chemotherapy in this large patient group. The test is designed to predict the likelihood of tumour recurrence within the first ten years of treatment, on the assumption that the patient will be taking tamoxifen for 5 years, giving a score between 0 and 100 and dividing the patients on an individual basis into Low, Intermediate or High Risk. The Oncotype DX test, which depends on PCR methodology, was initially developed for women with early-stage invasive node-negative breast cancer. However, analysis of tissue samples from a separate study, the large US-based SWOG 8814 clinical trial, showed that the Oncotype DX test also provided useful prognostic and predictive significance in women with either node-negative or positive early breast cancer receiving adjuvant endocrine treatment, and smaller studies with breast cancer patients receiving neoadjuvant treatment show similar results suggesting that the test may predict response to neoadjuvant hormonal therapy and also – admittedly from a smaller subset of data from the SWOG 8814 study – the likelihood of benefit from chemotherapy (the regimen used was CAF) – see Albain *et al.* [73]. The authors found that women whose tumours scored low on the genetic test appeared to gain little or no advantage from CAF chemotherapy added to tamoxifen, while those with higher scores seemed to derive major benefit. The disease-free survival hazards were strikingly different: for the low-risk group (recurrence score <18), 1.02 and for the high-RS group (recurrence score ≥31), 0.59. The 21-gene recurrence score test is now increasingly used for many patients with node-negative breast cancer to help determine whether a patient is likely to benefit from chemotherapy and may similarly predict chemotherapy benefit in node-positive patients. According to Dr Albain, when it comes to predicting likely relative benefit from chemotherapy, the data suggest that it does not seem to matter whether the lymph nodes are involved or not – the recurrence score on the genetic assay has greater prognostic impact – a potentially important departure from traditional belief.

How great is the risk of recurrent disease?
Risk has traditionally been defined by the pathological parameters of nodal involvement, grade and tumour size, modified by secondary parameters including receptor expression and vascular invasion.

Age
• Relative chemotherapy effect declines with age. The benefit of chemotherapy in a woman of 60–69 with ER-positive disease is approximately 50% of that of a woman of 40–49 with a similar tumour.
• Chemotherapy should not be offered routinely to women of 70 or older because of lack of evidence for efficacy, but could be considered for those at high risk, especially if ER and PR negative.
• Chemotherapy should be discussed with all women under 40 and be considered the norm for those under 35 as there is a disproportionate risk in this group of patients, especially those apparently low-grade diseases.

Receptor status
• Chemotherapy is relatively less effective for women with ER-positive and/or PR-positive disease over the age of 50. The situation in younger women is less clear-cut because of chemotherapy-induced ovarian failure. The 2000 overview suggests that steroid hormone receptor status is unimportant but several recent trials using chemotherapy not particularly likely to cause ovarian failure suggest an attenuated effect in hormone receptor-positive disease.
• The risk for women with HER2-positive disease is increased, with best estimates suggesting a relative risk of 1.5–1.7. Anthracycline chemotherapy produces an equal proportional benefit in HER2-positive and HER2-negative disease. There are no data on the interaction between steroid hormone receptor and HER2 status in terms of response to adjuvant chemotherapy.

Choice of chemotherapy
Patients should be offered effective chemotherapy. The standard recommended regimens in the North London Cancer Network (NLCN) are FEC100 and E-CMF. Higher risk patients with node-positive disease can be offered FEC100-docetaxel.

TNBC represents a particular challenge – see, for example, Carey [74]. TNBC, now recognized as a group of separate conditions of generally poor prognosis, shares morphological and genetic abnormalities with basal-like breast cancer, a subgroup of breast cancer defined specifically by gene-expression profiling. Breast cancers found in BRCA1 mutation carriers are also frequently triple-negative and basal-like. TNBC and basal-like breast cancer occur most frequently in young women, especially African Americans, and tend towards aggressive and metastatic behaviour. These tumours usually respond to conventional chemotherapy in the first instance, but relapse more frequently than hormone receptor-positive, luminal subtypes, and in general have a worse prognosis. New systemic therapies are urgently needed as most patients with TNBC and/or basal-like will relapse with distant metastases, and hormonal therapies and HER2-targeted agents are ineffective in this group of tumours. Poly (ADP-ribose) polymerase inhibitors, angiogenesis inhibitors, EGFR-targeted agents, and src kinase and mTOR inhibitors are among the therapeutic agents being actively investigated in clinical trials in patients with TNBC and/or BRCA1-associated tumours. Increased understanding of the genetic abnormalities involved in the pathogenesis of TNBC, basal-like and BRCA1-associated breast cancer is opening up several new therapeutic possibilities for these very difficult breast cancers.

Targeted therapies in breast cancer
A landmark study comparing the addition of the humanized monoclonal antibody trastuzumab (Herceptin) to chemotherapy in patients with high-risk or metastatic disease was published by Slamon and colleagues in 2001 [75] - and also see Slamon *et al.* [76], for subsequent work from this same group in the area of adjuvant therapy with trastuzumab, together with Chapter 6 for a fuller account of the biology of this crucially important targeted therapy. All patients were known to have tumours expressing the growth factor receptor gene *HER-2* (human epidermal

growth factor receptor), an adverse risk factor in breast cancer present in about 25% of all cases. Responses and survival were increased, with an impressive improvement in the progression-free interval, from 4.6 to 7.4 months, though at the cost of increased cardiotoxicity. The improvement may be small but the study clearly represents a real step forward in application of specific target-directed biological therapy. Several other studies have confirmed these observations and this agent is now widely used as part of initial adjuvant systemic therapy in selected high-risk patients, mostly with high-grade hormone receptor-negative tumours.

This new and exciting area of research (see Chapter 6) has resulted in extraordinarily rapid progress, and many new conceptual insights in the management of breast cancer. Until relatively recently, the dream of focussing cytotoxic therapy more precisely to the malignant cell had been a long-standing but unfulfilled ambition of oncologists over many years, and seemed destined to remain so. However, in both breast cancer and many other areas, we have witnessed a revolution in treatment approaches as a result of the increasing availability of active targeted agents. In breast cancer, the first of these, trastuzumab, almost immediately made a major impact in the management of early or localized disease. This humanized monoclonal antibody binds to the extracellular segment of the erb-B2 receptor, and tumour cells treated with trastuzumab appear to have significantly diminished angiogenic potential and therefore a sharply reduced tendency to metastasize (see also Chapter 6). Amplification of erb-B2 occurs in about 25% of patients with early breast cancer and encodes the transmembrane tyrosine kinase p185 ErbB2 glycoprotein.

It has clearly become imperative to assess HER-2 status in every patient, so that suitability for targeted therapy can be reliably identified. If the breast cancer does not over-express it, trastuzumab will have no beneficial effect and may even cause harm. The most commonly employed methods for this are immunohistochemistry (IHC) and the use of either silver, chromogenic or fluorescent in situ hybridisation (SISH, CISH or FISH). Several PCR-based methodologies have also been described in the literature. Treatment with trastuzumab is generally indicated in cases where HER2 expression is clearly amplified, with a score of 3+ on standard testing methods. FISH is often viewed as being the 'gold standard' technique but it is expensive, and requires fluorescence microscopy and an image capture system. Currently, the recommended assays are a combination of IHC and FISH, whereby IHC scores of 0 and 1+ are negative (no trastuzumab

treatment), scores of 3+ are positive (trastuzumab treatment), and score of 2+ (equivocal case) is referred for FISH, to aid the definitive treatment decision.

In a landmark prospectively randomized controlled study, the addition of trastuzumab (given every 3 weeks for 1 or 2 years) after adjuvant chemotherapy was shown to increase both survival and response rate, in comparison with chemotherapy alone [77,78]. In the long-term follow-up series of this trial [78], of a total of 5102 patients treated with or without trastuzumab, the number of deaths was clearly reduced by 1 year's administration of trastuzumab (59 vs 90 at a median of 2 years). As the authors pointed out, these long-term results reinforce the importance of early treatment with trastuzumab in HER2-positive patients. A number of other clinical trials have now given similarly impressive results, although the cardiotoxic potential of trastuzumab is an important consideration and 0.5% of patients in the study developed a cardiac-related side-effect described by the authors as 'severe'. Nonetheless, for patients with ErbB2-positive tumours, which clearly have a more adverse prognosis, the use of trastuzumab as part of the postoperative adjuvant treatment policy has dramatically improved the outlook. The optimum period for this expensive form of treatment remains unknown at present, but 1 year of treatment is generally recommended. Most authorities agree that simultaneous administration of the first part of the trastuzumab with the adjuvant chemotherapy programme is key to maximizing benefit. Although potentially serious cardiac side-effects have been widely reported, especially since both breast and/or chest wall irradiation as well [79], this problem is generally identifiable early, and manageable with contemporary cardiovascular monitoring and treatment. This issue will doubtless become increasingly highlighted as these newer agents pass into widespread adjuvant clinical use in patients with the potential for a lengthy lifespan, particularly since recent work strongly suggests that trastuzumab in combination with other targeted therapies offers important additional benefits even after relapse, clearly widening their potential for prolonged use (see O'Shaughnessy et al. in 'Further reading'). The recent development of cardio-oncology as an important discipline within cardiology is a welcome advance. Moreover, recent work suggests that the benefits of adjuvant trastuzumab may not be strictly limited to patients with ErbB2-positive tumours, a critically important issue with enormous biological and financial implications that requires urgent clarification (see Paik et al. in 'Further reading'). Interestingly, the HER2/neu peptide vaccine E75 triggers a strong immune response in breast cancer patients, regardless of the level of HER2/neu protein expression, raising the remarkable prospect of vaccine therapy as a realistic future hope.

Now that the case for adjuvant targeted antibody treatment has been made so convincingly, at least in selected cases, other monoclonal antibodies are currently under investigation, including bevacizumab, adecatumumab and pertuzumab, among others. In one large recent study that included over 720 patients [80], the use of bevacizumab in combination with paclitaxel in patients with advanced disease gave superior results to the use of paclitaxel alone – a prolonged progression-free survival of 11.8 months versus 5.9 months – although overall survival was no different. One fascinating aspect of this study was that most of the patients had HER2-negative disease, and therefore would not have been suitable for treatment with trastuzumab. In HER2-positive patients, NSABP is currently assessing the benefit of bevacizumab with a combination of docetaxel and carboplatin (BETH trial, still recruiting at the time of writing).

Not all these targeted agents share every detail of their mechanism of action. For example, adecatumumab appears to work essentially as a low-affinity IgG1 antibody targeting epithelial cell adhesion molecule (EpCAM)-positive cancer cells, high-level expression of EpCAM being associated with an unfavourable prognosis. Pertuzumab is a humanized antibody, the first in a new class of agents known as HER dimerization inhibitors (HDIs). These are known to block the ability of the HER2 receptor to collaborate with other HER receptor family members (HER1/EGFR, HER3, and HER4). In malignant cells, interfering with HER2's ability to collaborate with other HER family receptors blocks cell signalling, which may ultimately lead to cancer cell growth inhibition and the programmed death of the cancer cell. Because of their unique mode of action, HDIs have the potential to work in a wide variety of tumours, including once again those that do not overexpress HER2. Pertuzumab-trastuzumab combinations offer great promise and are currently being tested in a variety of settings including neoadjuvant use (without chemotherapy) prior to definitive surgery, and also for patients with metastatic disease. An important study showing benefit in this latter setting was recently reported from the CLEOPATRA trial, in which over 800 HER-2 positive patients with metastatic disease were randomly assigned to receive placebo plus trastuzumab plus docetaxel (control group), or pertuzumab plus trastuzumab plus docetaxel (pertuzumab group), as first-line treatment either until the time of disease progression, or the development of toxic effects that could not be effectively managed – see Baselga, Cortes *et al.* [81]. The primary endpoint was independently assessed progression-free survival, which was an impressive 12.4 months in the control group compared with 18.5 months in the pertuzumab group, with interim analysis of overall survival showing a strong trend in favour of combination pertuzumab/trastuzumab plus docetaxel. The combination of trastuzumab and pertuzumab is now widely used in appropriate patients with metastatic disease. As pointed out in a recent paper from the same group, this combination provides significant improvement in survival without additional major toxicity – see Swain *et al.* [82].

In addition to the increasing use of targeted antibody treatment, other approaches to the blocking of HER2-mediated adverse effects are now under detailed study. Lapatinib, an orally active small molecule that inhibits the tyrosine kinases of HER2 and epidermal growth factor receptor (EGFR) type 1, has been shown in preclinical studies to be non-cross-reactive with trastuzumab, and is now in clinical use. The mechanism of action appears to be via inhibition of downstream signalling pathways through blocking of the autophosphorylation sites on the receptors. The clinical activity of lapatinib in combination with capecitabine has now been demonstrated in progressive trastuzumab-resistant disease, and was further investigated in a study of over 320 patients by a large international group recruiting patients during 2004–2005; the 'control' arm of the study was with capecitabine alone [83]. For the combination-therapy group, median time to progression was 8.4 months compared with only 4.4 months in the control arm, a benefit achieved without an increase in serious toxic effects or symptomatic cardiac events. This landmark study in patients with advanced disease has now led to a number of trials in which lapatinib is being used in a more adjuvant fashion, a particularly exciting prospect since this agent clearly has a mechanism of action distinct from that of trastuzumab. Both preclinical and clinical studies have now suggested a potentially remarkable synergy between trastuzumab and lapatinib, offering the reality of a dual inhibition of HER2 in this important group of patients – about 20–25% of all patients with newly diagnosed breast cancer – see, for example, the NeoALTTO study: Baselga, Bradbury *et al.* [84]. In this important international trial, the neoadjuvant use of the combination more than doubled the pathological complete response rate at definitive surgery, from

21–29% with the single agents alone, to 51% with the dual inhibition.

Current guidelines for use of adjuvant trastuzumab in our department at University College Hospital are listed below.

Guidelines for adjuvant trastuzumab (Herceptin)

1 The indications for adjuvant trastuzumab as defined by the guidelines are as follows.

(a) HER2-positive primary breast cancer determined by an accredited laboratory which is compliant with NEQAS standards.

(b) Prior treatment with adjuvant chemotherapy.

(c) No contraindication to trastuzumab treatment, and specifically no contraindication as a result of cardiac history and a left ventricular ejection fraction (LVEF) of more than 55%.

2 The duration of trastuzumab treatment is 12 months (18 doses administered at 3-weekly intervals).

3 Treatment should commence at the time of chemotherapy – at least 3 weeks following the final dose of anthracycline chemotherapy (most patients then commence immediately on their taxane thaerapy) and within 6 months (12 months during the transitional period) of completion of chemotherapy.

4 Cardiac monitoring should be conducted in accordance with the NICE guidelines and manufacturer's recommendations. Trastuzumab should be suspended if LVEF falls by 10 percentage points from baseline and to below 50% and further cardiac assessment performed if resumption of treatment is considered.

5 The available evidence suggests that breast/chest wall radiotherapy does not increase the risk of cardiac complications of trastuzumab treatment and that there is no indication to delay treatment starting until the completion of radiotherapy.

6 NLCN advocates 3-weekly dosing of trastuzumab at 6 mg/kg. The current licensed dose and schedule for trastuzumab administration has been adapted from a pharmacokinetic model that has now been superseded [85]. Because of the consequent uncertainties about dosing, NLCN does not recommend the use of a trastuzumab loading dose and advises dose banding to the nearest nominal 50 mg (and measured to the nearest millilitre of reconstituted trastuzumab).

7 Medical review is not mandatory prior to each dose of trastuzumab once patients are established on treatment. For uncomplicated treatment, review is recommended prior to cycle 1, cycle 2, cycle 5 (with cardiac assessment),

cycle 9 (with cardiac assessment), cycle 13 (with cardiac assessment) and after cycle 18 (with end-of-treatment cardiac assessment).

A NICE technology assessment provides further guidance for adjuvant trastuzumab treatment [86] and additional advice on trastuzumab use in this setting is contained within National Cancer Research Institute (NCRI) guidelines [87].

Treatment of locally advanced and metastatic disease

In most patients with apparently localized breast cancer it is probable that the disease is in fact systemic or generalized at presentation and that metastatic disease will later develop. This view is supported both by the common occurrence of widespread metastases, often many years after mastectomy has been undertaken, and by long-term follow-up studies of patient cohorts (see Figure 13.6). In the classic study by Brinkley and Haybittle, the overall survival was only 20% after 25 years [88]. Even in women deemed suitable for mastectomy (the 'early' operable group), the survival was only 30%. The appearance of metastases usually proves fatal within 3 years, although many women who respond to treatment do live longer. The likelihood of dissemination is strongly linked to the presence or absence of histologically positive axillary lymph nodes at the time of operation, and a quantitative relationship between the number of positive axillary lymph nodes and the probability of metastatic disease has been established.

Although there is no clear-cut evidence for the use of primary (neoadjuvant) chemotherapy in improving overall survival, this approach has become increasingly employed in patients with locally advanced primary tumours. Wherever possible, such treatment should be followed by appropriate local treatment with surgery and/or radiotherapy. The obvious potential advantage is shrinkage of the primary tumour prior to the local treatment, hopefully providing a more secure and durable benefit. The current guidelines for use of primary chemotherapy in our department at University College Hospital are shown below, although primary endocrine therapy is also sometimes offered, especially to older or less me.

Guidelines for primary medical therapy

There is no evidence that the long-term outcome of patients treated with primary medical therapy followed by local treatment is any different from conventional treatment with initial surgery. Wherever possible, primary medical therapy should be followed by local treatment, especially for patients who have no overt metastatic disease. A core biopsy with receptor determination should be performed prior to initiation of primary medical treatment.

Patient selection

The following are absolute indications for the use of primary medical therapy:

- Inoperable/inflammatory primary tumour;
- Stage IV cancer.

The following are relative indications for the use of primary medical therapy:

- Local operable primary tumour where downstaging could potentially allow breast-conserving surgery;
- Patients unfit for surgery;
- Very high grade or rapidly growing tumours in which initial surgery would unacceptably delay systemic treatment;
- Patients who need time to decide about surgical options.

Treatment options (Box 13.1)

Chemotherapy is the preferred modality of primary medical treatment in younger patients and for patients with ER- and PR-negative disease. Anthracycline/taxane-containing chemotherapy should be considered the norm as this has been shown to be superior to simpler anthracycline regimens.

- EC90 ± docetaxel: epirubicin $90\,mg/m^2$ plus cyclophosphamide $600\,mg/m^2$ every 3 weeks for four cycles; then docetaxel $100\,mg/m^2$ every 3 weeks for four cycles.
- For women with HER2-positive disease receiving neoadjuvant taxane chemotherapy, concomitant therapy with trastuzumab should be considered provided the patient meets the other criteria for adjuvant trastuzumab. Coadministration of trastuzumab and neoadjuvant anthracyclines should only be done as part of a clinical trial.

Further treatment

- Good response to primary medical therapy in inflammatory/locally advanced breast cancer should be followed by surgery if possible.
- Radiotherapy may be used following primary systemic treatment but it is not an alternative to surgery for fit patients with operable disease.

- The optimum timing of radiotherapy in relation to surgery for locally advanced and inflammatory breast cancer is not established.
- Postoperative endocrine treatment should be given to patients with ER- or PR-positive disease.
- The role of postoperative chemotherapy in patients who receive neoadjuvant chemotherapy but who remain axillary node positive at the time of surgery is unclear. Cases should be considered on an individual basis by the relevant multidisciplinary team.

Important newer agents for relapsed, metastatic or locally progressive disease include a variety of exciting agents which clearly show considerable potential and are in some cases entering rapidly into clinical use. One of these, everolimus, is an oral agent, the 40-O-(2-hydroxyethyl) derivative of sirolimus which appears to work similarly to this parent agent, as an inhibitor of the mammalian target of rapamycin (mTOR). It was initially (and is still currently) used as an immunosuppressant to prevent rejection of organ transplants and treatment of renal cell cancer and other tumours. In an important recent international prospectively randomized study of over 720 patients (BOLERO-2 trial), it prolonged progression-free survival in patients with advanced or recurrent breast cancer (when given in conjunction with exemestane) by over 4 months (see Baselga, Campone *et al.* [89]). Secondly, eribulin, a recently approved i.v-administered synthetic macrocyclic ketone analogue of the marine sponge natural product halichondrin-B (a potent mitotic spindle or microtubule inhibitor) has shown real promise in refractory cases. In a recent large-scale randomized trial, it showed a trend towards better overall survival when compared to capecitabine, a widely used agent for patients with recurrent disease. It has yet to be approved by the NICE technology committee for use in the UK. Another newer agent, ixabepilone, a novel antitumour microtubule-stabilizing drug, has shown promise in single-agent studies in the neoadjuvant setting, and may possibly prove of particular value in ER-negative patients – see, for example, Saura *et al.* [90].

Options for hormonal manipulation (see also Chapter 6)

Since the first therapeutic oophorectomy by Beatson in 1896, it has become clear that at least one-third of patients with advanced disease gain symptomatic benefit from hormonal manipulation. A wide variety

Box 13.1 Chemotherapy for metastatic disease.

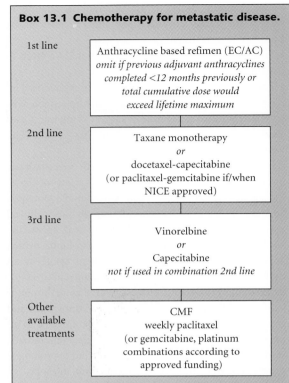

1st line

> Anthracycline based refimen (EC/AC)
> *omit if previous adjuvant anthracyclines*
> *completed <12 months previously or*
> *total cumulative dose would*
> *exceed lifetime maximum*

2nd line

> Taxane monotherapy
> *or*
> docetaxel-capecitabine
> (or paclitaxel-gemcitabine if/when
> NICE approved)

3rd line

> Vinorelbine
> *or*
> Capecitabine
> *not if used in combination 2nd line*

Other available treatments

> CMF
> weekly paclitaxel
> (or gemcitabine, platinum
> combinations according to
> approved funding)

When to use chemotherapy

Chemotherapy should be considered for treating patients with:
- hormone receptor-negative disease or
- patients with hormone receptor-positive tumours and visceral metastases or
- rapidly progressive disease or
- patients who have exhausted all hormonal options/failed to respond to two previous hormonal agents.

Choice of regimen

The most active chemotherapy regimens contain anthracyclines (EC or AC) or taxanes[a] (docetaxel recommended). Other agents/combinations with activity include vinorelbine*, capecitabine* and CMF. Some regimens are particularly suited to less fit patients (see below).

Combination vs. single agent

This question has not been convincingly answered. Docetaxel–capecitabine has shown a modest overall survival benefit over docetaxel alone (similarly for gemcitabine–paclitaxel vs. paclitaxel alone though full paper is awaited). However, this has not been compared with sequential single agents, and does carry significant toxicity in a palliative setting. For selected fit patients with aggressive disease, the risk-benefit ratio for the combination may still be favourable despite the increased toxicity.

Sequence of regimens

The following algorithm should be used as a general guide only. Consideration should be given to all the factors referred to at the beginning of the section on metastasis before deciding on therapy for individual patients.

Other therapies which can be considered

Gemcitabine–taxane combinations
- Full data from two key trials due: gemcitabine–paclitaxel versus paclitaxel as first-line therapy, phase III; docetaxel–gemcitabine versus docetaxel–capecitabine as first-line therapy.
- NICE appraisal. Document CG80, issued February 2009.

Single-agent gemcitabine
- Phase II data comparable to that for vinorelbine–capecitabine.

Platinum combinations
- Increasing body of phase II data on combinations of carboplatin/cisplatin usually with taxanes/gemcitabine (±trastuzumab for HER2-positive disease).
- Clinical trials are currently active for BRCA1/BRCA2-positive patients with metastatic disease.

Chemotherapy treatment of metastatic disease (HER2 amplified)

- HER2 positivity is defined as either immunohistochemistry (IHC) 3+ or fluorescence *in situ* hybridization (FISH) amplified ≥2.
- IHC 2+ cases must be confirmed with FISH testing.

Chemotherapy algorithm should be followed as above. Trastuzumab* may be added:
- in combination with a taxane (docetaxel–trastuzumab preferred) as first- or second-line therapy (depending on use of adjuvant anthracyclines);
- in combination with vinorelbine chemotherapy where taxanes are contraindicated or previously used;
- as monotherapy where chemotherapy options exhausted/inappropriate;
- currently no data to support the concurrent use of trastuzumab with hormonal therapy.

See also NLCN guidelines for the use of trastuzumab in metastatic disease.

Note that trastuzumab should not be used in combination with anthracycline chemotherapy because of high cardiotoxicity rates. It is still recommended that anthracyclines should not be started within 6 months of Herceptin administration because of the long half-life of trastuzumab and the high risk of cardiotoxicity. However, following data from the adjuvant trials where trastuzumab has been started as soon as 3 weeks after the last anthracycline injection, with acceptable cardiotoxicity rates, a long gap between finishing anthracyclines and starting trastuzumab is no longer considered necessary.

Chemotherapy options for frail patients/those with marrow failure or abnormal liver function

Frail but with normal haematology/liver function

- Vinorelbine
- Capecitabine
- Weekly paclitaxel
- 3-weekly docetaxel (60 mg/m^2)
- Single-agent mitoxantrone

Marrow failure/abnormal liver function (see NLCN guidelines on use of cytotoxic agents in patients with hepatic impairment)

- Single-agent dose reduced/weekly epirubicin
- Weekly paclitaxel
- Capecitabine
- Vinorelbine (not marrow failure)

Bisphosphonates for bony metastases

- Bisphosphonates can reduce the incidence of skeletal events and also reduce bone pain in patients with bony metastases.
- Their use should be considered in all patients with bony metastases and patients prioritized according to the Sheffield Guidelines (see www.yorkshire-cancer-net.org.uk). Patients scoring 7 or more should be considered for treatment (medium and high priority). Four bisphosphonates are currently available.
- Clodronate (800 mg b.d.), a first-generation oral bisphosphonate.

- Pamidronate (90 mg i.v. over 90 min every 3–4 weeks), a potent intravenous bisphosphonate.
- Zoledronate (4 mg i.v. over 15 min every 3–4 weeks), a potent intravenous bisphosphonate.
- Ibandronate, a potent bisphosphonate available in both oral and intravenous preparations.
  The choice of bisphosphonate will depend on the balance between:
- ease of administration;
- patient preference;
- cost;
- use of chemotherapy unit resources for intravenous formulations;
- toxicities;
- local funding.

Radiotherapy for metastatic disease

Radiotherapy can be an effective symptomatic treatment for:

- pain relief from bony metastases;
- spinal cord compression;
- brain metastases;
- leptomeningeal disease;
- superior vena caval obstruction;
- local control of primary tumour/local or chest wall recurrence;
- symptomatic skin metastases.

of procedures has been used, including oophorectomy, ovarian irradiation (sometimes referred to as 'artificial menopause'), treatment with oestrogens, antioestrogens, LHRH antagonists (e.g. goserelin), anabolic steroids, glucocorticoids and progesterones, surgical treatment by adrenalectomy or hypophysectomy, and treatment with aromatase inhibitors such as anastrozole or letrozole.

The conventional approach is largely based on the menstrual status of the patient. In most premenopausal and perimenopausal patients, surgical or radiation-induced ovarian ablation was traditionally employed for metastatic disease, but the advent of LHRH antagonists has led to these approaches being far less frequently employed nowadays since these agents provide adequate reduction of circulating oestrogen and render patients hormonally postmenopausal within 2 months of first administration. Goserelin is given monthly by intramuscular injection. Conversely, the use of laparoscopic oophorectomy, a safe and simple procedure requiring only a single night in hospital, has repopularized the surgical approach as a serious alternative. This is all the more true as patients are now much more carefully

selected on the basis of ER-positivity, filtering out those who could not benefit from oophorectomy. In postmenopausal patients, tamoxifen is still the most widely used agent throughout the world but is being supplanted in this setting by aromatase inhibitors such as anastrozole or exemestane, which are more effective and, on the whole, better tolerated. The important side-effects of aromatase inhibitors include osteopenia (leading to a higher frequency of fracture than is the case with tamoxifen), arthralgia (often quite severe in the first instance but tending to improve with time) and muscle stiffness. Side-effects of tamoxifen include flushing, nausea, hypercalcaemia, a disease 'flare', thrombocytopenia, fluid retention and menstrual disturbances. Many patients gain a pound or two in weight while taking tamoxifen, and some notice changes in the quality of their skin, hair or nails.

Patients with ER-positive tumours are very much more likely to demonstrate a significant response to hormonal manipulation; patients with ER-negative tumours rarely if ever respond and are no longer treated with hormonal agents, although 10 years ago this was not uncommon. Patients who are ER-positive have a different natural history from the ER-negative group, with a longer disease-free interval and overall survival. Simultaneous measurements of ER and PR give an even better prediction of response to hormone manipulation than measurement of ER alone (Table 13.5). PR-positivity is also correlated with a longer disease-free interval.

The site of metastatic disease may well influence responsiveness to hormonal treatment. Bone metastases are relatively likely to respond, although the ultimate outcome for such patients is poor, with a mean survival time of only about 12–15 months. Nevertheless, some patients with bone metastases from breast cancer do survive very much longer (sometimes several years) provided they are sufficiently hormone responsive.

In general, most premenopausal patients with recurrent disease, if known to be ER-positive, are treated either by LHRH therapy (goserelin is often preferred) or by radiation-induced menopause or laparoscopic oophorectomy in the first instance. Postmenopausal patients are more usually treated with tamoxifen if they have not already received it as adjuvant therapy (see below). In each case, at least 30% of patients can be expected to respond, the exogenous hormone continued indefinitely while the patient's response persists. Further hormone therapy should be reserved for patients who responded to the initial hormonal procedure. Following failure of the commonly used non-steroidal aromatase inhibitor anastrozole, a frequent treatment recommendation is to switch to the steroidal aromatase inhibitor exemestane. A further possibility following treatment failure is to use the ER downregulator fulvestrant (Faslodex). Several studies have shown that its effectiveness is similar to that of anastrozole in terms of overall survival in the second-line treatment of postmenopausal women with relapsed disease [91]. Unlike the oral aromatase inhibitors, fulvestrant is administered by subcutaneous or intramuscular administration at a dose of 250 mg monthly. One of its major benefits is its freedom from the partial oestrogen agonist side-effects of tamoxifen, without the oestrogen-depleting effects of the aromatase inhibitors.

When relapse occurs following these initial measures, other potentially useful agents, with at least some degree of activity, include anabolic steroids, progestogens and glucocorticoids. Anabolic steroids are more effective in postmenopausal women and seem particularly helpful for bone metastases. About 20% of untreated patients will respond, but side-effects of virilization can be troublesome. A convenient preparation is nandrolone decanoate (Deca-Durabolin) 50–100 mg given intramuscularly every 3–4 weeks. Progestational agents can be used if there has been a previous hormone response. The most commonly used drug is medroxyprogesterone acetate (Provera), which is often given at a dose of 100 mg three times daily by mouth, although weight gain may limit tolerability. Another frequently used progesterone, megestrol acetate (Megace), is equally effective.

The question of whether hormone manipulation should still be preferred to cytotoxic chemotherapeutic treatment of first relapse has been widely debated. Although, in quantitative terms, the choice lies between hormonal manipulation (which has a 30% likelihood of response) and combination chemotherapy (with a response rate of double this figure), this is an oversimplification of what is often a complex decision. Hormone-induced responses tend to be more durable and are usually accompanied by minimal toxicity to the patient. Chemotherapy-induced responses tend to be of shorter duration and are accompanied by a wider spectrum of physical and psychological difficulties. In the UK, there is no doubt that in suitable patients with receptor-positive disease, most clinicians prefer hormone manipulation first, and the routine availability of reliable ER assays makes this decision far more straightforward. Following the dramatic increase in the use of aromatase inhibitors over recent years, the twin problems of bone loss and skeletal health have become crucially important – how to recognize, prevent and treat the demineralization that so frequently accompanies extended use of these highly active agents. Useful algorithms have been produced to help the clinician towards a rational and hopefully reassuring approach for patients faced with these side-effects (Figure 13.7). See, for example, Johnston [92] and Johnston and Schiavon [93], for a comprehensive review of this rapidly-changing landscape.

Table 13.5 Response to endocrine therapy.

Receptor status	Response (%)
ER negative PR negative	<10
ER negative PR positive or ER positive PR negative	35
ER positive PR positive	70

ER, oestrogen receptor; PR, progesterone receptor.

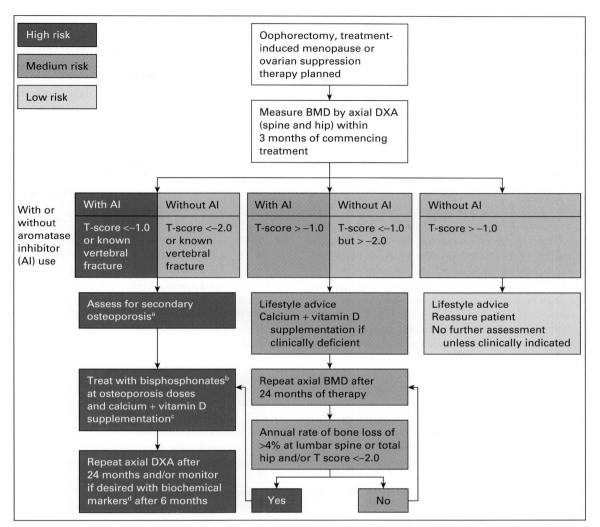

Figure 13.7 Management of bone loss in early breast cancer. a, Erythrocyte sedimentation rate, full blood count, bone and liver function (calcium, phosphate, alkaline phosphatase, albumin, aspartate aminotransferase/γ-glutamyltransferase), serum creatinine, endomysial antibodies, serum thyroid-stimulating hormone. b, Alendronate 70 mg/week, risedronate 35 mg/week, ibandronate 150 mg p.o. monthly or 3 mg i.v. 3-monthly, zoledronic acid 4 mg i.v. 6-monthly. c, To be given as calcium ≥1 g plus vitamin D ≥800 IU. d, Biochemical markers such as serum C-terminal telopeptide of type I collagen or urinary N-telopeptide of type I collagen. BMD, bone mineral density; DXA, dual-energy X-ray absorptiometry. (Based on Evaluation, Monitoring and Treatment of Bone Loss in Early Breast Cancer: Guidance from a UK Expert Group. Reviewed and Supported by the NCRI Breast Cancer Study Group and the National Osteoporosis Society. Access via www.tripdatabase.com or see *Cancer Treat Rev* 2008; 34 (Supplement 1): S3–S18.)

Treatment of special problems in metastatic disease

Radiotherapy is the treatment of choice for patients with painful bone metastases, offering relief of symptoms in over three-quarters of all cases, although objective radiological evidence of recalcification is much less common.

Some sites are particularly problematic, such as large cortical deposits in the femur or other weight-bearing bones, in which case it is often necessary to combine radiotherapy with internal orthopaedic fixation before a fracture occurs. Sternal metastases should be treated promptly since, if left untreated, the thoracic cage is unstable, leading to a mid-dorsal vertebral fracture which can be life-threatening.

Brain metastases occur in about 15% of all patients with breast cancer. Radiotherapy is beneficial in approximately two-thirds, often with control of symptoms until the patient's death. Spinal cord compression is also common, and its treatment is discussed in Chapter 8.

Pelvic irradiation to a relatively modest dose leads to complete and lasting amenorrhoea in premenopausal patients and radiation-induced menopause has, therefore, been used as an alternative to oophorectomy, particularly in patients whose general condition makes surgery inappropriate. The probability of total amenorrhoea is dose-dependent and fractionated treatment (12–15 Gy in five treatment fractions over 1 week) is usually given. Inducing a radiation-induced menopause appears as successful as oophorectomy for relief of symptoms. Clinical problems from metastases at other sites, such as skin, lymph node, pelvic or painful hepatic deposits, can often be alleviated by local radiotherapy even when systemic treatments have failed.

When local recurrence occurs after mastectomy, radiotherapy is undoubtedly the treatment of choice if not previously given. However, local recurrence often occurs in the context of systemic metastases, and if there is evidence of more widespread disease systemic treatment is often more appropriate. Even under these circumstances radiotherapy may be the best treatment for a troublesome local recurrence. If postoperative radiotherapy has previously been given, it may be difficult to give further treatment because of the radiation tolerance of local structures such as brachial plexus, skin and lung. Treatment by electron beam irradiation or hyperthermia can be helpful in this difficult situation.

A final, additional and beneficial type of treatment for metastatic disease involves the use of pamidronate and/or other bisphosphonates for patients with bone metastases [94]. The current estimated prevalence of bone metastases from breast cancer is 226 per 100 000 population – a much larger figure than with other solid tumours. Several studies have shown that pamidronate infusions, given monthly, together with hormonal therapy or chemotherapy, reduce skeletal complications such as fracture, and also provide useful palliation of pain. Zoledronic acid is increasingly selected as the bisphophonate of choice (see below), and is often regarded as more effective than pamidronate for metastatic bone disease from breast carcinoma [95]. It carries the advantage of requiring a less frequent treatment programme, perhaps as little as twice yearly, in selected cases. The NICE evaluation committee has recently updated its guidelines on the crucially important issue of how best to maintain adequate skeletal health in patients with breast cancer, an increasingly well-recognized part of holistic management since the prognosis has improved so rapidly and many patients – including those taking daily medication with aromatase inhibitor agents – have years or even decades of life ahead – see Coleman [96]. Until recently, zoledronic acid was regarded as the treatment of choice, but an important study comparing it with the newer agent denosumab (a fully human monoclonal antibody against receptor activator of nuclear factor κ B (RANK) ligand) demonstrated the superiority of the latter, with a HR of 0.82 for skeletal-related episodes, that is, a relative 18% reduction, without greater toxicity – see Stopeck et al. [97]. Osteoclasts resorb bone, releasing growth factors that may promote tumour cell proliferation, metastasis, and survival and perpetuating a vicious cycle of tumour expansion and bone resorption. Denosumab, given subcutaneously, appears to inhibit the osteoclast activity that results in reduced bone resorption, reversing this destructive cycle. In the UK, NICE has updated its guidelines (2012) for using this expensive agent recognizing its benefits and making it easier to prescribe, particularly in patients with breast cancer.

Prognosis of breast cancer

Overall, with advances in treatment and possibly the advent of screening, the prognosis in breast cancer has improved considerably in recent years. However, 5- and even 10-year survival rates do not give a true picture since relapses may occur well beyond this point (Figure 13.8), with a few additional deaths from relapse beyond 25 years. Prognosis is dependent on tumour stage, size of the primary (Figure 13.9) and tumour grade but independent of the extent of initial surgery, provided that adequate local control has been achieved (see also Figure 4.2). Axillary lymph node involvement is particularly important: of patients with stage I disease (T1–2N0) 80% are alive at 10 years, whereas with stage II disease (N2–3M0) 10-year survival is only 35%. An important recent study from the M. D. Anderson Hospital has confirmed how much better the overall prognosis for early breast cancer is nowadays, at least among the most favoured group with stage I node-negative cancer [98]. Over 50 000 patient records were accessed, with a median follow-up of over 5 years. Interestingly, with a median age at diagnosis of 65 years, the overall mortality was 24%, but the breast cancer-specific mortality was lower at 4%. In the group as a whole, only 1340 deaths were related directly to breast

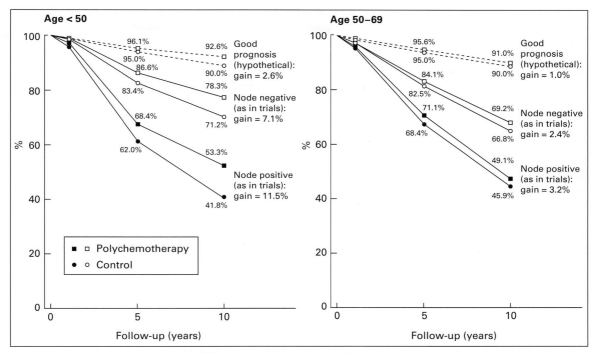

Figure 13.8 Estimated absolute survival advantages with prolonged polychemotherapy for populations of women with good, intermediate and poor prognosis (calculated by having the proportional risk reduction unaffected by prognosis). (Data from references [52,59].)

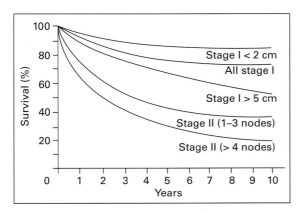

Figure 13.9 Survival in stages I and II operable breast cancer. In stage I, disease tumour size is an important prognostic determinant, as is degree of involvement of axillary nodes in stage II.

cancer whereas 5931 were caused by other 'competing' diagnoses such as cardiac and cerebrovascular disease.

The significance of the age of the patient at diagnosis is uncertain, but young patients do face an exceptional lengthy period at risk, and appear to have more to gain

from adjuvant chemotherapy [51]. Pregnancy in patients who have been treated for breast cancer during the premenopausal years does not appear to have a clear-cut adverse effect [99], in contrast to the traditionally held medical view that it should best be avoided. The question of HRT for breast cancer patients has also been addressed, notably by the HABITS (hormonal replacement therapy after breast cancer – is it safe?) study [100]. Sadly, this trial had to be discontinued early because of the apparent risks of HRT and an observed increased hazard rate, even though previous studies had been essentially negative. Although this study and its termination attracted worldwide interest, even the authors themselves are cautious about whether or not HRT should genuinely be regarded as unacceptably dangerous for breast cancer patients, an especially important question as so many now survive for such long periods, with the risk of severe and sometimes unremitting menopausal symptoms. Complete sequencing of the *p53* gene appears to provide useful prognostic information, mutations in certain regions of the gene carrying a significantly worse prognosis [101]. As far as genetic predisposition is concerned, a landmark study of *BRCA1* patients showed no evidence of a different prognosis as compared with sporadic cases [102]. This result was supported by a large nationwide study from Israel of all cases diagnosed within the 2-year period 1987–1988, assessing the long-term (10-year) outcome of treatment in *BRCA1* or *BRCA2* mutation carriers compared with non-carriers, and showing no convincing difference, with similar breast cancer-specific death rates [103]. However, there seems little doubt that *BRCA1*- or *BRCA2*-positive patients are at increased risk of developing a new contralateral cancer, judging from the results of a recent meta-analysis, which incidentally failed to confirm any other convincing predictive features [104]. Obesity appears to confer a real disadvantage in survival following initially successful treatment, with a clear-cut reduction in both disease-free and overall survival in patients with a body mass index of over 30 kg/m². Finally, there is increasing evidence that specialist breast cancer centres offer a standard of care that leads to an improved outcome, including survival [105]. Breast cancer should no longer be regarded as the province of the general surgeon.

The impressive late impact of adjuvant chemotherapy on overall survival has been reported by Bonadonna and colleagues, in a 30-year follow-up study using CMF [106]. Relapse and death rate were both significantly reduced, the latter by 21%, and with minimal long-term sequelae. Nonetheless, despite impressive response rates to chemotherapy, the expected lifespan for most patients with metastatic breast cancer has changed little as a result of the more widespread use of cytotoxic agents. More intensive chemotherapy regimens may possibly be associated with higher response rates, and it has even been claimed that high-dose chemotherapy with stem cell support may be justifiable, although recent results have been disappointing. Complete responders to chemotherapy certainly have a better prognosis than partial responders, but the adverse effects in non-responders must be weighed against these benefits. This may be one reason for the failure of combination chemotherapy to improve overall survival in patients with metastatic disease. Other reasons are that the responses are often short-lived (sometimes only a few months), and probably occur in patients with an intrinsically better prognosis than non-responders. A central problem, as with so many areas of cancer chemotherapy, is to select those who are likely to respond well, and avoid over-treating patients unlikely to be helped. Chemotherapy responses are more likely to be achieved in patients who are fit, have soft-tissue rather than bone metastases, have a small number of metastatic sites and have received no previous chemotherapy. ER status has little predictive value for chemotherapy response.

Cancer of the male breast

Breast cancer in men [107] is, at most, only 1% as common as in women (see Figure 13.2). Fewer than 250 cases are diagnosed each year in the UK, though it does seem to be becoming more common both in the UK and also the USA. The current incidence is about 0.86–1.08 per 100 000 men and the peak age at diagnosis is in the mid-60s. Relatively little is known of the aetiology, although a few family clusters have been reported, and it may be more common in patients who have had bilharzia with consequent liver damage and hyperoestrogenism. It has been reported as being about eight times more common than expected in radiation-exposed males who survived the Hiroshima atomic bomb blast, in patients with Klinefelter's syndrome, in which gonadotrophin levels are characteristically elevated, and in a small minority of men initially presenting with gynaecomastia – though there is no clear-cut causal link with this very common condition. In general, it is thought that there is probably a link with factors relating to androgen – a history of testicular maldescent or injury, mumps orchitis and possibly cirrhosis as this may lead to increased peripheral conversion of oestrogen from androgens – see Brinton *et al.* [108], for a good discussion. Breast cancer in males is also commoner in obese patients and also those taking exogenour oestrogens as part of a gender reassignment programme. It is far more common in those carrying the *BRCA1* or *BRCA2* gene [109], particularly the latter. Men carrying *BRCA2* also have an increased incidence of lymphoma, melanoma and cancers of the prostate, pancreas, gallbladder and stomach.

Most men diagnosed with breast cancer initially present with a tender indurated nipple, often with crusting or discharge, sometimes blood-stained. The disease involves the chest wall early. Routes of spread are similar to the disease in women, as is the pattern of metastasis. Most of the tumours are ER-positive.

Treatment is usually by mastectomy. Some surgeons prefer radical mastectomy because of the paucity of breast tissue in males and the possibility of early direct invasion, coupled with the lesser degree of mutilation and psychological distress following this operation in men. Local irradiation should be given when axillary lymph nodes are involved: the indications appear to be similar to those for female patients. Broadly speaking this is also true for adjuvant hormonal therapy and/or chemotherapy, although the information and data available are far sparser.

For recurrent disease orchidectomy is generally considered the treatment of choice, with responses in 60% of cases. The value of other endocrine manoeuvres is uncertain, but treatment with tamoxifen, aromatase inhibitors, progestogens, cyproterone or hypophysectomy has been employed. There have been few trials of chemotherapy, but it is often used when hormone treatments have failed and responses may be seen. Overall, the prognosis appears to be worse than in women [110], and male patients with breast cancer appear to have a higher risk of second malignancies than the general population.

References

1 McPherson K, Steel CM, Dixon JM. Breast cancer, epidemiology, risk factors and genetics. *Br Med J* 2000; 321: 624–8.

2 Kauff ND, Satagopan JM, Robson ME *et al.* Risk-reducing salpingo-oophorectomy in women with a *BRCA1* or *BRCA2* mutation. *N Engl J Med* 2002; 346: 1609–15.

3 Balmana J, Diez O, Rubio I T and Cardoso F, on behalf of the ESMO Guidelines Working Group. BRCA in breast cancer: ESMO clinical practice guidelines. *Ann Oncol* 2011; 22: vi31–34.

4 Lobb E, Meiser B. Genetic counselling and prophylactic surgery in women from families with hereditary breast or ovarian cancer. *Lancet* 2004; 363: 1841–2.

5 National Institute for Clinical Excellence. *Familial Breast Cancer: the Classification and Care of Women at Risk of Familial Breast Cancer in Primary, Secondary and Tertiary Care.* NICE Clinical Guideline No 14. London: NICE, 2004.

6 Writing Group for the Women's Health Initiative Investigators. Risks and benefits of estrogen plus progestin in healthy postmenopausal women. *JAMA* 2002; 288: 321–33.

7 Reeves GK, Beral V, Green J *et al.* for the Million Women Study Collaborators. Hormonal therapy for menopause and breast cancer risk by histologic type: a cohort study and meta-analysis. *Lancet Oncol* 2006; 7: 910–18.

8 Collaborative Group on Hormonal Factors in Breast Cancer. Breast cancer and breastfeeding: collaborative reanalysis of individual data from 47 epidemiological studies in 30 countries including 50302 women with breast cancer and 96973 women without disease. *Lancet* 2002; 360: 187–95.

9 Russo J, Russo IH. *Molecular Basis of Breast Cancer: Prevention and Treatment.* Berlin: Springer-Verlag, 2004: 448.

10 Eliassen AH, Colditz GA, Rosner B *et al.* Adult weight change and risk of postmenopausal breast cancer. *JAMA* 2006; 296: 193–201.

11 Khaw K-T. Dietary fats and breast cancer risk. *Brit Med J* 2013; 347: f4518.

12 Lavigne E, Holowaty EJ, Pan SY *et al.* Breast cancer detection and survival among women with cosmetic breast implants: systematic review and analysis of observational studies. *Brit Med J* 2013; 346: f2399.

13 Pharoah PD, Antoniou A, Easton DF, Ponder BAJ. Polygenes, risk prediction, and targeted prevention of breast cancer. *N Engl J Med* 2008; 358: 2796–803.

14 Smith JA. Treatment of ductal carcinoma-in-situ: new data refine the risk estimates associated with various treatments. *Brit Med J* 2011; 343: d5344.

15 Julien JP, Bijker N, Fentiman IS *et al.* Radiotherapy in breast-conserving treatment for ductal carcinoma in situ: first results of the EORTC randomized phase III trial 10853. *Lancet* 2000; 355: 528–33.

16 Fisher B, Dignam J, Wolmark N *et al.* Tamoxifen in treatment of intraductal breast cancer: NSABP B-24 randomized controlled trial. *Lancet* 1999; 353: 1993–2000.

17 Jones C, Mackay A, Grigoriadis A *et al.* Expression profiling of purified normal human luminal and myoepithelial breast cells: identification of novel prognostic markers for breast cancer. *Cancer Res* 2004; 64: 3037–45.

18 Metzger–Filho O, Tutt A, de Azambuja E *et al.* Dissecting the heterogeneity of triple-negative breast cancer. *J Clin Oncol* 2012; 30: 1879–87.

19 Cristofanilli M, Budd GT, Ellis MJ *et al.* Circulating tumor cells, disease progression, and survival in metastatic breast cancer. *N Engl J Med* 2004; 351: 781–91.

20 Van de Vijver MJ, Hey D, Van't Veer LJ *et al.* A gene-expression signature as a predictor of survival in breast cancer. *N Engl J Med* 2002; 347: 1999–2009.

21 Speirs V, Shaaban AM. Hormone receptors in defining breast cancer prognosis: time for a rethink? *Nat Clin Practice Oncol* 2007; 4: 204–5.

22 Gøtzsche PC, Olsen O. Is screening for breast cancer with mammography justifiable? *Lancet* 2000; 355: 129–34.

23 Brem RF. The never-ending controversies of screening mammography. *Cancer* 2004; 100: 1549–52.

24 Independent UK Panel on Breast Cancer Screening ("The Marmot Report"). Lancet published on-line 30 Oct 2012, 10.1016/S0140-6736(12)61611-0

25 Mukhtar TK, Yeates DR and Goldacre MJ. Breast cancer mortality trends in England and the assessment of the effectiveness of mammography screening: population-based study. *J Royal Soc Med* 2013; 106: 234–242.

26 Penston J, Steele R and Brewster D. Should we use total mortality rather than cancer specific mortality to judge cancer screening programmes? *Brit Med J* 2011; 343: d6397.

27 Zahl PH, Strand BH, Maehlen J. Incidence of breast cancer in Norway and Sweden during introduction of nationwide screening: prospective cohort study. *Br Med J* 2004; 328: 921–4.

28 Gotzche PC, Neilsen M. Screening for breast cancer with mammography. *Cochrane Database Syst Rev* 2006; 4: CD001877.

29 Moss SM, Cuckle H, Evans A *et al.* Effect of mammographic screening from 40 years on breast cancer mortality at ten years' follow-up: a randomized controlled trial. *Lancet* 2006; 368: 2053–60.

30 Advisory Committee on Breast Cancer Screening. *Screening for Breast Cancer in England: Past and Future*. NHSBSP Publication No. 61. London: Department of Health, 2006.

31 Hall FM. Breast imaging and computer-aided detection. *N Engl J Med* 2007; 356: 1464–6.

32 Schwartz LM, Woloshin S. Participation in mammography screening: women should be encouraged to decide what is right for them, rather than being told what to do. *Br Med J* 2007; 335: 731–2.

33 Banks E, Reeves G, Beral V *et al.* Influence of personal characteristics of individual women on sensitivity and specificity of mammography in the Million Women Study: cohort study. *Br Med J* 2004; 329: 477–84.

34 Bleyer A and Welch HG. Effect of three decades of screening mammography on breast cancer incidence. *New Engl J Med* 2012; 367: 1998–2005.

35 Cuzick J, Sestak I, Bonanni B *et al.* for the SERM Chemoprevention of Breast Cancer Overview Group. Selective oestrogen receptor modulators in prevention of breast cancer: an updated meta-analysis of individual participant data. *Lancet* 2013[a]; 381: 1827–34.

36 Cuzick J, Sestak I, Forbes JF *et al.* Anastrozole for prevention of breast cancer in high-risk postmenopausal women (IBIS-II): an international, double-blind, randomized placebo-controlled trial. *Lancet* 2013[b]; doi: 10.1016/S0140-6736(13)62292-8

37 Veronesi U, Paganelli G, Viale G *et al.* Sentinel lymph-node biopsy as a staging procedure in breast cancer: update of a randomized control study. *Lancet Oncol* 2006; 7: 983–90.

38 Osako T, Tsuda H, Horii R *et al.* Molecular detection of lymph node metastasis in breast cancer patients treated with preoperative systemic chemotherapy: a prospective multicentre trial using the one-step nucleic acid amplification assay. *Brit J Cancer* 2013; 109: 1693–98.

39 Early Breast Cancer Trialists' Collaborative Group. Favourable and unfavourable effects on long-term survival of radiotherapy for early breast cancer: an overview of the randomized trials. *Lancet* 2000; 355: 1757–70.

40 Fisher B, Bauer M, Margolese R *et al.* Five years' results of a randomized clinical trial comparing total mastectomy and segmental mastectomy with or without radiation in the treatment of breast cancer. *N Engl J Med* 1985; 312: 665–73.

41 Overgaard M, Hansen PS, Overgaard J *et al.* Postoperative radiotherapy in high-risk pre-menopausal women with breast cancer who receive adjuvant chemotherapy. *N Engl J Med* 1997; 337: 949–55.

42 Cancer Research Campaign (King's/Cambridge) working party trial for early breast cancer. A detailed update at the tenth year. *Lancet* 1980; 2: 55–62.

43 Haviland JS, Owen JR, Dewar JA *et al.* The UK Standardisation of Breast Radiotherapy (START) trials of radiotherapy hypofractionation for treatment of early breast cancer: 10-year follow-up results of two randomized controlled trials. *Lancet Oncol* 2013; 14: 1086–94.

44 Calle R, Pilleron JP, Schlienger P, Vilcoq JR. Conservative management of operable breast cancer. Ten years' experience at the Foundation Curie. *Cancer* 1978; 42: 2045–53.

45 Fisher B, Jeong JH, Dignam J *et al.* Findings from recent National Surgical Adjuvant Breast and Bowel Project adjuvant studies in stage 1 breast cancer. *J Natl Cancer Inst Monogr* 2001; 30: 62–6.

46 Tobias JS, Vaidya JS, Keshtgar M *et al.* Breast-conserving surgery with intra-operative radiotherapy: the right approach for the 21st century? *Clin Oncol* 2006; 18: 220–8.

47 Hughes KS, Schnaper LA, Berry D *et al.* Lumpectomy plus tamoxifen with or without irradiation in women 70 years of age or older with early breast cancer. *N Engl J Med* 2004; 351: 971–7.

48 Deutsch M, Land SR, Begovic M, Wieand HS, Wolmark N, Fisher B. The incidence of lung carcinoma after surgery for breast carcinoma with and without postoperative radiotherapy. Results of National Surgical Adjuvant Breast and Bowel Project (NSABP) clinical trials B-04 and B-06. *Cancer* 2003; 98: 1362–8.

49 Vaidya JS, Wenz F, Bulsara M, Tobias JS, *et al.* Risk-adapted targeted intraoperative radiotherapy versus whole-breast radiotherapy for breast cancer: 5-year results for local control and overall survival from the TARGIT-A randomized trial. *Lancet* 2014; 383, doi:10.1016/S0140-6736(13)61950-9

50 Veronesi U, Orecchia R, Maisonneuve P *et al.* Intraoperative radiotherapy versus external radiotherapy for early breast cancer (ELIOT): a randomized controlled equivalence trial. *Lancet Oncol* 2013; 14: 1269–77.

51 Early Breast Cancer Trialists' Collaborative Group (EBCTCG). Adjuvant chemotherapy in oestrogen-receptor-poor breast cancer: patient-level meta-analysis of randomized trials. *Lancet* 2008; 371: 29–40.

52 Early Breast Cancer Trialists' Collaborative Group. Effects of chemotherapy and hormonal therapy for early breast cancer on recurrence and 15-year survival: an overview of the randomized trials. *Lancet* 2005; 365: 1687–717.

53 Thiruchelvam PT, McNeill F, Jallali N *et al.* Postmastectomy breast reconstruction. *Brit Med J* 2013; 347: f5903.

54 Fisher B, Jeong J, Bryant J *et al.* Treatment of lymphnodenegative, oestrogen-receptor-positive breast cancer: long-term findings from National Surgical Adjuvant Breast And Bowel Project randomized clinical trials. *Lancet* 2004; 364: 858–68.

55 Gray R, Rea D et al. aTTom: Long-term effects of continuing adjuvant tamoxifen to 10 years versus stopping at 5 years in 6,953 women with early breast cancer. ASCO 2013: Abstract # 5.

56 Bergman L, Beelen ML, Gallee MPW et al. Risk and prognosis of endometrial cancer after tamoxifen for breast cancer. *Lancet* 2000; 356: 881–7.

57 Wysowski D, Honig S, Beitz J. Uterine sarcoma associated with tamoxifen use. *N Engl J Med* 2002; 346: 1832–3.

58 McCowan C, Wang S, Thompson AM et al. The value of high adherence to tamoxifen in women with breast cancer: a community-based cohort study. *Brit J Cancer* 2013; 109: 1172–80.

59 ATAC Trialists' Group. Effect of anastrozole and tamoxifen as adjuvant treatment for early-stage breast cancer: 100-month analysis of the ATAC trial. *Lancet Oncol* 2008; 9: 45–53.

60 Goss PE, Ingle JN, Martino S et al. A randomized trial of letrozole in postmenopausal women after five years of tamoxifen therapy for early-stage breast cancer. *N Engl J Med* 2003; 349: 1793–802.

61 Coombes RC, Kilburn LS, Snowden CF et al. Survival and safety of exemestane versus tamoxifen after 2–3 years' tamoxifen treatment (Intergroup Exemestane Study): a randomized controlled trial. *Lancet* 2007; 369: 559–70.

62 Jonat W, Gnant M, Boccardo F et al. Effectiveness of switching from adjuvant tamoxifen to anastrozole in postmenopausal women with hormone-sensitive early-stage breast cancer: a meta-analysis. *Lancet Oncol* 2006; 7: 991–6.

63 Kaufmann M, Jonat W, Blamey J et al. Survival analyses from the ZEBRA study: goserelin (Zoladex) versus CMF in premenopausal women with node-positive breast cancer. *Eur J Cancer* 2003; 39: 1711–17.

64 Goldhirsch A, Wood WC, Gelber RD et al. Meeting highlights: updated international expert consensus on the primary therapy of early breast cancer. *J Clin Oncol* 2003; 21: 3357–65.

65 LHRH-agonists in Early Breast Cancer Overview Group. Use of luteinising-hormone-releasing-hormone agonists as adjuvant treatment in premenopausal patients with hormone-receptor-positive breast cancer: a meta-analysis of individual patient data from randomized adjuvant trials. *Lancet* 2007; 369: 1711–23.

66 Nissen-Meyer R, Kjellgren K, Malmio K et al. Surgical adjuvant chemotherapy: results with one short course with cyclophosphamide after mastectomy for breast cancer. *Cancer* 1978; 41: 2088–98.

67 Recht A, Come SE, Henderson IC et al. The sequencing of chemotherapy and radiation therapy after conservative surgery for early stage breast cancer. *N Engl J Med* 1996; 334: 1356–61.

68 Poole CJ, Earl HM, Hiller L et al. Epirubicin and cyclophosphamide, methotrexate and fluorouracil as adjuvant therapy for early breast cancer. *N Engl J Med* 2006; 355: 1920–2.

69 Seidman AD, Reichmann BS, Crown JP et al. Paclitaxel as second and subsequent therapy for metastatic breast cancer: activity independent of prior anthracycline response. *J Clin Oncol* 1995; 13: 1152–9.

70 Henderson IC, Berry DA, Demetri GD et al. Improved outcomes from adding sequential paclitaxel but not from escalating doxorubicin dose in an adjuvant chemotherapy regimen for patients with node-positive primary breast cancer. *J Clin Oncol* 2003; 21: 976–83.

71 Hayes DF, Thor AD, Dressler LG et al. HER2 and response to paclitaxel in node-positive breast cancer. *N Engl J Med* 2007; 357: 1496–506.

72 Citron ML, Berry DA, Cirrincione C et al. Randomized trial of dose-dense versus conventionally scheduled and sequential versus concurrent combination chemotherapy as postoperative adjuvant treatment of node-positive primary breast cancer: first report of Intergroup Trial C9741/Cancer and Leukemia Group B Trial 9741. *J Clin Oncol* 2003; 21: 1431–9.

73 Albain KS, Barlow WE, Shak S et al. Prognostic and predictive value of the 21-gene recurrence score assay in postmenopausal women with node-positive, oestrogen-receptor-positive breast cancer on chemotherapy: a retrospective analysis of a randomized trial. *Lancet Oncol* 2010; 11: 55–65.

74 Carey LA. Novel targets for triple-negative breast cancer. *Clin Adv Hematol Oncol* 2011; 9: 678–80.

75 Slamon DJ, Leyland-Jones B, Shak S et al. Use of chemotherapy plus a monoclonal antibody against HER-2 for metastatic breast cancer that overexpresses HER-2. *N Engl J Med* 2001; 344: 783–92.

76 Slamon D, Eiermann W, Robert N et al. Adjuvant trastuzumab in HER-2 positive breast cancer. *New Engl J Med* 2011; 365: 1273–83.

77 Piccart-Gebhardt MJ, Procter M, Leyland-Jones B et al. Trastuzumab after adjuvant chemotherapy in HER-2 positive breast cancer. *N Engl J Med* 2005; 353: 1659–72.

78 Smith I, Procter M, Gelber RD et al. 2-year follow-up of trastuzumab after adjuvant chemotherapy in HER-2 positive breast cancer: a randomized controlled trial. *Lancet* 2007; 369: 29–36.

79 Perez EA, Suman VJ, Davidson NE et al. Cardiac safety analysis of doxorubicin and cyclophosphamide followed by paclitaxel with or without trastuzumab in the North Central Cancer Treatment Group 9831 adjuvant breast cancer trial. *J Clin Oncol* 2008; 26: 1231–8.

80 Miller K, Wang M, Gralow J et al. Paclitaxel plus bevacizumab versus paclitaxel alone for metastatic breast cancer. *N Engl J Med* 2007; 357: 2666–76.

81 Baselga J, Cortes J, Kim S-B et al. Pertuzumab plus trastuzumab plus docetaxel for metastatic breast cancer. *New Engl J Med* 2012; 366: 109–119.

82 Swain SM, Kim S-B, Cortes J *et al*. Pertuzumab, trastuzumab, and docetaxel for HER2-positive metastatic breast cancer (CLEOPATRA study): overall survival results from a randomized, double-blind, placebo-controlled, phase 3 study. *Lancet Oncol* 2013; 14: 461–71.

83 Geyer CE, Forster J, Lindquist D *et al*. Lapatinib plus capecitabine for HER-2 positive advanced breast cancer. *N Engl J Med* 2006; 355: 2733–43.

84 Baselga J, Bradbury I, Eidtmann H *et al*. Lapatinib with trastuzumab for HER2-positive early breast cancer (NeoALTTO): a randomized, open-label, multi-centre phase 3 trial. *Lancet* 2012; 379: 633–40.

85 Leyland-Jones B, Gelmon K, Ayoub JP *et al*. Pharmacokinetics, safety, and efficacy of trastuzumab administered every three weeks in combination with paclitaxel. *J Clin Oncol* 2003; 21: 3965–71.

86 National Institute for Clinical Excellence. *Trastuzumab for the Adjuvant Treatment of Early-stage HER2-positive Breast Cancer*. NICE Technology Assessment TA107. Available at http://www.nice.org.uk/page.aspx?o=TA107guidance.

87 National Cancer Research Institute. *UK Clinical Guidelines for the Use of Adjuvant Trastuzumab (Herceptin) With or Following Chemotherapy in HER2-positive Early Breast Cancer*. Available at http://www.dh.gov.uk/assetRoot/04/12/63/84/04126384.pdf

88 Brinkley D, Haybittle JL. The curability of breast cancer. *Lancet* 1975; 2: 95–7.

89 Baselga J, Campone M, Piccart M *et al*. Everolimus in postmenopausal hormone-receptor-positive advanced breast cancer. *New Engl J Med* 2012; 366: 520–29.

90 Saura C, Tseng L-M, Chan S *et al*. Neoadjuvant doxorubicin/cyclophosphamide followed by ixabepilone or paclitaxel in early stage breast cancer and evaluation of betaIII-tubulin expression as a predictive marker. *Oncologist* 2013; 18: 787–94.

91 Howell A, Pippen J, Elledge RM *et al*. Fulvestrant versus anastrozole for the treatment of advanced breast carcinoma: a prospectively planned combined survival analysis of two multi-center trials. *Cancer* 2005; 104: 236–9.

92 Johnston SR. The role of chemotherapy and targeted agents in patients with metastatic breast cancer. *Eur J Cancer* 2011; 47 Suppl 3: S38–47.

93 Johnston SR and Schiavon G. Treatment algorithms for hormone-receptor-positive advanced breast cancer. *Am Soc Clin Oncol Educ Book*. 2013; 2013: 28–36.

94 Lipton A, Theriault RL, Hortobagyi GN *et al*. Pamidronate prevents skeletal complications and is effective palliative treatment in women with breast carcinoma and osteolytic bone metastases. *Cancer* 2000; 88: 1082–90.

95 Rosen LS, Gordon D, Kaminsky M *et al*. Long-term efficacy and safety of zoledronic acid compared with pamidronate sodium in the treatment of skeletal complications in patients with advanced multiple myeloma or breast carcinoma: a randomized, double-blind, multicenter comparative trial. *Cancer* 2003; 98: 1735–44.

96 Coleman RE. Adjuvant bone-targeted therapy to prevent metastasis: lessons from the AZURE study. *Curr Opin Support Palliat Care* 2012; 6: 322–29.

97 Stopeck AT, Lipton AL, Body J-J *et al*. Denosumab compared with zoledronic acid for the treatment of bone metastases in patients with advanced breast cancer: a randomized, double-blind study. *J Clin Oncol* 2010; 28: 5132–39.

98 Hanrahan EO, Gonzalez-Angulo AM, Giordano SH *et al*. Overall survival and cause-specific mortality of patients with stage 1a, bN0M0 breast carcinoma. *J Clin Oncol* 2007; 25: 4952–60.

99 Ives A, Saunders C, Bulsara M, Semmens J. Pregnancy after breast cancer: population based study. *Br Med J* 2007; 334: 194–6.

100 Holmberg L, Anderson H, for the HABITS steering and data monitoring committees. HABITS (hormonal replacement therapy after breast cancer: is it safe?), a randomized comparison: trial stopped. *Lancet* 2004; 363: 453–5. [Correspondence *Lancet* 2004; 363: 1476–8.]

101 Bergh J, Norberg T, Sjogren S *et al*. Complete sequencing of the *p53* gene provides prognostic information in breast cancer patients, particularly in relation to adjuvant systemic therapy and radiotherapy. *Nature Med* 1995; 1: 1029–34.

102 Verhoog LC, Brekelmans CTM, Seynaevy C *et al*. Survival and tumour characteristics of breast-cancer patients with genetic mutations of BRCA1. *Lancet* 1998; 351: 316–21.

103 Rennert G, Bisland-Naggan S, Barnett-Griness O *et al*. Clinical outcomes of breast cancer in carriers of BRCA1 and BRCA2 mutations. *N Engl J Med* 2007; 357: 115–23.

104 Liebens FP, Carly C, Pastijn A, Rozenberg S. Management of BRCA1/2 associated breast cancer: a systematic qualitative review of the state of knowledge in 2006. *Eur J Cancer* 2007; 43: 238–57.

105 Gillis CR, Hole DJ. Survival outcome of care by specialist surgeons in breast cancer: a study of 3786 patients in the West of Scotland. *Br Med J* 1996; 312: 145–8.

106 Bonadonna G, Moliterni A, Zambetti M *et al*. 30 years' follow up of randomized studies of adjuvant CMF in operable breast cancer: cohort study. *Br Med J* 2005; 330: 217–20.

107 Nahleh Z, Girnius S. Male breast cancer: a gender issue. *Nat Clin Pract Oncol* 2006; 3: 428–37.

108 Brinton LA, Carreon JD, Gierach GL *et al*. Etiologic factors for breast cancer in the US Veterans' Affairs medical care symptom database. *Breast Cancer Res Treat* 2010; 119: 185–219.

109 Basham VM, Lipscombe JM, Ward JM *et al*. BRCA1 and BRCA2 mutations in a population-based study of male breast cancer. *Breast Cancer Res* 2002; 4: R2.

110 Gennari R, Curigliano G, Jereczek-Fossa BA *et al*. Male breast cancer: a special therapeutic problem. Anything new? *Int J Cancer* 2004; 24: 663–70.

111 Sobin LH, Gospodarowicz MK, and Wittekind Ch, eds. *TNM Classification of Malignant Tumours*, 7th edn. Chichester: Wiley-Blackwell, 2009.

Further reading

Agrawal A, Gutteridge E, Gee JM, Nicholson RI, Robertson JF. Overview of tyrosine kinase inhibitors in clinical breast cancer. *Endocr Relat Cancer* 2005; 12 (Suppl. 1): S135–44.

Armstrong AC, Evans GD. Management of women at high risk of breast cancer. *Brit Med J* 2014; 348: g 2756.

Banerjee S, Dowsett M, Ashworth A, Martin L-A. Mechanisms of disease: angiogenesis and the management of breast cancer. *Nat Clin Pract Oncol* 2007; 4: 536–50.

Biller-Adorno N, Juni P. Abolishing mammography screening programmes ? A view from the Swiss medical Board. *New Engl J Med* 2014; 370: 1965–67.

Bonnefoi H, Potti A, Delorenzi M et al. Validation of gene signatures that predict the response of breast cancer to neoadjuvant chemotherapy. *Lancet Oncol* 2007; 8: 1071–8.

Bowen RL, Duffy SW, Ryan DA et al. Early onset of breast cancer in a group of British black women. *Br J Cancer* 2008; 98: 277–81.

Buchholz TA. Radiation therapy for early-stage breast cancer after breast-conserving surgery. *N Engl J Med* 2009; 360: 63–70.

Cancer Research UK. *CancerStats*. Breast Cancer Statistics, 2009. Available at www.cancerresearchuk.org.

EJC Supplements (various authors). VEGF inhibition: changing the face of breast cancer management. *Eur J Cancer* 2008; 6 (Suppl. 6): 1–50.

Ellis P, Barrett-Lee P, Johnson L et al., for the TACT Trialists. Sequential docetaxel as adjuvant chemotherapy for early breast cancer (TACT): an open-label, phase III, randomized controlled trial. *Lancet* 2009; 373: 1681–92. Comment in: *Lancet* 2009; 373: 1662–3.

Gigerenza G. Breast cancer screening pamphlets mislead women. *Brit Med J* 2014; 348: g 2636.

Gilbert FJ, Astley SM, Gillan MG et al. Single reading with computer-aided detection for screening mammography. *N Engl J Med* 2008; 359: 1675–84.

Gnant M, Mlineritsch B, Schippinger W et al. for ABCSG-12 Trial Investigators. Endocrine therapy plus zoledronic acid in premenopausal breast cancer. *N Engl J Med* 2009; 360: 679–91.

Hannaford PC, Selvaraj S, Elliott A et al. Cancer risk among users of oral contraceptives: cohort data from the Royal College of General Practitioners' oral contraception study. *Br Med J* 2007; 335: 651–4

Hudis CA. Trastuzumab: mechanism of action and use in clinical practice. *N Engl J Med* 2007; 357: 39–51.

Jordan VC. Tamoxifen: catalyst for the change to targeted therapy. *Eur J Cancer* 2008; 44: 30–8.

Kell MR. Management of breast cancer in women with BRCA gene mutation. *Br Med J* 2007; 334: 437–8.

Kumle M. Declining breast cancer incidence and decreased HRT use. *Lancet* 2008; 372: 608–10.

LHRH-Agonists In Early Breast Cancer Overview Group. Use of luteinising-hormone-releasing hormone agonists as adjuvant treatment in premenopausal patients with hormone-receptor-positive breast cancer: a meta-analysis of individual patient data from randomized adjuvant trials. *Lancet* 2007; 369: 1711–23.

Li CI, Malone KE, Porter PL et al. Relationship between menopausal hormone therapy and risk of ductal, lobular, and ductal-lobular breast carcinomas. *Cancer Epidemiol Biomarkers Prev* 2008; 17: 43–50.

Lin NU, Winer EP. Optimal use of aromatase inhibitors: to lead or to follow? *J Clin Oncol* 2007; 25: 2639–41.

Moore A. Breast-cancer therapy: looking back to the future. *N Engl J Med* 2007; 357: 1547–9.

Muss HB, Berry DA, Cirrincione CT et al. Adjuvant chemotherapy in older women with early-stage breast cancer. *N Engl J Med* 2009; 360: 2055–65.

O'Shaughnessy KL, Blackwell H, Burstein AM et al. A randomized study of lapatinib alone or in combination with trastuzumab in heavily pretreated HER2+ metastatic breast cancer progressing on trastuzumab therapy. *J Clin Oncol* 2008; 26: 1015.

Pagani O, Regan MM, Walley BA et al. Adjuvant exemestane with ovarian suppression in premenopausal breast cancer. *New Engl J Med* 2014; 371: 107–18.

Paik S, Kim C, Wolmark N. *HER2* status and benefit from adjuvant trastuzumab in breast cancer. *N Engl J Med* 2008; 358: 1409–11.

Pegram MD, Konecny GE, O'Callaghan C et al. Rational combinations of trastuzumab with chemotherapeutic drugs used in the treatment of breast cancer. *J Natl Cancer Inst* 2004; 96: 725–7.

Pharoah PD, Antoniou AC, Easton D, Ponder BA. Polygenes, risk prediction, and targeted prevention of breast cancer. *N Engl J Med* 2008; 358: 2796–803.

Rabaglio M, Aebi S, Castiglioni-Gertsch M. Controversies of adjuvant endocrine treatment for breast cancer and recommendations of the 2007 St Gallen conference. *Lancet Oncol* 2007; 8: 940–9.

Ravdin PM, Cronin KA, Howlader N et al. The decrease in breast-cancer incidence in 2003 in the United States. *N Engl J Med* 2007; 356: 1670–4. [Correspondence *N Engl J Med* 2008; 357: 509–13.]

Rugo HS. Hormone therapy in premenopausal women with early-stage breast cancer. *New Engl J Med* 2014; 371: 175–6.

Sims AH, Howell A, Howell SJ, Clarke RB. Origins of breast cancer subtypes and therapeutic implications. *Nat Clin Pract Oncol* 2007; 4: 516–25.

Sotiriou C, Pusztai L. Gene-expression signatures in breast cancer. *N Engl J Med* 2009; 360: 790–800.

Sparano JA, Wang M, Martino S et al. Weekly paclitaxel in the adjuvant treatment of breast cancer. *N Engl J Med* 2008; 358: 1663–71.

Sprague BL, Trentham-Dietz A, Egan KM et al. Proportion of invasive breast cancer attributable to risk factors modifiable after menopause. *Am J Epidemiol* 2008; 168: 404–11.

START Trialists Group. The UK standardisation of breast radio-therapy (START) trial B of radiotherapy hypofractionation for treatment of early breast cancer: a randomized trial. *Lancet* 2008; 371: 1098–107.

Turner NC, Jones AL. Management of breast cancer. Parts I and II. *Br Med J* 2008; 337: 107–10 and 164–9.

Welch HG. Overdiagnosis and mammography screening: the question is no longer whether, but how often, it occurs. *Br Med J* 2009; 359: 182–3.

Xu F, Michaels KB. Intrauterine factors and risk of breast cancer: a systematic review and meta-analysis of current evidence. *Lancet Oncol* 2007; 8: 1088–100.

Yarnold J. Early and locally advanced breast cancer: diagnosis and treatment. National Institute for Health and Clinical Excellence Guideline 2009. *Clin Oncol* 2009; 21: 159–60.

Yeo B, Turner NC, Jones A. Medical management of breast cancer. *Brit Med J* 2014; 348: g 3608.

14 Cancer of the oesophagus and stomach

Carcinoma of the oesophagus

Incidence and aetiology

Oesophageal cancer has a male to female ratio of over 2:1 and a peak incidence in the 60–80 age group (Figure 14.1) [1]. In the United Kingdom, United States and elsewhere the incidence of adenocarcinoma of the oesophagus has increased significantly. In parts of Scandinavia, carcinoma of the oesophagus is as common in women as in men. There are marked geographical variations in incidence, with very high levels near the Caspian Sea, in Central Asia and in the Far East (Figure 14.2); in the United States it is commoner in less advantaged socioeconomic groups and is diagnosed three times more frequently in African-Americans. Aetiological factors include cigarette smoking, excessive alcohol intake and poor nutrition. Repeated oral infection, development of benign oesophageal stricture or achalasia and a history of syphilis are also thought to be contributory. The Plummer–Vinson (Paterson–Kelly) syndrome of a congenital web in the upper oesophagus, with glossitis and iron-deficiency anaemia, is a predisposing factor, more common in women. There is a significant incidence of oesophageal carcinoma developing within long-standing achalasia, and Barrett's oesophagus should also be regarded as a potentially premalignant condition, particularly in patients with dysplasia [2]. Although surgical excision has in the past been recommended as a prophylactic measure for high-grade dysplasia, there is an increasing interest in newer strategies such as endomucosal resection and photodynamic therapy in this condition. This group of patients must be kept in a strict surveillance programme. Finally, oesophageal cancer is reportedly more common in breast cancer patients who have received radiation therapy (relative risk for squamous oesophageal cancer 5.42 and for adenocarcinoma 4.22), presumably due directly to radiation carcinogenesis.

Pathology

The oesophagus can be conveniently divided into cervical oesophagus (distal limit 18 cm from upper incisors), mid-third (distal limit 30–31 cm from incisors) and lower third (distal 10 cm of oesophagus). The most frequent sites for oesophageal cancer are the narrowed areas in the cricopharyngeal region, adjacent to the bifurcation of the trachea, and in the lowest part of the oesophagus near the sphincter. Lower-third lesions are commonest (40–45%), followed by mid-third (35–40%) and cervical oesophageal cancers (10–15%). Both squamous carcinomas and adenocarcinomas occur, the histology varying with the level in the oesophagus. Cervical oesophageal and upper-third lesions are always squamous cell in origin. Adenocarcinomas are occasionally seen in the mid-third and are increasingly common in the lower

Cancer and its Management, Seventh Edition. Jeffrey Tobias and Daniel Hochhauser.
© 2015 John Wiley & Sons, Ltd. Published 2015 by John Wiley & Sons, Ltd.

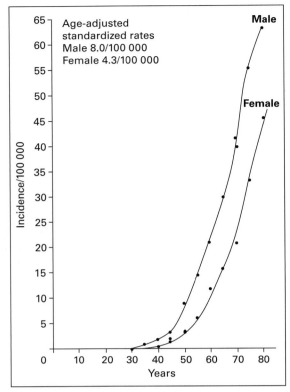

Figure 14.1   Age-specific incidence of carcinoma of the oesophagus.

third. Adenocarcinoma of the oesophagus is rising in incidence [1] and now accounts for an increasing proportion of cases, particularly in the gastro-oesophageal junction. The recent fivefold increase in adenocarcinoma of the oesophagus remains unexplained, the only known predisposing features being Barrett's oesophagus and duodenal ulcer (and occasionally in previously irradiated patients; see above).

Tumour spread (Figure 14.3) occurs chiefly by direct extension and by lymphatic metastases. Direct extension occurs early, both intramurally in the craniocaudal direction and circumferentially. Submucosal spread is almost universal and carries important implications for treatment. Direct mediastinal involvement occurs, usually later in the disease, by penetration of the muscular coat. Fistulous connection to the trachea may occur.

Cancers of the upper or cervical oesophagus chiefly drain to the deep cervical nodes either directly or via paratracheal or retropharyngeal lymphatics. Mid- and lower-third lesions drain to the posterior mediastinal

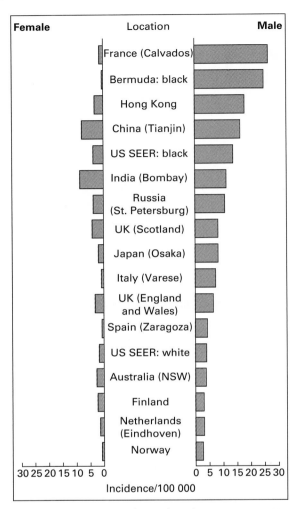

Figure 14.2   Incidence of oesophageal cancer, 1983–1987. Directly standardized rates per 100 000 (world population). These international comparisons show a high incidence stretching from the Caspian Sea across Mongolia and northern China. European rates are generally low, with the remarkable exception of the Calvados region in northern France.

nodes and abdominal nodes, sometimes traversing the diaphragm. Haematogenous spread characteristically occurs later, although unexpected hepatic metastases may be encountered at laparotomy in cases thought to be suitable for radical surgery. The liver is much the commonest site of haematogenous spread, though bone, lung and brain deposits also occur.

The patterns of drainage are important in defining clinical stage. For example, involvement of coeliac nodes

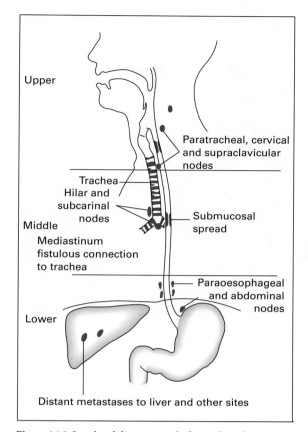

Figure 14.3 Local and distant spread of oesophageal cancer.

would be defined as local lymph node involvement for a carcinoma of the lower oesophagus but would be regarded as metastatic in relation to cancers of the upper and mid-third oesophagus.

Clinical features

The risk of oesophageal adenocarcinoma is almost eight times higher in persons with symptoms of gastro-oesophageal reflux (heartburn, regurgitation) [3]. When the disease becomes established, dysphagia is the commonest symptom, frequently accompanied by weight loss, often amounting to 10% or more of body weight. The dysphagia is more pronounced for solids than liquids, and patients often find that a soft or liquidized diet is the only means of securing a regular intake of food. Typically, the dysphagia becomes more severe, and some patients progress to complete dysphagia with inability even to swallow their own saliva. Many are able to point to the site at which the food lodges. Pain is a relatively late symptom, usually felt retrosternally. Spillover or aspiration of oesophageal contents into the larynx or lung may cause coughing, and involvement of the recurrent laryngeal nerve may lead to hoarseness. Haematemesis and melaena are unusual.

On examination there may be no abnormality apart from obvious weight loss and malnourishment. Occasionally, patients present with metastatic symptoms, usually from liver metastases, with only minimal dysphagia. Evidence of metastases may be found on examination, with enlarged supraclavicular nodes or hepatomegaly.

Investigation and staging

Patients with dysphagia should be urgently investigated with endoscopy or barium swallow and meal. In general, endoscopy is the investigation of choice, wherever possible. Radiologically, the characteristic appearance is of an obvious area of irregular narrowing (Figure 14.4). The narrowed segment may be long, often with an irregular 'shoulder'. Patients with severe dysphagia may be difficult to investigate because of the danger of aspiration of contrast material into the lungs. Paratracheal or other mediastinal node enlargement is common, and is generally a contraindication to radical surgery. Figure 14.5 shows the typical computed tomography (CT) appearances (sagittal view), with concentric thickening at the lower end of the oesophagus, together with food debris within. The cause of the dysphagia is sometimes due to secondary mediastinal lymphadenopathy.

Endoscopic oesophagoscopy and biopsy are mandatory in all patients who are fit enough to undergo the procedure. Intraluminal endoscopic ultrasonography gives additional internal anatomical detail that allows more accurate assessment of nodal involvement. About two-thirds of patients have lymphatic involvement at the time of diagnosis. The extent of the primary tumour may be difficult to determine even under direct vision, and positron emission tomography (PET) or PET/CT fusion scans, if available, may provide the most reliable information. It can sometimes be difficult to pass the endoscope so the lower border may be inaccurately determined.

Treatment

It is generally agreed that adenocarcinoma of the oesophagus (almost always lower-third lesions) is best treated by surgery for attempted cure if the lesion is technically operable. In other cases, particularly squamous cancers of upper-third and cervical oesophagus, combinations of

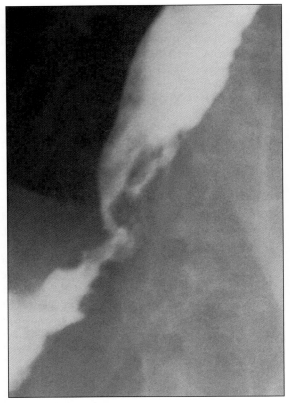

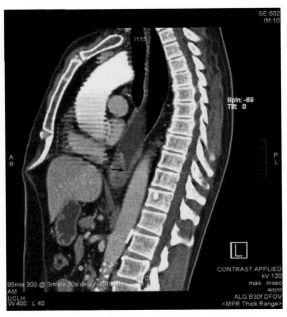

Figure 14.5 Sagittal CT view of a lower-third oesophageal carcinoma that proved at biopsy to be an adenocarcinoma, potentially surgically resectable. (Courtesy of Dr Chris Hare.)

Figure 14.4 Barium swallow showing carcinoma of distal oesophagus. A long irregular stricture is shown, with dilation above.

chemotherapy and radiotherapy are probably equivalent. Before embarking on local treatment, the surgeon or radiotherapist must be clear as to whether the aim of treatment is radical or palliative. The management of oesophageal cancer is optimally achieved by a multidisciplinary team including surgeon, gastroenterologist, radiologist, and radiation and medical oncologists.

Radical treatment

When radical surgical treatment is contemplated in patients who are generally fit and with no evidence of distant disease, it is important to determine the extent of the lesion before definitive resection is attempted. Exploratory laparoscopy is often advocated to determine if there is occult peritoneal dissemination undetected on imaging. Radical removal of the oesophagus is usually performed as a single-stage procedure with oesophagogastric anastomosis or colonic interposition. Only a

minority of patients with oesophageal cancer are suitable for radical surgery, and the commonest indication is a mid- or lower-third lesion, particularly where the histology is adenocarcinoma, in a fit patient with no demonstrable evidence of metastases.

In patients with squamous carcinomas of the oesophagus, chemoradiation is usually considered, though surgical treatment is preferred by some. No randomized comparison has been made. Combinations of chemotherapy and radiotherapy are more effective than radiation therapy alone [4,5].

The upper third of the oesophagus is technically a difficult area to irradiate because of the length of the treatment field and the proximity of the spinal cord (Figure 14.6). Radiation fields should ideally extend for at least 5 cm above and below the known limits of disease, in order to treat adequately the presumed submucosal extension. As with postcricoid carcinomas, sophisticated planning techniques are often required, using twisted, wedged, oblique, multiple fields, often with compensators, and careful radiation planning at two or three levels so that a cylinder of tissue is irradiated to a uniform high dose without over-irradiation of the adjacent spinal cord.

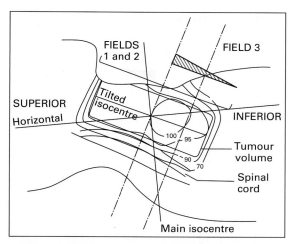

Figure 14.6 Radical radiotherapy for carcinoma of the cervical oesophagus. The irregular anatomy necessitates a complex multi-field treatment plan.

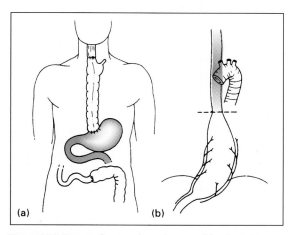

Figure 14.7 Surgery for oesophageal cancer: (a) colonic interposition following total oesophagectomy; (b) gastric mobilization and pull-through for carcinoma of the lower third.

With tumours of the mid-third of the oesophagus preoperative or radical is technically simpler than with tumours of the upper third. For cancer of the lower third of the oesophagus, surgery is often preferable and reconstruction, usually employing mobilized stomach (see Figure 14.7), less difficult.

At all sites, complications of treatment can be troublesome or even severe, for both radiotherapy and surgery. Radical radiotherapy, when surgery is not indicated, is often accompanied by radiation oesophagitis, requiring

treatment with alkaline or aspirin-containing suspensions to act locally on the inflamed oesophageal mucosa. Potential later complications include radiation damage to spinal cord (see Chapter 11) or lung, leading to radiation pneumonitis and occasionally dyspnoea, cough and reduction in respiratory capacity, although in day-to-day practice these are rarely seen. Oesophageal fibrosis and scarring can lead to stricturing of the oesophagus, which may require dilatation to retain oesophageal patency. Despite these concerns, most patients tolerate this treatment surprisingly well, even when chemotherapy is used. Surgical complications include oesophageal stricture and anastomotic leak, resulting in mediastinitis, pneumonitis and septicaemia, which can be fatal.

For patients with high-grade dysplasia within Barrett's oesophagus, photodynamic therapy has shown considerable promise. Although current evidence is based on small patient numbers, this form of treatment is appropriate in selected cases [6]. However, a study comparing radiofrequency ablation with surveillance in patients with Barretts and dysplasia, showed complete eradication of dysplasia in 77.4% of the treated group versus 2.3% in the surveillance group [7]. Additionally there were significantly fewer cancers arising in the treated group (1.2% vs 9.3%).

Neoadjuvant therapy

In view of the poor results obtained from surgical treatment alone there has been increased interest in preoperative (neoadjuvant) treatment with chemotherapy or chemoradiation in selected patients. The objective of this treatment is to reduce the size of the primary tumour and to eradicate distant metastases. Until recently there was little, if any, evidence that preoperative radiotherapy or chemotherapy influences resection rate, operative mortality rate or overall survival, but a large-scale study from the UK (OEO2) showed a striking improvement using a preoperative combination of chemotherapy (cisplatin and 5-FU) [8]. The 2-year survival rates were 43% and 34% (with or without chemotherapy); median survival rates were 16.8 months compared with 13.3 months. This has made preoperative chemotherapy the standard of care in the United Kingdom, although it should be noted that a similarly designed US study failed to show benefits using this approach [9].

Palliative treatment

Palliative treatment [10] is critical in oesophageal cancer for relief of dysphagia, malnutrition, pain and intra-luminal tumour bleeding, using either a stent or other indwelling prosthesis, radiotherapy or laser treatment. Patients unsuitable for radical surgery or radiotherapy should always be considered for palliative treatment, particularly if the dysphagia is severe. Modest doses of radiation can result in impressive clinical improvements. In experienced hands, passage of a stent or expandable metallic mesh endo-oesophageal tube is relatively safe and effective, and can be combined with radiation therapy. Common problems associated with tube insertion include migration of the tube, gastro-oesophageal reflux (sometimes associated with lung aspiration of gastric contents) and retrosternal pain or discomfort. Complications from palliative irradiation should be minimal since dosage is low: treatment to a dose of 30 Gy in daily fractions over a 2-week period is usually beneficial, provided the dysphagia is not total, and high doses are rarely warranted. Endo-oesophageal brachytherapy offers a simple and rapid alternative.

Laser therapy has a role [10] in restoration of swallowing, even sometimes after a single session, and is easily repeatable. For patients with unresectable tumours it may offer the best and least traumatic form of palliation.

The use of systemic chemotherapy has been shown to produce improved survival and palliation of symptoms in both oesophageal and gastric cancers (see below). Dysphagia can usually be significantly improved following treatment, particularly with squamous cancers of the oesophagus.

Carcinoma of the stomach

Incidence and aetiology

Fifty years ago, stomach cancer was the leading cause of cancer death in the United Kingdom. It has sharply declined in incidence but still remains an important cause of mortality worldwide [11], with an estimated 790 000 new cases occurring annually. High incidence rates (30–80 per 100 000) occur in the Far East, Russia and Eastern Europe. The overall incidence in the United Kingdom is 29 per 100 000 (men) and 19 per 100 000 (women). Incidence rises steeply with age, to over 200 per 100 000 men aged over 80. In both the UK and USA, there has been a gradual reduction of death rate in the last 20 years. In other countries the incidence is far higher, for example, 80 per 100 000 in Japan and Korea and 70 per 100 000 in Chile (Figure 14.8). Environmental causes are suggested by the fact that Japanese migrants to the USA show a reduction in incidence but still retain a higher risk than the indigenous population. The likelihood of

developing gastric cancer is also related to socioeconomic class, the disease being twice as common in classes 4 and 5 as in classes 1 and 2 (Figures 14.9 and 14.10).

The causes of carcinoma of the stomach are unknown, but genetic, environmental, dietary, infective and premalignant factors have been implicated (Table 14.1) Gastric carcinoma is three to six times as common in patients with pernicious anaemia, which is itself an inherited disorder. The cancer is slightly more common in people with blood group A than in the general population, and possibly in patients who have had a Polya partial gastrectomy. Patients with inherited hypogammaglobulinaemia have a greatly increased risk of gastric cancer.

Table 14.1 Risk factors positively associated with stomach cancer.

Diet
Low intake of animal fats and protein
High intake of carbohydrates, mainly from grains and
    starchy roots
High salt intake
High dietary nitrate intake (from water or foodstuffs)
Low intake of fresh fruits
Low intake of raw vegetables and salads
Smoking
Alcohol

Socioeconomic
Overcrowded housing
Low socioeconomic status
Low income
Large families
Dusty occupations, for example, pottery industry

Geographical
North Wales
Staffordshire

Genetic
Blood group A
Hereditary non-polyposis colon cancer

Medical
Pernicious anaemia
Chronic atrophic gastritis
Helicobacter pylori infection
Gastric surgery
Hypogammaglobulinaemia

Source: Data from Cancer Research
(http://www.cancerresearchuk.org/cancer-info/cancerstats/
types/stomach/riskfactors/, accessed April 2014).

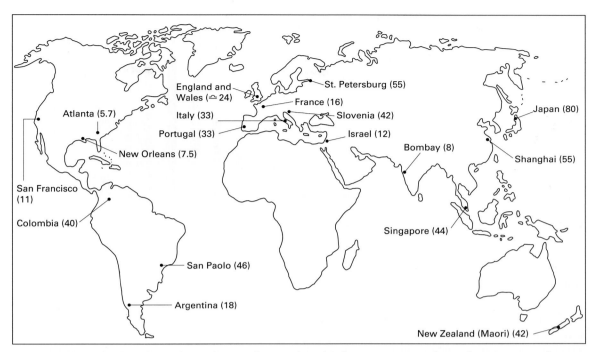

Figure 14.8 Geographical incidence of stomach cancer figures indicate incidence per 100 000 male population. American figures are for the white population only; rates are approximately double in the black population. Stomach cancer probably remains the second commonest cancer worldwide, despite the recent decline in incidence.

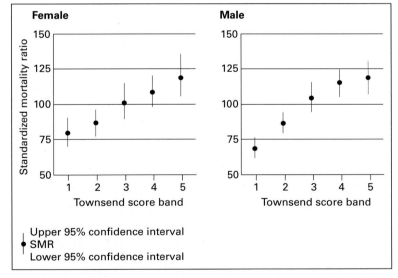

Figure 14.9 Gastric cancer mortality related to socioeconomic class. Figures are for men aged 15–64 for the years 1970–1972 in England and Wales. Values for each social class are in proportion to 100, which represents all social classes combined. 'Townsend score band' refers to what was previously regarded as 'social class' but is now more clearly defined with respect to socioeconomic status. (Figures from data from the Office of Population Censuses and Surveys, 1978.)

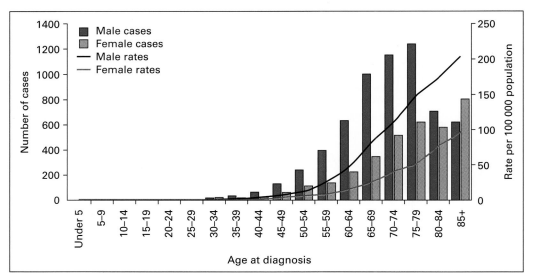

Figure 14.10 Number of new cases and rates by age and sex, stomach cancer, UK, 1999.

There is an increased incidence of carcinoma of the stomach in patients with chronic atrophic gastritis. The increased risk in patients with pernicious anaemia and atrophic gastritis is approximately threefold. Gastric atrophy may be followed by intestinal metaplasia and it has been postulated that dietary carcinogens might provoke this change. Dietary characteristics of populations at high risk for gastric cancer include high intake of salt, dietary nitrates, starches and carbohydrates, and low intake of raw vegetables, salads, fresh fruit and animal protein. A hypothesis for the stepwise causation of gastric carcinoma is shown in Figure 14.11 together with a summary of known aetiological features. It is likely that gastric atrophy leads to a rise in pH in the stomach and subsequent bacterial colonization which cannot occur at low pH. Gastric atrophy appears to relate to malnutrition in countries where there is a high risk of gastric cancer. Bacterial colonization of the stomach is much more common below 50 years of age in these regions. Pernicious anaemia is also accompanied by gastric atrophy, and hypoacidity may occur following Polya partial gastrectomy, both being situations where the risk of gastric cancer may be increased. The result of bacterial colonization may be to reduce dietary nitrates (present in water, vegetables and cured meats) to nitrites, which in turn react with amino acids to form N-nitroso compounds. These are carcinogens in animals (causing intestinal metaplasia of the gastric mucosa in rats) and may be so in humans.

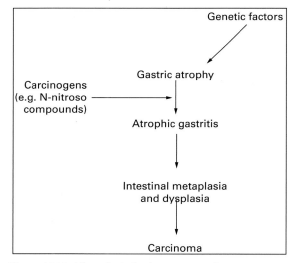

Figure 14.11 A hypothesis for the causation of gastric cancer.

The association of gastric cancer with *Helicobacter pylori* infection is compelling [12]. *H. pylori* infection is associated with the development of gastritis, with associated cell proliferation and DNA damage; 65–80% of non-cardia gastric cancers may be attributable to infection. The preventive implications of this association, if confirmed, are of great potential importance, since the infection affects 30–50% of European adults and over 80% in parts of the developing world. These figures do not explain the worldwide male preponderance of gastric cancer. Overall, studies suggests that successful eradication of chronic *H. pylori* reduces the risk of gastric cancer [13]. This has led to the suggestion of population-based screening and eradication of *H. pylori* for high-risk populations such as the Asia-Pacific region.

Up to 10% of gastric cancers may have a familial predisposition, particularly the hereditary diffuse form. The only clearly identified genetic link is in mutations of the E-cadherin gene [14]. Referral of suspected familial gastric cancer patients to specialized genetic clinics is essential to allow the screening and identification of mutations [15]. In some cases prophylactic gastrectomy will be warranted and has been demonstrated to result in the removal of early, clinically undetectable cancers.

The association between gastric cancer and peptic ulceration remains uncertain as is the relationship between gastric polyps and malignancy. Gastric polyps are relatively common and 10% show evidence of carcinoma *in situ*. This change has doubtful prognostic significance, and the lesion which seems most likely to be premalignant is the villous adenoma (Figure 14.12).

Pathology

Over 95% of gastric carcinomas are adenocarcinomas. Carcinoid tumours, squamous carcinoma, adenoacanthoma and leiomyosarcoma make up the rest. Early gastric cancer is defined as a tumour confined to the mucosa and submucosa, irrespective of lymph-node invasion. Histological differentiation from 'precancerous' lesions can be difficult, even with gastric biopsy. Symptoms are minimal and the diagnosis is often made at endoscopy for screening (see below) or for an unrelated symptom. The lesions are usually adenocarcinomas with features similar to those for advanced cancers.

The commonest type of gastric cancer is a diffuse infiltrating lesion which varies in size from 1 cm to a tumour that may occupy most of the stomach. It often invades through the stomach wall, spreading into the pancreas and omentum, metastasizing to regional lymph nodes, liver and peritoneal cavity. Some tumours exhibit a polypoid growth with projection into the lumen of the stomach, later invading the stomach wall and adjacent tissues. Others spread superficially through the mucosa, sparing regional lymph nodes until late in the disease and with a better prognosis. In other cases there is a diffuse sclerosis involving the whole of the stomach wall (linitis plastica). The stomach is small and contracted and will not distend. This tumour has a particularly poor prognosis. Cancers tend to arise in the antrum or lower third of the stomach and are more common on the lesser curvature. Some of these tumours are multicentric. The location of these tumours appears to be changing with time, with an increase in proximal tumours and

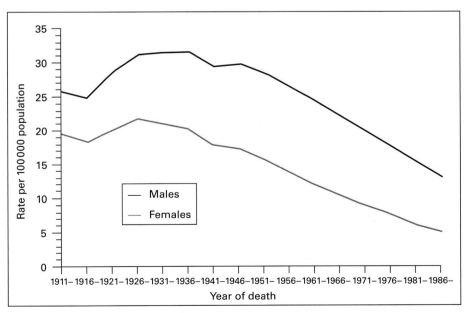

Figure 14.12 World-standardized mortality rates, males and females, England and Wales 1911–1990.

a decline in those in the antrum, both in the West and in Japan.

Microscopically, the most useful division is made between those carcinomas where the cells resemble intestinal cells and there is intestinal metaplasia surrounding the tumour (intestinal type) and those which tend to infiltrate the gastric wall and are surrounded by normal mucosa (diffuse type). Tumours of the intestinal type are associated with a better survival, tend to occur in older patients and are more likely to be preceded by atrophic gastritis. In high-risk populations (such as Japan) most tumours are of this type. Diffuse carcinomas occur more frequently in women, are associated with blood group A and have a worse overall survival. Parietal cell tumours are an uncommon variant.

In Japan, screening programmes have resulted in many tumours being diagnosed early, and the term 'early gastric cancer' has been introduced for tumours limited to the mucosa or submucosa. These can be of the intestinal or diffuse types with varying degrees of differentiation. At this stage the prognosis is excellent with over 90% of patients alive at 5 years. Lymphatic spread of the tumour (Figure 14.13) is via the superficial lymphatic networks into nodes in the left gastric chain and the splenic and hepatic chains along the lines of major vascular supply to the stomach. Spread is then to nodes in the coeliac plexus, the splenic chain and into the hepatic chain around the porta hepatis. There is sometimes enlargement of nodes in the left supraclavicular region deep to the sternomastoid insertion (Virchow's node). Cancer of the stomach also spreads locally through the stomach wall into the omentum, liver and pancreas. Tumours can seed through the peritoneal cavity, causing malignant ascites and Krukenberg tumours on the surface of the ovary. Blood-borne metastases are particularly common in the liver but pulmonary metastases also occur. Bone metastases are uncommon and central nervous system metastases are rare.

Clinical features

Initial symptoms are often mild and indefinite resulting in late diagnosis. These include anorexia, nausea and vague upper abdominal pain, but many patients are only diagnosed at the time a large epigastric mass is palpable (sometimes with ascites), making curative resection clearly impossible. Other symptoms include dysphagia (particularly with proximal tumours) and vomiting if there is outflow obstruction. Massive gastrointestinal bleeding does occur but is unusual. Low-grade bleeding is common and presentation with iron-deficiency

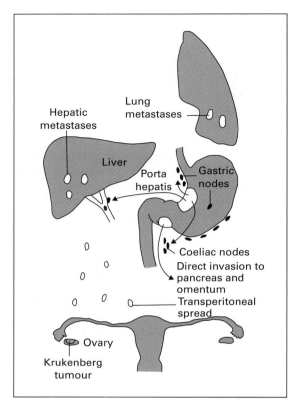

Figure 14.13 Common paths of spread in gastric cancer.

anaemia not infrequent. Non-metastatic manifestations of malignancy are unusual, with the exception of acanthosis nigricans (see Chapter 9).

Clinical signs are minimal except in the late stages. The patient will usually appear to have lost weight, and may be anaemic. Virchow's node may be palpable in the left supraclavicular region and there may be an epigastric mass or hepatomegaly from metastases. Tumour masses may be felt on abdominal or pelvic examination and ascites may be present. These signs indicate inoperable advanced cancer.

Diagnosis

The standard diagnostic investigation was the double-contrast barium meal examination (Figure 14.14) but this has been almost totally replaced by endoscopy. At endoscopy, multiple biopsies from the ulcer or tumour are obtained. A positive biopsy or cytology is obtained in around 90% of patients, except in the infiltrative forms of gastric carcinoma where the diagnosis can be missed on both endoscopic appearance and cytological

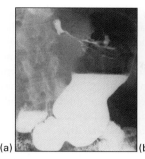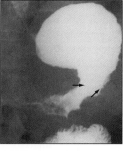

Figure 14.14 Barium meal appearances in carcinoma of the stomach. (a) Carcinoma at cardio-oesophageal junction showing tumour infiltration with mucosal irregularity. (b) Linitis plastica. The tumour infiltrates extensively (arrow).

Table 14.2 TNM staging system for gastric carcinoma.

T stage			
T1	Limited to mucosa or submucosa		
T2	Extension to serosa		
T3	Extension through serosa		
T4	Invasion of local structures		
N stage			
N0	No nodes		
N1	Local node involvement within 8 cm		
N2	Node involvement more than 3 cm, but resectable		
N3	Distant node involvement		
M stage			
M0	No metastases		
M1	Distant metastases		
Stage grouping			
Stage I	T1	N0	M0
Stage II	T2–3	N0	M0
Stage III	T1–3	N1–2	M0
	T4a	N0	M0
Stage IV	T1–3	N3	M0
	T4a	N1–3	M1

examination. Liver function tests and full blood count should be carried out. CT scanning defines nodal or hepatic metastases and extent of local spread such as involvement of the lesser sac or liver. PET scanning is indicated to define possible metastatic disease. Tumour node metastasis (TNM) staging system is shown in Table 14.2. In the United Kingdom, the majority of patients present at stages III and IV. Tumours demonstrating local invasion (T4) or distant metastases (M1) are typically not amenable to curative treatment. Patient fitness is defined by physical activity status, biological age and comorbidities, and is measured objectively by lung function and cardiopulmonary exercise testing, where indicated.

Early diagnosis of gastric carcinoma

Because so many patients present with inoperable disease, programmes have been devised to screen for the disease in countries such as Japan where there is a very high incidence. A high incidence (31%) of early carcinomas has been found, with excellent survival following surgery. It is not clear if early gastric cancer will always develop into advanced disease but it is reasonable to assume that this will usually occur. Unfortunately in the United Kingdom (Table 14.3), late diagnosis is the rule, with only 20% of patients proving surgically operable, though increased awareness in primary care should result in improvements. Screening asymptomatic populations, especially in low-risk countries, has not proved cost-effective, although screening of patients with upper abdominal symptoms has been suggested as a compromise since 50% of cases of early gastric cancer diagnosed by screening had such symptoms. In countries such as the UK, such an approach is the only practical possibility in view of declining incidence, and may become increasingly

Table 14.3 Accuracy of four diagnostic methods to assess TNM features in patients with gastric carcinoma.

	CT (%)	EUS (%)	Hydro-CT (%)	Lap. (%)
T category	25–66	71–92	51	47
N category	25–68	55–87	51	60–90
M category	65–72	–	79	80–90

EUS, endogastric ultrasonography; Lap., laparoscopy (with laparoscopic ultrasonography).
Source: Reproduced from Hohenburger & Gretschel [16] with permission from Elsevier.

justifiable in view of the rapidly rising incidence of carcinoma at the gastro-oesophageal junction.

Treatment

Surgical treatment of gastric carcinoma

Surgical resection is the only curative treatment for gastric carcinoma. A variety of procedures can be performed, depending on the localization of the tumour and the degree of local extension. The most radical surgery involves total gastrectomy (Figure 14.15), although for relatively localized tumours a partial gastrectomy can be performed. Some form of subtotal gastrectomy is the most generally employed surgical procedure. Total gastrectomy, if required, involves removal of the entire stomach, the greater omentum, usually removal of the spleen and occasionally of the lower portion of the oesophagus if the tumour is proximal. In a radical subtotal gastrectomy 80% of the stomach is removed with the omentum and part of the duodenum. Following gastrectomy, there is now a wide variety of options for surgical restoration of gastrointestinal continuity. Furthermore, the extent of the regional lymphadenectomy has been the subject of intense debate over the past few years [17]. A

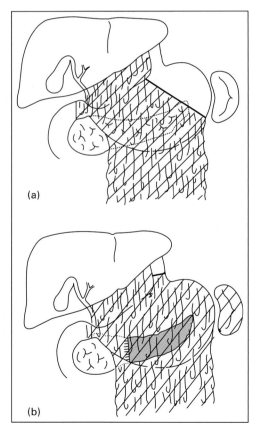

Figure 14.15 Operations for gastric carcinoma: (a) radical subtotal gastrectomy; (b) extended total gastrectomy.

large Dutch group recently reported additional operative complications and mortality with the more radical Japanese approach of extended gastrectomy with regional node dissection – though this procedure is performed routinely in Japan – without necessarily adding to overall survival. Recent randomised controlled trials have advocated D2 lymph node dissection (perigastric nodes and nodes along the coeliac trunk) over D1 dissection (perigastric nodes only) because D2 dissection results in lower rates of locoregional recurrence and cancer related death, despite increased rates of early morbidity and mortality [18] The morbidity of total gastrectomy is considerable, with difficulty in maintaining body weight and, if the patient survives, the issues of iron- and vitamin B_{12}-deficient anaemia that requires lifelong treatment.

Patients presenting with a large intra-abdominal mass, malignant ascites, demonstrable nodal deposits, fixity of the tumour, or liver metastases are generally inoperable. In inoperable cases, bypass procedures are usually unrewarding.

The results of surgery remain poor despite repeated attempts at more extensive resections. In European studies only 60–70% of patients undergoing surgery prove to have resectable tumours. Of these, in some series only 20–25% will be alive at 5 years. In Japan the results are much better, with a higher surgical resectability rate (70–75%). Of those resected, 55% are alive at 5 years, and the 5-year postoperative survival rate is about 30%. In Japanese studies 15% of cases have early gastric cancer, compared with 2.5% in the West. There is evidence that these results may now be reproducible in Western populations with optimal surgery in specialised centres [19].

Radiation treatment
Palliation of some of the symptoms of gastric carcinoma can occasionally be achieved with radiation. Treatment is difficult since there are numerous radiosensitive organs in the upper abdomen, namely, the small intestine, liver, spinal cord and kidneys. A dose of 40 Gy can usually be administered safely in 4–5 weeks. Anorexia and nausea are frequent and patients usually lose weight during the procedure. The intention is palliative, although occasional long-term survival has been noted.

Chemotherapy for cancer of the stomach
In advanced gastric cancer, chemotherapy may produce response rates of greater than 50% responses are partial, lasting for only a few months. There is evidence

that survival is prolonged by the use of chemotherapy either as single agents or in combination. Additionally, randomised trials have demonstrated improved quality of life benefit from chemotherapy over BSC alone for patients with metastatic gastric cancer [20]. The results of combination chemotherapy are superior to single-agent regimens and now represent the standard of care. In advanced gastric cancer several combination chemotherapy regimens have been used. In the past, the most widely used was the combination of 5-FU, doxorubicin and mitomycin (FAM) with a response rate of about 40%, but more intensive regimens have produced response rates as high as 62%. Epirubicin is now more frequently used instead of doxorubicin, often in combination with cisplatin and infusional 5-FU (ECF regimen) which showed optimal activity in comparison with a number of other regimens [21]. The tolerability of this regimen has been improved by the substitution of oxaliplatin for cisplatin and the orally bioavailable capecitabine for 5-FU. A large randomized study (REAL2) indicated equivalent efficacy for this combination [17]. There are modest benefits for second line chemotherapy with irinotecan and paclitaxel as second line therapy following progression [22].

Adjuvant chemotherapy

There has been recent interest in the use of chemotherapy as an adjuvant to surgical removal of the tumour with either a small or no improvement found in a several studies. Although most studies have failed to show a significantly improved survival in the chemotherapy-treated group compared with surgery alone a recent meta-analysis suggests a significant benefit of around 6% improvement in overall survival [23]. In a Japanese study use of the oral fluoropyrimidine S-1 resulted in a significant improvement in survival over surgery alone of 80% versus 70% at 3 years [24]. It remains unclear as to whether this approach might be more widely beneficial especially noting the excellent survival in the surgery-only arm but the significant benefit was still apparent on 5-year survival rates [25].

However, a randomized study in over 500 patients provided a strongly positive result for adjuvant chemoradiotherapy used postoperatively in high-risk adenocarcinoma of the stomach or gastro-oesophageal junction [26]. The median survival for patients treated with surgery alone was 27 months as compared with 36 months for those treated additionally with chemoradiation. There were substantial toxicities in the chemoradiation arm with a 1% mortality and, additionally, concerns were raised about survival in the surgery-alone arm as compared with expected median survival for this group. However, this result has altered clinical practice in the United States. The issue of adjuvant chemotherapy in gastric cancer has been controversial. Several small studies have suggested a benefit and this has now been confirmed in meta-analyses.

Neoadjuvant treatment of gastric cancer

The rationale for systemic treatment administered prior to definitive surgery (neoadjuvant) or following resection (adjuvant) is to treat micro-metastases and hence improve outcome. The pivotal Medical Research Council Adjuvant Gastric Infusional Chemotherapy (MAGIC) study of over 500 patients with operable gastric and oesophagogastric junction cancers confirmed a major benefit for perioperative (i.e. treatment before and after surgery) chemotherapy [27]. This has become the standard of care for resectable gastric cancer in the United Kingdom. Using the ECF regimen, the survival rate at 5 years was 36% in patients treated with chemotherapy as compared with 23% in the surgery-alone group. In conclusion, there is a clear role for adjuvant therapy in gastric cancer (and tumours of the oesophagogastric junction). In terms of tolerability and long-term survival, chemotherapy is a more attractive option especially where the quality of surgery is good. Research is currently focusing on alternative strategies with differing combinations of chemotherapeutic agents and addition of novel biological therapies.

Targeted agents in gastric cancer

There has thus far been only moderate success in the development of biological agents for treatment of gastric cancer. However approximately one-fifth of patients with gastric cancer have tumours which show amplification for HER2 (erbB2), more frequently amplified in breast cancer. The randomised ToGA (Trastuzumab with Chemotherapy in HER2-Positive Advanced Gastric Cancer) study involving nearly 600 patients, demonstrated that herceptin (trastuzumab) plus chemotherapy (cisplatin with capecitabine or 5-FU) was superior to chemotherapy alone in this group of patients [28]. For patients whose tumours showed high HER2 expression, median overall survival was 16.0 months in those assigned to trastuzumab plus chemotherapy compared with 11.8 months in those assigned to chemotherapy alone. The ToGA trial has established this treatment as standard for HER2 positive patients with advanced cancer. Another area of progress is through targeting the angiogenesis pathway. Additionally, recent randomized study demonstrated that ramucirumab, a monoclonal antibody VEGFR-2 antagonist, prolonged survival in patients with advanced gastric cancer. Although this was only a modest effect, the study illustrates that targeted agents may play a role in treatment of gastric cancer [29].

References

1 Pennathur A, Gibson MK, Jobe BA *et al.* Oesophageal carcinoma. *Lancet* 2013; 381: 400–12.

2 Bird-Lieberman EL, Fitzgerald RC. Early diagnosis of oesophageal cancer. *Br J Cancer* 2009; 101(1): 1–6.

3 Lagergren J, Bergstrom R, Linogren M, Nyren O. Symptomatic gastroesophageal reflux as a risk factor for esophageal adenocarcinoma. *N Engl J Med* 1999; 340: 825–83.

4 Al-Sarraf M, Martz K, Herskovic A *et al.* Progress report of combination chemoradiotherapy versus radiotherapy alone in patients with esophageal cancer: an intergroup study. *J Clin Oncol* 1997; 15: 227–84.

5 Cooper JS, Guo MD, Herskovic A *et al.* Chemoradiotherapy of locally advanced esophageal cancer. *JAMA* 1999; 281: 1623–27.

6 Allum WH, Blazeby JM, Griffin SM *et al.* Guidelines for the management of oesophageal and gastric cancer. *Gut* 2011; 60(11): 1449–72.

7 Shaheen NJ, Sharma P, Overholt BF *et al.* Radiofrequency ablation in Barrett's esophagus with dysplasia. *N Engl J Med* 2009; 360: 2277–88.

8 MRC Oesophageal Cancer Working Party. Surgical resection with or without preoperative chemotherapy in oesophageal cancer: a randomised controlled trial. *Lancet* 2002; 359: 1727–33.

9 Kelsen DP, Ginsberg R, Pajak TF *et al.* Chemotherapy followed by surgery compared with surgery alone for localized oesophageal cancer. *N Engl J Med* 1998; 339: 1979–84.

10 Freeman RK, Ascioti AJ, Mahidhara RJ. Palliative therapy for patients with unresectable esophageal carcinoma. *Surg Clin North Am.* 2012; 92(5): 1337–51.

11 Thrumurthy SG, Chaudry MA, Hochhauser D, Mughal M. The diagnosis and management of gastric cancer. *BMJ* 2013; 347: f6367.

12 Eurogast Study Group. An international association between *Helicobacter pylori* infection and gastric cancer. *Lancet* 1993; 341: 1359–62.

13 Fuccio L, Zagari RM, Eusebi LH *et al.* Meta-analysis: can Helicobacter pylori eradication treatment reduce the risk for gastric cancer? *Ann Intern Med* 2009; 151: 121–8.

14 Guilford P, Hopkins J, Harraway J *et al.* E-cadherin germline mutations in familial gastric cancer. *Nature* 1998; 392: 402–5.

15 Fitzgerald RC, Hardwick R, Huntsman D *et al.* Hereditary diffuse gastric cancer: updated consensus guidelines for clinical management and directions for future research. *J Med Genet* 2010; 47(7): 436–44.

16 Hohenburger P, Gretschel S. Gastric cancer. *Lancet* 2003; 362: 305–15.

17 Cunningham D, Starling N, Rao S, *et al.* Capecitabine and oxaliplatin for advanced esophagogastric cancer. *N Engl J Med* 2008; 358: 36–46.

18 Songun I, Putter H, Kranenbarg EM, Sasako M, van de Velde CJ. Surgical treatment of gastric cancer: 15-year follow-up results of the randomised nationwide Dutch D1D2 trial. *Lancet Oncol* 2010; 11: 439–49.

19 Hanna GB, Boshier PR, Knaggs A, Goldin R, Sasako M. Improving outcomes after gastroesophageal cancer resection: can Japanese results be reproduced in Western centers? *Arch Surg* 2012; 147(8): 738–45.

20 Wagner AD, Unverzagt S, Grothe W *et al.* Chemotherapy for advanced gastric cancer. *Cochrane Database Syst Rev* 2010; 3: CD004064.

21 Webb A, Cunningham D, Scarffe JH, *et al.* Randomized trial comparing epirubicin, cisplatin, and fluorouracil versus fluorouracil, doxorubicin, and methotrexate in advanced esophagogastric cancer. *J Clin Oncol* 1997; 15: 261–7.

22 Kang JH, Lee SI, Lim do H *et al.* Salvage chemotherapy for pretreated gastric cancer: a randomized phase III trial comparing chemotherapy plus best supportive care with best supportive care alone. *J Clin Oncol* 2012; 30: 1513–8.

23 Paoletti X, Oba K, Burzykowski T *et al.* Benefit of adjuvant chemotherapy for resectable gastric cancer: a meta-analysis. GASTRIC (Global Advanced/Adjuvant Stomach Tumor Research International Collaboration) Group, *JAMA.* 2010; 303: 1729–37.

24 Sakuramoto S, Sasako M, Yamaguchi T *et al.* Adjuvant chemotherapy for gastric cancer with S-1, an oral fluoropyrimidine. *N Engl J Med* 2007; 357: 1810–20.

25 Sasako M, Sakuramoto S, Katai H *et al.* Five-year outcomes of a randomized phase III trial comparing adjuvant chemotherapy with S-1 versus surgery alone in stage II or III gastric cancer. *J Clin Oncol* 2011; 29(33): 4387–93.

26 Macdonald JS, Smalley SR, Benedetti J *et al.* Chemoradiotherapy after surgery compared with surgery alone for adenocarcinoma of the stomach or gastroesophageal junction. *N Engl J Med* 2001; 345: 725–30.

27 Cunningham D, Allum WH, Stenning SP *et al.*, for the MAGIC Trial Participants. Perioperative chemotherapy

versus surgery alone for resectable gastroesophageal cancer. *N Engl J Med* 2006; 355: 11–20.

28 Bang YJ, Van Cutsem E, Feyereislova A *et al.* Trastuzumab in combination with chemotherapy versus chemotherapy alone for treatment of HER2-positive advanced gastric or gastro-oesophageal junction cancer (ToGA): a phase 3, open-label, randomised controlled trial. *Lancet* 2010; 376: 687–97.

29 Fuchs CS, Tomasek J, Yong CJ *et al.* Ramucirumab monotherapy for previously treated advanced gastric or gastro-oesophageal junction adenocarcinoma (REGARD): an international, randomised, multicentre, placebo-controlled, phase 3 trial. *Lancet* 2013; pii: S0140-6736(13) 61719-5.

15 Cancer of the liver, biliary tract and pancreas

Primary liver cancer

Primary cancer of the liver (predominantly hepatocellular carcinoma, HCC) is a major global health problem, being the fifth most common cancer in men and the seventh in women. [1]. It arises from a complex variety of genetic and environmental interactions [2]. There are several types of carcinoma arising in the liver, the most frequent being HCC. In recent years, there has been an increasing incidence of cholangiocarcinoma arising from within the intrahepatic bile ducts, and rarely, angiosarcoma and hepatoblastoma occur in adults.

Hepatocellular carcinoma (hepatoma)
Incidence
There are over 500 000 new cases a year worldwide [1]. In the UK and the USA, the incidence is approximately 1.8 per 100 000 for men and 0.7 per 100 000 for women (Figure 15.1). The tumour can arise in childhood. Worldwide the incidence (per 100 000) varies greatly: 104 in Mozambique, 29 in South Africa and 12 in Nigeria.

Aetiology
In the West, most cases of HCC (about 90%) arise in cirrhotic livers. The causes of cirrhosis with the highest risk of developing hepatoma are chronic hepatitis associated with alcohol, hepatitis B virus (HBV), hepatitis C virus (HCV) and haemochromatosis. Hepatoma is much more common in alcoholic cirrhosis where there is evidence of previous HBV infection. Patients with primary biliary cirrhosis and hepatitis B surface antigen (HBsAg)-negative chronic active hepatitis are less at risk (although more likely to develop the cancer than the non-cirrhotic population). The carcinoma is more likely to develop in men (male to female ratio 11:1) and in patients with long-standing cirrhosis over the age of 50. The association with cirrhosis is found in both high- and low-incidence areas. Duration of cirrhosis is more important than the aetiology. The 5-year cumulative risk for the development of HCC in patients with cirrhosis ranges between 5% and 30%, depending on the cause (with the highest risk among those infected with HCV), region or ethnic group (17% in the USA and 30% in

Cancer and its Management, Seventh Edition. Jeffrey Tobias and Daniel Hochhauser.
© 2015 John Wiley & Sons, Ltd. Published 2015 by John Wiley & Sons, Ltd.

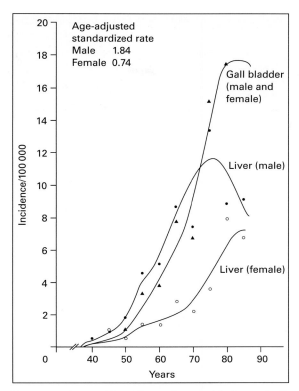

Figure 15.1 Age-specific incidence of cancer of the liver and gall-bladder (UK figures).

Japan), and stage of cirrhosis (with the highest risk among patients with decompensated disease) [1,3]. Increased prevalence of obesity in the population with resultant fatty liver may result in a further increase in incidence of HCC, although the extent of this emerging problem remains unclear [4].

The geographical variations in incidence may reflect different causal factors. Cirrhosis from any cause is associated with hepatoma. In low-incidence areas (Europe and North America) alcoholic cirrhosis is a more frequent association than in high-incidence areas where macronodular cirrhosis associated with HBV is the main association. Exposure to aflatoxin, derived from the *Aspergillus flavus* mould on stored grain, is more frequent in high-incidence areas. The toxin may be one of the factors which act as tumour promoters.

There is a strong causal association with HBV. In high-incidence areas 80% of cases are associated with serological evidence of HBV, with a risk of 230:1 in HBsAg-positive individuals. In the West 15–20% are HBsAg-positive. Viral DNA sequences have

been demonstrated in the genome of liver cells of HBsAg-positive individuals. HCV is an RNA virus that is not incorporated into the host DNA, but HCV proteins activate cell genes. Like HBV it is associated with HCC. Treatment of HCV chronic hepatitis with interferon alpha reduces the risk of subsequent HCC [5]. The carrier rate of HCV is 0.2% in northern Europe and 5% in the Far East. It can be transmitted by parenteral inoculation. HCV appears to be the most important causal association in the USA, Europe and Japan.

Pathology

In 60% of cases, the liver contains multiple nodules of cancer. In 30% of cases, there is a large single mass of cancer, often with surrounding lesions; in the remaining cases, the liver is diffusely infiltrated. In 80% of cases the surrounding liver is cirrhotic. In the group of patients where it is not, the sex ratio is equal and the average age is lower. In a small subgroup of the patients without cirrhosis, the tumour forms cords with collagen strands (fibrolamellar carcinoma). In cholangiocarcinoma of the intrahepatic ducts, the tumour cells form a tubular pattern, usually with extensive fibrosis.

Clinical features

The usual presentation is with right upper quadrant pain, weight loss and a palpable liver mass. In a cirrhotic patient this is often accompanied by a rapid deterioration in liver function. Usually, the cirrhosis is advanced and long-standing. Presentation may, therefore, be accompanied by ascites. Ascites may be due to cirrhosis, or due to the sudden onset of Budd–Chiari syndrome due to hepatic vein occlusion.

On examination, there may be evidence of cirrhosis and liver failure. The liver is enlarged with a palpable mass over which there may be a bruit. Frequently the tumour is asymptomatic and diagnosed on routine imaging.

Diagnosis

The presence of a focal liver mass greater than 2 cm with pre-existing cirrhosis confers a 95% probability of HCC. Elevated α-fetoprotein (AFP) is sufficient to make the diagnosis without confirmatory biopsy, which may be hazardous. If AFP is normal, computed tomography (CT), magnetic resonance imaging (MRI) or lipiodol angiography will facilitate diagnosis without the need for a biopsy. In selected cases including focal masses arising in the background of a normal liver and to differentiate from metastatic disease, biopsy may be indicated. Liver function tests have no diagnostic pattern or value but are generally abnormal. The tumour may produce erythropoietin and secondary polycythaemia may therefore be present. Other non-metastatic manifestations include hypoglycaemia, hypercalcaemia, gonadotrophin production, ectopic adrenocorticotrophic hormone (ACTH) and elevated plasma calcitonin (see also Chapter 9).

The malignant hepatocytes in most hepatomas produce AFP that can be detected in the serum. With sensitive methods, the serum AFP can be of diagnostic help. Levels below 10 ng/mL make the diagnosis very unlikely in a cirrhotic patient, although over half of non-cirrhotic patients do not have an elevated serum AFP. Levels of 10–500 ng/mL make the diagnosis probable, but cirrhosis due to chronic hepatitis may be associated with levels of this magnitude (as may metastases from the gastrointestinal tract). In the West, levels above 500 ng/mL in a cirrhotic patient make the diagnosis of HCC likely.

CT scans and ultrasound liver scans usually show a large lesion or multiple lesions, but in the presence of cirrhosis the appearances may not be diagnostic and care must be taken in interpretation. CT angiography may show a tumour circulation but is usually carried out only if there is diagnostic doubt or if there is a possibility of surgical resection or intra-arterial chemotherapy or embolization.

A biopsy of the lesion will help in diagnosis but may not be possible if liver function has deteriorated. If the prothrombin time is prolonged by more than 4 s, the procedure is unsafe since the tumours are vascular. Even with a biopsy, the histological distinction from metastatic tumours (such as hypernephroma) may be difficult.

Treatment

Treatment of HCC requires multidisciplinary management with specialist hepatology, surgery, oncology, radiology and pathology input. Resection of the tumour offers the only possibility of cure [6]. It must be considered particularly in a non-cirrhotic patient because the liver will regenerate even if three-quarters of the organ is removed. In a cirrhotic patient, resection may precipitate deterioration of liver function. Curative resection is possible in less than 10% of patients (Table 15.1). Liver transplantation is indicated for highly selected cirrhotic patients based on the Milan criteria. According to these criteria, transplantation can be considered only for patients with a single tumour <5 cm in diameter or for patients with up to 3 tumours <3 cm without macrovascular invasion.

Table 15.1 Indications for surgery in hepatocellular carcinoma.

No extrahepatic spread
No vascular invasion
Adequate liver function

Local ethanol injection has been used for palliation, although there is no evidence of efficacy from randomized studies. Embolization or ligation of the hepatic artery has been used, but these procedures also cause deterioration of function in the cirrhotic patient. Selective hepatic artery embolization may be attempted in a cirrhotic patient if the tumour is localized. The value of this technique has not been adequately assessed, but pain may be relieved and survival may possibly be improved. There is increased interest in combinations of chemotherapy and embolization and randomized trials are underway to assess the benefit of this approach.

Despite numerous phase II studies using a variety of agents, there is no evidence from randomized studies of a beneficial effect on survival from chemotherapy in advanced HCC. Doxorubicin has been the most widely used cytotoxic agent although there is little objective evidence of efficacy [7]. A pivotal placebo-controlled phase III study using sorafenib, an inhibitor of the vascular endothelial growth factor receptor cascade and raf kinase, was the first to show a significant survival advantage in this condition [8]. Overall survival was 10.7 months in the sorafenib arm compared with 7.9 months in the placebo arm. A subsequent randomized trial demonstrated that the combination of sorafenib with doxorubicin showed significantly improved overall survival compared with doxorubicin monotherapy (13.7 months versus 6.5 months) [9] but it will be important to demonstrate if chemotherapy improves efficacy when combined with sorafenib in ongoing studies. Future studies will build on this important result in the development of combinations of sorafenib with chemotherapy and embolization.

The liver does not tolerate radiotherapy to high dose. Fatal hepatic damage occurs when the dose to the whole liver is above 38 Gy. Locoregional radiotherapy may produce regression with less toxicity. An exception to the general chemoresistance of HCC is the infrequent histological subtype of fibrolamellar cancer. It is important to diagnose this condition, as it is sensitive to cisplatin-based chemotherapy [10].

Prognosis

When hepatoma arises in advanced cirrhotic liver the prognosis is poor; 50% of all patients are dead in 3 months, with 10% survivors at 12 months. The prognosis is better in patients with small tumours, that is, in those who are suitable for complete surgical resection or in those who show a complete response to chemotherapy. Overall 5-year survival after surgical resection is 15%, although if the tumour is less than 3 cm the figure rises to 50%. These figures have suggested that the results might be improved if patients with cirrhosis are screened regularly with ultrasound and AFP measurement. The impact of such a policy on survival is not known.

Angiosarcoma

These malignant vascular tumours arise in normal livers. They are rare, but of interest since they are known to occur in workers who have been chronically exposed to polyvinylchloride (PVC). The tumours develop 15–20 years after exposure to PVC. They have also been reported in patients who received thorotrast (a radioactive contrast agent used diagnostically between 1930 and 1950). The presentation is of a painful hepatic mass, and diagnosis is made by biopsy. Surgical resection may be possible.

A very rare, indolent, vascular tumour termed *epithelioid haemangioendothelioma* may occur in the liver. Treatment is by local excision if possible.

Hepatoblastoma

This rare tumour occurs in childhood. The tumour is associated with anomalies such as hemihypertrophy, and with storage diseases and Fanconi's syndrome. The pathological features are of immature hepatic epithelial cells or a mixture of these cells with mesenchymal elements.

It usually arises in the right lobe and presents with a visible asymptomatic mass, which later causes pain and weight loss. Like HCC (which can also occur in children over 5 years of age) the tumour produces AFP. It can be demonstrated by isotopic ultrasound and CT scanning but arteriography gives the best localization and is essential if resection is to be attempted.

The tissue diagnosis is usually made at operation when an attempt at resection is made. The chance of cure is greater if there is complete surgical excision. Up to 75% of the liver can be removed but haemorrhage can be severe and great skill is necessary. The tumour may respond to chemotherapy with alkylating agents and is frequently administered in the adjuvant and advanced settings; the rarity of this condition prevents design of appropriately powered randomized studies.

Cancer of the gallbladder and biliary tract

Incidence and aetiology

Cancer of the gallbladder and biliary tract (cholangiocarcinoma) has an equal incidence in men and women, most cases occurring after the age of 65 (see Figure 15.1), when it is commoner than HCC. Conversely, carcinoma of the gallbladder itself is a highly lethal disease, with a 10% 5-year survival [10]. Carcinoma of the gallbladder has a particularly high incidence in Chile, Japan and northern India. Gallstones are an important predisposing cause, but the incidence of gallbladder cancer in patients with untreated cholelithiasis is probably not more than 2%, which does not justify surgery for asymptomatic gallstones. Worldwide, liver flukes are the major predisposing cause (*Clonorchis sinensis, Opisthorchis felineus*). These flukes produce a chronic sclerosing cholangitis that appears to be premalignant. Cholangiocarcinoma is associated with ulcerative colitis, primary sclerosing cholangitis and choledochal cysts. 'Porcelain gallbladder', with characteristic brittle and bluish discoloration, is also closely associated with malignant change, as is the presence of gallbladder polyp(s) especially if larger than 1 cm in size (these should be removed).

Pathology

Carcinoma of the gallbladder, usually arises in the body and only rarely in the cystic duct (4% of cases). The tumours are usually adenocarcinomas (85%) but anaplastic (6%) and squamous (5%) histologies occur. There appears to be a genuine progression from dysplasia to *in situ* carcinoma and then invasive change in substantial number of cases.

Half of all bile duct cancers develop in the distal common duct, with carcinoma of the ampulla of Vater being the second commonest biliary cancer. The cancers arise in the proximal duct in 30% of cases and proximal to the porta hepatis in a further 20%. They are almost always adenocarcinomas, usually well differentiated and sometimes with a fibrous stroma.

These tumours spread locally and to regional lymph nodes and there may be multiple primary bile duct tumours. From these nodes, lymphatic spread is to the coeliac and aortic nodes. Hepatic metastases are common. Gallbladder cancer may seed into the peritoneum, and both types of cancer may directly invade the liver. Carcinomas of the ampulla may be slow-growing and causes obstructive jaundice early before it has spread widely. The tumour often ulcerates and sometimes bleeds,

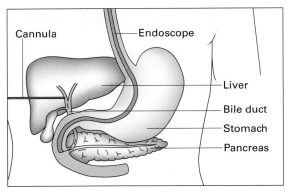

Figure 15.2 Percutaneous cholangiography and endoscopic retrograde cholangiopancreatography.

and the jaundice may fluctuate if the tumour sloughs. This form of biliary tract cancer has the best prognosis.

Clinical features

Cancer of the gallbladder is frequently diagnosed after routine histological analysis of a resected gallbladder specimen. Symptoms include right upper quadrant pain, and in advanced cases nausea, vomiting, weight loss and obstructive jaundice. Diagnostic delay is often due to attributing symptoms to pre-existing gallstones.

Cancer of the biliary tree more frequently presents with obstructive jaundice. At this stage, the tumour is often advanced. The gallbladder may be enlarged and palpable if the distal duct is obstructed.

Diagnosis

The diagnosis of early gallbladder carcinoma is difficult because the symptoms suggest gallstone disease. By the time a mass is palpable surgical resection may be impossible. Ultrasound and CT scanning may show a mass, but in the majority of cases the diagnosis is only made at laparotomy for presumed gallstone disease. In carcinoma of the extrahepatic bile ducts, obstructive jaundice leads to investigation. Percutaneous transhepatic cholangiograms may give an outline of the proximal ducts, and endoscopic retrograde cholangiopancreatography (ERCP) may demonstrate the lower end of the block and provide material for cytological examination (Figures 15.2 and 15.3), as well as permitting a stent to be inserted. The transhepatic route may also allow a catheter to be placed past the lesion with relief of jaundice either preoperatively or as a palliative procedure. Surgical resection requires additional diagnostic evaluation (see below).

The TNM staging system (Table 15.2) is now widely used.

Treatment
Surgery

When a gallbladder carcinoma is found at laparotomy, the surgeon must decide if it can be resected. The results of simple cholecystectomy are not good since the tumour may be locally extensive. Liver resection may be indicated for complete excision. Distant lymph node spread may have occurred and surgical excision deemed unwise, and

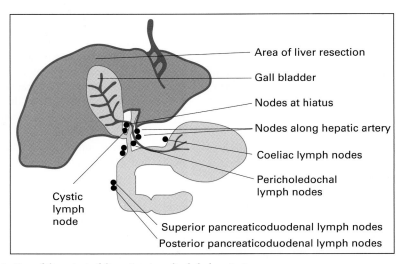

Figure 15.3 An illustration of the extent of dissection in radical cholecystectomy.

Table 15.2 TNM classification* and staging of gallbladder carcinoma.

Primary tumour (T)

TX	Primary tumour cannot be assessed
T0	No evidence of primary tumour
Tis	Carcinoma *in situ*
T1	Tumour invades lamina propria or muscle layer
T1a	Tumour invades lamina propria
T1b	Tumour invades muscle layer
T2	Tumour invades perimuscular connective tissue, no extension beyond serosa or into liver
T3	Tumour perforates serosa (visceral peritoneum) or directly invades the liver and/or one other adjacent organ or structure, e.g. stomach, duodenum, colon, pancreas, omentum, extrahepatic bile ducts
T4	Tumour invades main portal vein or hepatic artery, or invades two or more extrahepatic organs or structures

Regional lymph nodes (N)[†]

NX	Regional lymph nodes cannot be assessed
N0	No regional lymph-node metastasis
N1	Regional lymph-node metastasis

Distant metastasis (M)

MX	Distant metastasis cannot be assessed
M0	No distant metastasis
M1	Distant metastasis

Table 15.2 (continued)

Stage grouping

Stage 0	Tis	N0	M0
Stage IA	T1	N0	M0
Stage IB	T2	N0	M0
Stage IIA	T3	N0	M0
Stage IIB	T1, T2, T3	N1	M0
Stage III	T4	Any N	M0
Stage IV	Any T	Any N	M1

AJCC Cancer Staging Manual, 6th edn. New York: Springer-Verlag, 2002.
[†]The regional lymph nodes are the cystic duct node and the pericholedochal, hilar, peripancreatic, periportal, coeliac and superior mesenteric nodes.
Source: Reprinted from Misra *et al.* [10] .Reproduced with permission from Elsevier.

a palliative procedure is then undertaken, if possible with biliary decompression.

In the surgical management of cholangocarcinoma, it is critical to determine the extent of the tumour preoperatively radiologically by CT to exclude metastatic disease (possibly including PET-CT), and detailed MRI. Biliary decompression preoperatively may be needed preoperatively using ERCP or percutaneous transhepatic cholangiography (PTC). Involvement of the hepatic artery or portal vein is now not considered a contraindication to resection as *en bloc* resection of vascular structures with vascular reconstruction can be carried out. Contraindications to surgery include extension of the tumour to segmental bile ducts of both right and left liver lobes, and significant pre-existing lobar atrophy [11]. Diffuse intraductal spread cannot be resected. Spread into the intrahepatic ducts, invasion of blood vessels and distant lymph nodes, and peritoneal and hepatic metastases are also indications of unresectability. Microscopic examination of bile duct carcinomas often reveals intramural spread. Despite formidable surgical difficulties, tumours at the junction of the right and left hepatic ducts can sometimes be removed, as can mid and distal duct tumours, the latter by radical pancreaticoduodenectomy (Figure 15.4).

In a different series, between 13% and 55% of cholangiocarcinomas have been found to be operable, and major resections have high mortality and morbidity. A surgical algorithm for management has been proposed, basing decisions on the TNM staging system (Figure 15.5).

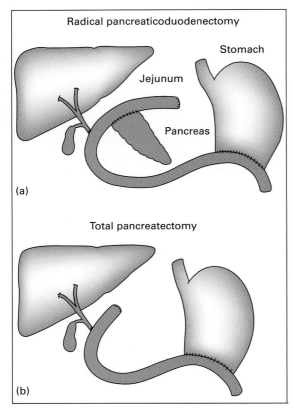

Figure 15.4 Surgical operations for cancer of the (a) bile ducts and (b) pancreas.

Palliative relief of obstruction may be obtained by bypass operation but internal bile duct drainage by non-surgical procedures is now becoming a preferred method of palliation. Carcinoma of the ampulla has the most favourable prognosis, with a 5-year survival of 25–30% after radical pancreaticoduodenectomy. There has been interest in the use of neoadjuvant chemotherapy and preoperative chemoembolization to optimize results of surgical resection of cholangiocarcinoma.

Radiotherapy

Many patients with biliary tract cancer have a localized but unresectable tumour. In these cases, effective control can be achieved temporarily with radiotherapy. The dose is usually 40–50 Gy in daily fractions, but the treatment details depend on the volume and site of the irradiation. Relief of pain and obstructive jaundice may be achieved.

Chemotherapy

Until recently, there were no proven chemotherapy regimens for cholangiocarcinoma and gallbladder cancer. Gemcitabine has been increasingly used for treatment of advanced disease. A major study in over 300 patients comparing gemcitabine alone and in combination with cisplatin for the treatment of advanced gall bladder and cholangiocarcinoma resulted in improved survival of the combination chemotherapy arm (11.7 months) as compared with gemcitabine monotherapy (8.2 months) [12]. It is likely that this will now be the standard of care. Chemotherapy may be used in the neoadjuvant setting in an attempt to increase the possibility of resection but this remains unproven.

Cancer of the exocrine pancreas

Incidence and aetiology

Pancreas cancer remains a major cause of morbidity and mortality with only modest improvement in outcome over the past decades and an overall 5-year survival around 5% [13]. Globally, the incidence of carcinoma of the pancreas is slowly rising, although in many parts of the UK this increase seems to have levelled out over the past decade. At present it is 15 per 100 000 in men and 13 per 100 000 in women (Figure 15.6). The condition has a high mortality, less than 1% of patients surviving 5 years. The disease is twice as common in diabetes mellitus. It also appears to be a smoking-related cancer with a 2.5–3.6 increased rate in smokers compared with non-smokers. There is an increased incidence in patients with chronic pancreatitis which, in turn, is frequently associated with excessive alcohol consumption. An increased risk has also been reported in metal, mine, chemical and sawmill workers. Wide variance in incidence has been noted across the world, from 2.2 cases per 100 000 in India, Kuwait and Singapore to 12.5 per 100 000 in parts of Scandinavia (Figure 15.7). Urban and socioeconomically disadvantaged populations have a higher incidence in the developed world. Between 5 and 10% of pancreatic cancers have a family history of the disease. The genetic basis for familial pancreas cancer syndromes remains unclear. There are some well-defined predisposition syndromes including the PALB2, BRCA1 and BRCA 2 genes [14].

Pathology

The great majority of histologically verified tumours are adenocarcinomas (Table 15.3) arising from the

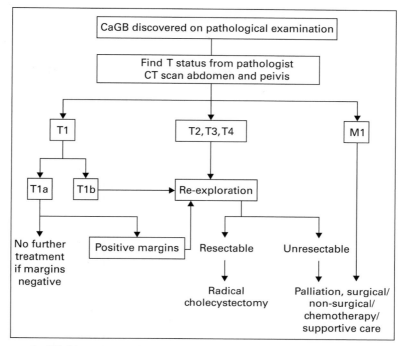

Figure 15.5 Management of gallbladder carcinoma (CaGB) discovered after pathological examination of excised tissue. (Source: Modified from Misra *et al*. [10]. Reproduced with permission from Elsevier)

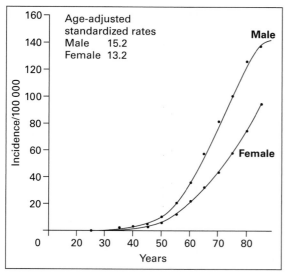

Figure 15.6 Age-specific incidence of cancer of the exocrine pancreas (UK figures.)

ductal epithelium. An intense fibrotic reaction often accompanies the tumour. Cystadenocarcinoma (1%) has a particularly good prognosis. Acinar cell tumours constitute 5% of the total. Sarcoma of the pancreas is a rare disease, usually occurring in childhood.

The exocrine pancreas has an extensive lymphatic drainage along blood vessels. Spread to local nodes has usually occurred by the time of presentation in tumours of both the body and tail.

The head of the pancreas is the site of the tumour in 65% of cases, the body and tail in 30% and the tail alone in 5%. Local spread occurs and accounts for many of the clinical features (Figure 15.8). Tumours in the head spread into the duodenum, obstruct the bile duct, and spread back into the retroperitoneal space and forward into the lesser sac and peritoneal cavity. The portal vein may be infiltrated, and tumours of the body and tail may occlude the splenic vein and extend into the transverse colon and spleen. Metastatic spread to the peritoneum, liver and lung is frequent.

Pain and weight loss are frequent symptoms. With tumours of the head the pain is usually epigastric, and with the tail it may be in the left upper quadrant. The

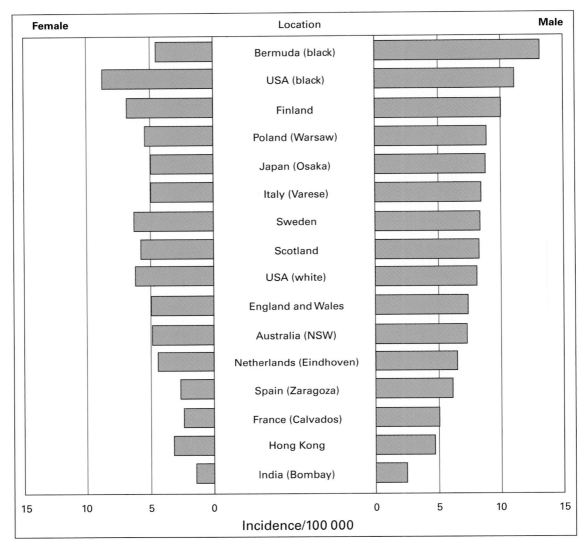

Figure 15.7 Geographic incidence of cancer of the exocrine pancreas.

pain gradually becomes severe and unremitting, is often nocturnal and extends into the back as retroperitoneal structures are invaded. Acute exacerbations may be due to episodes of pancreatitis. Left-sided abdominal pain and altered bowel habit may be caused by infiltration of the colon by tumours of the body or tail. Acinar cell carcinoma may be accompanied by a syndrome of patchy inflammation and necrosis of subcutaneous fat with polyarthralgia and eosinophilia. There are high levels of lipase in serum. The syndrome resembles relapsing panniculitis (Weber–Christian disease). Another

non-metastatic manifestation of pancreatic carcinoma is superficial migratory thrombophlebitis. Diabetes mellitus may be the presenting feature and carcinoma of the pancreas must be kept in mind in elderly patients developing glycosuria.

Obstructive jaundice is frequent and eventually occurs in 90% of patients with tumours of the head. It is usually progressive, although fluctuations may occur if the tumour sloughs. It is much less common in tumours of the body and tail. Fever may occur due to cholangitis. The gallbladder is not usually palpable, unlike in bile duct

Table 15.3 Benign and malignant pancreatic tumours.

	Malignant (%)
Tumours of exocrine pancreas	
Adenocarcinoma	
Acinar cell tumour	
Sarcoma	
Tumours of endocrine pancreas	
Islet cell tumours	20
Gastrinoma	70
Glucagonoma	60
Vipoma	90
Carcinoids	Not known
Somatostatinoma	90

or ampullary carcinoma. Peritoneal dissemination leads to malignant ascites, which is present in 15% of cases at diagnosis.

Investigation and diagnosis

It is difficult to diagnose early pancreatic carcinoma at the stage before obstruction of the bile duct or infiltration of the duodenum. It should be considered in any patient with unexplained continued upper abdominal pain.

The key investigations in diagnosis of pancreatic cancer are ultrasound and CT scanning. Endoscopic ultrasonography can be valuable in selected cases. CT may show a pancreatic mass or extension of the pancreas into the fat space surrounding it, and there may also be evidence of metastatic spread to adjacent nodes and the liver (Figure 15.8). If a mass is found, fine-needle aspiration may give a cytological diagnosis although this is usually avoided if there is a planned surgical resection in view of the potential risk of tumour seeding the needle track.

Following presentation with obstructive jaundice, ERCP will usually be performed (see Figure 15.2). This will often demonstrate the site of obstruction and help to distinguish the tumour from carcinoma of the gallbladder, ampulla or bile ducts. Additionally, there may be stenosis of the main pancreatic duct or compression of the common bile duct by tumour. Specimens for cytology can be taken from the pancreatic duct. ERCP has a high diagnostic accuracy (75–85%), but early diagnosis, before biliary obstruction has occurred, remains the clinical problem because symptoms are often late or non-specific. Significant elevation of the tumour marker CA-19-9 is frequent but too non-specific to allow diagnosis.

Treatment

It is essential that the diagnosis and treatment of pancreatic cancers is carried out in a multidisciplinary setting encompassing gastroenterology, surgical, oncological, radiological and pathological expertise. The crucial decision is to identify patients for surgical resection or for palliative modalities including radiation and chemotherapy. In view of the frequency of pain, access to specialists in symptom control is important.

Surgery

Surgical resection offers the only possibility of cure. Radical pancreaticoduodenectomy and total pancreatectomy are major surgical procedures (see Figure 15.4). Preservation of part of the pancreas is desirable but there may be problems with fistula formation at the

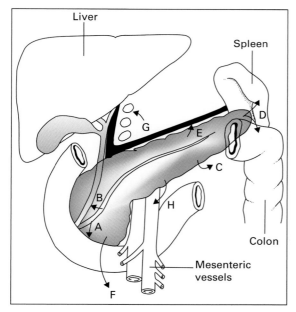

Figure 15.8 Sites of spread and production of symptoms in adenocarcinoma of the pancreas: (A) to duodenum, with pain, vomiting, obstruction; (B) to bile duct and pancreas, with jaundice, pancreatitis; (C) to retroperitoneum, with back pain; (D) to spleen and colon, with left upper quadrant pain; (E) to portal and splenic vein, with varices, splenomegaly, hepatic disorders; (F) to peritoneal cavity, with ascites; (G) to lymph nodes, with obstructive jaundice; and (H) to bloodstream, with distant metastases.

anastomotic site. Total pancreatectomy leads to diabetes and lack of exocrine function.

Only a minority of patients are suitable for surgery, because at the time of diagnosis there are often nodal or distant metastases or vascular involvement. Careful definition of the extent of the tumour preoperatively is essential and many centres carry out laparoscopy prior to definitive surgery to define the extent of tumour and exclude peritoneal involvement. PET scanning may be used to stage disease more accurately. If the tumour cannot be removed, the obstruction can be relieved by a biliary bypass procedure. This may be achieved surgically, but it is more common and optimal to place catheters in the biliary tree endoscopically or via the percutaneous transhepatic route if that is not possible.

Radiotherapy

Palliation, especially of pain, can be achieved by radiotherapy. With external beam irradiation, the dose required is high (50–60 Gy). Some reports have suggested that a few patients may achieve long-term remission. The synchronous administration of 5-FU or gencitabine as a radiation sensitizer appears to improve local control and possibly survival, although there are still no convincing data from randomised studies. Radiation therapy is most often used for locally advanced disease in which the prognosis is considerably better than for metastatic disease. In view of the frequency of metastatic disease at presentation, even where the appearance is of locally advanced disease, a reasonable strategy is to initiate treatment with a course of chemotherapy and consolidate with chemoradiation if there is no evidence of dissemination subsequent to this.

Chemotherapy

Despite many trials of chemotherapy, few cytotoxic drugs have demonstrated effectiveness in pancreatic cancer. The most widely used agent is gemcitabine, an anti-metabolite nucleoside analogue that showed superiority to 5-FU in a randomized study [15]. Although responses are often of short duration and there is only a modest improvement in survival, this agent was approved because of an increased clinical benefit as evidenced by increased appetite and decreased requirement for analgesia. However, two recent studies have demonstrated a significantly improved survival with chemotherapeutic agents for metastatic pancreatic adenocarcinoma. In the randomized study, the use of FOLFIRINOX (a chemotherapy combination of irinotecan, oxaliplatin, folinic acid

and 5-fluorouracil) was compared with gemcitabine monotherapy [16]. Median overall survival was 11.1 months in the FOLFIRINOX group as compared with 6.8 months in the gemcitabine group (hazard ratio for death, 0.57; P < 0.001). Although the FOLFIRINOX regimen was associated with significantly increased survival, this was at the cost of markedly increased toxicities. This regimen is now the 'gold standard' for advanced pancreas cancer but as with other chemotherapy protocols, the patient's comorbidities, performance status and quality of life issues are crucial before treatment decisions. More recently, the addition of the albumin-bound paclitaxel (nab-paclitaxel) was compared in a randomized study with gemcitabine monotherapy [17]. There was a modest improvement in median overall survival with 8.5 months in the nab-paclitaxel-gemcitabine group as compared with 6.7 months in the gemcitabine group (hazard ratio for death, 0.72; P < 0.001). The survival rate was 35% in the nab-paclitaxel-gemcitabine group versus 22% in the gemcitabine group at 1 year, and 9% versus 4% at 2 years. Toxicity of the nab-paclitaxel-gemcitabine does not appear to be as marked as with FOLFIRINOX though as yet these two regimens have not been directly compared.

These studies indicate that pancreatic cancer may not be as resistant to chemotherapy as generally thought and permeability may be a key factor. It will be important to define the role of these regimens in the adjuvant and neoadjuvant settings.

Several randomized studies have investigated the use of novel biological agents in combination with chemotherapy. A modest improvement in median survival of around 3 weeks was found with the combination of gemcitabine and the epidermal growth factor receptor inhibitor erlotinib [18]. Although there was an increase in 1-year survival from 17 to 23%, increased adverse events occurred in the combination-treated group.

A large randomized study has found that adjuvant chemotherapy using 5-FU plus folinic acid provides benefit in patients with resected pancreatic cancer [19]. Gemcitabine is equally efficacious as an adjuvant and randomised trials are under way to determine if combinations with other agents such as capecitabine improves outcome. Adjuvant radiotherapy was not beneficial and possibly harmful in the large ESPAC trial although other studies have suggested that there may be a benefit for radiation. The 5-year survival rate was 21% for patients who received chemotherapy but only 8% in patients who did not, the benefit persisting even after adjustment for major prognostic factors.

Palliative treatment and prognosis

Pain may be relieved by analgesics, but radiotherapy may be helpful in preventing the need for opiates for several months. Chemical block by injecting alcohol into the coeliac plexus is difficult but sometimes very helpful in relieving pain. Percutaneous drainage of the biliary tree may relieve itching and steatorrhoea due to obstructive jaundice. Steroids may help improve appetite for a while. Overall, the prognosis is very poor, with treatment making a minor long-term impact. For both men and women, the median survival time is well under 1 year, and less than 2% of all patients survive for 5 years.

Neuroendocrine tumours of the gastrointestinal tract

Neuroendocrine tumours of the gastrointestinal tract [20] are rare tumours with an incidence of 6 per 100 000 that can be divided into carcinoid tumours more commonly affecting the small bowel and pancreatic neuroendocrine tumours (incidence 0.4 per 100 000). They are derived from the 'diffuse endocrine system' and are divided into 'functional', hormone secreting with associated syndrome, or 'non-functional' with no associated syndrome. Classically carcinoids are often divided into their embryological site of origin from the foregut, midgut or hindgut. The endocrine pancreatic tumours are classified according to the hormonal syndrome they produce. The carcinoid syndrome is produced by tumours of the foregut and midgut, especially in the presence of hepatic metastases. Most neuroendocrine tumours are non-functional. These tumours often present late and are advanced at diagnosis [21]. With the advent of whole-exome sequencing there has been extensive progress in the in understanding of the molecular pathology of these tumours. A study of pancreatic NET indicated mutations in ATR/DAXX and the MEN1 (the causative mutation of multiple endocrine neoplasia, MEN, type 1) in around 45% of tumours [22]. These genes are involved in remodelling of chromatin and this may have implications in treatment.

Carcinoid tumours

The curious name of these tumours was coined in 1907 to emphasize the benign course which they generally follow, although a proportion are malignant at the outset and others become so with time.

Pathology

Localized intestinal carcinoids are present in 0.5% of autopsies, usually in the appendix. They may be found incidentally in the stomach or rectum at endoscopic assessment. There are, however, many other sites at which carcinoids may occur: bronchus, thymus, as well as any part of the gastrointestinal tract, ovary and testis.

Appendiceal carcinoids are usually located near the tip. The tendency to metastasize is related to size; tumours less than 1 cm in size are rarely associated with metastases, while 80% of those greater than 3 cm have metastasized. Metastases are much more common with small-bowel (jejunal–ileal) carcinoids than with appendiceal tumours.

Macroscopically, carcinoid tumours are often yellow or orange in colour. Microscopically, they consist of densely packed epithelial cells that stain using immunocytochemistry with chromogranin or synaptophysin. An important histological marker is the Ki67 proliferation index, which assesses the number of cells in cycle. Ki67 is a prognostic marker: more often the higher the proliferation index the worse the prognosis. Intestinal carcinoids are derived from enterochromaffin cells in the small-bowel mucosa but the cell of origin of many of the pancreatic tumours is not known. Most patients have elevated levels of chromogranin A in the serum, which can be an aid in diagnosis. The hormones produced by the tumours are responsible for the carcinoid syndrome. Both primary and secondary tumours are often slow-growing. The commonest metastatic site is the liver. Lung and bone are less frequently involved. There is an associated adenocarcinoma in 15% of patients. Neuroendocrine tumours, particularly pancreatic, are occasionally associated with hereditary syndromes, for example, MEN type 1, von Hippel Lindau, Neurofibromatosis and Tuberous sclerosis.

Clinical features

Management of these complex tumours requires a multidisciplinary approach with input from gastroenterologists, surgeons, radiologists (including nuclear medicine expertise), oncologists and pathologists.

Local symptoms

Patients may present with local symptoms due to metastases. Pain in the right-upper quadrant, due to distension of the liver by metastases, is a frequent symptom; weight loss, anorexia and malaise occur later as liver function deteriorates. Primary intestinal carcinoids are seldom diagnosed during life unless they cause obstruction, intussusception or pain in the right iliac fossa leading to appendicectomy.

The carcinoid syndrome

This syndrome occurs in about 50% of all patients with hepatic metastases from intestinal carcinoid tumours. A variety of chemicals are produced by the tumour and their release is accompanied by symptoms that may dominate the clinical picture. The syndrome is particularly likely to occur with bronchial carcinoid even without hepatic metastases, since the venous drainage is into the systemic circulation and not via the liver, which metabolizes the pharmacological mediators liberated by intestinal carcinoids.

In normal individuals, tryptophan is converted into nicotinic acid. In carcinoid syndrome, 5-hydroxy-tryptamine also known as serotonin (5-HT) is produced instead and, occasionally, pellagra occurs due to nicotinic acid deficiency. A metabolite of 5-HT, 5-hydroxyindoleacetic acid (5-HIAA), is excreted in the urine. When present in excess it confirms the diagnosis. 5-HT is quickly inactivated in the lungs and liver, so large quantities must be produced to cause symptoms. The release of 5-HT is probably responsible for diarrhoea. The diarrhoea is typically episodic, watery and may be explosive, leading to incontinence. It is often accompanied by noisy borborygmi and cramping pains. Excess 5-HT is probably responsible for endocardial fibrosis, which can lead to tricuspid incompetence, which in turn may cause right-sided heart failure with ascites. Bradykinin is produced by some tumours and may be partly responsible for the flushing that is characteristic of the syndrome. The flush is at first intermittent, often being precipitated by emotion and alcohol. The face and neck become red and the patient may perspire. It lasts a few minutes and is reminiscent of the flushing of menopausal women. Later the flushing becomes more frequent and some patients become almost permanently flushed. Telangiectases occur on the face, and skin may become thickened. Prostaglandins are liberated from some tumours and may contribute to both the flushing and the diarrhoea. Bronchospasm occurs and has been variously attributed to histamine, bradykinin and prostaglandins. It is episodic at first but permanent wheezing dyspnoea may develop. Episodes of hypotension are sometimes seen and are thought to be caused by 5-HT. A carcinoid crisis is a combination of hypotension, wheezing and flushing. It is treated by intravenous octreotide.

Other clinical features

The tumours are slow-growing and the diagnosis is often missed or delayed for months or years. If all the symptoms are present the diagnosis is easy to make, but if the complaint is of diarrhoea alone, negative investigations may lead to the diagnosis of 'irritable bowel syndrome'. Bronchial carcinoids usually present with unilateral airways obstruction and haemoptyses. Carcinoids in the bronchus, thymus and pancreas occasionally cause Cushing's syndrome, due to production of ACTH by the tumour, leading to bilateral adrenal hyperplasia. The primary tumour may be small. They may also secrete antidiuretic hormone and growth hormone-releasing peptide.

Diagnosis

The tumours can be visualized preoperatively by CT and MRI. Scintigraphy using Indium-111 labelled octreotide (which demonstrates the somatostatin type 2 receptor) is positive in 70–80% of patients, and is especially useful in demonstrating distant metastases. It is considered an essential modality in patients with metastatic neuroendocrine tumour. New positron emission tomography (PET) agents look to be very promising such a Gallium-68 labelled Octreotate. About 60% of tumours take up meta-iodobenzylguanidine (mIBG), usually carcinoids of small bowel origin. Iodine-131-labelled mIBG is thus sometimes used for scintigraphic diagnostic imaging.

In patients without the carcinoid syndrome the diagnosis is made as a result of the primary tumour in the bowel causing abdominal symptoms or, in the lung, symptoms of a bronchial tumour. Secondary deposits in the liver are usually diagnosed by liver biopsy.

In patients with the carcinoid syndrome, the 24-hour urinary 5-HIAA is usually elevated. False-positive results can be obtained with 5-HT-containing foods (bananas contain 4 mg of 5-HT). In some patients, the urinary 5-HIAA excretion may vary from day to day and this leads to false-negative results and makes 5-HIAA excretion an unreliable guide to treatment. Foregut carcinoids may produce 5-HT and not 5-HIAA; they may also produce histamine.

Management

Localized intestinal, bronchial or foregut carcinoids should be removed surgically. In metastatic carcinoids, surgery should be considered if liver secondaries are found that are well localized and which are resectable. This may relieve symptoms for months or years because the tumour is slow-growing. Another effective means of reducing the tumour mass is hepatic artery embolization. These surgical approaches may result in a sudden release of large quantities of pharmacologically active agents, resulting in hypotension and bronchospasm. Some patients with hepatic metastases may be suitable for liver transplantation.

In patients with metastatic carcinoid syndrome that cannot be treated surgically, the usual approach is to attempt to block the pharmacological effects of the tumours in the first instance. However, this is usually only partially successful since each symptom may be produced by more than one agent and pharmacological antagonists are partially effective against some tumour products and do not exist for others.

• The somatostatin analogues octreotide or Lanreotide are the most effective agents [23]. They control flushing and diarrhoea in 70% of patients. Short acting Octreotide may be started but often patients are switched to the long-acting monthly preparations such as octreotide LAR. Somatostatin analogues may contribute to tumour stabilization but rarely cause regression. A recent study indicated a significant improvement in progression-free survival for patients with advanced neuroendocrine tumours associated with carcinoid syndrome treated with everolimus plus octreotide LAR, compared with placebo plus octreotide [24].

• Diarrhoea may be mitigated by simple measures such as codeine phosphate, diphenoxylate or loperamide. Patients who have undergone a right hemi-colectomy may require bile-salt binding with cholestyramine.

• Bronchospasm may be helped by somatostatin analogues as well as agents that block histamine (cyproheptadine) or bradykinin (phenothiazines), as can conventional bronchodilators.

Chemotherapy is usually ineffective against carcinoid tumours. However, there is activity in other tumour types, especially pancreatic and high grade or poorly differentiated neuroendocrine tumours. The agents with activity include combinations of streptozotocin, 5-FU, doxorubicin, and cisplatin with reported response rates of 30–40% [25]. Response duration is of the order of 6 months. Combinations of temozolomide and capecitabine are currently being assessed with some promising results.

Transarterial embolization of the hepatic artery supplying the liver metastases is a common therapeutic modality. Sometimes a chemotherapy agent is also added – chemoembolisation. The acute effect of cutting off the blood supply to the tumour may result in the release of tumour products resulting in carcinoid crisis; hence, such procedures need to be covered with an intravenous infusion of Octreotide.

IFN-α has been used alone or with chemotherapy. Some of the responses have been very durable. About 50% of cases show improvement biochemically, although tumour shrinkage occurs in less than 15%. The toxicity of IFN-α is considerable but symptoms of carcinoid syndrome may be greatly relieved. Further progress may be achieved by combinations of octreotide, IFN and chemotherapy.

Radionuclide targeted therapy with radioactive beta-emitting agents such as Iodine-131 mIBG, Yttrium-90 DOTA Octreotide or Lutetium-177 DOTA Octreotate have shown promise in reducing tumour symptoms as well as inhibiting tumour growth. Such therapies can be used in patients who have avid uptake on their diagnostic scan. Anti-angiogenesis agents such as tyrosine kinase inhibitors are currently being assessed.

In terms of molecular targeting, two pivotal large-scale randomized controlled trials demonstrated significantly improved progression-free survival with the use of sunitinib, a multikinase inhibitor (targeting VEGFR, PDGF, c-kit, RET and FLT3) [26] and everolimus (targeting mTOR) [27] in the treatment of selected patients with low and intermediate grade pancreatic neuroendocrine tumours. These critical studies suggest a major new approach to these cancers by molecular targeting, which will be informed by improved understanding of genetic alterations.

Endocrine tumours of the pancreas

A variety of endocrine tumours may develop in the pancreas (see Table 15.3). Although they are uncommon, they are of importance both because they present with symptoms due to the excess hormone production and because they shed light on the normal function of the endocrine pancreas It is not uncommon for patients with such tumours to initially be mislabelled as pancreatic cancer. The amine precursor uptake and decarboxylation (APUD) system was proposed as the cell of origin in medullary carcinoma of the thyroid, carcinoid tumours, small-cell lung cancer, endocrine tumours of the pancreas, phaeochromocytoma, neuroblastoma and others. There is debate as to whether the concept can be used to account for the origin of these tumours. Currently it is felt that these tumours are derived from multipotent stem cells, which undergo endocrine differentiation within, for example, the pancreas. However, the hypothesis does help to explain the syndromes of MEN. About 70% of the tumours are malignant and a similar proportion produce hormone. Metastases are usually to liver and adjacent nodes.

Multiple endocrine neoplasms

These inherited syndromes have been the subject of intense genetic studies in recent years [28]. The locus of the MEN-1 gene is on the long arm of chromosome 11 (11q13) and tumour development is associated with loss of heterozygosity at this site. MEN-2 syndromes are associated with a germline mutation in the *RET* proto-oncogene which codes for a tyrosine kinase. The mutation is dominant.

Three syndromes are recognized.

1 *MEN-1 (Wermer's syndrome).* This consists of hyperplasia or adenomas of parathyroids and tumours of islet cells, pituitary, adrenal cortex and thyroid (in order of frequency). Patients usually present with hypercalcaemia. Hypoglycaemia and pituitary tumours are less common. The pancreatic islet cell tumour may be malignant. It is usually an insulinoma but gastrinoma, glucagonoma or vipoma may occur (see below). The condition is inherited in an autosomal dominant fashion, and usually presents at age 20–60.

2 *MEN-2 (Sipple's syndrome).* This consists of medullary carcinoma of the thyroid, phaeochromocytoma and parathyroid hyperplasia. The phaeochromocytoma is often bilateral. About 10% of all cases of medullary carcinoma of the thyroid are part of the MEN-2a or MEN-2b syndrome. The syndrome usually presents with symptoms of a phaeochromocytoma or with a lump in the neck. It can occur at any age. The plasma calcitonin is elevated if medullary carcinoma of the thyroid is present and since C-cell hyperplasia precedes the development of malignancy, siblings of patients should have their plasma calcitonin measured. DNA analysis of potential carriers of MEN-2a provides unequivocal identification prior to symptoms [22]. Treatment of these tumours is discussed in Chapter 20. The condition is also autosomal dominant.

3 *MEN-2b (mucosal neuroma syndrome).* In this condition, phaeochromocytoma and medullary carcinoma of the thyroid also occur (as in MEN-2a) but patients also have neuromas of the lips, tongue, mouth and entire gut. The underlying genetic abnormality is a mutation in the *RET* proto-oncogene, which codes for a tyrosine kinase receptor. There may be hyperextensible joints, pes cavus and soft-tissue prognathism. The management is of the thyroid carcinoma and phaeochromocytoma as in MEN-2a. Parathyroid hyperplasia is less frequent than in MEN-2a. The disease presents earlier than MEN-2a. It is also due to a mutation in *RET*.

Von Hippel Lindau is an autosomal, dominant, inherited condition with a mutation found on chromosome 3p25-26. It is characterized by retinal or central nervous system haemangioblastomas, clear cell renal carcinomas, pancreatic cystic tumours and pancreatic endocrine tumours, the latter being found in 15–20% of cases.

Neurofibromatosis is an autosomal dominantly inherited disorder with a mutation found on chromosome 17q11.2. It is characterized by café au-lait spots, cutaneous or subcutaneous neurofibromas, optic gliomas, hamartomas and bone lesions. A minority will also develop ampullary endocrine tumours.

Insulinoma

Pathology

These are tumours of the α cells of the islets. They produce proinsulin, which is converted to insulin. The insulin is secreted with its connecting C-peptide (which joins the two chains). The tumours are often small and arise with equal frequency in head, body and tail, and 20% are multiple and an equal number malignant. About 5% are associated with MEN-1 syndrome. The diagnosis of malignancy is difficult histologically but metastases occur to liver and adjacent nodes in about 10% of cases.

Clinical features

The patient presents with symptoms of excess insulin production: loss of consciousness, dizziness, episodic mental confusion and weakness. As the condition progresses, mental confusion is present most of the time and irreversible dementia may occur. It usually presents in mid-life but can occur at any age. Other symptoms of MEN-1 may be present. The vagueness of the presentation often leads to considerable diagnostic delay.

Diagnosis

A fasting blood sugar of below 2.8 mmol/L is the characteristic finding. The fasting test must be carefully controlled, and blood is taken for both sugar and insulin measurements. In a normal person, fasting lowers the blood sugar (but seldom below 2.8 mmol/L) but the plasma insulin then falls. By contrast, with insulinoma the plasma insulin is either very high or inappropriately raised or maintained while the blood sugar falls. The main differential diagnosis is from self-induced (factitious) hypoglycaemia, which should be suspected, particularly in medical staff. However, exogenous insulin is associated with a low C-peptide level, while insulinoma is not. Surreptitious taking of a sulphonylurea can also cause diagnostic difficulty.

Selective arteriography mat be helpful in determining whether the lesions are single or multiple. More recently endoscopic ultrasound (EUS) has been shown to be a less invasive and sensitive imaging modality for insulinomas. The Indium-111 labelled Octreotide scan is only positive in 50% of cases. CT scanning using an early arterial phase contrast injection protocol is complementary in identifying the tumours.

Treatment

After localization, a partial pancreatectomy is performed, leaving the head of the pancreas wherever possible. When the tumour has not been localized preoperatively, it may nonetheless be palpable at operation. The plasma insulin is monitored during the operation. If no tumour is found, a subtotal pancreatectomy is usually performed. Chemotherapy is discussed below.

Metastases are uncommon but if they occur they may respond to streptozotocin, 5-FU or doxorubicin. A combination of all three has also been used, with response rates of 50–60%. Diazoxide can be used to treat hypoglycaemia. Glucagon is of little value. Somatostatin analogues may also be useful. Recently, radionuclide targeted therapy with Yttrium-90 Octreotide or Lutetium-177 Octreotate have been shown to be useful although still considered experimental.

Gastrinoma (Zollinger–Ellison syndrome)
Incidence and pathology

These tumours arise from the δ or D cells of the islets and are often malignant. They usually present at age 20–45 and probably account for 0.1% of all peptic ulcer disease; 35% occur in the pancreas, 60% in the duodenum and others occur in the stomach and, very rarely, in the thyroid and ovary. They may be single or multiple and vary greatly in size (less than 5 mm to 15 cm). Rarely there may be co-secretion of other peptide hormones (ACTH, vasoactive intestinal polypeptide, VIP, glucagon). In 60–70% of patients metastases have occurred at diagnosis, usually to adjacent nodes and liver, but more distant spread is not uncommon.

Most of the gastrin produced in the tumour is a peptide of 17 amino acids (G-17) but a larger molecule (G-34) is also formed. Circulating gastrin is mainly G-34. The constant stimulation of the gastric parietal cells leads to a great increase in their mass. In 20–25% of patients other

features of the MEN-1 syndrome are present, usually hyperparathyroidism.

Clinical features

The dominant symptom is peptic ulceration. Usually the ulcer is in the first part of the duodenum or in the stomach. Occasionally there are multiple ulcers that extend down the proximal duodenum. Recurrence soon after medical treatment, perforation and haemorrhage all occur. The symptoms of ulceration are severe and response to medical treatment is limited, although histamine H_2-receptor antagonists are effective for a while.

Diarrhoea occurs in 30–50% of cases, due to the large volume of acid produced by the stomach. Pancreatic lipase is inactivated at low pH, leading to steatorrhoea. The low pH also interferes with bile salt function and with the activity of intrinsic factor.

Investigation and diagnosis

The history of recurrent severe peptic ulceration with diarrhoea in a young person should point to the possible diagnosis. There is occasionally a family history of endocrine neoplasia. Acid output is raised, but not necessarily to levels above than that found in some patients with duodenal ulcer. The diagnosis is confirmed by finding an elevated plasma gastrin level. Most radioimmunoassay antibodies will detect all types of gastrin molecule produced by gastrinomas. The secretin stimulation test is often diagnostic in inducing a significant rise in serum gastrin and acid output.

When the diagnosis has been made, attempts are usually made to locate any tumour. Contrast enhanced CT scanning may be helpful in showing metastases but usually fails to demonstrate the primary. EUS and sometimes angiography are used to locate the primary tumour when surgery is being considered. The indium-111-labelled Octreotide scan is the most sensitive imaging modality for metastatic disease.

Management

Duodenectomy or pancreatectomy is seldom practicable. The tumours are often multifocal and have frequently metastasized. Histamine antagonists were originally used as anti-acid therapy, but now the mainstay is high-dose proton pump inhibitor. Before their introduction, total gastrectomy was the preferred treatment for intractable ulceration. Somatostatin analogues may be considered to aid control of disease and acid therapy. Chemotherapy and radionuclide targeted therapies are also sometimes used. About 60% of patients are alive 5 years after diagnosis.

Vipoma (Verner–Morrison syndrome)

This rare syndrome of profuse watery diarrhoea, facial flushing, hypokalaemia, hypochlorhydria and hypertension is caused by the secretion of VIP by tumours of the pancreatic islets [26]. VIP (and the syndrome) can be produced by phaeochromocytomas, ganglioneuroblastomas and bronchogenic (small-cell) carcinoma. Hyperglycaemia and hypercalaemia may also rarely occur and can be caused by VIP.

The tumours are usually solitary and can sometimes be shown angiographically. They may be shown on an Indium-111-labelled Octreotide scan. Treatment is by surgical removal. There is a high risk of malignancy. For patients with advanced disease, somatostatin analogues can be life-saving and are often required in high doses.

Glucagonoma

These are tumours of the pancreatic α cell and usually affect postmenopausal women. The clinical syndrome is characterized by a severe skin eruption with migratory erythema, bullous ulceration and scabbing on the legs, trunk, genital area and face (migratory necrolytic erythema). In addition, there is normochromic anaemia, stomatitis, diarrhoea and hypokalaemia. Most of the tumours are in the body and tail and are often malignant (60%) but with a slow growth rate. Metastasis is usually to the liver.

The diagnosis is made by the typical rash and raised plasma glucagon levels. Glucagon causes gluconeogenesis and glycogenolysis, elevating the blood sugar. The mechanism of production of the skin rash is not known. Treatment is by surgical removal wherever possible. In patients with advanced disease, somatostatin analogues are often used.

Somatostatinoma

This rare islet cell tumour is usually malignant. The syndrome consists of steatorrhoea and diarrhoea due to suppressed pancreatic exocrine function, gallstones due to decreased gallbladder contractility, diabetes from suppression of insulin, and hypochlorhydria from suppression of gastrin.

Plasma somatostatin and calcitonin are elevated. Diagnosis is late because the symptoms are not specific. The tumours should be removed if metastases have not yet occurred.

Treatment of advanced neuroendocrine (enterohepatic) tumours

There are few controlled trials of the value of chemotherapy in these diverse tumours. It is still considered the first line option in patients who have progressive tumour growth. More recent evidence suggests that treatment of patients with locally advanced or metastatic neuroendocrine cancers with chemotherapy combination of fluorouracil, doxorubicin and streptozocin may result in response rates of 30–40% with prolonged stable disease in a significant number of patients [29,30]. It does seem that these tumours, unlike midgut carcinoids, do show chemosensitivity.

The somatostatin analogues Octreotide and Lanreotide bind to the tumour cell somatostatin receptor and inhibit hormone release downregulating cell growth. Biochemical parameters improve in 30% of patients but only 10% show reduction in tumour size. However, subjective improvement is common. Side-effects are mainly of gastrointestinal disturbance. They can potentiate hypoglycaemia, but is nonetheless of value in islet cell tumours. IFN-α produces biochemical response in 50% of cases and objective shrinkage in 10%. Radionuclide targeted therapies including either Yttrium-90 Octreotide or Lutetium-177 Octreotate have been shown to be useful in non-randomized studies. There may also be a role for chemoembolization in patients with hepatic predominant disease.

An important recent study has clearly shown that treatment with Lanreotide significantly prolonged progression-free survival among patients with metastatic enteropancreatic neuroendocrine tumours of grade 1 or 2 [31]. The estimated rates of progression-free survival at 24 months were 65.1% in the Lanreotide group and 33.0% in the placebo group. This emphasises the importance of inhibition of somatostatin pathways for therapy of these tumours.

References

1 El-Serag HB. Hepatocellular carcinoma. *N Engl J Med.* 2011; 365(12): 1118–27.

2 Farazi PA, DePinho RA. Hepatocellular carcinoma pathogenesis: from genes to environment. *Nat Rev Cancer* 2006; 6: 674–87.

3 Fattovich G, Stroffolini T, Zagni I, Donato F. Hepatocellular carcinoma in cirrhosis: incidence and risk factors. *Gastroenterology* 2004; 127(Suppl 1): S35–S50.

4 White DL, Kanwal F, El-Serag HB. Association between nonalcoholic fatty liver disease and risk for hepatocellular

cancer, based on systematic review. *Clin Gastroenterol Hepatol* 2012; 10(12): 1342–59.

5 International Interferon α Hepatocellular Carcinoma Study Group. Effect of interferon α on progression of cirrhosis to hepatocellular carcinoma: a retrospective cohort study. *Lancet* 1998; 351: 1535–9.

6 Vivarelli M, Montalti R, Risaliti A. Multimodal treatment of hepatocellular carcinoma on cirrhosis: an update. *World J Gastroenterol* 2013; 19(42): 7316–26.

7 Asghar U, Meyer T. Are there opportunities for chemotherapy in the treatment of hepatocellular cancer? *J Hepatol* 2012; 56: 686–95.

8 Llovet JM, Ricci S, Mazzaferro V *et al.*, SHARP Investigators Study Group. Sorafenib in advanced hepatocellular carcinoma. *N Engl J Med* 2008; 359: 378–90.

9 Abou-Alfa GK, Johnson P, Knox JJ *et al.* Doxorubicin plus sorafenib vs doxorubicin alone in patients with advanced hepatocellular carcinoma: a randomized trial. *JAMA.* 2010; 304: 2154–60.

10 Misra S, Chaturvedi A, Misra NC, Sharma ID. Carcinoma of the gallbladder. *Lancet Oncol* 2003; 4: 167–77.

11 Review article: surgical, neo-adjuvant and adjuvant management strategies in biliary tract cancer. *Aliment Pharmacol Ther* 2011; 34(9): 1063–7811

12 Valle J, Wasan H, Palmer DH *et al.* Cisplatin plus gemcitabine versus gemcitabine for biliary tract cancer. *N Engl J Med* 2010; 362: 1273–81.

13 Hidalgo M. Pancreatic cancer. *N Engl J Med* 2010; 362(17): 1605–17.

14 Klein AP. Genetic susceptibility to pancreatic cancer. *Mol Carcinog* 2012; 51(1): 14–24.

15 Burris HA, III,, Moore MJ, Andersen J *et al.* Improvements in survival and clinical benefit with gemcitabine as first-line therapy for patients with advanced pancreas cancer: a randomized trial. *J Clin Oncol* 1997; 15: 2403–13.

16 Conroy T, Desseigne F, Ychou M *et al.* FOLFIRINOX versus gemcitabine for metastatic pancreatic cancer. *N Engl J Med* 2011; 364: 1817–25.

17 Von Hoff DD, Ervin T, Arena FP *et al.* Increased survival in pancreatic cancer with nab-paclitaxel plus gemcitabine. *N Engl J Med* 2013; 369(18): 1691–703.

18 Moore MJ, Goldstein D, Hamm J *et al.* Erlotinib plus gemcitabine compared with gemcitabine alone in patients with advanced pancreatic cancer: a phase III trial of the National Cancer Institute of Canada Clinical Trials Group. *J Clin Oncol* 2007; 25: 1960–6.

19 Neoptolemos JP, Stocken DD, Friess H *et al.* A randomised trial of chemoradiotherapy and chemotherapy after resection of pancreatic cancer. *N Engl J Med* 2004; 350: 1200–10.

20 Modlin IM, Oberg K, Chung DC *et al.,* Gastroenteropancreatic neuroendocrine tumours. *Lancet Oncol.* 2008; 9: 61–72.

21 Plöckinger U, Wiedenmann B. Treatment of gastroenteropancreatic neuroendocrine tumors. *Virchows Arch* 2007; 451: S71–80.

22 Jiao Y, Shi C, Edil BH *et al.* DAXX/ATRX, MEN1, and mTOR pathway genes are frequently altered in pancreatic neuroendocrine tumors. *Science* 2011; 331: 1199–203.

23 Toumpanakis C, Caplin ME. Update on the role of somatostatin analogs for the treatment of patients with gastroenteropancreatic neuroendocrine tumors. *Semin Oncol* 2013; 40(1): 56–68.

24 Pavel ME, Hainsworth JD, Baudin E *et al.* Everolimus plus octreotide long-acting repeatable for the treatment of advanced neuroendocrine tumours associated with carcinoid syndrome (RADIANT-2): a randomised, placebo-controlled, phase 3 study. *Lancet* 2011; 378: 2005–12.

25 Karpathakis A, Caplin M, Thirlwell C. Hitting the target: where do molecularly targeted therapies fit in the treatment scheduling of neuroendocrine tumours? *Endocr Relat Cancer.* 2012; 19(3): R73–92.

26 Raymond E, Dahan L, Raoul J-L *et al.* Sunitinib malate for the treatment of pancreatic neuroendocrine tumors. *N Engl J Med* 2011; 364: 501–13.

27 Yao JC, Shah MH, Ito T *et al.* Everolimus for advanced pancreatic neuroendocrine tumors. *N Engl J Med* 2011; 364: 514–23.

28 Zhang J, Francois R, Iyer R *et al.* Current understanding of the molecular biology of pancreatic neuroendocrine tumors. *J Natl Cancer Inst* 2013; 105: 1005–17.

29 Kouvaraki MA, Ajani JA, Hoff P *et al.* Fluorouracil, doxorubicin, and streptozocin in the treatment of patients with locally advanced and metastatic pancreatic endocrine carcinomas. *J Clin Oncol* 2004; 22: 4762–71.

30 Turner NC, Strauss SJ, Sarker D *et al.* Chemotherapy with 5-fluorouracil, cisplatin and streptozocin for neuroendocrine tumours. *Br J Cancer* 2010; 102: 1106–12.

31 Caplin ME, Pavel M, Ćwikła JB *et al.* Lanreotide in metastatic enteropancreatic neuroendocrine tumors. *N Engl J Med.* 2014; 37: 224–33.

16 Tumours of the small and large bowel

Tumours of the small bowel

Incidence, aetiology and pathology

The small bowel includes 90% of the surface area of the gastrointestinal tract, but small-bowel tumours account for under 5% of all gastrointestinal tumours [1]. Although malignant lesions occur most frequently in the duodenum and jejunum, benign adenomas and fibromas are more common in the ileum. The incidence of adenocarcinoma is more common in patients with familial adenomatous polyposis (FAP), Peutz–Jeghers syndrome and Crohn's disease, and generally diagnosed over the age of 60 years. Long-standing coeliac disease predisposes to the development of small-bowel lymphoma.

The commonest malignancies are adenocarcinomas (45%), carcinoid tumours (30%), lymphomas (10%) and sarcomas (mostly leiomyosarcomas). Metastatic deposits (most frequently from ovary or pancreas) may also occur.

Adenocarcinomas of the small bowel generally metastasise to the liver and regional nodes. Characteristically these are raised ulcerating neoplasms; histologically they are usually mucin-secreting adenocarcinomas. Small-bowel lymphomas are usually diffused and poorly differentiated. The small bowel is an important site of non-Hodgkin's lymphoma in childhood. The management of small-bowel lymphoma is discussed in Chapter 26.

Carcinoid tumours arise principally in the ileum, caecum, appendix and duodenum. They appear as small yellowish nodules in the bowel wall, arising from the chromaffin cells, which probably belong to the amine precursor uptake and decarboxylation (APUD) system and which secrete small polypeptide hormones and amines. The management of the carcinoid syndrome is discussed in Chapter 15. Gastrointestinal stromal tumours arise in supporting tissue in both small and large bowel. Both epithelioid and spindle cell forms occur.

Clinical features

Clinical diagnosis is difficult. Patients often present late with abdominal obstruction or intermittent pain, often with melaena. Intussusception may be a cause of the obstruction and pain.

Chronic anaemia, weight loss, diarrhoea and steatorrhoea may occur, particularly with lymphomas. Some patients develop a palpable abdominal mass, with abdominal distension if there is intestinal obstruction. Commonly, there are no abnormal physical signs. Perforation is rare with adenocarcinoma, but commoner with lymphoma. There is commonly disseminated disease at the time of diagnosis.

Cancer and its Management, Seventh Edition. Jeffrey Tobias and Daniel Hochhauser.
© 2015 John Wiley & Sons, Ltd. Published 2015 by John Wiley & Sons, Ltd.

Diagnosis

Contrast radiographic studies are essential. In proximal tumours, a barium follow-through is required, whereas in distal lesions causing ileocolic intussusception the barium enema is usually more useful. Hypotonic duodenography may give better visualization of duodenal lesions and small-bowel enemas are helpful with lower tumours. Ultrasound and computed tomography (CT) are helpful in delineating masses. Duodenal lesions can usually be seen endoscopically, and biopsy and cytological specimens can be obtained.

Treatment and prognosis

Surgical resection is the only curative treatment. Benign tumours can usually be removed by resection, but adenocarcinomas require wider excision including removal of the lymph node drainage area since lymphatic invasion is common. Only 70% of tumours are resectable. For duodenal cancers, pancreaticoduodenectomy may be required. In view of the low incidence of small-bowel cancers, no definitive randomized trials have been performed to confirm efficacy of systemic chemotherapy in either the adjuvant or advanced settings. Regimens validated for colorectal cancer including oxaliplatin, irinotecan and fluoropyrimidines are used in many centres, but there is no objective evidence of efficacy.

Lesions of the terminal ileum are often best treated by hemicolectomy, in order to achieve an adequate resection of regional lymphatics. With leiomyosarcomas, regional node involvement is less frequent and removal of the lymph node drainage area may not be necessary. For lymphomas of the small bowel, multiple-site involvement including liver or spleen is common. Wide resection of the involved area is necessary, with removal of adjacent nodes. Further treatment with chemotherapy or radiotherapy is usually indicated (see Chapter 26). In any lesion larger than 2 cm, a more widespread excision seems justified because of the risk of spread beyond the primary site.

Only 20% of patients with small-bowel adenocarcinomas survive 5 years, probably because of the delay in diagnosis. For localized carcinoid tumours, 5-year survival rates of up to 90% have been reported. The prognosis for metastatic disease is discussed in Chapter 15.

Tumours of the appendix

These are uncommon, and 90% are carcinoids which are treated by local resection. Tumours greater than 2 cm in size are generally treated with a right hemicolectomy in view of the high risk of metastasis. The remainder are either adenocarcinomas or mucoceles, which contain a gelatinoid mucoid material and can undergo malignant change to become papillary mucinous cystadenocarcinomas. Rupture of these lesions leads to the condition of *pseudomyxoma peritonei*, a gelatinous, ascitic, implanting tumour that can coat the entire peritoneal surface, resulting in progressive abdominal enlargement, often mimicking ovarian carcinoma. Treatment of pseudomyxoma involves surgical evacuation, though repeated operations are usually required. There is no documented evidence for the efficacy of systemic chemotherapy although 5-fluorouracil (5-FU)-containing regimens are often used.

Gastrointestinal stromal tumours

Although uncommon, these tumours are increasingly diagnosed, perhaps due to development of more effective treatment [2]. The tumours arise in the supporting stroma of the bowel. Many of these tumours have an activating mutation in the receptor tyrosine kinase gene c-*KIT*. Exon 11 of the gene is the commonest site of mutation.

The tumours present with bowel obstruction and may be metastatic or unresectable at presentation. In these cases the tyrosine kinase inhibitor imatinib mesilate has been shown to produce responses that are frequently complete and durable for several years. Not all tumours respond, but the response rate reaches 80% in those with c-*KIT* mutations in exon 11. The role of the drug in the treatment of earlier stage tumours is now under investigation. If progression occurs while on therapy, it appears that continuing the drug or increasing the dose may slow the rate of progress of the disease. The multitargeted tyrosine kinase inhibitor sunitinib has shown activity in imatinib-resistant GIST. Resection of tumour progressing at a single site may also be indicated.

Tumours of the large bowel

Incidence, aetiology and genetics

Cancers of the large bowel (colon and rectum) are common (third in the UK after lung and breast), and represent the second largest cause of death from cancer in the Western world. In the UK, over 30,000 people develop colorectal cancer each year. Cancers of the colon outnumber rectal carcinomas by 3:2 (Figure 16.1), and the two sites together constitute 10–15% of all cancers. The disease is uncommon in Africa, Asia and South America,

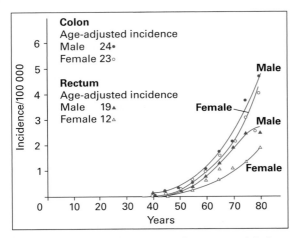

Figure 16.1 Age-specific incidence of carcinoma of the large bowel.

suggesting a possible dietary aetiology. High intake of animal fat may increase the risk of colon cancer and, although previous studies have overemphasised the risk [3], this could contribute to the high incidence of colorectal carcinoma (30–60 per 100,000) in North America, western Europe and Australia. Other dietary components of aetiological importance include vegetables, fibre and vitamin C (all of which probably lower the risk), whereas high alcohol consumption appears to increase it. A number of reports have suggested that regular use of aspirin and/or non-steroidal anti-inflammatory drugs (NSAIDs) such as aspirin or celecoxib may be protective [4], but recent studies of high-fibre supplements have been disappointing. Evidence of an increase in cardiac events in patients receiving the NSAID rofecoxib resulted in closure of pivotal studies determining potential role in prevention [5].

According to the model developed by Vogelstein [6], step-wise genetic alterations result in the accumulation of mutations in tumour-suppressor genes or negative regulators of cell proliferation that trigger their progression to a full-blown invasive phenotype. Several conditions predispose to the development of colonic cancers. In ulcerative colitis, the risk increases with length of history and extent of involvement [7]. In the past some physicians recommended total colectomy if the disease is active for more than 10 years since these patients often develop multicentric or poorly differentiated carcinomas. Recent studies suggest that a close surveillance policy is sufficient in patients with well-controlled inflammatory bowel disease.

FAP also predisposes to malignant change. The distal colon tends to be most severely involved and the similarity of symptoms of familial polyposis and true carcinoma makes diagnosis of the development of malignancy extremely difficult. Most surgeons now recommend restorative proctocolectomy (in which a 'pouch' is fashioned from small bowel to replace the rectum), a procedure now considered safe, generally well tolerated and with a good prognosis. The persistent excess mortality is due to the occurrence of upper gastrointestinal (duodenal and gastric) cancers and intra-abdominal desmoid tumours.

Non-familial (sporadic) adenomatous polyps are also premalignant. Most cancers apparently arise from them although, in contrast, not all adenomas become cancerous. Such lesions are found increasingly with age, and residual evidence of an adenomatous polyp occurs in a small percentage of patients with bowel cancer. The risk of malignant change increases greatly with increasing size of the polyp [8]. Routine removal of polyps found at sigmoidoscopy is recommended, particularly since two-thirds of large-bowel cancers are found in the rectum and sigmoid colon (see below). Villous adenomas at any site in the bowel may be pre-malignant. The risk relates to size and histology; villous lesions are more likely to become malignant than tubulovillous or tubular adenomas. They can present with diarrhoea, rectal bleeding or a characteristic picture of fluid and electrolyte loss, often with severe hypokalaemia. The incidence of malignant change is at least 15%, and these lesions should always be removed even if this necessitates an extensive operation. Other familial syndromes known to be associated with an increased incidence of colorectal carcinoma include Gardner's, Turcot's, Peutz–Jeghers and Lynch syndromes.

The last few years have seen a major advance in our understanding of chromosomal changes in FAP. The familial polyposis gene is located on chromosome 21 (5q). Loss of an allele at this site has been found in 40% of cases of sporadic carcinoma of the colon, implicating the FAP gene in the pathogenesis of the disease. Allelic loss has also been found for the *p53* gene on chromosome 17 and another gene on 18q named *DCC* (deleted in colorectal carcinoma) although it remains unclear as to whether DCC loss is itself oncogenic or a marker of progression. A model of the genetic changes in the development of the adenoma–carcinoma sequence is shown in Figure 16.2.

Mismatch repair genes are the genetic basis for hereditary non-polyposis colon cancer (HNPCC). The genes are *hMSH2* on chromosome 2p, *hMLH1* on 3p, *hPMS1* on

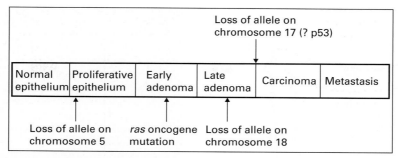

Figure 16.2 The genetic changes in the development of the adenoma–carcinoma sequence.

2q and *hPMS2*. Thus four separate genes have now been located, mutations of which predispose to colonic cancer by decreasing the efficiency of mismatch repair in DNA, presumably allowing defects induced by carcinogens to cause genetic damage [9]. An additional exciting prospect for colorectal cancer control is the potential use of NSAIDs, which are known to inhibit colorectal carcinogenesis [10]. Drugs such as sulindac and celecoxib both reduce the incidence of cancer in patients with FAP and of existing polyps in patients with FAP, though the mechanisms remain unclear. There is evidence from a large randomised study of a significant reduction in the incidence of colorectal cancer following use of aspirin in carriers of the Lynch syndrome [11].

Other genes may also contribute to hereditary cancer syndromes such as the base excision repair gene MYH, in which loss of expression results in multiple colorectal polyps [12]. Extensive work is in progress to identify other genes involved in hereditary predisposition syndromes as well as genes which confer increased risk to colon cancer.

Screening for colorectal cancers

Since early or precancerous lesions can be resected if identified, prompt management should lead to reduced incidence and mortality from bowel cancer [13]. The high prevalence of colorectal cancer in the Western world is sufficient for screening to be a realistic proposition, using relatively inexpensive and reliable investigations such as faecal occult blood testing (FOBT) and sigmoidoscopy. However, there are significant barriers to widespread adoption of population-wide screening programmes including specificity and sensitivity of the various diagnostic techniques, as well as the small but important risk of complications from procedures such as colonoscopy [14].

Patients with a family history of, or those with, FAP are candidates for more intensive screening. Randomized controlled trials have shown that screening by FOBT every 2 years may significantly reduce mortality. The technique has a sufficiently high sensitivity to warrant further study [13]. Almost half a million people were invited to take part in a screening programme using FOBT, with a final uptake of almost 57%, a positive result in 1.9% and a cancer detection rate of 1.62 per 1000 screened. The positive predictive value was 10.9% for cancer and 35% for adenomas. A total of 552 cancers were detected, of which 48% were early stage (Dukes A). Only 1% had metastasized at the time of diagnosis. Clearly these results justify wider application, particularly since an estimate of costs showed that the financial burden was under £6000 per life-year saved, a figure regarded as well below the threshold most European countries are willing to pay. Successful pilot studies have resulted in a major national initiative extending the programme [15]. The NHS Bowel Cancer Screening Programme offers screening every two years to all men and women aged 60–69 and is currently being extended to 60–74. This extensive programme which is heavily supported with a widely distributed information package on a population basis should impact significantly on UK morbidity and mortality from this disease. Colonoscopy is offered to those who have FOBT positivity. American Cancer Society recommendations for early detection of colorectal cancer begin at age 50. Men and women who are at average risk for developing colorectal cancer should have one of the screening options listed below [16]:
• FOBT or faecal immunochemical test (FIT) every year or;
• flexible sigmoidoscopy every 5 years or;
• annual FOBT (or FIT) and flexible sigmoidoscopy every 5 years or;
• double-contrast barium enema every 5 years or;
• colonoscopy every 10 years.

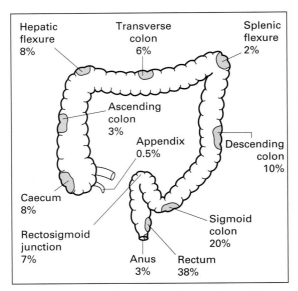

Figure 16.3 Cancer of the large bowel: proportion of all cases arising at each site.

Pathology and surgical staging

The distal large bowel is the commonest site of malignancy: approximately 20% occur in the sigmoid colon and 40% in the rectum (Figure 16.3). The typical lesion is either polypoid with a fleshy protuberance on a narrow base, or sessile with a broader base and a generally flatter appearance. The most characteristic form is a well-demarcated polypoid mass with ulceration in its centre, involving part or all of the bowel circumference. The tumour may have breached the full thickness of the bowel wall, although lateral spread beyond 3 cm is unusual. Local lymphatic invasion is common and about one-third of these patients have evidence of nodal metastases at presentation. Blood-borne metastases are usually via the portal vein and the liver is the commonest site of distant spread. Systemic haematogenous dissemination to the brain and skeleton occurs less frequently although rectal tumours show an increased propensity for lung metastases. Local recurrence can be a major problem, often leading to intestinal or ureteric obstruction, or fistula formation.

The Dukes staging system is widely employed and remains a valuable predictor of survival in both colonic and rectal lesions (Table 16.1); extensive regional node involvement has a particularly adverse prognosis. Tumour grade and depth of penetration are also important. There is increasing evidence that the number of

Table 16.1 Dukes staging system for rectal cancer

Stage	Description
A	Confined to bowel wall, i.e. mucosa and submucosa, or early muscular invasion
B	Invasion through the muscle wall but no lymph node involvement
C1	Lymph node involvement but not up to highest point of vascular ligation
C2	Nodes involved up to highest nodes at the point of ligation

lymph nodes harvested at surgery may be an important prognostic factor. The rationale for this observation could be a correlation of increased lymph nodes harvested with surgical proficiency as well as more accurate staging but remains unclear.

Clinical features and diagnosis

The symptoms of colorectal cancer vary with the site of the primary tumour (Figure 16.4). In the caecum and right side of the colon, the main complaint is frequently ill-defined abdominal pain that may be mistaken for gallbladder or peptic ulcer disease. Chronic iron-deficiency anaemia from occult blood loss is a common presenting feature. Frank melaena may occur, and an abdominal mass may be palpable.

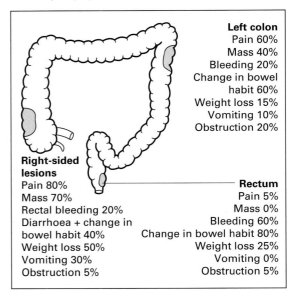

Figure 16.4 Symptoms of colorectal cancer according to site.

In left-sided colonic lesions the pain is often cramping and patients are more likely to present with alteration of bowel habit and intestinal obstruction. Abdominal distension may be present. Constipation, occasionally alternating with diarrhoea, is a frequent complaint and symptomatic rectal bleeding occurs in 20% of patients. Rectal carcinoma is often accompanied by passage of bright red blood. However, this is a common symptom in the normal population since haemorrhoids are very frequent. Change in bowel habit with tenesmus and constipation are later symptoms. It is crucial that rectal bleeding is not diagnosed as secondary to haemorrhoids until a cancer has been excluded.

Rectal examination is essential. Sigmoidoscopy allows examination of the distal 25 cm of large bowel and the majority of rectal tumours can be diagnosed in this way. The introduction of flexible sigmoidoscopy and colonoscopy gives a more accurate preoperative diagnosis of the majority of large-bowel cancers. Radiologically, the double-contrast enema has improved diagnostic accuracy, giving better resolution of small tumours. The characteristic appearance is of a narrowed or strictured segment, or a mass indenting the contrast medium (Figure 16.5). On the right side of the colon, tumours are more easily missed, particularly in the caecum, which may be poorly demonstrated by the examination. However, flexible sigmoidoscopy, colonoscopy and CT scanning with air contrast (CT pneumocolon) have become the procedures of choice. 'Virtual colonoscopy', a technique

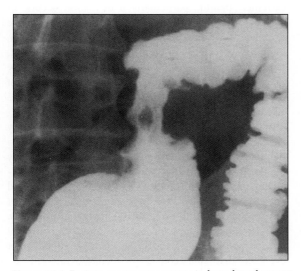

Figure 16.5 Barium enema appearances in large-bowel cancer showing carcinoma of the rectosigmoid.

employing helical CT with fine-slice imaging, provides a high concordance with conventional colonoscopy [17].

Carcinoembryonic antigen (CEA) is a tumour marker often elevated in colorectal cancer but is insufficiently specific to be a reliable indicator of disease since it can also be elevated in pancreatitis, inflammatory bowel disease and in heavy smokers. Additionally it may not be elevated in all cases. The differential diagnosis of large-bowel cancer includes diverticular disease, ulcerative or ischaemic colitis and irritable bowel syndrome. Other causes of rectal bleeding, such as haemorrhoids and polyps, may cause diagnostic difficulty. Abdominal pain may suggest biliary tract disease or peptic ulceration. Radiologically, it may be difficult to distinguish left-sided neoplasms from diverticular disease, and benign tumours such as lipomas and neurofibromas may occur at any site, although these are extremely rare.

Prognostic factors

Adverse factors include high pathological stage, degree of penetration of the primary tumour and lymph node involvement. Undifferentiated tumours, mucinous or 'signet-ring' forms, inadequate resection margins, vascular or lymphatic invasion or large-bowel obstruction are also considered prognostically important. There has been a revolution in the understanding of both prognostic and predictive markers in colorectal cancer [18]. However, although intriguing, molecular markers have not thus far been sufficiently robust to allow prognostic stratification, though it is likely that a gene signature will be developed in the future to refine prediction.

Management
Surgery

Surgery remains the foundation of treatment and the only curative modality. Wide removal of the involved segment should include resection of the local lymphatic drainage area (Figure 16.6). Even in patients with hepatic or peritoneal metastases, surgical resection may offer palliation.

There have been a number of reports suggesting that centres with a high volume of work have better survival outcomes [19]. Recent reports have suggested that laparoscopically assisted resection for colonic cancers may offer a better outcome with respect to reduction in surgical complications and hospital stay. One large randomized study from 48 collaborating hospitals in the USA showed a 3-year recurrence rate similar in the two groups, whether surgically resected using conventional techniques or by laparoscopic intervention. Recovery is more rapid in the laparoscopic group, with a shorter

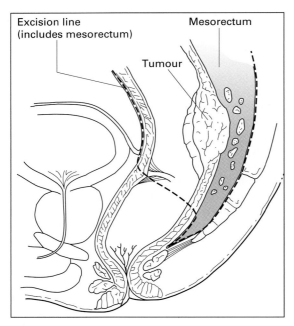

Figure 16.6 Mesorectal excision.

hospital stay and briefer use of analgesia [20]. The same appears to be true for rectosigmoid cancers.

In rectal cancer the type and extent of the excision depend on the site of the tumour. For low rectal lesions, abdominoperineal resection is still widely performed (Figure 16.6). Sphincter-preserving surgery, first performed in the late 1930s, is now performed on over 50% of surgically resectable rectal cancers. Local resection is sometimes performed for small mobile polypoid lesions of favourable histological grade. Patients who are unwell through obstruction, cachexia or perforation may benefit from an initial defunctioning colostomy before tumour removal is attempted. Even in totally unresectable lesions, a colostomy should generally be performed since this will at least allow a reasonable quality of life and makes high-dose radiotherapy for the primary tumour a feasible proposition (see below).

Surgical mortality has rapidly diminished in recent years and is now below 3% in experienced hands. Complications include anastomotic leaks, postoperative infection and urinary dysfunction, particularly if nerve damage has occurred during the operation. The major advance in rectal cancer has been the widespread adoption of total mesorectal excision in which the entire rectum is dissected *en bloc* without violating the fascial plane. The adoption of careful surgery with fine

dissection has been the major factor in reducing local recurrence. The key to successful outcome is careful preoperative clinical assessment and evaluation with magnetic resonance imaging (MRI). This allows the critical identification of lesions with a good probability of complete resection and allows decisions on the preoperative radiotherapy regimen (Figure 16.6). High-grade rectal lesions are particularly likely to recur locally, especially where regional node metastases have been demonstrated. Detailed pathological description of the surgical specimen is extremely important and should include the gross and microscopic extent of surgical margins, depth of penetration, number of nodes removed (and involved) and, in particular, whether the apical node (highest level) is positive. Characteristics such as venous or lymphatic invasion, perineural invasion, histological subtype and grade should also be documented.

Radiotherapy

This modality of treatment is widely employed in rectal cancer [21], especially in carcinomas below the mid-sigmoid region. Radiation therapy given preoperatively, frequently downstages tumours facilitating complete excision, but even in cases in which a complete response occurs clinically and radiologically, surgical excision is still recommended [22]. Radiotherapy can also be useful for inoperable or recurrent cancers. Troublesome symptoms of pain or rectal bleeding can usually be palliated and long survival occasionally achieved. Perineal, anastomotic or wound recurrences can be extremely painful, particularly if ulceration occurs. In such cases, and indeed when the surgeon cannot achieve complete operative removal of the primary lesion, radiotherapy is likely to be the most effective treatment. Doses in the range of 40–50 Gy in 4–5 weeks are usually recommended. As a result of this experience, studies of preoperative irradiation, usually to modest doses, have also been carried out.

In the UK, the Medical Research Council (CR-07) study randomised patients to short-course preoperative radiotherapy and selective postoperative chemo-radiotherapy for patients with involved circumferential margins following surgery [23]. The study involved 1350 randomised patients and resulted in a 61% reduction in the risk of local recurrence in those receiving preoperative therapy. This corresponds to a 6% absolute reduction in local recurrence rate and provided convincing and consistent evidence that short-course preoperative radiotherapy is an effective treatment for patients with operable rectal cancer. For cancers threatening circumferential margins, or which are fixed and bulky, long-course chemo-radiation is mandatory in optimizing the chance of a complete surgical excision with uninvolved margins.

Chemotherapy and other systemic treatment

There has been great progress in chemotherapy for colorectal cancer over the past decade in terms of improvements in response rates and survival. The addition of biological therapies and the range of therapeutic options have increased greatly the scope and complexity of treating colorectal cancer. Chemotherapy is used primarily in the adjuvant and advanced settings [24]. However, recent studies demonstrate an important role for neoadjuvant chemotherapy whereby unresectable metastatic disease can be downstaged resulting in potentially curative resection [25].

5-FU has been the mainstay of treatment for colon cancers for many years (Figure 16.7). This agent can produce symptomatic improvement, although objective responses are usually incomplete and transient, and occur

in around 20% of all patients. A meta-analysis of 5-FU in the setting of advanced colorectal cancer suggested a 3-month improvement in survival over supportive care alone, although the benefits are probably greater than this [26]. Treatment with 5-FU can be given in several ways including bolus and infusion and evidence suggests that infusional regimens are associated with decreased toxicity and improved response rates. However, infusional regimens require implantation of an indwelling peripheral or central venous catheter, with attendant inconvenience and complications, for example, sepsis and thrombosis. The response to 5-FU in metastatic colorectal cancer can be increased by concomitant administration with folinic acid (see Chapter 6). Oral capecitabine, a fluoropyrimidine, is chiefly metabolized in the liver, then converted in tumour tissue to 5-FU by the enzyme thymidine phosphorylase which is present in higher concentration in tumour cells than normal cells. Both effectiveness and tolerability are at least equivalent to 5-FU, with the benefit of oral therapy [27].

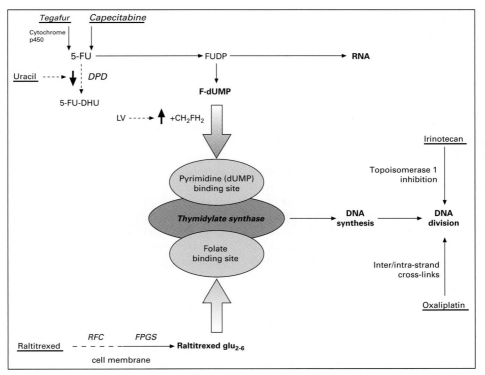

Figure 16.7 Mechanism of action of the common chemotherapeutic agents used in colorectal cancer. DPD, dihydropyrimidine dehydrogenase; LV, leucovorin (folinic acid); FPGS, folylpolyglutamate synthesase; RFC, reduced folate carrier; F-dUMP, 5-fluoro-2′-deoxyuridine-5′-monophosphate. (Source: Thomas *et al.* (2003). Reproduced with permission from Elsevier.)

Management in both adjuvant and advanced settings of colorectal cancer has been significantly altered by the introduction of two new chemotherapeutic agents, irinotecan and oxaliplatin [24]. Irinotecan is a topoisomerase I poison that converts the single-strand DNA breaks produced as reaction intermediates into irreversible cytotoxic lesions. The combination of irinotecan and 5-FU is active in advanced colorectal cancer and a mainstay of treatment. The major toxicity of this treatment is potential delayed onset of severe diarrhoea. Oxaliplatin also produces high response rates and prolongation of survival in colon cancer when used in combination with 5-FU.

Adjuvant treatment

In view of the risk of metastatic disease, particularly in node-positive disease, a number of large randomized studies have been performed to determine the benefits of additional therapy following potentially curative surgical resection. The pivotal study by Moertel demonstrated a significant reduction in recurrence following 12 months of treatment with 5-FU and levamisole (an antihelminthic agent) in node-positive patients [28]. Subsequent large randomized studies have confirmed this result [29,30] and demonstrated that treatment for 6 months is adequate. Levamisole is not used but 5-FU is administered in combination with folinic acid (leucovorin). The benefit of adjuvant chemotherapy for patients with Dukes B is less clear. The QASAR study suggests that this may result in an absolute improvement in survival of 3.6%.

There is now evidence from a large randomized study that combining oxaliplatin with 5-FU results in a significant reduction in the risk of recurrence for patients with Dukes C disease but no benefit was found for Dukes B patients [31]. Disease free survival was 78.2% at 3 years in the arm receiving oxaliplatin with 5-FU, as compared with 72.9% in the 5-FU alone group. As this regimen is associated with increased toxicity attributable to oxaliplatin, notably neuropathy and myelosuppression, its use in older patients or those with significant comorbidities needs careful consideration. However, this important study has had important implications for adjuvant treatment and, crucially, has translated into improvement in overall survival at 6 years in Stage 3 patients with 72.9% in the combination arm versus 68.7% in the fluorouracil arm [32].

The situation following resection of Dukes B cancer is less clear. The UK QUASAR study showed benefit for treatment with a fluoropyrimidine [29], but this is less than 5%. Factors which have been suggested to favour use of chemotherapy in this setting by subgroup analysis include bulky or obstructing tumours and T4 stage, although this approach is also used in younger patients and those with vascular invasion histologically.

Treatment of advanced colorectal cancer

The use of combination regimens in advanced colorectal cancer has made a significant difference to median overall survival, which has improved from 6 months to over 22 months with the use of drug combination therapies. This is associated with maintenance of good quality of life, although there are substantial issues in relation to cost. The recent development of targeted therapies in colorectal cancer has increased the options available for treatment of advanced disease.

Bevacizumab is a monoclonal antibody directed against vascular endothelial growth factor (VEGF). In a large randomized trial from the USA, including over 800 patients, addition of bevacizumab to irinotecan and 5-FU improved the survival rate from just over 15 months to over 20 months, a highly significant difference [33].

Cetuximab is a monoclonal antibody that binds the epidermal growth factor receptor (EGFR). EGFR is relevant in colorectal cancer because expression or up-regulation of the EGFR gene occurs in up to 80% of patients, and gene expression is associated with poor survival. The EGFR signalling pathway regulates cell differentiation, proliferation, angiogenesis and apoptosis. Cetuximab is a monoclonal antibody that binds EGFR with high specificity and affinity, blocking ligand-induced phosphorylation of EGFR. Responses were documented in a study in which this agent was combined with irinotecan in patients who were previously documented as being resistant to irinotecan [34]. Although the effect on overall survival was small, there have now been several randomised studies in which EGFR antibodies have been assessed in combination with chemotherapy [35]. Although there is clear benefit when cetuximab and panitumumab are added to irinotecan-based chemotherapy, there was no benefit for oxaliplatin-based regimens with cetuximab [36]. The appearance of an acneiform skin rash indicates response, although it can be debilitating.

The identification of patients likely to benefit from these costly therapies is a major priority. Interestingly, there is no clear relationship between the efficacy of this agent and levels of EGFR in the tumour. Indeed cetuximab may even be effective in patients in whom no EGFR can be detected by immunohistochemistry [37]. Responses to antibodies targeting EGFR are found only in patients without mutations in K-ras (i.e. expressing wild type K-ras) [38]. Treatment of patients with mutations results in no benefit [39]. Emerging evidence indicates that other genes in this pathway, such as BRAF may also be critical determinants of response to EGFR inhibition. Characterisation of K-ras status is now considered mandatory prior to a decision on treatment with antibodies targeting EGFR. The situation in relation to other mutations found in genes downstream of EGFR is less clear. A recent large retrospective study demonstrated that apart from K-ras, mutations in the N-ras and B-raf genes conferred resistance to panitumumab when administered in combination with chemotherapy [40]. Although other studies have suggested that other molecular markers such as PI3 - kinase mutations or deletions of the tumour suppressor gene PTEN may also be useful - these are not yet definitively validated.

The multikinase inhibitor regorafenib showed small benefit in a randomised study in patients progressing through multiple lines of treatment (median overall survival 6.4 months in the regorafenib group versus 5.0 months in the placebo group) [41]. Newer targets being evaluated include mutated B-raf of patients although an initial study of the B-raf inhibitor venflurafamib which is highly effective in b-raf mutated melanoma showed no benefit. Combination of these agents with EGFR inhibitors may be effective and is the focus of a current clinical trial [42].

With the development of whole exome sequencing and integrative analysis, the molecular architecture of colorectal cancer is becoming clearer [43]. These findings suggest a number of therapeutic approaches to CRC including WNT-signalling inhibitors and small-molecule β-catenin inhibitors, which are showing initial promise. Proteins in the RTK – RAS and PI3K pathways, including IGF2, IGFR, ERBB2, ERBB3, MEK, AKT and MTOR could also be targets for inhibition. This study illustrates the major potential for detailed genetic studies to inform novel targeting studies for colorectal and other cancers.

The only curative modality for patients with hepatic metastases is surgical resection. Although there have been no randomized studies comparing resection with non-surgical regimens, many published studies indicate survival of up to 40% for patients with liver metastases. There has been a trend towards a more aggressive approach, with resection of bilobar disease, multiple metastases and extrahepatic disease such as pulmonary lesions [44]. Neoadjuvant chemotherapy can be used to downstage disease and allow resection. There are no randomized studies allowing unequivocal endorsement

of the more aggressive approaches but it does seem that colorectal cancer metastases may be limited and potentially curable as compared with other solid tumours such as pancreatic and oesophagogastric cancers in which localized resection does not confer benefit. In patients with limited disease in whom surgical resection is not feasible because of co-morbidities, radiofrequency ablation and other local ablative techniques may control disease.

Living with a colostomy

Patients faced with the prospect of a permanent colostomy need sympathetic support. Quite apart from worrying about its appearance and the possibility of spillage and odour, most patients are concerned that they will find it impossible to manage the colostomy themselves without skilled help. They may need reassurance that the presence of the colostomy does not imply that residual cancer has been left behind and also that it will be possible to return to a normal active life. Despite enthusiastic help, many patients will develop depressive symptoms and, in a proportion, agoraphobia or fear of social contact may become a disability. The value of a skilled stoma therapist cannot be overestimated, and the same is true of the well-informed self-help groups such as the British Colostomy Association.

It is often valuable for the patient with cancer of the large bowel to meet a colostomy patient before the definitive surgery is performed. In many instances this has been crucial in persuading a hesitant patient to undergo what subsequently proves to be curative surgery.

Screening following curative surgery

There are few randomised studies demonstrating the benefits of specific follow-up pathways for early diagnosis of metastatic disease although general guidelines have been developed [45]. With a more aggressive approach to resection of metastatic disease, the case for surveillance appears better founded. A meta-analysis demonstrated the cost utility of this approach [46]. As most metastases develop within 2 years of diagnosis, most centres have a policy of repeat imaging at six-monthly intervals with CT or ultrasound. It can be useful in monitoring disease in patients with a preoperatively raised CEA that has fallen following successful surgery, in whom a rise in CEA may be the first sign of recurrence. Although there is no evidence that monitoring CEA levels affect survival, the 2013 American Society for Clinical Oncology recommendations on surveillance following resection of colorectal cancer suggest 3 – 6 monthly testing for 5 years [45].

Carcinoma of the anus
Pathology and clinical features

Fortunately these tumours are rare, accounting for about 2% of all large-bowel cancers. They are slightly more common in women and may occur in association with carcinoma of the cervix or vulva. Carcinoma of the anus is reportedly more common in anoreceptive male homo-sexuals and is recognized as an AIDS-related (though not AIDS-defining) malignancy. It is also commoner in immunosuppressed organ allograft transplant recipients. There is evidence to suggest an infectious aetiology most likely via human papillomavirus (HPV), notably HPV16, which is generally considered causative for cancer of the cervix as well. There are consistent and statistically sig-nificant associations between measures of sexual activity and the risk of anal cancer for both men and women. For example, the risk in women with 10 or more sexual partners was nearly 5 times that of women with only one lifetime partner. Strong associations with a variety of venereal diseases were also confirmed. Screening for anal carcinoma in high-risk populations (homosexual and bisexual males, using exfoliative cytology) has been suggested as being cost-effective (comparable to cervical screening in females) [47].

The tumour may present as small firm nodules that may be confused with haemorrhoids, the true nature of the lesion becoming apparent only after histological review of the surgical specimen. Rectal bleeding and pain are common symptoms. The diagnosis is often delayed since the symptoms are attributed to haemorrhoids or fissure *in ano*. Other lesions producing occasional diagnostic confusion include leucoplakia, Bowen's disease or Paget's disease of the anus. Local invasion of the anal sphincter and rectal wall is not uncommon, with more advanced local spread involving the prostate, bladder or cervix. Although these cancers are mostly of squamous origin, other histological types occur including basal cell carcinoma and melanoma. It is important, if possible, to distinguish tumours above the pectinate line from those below since the latter tend to have a better prognosis.

Treatment

Surgical resection is now no longer appropriate as first-choice therapy since non-surgical sphincter-conserving treatment with radiotherapy and chemother-apy is generally curative and has become standard treatment [48,49]. This represents an important and exciting change from traditional teaching. However, surgery may be required for postradiation recurrence.

In cases initially treated by surgery or radiotherapy but subsequently developing inguinal node metastases, block dissection of the nodes is usually required, though additional postoperative irradiation can be useful if the dissection is incomplete. Prophylactic block dissection of the inguinal nodes is not usually recommended. Chemoradiotherapy is clearly superior to radiation ther-apy alone, particularly in terms of local recurrence; overall survival may also be improved. In a large-scale multicen-tre UK study of nearly 600 patients randomly assigned to treatment by radiation therapy alone or with synchronous 5-FU and mitomycin-C, the local failure rate was reduced from 61% to 39% [48], resulting in a fall of almost 50% in the number of patients requiring radical salvage surgery with permanent colostomy. Radiation fields should be generous, to include local lymph node drainage sites as well as the primary carcinoma with an adequate margin, all irradiated to a minimum dose of 50 Gy. In an impor-tant large randomised trial the use of this combination approach was confirmed as superior to that achieved with a cisplatin-based chemoradiation regimen [50].

Prognosis

Prognosis in carcinoma of the anus depends on the location and tumour grade. The 5-year survival rate in patients undergoing abdominoperineal resection is 30–50%. Results from radical radiochemotherapy are at least as good, reportedly as high as 67% (5-year survival rate), with excellent functional preservation in the majority of cases. In the recent UK-based multicentre randomized study, 3-year survival was 58% for the radiotherapy group and 65% for the combined modality group [44]. For tumours of the anal verge, the 5-year survival rate is of the order of 60%. If inguinal nodes are involved at diagnosis, 5-year survival falls to 15%.

References

1 Schottenfeld D, Beebe-Dimmer JL, Vigneau FD. The epidemiology and pathogenesis of neoplasia in the small intestine. *Ann Epidemiol* 2009; 19: 58–69.

2 Judson I, Demetri G. Advances in the treatment of gastroin-testinal stromal tumours. *Ann Oncol* 2007; 18: 20–4.

3 Giovannucci E. Modifiable risk factors for colon cancer. *Gastroenterol Clin North Am* 2002; 31: 925–43.

4 Marshall JR. Prevention of colorectal cancer: diet, chemopre-vention, and lifestyle. *Gastroenterol Clin North Am* 2008; 37: 73–82.

5 Bresalier RS, Sandler RS, Quan H *et al*. Cardiovascular events associated with rofecoxib in a colorectal adenoma chemo-prevention trial. *N Engl J Med* 2005; 352: 1092–102.

6 Kinzler KW, Vogelstein B. Lessons from hereditary colorectal cancer. *Cell* 1996; 87: 159–70.

7 Ekbom A, Helmick C, Zack M *et al.* Ulcerative colitis and colorectal cancer: a population-based study. *N Engl J Med* 1990; 323: 1228–33.

8 Scholefield JH, Moss S. Screening sigmoidoscopy for colorectal cancer. *Lancet* 2003; 362: 1167–8.

9 Lynch HT, Lynch JF, Lynch PM, Attard T. Hereditary colorectal cancer syndromes: molecular genetics, genetic counselling, diagnosis and management. *Fam Cancer* 2008; 7: 27–39.

10 Huls S, Koornstra JJ, Kleibeuker JH. Non-steroidal anti-inflammatory drugs and molecular carcinogenesis of colorectal carcinomas. *Lancet* 2003; 362: 230–2.

11 Burn J, Gerdes AM, Macrae F *et al.* Long-term effect of aspirin on cancer risk in carriers of hereditary colorectal cancer: an analysis from the CAPP2 randomised controlled trial. *Lancet* 2011; 378: 2081–7.

12 Sieber OM, Lipton L, Crabtree M, *et al.* Multiple colorectal adenomas, classic adenomatous polyposis, and germ-line mutations in MYH. *N Engl J Med* 2003; 348: 791–9.

13 Ransohoff DF, Sandler RS. Screening for colorectal cancer. *N Engl J Med* 2002; 346: 40–4.

14 Thompson MR, Steele RJ, Atkin WS. Effective screening for bowel cancer: a United Kingdom perspective. *Dis Colon Rectum* 2006; 49: 895–908.

15 Rees CJ, Bevan R. The National Health Service Bowel Cancer Screening Program: the early years. *Expert Rev Gastroenterol Hepatol* 2013; 7: 421–37.

16 Levin B, Lieberman DA, McFarland B *et al.* Screening and surveillance for the early detection of colorectal cancer and adenomatous polyps, 2008: a joint guideline from the American Cancer Society, the US Multi-Society Task Force on Colorectal Cancer, and the American College of Radiology *CA Cancer J Clin* 2008; 58: 130–60.

17 Fenlon HM, Nunes DP, Schroy PC *et al.* A comparison of virtual and conventional colonoscopy for the detection of colorectal polyps. *N Engl J Med* 1999; 341: 1496–503.

18 Walther A, Johnstone E, Swanton C, *et al.* Genetic prognostic and predictive markers in colorectal cancer. *Nat Rev Cancer* 2009; 9: 489–99.

19 Meyerhardt JA, Catalano PJ, Schrag D *et al.* Association of hospital procedure volume and outcomes in patients with colon cancer at high risk for recurrence. *Ann Intern Med* 2003; 139: 649–57.

20 Clinical Outcomes of Surgical Therapy Study Group. A comparison of laparoscopically assisted and open colectomy for colon cancer. *N Engl J Med* 2004; 350: 2050–9.

21 Colorectal Cancer Collaborative Group. Adjuvant radiotherapy for rectal cancer: a systematic overview of 8507 patients from 22 randomised trials. *Lancet* 2001; 358: 1291–304.

22 Kapiteijn E, Marijnen CA, Nagtegaal ID *et al.* for the Dutch Colorectal Cancer Group. Preoperative radiotherapy combined with total mesorectal excision for resectable rectal cancer. *N Engl J Med* 2001; 345: 638–46.

23 Sebag-Montefiore D, Stephens RJ, Steele R *et al.* Preoperative radiotherapy versus selective postoperative chemoradiotherapy in patients with rectal cancer (MRC CR07 and NCIC-CTG C016): a multicentre, randomised trial. *Lancet* 2009; 373: 811–20.

24 Chau I, Cunningham D. Treatment in advanced colorectal cancer: what, when and how? *Br J Cancer* 2009; 100: 1704–19.

25 Brouquet A, Nordlinger B, Neoadjuvant and adjuvant therapy in relation to surgery for colorectal liver metastases. *Scand J Gastroenterol* 2012; 47: 286–95.

26 Simmonds PC. Palliative chemotherapy for advanced colorectal cancer: systematic review and meta-analysis. Colorectal Cancer Collaborative Group. *BMJ* 2000; 321: 531–5.

27 Hoff PM, Ansari R, Batist G, *et al.* Comparison of oral capecitabine treatment in 605 patients with metastatic cancer: results of a randomised phase III study. *J Clin Oncol* 2001; 19: 2282–92.

28 Moertel CG, Fleming TR, MacDonald JS *et al.* Levamisole and fluorouracil for adjuvant therapy of resected colon carcinoma. *N Engl J Med* 1990; 322: 352–8.

29 Krook JE, Moertel CG, Gunderson LL *et al.* Effective surgical adjuvant therapy for high risk rectal carcinoma. *N Engl J Med* 1991; 324: 709–15.

30 Quasar Collaborative Group, Gray R, Barnwell J, McConkey C *et al.* Adjuvant chemotherapy versus observation in patients with colorectal cancer: a randomised study. *Lancet* 2007; 370: 2020–9.

31 André T, Boni C, Mounedji-Boudiaf L *et al.* Oxaliplatin, fluorouracil, and leucovorin as adjuvant treatment for colon cancer. Multicenter International Study of Oxaliplatin/5-Fluorouracil/Leucovorin in the Adjuvant Treatment of Colon Cancer (MOSAIC) Investigators. *N Engl J Med* 2004; 350: 2343–5.

32 André T, Boni C, Navarro M *et al.* Improved overall survival with oxaliplatin, fluorouracil, and leucovorin as adjuvant treatment in stage II or III colon cancer in the MOSAIC trial. *J Clin Oncol* 2009; 27: 3109–16.

33 Hurwitz H, Fehrenbacher L, Novotny W *et al.* Bevacizumab plus irinotecan, fluorouracil and leucovorin for metastatic colorectal cancer. *N Engl J Med* 2004; 350: 2335–42.

34 Cunningham D, Humblet Y, Siena S *et al.* Cetuximab monotherapy and cetuximab plus irinotecan in irinotecan-refractory metastatic colorectal cancer. *N Engl J Med* 2004; 351: 337–45.

35 Jain VK, Hawkes EA, Cunningham D. Integration of biologic agents with cytotoxic chemotherapy in metastatic colorectal cancer. *Clin Colorectal Cancer* 2011; 10: 245–57.

36 Maughan TS, Adams RA, Smith CG *et al.* Addition of cetuximab to oxaliplatin-based first-line combination chemotherapy for treatment of advanced colorectal cancer: results of the randomised phase 3 MRC COIN trial. *Lancet* 2011; 377: 2103–14.

37 Chung KY, Shia J, Kemeny NE *et al.* Cetuximab shows activity in colorectal cancer patients with tumors that do not express the epidermal growth factor receptor by immunohistochemistry. *J Clin Oncol* 2005; 23: 1803–10.

38 Karapetis CS, Khambata-Ford S, Jonker DJ *et al.* K-ras mutations and benefit from cetuximab in advanced colorectal cancer. *N Engl J Med* 2008; 359: 1757–65.

39 Evaluation of Genomic Applications in Practice and Prevention (EGAPP) Working Group. Recommendations from the EGAPP Working Group: can testing of tumor tissue for mutations in EGFR pathway downstream effector genes in patients with metastatic colorectal cancer improve health outcomes by guiding decisions regarding anti-EGFR therapy? *Genet Med* 2013; 15: 517–27.

40 Douillard JY, Oliner KS, Siena S *et al.* Panitumumab-FOLFOX4 treatment and RAS mutations in colorectal cancer. *N Engl J Med* 2013; 369: 1023–34.

41 Grothey A, Van Cutsem E, Sobrero A *et al.* Regorafenib monotherapy for previously treated metastatic colorectal cancer (CORRECT): an international, multicentre, randomised, placebo-controlled, phase 3 trial. *Lancet* 2013; 381: 303–12.

42 Prahallad A, Sun C, Huang S *et al.* Unresponsiveness of colon cancer to BRAF(V600E) inhibition through feedback activation of EGFR. *Nature* 2012; 483: 100–3.

43 Cancer Genome Atlas Network. Comprehensive molecular characterization of human colon and rectal cancer. *Nature* 2012; 487: 330–7.

44 Adam R, De Gramont A, Figueras J *et al.* The oncosurgery approach to managing liver metastases from colorectal cancer: a multidisciplinary international consensus. *Oncologist* 2012; 17: 1225–39.

45 Renehan AG, O'Dwyer ST, Whynes DK. Cost effectiveness analysis of intensive versus conventional follow up after curative resection for colorectal cancer. *BMJ* 2004; 328: 81.

46 Meyerhardt JA, Mangu PB, Flynn PJ *et al.* Follow-up care, surveillance protocol, and secondary prevention measures for survivors of colorectal cancer: American Society of Clinical Oncology clinical practice guideline endorsement. *J Clin Oncol* 2013; 31: 4465–70.

47 Tanum G, Tveit K, Karlsen K *et al.* Chemotherapy and radiation therapy for anal carcinoma: survival and later morbidity. *Cancer* 1991; 67: 2462–6.

48 UKCCCR Anal Cancer Trial Working Party. Epidermoid anal cancer: results from the UKCCCR randomised trial of radiotherapy alone vs. radiotherapy, 5-fluorouracil and mitomycin. *Lancet* 1996; 348: 1049–54.

49 Glynne-Jones R, Renehan A. Current treatment of anal squamous cell carcinoma. *Hematol Oncol Clin North Am* 2012; 26: 1315–50.

50 James RD, Glynne-Jones R, Meadows HM *et al.* Mitomycin or cisplatin chemoradiation with or without maintenance chemotherapy for treatment of squamous-cell carcinoma of the anus (ACT II): a randomized, phase 3, open-label, 2 × 2 factorial trial. *Lancet Oncol* 2013; 14: 516–24.

17 Gynaecological cancer

Gynaecological cancers account for approximately one-quarter of all malignant disease in women, with striking differences in incidence for each of the major primary sites (Figure 17.1). Worldwide incidence rates differ greatly (Figure 17.2). Endometrial carcinoma has become more prevalent with increasing average body weight and is now both the commonest and most frequently cured of gynaecological malignancies [1]. Tumours of the female genital tract are important not only because of their high incidence, but also because many can be diagnosed while still relatively localized. Standard screening techniques can detect both early and even premalignant stages of disease (see below). Management requires the combined skills of surgeons, radiotherapists and medical oncologists; many women with gynaecological cancer are best treated with a combination of these approaches.

The overall incidence rates of carcinomas of cervix, corpus uteri and ovary are approximately equal, but because curative treatment is much less likely in ovarian carcinoma, the mortality from this disease now exceeds the combined death rate from carcinomas of the cervix and corpus [1,2]. There are a number of known aetiological factors for gynaecological cancer. Epidemiological studies have shown, for example, that the low incidence of carcinoma of the ovary in Japanese women rapidly rises within a generation or two when they emigrate to the USA – a six-fold increase that strongly suggests environmental factors predominating over genetic ones. The importance of family history in ovarian cancer is increasingly recognized; a meta-analysis of 15 cohort and case–control studies gave a relative risk of 3.8 for sisters, and 6.0 for daughters of cases [3]. In addition, the daughter's social behaviour is also important as a risk factor: good examples include the high risk of ovarian cancer among nulliparous or subfertile women and the close relationship between *in situ* invasive carcinoma of

Cancer and its Management, Seventh Edition. Jeffrey Tobias and Daniel Hochhauser.
© 2015 John Wiley & Sons, Ltd. Published 2015 by John Wiley & Sons, Ltd.

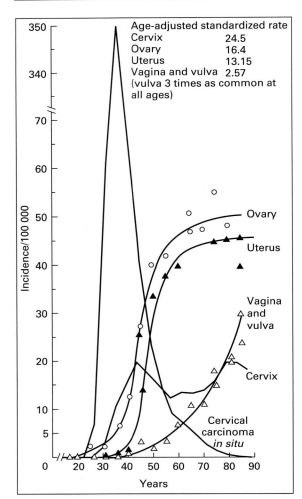

Figure 17.1 Age-specific incidence of gynaecological cancers. The high incidence of carcinoma of the cervix below the age of 40 is chiefly due to *in situ* cases.

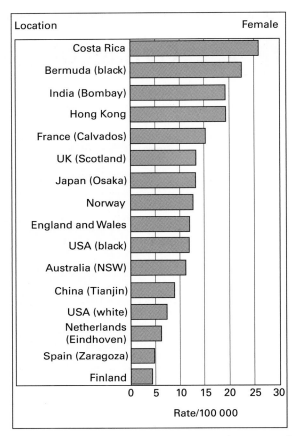

Figure 17.2 Geographic variation in incidence of carcinoma of the cervix per 100 000 (excluding *in situ* cases). Total new cases annually, 370 000.

the cervix and early sexual experience and social class (Figure 17.3). Screening programmes have undoubtedly helped to reduce the frequency of invasive carcinoma of the cervix, which has fallen sharply during the 1990s. A recent publication from the UK confirms the remarkable success of our national screening programme introduced in 1988 [4]. The estimate was that cervical screening had prevented an epidemic that would have killed about 1 in 65 of all British women born since 1950, culminating in about 6000 deaths per annum in the UK. At the current time, women in the UK are first invited for screening at the age of 25 years. At present, it is thought that some

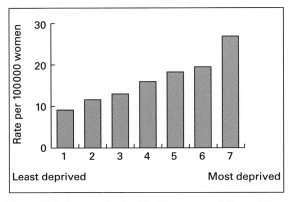

Figure 17.3 Age-standardized incidence rates of Cervical Cancer by Carstairs deprivation category (broadly equivalent to socioeconomic status). (Source: Cancer Research UK 2006.)

4500 lives are saved each year in the UK as a result of screening, although nearly 3000 women are newly diagnosed each year, of whom about 1100 die from the disease. In 2005, over 3.5 million women were screened in England. Nonetheless, current concerns about the national screening programme centre on the worrying fall in the rate of uptake, from 82% in 2000 to 80.3% in 2005, with even lower figures for younger women in their twenties. Even with lowered incidence rates of invasive disease, national screening will remain necessary for the foreseeable future, because of the high prevalence of human papillomavirus (HPV) infection (see below). An important and startling statistic is that about 8 of every 10 sexually active women can expect to develop an HPV infection at some point in their lives. Some authorities believe that it is logical, and would be even more effective, to start screening programmes earlier in a woman's life [5], and great concern has recently been expressed about the rising cost of this essential public-health requirement – see, for example, the impassioned plea from Bettigole [6].

The question remains as to the risk of invasive cervical cancer following treatment of cervical intraepithelial neoplasia (CIN), with recent studies suggesting that not only CIN III but also earlier stages, both CIN I and CIN II (see below), may confer a continuing risk. In one large study from Finland, over 7500 women treated for CIN (various grades) from the 1970s were followed up until 2003 [7]. The risk of an invasive cancer developing remains higher for the 20-year period following treatment, strongly suggesting that close follow-up even of low-grade (CIN I and CIN II) lesions is essential, and may have been inadequate in the past.

Carcinoma of the cervix

Incidence and aetiology

The aetiology of carcinoma of the cervix, which is essentially viral, remains a subject of great interest. The viral transmission of cervical cancer is clearly related to sexual intercourse and multiple partners.

Preinvasive lesions

It is widely accepted that invasive carcinoma of the cervix is preceded by premalignant lesions that are benign [8]. There are currently well over 25 000 new registrations of carcinoma *in situ* of the cervix uteri in the UK. Most cases (90%) are registered in women under 45, with peak incidence in the 25–29 age group.

Invasive carcinoma

Over 3000 new cases of invasive carcinoma are diagnosed annually in the UK, making it the eleventh most common cancer in women and accounting for around 2% of all female cancers. The European age-standardized annual incidence rate in the UK is 9.7 per 100 000 women (crude rate 10.8 per 100 000 women). Worldwide, the burden of newly diagnosed disease is about 500 000 new cases annually, with over 275 000 deaths recorded in 2002 or one-tenth of all female cancer deaths globally [9]. More than 80% of these deaths occur in developing countries, and this figure is likely to increase further. Cervical cancer is the second most common cancer after breast cancer in the under-35 age group, with around 600 new cases diagnosed annually in the UK. More than with any other type of cancer, cervical cancer reflects striking global health inequity [10].

More women with cervical cancer have been sexually active under age 20 than matched controls. Race and social class may not be independent factors since sexual behaviour may differ in these groups. It has frequently been suggested that the low incidence of carcinoma of the cervix among Jewish women may be the result of male circumcision, although more recent studies suggest that circumcision of the male partner may be less important than was previously thought [11]. It is likely that such women start intercourse later in life and have fewer partners. There is some evidence that the peak age of onset is falling, possibly because of changes in social habits (see below). In recent years there has been a significant reduction in invasive carcinoma of the cervix, coupled with an increase in microinvasive or *in situ* disease. Of the 3000 new cases diagnosed annually in the UK, about two-thirds of patients will be cured, resulting in an annual death rate of over 1000. Prior to screening, the cervical cancer death rate rose from 0.7 per 100 000 in 1963–1967 to 2.2 per 100 000 in 1983–1987. An important recent meta-analysis has suggested that using oral contraceptives is itself a further risk factor: taking an oral contraceptive for about 10 years from age 20–30 years was estimated to increase the cumulative risk by age 50 from 7.3 to 8.3 per 1000 in less developed countries and from 3.8 to 4.5 per 1000 in more developed countries [12]. However, such women would of course be likely to be more sexually active than others, and use condoms less regularly, thereby avoiding a mechanical barrier to viral transmission during intercourse and somewhat confounding the results.

The aetiology has now been unequivocally linked to sexually transmitted infection by HPV, particularly types 11, 16 and 18, which have been shown to produce morphological changes in human vaginal cells [13]. It is clear that HPV-16 and HPV-18 cause approximately 70% of cervical cancers worldwide, and as recently pointed out in an influential review, "Virtually all cases of cervical cancer are caused by persistent infection with one of about a dozen carcinogenic HPV genotypes – specifically, HPV types 16, 18, 31, 33, 35, 39, 45, 51, 52, 56, 58, 59, and 68" – see Ref. [14]. Although HPV-16 is strongly linked with squamous cell carcinoma (much the commonest histological variety). More than 80% of the deaths occur in developing countries, HPV-18 is particularly linked with adenocarcinoma. Apart from the known link with sexual activity and deprivation score, important additional non-viral cofactors include smoking and a history of cervical dysplasia. Tobacco smoking has now been classified as a clear-cut cause of cervical cancer, with an increased relative risk for squamous cell carcinoma in current smokers approaching 60%. The risk appeared to increase with the number of cigarettes smoked per day, and also with younger age at starting smoking [15]. However, there is no known link between smoking and the less common adenocarcinoma. Women in developing countries also have a much higher risk. In addition, there is a substantial incidence in women over age 65 years who are not routinely screened in most Western countries [16]. Older women often present with late stages of disease, and a more active screening programme in older women in the UK would doubtless result in hundreds of lives saved every year. One extremely promising approach recently publicized at the 2013 ASCO conference was the use of acetic acid staining (using simple vinegar!) with biennial screening by inspection, employing well-trained (4 weeks training was all that was required) non-medical health-workers (see Ref. [17]). This was a randomized trial of over 150 000 women in deprived slum areas of Mumbai over a 15-year period, and showed a clear-cut benefit, namely, a diagnosis of cervical carcinoma not made more frequently overall, but at an earlier stage of disease, thus improving the likelihood of overall survival. In each group, approximately 27 cases were diagnosed in 100 000 women-years of observation, but with a dramatic 31% fall in the disease-specific death rate – from 16 to 11 per 100 000 women-years observation. This key finding is likely to lead to a far more widespread use of this approach in developing countries.

HPV testing of cervical smears is more sensitive but less specific than cytology in detecting high-grade CIN (II+) (Figure 17.4). HPV testing has been carefully assessed in comparison with standard cytology [18,19]. In a study of 825 randomized women, HPV testing was confirmed to be valuable as primary screening in women older than 30 years, with cytology useful for triage in HPV-positive women. HPV-positive women with normal or borderline cytology (about 6% of the screened patients) could be managed by repeat testing after 12 months, potentially improving detection rates in high-risk cases without increasing the colposcopy referral rate. Recent work has suggested that the degree of abnormality in a squamous intraepithelial lesion may depend closely on the known risk rate of the associated HPV type, high-grade squamous lesions being associated with high-risk HPV and low-grade lesions with low-risk HPV types, with little or no risk of progression [20]. Only a subset of HPV genotypes commonly considered to be oncogenic were closely associated, at least in this series of over 280 preinvasive lesions, with a tendency towards frank invasion.

Although conventional Papanicolaou screening for cervical cancer has been used for over 30 years, concerns have emerged about its reliability and predictive value. Liquid-based cytology, rinsing the sampling tool into a vial of liquid to produce a suspension of cells from which a monolayer is prepared for the microscope slide, has been advocated as superior. Slides produced in this way can be read more quickly, and the liquid sample used for HPV testing. There remains a clear need for a large-scale randomized study to assess what must still be regarded as a promising yet unproven technique, although a recent Italian study (nine screening centres) did suggest that the rate of unsatisfactory smears can certainly be reduced by switching to this methodology [21], but a lively debate continues as to the pros and cons of each method [22]. Work from centres in the developing world has suggested that visual screening with visual inspection using 4% acetic acid can be an effective form of early diagnosis, with a corresponding fall in mortality at relatively low cost [23].

Because of the viral causation of squamous carcinoma of the cervix, generally by HPV-16 and HPV-18, the possibility of a therapeutic vaccine has been under serious consideration since the 1980s – see, for example, Ref. [24]. It was recognized in the early 1990s that it might be possible to achieve this, but it took a further 10 years before the phase II published trial confirmed that this could become a clinical reality [25–27]. Several large-scale studies have now proven equally successful. Two vaccines, initially created using the L1 protein of the viral capsid, give prolonged protection against HPV: the quadrivalent Gardasil protects against HPV-6, HPV-11, HPV-16 and HPV-18; the bivalent Cervarix protects

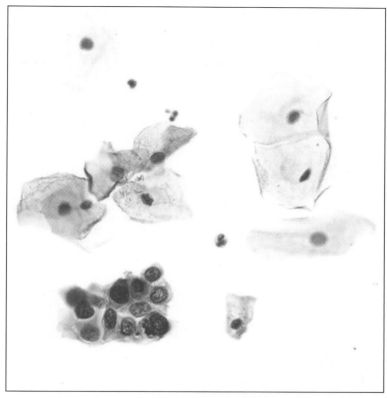

Figure 17.4 This cervical smear shows moderate/severe dyskaryosis. In the group of cells on the bottom left the nuclei are very large, highly irregular, highly stained and take up most of the cell (with very little normal cytoplasmic content.

against HPV-16 and HPV-18, which together cause the large majority of cervical cancers. These have now been approved for use in both the UK and USA, for females aged 9–26 years, and current studies have demonstrated long-term protection for at least 5 years and almost certainly considerably longer. We finally appear to have an opportunity to eliminate the majority of cases of this potentially fatal condition which worldwide still remains the second commonest of all female cancers. Gardasil is a recombinant vaccine that contains no live virus and is given as three injections over a 6-month period in the presexual phase of life. Since it does not protect against less common HPV types, routine and regular screening remain critically important, exactly as at present. However, it is worth mentioning that it also offers protection against genital warts and HPV-related anal carcinoma caused by HPV-16 and HPV-18, and that the additional protection against genital warts afforded by Gardasil, though not Cervarix, is emerging as a political issue in the UK, where the Cervarix vaccine has

been selected for national use on grounds of cost. For adenocarcinoma of the cervix, there is increasing evidence that, as with adenocarcinoma of the endometrium, obesity is an important potential risk factor [28]. HPV-18 is particularly associated with this malignancy.

In the USA, the Advisory Committee on Immunization Practices of the Centers for Disease Control and Prevention (CDC) has now unanimously recommended that girls of 11 and 12 years of age receive the vaccine, and the CDC has added Gardasil to its Vaccines for Children Program, which provides free immunizations to impoverished children [29], a move that will inevitably place the decision in the political arena and has already been attacked on moral grounds by some religious groups and parent bodies. In England and Wales, vaccination will be offered to girls of a slightly older age group (12–13 years, with a catch-up campaign up to age 18 years) from September 2008. The new policy is expected to save hundreds of lives each year, and initial uptake of the vaccine appears to be encouraging.

Pathology and spread

Routine Papanicolaou screening cytology has taught us a great deal about precancerous lesions in the cervix. These changes, collectively known as CIN, can be graded according to the degree of cytological abnormality. Carcinoma *in situ* (CIN III) represents the most severe of the preinvasive intraepithelial changes, and a large proportion (possibly 30–40%) will develop into true invasive carcinomas if left untreated.

The usual invasive lesion is a squamous carcinoma (85% of all cases). Microscopically, these are arranged in nests and sheets, invading the cervical stroma. Adenocarcinomas account for a further 5–10%, and the remainder are much rarer lesions including mixed adenosquamous tumours, adenoacanthomas, small-cell cancers and sarcomas. The majority of adenocarcinomas of the cervix arise from the endocervical canal.

The major routes of spread are predictable, forming the basis of standard surgical and pathological staging (Table 17.1 and Figure 17.5). Direct and lymphatic spread occur much earlier than haematogenous

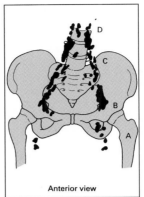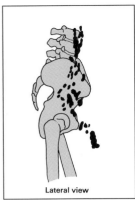

| Anterior view | Lateral view |

Figure 17.5 Lymphatic drainage of the cervix. Lymphatic involvement in carcinoma of the cervix generally occurs in an orderly progression. The sequence is (A) obturator; (B) internal, external and common iliac; (C) lateral sacral; (D) para-aortic.

dissemination. The most important direct routes of spread are downwards into the vaginal vault (often extending microscopically beyond the limits of visible disease) and laterally beyond the paracervical tissues to the parametria, resulting in extension to the lateral pelvic wall.

Lymphatic spread is via the paracervical lymphatics, to pelvic and para-aortic groups which follow the course of the major vessels. There is a high incidence of nodal spread even in patients with localized disease, and lymph node involvement occurs in almost 20% of these 'early' cases. Sites of blood-borne metastases include the lungs, liver and bone (rarely, and chiefly by local extension).

Clinical features

Women with dysplasia or CIN of all grades are asymptomatic but coexisting other conditions such as cervical erosion may produce incidental symptoms.

Invasive cancers present with vaginal bleeding (80%) and/or discharge, often offensive and discoloured. Some women consider these symptoms a normal feature of their lives and fail to seek advice for many months. Vaginal bleeding often follows intercourse. Abdominal pain, dyspareunia or low back pain also occur, and suggest a bulky or advanced lesion. Urinary and rectal symptoms suggest locally extensive disease. The tumour is usually visible with simple speculum techniques. *Exophytic* lesions are bulky, often forming large friable polypoid growths, making them easy to diagnose. *Infiltrative* tumours show little in the way of visible ulceration as the abnormal growth is often directed inwards towards the body of the uterus, often replacing the cervix and upper

---

Table 17.1 Simplified clinical staging for carcinoma of the cervix based on TNM classification (7th edn) and FIGO criteria.

Stage	Description
Preinvasive carcinoma	
Stage 0	Carcinoma *in situ*
Invasive carcinoma	
Stage I	Disease confined to the cervix
Ia	Microinvasive carcinoma
Ib	All other cases of stage I
Stage II	Disease beyond cervix but not to pelvic wall. Upper two-thirds of vagina may be involved
IIa	No parametrial involvement evident
IIb	Parametrial involvement
Stage III	Extension to pelvic side-wall and/or lower third of vagina. Includes cases with hydronephrosis or non-functioning kidney (unless other known cause exists)
IIIa	No extension to pelvic side-wall
IIIb	Extension to pelvic side-wall and/or hydronephrosis or non-functioning kidney
Stage IV	Carcinoma beyond true pelvis or involving mucosa of bladder or rectum
IVa	Spread to local organs
IVb	Spread to distant organs

vagina by a large confluent malignant ulcer. If the disease recurs following treatment, a characteristic clinical syndrome usually occurs, with pelvic, back and buttock pain, bowel disturbance, and unilateral leg oedema due to lymphatic and venous obstruction.

Staging

Careful staging is essential, yielding important prognostic information and allowing comparison of results in centres using different approaches. The International Federation of Gynaecology and Obstetrics (FIGO) staging system is in common use (Table 17.1), and the current tumour node metastasis (TNM) system is less popular. Staging is based on colposcopy, inspection, palpation, curettage and biopsy, together with investigations such as chest radiography and computed tomography (CT) or magnetic resonance imaging (MRI). Colposcopy is indispensable, capable of diagnosing stage 0 and Ia cancers that might otherwise escape detection. Wherever possible, examination is performed under anaesthesia. Using these criteria, the reproducibility of assessment is excellent. There is an increasing incidence of nodal metastases with advancing stage, with involvement in almost 20% of patients with stage Ib disease, and over 60% of patients with stage III disease.

Management

For patients with CIN III, therapeutic cone biopsy usually results in complete excision and cure, with preservation of reproductive function. However, newer approaches, particularly laser surgery or cryotherapy, can be expected to cure 70% of cases without cone biopsy [30]. Occasionally, hysterectomy is performed in women beyond child-bearing age or in those who have no wish for further children.

For patients with frankly invasive disease, the most important modalities of treatment are surgery and radiotherapy. Management details vary from one institution to another, and it would be unrealistic to deny that local expertise and facilities play an important part in these decisions. Most centres rely on the FIGO staging system to provide guidelines for management.

Stage Ib and IIa cancers now account for over half of all carcinomas of the cervix. In some patients, the invasive nature of the disease is more limited than was previously recognized. For this group, with microinvasive or non-confluent early invasive disease, therapeutic intervention may perhaps be more conservative. It is important to distinguish true microinvasive lesions from those with microscopic evidence of lymphovascular involvement. Surgery and radiotherapy are equally effective, with high 5-year survival rates (over 85–90% in patients with stage Ib disease) following either method. Although radiotherapy has become standard treatment in many institutions, few direct comparisons are available from the same source. Surgical series tend to be more highly selective: in some series, the operability rate of patients with stage Ib disease is not much more than half of all patients referred for consideration of surgery. In patients who are suitable, a radical (Wertheim's) hysterectomy is usually recommended. This involves total abdominal hysterectomy, with removal of a 2–3 cm cuff of vagina and all supporting tissues within the true pelvis. A complete pelvic lymphadenectomy is performed because 20% of patients have lymph node involvement. Bilateral oophorectomy is often performed but is not mandatory since the tumour rarely metastasizes to the ovary. Indeed, in young women, conservation of the ovaries is one of the advantages which surgery has over radical radiotherapy.

Care must be taken not to damage the ureters, and operations as extensive as this require great skill. It is better for a limited number of gynaecologists to maintain the technique and to practise it frequently than for all gynaecologists to perform this sort of operation infrequently. An important advantage of surgery is the definition of the true state of spread in order to allow more accurate overall planning of treatment; the radiotherapist will never have such complete information. Although early surgical morbidity is greater than that from radiotherapy in the younger age group, there are undoubtedly fewer late complications. Surgery is certainly the treatment of choice for young women in whom avoidance of late radiation reactions is particularly desirable. It is often possible to conserve at least one ovary in an otherwise radical operation.

In older patients, there is little dispute that radical irradiation (or chemoirradiation, see below) is the most appropriate form of treatment. A large randomized study from Italy confirmed identical results for both surgery and radical radiation therapy: 83% overall survival and 74% disease-free survival at 5 years [31]. However, in these older patients, late or 'severe' morbidity was more frequent in the surgical group (28% vs 12%). Late-onset problems, particularly relating to chronic gastrointestinal toxicity, occur regularly in heavily irradiated patients, and the management of these complications demands particular diagnostic and treatment expertise [32].

For patients presenting with more *advanced stages of disease (IIb–IV)*, radiotherapy is clearly the treatment of choice. In some centres (mostly in North America), radical lymphadenectomy is performed in selected cases, but its therapeutic contribution is uncertain and it has no place in routine management. The claim that radiotherapy cannot deal with node-positive cases seems unfounded. The number of histologically positive nodes is as low as one-third of the expected number treated by surgery alone, suggesting that radiation therapy can successfully 'downstage' in individual cases. An extremely important observation, confirmed in several randomized studies, is the improved results from combined chemoradiation therapy [33,34]. Various chemotherapy regimens have been used, generally cisplatin-based, given synchronously with radical radiation therapy. This has rapidly become the current standard of care for patients with advanced carcinoma (see below).

Radiation technique and dosage, and radical chemoradiation therapy

Radiotherapy is the most important single treatment for carcinoma of the cervix, and can cure a large proportion of patients, even including some with advanced disease and those who relapse following surgery. Both internal (intracavitary) and external treatments are used. Intracavitary radium treatment is of considerable historic importance in the evolution of modern radiotherapy techniques, but with improvements in equipment, external irradiation has assumed an increasing role. In general, intracavitary treatment is of greater importance in early disease and external beam treatment makes the greater contribution in advanced cases. Some patients with early disease are initially unsuitable for intracavitary treatment, particularly where there is distortion of local anatomy, where the vaginal vault is narrow or the cervical os is obliterated by tumour, making it impossible in the first instance.

Intracavitary treatment consists of placement of an intrauterine source (usually radioactive caesium rather than radium, because of its more suitable characteristics; see Chapter 5) together with radioactive sources adjacent to the cervix in the lateral vaginal fornices (Figure 17.6). Most centres perform these insertions under general anaesthesia, though local or epidural anaesthesia may be sufficient. Radiotherapy departments now mostly employ after-loading techniques, whereby the plastic housing for both the intrauterine and vaginal fornix containers is introduced first and the active source inserted only when the geometrical placement is perfect. These techniques produce a typical pear-shaped isodose distribution (Figure 17.7). In this way the uterus, cervix

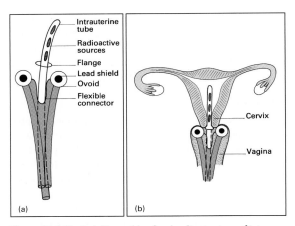

Figure 17.6 Typical disposable after-loading system of intracavitary irradiation in carcinoma of the cervix: (a) components; (b) in position. After placement, these sources act as a single irradiation source, and the components are packed into position to retain their location.

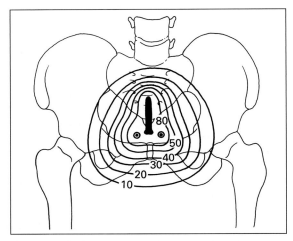

Figure 17.7 Typical isodose curves following intracavitary placement of caesium sources for carcinoma of the cervix. The numbers refer to the dose in greys.

and upper vagina all receive a high dose of radiation, with a decreasing but significant dosage to the paracervical and parametrial tissues including at least some of the regional lymphatics. Traditionally, two points, designated A and B, are used as a guide to dosimetry ('Manchester Applicator System') – see Figure 17.8.

Although variability in both normal and abnormal gynaecological anatomy necessarily makes dosimetry based on these arbitrary points difficult, they are widely

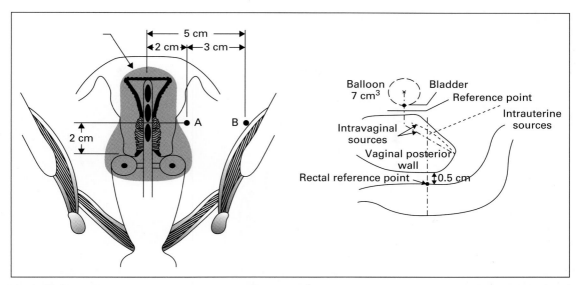

Figure 17.8 Classical Manchester system for intracavitary irradiation for carcinoma of the cervix. (Source: Reproduced by permission of Oxford University Press.)

used as a basis for dose calculation. Point A is located 2 cm from the midline of the cervical canal and 2 cm superior to the lateral vaginal fornix. Point B is 3 cm lateral to point A (i.e. 5 cm from the midline along the same lateral axis). However, in Europe and elsewhere the GEC-ESTRO recommendations for radiation dosimetry are being increasingly preferred, taking greater note of expected and tolerance doses to normal surrounding structures vulnerable to radiation injury, especially the rectum and bladder – see Figure 17.9.

Combinations of intracavitary and external beam treatment are often employed, though the emphasis varies in different departments. For patients with early stages of disease, intracavitary irradiation is of the greatest importance; for more advanced cases, particularly with lateral spread to the pelvic side-wall, external radiation therapy to the whole pelvis contributes more to the final probability of cure. When both methods are employed, as in the majority of patients, some radiotherapists prefer the traditional approach of using intracavitary irradiation first, whereas an increasing number always use external beam treatment initially. Additionally, intracavitary treatment may become possible as a result of tumour shrinkage, since there will always be cases where the attempt to insert radioactive tubes at the outset is unsuccessful, because of tumour bulk – an unfortunate situation which to a large extent can be reduced by treating with external irradiation first.

Although the complications of irradiation have been substantially reduced by improved technique and understanding of radiation pathology, they cannot be avoided entirely. Early problems include diarrhoea, anorexia, nausea, erythema, dry and (less frequently) moist desquamation of the skin, mostly easily controllable with symptomatic measures. Intracavitary treatment may produce proctitis and/or cystitis. Late complications are more important and include chronic proctosigmoiditis, small-bowel damage and rectovaginal or vesicovaginal fistulae, which can require urinary or colonic diversion. Chronic skin changes (excessive fibrosis, depigmentation, telangiectasia) are common though rarely cause serious problems. After radiotherapy, the upper vagina usually becomes stenosed and dry. Sexual intercourse is certainly possible but additional lubrication is often required. Conversely, radical surgery leads to a short but normally lubricated vagina. The frequency of radiation sequelae is dependent on dose and technique.

Radiation damage occurs even in the most experienced hands since malignant tumours are only marginally more sensitive to radiation than normal tissues and radiation dosage is therefore limited by the tolerance of surrounding normal tissues such as bladder, bowel, kidneys and skin (see Chapter 5). Fortunately, with increasingly sophisticated planning and treatment techniques, severe complications such as fistulae and bowel necrosis are now seen far less frequently than in the past.

• Delineation of GTV and high risk CTV so that D90 and D100 can be calculated, moving away from Point A prescription.

• Eventually aiming to use interstitial needles to treat GTV more conformally

• Bladder and rectum outlining to calculate D2cc {minimum dose to the most irradiated 2 cm³}

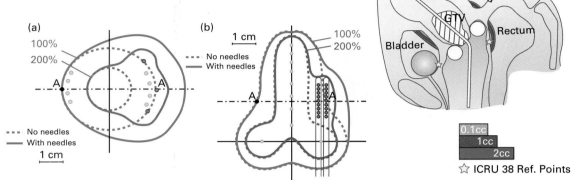

Figure 17.9 (a and b) GEC-ESTRO recommendations. Source: Pötter *et al.* [35]. Reproduced by permission of Elsevier.

In recent years, the widespread use of concurrent chemoradiation for locally advanced cancers of the cervix has dramatically improved the prognosis [32–34]. The most widely used schedule in the UK involves weekly cisplatin, which is well tolerated in modest dosage by most patients, as outpatient therapy. Several randomized studies have now been performed. The advantages are clear-cut, despite an acceptable increase in short-term toxicity.

Although the practice in the UK is to prefer either radical surgery alone (in good-risk or even selected intermediate-risk patients) or radical non-surgical treatment in more advanced cases, surgery combined with postoperative radiotherapy is often employed elsewhere. For example, in the USA-based GOG 92 study, the role of postoperative radiotherapy was investigated in patients with at least two of the following risk factors: greater than one-third stromal invasion, lymphovascular space invasion, or large tumour diameter beyond 4 cm [36]. In these circumstances, the benefits of adjuvant radiotherapy were clear: a 46% reduction in recurrence risk, both local and distal, particularly for patients with adenocarcinomas and adenosquamous carcinomas. The use of chemoradiation in these circumstances is probably even more effective, with an improvement in survival for the combination arm (cisplatin/5-fluorouracil) of 81% at 4 years, compared with 71% for radiotherapy alone [37].

The survival advantage was particularly impressive for patients who were node-positive.

Treatment of recurrent disease

In patients with recurrent post-irradiation local disease, without evidence of distant metastases, pelvic exenteration represents the only chance of cure. This is a major operation, with complete removal of the pelvic contents usually including the rectum and bladder, and with a permanent colostomy and ileostomy. Few surgeons are prepared to undertake this formidable procedure, and very careful selection of patients is essential.

Chemotherapy

The most important use of chemotherapy is clearly in conjunction with radiation for primary treatment. Several agents have now been identified with significant response rates. For treatment of recurrent disease, multiagent regimens are preferred since the response rates are clearly higher, for example, the combination of bleomycin, ifosfamide and cisplatin has a response rate of over 70% in previously untreated patients with advanced disease [38]. Many patients do at least enjoy a subjective improvement, often including substantial and worthwhile relief of pain. In an important recent study of over 450 patients from the Gynecologic Oncology Group (study GOG 240), patients with recurrent disease undergoing treatment with chemotherapy (combinations of cisplatin/paclitaxel or topotecan/paclitaxel) were randomized to receive three-weekly bevacizumab (see Ref. [39]). The overall survival time was increased from 13.3 to 17 mths – hazard ratio (HR) for death 0.71, with corresponding improvement in the progression-free survival – a result likely lead to a change in practice.

An additional important role for chemotherapy relates to its use in small-cell carcinoma of the cervix, which accounts for about 3% of all cervical cancers. This poor-prognosis tumour is characterized by early haematogenous spread, and is probably best treated by concurrent chemoirradiation, without surgery [40]. Reliable reports of treatment and outcome are few in number, but treatment principles are similar to those for small-cell carcinoma of the bronchus. Some authorities have even advocated the use of prophylactic cranial irradiation, based on experience with the far more common lung primary.

Prognosis

In the developed world, there has been a continuous fall in the overall death rate from carcinoma of the cervix during the past 40 years, partly due to the 100% curability of CIN III which, in recent years, has been diagnosed more frequently as a result of routine cervical smear testing. For *invasive* carcinoma there has also been a real improvement in overall survival over the same time period, particularly in older women, in the period 1950–2000. Current age-specific mortality is shown in Fig 17.10.

The 5-year survival rates reflect the final outcome in the majority of patients, since most will recur before 5 years or not at all. Tumour stage is the most important prognostic factor, and patients with stage I disease have a 5-year survival rate of 80–90%; the 10–20% who fail are probably those who have occult abdominal nodal disease. For patients with stage III disease, the 5-year survival rates are around 25% and stage IV disease has a particularly bad prognosis.

Cancer of the cervix and pregnancy

Diagnosis of cancer of the cervix complicates 1 in 2500 pregnancies. Moreover, in about 1% of cases of cervical cancer, the diagnosis is made during pregnancy, and this proportion will rise as the mean age of diagnosis of cervical cancer falls. Management depends on the stage of disease at diagnosis, and also the stage of the pregnancy and the mother's wishes regarding termination.

If carcinoma *in situ* is diagnosed in a young woman, it is usually safe to allow the pregnancy to continue, though regular cervical smears and colposcopy should

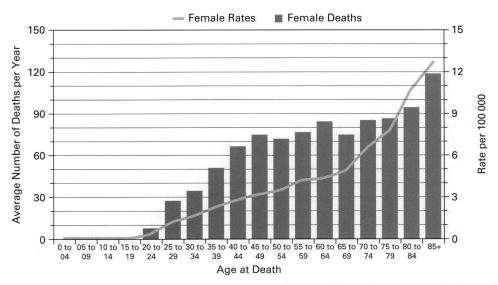

Figure 17.10 (a) Cervical cancer average number of deaths per year and age-specific mortality rates per 100 000 population, UK (2009–2011). (b) Cervical cancer; average number of deaths per year and age-specific mortality rates, UK, 2009–2011. Source: http://www.cancerresearchuk.org/cancer-info/cancerstats/types/cervix/mortality/#age accessed March 2014. © 2014 Cancer Research UK, Reproduced with permission.

be undertaken throughout the pregnancy. In older women, early surgical treatment (cone biopsy) has in the past been considered advisable though there is a 20% complication rate, particularly from haemorrhage. It is no longer considered necessary, as long as regular colposcopy is undertaken.

For invasive carcinoma, treatment during the first and second trimester should generally be undertaken without regard to the fetus, providing the patient is prepared to accept termination. Pelvic irradiation causes fetal death and inevitable abortion within 6 weeks. Following evacuation of the uterus, intracavitary treatment can be undertaken in the usual way. If the diagnosis is made in the final trimester, treatment can safely be delayed, with elective caesarean section before the 38th week. Treatment is by surgery (sometimes performed at the time of caesarean section) or by irradiation following healing of the surgical wound. Unfortunately, delayed treatment cannot always be recommended in the third trimester, for example, where severe haemorrhage presents a real threat to the mother's health. Provided that diagnosis and treatment are prompt, the results are as good as those obtained in non-pregnant patients.

Carcinoma of the uterus

Aetiology

Endometrial carcinoma is commonest among women aged 50–70, with a mean age at diagnosis of 63 years. Its incidence has risen slightly in the past 20 years, although the reasons are not entirely clear (see below). There are wide variations in incidence (Table 17.2), and it is common in Jewish women. The death rate is low since this is a relatively slow-growing and well-localized malignancy. Obesity, hypertension and diabetes have long been considered to be risk factors and are directly or indirectly associated with excess oestrogen exposure. It seems likely that there is peripheral conversion of oestrogen precursors in fat, which may account at least for the role of obesity. Diabetes and hypertension appear to be risk factors only by virtue of their association with obesity. A widely discussed aetiological factor is the presence of endometrial hyperplasia, particularly in relation to oestrogenic hormone replacement therapy (HRT) at the menopause, which frequently produces such change. Of the two major types of hyperplasia, cystic glandular hyperplasia has a low rate of progression, while in the other type, atypical adenomatous hyperplasia, at least 10% of patients progress to develop endometrial

Table 17.2 World age-standardized incidence and mortality rates of corpus uteri cancer, selected regions, 2008 estimates.

World Region	Incidence Rate	Mortality Rate
Northern America	16.4	2.4
Central and Eastern Europe	14.6	3.4
Northern Europe	13.8	2.2
Australia/New Zealand	11.5	1.6
Western Europe	11.2	1.8
Southern Europe	10.4	1.9
Caribbean	10.3	2.2
Southern Africa	9	3.3
Central America	6.1	2.5
South-Eastern Asia	5.7	2
Western Asia	5.6	1.5
South America	4.4	1.7
Eastern Africa	2.4	0.8
Northern Africa	2.2	0.7
South-Central Asia	2.1	1.1
Middle Africa	1.9	0.7
Western Africa	1.9	0.7

Data from Cancer Research UK; http://www.cancer-researchuk.org/cancer-info/cancerstats/types/uterus/ accessed February 2014.

carcinoma, higher still in some studies. Late menopause is a risk factor because of excess and prolonged oestrogen exposure and also the frequency of late anovulatory (oestrogenic) cycles and the presence of metropathia.

A number of studies have suggested an increased incidence (up to five-fold) of carcinoma of the endometrium in patients taking exogenous oestrogens. However, there are a number of criticisms, including the frequency with which control cases and patients taking oestrogen were examined, as well as the possibility that hyperplasia can be difficult to distinguish from frank malignancy, even by experienced pathologists. Unopposed continuous oestrogen replacement is more dangerous in this respect than cyclical oestrogen used in conjunction with a progestogen. Low-dose oestrogen probably carries little risk. In a recent large questionnaire study of over 700 000 postmenopausal British women, there appeared to be a benefit from continuous combined HRT [41], although the incidence of uterine cancer was not significantly reduced in women taking cyclic combined HRT (i.e. with progesterone added to oestrogen only on some days of the month). The potential importance of HRT remains somewhat confusing, particularly bearing in mind that the incidence of breast cancer also varies according to the regimen of HRT used, with breast cancer far more common than endometrial carcinoma, therefore dominating the overall risk of malignancy. Tamoxifen is clearly associated with a small additional risk of endometrial carcinoma [42] (see Chapter 13), whereas progesterone, the major component of most contemporary oral contraceptive agents, generally confers a protective effect against the development of endometrial cancer, persisting at least a decade beyond regular use.

Finally, uterine carcinoma is the commonest non-colonic type of malignancy in female patients with hereditary nonpolyposis colorectal cancer (Lynch syndrome II), these patients also having a high incidence of breast and ovarian cancer. The lifetime risk for these patients is approximately 40–60% for endometrial cancer and about 10–12% for ovarian cancer. A recent large-scale study has strongly suggested that prophylactic gynaecological surgery is beneficial in this group [43]. Of 315 women with documented germline mutations, those undergoing prophylactic hysterectomy (with or without bilateral salpingo-oophorectomy) had zero incidence of both endometrial and ovarian cancer, compared with 69 women in the control group developing endometrial carcinoma and a further 12 patients with ovarian cancer, a remarkable 'prevented fraction' of 100% with an average follow-up period over 11 years. This form of prophylactic surgery is likely to become a standard recommendation for women with Lynch syndrome II, particularly after they have completed their families.

A recent study from China has suggested that regular consumption of soya foods appears to be inversely associated with the risk of endometrial cancer, particularly in women with high body mass index, i.e. the typical bodily morphology of patients with this type of gynaecological cancer [44].

Pathology and staging

By far the commonest of tumours of the body of the uterus is endometrial adenocarcinoma, which constitutes 95% of all endometrial neoplasms. The next largest group is adenoacanthoma, an adenocarcinoma with areas of benign squamous metaplasia. Mixed mesodermal tumours also occur, as well as adenosquamous carcinoma and a variety of soft-tissue sarcomas (chiefly leiomyosarcoma), arising from the muscle wall. Malignant mixed Mullerian tumours, initially classified as sarcomas and often also termed carcinosarcoma, (the descriptive title most in use with important co-operative study groups such as the US-based GOG), have been re-classified by

WHO as a variety of endometrial carcinoma since these tumours have genetic alterations common to both the epithelial and mesenchymal components which characterize this histologically 'biphasic' type of gynaecological malignancy. These include a high frequency of TP53 mutations, amplification of *HER2* and *KRAS* mutations, and a variety of other chromosomal aberrations. The carcinomatous component is almost invariably of high grade (see below) and there is no transition between the epithelial and mesenchymal components.

For the common type of endometrial adenocarcinoma, three grades or histological differentiations are recognized. The commonest group is the well-differentiated (grade I) adenocarcinoma. Lymphatic spread is chiefly to pelvic nodes, particularly the external and common iliac groups (and thence to the para-aortic nodes), as well as the paracervical and obturator nodes. Lymph node 'skipping' (i.e. with metastatic involvement of para-aortic nodes bypassing the pelvic node groups) is well described. Inguinal node metastases are also encountered. Both tumour grade and depth of myometrial invasion are predictors for nodal involvement (Table 17.3), and it seems clear that local nodal metastases are almost as common in endometrial carcinoma as in cancer of the cervix [45].

Because the histological grade, depth of invasion, nodal involvement and likelihood of local recurrence are interrelated variables, it is difficult to assess the separate contributions to prognosis. Histological grade does not form part of the current staging notation (Table 17.4). Myometrial invasion is important since its depth correlates closely with the incidence of recurrence. Patients whose tumour shows only superficial invasion have a local recurrence rate of well below 10%, whereas with deep invasion the recurrence rate is approximately 25%. Direct spread to the cervix and vagina also occurs, though vaginal 'satellite' metastases (i.e. not as part of direct extension) are unusual at presentation. They are commoner in patients with recurrent disease, and occur predominantly in those who have not been treated with radiotherapy. Local spread to other pelvic structures such as the broad ligament, fallopian tubes and ovaries also occurs.

Blood-borne metastases are unusual, though more common than with carcinoma of the cervix. Peritoneal involvement, pulmonary deposits and even ascites are features of advanced disease. Late metastases to para-aortic nodes, lung, bone and supraclavicular nodes are increasingly encountered with greater survival time.

Routes of spread and current staging systems are summarized in Figure 17.11 and Table 17.5. The FIGO staging system developed from a clinical to a surgical/

Table 17.3 Tumour grade, depth of myometrial invasion, and pelvic or para-aortic nodal metastasis in patients with uterine cancer.*

Depth of invasion	Number (%) with pelvic nodal metastasis			Number (%) with para-aortic nodal metastasis		
	Grade 1 ($N = 180$)	Grade 2 ($N = 288$)	Grade 3 ($N = 153$)	Grade 1 ($N = 180$)	Grade 2 ($N = 288$)	Grade 3 ($N = 153$)
Endometrium only ($N = 86$)	0	1 (3)	0	0	1 (3)	0
Inner ($N = 281$)	3 (3)	7 (5)	5 (9)	1 (1)	5 (4)	2 (4)
Middle ($N = 115$)	0	6 (9)	1 (4)	1 (5)	0	0
Deep ($N = 139$)	2 (11)	11 (19)	22 (34)	1 (6)	8 (14)	15 (23)

*Percentages represent the proportion of women who had metastases in each subgroup defined by both tumour grade and depth of invasion.
Data from Creasman *et al.* [45].

Table 17.4 The 1988/1997 system for surgical staging of carcinoma of the uterus.

Stage	Description
IA	Tumour limited to endometrium
IB	Invasion of less than half the myometrium
IC	Invasion of more than half the myometrium
IIA	Endocervical glandular involvement only
IIB	Cervical stromal invasion
IIIA	Tumour invading serosa or adnexa, or malignant peritoneal cytology
IIIB	Vaginal metastasis
IIIC	Metastasis to pelvic or para-aortic lymph nodes
IVA	Tumour invasion of the bladder or bowel mucosa
IVB	Distant metastasis including intra-abdominal or inguinal lymph nodes

Data from American Joint Committee on Cancer (AJCC). *AJCC Cancer Staging Manual*, 5th edn.

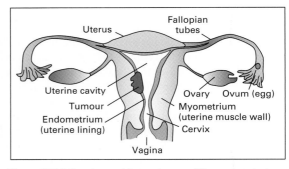

Figure 17.11 Local spread in carcinoma of the corpus uteri.

adenocarcinomas [46]. Several prognostic factors have been identified, including a high mitotic count, advanced stage at presentation, high tumour grade and presence of lymphovascular space invasion. These tumours and their management are discussed more fully in Chapter 23, pages 422–429.

Clinical features and treatment

Postmenopausal bleeding is the cardinal symptom and is an indication for dilatation and curettage even if the bleeding is mild; 20% of cases occur in perimenopausal patients, so intermenstrual bleeding is also important. About 5% of all cases occur in patients below the age of 40. Other symptoms such as pain and vaginal discharge are uncommon and suggestive of more advanced disease. The uterus may be enlarged clinically and these patients should be investigated with particular urgency. The diagnosis is established by curettage, the differential diagnosis

pathological (including cytological) assessment, formalized in 1988 and subsequently refined. The large majority of patients with endometrial carcinoma have localized disease, potentially curable by surgery. The commonest clinical stage at presentation is Ia or Ib. Surgical staging at laparotomy is particularly important, often dictating which patients require additional treatment, using information that cannot be determined preoperatively.

Uterine sarcomas, though far less common than adenocarcinoma, are a histologically variable group of tumours, far more difficult to cure than endometrial

Table 17.5 FIGO staging system in carcinoma of the ovary.

Stage I

The cancer is still contained within the ovary (or ovaries)

Stage IA (T1aN0M0): cancer has developed in one ovary, and the tumour is confined to the inside of the ovary. There is no cancer on the outer surface of the ovary. Laboratory examination of washings from the abdomen and pelvis did not find any cancer cells.

Stage IB (T1bN0M0): cancer has developed within both ovaries without any tumour on their outer surfaces. Laboratory examination of washings from the abdomen and pelvis did not find any cancer cells.

Stage IC (T1cN0M0): the cancer is present in one or both ovaries and one or more of the following are present:
• Cancer on the outer surface of at least one of the ovaries
• In the case of cystic tumours (fluid-filled tumours), the capsule (outer wall of the tumour) has ruptured (burst)
• Laboratory examination found cancer cells in fluid or washings from the abdomen

Stage II

The cancer is in one or both ovaries and has involved other organs (such as uterus, fallopian tubes, bladder, sigmoid colon, or rectum) within the pelvis.

Stage IIA (T2aN0M0): the cancer has spread to or has actually invaded (grown into) the uterus or the fallopian tubes, or both. Laboratory examination of washings from the abdomen did not find any cancer cells.

Stage IIB (T2bN0M0): the cancer has spread to other nearby pelvic organs such as the bladder, sigmoid colon, or rectum. Laboratory examination of fluid from the abdomen did not find any cancer cells.

Stage IIC (T2cN0M0): the cancer has spread to pelvic organs as in stages IIA or IIB and laboratory examination of the washings from the abdomen found evidence of cancer cells.

Stage III

The cancer involves one or both ovaries, and one or both of the following are present: (1) cancer has spread beyond the pelvis to the lining of the abdomen; (2) cancer has spread to lymph nodes

Stage IIIA (T3aN0M0): during the staging operation, the surgeon can see cancer involving the ovary or ovaries, but no cancer is grossly visible (can be seen without using a microscope) in the abdomen and the cancer has not spread to lymph nodes. However, when biopsies are checked under a microscope, tiny deposits of cancer are found in the lining of the upper abdomen.

Stage IIIB (T3bN0M0): there is cancer in one or both ovaries, and deposits of cancer large enough for the surgeon to see, but smaller than 2 cm across, are present in the abdomen. Cancer has not spread to the lymph nodes.

Stage IIIC: the cancer is in one or both ovaries, and one or both of the following are present:
• Cancer has spread to lymph nodes (any T, N1, M0)
• Deposits of cancer larger than 2 cm across are seen in the abdomen (T3cN0M0)

Stage IV (any T, any N, M1) (metastases to distant sites including hepatic parenchymal disease)

This is the most advanced stage of ovarian cancer. In this stage the cancer has spread to the inside of the liver, the lungs, or other organs located outside the peritoneal cavity. (The peritoneal cavity, or abdominal cavity, is the area enclosed by the peritoneum, a membrane that lines the inner abdomen and covers most of its organs.) Finding ovarian cancer cells in the fluid around the lungs (called pleural fluid) is also evidence of stage IV disease.

Recurrent ovarian cancer

This means that the disease has come back (recurred) after completion of treatment

Source: http://www.cancer.org/acs/groups/cid/documents/webcontent/003130-pdf.pdf, accessed February 2014. © American Cancer Society, Inc.

including postmenopausal bleeding from other causes, of which the most common is probably atrophic vaginitis.

Surgery is the most important treatment for endometrial carcinoma [1]. Total abdominal hysterectomy with bilateral salpingo-oophorectomy is the operation of choice. Because of the success of surgical treatment in localized cancers, the role of radiotherapy as a routine additional treatment has been questioned [47]. There seems little need for irradiation for localized well-differentiated tumours without evidence of myometrial invasion. Conversely, where the histology is poorly differentiated or anaplastic, radiation is often offered because of the risk of local recurrence, particularly with evidence of myometrial invasion beyond one-third of the thickness of the uterine wall. With myometrial penetration, or involvement of the cervix, the risk of node metastases is also high, at least 30% in a high-grade tumour. A very large recent US-based retrospective survey of the use of postoperative radiotherapy for early-stage disease has supported the role of radiotherapy for stage IC tumours, i.e. those with significant myometrial invasion [48].

Additional radiotherapy treatment can be either preoperative, usually by means of intrauterine radioactive caesium insertion, or by external beam irradiation to the true pelvis. Preoperative intracavitary irradiation reduces the volume of tumour and also reduces the probability of subsequent vaginal metastases. However, preoperative treatment may be technically difficult because of enlargement of the uterus and/or widespread intrauterine involvement by the tumour. It may be necessary to pack the uterus with several irradiating sources, rather than relying on the arrangement usually employed for carcinoma of the cervix. Our own practice is to recommend postoperative external irradiation in selected cases with adverse risk factors (see above). In most patients, a dose of 45–50 Gy in daily fractions over 4.5–5.5 weeks is well tolerated and effective. In patients with stage I disease it seems likely that long-term pelvic control can be achieved as effectively by external beam irradiation as by vaginal brachytherapy [49].

In patients with recurrent disease, the use of further irradiation, endocrine therapy with progestogens, or chemotherapy can all be worthwhile. Vaginal recurrences, usually seen in previously unirradiated patients, respond to local therapy with intravaginal caesium, although some oncologists prefer interstitial radiotherapy (usually with ^{192}Ir). The most valuable form of systemic therapy is progestogen treatment, particularly valuable for patients with distant metastatic disease. About one-third of patients have an objective response, often remarkably durable. Conversely, progestogen as an adjuvant to surgery has not been shown to prolong survival. The most popular drug is medroxyprogesterone acetate, given by mouth in doses of the order of 100 mg three times daily. Pulmonary metastases seem particularly likely to respond.

In patients who fail to respond to progestogen therapy, chemotherapy has sometimes been of value. The most useful agents appear to be taxanes, 5-fluorouracil (5-FU), cyclophosphamide, doxorubicin and cisplatin or carboplatin. Combination chemotherapy produces more responses than treatment with single agents, but at the cost of increased toxicity. There is no place for chemotherapy in the routine treatment of early endometrial carcinoma [50].

For further discussion of uterine sarcomas and their management, see Chapter 23.

Prognosis

The age-adjusted death rate is 1.4 per 100 000, far below the incidence rate. About two-thirds of patients are cured by surgery (or occasionally radiotherapy in inoperable cases). Survival rates fall with extrauterine spread, poorly differentiated (high-grade) tumours and deep myometrial invasion. Taking together the large series of patients treated with preoperative radiotherapy and surgery, the 5-year survival rate is over 75%. Indeed, the results of radiotherapy alone have often surprised those who feel surgery to be essential. In Kottmeier's classic series of almost 1500 patients treated by radiation in Stockholm, the 5-year survival was 63%. The survival of 'operable lesions' (809 patients) was 79%, comparable to or better than many of the surgical series. These reports have been updated by Einhorn [51].

The relatively favourable prognosis of endometrial carcinoma is largely due to the preponderance of localized disease, itself probably a reflection of the slow-growing nature of the tumour and the early concern aroused by its major symptom, postmenopausal bleeding.

The increasing incidence of adenosquamous carcinomas is worrying since this group of tumours has a poor prognosis. The 5-year survival rate is less than 20%, compared with over 70% for well-differentiated adenocarcinomas and adenoacanthomas. Patients with sarcomas of the uterus also do far less well, with reported 5-year survival rates of 15–32%. If leiomyosarcoma is discovered as an incidental finding following removal of a uterine fibroid, the survival rate is over 80%, whereas in patients with invasive leiomyosarcomas survival is very poor indeed.

Carcinoma of the ovary

Little is known of the aetiology of this disease, the sixth commonest female cancer worldwide, and slightly commoner – fifth position – in most parts of the Western world. It is more prevalent in women carrying both the BRCA1 and BRCA2 genes; these patients appear to have a 16–40% lifetime risk of developing it [52]. Women of Ashkenazi Jewish heritage, regardless of their BRCA1 or BRCA2 carrier status, also appear to be at increased risk.

It is also unequivocally more common in nulliparous and subfertile women. An increasing number of pregnancies seem to be protective, and recent large-scale epidemiological studies have strongly suggested that use of the oral contraceptive pill also confers long-term protection against ovarian cancer [53]. There are wide demographic differences in mortality, for example, the rate in Denmark is six times as great as in Japan. There is both a familial incidence and an apparent link with breast cancer, perhaps related to nulliparity and *BRCA1*. Early menopause seems to reduce the risk, raising the possibility – as seems convincingly the case with most breast cancers – that oestrogen exposure is a likely risk factor. This suggestion is further supported by the recent confirmation of an increased incidence of breast cancer in the Million Women Study [54], which clearly demonstrated a higher risk of ovarian carcinoma in women taking HRT. This was a large cohort study, following women who enrolled during 1996–2001, about half of whom were taking (or had taken in the past) some form of HRT. Although the absolute additional risk was small, the authors concluded that in the UK, since the planning and inception of the study in 1991, there had been an extra 1300 cases of ovarian cancer due to HRT and about 1000 additional deaths. Obesity is also emerging as an independent risk factor, with 24 of 28 recent studies reporting a positive association [55]. Use of talc, especially around the genital area, has also been found in a number of case-control studies to be a possible significant aetiological factor. In addition there is a 10% risk of ovarian tumours in patients with Peutz–Jeghers syndrome.

Ovarian cancer has become the commonest pelvic malignancy in many Western countries, and is the fourth commonest female cancer in the UK, with a crude yearly rate of 17.5 per 100 000. In 2003 in the USA, almost 20 000 patients were diagnosed with this disease, with over 14 600 deaths. The figure appears to be rising, with 21 550 women expected to be diagnosed in the USA during 2009 (data from the National Cancer Institute, www.cancer.gov). In the UK, there are about 7000 new cases annually (mostly presenting with advanced disease), and some 4600 deaths. In these, the overall 5-year survival rate is below 15%, despite many advances in management techniques (see below). As recently pointed out by Kemp and Ledermann (see Ref. [56]), the survival figures for ovarian cancer are the poorest among all of the gynecological cancers, though the overall results of treatment appear to have improved over the past decade, with recent statistics from the UK, for example, of 3820 deaths from this disease in 2001 falling to 3453 in 2010,

a reduction of about 20% (11.2 per 100 000 women to 8.8 per 100 000) – see the important report from the UK National Cancer Intelligence Network [57]. In Europe, for example, there are an estimated 65 697 new cases and 41 448 deaths each year. Only a minority of women (approximately 15%) present with disease confined to the ovaries, and following surgery their 5-year survival is more than 90%. For those presenting with advanced disease (FIGO stage III–IV), the prognosis is far worse, with the probability of surviving 5 years being less than 30%. Early diagnosis of ovarian cancer is therefore highly desirable but confounded by the lack of clearly defined symptoms. Trials have been undertaken to assess the efficacy of screening asymptomatic women with annual CA 125 and transvaginal ultrasound but, to date, these have failed to demonstrate a reduction in mortality though the ongoing UK Collaborative Trial of Ovarian Cancer Screening will report in the next 2 years. In the 80% of women in whom the diagnosis is made at a late stage, the 5-year survival rate falls to about 30% [52,58]. With an *overall* 5-year survival rate of about 55%, it is now the most lethal gynaecological cancer worldwide. Factors that reduce the risk of developing ovarian cancer include the oral contraceptive pill (odds ratio about 0.7, with increasing protection with extended use beyond 3 years), pregnancy and lactation.

Because of the relative frequency and lethality of this disease, particularly the advanced stages, screening programmes are currently under active trial [59,60]. The largest study of 22 000 women used CA-125 and ultrasound detection techniques, and detected 11 ovarian cancers of which four were stage I, but no advantage has yet been seen in overall survival. Several other studies are now in progress, both in the UK and USA [61], and Lu and colleagues from Houston, Texas have recently reported on an important though relatively small study of over 4000 post-menopausal women followed over an 11-year period (see Ref. [62]). They used a 2-step screening approach: initial CA-125 estimation annually, but followed by a 3-month repeat for intermediate-risk cases (which turned out to be necessary in 5.8% of cases per year) or immediate referral for transvaginal ultrasound and an expert clinical opinion (average annual rate of referral 0.9%) in the high-risk woman – based on the level of CA-125. On this basis, 10 women underwent exploratory surgery, and four invasive cancers were detected (1 with stage IA disease, 2 with stage IC disease, and 1 with stage IIB disease), plus two ovarian tumours of low malignant potential (both stage IA), one endometrial cancer (stage I), and three benign ovarian tumours, providing a positive predictive value of 40% for detecting invasive ovarian cancer and with an impressive specificity of 99.9%. All four women with invasive ovarian cancer had been enrolled in the study for at least 3 years, with low-risk annual CA125 test values prior to rising CA125 levels. Clearly, it is still not yet fully understood how best to use the known risk factors for ovarian cancer as part of a screening strategy. With respect to CA-125, by far the most widely used tumour marker at present, the definition of an abnormal value varies with menopausal status, and a raised level is far from diagnostic since it can be elevated in other conditions including fibroids, endometriosis, pregnancy, cardiac disorders and even appendicitis. Nonetheless, there may now finally be cautious grounds for optimism since the tumour appears to be becoming more common, is potentially curable when identified early, but despite modern expert and aggressive treatment, so frequently fatal when diagnosed in its advanced stages. The results of the large UK-based UKCTOCS study of 300 000 women, due to be reported in 2015, are awaited with great interest.

Clinical features

These tumours usually present late and only one-third are localized at the time of diagnosis. Early ovarian cancer is often asymptomatic. When symptoms occur they are often vague and are overlooked by patients, even when the tumour is locally advanced and abdominal distension has become obvious. Lower abdominal pain, bloating and anorexia are common, but often insufficient to raise suspicion. A recent statement from major gynaecological organizations in the USA (including the Gynecologic Cancer Foundation, the Society of Gynecologic Oncologists and the American Cancer Society) stressed that symptoms such as abdominal bloating, pelvic or abdominal pain and difficulty eating or early satiety must be taken more seriously [63]. Signs such as ascites or palpable pelvic masses often indicate advanced disease. Even with more widespread use of cervical smear tests and annual examination, the proportion of early diagnoses has not risen. There is no evidence that routine screening uncovers a significant number of women with early disease. Possibilities for the future include pelvic ultrasound, which is rapidly improving its resolving power; transvaginal aspiration with cytology of washings; and the increasing use of CA-125, a moderately specific tumour antigen detected by a simple blood test and with a semi-quantitative relationship with tumour response. So far, the rate of diagnosis in asymptomatic women is low, but screening may prove valuable in the future, particularly perhaps if these tests are used in combination.

Pathology, staging and prognosis

There is great histological variety and the World Health Organization lists 27 subtypes. About 90% of ovarian carcinomas originate from the epithelial surface of the ovary, the remainder comprising the much less common group of germ-cell tumours (both teratomas and dysgerminomas), ovarian sarcomas, granulosa cell tumours, thecomas, and Leydig and Sertoli cell tumours. Most epithelial ovarian carcinomas stain for CA-125 and some also, curiously, for WT-1, a Wilms' tumour-derived antigen, which interestingly is also positive in many cases of mesothelioma, the other human cancer, apart from ovarian cancer, which so characteristically spreads across tissue planes and surfaces. Carcinosarcomas (also termed malignant mixed Müllerian tumours or sarcomatoid carcinomas) are an important small group (up to 4% of all ovarian tumours), and are generally regarded as being aggressive in their clinical behaviour – worse, stage for stage, than the more common types of epithelial cancer.

Of the epithelial carcinomas, the major types include serous cystadenocarcinoma, mucinous, endometrioid, clear-cell (mesonephroid) and undifferentiated adenocarcinomas. The tumour grade, or degree of differentiation, is of great prognostic importance [64], at least in serous tumours, in which the grade can vary from barely malignant to highly undifferentiated invasive tumours. Ovarian tumours of low malignant potential form a special group where it may be possible to preserve fertility by undertaking conservative surgical resection [65]. No adjuvant therapy has been shown to prolong survival in this important population of patients, reported to comprise 4–14% of all ovarian neoplasms. In general, tumours which are relatively well differentiated are more likely to be operable. Mucinous tumours appear to be associated with improved survival. Recent work from the Ovarian Tumour Tissue Analysis consortium study has suggested a benefit for certain sub-groups of patients with tumours expressing positivity for hormonal immunophenotype markers – oestrogen – and progesterone receptors (see Ref. [66]). They studied a large panel of cases – 2933 patients. Those with endometrioid carcinoma had improved disease-specific survival if the tumour carried ER-positive or PR-positive markers; those with high-grade serous carcinoma had improved prognosis if the tumour carried PR-positivity. No other significant associations were noted, and the authors felt that this intriguing result should lead to better

Table 17.6 Relationship between FIGO stage and prognosis in carcinoma of the ovary.

Stage	Relative 5-year survival rate (%)
Ia	92.7
Ib	85.4
Ic	84.7
IIa	78.6
IIb	72.4
IIc	64.4
IIIa	50.8
IIIb	42.4
IIIc	31.5
IV	17.5

By comparison with Tobias & Griffiths [58], these results have improved.
Source: Data from American Cancer Society, Inc.

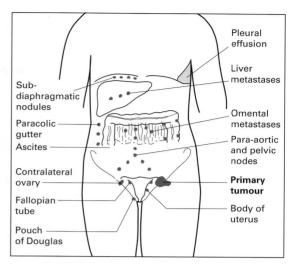

Figure 17.12 Common sites of metastasis in carcinoma of the ovary.

stratification of cases in randomized trials, in order to pursue the goal of a more personalized approach to treatment for ovarian cancer.

Clinicopathological staging is of the greatest importance and remains the most important indicator of prognosis [58,67]. The FIGO staging system is widely accepted (Table 17.5), and Table 17.6 shows the relation between stage and prognosis. Patients with disease localized to the ovaries have an overall survival rate of 60%. However, even within this group, further risk factors have been identified. For example, intracystic tumours have a 5-year survival rate of almost 100%, whereas in those with adherence of the tumour to surrounding structures, the 5-year survival is reduced by half. When the disease has spread outside the ovary but still confined to the pelvis, there is an important distinction between tumours with minimal local spread to adjacent gynaecological organs (stage IIa, carrying a 5-year survival rate almost as good as stage I tumours) and those which have spread more widely (stage IIb), which carry a very much poorer prognosis.

Once the tumour has disseminated into the peritoneal cavity, the outlook is very much worse, particularly with bulky abdominal disease. Common sites include the omentum, peritoneal surface (often the site of multiple seedlings) and undersurface of the diaphragm, a particularly important area for inspection at the initial operation (Figure 17.12). Beyond the peritoneal cavity, important sites include liver, lungs and occasionally the central nervous system. Lymph node spread is chiefly

to pelvic and para-aortic nodes, and less commonly to supraclavicular, neck and inguinal nodes. Bone marrow dissemination is extremely unusual.

For women below the age of 65 years, ovarian cancer is a significant cause of death, particularly since the majority present with advanced stages (Table 17.6). Survival has improved little if at all in recent years, with over 4000 deaths per annum in the UK making it the fourth most lethal female cancer (after breast, lung and large bowel) and accounting for 1000 more deaths than all other gynaecological cancers combined. The average 5-year survival is only of the order of 30%; overall, death from ovarian cancer accounts for 6% of all cancer deaths in women. The age-specific mortality increases from 0.8 (per 100 000) at age 25–34 years, 17.7 at 45–54 years to 35.0 at 55–64 years.

Surgical management [58,68–70]

Operative treatment has always been the cornerstone of successful management. The initial operation has a greater bearing on outcome than any subsequent therapy, and the success of postoperative treatment largely depends on careful operative assessment and adequate tumour removal.

Careful inspection of the whole of the abdominal cavity is essential before surgical resection. In particular, the infra-diaphragmatic surfaces and paracolic gutters should be carefully assessed, since these are common but often overlooked sites of spread. Even when subdiaphragmatic seedlings are not visible, peritoneal lavage may reveal malignant cells from this and other sites. A substantial proportion of patients, initially thought to have localized disease, may have evidence of more widespread dissemination, making local treatment inappropriate.

For stage I disease, surgery is often adequate, and consists of total abdominal hysterectomy and bilateral salpingo-oophorectomy. Even with unilateral tumours, the opposite ovary is normally removed as there is a 20% frequency of bilateral tumours or occult metastases. In young women, particularly those anxious to retain one of the ovaries, conservative operations are occasionally performed. In tumours of borderline malignancy, conservative operations can be recommended with greater confidence, though most gynaecologists understandably prefer to perform a full operation unless the patient is particularly anxious to become pregnant.

In patients with more advanced disease (stages II–IV) the consensus of opinion favours excision of as much tumour as possible at the time of initial operation. Good palliation may be achieved by the reduction of a heavy tumour burden but there is little evidence that surgical debulking procedures substantially improve survival unless all or nearly all of the tumour can be excised. Many technically operable tumours are of relatively low grade, which will itself imply a more favourable prognosis. Nevertheless, the size of the largest postoperative residual tumour nodule is a good predictor of responsiveness to subsequent chemotherapy and also of the ultimate outcome [69]. Using a multiple linear regression equation with survival as the end-point, only histological tumour grade and size of the largest postoperative residual mass were factors of real importance; the operation itself contributed nothing, unless it reduced the size of the largest tumour mass to 1.6 cm (or less) in diameter.

Postoperative chemotherapy or radiotherapy in patients with residual palpable masses is extremely unlikely to be curative. For this reason a second operative procedure by an expert surgeon, at least in selected patients, may be needed. Lengthy operations, including removal of pelvic contents, omentectomy, bowel resection and excision of the entire parietal pelvic peritoneum, are now performed more frequently. A large-scale European cooperative study (319 patients prospectively randomized, after initial surgery and chemotherapy, to undergo further debulking or no additional surgery) confirmed the advantages of additional surgery [69]. Both progression-free interval and overall survival were lengthened in patients undergoing postchemotherapy surgical debulking (so-called second-look laparotomy).

Despite the advent of ultrasonography, CT and MRI, there is no reliable guide to the effectiveness of treatment in advanced ovarian cancer short of a further exploratory procedure, so further surgery – even beyond the 'second-look' – is sometimes advocated. Laparotomy is often justifiable in cases where laparoscopic examination has failed to show residual disease and peritoneal washings are clear. It is difficult to demonstrate beyond doubt that second-look laparotomy (sometimes termed 'interval debulking surgery') has contributed to improved survival in ovarian cancer, but important treatment decisions have become more logical as a result. It is now widely accepted that second-look laparotomy has its most clear-cut role when the results of the surgery could reasonably be expected to influence further treatment.

The role of the gynaecological surgeon in the management of ovarian cancer has changed, and continues to evolve. The initial assessment and operative procedure is critically important, for both localized and generalized disease. The surgeon has a crucially important role in evaluation of treatment. Although second-look laparotomy is the most reliable means of judging response, there remains considerable doubt about its true therapeutic value. However, there is no longer any disagreement that ideal management of ovarian carcinoma involves a multidisciplinary team, with well-trained gynaecological surgeons, pathologists, radiologists, medical oncologists and clinical oncologists working together to achieve the best possible result.

Chemotherapy

After surgical excision, chemotherapy is the most important modality of treatment for ovarian cancer. It is essential for patients who present with disease outside the true pelvis (FIGO stages III and IV) and is increasingly offered to selected patients with more limited disease, notably with high-grade tumours, adherence or incomplete resection. Ovarian cancer is moderately sensitive to cytotoxic agents but, for most drugs, information regarding response rates was gained at a time when no attempt was made to reduce tumour bulk before starting treatment. Since massive disease so clearly reduces responsiveness (see Chapter 6), the reported response rates may be lower than those which could be achieved under more favourable conditions. Nowadays response data should be based on careful pre- and post-treatment assessment of tumour size, including suitable imaging techniques and, if appropriate, second-look laparotomy.

Since the 1970s, the standard of care for the management of advanced ovarian cancer has been maximum cytoreductive surgery and platinum-based chemotherapy, with carboplatin combinations replacing cisplatin-based chemotherapy over the last 15 years.

Single-agent chemotherapy is no longer recommended, as treatment with two agents ('doublets') or more clearly offer superior response rates (see below). Cisplatin, carboplatin and paclitaxel are regarded as the most active agents (with 50–70% response rates), but in the past alkylating agents were widely employed, including chlorambucil, cyclophosphamide and melphalan, with response rates of around 40%. However, it is now widely accepted that cisplatin and carboplatin are more effective agents, though cisplatin is even nowadays an agent with considerable toxicity although advances in antiemetic therapy, particularly with 5-hydroxytryptamine (5-HT)$_3$ antagonists such as ondansetron and granisetron, have made it far more acceptable. Carboplatin has similar activity to the parent compound, but reduced toxicity (see Chapter 6). Unfortunately, despite the lesser degree of gastrointestinal toxicity, carboplatin is a more myelosuppressive agent than cisplatin and is less easy to use in combination regimens. Paclitaxel, the first in a group of taxane cytotoxic agents, clearly has considerable activity, even in cisplatin-resistant disease (see below). It is now widely used as first-line treatment, generally in combination with cisplatin or carboplatin (see below for further details) [71,72].

Doxorubicin is frequently used in its pegylated liposomal form (Caelyx). This preparation involves encapsulation of the parent agent in a specifically engineered liposome consisting of a double layer of phospholipid, with an outer layer permitting the liposome to avoid uptake and degradation, thus increasing the half-life of the cytotoxic agent whilst ingeniously decreasing systemic exposure to its many side-effects. It has been directly compared with other agents such as topotecan (a topoisomerase inhibitor) in both platinum-sensitive and platinum-resistant patients, mostly with a favourable outcome [73,74].

Combination chemotherapy

As in other malignancies, there has been an increasing tendency to use combinations of drugs for advanced ovarian cancer. In previously untreated patients, higher response rates have regularly been achieved than with single agents (Table 17.7). Most of these studies have not made any formal comparison with a single agent so that an advantage in *survival* over simple alkylating agent therapy has been difficult to confirm. A large Italian study suggested an improvement with combined use of

Table 17.7 Novel and combination chemotherapy in advanced ovarian cancer.*

Drug	Dose	Response rate (%)
Paclitaxel	135 mg/m² by i.v. infusion over 24 hours every 3 weeks	25[†]
Doxorubicin	40 mg/m² day 1	55
Cyclophosphamide (AC)	500 mg/m² day 1 every 4 weeks	
Hexamethylmelamine	150 mg/m² daily × 14	65
Cyclophosphamide	150 mg/m² daily × 14	
Methotrexate	40 mg/m² day 1, 8	
5-Fluorouracil (Hexa-CAF)	600 mg/m² day 1, 8 every 4 weeks	
Cyclophosphamide	300 mg/m² day 1	75
Doxorubicin	30–40 mg/m² day 1	
Cisplatin (CAP)	50 mg/m² day 1 every 3 weeks	
Paclitaxel	135 mg/m² as 24-hour i.v. infusion	70–75
Cisplatin	75 mg/m² i.v. (rate 1 mg/min) every 3 weeks	
Pegylated doxorubicin	50 mg/m²	
Topotecan	1.5 mg/m² × 5 days	

*Schedules and administration vary widely. Reported response rates also differ and figures are approximate.
[†]In cisplatin-resistant patients.

cyclophosphamide and cisplatin (compared with cisplatin alone), although the addition of a third drug, doxorubicin, was unhelpful. A widely publicized study from the Gynecological Study Group in the USA concluded that cisplatin–paclitaxel is a superior combination to the widely used cisplatin–cyclophosphamide for patients with advanced disease [71]. Nevertheless, overall median survival remained disappointing at 38 months even for the cisplatin–taxane group (compared with 24 months for the remainder). The hope for improvement in survival rate with carboplatin–paclitaxel (probably the two most active agents) has not so far been realized though carboplatin and paclitaxel have become the established standard of care in most centres.

Although the response rate for first-line carboplatin and paclitaxel is 70–80%, with more than 50% achieving complete remission after surgery and chemotherapy, the majority of women with advanced ovarian cancer will subsequently relapse or progress and eventually develop chemotherapy-resistant disease. A number of randomized trials have sought to improve survival by addition of a third agent, but again, no real consensus has emerged. The largest of these studies was GOG 182/ICON-5, an international collaboration which sought to evaluate three drugs with well defined activity – topotecan, gemcitabine, and pegylated liposomal doxorubicin (Bookman *et al.*, [75]). However, at the planned interim analysis in 2004, none of the experimental arms had met the prespecified reduction in progression-free survival compared with the reference arm, and the study was closed.

In future studies of combination chemotherapy, it will be essential to compare newer combinations after 'debulking' surgery has been carried out. Studies which include a majority of patients with a poor prognosis (including those in whom the operation did not result in worthwhile removal of bulk disease) may obscure the potential benefits of intensive chemotherapy in the others. For patients with a poor prognosis, the substantial toxicity of combination chemotherapy may not be justified by the few extra months of life. The current position is that surgical removal of as much of the tumour mass as possible, followed by an effective single agent, usually cisplatin or carboplatin, or a combination regimen including paclitaxel will result in a minority of patients being free of tumour 1–2 years after the initial treatment, as judged by subsequent laparotomy or laparoscopy. The ultimate prognosis of these patients remains to be determined, but there is little doubt that cure is possible, albeit in a disappointingly small proportion. The results of the international ICON-4 trial, which compared a single-agent platinum compound to a platinum-based combination with paclitaxel in platinum-sensitive patients at relapse, have been much discussed [72]. The study reported a HR of 0.76 ($P = 0.0004$) in favour of the combination for progression-free survival, and an HR of 0.82 ($P = 0.023$) in favour of the combination for overall survival. This resulted in a 10% improvement in the 1-year progression-free survival (40% vs 50%), and a 7% improvement in 2-year overall survival (50% vs 57%). However, the combination was associated with significantly greater grade 2–4 neurotoxicity (20% vs 1%). Many gynaecological oncologists feel that the combination offers a better chance for most patients, though the additional toxicities still represent a major drawback, particularly in those with poor performance status. Important work recently published from the large

co-operative Japanese group (85 collaborating centres) has suggested that dose-dense treatment with paclitaxel and carboplatin offers a better overall likelihood of survival than treatment at conventional doses – see Ref. [76]. They studied 637 patients, and with a median follow-up of 77 months noted a considerable survival advantage for this group – 100 months versus 62 months. There is also a possible role, in very selected patients, for hormonal therapy in the management of these patients. Tamoxifen, progestogens, aromatase inhibitors and others have all been employed, probably with an overall response rate of about 5–10%, presumably in patients whose cancers exhibit functional oestrogen and/or progesterone receptors. These agents are chiefly used in patients felt to be too frail for a serious attempt at controlling the disease with chemotherapy.

Treatment of relapsed ovarian cancer remains unsatisfactory, with no long-term cures despite useful and clinically worthwhile responses to chemotherapy, at least in selected patients [73,74]. One relatively well-tolerated cytotoxic regimen is the combination of gemcitabine with carboplatin for patients with advanced pretreated ovarian cancer, a combination now approved by the Food and Drug Administration (FDA) in the USA, despite the absence of a substantial survival advantage. Nonetheless, one recent large intergroup study confirmed a definite improvement in disease-free survival, compared with carboplatin given as a single agent [77]. The main objectives of further treatment are symptom control and, wherever possible, an improvement in quality of life. Further intervention such as additional chemotherapy and debulking surgery needs careful consideration, particularly in patients who have relapsed only a few months beyond the initial first-line chemotherapy. Biological and targeted therapies have also been employed, but with limited success. Current trials are in progress with the vascular endothelial growth factor (VEGF) receptor and epidermal growth factor receptor inhibitors bevacizumab and erlotinib, used together with carboplatin–paclitaxel combinations. In the large-scale prospectively randomized ICON-6 study, the proposal is to use the novel targeted agent cediranib (also known as AZD2171) for patients with recurrent disease. This is a once daily, orally available, highly potent and selective VEGF signalling inhibitor that inhibits all three VEGF receptors. In the international ICON-7 study of over 1500 previously untreated patients from 11 countries, the novel agent under study was bevacizumab (Avastin), in combination with carboplatin–paclitaxel. The overall results showed a small benefit – progression-free survival increasing from 20.3 months to 21.8 months but with additional toxicity, though in patients with high risk of recurrence the benefit was greater – see Ref. [78]. For a review of the current position regarding the use of bevacizumab, also see Ref. [79]. Recent work from a UK-based group has confirmed the benefit of maintenance therapy with olaparib, a novel oral poly(adenosine diphosphate [ADP]-ribose) polymerase inhibitor, in a study investigating 265 patients with platinum-sensitive but relapsed ovarian cancer and demonstrating an improvement in progression-free survival from 4.8 mths to 8.4 mths (see Ref. [80]).

One important recent study assessing the value of intraperitoneal chemotherapy has suggested that, despite many failures in the past, this form of treatment might now have an important role [81]. This was a large multicentre study from the USA, in which 429 patients with stage III ovarian carcinoma, surgically debulked to a residual mass of 1.0 cm or less, received intravenous chemotherapy (paclitaxel–cisplatin or intravenous paclitaxel) with additional cisplatin–paclitaxel given by the intraperitoneal route. Although the latter group had more side-effects, the duration of overall survival was 50 months (intravenous group) versus 66 months (intraperitoneal group), a significant difference. Since escalating doses of intravenous chemotherapy has been largely unsuccessful, the higher local drug concentration achieved by the intraperitoneal route clearly represents an attractive approach, since ovarian cancer generally remains contained within the abdominal cavity, at least for most of its natural history.

Radiotherapy

Radiotherapy has historically been used as definitive therapy, as an adjuvant to surgery, for recurrent disease, and occasionally as preoperative treatment [82]. In the past it was sometimes recommended as postoperative treatment for patients with disease confined to the pelvis. Two main techniques have been used: first, pelvic irradiation (for patients with stage I or II disease) usually to a dose of 40–50 Gy over 4–5.5 weeks, using either anteroposterior or multifield techniques; and second, whole-abdominal irradiation. The latter is technically one of the most difficult techniques in clinical radiotherapy, always difficult to achieve in view of the very large treatment volume. Adequate irradiation, including the subdiaphragmatic areas, results in a treatment volume extending from the pelvic floor to the domes of the diaphragm. The dose rate has to be low (usually 1 Gy daily) for patients to be able to tolerate this treatment without developing severe nausea

and myelosuppression. It is especially difficult to deliver after chemotherapy because of the risk of radiation nephritis and hepatitis. The kidneys and liver are shielded after doses of 15–20 Gy, and the total elsewhere has to be limited to doses of the order of 25 Gy (usually taking about 5 weeks of daily treatment) together with boosting of the pelvis alone to a dose of 40–50 Gy.

In FIGO stage I disease, retrospective studies of surgery alone compared with surgery plus postoperative irradiation have suffered from the usual difficulty that the two study groups may not have been similar enough for valid comparison. In many of these retrospective studies, the group receiving postoperative radiotherapy did less well than the group receiving surgery alone, implying that patients selected for postoperative irradiation were, in general, a higher-risk group, because of cyst rupture at operation or other unspecified features. The 5-year survival rates in patients with stage I disease vary from 50 to 65%, regardless of whether or not radiotherapy is given. Survival figures from prospective studies (surgery alone vs surgery plus local irradiation) are beginning to emerge, though no clear differences have so far been demonstrated.

In stage II disease, it seems possible that there is a genuine benefit from the use of postoperative pelvic irradiation [58,82], although chemotherapy is now much more commonly used and is clearly the treatment of choice. In almost all series, admittedly retrospective, the 5-year survival rate was improved, particularly where adequate surgery had already been undertaken (see pages 314–315). Since these studies were performed before careful operative staging was a routine part of the initial assessment, many of these patients would in fact have had stage III disease. In patients with more advanced disease (stages III–IV) the value of postoperative irradiation is unconvincing. Although postoperative whole-abdominal irradiation has been claimed to produce modest improvement in 5-year survival from about 5 to 10%, this was largely before the era of more effective chemotherapy. In the 1970s, work from Toronto reawakened interest in radiation therapy for ovarian carcinoma. There was a clear survival advantage for patients receiving abdominopelvic irradiation (stages IIa–III), despite the difficulties in achieving more than a low dose of irradiation to such a large area. There seems little doubt that the superior results from this study largely reflected the adequacy of initial surgical treatment, with a highly significant survival difference in favour of patients without palpable postoperative tumour, regardless of whether chemotherapy or radiotherapy was used postoperatively. Clearly, with increased emphasis on surgical debulking at the initial operation and, if necessary, after chemotherapy, the role of pelvic or abdominal irradiation has diminished. Moreover, the incidence of recurrent bowel obstruction appears to be increased by the use of abdominal radiation therapy.

An alternative form of radiotherapy is the use of intraperitoneal radioactive colloids such as gold (^{198}Au) or phosphorus (^{32}P). Originally used for treatment of malignant effusions, this has also largely been replaced by systemic treatment with chemotherapy.

Unresolved controversies in epithelial ovarian cancer

Several important issues in management remain extremely contentious.

1 The contribution (and timing) of debulking surgery to improving response rates to chemotherapy, and to overall survival.

2 The contribution from second-look laparotomy or interval debulking surgery. It seems unlikely that there is a major therapeutic benefit, although it has value as a staging procedure and as an aid to further therapy. In selected cases, where further treatment decisions might depend initially on the presence of microscopic disease, it may be valuable; it may also be justified within the context of prospective clinical trials.

3 Is second-line chemotherapy of real and lasting value in patients who fail to achieve complete remission or who relapse after treatment? What are the most useful agents?

4 In view of GOG (Gynecologic Oncology Group) results [and others] with intraperitoneal chemotherapy, should this be more widely offered?

5 What is the role of promising new therapies with novel chemotherapy, VEGF receptor inhibitors or reactors, intraperitoneal radioimmunotherapy, etc? Are these expensive new therapies ever justifiable outside the context of clinical trials? Which of the many novel agents offers the greatest promise? Does dose-dense therapy really offer a better outcome?

Germ-cell tumours of the ovary

A pathological classification of these unusual tumours is shown in Table 17.8. Benign dermoid cysts are relatively common and cured by surgical excision. Occasionally, they consist largely of thyroid tissue, *struma ovarii*, which may even be functioning. Less than 5% of strumas are malignant, so-called *monomorphic* or *monodermal*

Table 17.8 Germ-cell tumours of the ovary.

Tumour	Percentage of all malignant germ-cell tumours
Benign (20% of all ovarian tumours)	
Dermoid cyst: mature cystic teratoma	
Malignant (3% of all ovarian tumours)	
Dysgerminoma	50
Endodermal sinus tumour or yolk sac tumour	20
Embryonal carcinoma	3
Malignant (immature) teratoma (includes malignant monodermal teratomas and carcinoids)	20
Mixed germ-cell tumours	7
Choriocarcinoma	Rare
Gonadoblastoma	Rare

teratomas. Very rarely they develop secondary malignant change, most commonly squamous carcinoma.

Of the malignant tumours, *dysgerminoma* is much the commonest; histologically it is a uniform clear-cell tumour resembling seminoma in males. Lymphocytic infiltration is common. The endodermal sinus tumour (*yolk sac tumour*) is a highly malignant tumour that produces α-fetoprotein (AFP), demonstrable in the tumour and detectable in the blood. Rupture of the tumour occurs early. *Embryonal carcinoma* consists of glandular and papillary masses, often with trophoblastic elements that secrete human chorionic gonadotrophin (HCG). It may occur in childhood and produce sexual precocity. AFP may also be produced by yolk sac elements. *Immature teratoma* is a mainly solid tumour containing a multiplicity of different tissues. Primitive neuroectoderm often predominates, but monomorphic forms consisting of thyroid tissue or malignant carcinoid also occur. Even when the tumour has not metastasized, carcinoid syndrome may occur because of the large size. The *mixed germ-cell tumour* contains mixtures of the previous histological types. *Gonadoblastoma* is a small tumour arising in childhood, usually composed of several of the elements of the developing gonad. It may calcify, rarely metastasizes, but might cause virilization as it sometimes contains functioning Leydig cells.

Clinical features

In dysgerminoma, as with other malignant ovarian tumours, the presentation is with an abdominal mass and pain, but the mean age is far lower; 75% of patients are between 10 and 30 years old (median 20 years). They do not usually produce marker hormones unless teratomatous elements are present, and they not infrequently present during or shortly after pregnancy. Other germ-cell tumours (yolk sac, endodermal sinus tumours, teratoma, mixed germ-cell tumour) also occur in adolescents and young women. Many of these patients have precocious puberty, menstrual disturbance and a positive pregnancy test (with pregnancy as a differential diagnosis of the pelvic mass!). These tumours usually grow rapidly, causing abdominal pain.

Management

In dysgerminoma, management depends on stage. Of patients with FIGO stage I, 90% are cured by unilateral oophorectomy, but the recurrence rate is higher with large tumours, positive peritoneal washings at operation, or if the tumour contains mixed germ-cell elements. If recurrence occurs or if there are metastases, patients are usually treated with chemotherapy as for teratoma (see below), or by whole-abdominal irradiation. Yolk sac, endodermal sinus and mixed germ-cell tumours have a much worse prognosis with surgical treatment than dysgerminoma, even in stage I disease. The use of serum AFP and β-HCG as markers has greatly improved the monitoring of chemotherapy, which is now an essential part of treatment for most patients (exceptions are discussed below).

The use of platinum-based regimens has followed the outstanding success achieved in testicular teratoma. Since the tumours are unilateral they can be managed by unilateral salpingo-oophorectomy followed by chemotherapy, with the possibility of preservation of fertility. Exceptions to the use of chemotherapy include teratomas, which have low mitotic activity, those with no embryonal or trophoblastic elements and where there are no detectable tumour markers after surgery. Such patients can be treated by surgery alone, but do need careful follow-up. Ovarian choriocarcinoma is usually treated with chemotherapy as for other non-dysgerminomatous ovarian germ-cell tumours. Combinations of cisplatin, etoposide and bleomycin are used, in regimens identical to those used for testicular non-seminomatous germ-cell tumours (see Chapter 19), and with excellent results, the cure rate with current chemotherapy protocols approaching 90% [83].

Ovarian carcinoid tumours and struma ovarii are treated by unilateral oophorectomy.

Granulosa cell tumours of the ovary

These tumours account for 3–5% of malignant ovarian tumours. The cell of origin is unclear. They are frequently hormone-producing. The granulosa–theca tumour is composed of cells which resemble the normal granulosa cell of the follicle. It may be difficult to decide whether the tumour is malignant or not because it often lacks the typical cellular features of malignancy. Capsular invasion and cellular atypia are the most reliable signs of malignancy, and influence prognosis. Granulosa–theca cell tumours produce oestrogen (mainly from theca cells), androgens and progesterone. Oestrogen-related symptoms include postmenopausal bleeding, menorrhagia and breast tenderness. Virilizing symptoms, which are rarer, include hirsutism and oligomenorrhoea. The prognosis is excellent as they are mostly cured by conservative surgery (unilateral salpingo-oophorectomy). Responses to chemotherapy have been recorded in patients with recurrence.

Sertoli–Leydig cell tumours of the ovary

These rare tumours, representing 0.5% of ovarian cancers, are seen at age 20–40, and are sometimes termed *arrhenoblastomas*; 80% of them are associated with virilization. The histological appearance varies and some are poorly differentiated, though all contain Leydig cells identical to the male testicular cell. Occasionally, teratomatous elements are present.

Following surgical removal, the prognosis is excellent and over 90% of patients are alive at 10 years. The tumours are rarely bilateral so unilateral oophorectomy is usually adequate.

Carcinoma of the fallopian tube

This uncommon gynaecological malignancy is sometimes considered a 'variant' of ovarian carcinoma since the two diseases share the common aetiological feature of low fertility or nulliparity, with adenocarcinoma (solid, cystic or mixed) as the commonest histological type. Clinical symptoms include pelvic pain and vaginal discharge, which is sometimes profuse and often blood-stained. Other symptoms, similar to those found in ovarian carcinoma, include abdominal distension, altered bowel habit or, in occasional cases, dyspareunia.

Staging and treatment are similar to the recommendations for ovarian cancer (see above). Where a carcinoma of the fallopian tube is encountered at the initial laparotomy, it is much more likely to be due to secondary involvement from a carcinoma of the ovary than a true primary fallopian tube cancer. As for ovarian cancer generally, stage is an important prognostic determinant.

Carcinoma of the vulva

This uncommon tumour accounts for about 5–6% of all gynaecological cancers (1% of all cancers), with about 1000 new cases annually in the UK, chiefly affecting the older age group. Invasive carcinoma is distinctly uncommon in patients under 50 years (see Figure 17.1), while carcinoma *in situ*, now generally referred to as vulval intraepithelial neoplasia (VIN) III (analogous to CIN III), typically occurs in younger women (median age 50). As with both preinvasive and invasive squamous cell carcinomas of the cervix, it seems increasingly likely that subtypes of the HPV family, notably HPV-6, HPV-11, HPV-16 and HPV-18, are the major cause of squamous malignancies of the vulva and also other anogenital areas. This observation is the basis for the FUTURE I study, which in a large prospective trial of 5455 women has now demonstrated the effectiveness of a quadrivalent vaccine against HPV-6, HPV-11, HPV-16 and HPV-18 in reducing the incidence of these lesions, at least for the first 3 years of follow-up [84].

Aetiology, pathogenesis and diagnosis

Leucoplakia and other dystrophic changes in vulval skin can predispose to carcinoma. These can be hypoplastic, including lichen sclerosus and atrophic vulvitis, or hyperplastic, including leucoplakia as well as hypertrophic vulvitis. The hypoplastic form of dystrophic change is not usually regarded as premalignant, although there are certainly instances on record where this appears to have been the case. These are distinct from true intraepithelial neoplasia, which is a group including carcinoma *in situ* (often multifocal) and Paget's disease. Most vulval cancers are squamous cell carcinomas, though other types are occasionally seen, including adenocarcinoma (usually arising in a Bartholin's gland), melanoma, basal cell carcinoma, fibrosarcoma and adenoid cystic carcinoma. Diabetes is not infrequently associated with carcinoma of the vulva.

Pruritus vulvae, pain, ulceration, bleeding or discharge are the usual symptoms, although some patients are unaware of a vulval problem and seek advice about a lymph node in the groin. The most common sites are the labia majora, although the labia minora and clitoris can be primary sites. All thickened, fissured, ulcerated or sloughing lesions should be viewed with great suspicion, particularly in elderly patients, and biopsied. Histological distinctions between leucoplakia, lichen sclerosus et atrophicus and frank invasive carcinoma can be difficult, particularly since intraepithelial cancer can occur in areas of hypertrophic leucoplakia. Vulval carcinomas are almost always visible, so careful follow-up of suspicious lesions should not be difficult. Clinical photographs are useful to document slowly evolving changes.

Benign lesions can cause diagnostic confusion. These include chronic vulvitis, vulval condylomas of tuberculous, syphilitic, viral or unknown aetiology, lymphogranuloma inguinale, lymphogranuloma venereum (chiefly in younger patients) and vulval abscesses. The vulva is occasionally a site of secondary spread from carcinoma of the endometrium, cervix and large bowel.

Patterns of spread and clinical staging

The FIGO system is widely used (Table 17.9) and is based on the predictable behaviour of vulval carcinoma. Dissemination is chiefly via direct and lymphatic routes, and haematogenous spread is very unusual [85]. Local spread occurs to contiguous areas of the vulva, vagina and urethra, or to the perineum and/or anus (Figure 17.13). Local pubic tenderness may result from infection and periostitis, though malignant bone erosion has been described. Nodal involvement may be unilateral or bilateral, first to the inguino-femoral group, then more deeply (including contralateral node sites). Clitoral lesions may spread to either groin but do not directly involve deeper node groups without superficial node involvement in the first instance. Overall, nearly half of all vulval cancers have evidence of local lymphatic involvement.

Table 17.9 FIGO staging of carcinoma of the vulva. Stage 0 has been dropped from the FIGO classification but remains in the latest (seventh) edition of the UICC/TNM manual (2009).

Stage 0	Carcinoma *in situ*
Stage I	Tumour confined to vulva (<2 cm) No palpable nodes
Stage II	Tumour confined to vulva (>2 cm) No palpable nodes
Stage III	Tumour spread to urethra, vagina, or perineum Palpable mobile nodes
Stage IV	Tumour infiltrates bladder or rectum Fixed nodes

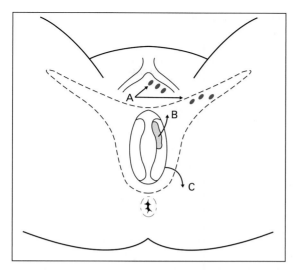

Figure 17.13 Local and nodal spread in carcinoma of the vulva. (A) Nodal involvement: inguinal, femoral, deep pelvic and common iliac nodes. Bilateral spread is common. (B) Anteriorly to contiguous parts of the vulva, clitoris, vagina, urethra and bladder. (C) Posteriorly to posterior vulva and rectum. Dotted line shows incision and resection in radical vulvectomy.

Investigation and management

Routine investigation should include full blood count, chest radiography and electrolyte estimation. MRI is useful in delineating pelvic and para-aortic nodes, particularly in patients where there is doubtful clinical evidence of involvement and the gynaecologist is uncertain whether to proceed with surgery. Needle aspiration of enlarged superficial nodes may occasionally help to decide whether surgery is appropriate.

Treatment

Treatment is by surgical excision, preferably of the primary carcinoma and lymphatic drainage *en bloc*. Even in patients who are elderly or have advanced local disease, surgery is generally the treatment of choice. Wide excision of vulval skin has traditionally been considered necessary since contiguous subdermal lymphatic spread is common; however, many gynaecologists are now less radical in their approach. Removal of the lower part of the urethra may also be necessary in more advanced stages. Because of the laxity of skin and subcutaneous tissue in this area, primary closure is usually possible despite the wide excision. Although postoperative infection is not uncommon and is the major surgical complication, most patients rehabilitate well. Surgical

excision is generally regarded as the treatment of choice although a few patients are unfit for these procedures, and palliative local irradiation can be extremely valuable, particularly in those with pain and ulceration. Radiation tolerance in these elderly patients is limited by bladder, bowel and other local structures. It is usually possible to achieve a total dose of at least 45–55 Gy, in 4–5.5 weeks, to the perineum and/or nodal sites. Treatment to a radical dose of 60 Gy should be attempted in younger, fit patients. In some patients with extensive nodal disease, a combination of primary resection with groin exploration and postoperative radiotherapy (to the nodal areas) represents the best means of achieving local control. The role of chemotherapy remains to be defined, though recent reports using synchronous chemoradiation therapy in selected patients have been encouraging, and radical chemoirradiation has been suggested as a serious alternative to surgery [86].

Prognosis

The survival rate depends largely on whether or not there is nodal involvement. About 75% of operable patients without lymphatic metastases are alive and disease-free at 5 years, whereas the 5-year survival of patients with inguinal or femoral node deposits is 30–40%, and less than 20% in patients with pelvic node involvement, even where pelvic lymph node dissection has been performed. Very occasionally further surgery (including pelvic exenteration) may be considered for patients with recurrent disease, though the end-results are generally poor.

Carcinoma of the vagina

This is a rare tumour, accounting for less than 1% of all gynaecological malignancy (i.e. about one-fiftieth as common as carcinoma of the cervix) and chiefly occurring in the 50–70 year age group. Little is known of the aetiology, but prolonged irritation from a vaginal ring pessary sometimes appears to predispose to malignant change. Vaginal carcinoma is almost invariably a squamous cell carcinoma, most frequently arising in the upper vagina, sometimes extensively involving the vaginal wall. Clear cell adenocarcinoma of the vagina has been reported in girls and young women whose mothers were taking exogenous diethylstilbestrol in pregnancy, an example of a transplacental carcinogen with a latent period of 15–30 years. Secondary deposits are occasionally encountered in the vagina, usually as a result of lymphatic spread from endometrial carcinoma (often thought to occur at operation); vaginal deposits from malignant melanomas are also well recognized, and on rare occasions the vagina is the primary site of a melanoma. Direct extension may occur from carcinoma of the cervix or bladder.

Symptoms, diagnosis and staging

A painless blood-stained vaginal discharge is the commonest symptom. In view of the typical age group, vaginal bleeding, when it occurs, is usually postmenopausal. Urinary complaints (frequency, nocturia and haematuria) or rectal discomfort occur with advanced disease. As with carcinoma of the cervix, spread of the disease tends to take place chiefly by direct and lymphatic invasion (Figure 17.14), to the parametria, pelvic side-wall and bladder. The lymphatic route varies with the site of the lesion. Lymphatic drainage of the upper part of the vagina is similar to that of the cervix, i.e. via external, internal and common iliac nodes. Lesions situated lower in the vagina drain to pelvic, inguinal and femoral nodes. Posteriorly placed lesions may spread towards the rectum because the lymphatic drainage of the posterior vaginal

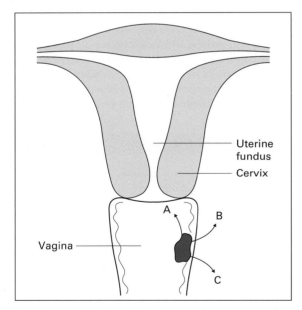

Figure 17.14 Local and lymph node spread in carcinoma of the vagina. (A) Submucosal spread to adjacent parts of vagina and cervix. (B) Parametrial tissues, bladder, rectum and eventually to pelvic side-wall. (C) Lymphatic spread: upper vagina as for cervix (see Figure 17.5); posterior vagina as for rectal lymphatics; anterior wall, towards lateral pelvic wall nodes; lower vagina, to pelvic and inguino-femoral nodes.

wall is to deep pelvic nodes (sacral, rectal and lower gluteal). As with carcinoma of the cervix, haematogenous spread is uncommon, and local control of disease tends to be the major clinical problem.

Careful vaginal examination should always be performed in patients presenting with vaginal bleeding and discharge, with direct inspection using a vaginal speculum. Colposcopy and biopsy can be extremely valuable, particularly where the speculum examination is inconclusive. Cytology of vaginal smears can be diagnostic. Where there is no obvious visible lesion, but definite cytological abnormalities are present, carcinoma *in situ* (now often termed vaginal intraepithelial neoplasia or VAIN) of the vagina must be suspected. This condition should also be considered where cervical cytology has yielded malignant cells but colposcopy-directed biopsy of the cervix has proved negative, particularly where subsequent high vaginal smears are still abnormal. Although an annual smear test is often performed after hysterectomy for benign disease, particularly in the USA, this method of screening for vaginal carcinoma is unrewarding and cannot be recommended.

Important investigations for symptomatic patients include examination under anaesthesia with cystoscopy, cervical dilatation and biopsy, and uterine curettage to exclude a primary carcinoma of the cervix. CT or MRI, sigmoidoscopy and peritoneal cytology may help to confirm the extent of spread in doubtful cases.

The FIGO staging system is generally used. This clinical staging system (Table 17.10) has been in use for over 10 years.

Treatment

Surgery and radiotherapy can both be effective, though surgical resection has to be very radical to stand a real chance of success and is not often employed as a primary procedure. Total vaginectomy, pelvic lymphadenectomy and abdominal hysterectomy would be necessary, with

Table 17.10 FIGO staging of carcinoma of the vagina.

Stage 0	Carcinoma *in situ*
Stage I	Vaginal wall only
Stage II	Subvaginal tissue involved
Stage III	Extension to pelvic side-wall
Stage IV	Spread beyond true pelvis:
IVa	to adjacent organs
IVb	to distant organs

reconstruction of the perineum and vagina where possible. This operation is only suitable for early lesions (stage I) or in a few highly selected cases following radiation failure. For most patients, radiotherapy is considered to be the treatment of choice. The 5-year disease-specific survival rates are 45% overall and about 75% for stage I cases [87].

Vaginal intraepithelial neoplasia

For stage I tumours, surgery is sometimes recommended, particularly in younger patients with more distal lesions (lower third of vagina). For the large majority of patients, however, treatment by intracavitary caesium insertion is combined with external beam irradiation as for carcinoma of the cervix (see above), particularly with tumours of the upper part of the vagina. Irradiation of the whole pelvis, using external beam multifield techniques, may be the best means of achieving homogeneous treatment to the primary and local node groups. In patients with more advanced disease (FIGO stages II–IV), a dose of 45–50 Gy, given in daily fractions over 4.5–5 weeks, is usually well tolerated and generally considered adequate for sterilizing microscopic direct or local lymphatic extension, although it is essential to give additional irradiation to the primary site and to any area which is obviously clinically involved. This is achieved either by intracavitary treatment or by additional external beam radiotherapy to encompass the whole of the vagina, treating the primary site if possible to a total of 60 Gy in daily fractions over 6 weeks.

Side-effects include acute proctitis in a substantial proportion of patients. Late radiation-induced rectal stricture may follow. Other complications include increased urinary frequency with cystitis and, in the longer term, local fistula formation, proctitis or sigmoid colitis, which may require bowel diversion, although local intrarectal steroid preparations may be adequate if the bowel is sufficiently viable. In view of the poor results and high complication rate with very advanced (stage IV) disease, treatment of these patients is usually palliative and lower doses, consistent with symptom relief, are generally more appropriate. Overall, the results of treatment are disappointing. Even with a radical approach, the 5-year survival rate falls from 75% with stage I disease to 25% with stage II and less than 5% for patients with stage IV tumours.

Carcinoma *in situ*

The whole of the vaginal mucosa is usually irradiated using a vaginal applicator containing radioactive sources (often termed Dobbie applicators, after their originator).

The intravaginal mould can be differentially loaded to treat the area at greatest risk to a higher dose, but irradiation of the whole mucosa is usually advised as there may be more than one neoplastic site. Complications of treatment include vaginal stenosis, lack of lubrication and proctitis. A radical dosage of at least 60 Gy mucosal dose is usually recommended.

Alternatively, laser therapy with colposcopy may be adequate for well-localized lesions. Occasionally, treatment by topical chemotherapy (generally with 5-FU) may be valuable, sometimes in conjunction with local irradiation.

Choriocarcinoma

This rare tumour has received considerable attention because of its extreme chemosensitivity, placing it in the small group of solid tumours that can be cured even when metastatic [88–91]. In addition, the secretion of a tumour marker, HCG (see Chapter 4), in 100% of cases of choriocarcinoma, permits a logical treatment approach based on a reliable index of tumour bulk.

The tumour most frequently follows pregnancies which have resulted in a complete or even a partial hydatidiform mole (occurring in approximately 1 in 1400 normal pregnancies in the UK), though it may rarely accompany a normal or ectopic pregnancy, or even a termination. It seems increasingly probable that most, or even all, carcinomas following an apparently normal pregnancy are, in reality, metastases from an undetected small intraplacental carcinoma, easily overlooked unless the placenta is minutely examined. It is more common in Asia than in Europe or the USA, and following pregnancy in 'elderly' subjects (> 40 years).

Pathology

Histopathologically, the tumour consists of malignant syncytiotrophoblast or cytotrophoblast cells, which can be shown immunocytochemically to contain HCG. Following successful evacuation of a hydatidiform mole, sequential determination of plasma HCG provides reliable information as to the completeness of the evacuation. In some cases, the HCG level falls more slowly to normal than would be predicted by the half-life of HCG (24–36 hours), suggesting that spontaneous regression of a tumour may have occurred. In others, local or distant invasion of tumour supervenes and the HCG level remains elevated.

The traditional classification of trophoblastic tumours, namely *hydatidiform moles*, *invasive moles* and *true choriocarcinomas*, was based on morphology. However, the availability of the quantitative HCG assay has largely supplanted these terms, since the diagnosis is made as a result of persistently raised HCG and tissue is now rarely available. It is probably better to use the term 'gestational trophoblastic tumour' instead. Abnormalities such as mitotic activity, degree of cellular atypia and local invasiveness appear to correlate fairly closely with prognosis.

Although the tumour may remain localized within the uterus, local extension into the myometrium or even the serosal surface or vagina may take place, sometimes causing severe intrauterine or intraperitoneal bleeding. More distant blood-borne secondary deposits occur, chiefly to lung, liver and brain, with a frequency that depends on the antecedent history – possibly as many as 1 in 20 molar pregnancies, but very rarely following normal or ectopic pregnancy.

Diagnosis and staging

Vaginal bleeding during or after pregnancy should be regarded with suspicion. Some patients appear to suffer from particularly marked symptoms of pregnancy, or pre-eclampsia. Ultrasound examination may lead to an almost certain diagnosis of a molar pregnancy before delivery. In the UK, evacuation of a hydatidiform mole and/or persistent elevation of postpartum HCG levels should result in registration of the patient at a reference centre (Charing Cross Hospital, London in the southern UK, and Sheffield in the north). The patient will then be followed closely, with regular samples of blood and/or urine sent to the designated centre. Staging investigations include repeat estimations of β-HCG, with chest and abdominopelvic CT scanning. Pelvic ultrasound may also be valuable.

Risk classification is important since optimal treatment is different for patients at varying risk of drug resistance [91]. Important prognostic factors include age (older patients do worse), interval between antecedent pregnancy and start of chemotherapy, initial HCG level, number and sites of metastases (the brain is a particularly adverse site) and previous administration of chemotherapy.

Treatment

Patients with *low-risk* disease are treated either by chemotherapy (generally single-agent chemotherapy with methotrexate) or by hysterectomy in patients who have no wish for further children. Where surgery is performed, it is often recommended that the hysterectomy be 'covered' by administration of methotrexate. If methotrexate is the definitive method of treatment, it is usually given daily or every other day for 1 week, the treatment repeated until the HCG marker has been undetectable in the serum for 6–8 weeks. Patients should be advised to avoid further pregnancy for at least 1 year.

Patients with more advanced *moderate-risk* disease are treated with combination chemotherapy, once again using serial HCG assays as a means of monitoring response. Surgery (hysterectomy) may be necessary if vaginal bleeding is troublesome.

Most drug regimens include methotrexate, actinomycin D and an alkylating agent (cyclophosphamide or chlorambucil). Newer regimens include vinca alkaloids, cisplatin and etoposide. All patients in this category respond to combination chemotherapy, usually resulting in cure, and high-risk patients or those with drug resistance to 'conventional' regimens usually respond to more aggressive regimens [90]. In patients with pulmonary metastases but no other adverse features, single-agent chemotherapy with methotrexate and folinic acid is probably still the treatment of choice.

Prognosis

Before chemotherapy was available, patients with localized disease were treated by surgery and/or pelvic irradiation and the cure rate was 40%. Patients with advanced disease were virtually never cured. With current treatment, 100% of patients with localized disease should be cured, and over 70% of patients with more advanced stages. Even with stage IV disease, the majority survive, and the number of tumour deaths in England and Wales is now under 10 per annum. For the most part, fertility of choriocarcinoma survivors is well maintained.

References

1 Rose PG. Medical progress: endometrial carcinoma. *N Engl J Med* 1996; 335: 640–9.

2 Parker SL, Tong T, Bolden S *et al*. Cancer statistics, 1996. *CA Cancer J Clin* 1996; 46: 5–27.

3 Stratton JF, Pharoah P, Smith SK, Easton D, Ponder BA. A systematic review and meta-analysis of family history and risk of ovarian cancer. *Br J Obstet Gynaecol* 1998; 105: 493–9.

4 Peto J, Gilham C, Fletcher O, Mathews FE. The cervical cancer epidemic that screening has prevented in the UK. *Lancet* 2004; 364: 249–56.

5 Sigurdsson K, Sigvaldason H. Is it rational to start population-based cervical cancer screening at or soon after age 20? Analysis of time trends in preinvasive and invasive diseases. *Eur J Cancer* 2007; 43: 769–74.

6 Bettigole C. The thousand-dollar pap smear. *New Engl J Med* 2013; 369: 1486–87.

7 Kalliala I, Anttila A, Pukkala E, Nieminen P. Risk of cervical and other cancers after treatment of cervical intra-epithelial neoplasia: retrospective cohort study. *Br Med J* 2005; 331: 1183–5.

8 Lawrence G, Man S for Cancer Research UK. *Cancer Stats – Cervical Cancer*, 2003. Available at www.cancerresearchuk. org, accessed 15 May 2006.

9 Schiffman M, Castle PE, Jeronimo J *et al.* Human papillomavirus and cervical cancer. *Lancet* 2007; 370: 890–907.

10 Agosti JM, Goldie SJ. Introducing HPV vaccine in developing countries: key challenges and issues. *N Engl J Med* 2007; 356: 1908–10.

11 Castellsagué X, Bosch FX, Muñoz N *et al.* Male circumcision, penile human papillomavirus infection, and cervical cancer in female partners. *N Engl J Med* 2002; 346: 1105–12.

12 International Collaboration of Epidemiological Studies of Cervical Cancer. Cervical cancer and hormonal contraceptives: collaborative reanalysis of individual data for 16 573 women with cervical cancer and 35 509 women without cervical cancer from 24 epidemiological studies. *Lancet* 2007; 370: 1609–21.

13 Ferenczy A, Franco E. Persistent human papillomavirus infection and cervical neoplasia. *Lancet Oncol* 2002; 3: 11–16.

14 Schiffman M and Solomon D. Cervical-cancer secreening with human papillomavirus and cytologic cotesting. *New Engl J Med* 2013; 369: 2324–2331.

15 International Collaboration of Epidemiological Studies of Cervical Cancer. Carcinoma of the cervix and tobacco smoking: collaborative re-analysis of individual data on 13 541 women with carcinoma of the cervix and 23 017 women without carcinoma of the cervix from 23 epidemiological studies. *Int J Cancer* 2006; 118: 1481–95.

16 Manetta A (ed.). *Cancer Prevention and Early Diagnosis in Women*. Philadelphia: Mosby, 2004.

17 Shastri S, Mittra I, Mishra G *et al.* Effect of visual inspection with acetic acid (VIA) screening by primary health workers on cervical cancer mortality: A cluster randomized controlled trial in Mumbai, India. *J Clin Oncol* 2013; 31 (suppl; abstr 2).

18 Goodman A, Wilbur DC. Case records of the Massachusetts General Hospital. Weekly clinicopathological exercises. Case 32-2003. A 37-year-old woman with atypical squamous cells on a Papanicolaou smear. *N Engl J Med* 2003; 349: 1555–64.

19 Cuzick J, Szarewski A, Cubie H *et al.* Management of women who test positive for high-risk types of human papillomavirus: the HART study. *Lancet* 2003; 362: 1871–6.

20 Zuna RE, Allen RA, Moore WE *et al.* Distribution of HPV genotypes in 282 women with cervical lesions: evidence of three categories of intra-epithelial lesions based on morphology and HPV type. *Mod Pathol* 2007; 20: 167–74.

21 Ronco G, Cuzick J, Pierotti P *et al.* Accuracy of liquid based versus conventional cytology: overall results of new technologies for cervical cancer screening: randomised controlled trial. *Br Med J* 2007; 335: 28–31.

22 Various authors. Human papillomavirus DNA versus Papanicolaou screening tests for cervical cancer. [Correspondence] *N Engl J Med* 2008; 358: 641–4.

23 Sankaranarayanan R, Okkuru Esmy P, Raijkumar R *et al.* Effect of visual screening on cervical cancer incidence and mortality in Tamil Nadu, India: a cluster-randomised trial. *Lancet* 2007; 370: 398–406.

24 Kitchener HC, Denton K, Soldan K and Crosbie EJ. Developing role of HPV in cervical cancer prevention. *Brit Med J* 2013; 347: f4781.

25 Harper DM, Franco EL, Wheeler CM *et al.* Sustained efficacy up to 4.5 years of a bivalent L1 virus-like particle vaccine against human papilloma virus types 16 and 18: follow up – from a randomised control trial. *Lancet* 2006; 367: 1247–55.

26 Mau C, Koutsky LA, Ault KA *et al.* Efficacy of human papilloma virus-16 vaccine to prevent cervical intraepithelial neoplasia: a randomised controlled trial. *Obstet Gynecol* 2006; 107: 18–27.

27 FUTURE II Study Group. Quadrivalent vaccine against human papillomavirus to prevent high-grade cervical lesions. *N Engl J Med* 2007; 356: 1915–27.

28 Lacey JV Jr, Swanson CA, Brinton LA *et al.* Obesity as a potential risk factor for adenocarcinomas and squamous cell carcinomas of the uterine cervix. *Cancer* 2003; 98: 814–21.

29 Charo RA. Politics, parents, and prophylaxis: mandating HPV vaccination in the United States. *N Engl J Med* 2007; 356: 1905–8.

30 Cox JT. Management of cervical intraepithelial neoplasia. *Lancet* 1999; 353: 857–90.

31 Landoni F, Maneo A, Colombo A *et al.* Randomised study of radical surgery versus radiotherapy for stage Ib–IIa cervical cancer. *Lancet* 1997; 350: 535–40.

32 Andreyev HJN. Gastrointestinal problems after pelvic radiotherapy: the past, the present and the future. *Clin Oncol* 2007; 19: 790–9.

33 Thomas GM. Improved treatment for cervical carcinoma: concurrent chemotherapy and radiotherapy. *N Engl J Med* 1999; 340: 1198–9.

34 Green J, Kiwan J, Tierney J *et al.* Survival and recurrence after concomitant chemotherapy and radiotherapy for cancer of the uterine cervix: a systematic review and meta-analysis. *Lancet* 2001; 358: 781–6.

35 Pötter R, Haie-Meder C, Van Limbergen E, Barillot I, De Brabandere M, Dimopoulos J *et al.* Recommendations from gynaecological (GYN) GEC ESTRO working group (II): Concepts and terms in 3D image-based treatment planning in cervix cancer brachytherapy – 3D dose volume parameters and aspects of 3D image-based anatomy, radiation physics, radiobiology. *Radiother Oncol* (2006); 78: 67–77.

36 Rotman M, Sededlis A, Piedmonte MR *et al.* A phase III randomized trial of post-operative pelvic irradiation in stage IB cervical carcinoma with poor prognostic features: follow-up of a Gynecologic Oncology Group study. *Int J Radiat Oncol Biol Phys* 2006; 5: 169–76.

37 Monk BJ, Wang J, Im S *et al.* Rethinking the use of radiation and chemotherapy after radical hysterectomy: a clinical-pathologic analysis of a Gynecologic Oncology Group/Southwest Oncology Group/Radiation Therapy Oncology Group Trial. *Gynecol Oncol* 2005; 96: 721–8.

38 Blackledge F, Buxton EJ, Mould JJ *et al.* Phase II studies of ifosfamide alone and in combination in cancer of the cervix. *Cancer Chemother Pharmacol* 1990; 26 (Suppl.): 512–16.

39 Tewari KS, Sill M, Long HJ *et al.* Incorporation of bevacizumab in the treatment of recurrent and metastatic cervical cancer: a phase III randomized trial of the Gynecologic Oncology Group. *J Clin Oncol* 2013; 31 (suppl; abstr 3).

40 Hoskins PJ, Swenerton KD, Pike JA *et al.* Small-cell carcinoma of the cervix: fourteen years of experience at a single institution using a combined-modality regimen of involved-field irradiation and platinum-based combination chemotherapy. *J Clin Oncol* 2003; 21: 3495–501.

41 Beral V, Bull D, Reeves G *et al.* Endometrial cancer and hormone-replacement therapy in the Million Women Study. *Lancet* 2005; 365: 1543–51.

42 Bergman L, Beelen ML, Gallee MP *et al.* Risk and prognosis of endometrial cancer after tamoxifen for breast cancer. *Lancet* 2000; 356: 881–7.

43 Schmeler KM, Lynch HT, Chen L-M *et al.* Prophylactic surgery to reduce the risk of gynecologic cancers in the Lynch syndrome. *N Engl J Med* 2006; 254: 261–9.

44 Xu WH, Zheng W, Xiang YB *et al.* Soya food intake and risk of endometrial cancer among Chinese women in Shanghai: population based case-control study. *Br Med J* 2004; 328: 1285–8.

45 Creasman WT, Morrow CP, Bundy BN *et al.* Surgical pathologic spread patterns of endometrial cancer. *Cancer* 1987; 60 (Suppl.): 2035–41.

46 Giuntoli RL, Metzinger DS, DiMarco CS *et al.* Retrospective review of 208 patients with leiomyosarcoma of the uterus: prognostic indicators, surgical management, and adjuvant therapy. *Gynecol Oncol* 2003; 89: 460–9.

47 Creutzberg CL, Van Putten WL, Koper PC *et al.* Surgery and postoperative radiotherapy vs surgery alone for patients with Stage 1 endometrial carcinoma: multicentre randomised trial. *Lancet* 2000; 355: 1404–11.

48 Lee CM, Szabo A, Shrieve DC *et al.* Frequency and effect of adjuvant radiation therapy among women with stage I endometrial adenocarcinoma. *JAMA* 2006; 295: 389–97.

49 Rush S, Gal D, Potters L *et al.* Pelvic control following external beam radiation for surgical stage I endometrial adenocarcinoma. *Int J Radiat Oncol Biol Phys* 1995; 33: 851–4.

50 Randall ME, Filiaci VL, Muss H *et al.* Randomized phase III trial of whole-abdominal irradiation versus doxorubicin and cisplatin chemotherapy in advanced endometrial carcinoma: a Gynecologic Oncology Group Study. *J Clin Oncol* 2006; 24: 36–44.

51 Einhorn N. Role of radiation therapy in carcinoma of the endometrium. In: Tobias JS, Thomas PRM, eds. *Current Radiation Oncology*, Vol. 2. London: Edward Arnold, 1996: 350–67.

52 Cannistra SA. Cancer of the ovary. *N Engl J Med* 2004; 351: 2519–29.

53 Collaborative Group on Epidemiological Studies of Ovarian Cancer. Ovarian cancer and oral contraceptives: collaborative reanalysis of data from 45 epidemiological studies including 25 257 women with ovarian cancer and 87 303 controls. *Lancet* 2008; 371: 303–14.

54 Million Women Study Collaborators. Ovarian cancer and hormone replacement therapy in the Million Women Study. *Lancet* 2007; 369: 1703–10.

55 Olsen CM, Green AC, Whiteman DC *et al.* Obesity and the risk of epithelial ovarian cancer: a systematic review and meta-analysis. *Eur J Cancer* 2007; 43: 690–709.

56 Kemp Z and Ledermann JA. Update on first-line treatment of advanced ovarian carcinoma. *Int J Womens Health* 2013; 5: 45–51.

57 National Cancer Intelligence Network, UK. *Overview of Ovarian Cancer in England: Incidence, Mortality and Survival.* London, UK: NCIN, 2012 – enquries@ncin.org.uk

58 Tobias JS, Griffiths CT. Management of ovarian carcinoma: current concepts and future prospects. *N Engl J Med* 1976; 294: 818–23 and 877–82.

59 Jacobs IJ, Skates SJ, MacDonald N *et al.* Screening for ovarian cancer: a pilot randomised controlled trial. *Lancet* 1999; 353: 1207–10.

60 Menon U. Ovarian cancer: challenges of early detection. *Nat Clin Pract Oncol* 2007; 4: 498–9.

61 Anon. An experiment in earlier detection of ovarian cancer. [Editorial] *Lancet* 2007; 369: 2051.

62 Lu KH, Skates S, Hernandez MA, *et al.* A 2-stage ovarian cancer screening strategy using the Risk of Ovarian Cancer Algorithm (ROCA) identifies early-stage incident cancers and demonstrates high positive predictive value. *Cancer* 2013; 119: 3454–61.

63 Black SS, Butler SL, Goldman PA, Scroggins MJ. Ovarian cancer symptom index: possibilities for earlier detection. *Cancer* 2007; 109: 167–9.

64 Vergote I, de Brabanter J, Fyles A *et al.* Prognostic importance of degree of differentiation and cyst rupture in Stage 1 invasive epithelial ovarian carcinoma. *Lancet* 2001; 357: 176–82.

65 Trimble CL, Trimble EL. Ovarian tumors of low malignant potential. *Oncology* 2003; 17: 1563–75.

66 Sieh W, Kobel M, Longacre TA *et al.* Hormone-receptor expression and ovarian cancer survival: an Ovarian Tumor Tissue Analysis consortium study. *Lancet Oncol* 2013; 14: 853–861.

67 Bristow RE, Berek JS. Surgery for ovarian cancer: how to improve survival. *Lancet* 2006; 367: 1558–9.

68 Griffiths CT. Surgical resection of bulk tumor in the primary treatment of ovarian carcinoma. *Natl Cancer Inst Monogr* 1975; 42: 101.

69 Van der Burg MEL, van Lent M, Buyse M *et al.* The effect of debulking surgery after induction chemotherapy on the prognosis in advanced epithelial ovarian cancer. *N Engl J Med* 1995; 332: 629–34.

70 Berek JS, Bertelsen K, du Bois A *et al.* Advanced epithelial ovarian cancer: 1998 consensus statements. *Ann Oncol* 1999; 10: 91–6.

71 McGuire WP, Hoskins WJ, Brady MF *et al.* Cyclophosphamide and cisplatin compared with paclitaxel and cisplatin in patients with stage III and stage IV ovarian carcinoma. *N Engl J Med* 1996; 334: 1–6.

72 ICON and AGO Collaborators. Paclitaxel plus platinum-based chemotherapy versus conventional platinum-based chemotherapy in women with relapsed ovarian cancer: the ICON4/AGO-OVAR-2.2trial. *Lancet* 2003; 361: 2099–106.

73 Gordon AN, Flegle JT, Gutherie D *et al.* Recurrent epithelial ovarian carcinoma: a randomised phase III study of pegylated liposomal doxorubicin versus topotecan. *J Clin Oncol* 2001; 19: 3312–22.

74 National Institute of Clinical Excellence. Paclitaxel, pegylated liposomal doxorubicin hydrochloride and topotecan for second-line or subsequent treatment of advanced ovarian cancer. A review of Technology Appraisal Guidance 28, 45 and 55. Technology Appraisal 91. London: NICE, 2005.

75 Bookman MA, Brady MF, McGuire WP *et al.* Evaluation of new platinum-based treatment regimens in advanced-stage ovarian cancer: a phase III trial of the Gynecologic Cancer InterGroup. *J Clin Oncol* 2009; 27: 1419–25.

76 Katsumata N, Yasuda M, Isonishi S *et al.* Long-term results of dose-dense paclitaxel and carboplatin versus conventional paclitaxel and carboplatin for treatment of advanced epithelial ovarian, fallopian tube or primary peritoneal cancer (JGOG 3016): a randomized, controlled, open-label trial. *Lancet Oncol* 2013; 14: 1020–1026.

77 Pfisterer J, Plante M, Vergote I *et al.* Gemcitabine plus carboplatin compared with carboplatin in patients with platinum-sensitive recurrent ovarian cancer: an intergroup trial of the AGO-OVAR, the NCIC CTG, and the EORTC GCG. *J Clin Oncol* 2006; 24: 4699–707.

78 Perren TJ, Swart AM, Pfisterer J *et al.* A Phase 3 Trial of bevacizumab in ovarian cancer. *New Eng J Med* 2011; 365: 2484–2496.

79 Burger RA, Brady MF, Bookman MA *et al.* Incorporation of bevacizumab in the primary treatment of ovarian cancer. *New Eng J Med* 2011; 365: 2473–83.

80 Ledermann JA, Harter B, Gourley C *et al.* Olaparib maintenance therapy in platinum-sensitive relapsed ovarian cancer. *New Engl J Med* 2012; 366: 1382–1392.

81 Armstrong DK, Bundy B, Wenzel L *et al.* Intra-peritoneal cisplatin and paclitaxel in ovarian cancer. *N Engl J Med* 2006; 354: 34–43.

82 Einhorn N, Lundell M, Nilsson B *et al.* Is there a place for radiotherapy in the treatment of advanced ovarian cancer? *Radiother Oncol* 1999; 53: 213–18.

83 Bower M, Fife K, Holden L *et al.* Chemotherapy for ovarian germ cell tumours. *Eur J Cancer* 1996; 32A: 593–7.

84 Garland SM, Hernandez-Avila M, Wheeler CS *et al.* For the FUTURE I Investigators. Quadrivalent vaccine against human papillomavirus to prevent anogenital diseases. *N Engl J Med* 2007; 356: 1928–43.

85 Oonk MH, Hollema H, de Hullu J, van der Zee AG. Prediction of lymph node metastases in vulvar cancer: a review. *Int J Gynecol Cancer* 2006; 16: 963–71.

86 Wahlen SA, Slater JD, Wagner RJ *et al.* Concurrent radiation therapy and chemotherapy in the treatment of primary squamous cell carcinoma of the vulva. *Cancer* 1995; 75: 2289–94.

87 Hellman K, Lundell M, Silfversward C *et al.* Clinical and histopathologic factors related to prognosis in primary squamous cell carcinoma off the vagina. *Int J Gynecol Cancer* 2006; 16: 1201–11.

88 El-Helw LM, Hancock BW. Treatment of metastatic gestational trophoblastic neoplasia. *Lancet Oncol* 2007; 8: 715–24.

89 Fox H. Gestational trophoblastic disease: neoplasia or pregnancy failure? *Br Med J* 1997; 314: 1363–4.

90 Bower M, Newlands ES, Holden L *et al.* EMA/CO for high-risk gestational trophoblastic tumours: results from a cohort of 272 patients. *J Clin Oncol* 1997; 15: 2636–43.

91 Papadopoulos AJ, Soskett M, Seckl MJ *et al.* Twenty five years' clinical experience of placental site trophoblastic tumours. *J Reprod Med* 2002; 47: 460–4.

Further reading

Carter J. Laparoscopy or laparotomy for early endometrial cancer? *Lancet Oncol* 2010; 11: 1021–1022.

Chemoradiotherapy for Cervical Cancer Meta-analysis Collaboration. Reducing uncertainties about the effects of chemoradiotherapy for cervical cancer: a systematic review and metaanalysis of individual patient data from 18 randomized trials. *J Clin Oncol* 2008; 26: 5802–12.

Khan JA. HPV vaccination for the prevention of cervical intra-epithelial neoplasia. *N Engl J Med* 2009; 361: 271–8.

Menon U, Gentry-Maharaj A, Hallett R *et al.* Sensitivity and specificity of multimodal and ultrasound screening for ovarian cancer, and stage distribution of detected cancers: results of the prevalence screen of the UK Collaborative Trial of Ovarian Cancer Screening (UKCTOCS). *Lancet Oncol* 2009; 10: 308–16.

Roehr B. Routine screening for ovarian cancer harms more than it helps, says US preventative health authority. *Brit Med J* 2012; 345: e6203.

Sanjose S, Quint WGV, Alemany L *et al.* Human papillomavirus genotype attribution in invasive cervical cancer: a retrospective cross-sectional worldwide study. *Lancet Oncol* 2010; 11: 1048–56.–9.

Sebire NJ, Seckl MJ. Gestational trophoblastic disease: current management of hydatidiform mole. *Br Med J* 2008; 337: 453–8.

Sobin LH, Gospodarowicz MK, Wittekind Ch, eds. *TNM Classification of Malignant Tumours*, 7th edn. Chichester: Wiley-Blackwell, 2009.

Over one-quarter of all cancers in males are due to tumours of the kidney, bladder or prostate. Testicular tumours are dealt with separately in Chapter 19. Other rare sites of cancer include the urethra, penis and epididymis. Although surgery has traditionally been the cornerstone of treatment, both radiotherapy and cytotoxic chemotherapy are assuming increasing importance. Management approaches and guidelines have changed markedly during the past 25 years.

Tumours of the kidney

Incidence and aetiology

Tumours of the kidney account for about 2–3% of all cancers (Figure 18.1). The incidence has increased by over 40% during the past three decades [1]. Clinical evolution is sometimes measured over many years, with apparent success followed by late recurrence, often several years later. In adults, the commonest type of renal tumour is the *renal cell carcinoma* (*hypernephroma*), which accounts for 75% of adult cases. Tumours of the renal pelvis are uncommon (10%) and are discussed

later. In children, *nephroblastoma* (*Wilms' tumour*) is among the commonest of malignant paediatric tumours, and is discussed in Chapter 24. About two-thirds of all patients presenting with renal cell carcinoma fortunately have a localized disease that is potentially curable by surgical nephrectomy, even though about one-third of these patients will relapse at a later stage, with metastatic disease. Although traditionally, chemotherapy has been disappointing for renal cell carcinoma, targeted therapy represents an important new modality of treatment in this group of patients – this is discussed more fully below.

Renal cell carcinoma is about twice as common in men (Figure 18.1), is aetiologically related to cigarette smoking, and has a median age at diagnosis of around 65 years. There is considerable variation in incidence throughout the world (Figure 18.2), and apart from cigarette smoking (which doubles the likelihood of renal cell carcinoma), obesity also appears to be a risk factor [2]. Although only a small proportion of patients have an affected family member, the risk is increased fourfold in first-degree relatives of patients. Little else is known about its pathogenesis, although it is common in patients with the Von Hippel–Lindau (VHL) syndrome (characterized

Cancer and its Management, Seventh Edition. Jeffrey Tobias and Daniel Hochhauser.
© 2015 John Wiley & Sons, Ltd. Published 2015 by John Wiley & Sons, Ltd.

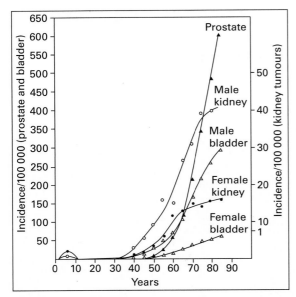

Figure 18.1 Age-specific incidence of renal, bladder and prostatic cancer.

by haemangioblastomas in the cerebellum and retina, associated with phaeochromocytoma), occurring in some 40% of all patients and frequently proving fatal. Stone formation in the renal pelvis, carcinogenic derivatives of aromatic amines or tryptophan, and phenacetin abuse are all thought to be important causes of renal pelvic tumours.

The *VHL* gene is a classic tumour-suppressor gene whose inactivation leads to tumour development, often with bilateral involvement. The gene has been localized to chromosome 3p25. One of the consequences of mutation of the *VHL* gene is the overproduction of vascular endothelial growth factor (VEGF) through a mechanism involving a hypoxia-inducible factor [3]. By its regulation of VEGF, the VHL protein is tightly linked to angiogenesis. This has had important therapeutic implications, notably the use of the 'humanized' anti-VEGF (initially a murine antibody) bevacizumab for metastatic renal cancer (see pages 360–361).

Renal cell adenocarcinoma (hypernephroma)
Pathology and staging
Stone formation in these tumours arises from the epithelium of the renal tubules themselves. For this reason, the term 'renal cell adenocarcinoma' is now increasingly preferred to the previously used 'hypernephroma'. A new

histological classification was introduced in 1986, based on histological and morphological criteria and subsequently validated on a molecular basis. The commonest variety, clear-cell carcinoma, makes up three-quarters of all cases and is characterized by deletion or inactivation of the *VHL* gene. Most of the remaining cases are chromophilic (also called papillary) carcinomas (12% of the total).

Local, lymphatic and haematogenous spread are all relatively common, making surgery unwise or technically impossible in about one-third of all cases. It is estimated that about 30% of patients have metastases at the time of initial diagnosis.

Direct invasion into perirenal tissues occurs in over 20% and local lymph node metastases in 8%. Renal vein invasion is also common, with cords of tumour cells sometimes growing directly into the inferior vena cava, although this is often undetectable preoperatively. Likelihood of dissemination correlates with histological differentiation. In patients with low-grade carcinoma the incidence of metastatic disease at presentation is very low.

The current tumour node metastasis (TNM) staging system chiefly relies on information obtained at operation [4] (Table 18.1). Prognosis is closely related to stage (see page 361). About 2–3% of all renal cell carcinomas are bilateral at presentation.

Clinical features
These tumours present with a wide variety of symptoms. Approximately 50% of patients have haematuria, often very slight but occasionally sufficiently severe to produce anaemia. Fortunately, with the widespread advent of haematuria clinics, earlier diagnosis is now becoming a reality though renal carcinoma will be a relatively unusual diagnosis from such a setting – bladder cancer is most likely and of course, non-malignant diagnoses likelier still. Loin pain and a palpable mass are classical features, and a large mass may be palpable. Fatigue and weight loss are common and many patients present with complaints resulting from metastases, such as pathological fracture through a bone deposit, dyspnoea and cough from mediastinal, hilar or lung metastases, or even epilepsy from an intracerebral deposit. Approximately one-quarter of patients have evidence of distant metastases at presentation. Renal cell tumours are a well-known cause of pyrexia; fever without other symptoms is not uncommon. Hypertension, polycythaemia and hypercalcaemia also occur in about 5% of patients. About 2% of male patients present with a varicocele, usually left-sided, due to obstruction of the testicular vein. Liver function tests

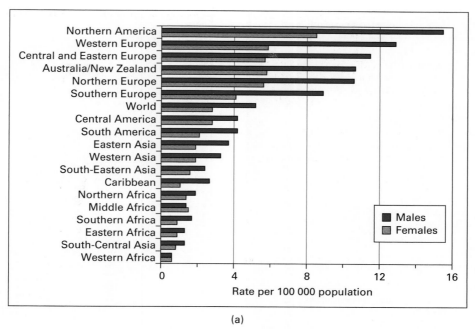

(a)

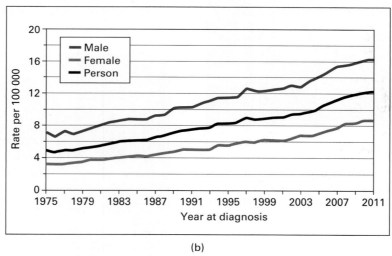

(b)

Figure 18.2 (a) World age-standardized incidence rates for kidney cancer, world regions, 2008 estimates. (b) Kidney Cancer (C64-C66 and C68), European Age-Standardized Incidence Rates, Great Britain, 1975–2011. Source: http://info.cancerresearchuk.org/cancerstats/types/kidney/incidence/?a=5441 accessed Feb 2014. © 2014 Cancer Research UK, Reproduced with permission.

may be abnormal even in patients without metastatic disease, although they are unreliable as tumour markers.

Even when a renal cell carcinoma is suspected, the diagnosis can be difficult. Intravenous urography (IVU), ultrasound or computed tomography (CT) usually demonstrates a space-occupying mass in the renal cortex,

often with distortion of the calyceal system (Figures 18.3 and 18.4).

Renal calcification, particularly if 'rim-like', is a common finding. Further radiological investigations using magnetic resonance imaging (MRI) may give additional information. Before surgery, chest radiography is essential

Table 18.1 TNM classification of malignant tumours.

Primary tumour (T)

TX	Primary tumour cannot be assessed
T0	No evidence of primary tumour
T1	Tumour 7.0 cm or less in greatest dimension, limited to the kidney
T2	Tumour more than 7.0 cm in greatest dimension, limited to the kidney
T3	Tumour extends into major veins or invades adrenal gland or perinephric tissues but not beyond Gerota's fascia
T3a	Tumour invades adrenal gland or perinephric tissues but not beyond Gerota's fascia
T3b	Tumour grossly extends into renal vein(s) or vena cava below diaphragm
T3c	Tumour grossly extends into vena cava above diaphragm
T4	Tumour invades beyond Gerota's fascia

Regional lymph nodes (N)

NX	Regional lymph nodes cannot be assessed
N0	Regional lymph node metastasis
N1	Metastasis in a single regional lymph node
N2	Metastasis in more than one regional lymph node

Distant metastasis (M)

MX	Distant metastasis cannot be assessed
M0	No distant metastasis
M1	Distant metastasis

Source: Sobin and Wittekind [4]. Reproduced with permission from John Wiley and Sons.

in case pulmonary metastases are already present, and CT scanning is advisable since pulmonary metastases have to be at least 2 cm in diameter to be visible on a standard chest radiograph. Isotope bone scanning may reveal unsuspected bone metastases, particularly in patients whose primary lesion is palpable. Biochemical tests of renal and liver function are important, and it is also wise to perform isotope renography preoperatively to assess the function of the contralateral kidney.

Management

Surgical resection is the most effective method of treatment, though over 25% of renal carcinomas are technically unresectable. *En bloc* resection of the kidney with as little disturbance as possible is probably the best approach, coupled with a dissection from the aortic bifurcation to the diaphragm and with prevention of tumour dissemination by early ligation of the renal artery and vein. Although still controversial, lymph node dissection

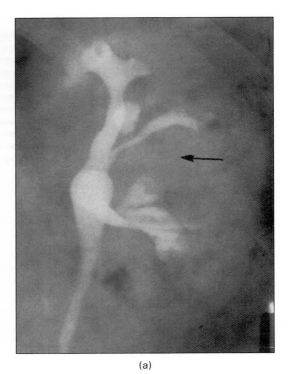

(a)

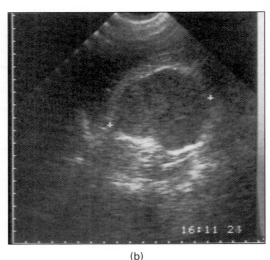

(b)

Figure 18.3 (a) Intravenous urogram in renal carcinoma. The left kidney contains a tumour (arrow) which displaces the calyces. (b) Transverse ultrasound scan showing a large renal carcinoma below the liver. (c) Line drawing of (b).

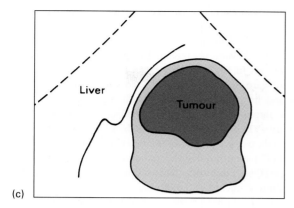

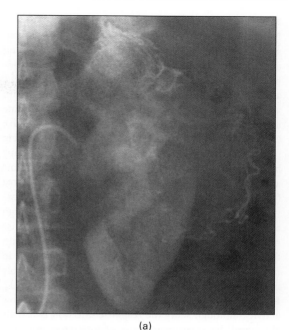

(a)

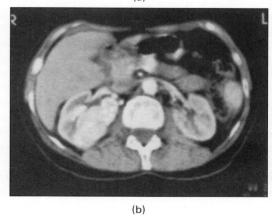

(b)

(c)

Figure 18.3 (*continued*)

seems advisable since the incidence of regional lymph node involvement is around 15%. In cases where the tumour is large, or difficult to remove, it may be necessary to perform nephroureterectomy, with removal of part of the bladder if indicated. Radical surgery is usually the best way forward even where extension of the tumour to the renal vein or inferior vena cava has occurred. Difficulties arise where a renal carcinoma occurs in a solitary or horseshoe kidney, and the commonest approach is to perform a partial nephrectomy. Occasionally, if the tumour is too large for a conservative resection, total nephrectomy is unavoidable, with transplantation of an allogeneic kidney (if available) at a later procedure.

In patients with obvious clinical or radiological evidence of metastases elsewhere, the choice of initial treatment is more difficult [5]. The primary lesion may be technically operable, and providing the patient's condition is reasonably good, nephrectomy is by far the most effective and simplest means of securing control of the primary, particularly when there are troublesome symptoms such as renal pain or haematuria [1]. Although there are sporadic case reports of regression of secondary lung deposits following resection of the primary tumour [6], this phenomenon is in fact very rare and the possibility of its occurrence should never be used as the sole rationale for surgery [7]. Since this capricious tumour can remain quiescent for many years (even decades) before metastases become apparent, it is sometimes recommended that solitary metastases be surgically removed. In symptomatic patients with obvious widespread metastatic disease, in whom nephrectomy seems unwise, renal artery embolism or occlusion is worth considering since it leads to partial or complete infarction of the kidney and offers a reasonable chance of temporary

Figure 18.4 Renal arteriogram (late arterial phase). (a) A tumour circulation is seen due to a large carcinoma occupying the upper two-thirds of the kidney. (b) CT scan of the abdomen (with contrast) in a patient with a carcinoma of the right kidney.

control. It should probably be used only in symptomatic patients since it can be painful and hazardous, though some urologists use it routinely as a preoperative adjunct to nephrectomy. Several other methods of occlusion are currently in use, including intra-arterial balloon catheter occlusion, induction of autologous local thrombus, or insertion of foreign material such as gelatine sponge or polyacrylamide gel. Radiotherapy is no longer used in primary management [8].

Systemic treatments and palliative therapy

Despite early reports of response to hormone preparations, the overall response rate to progestogens and androgens is very low, of the order of 5%. Notwithstanding this disappointing figure, these agents are non-toxic and therefore worth considering in patients with widespread metastases. Medroxyprogesterone acetate is widely used (100 mg three times daily by mouth). Other hormonal agents, such as flutamide and tamoxifen, probably have similar response rates [9]. Chemotherapy has had little success [10]. The most widely used agents are vinblastine, cisplatin *cis*-chloroethyl nitrosourea (CCNU), doxorubicin, cyclophosphamide and hydroxycarbamide (hydroxyurea). None of these has high activity on its own, and in combination the response rate is still very low (20% at best). Dissatisfaction with these poor results has led to increasing interest in newer therapies in metastatic renal cancer, notably immunotherapy using cytokines and other agents [1,11]. In 1983, human interferon was first reported to show activity, although sadly the response duration is usually short and the experimental use of interferons together with chemotherapy does not appear promising. Use of interleukin (IL)-2, lymphokine-activated killer (LAK) cells and other types of interferon seems less encouraging despite the initial euphoria aroused by Rosenberg's contention [12] that metastatic renal cell carcinoma was frequently responsive. Although there are now more potentially valuable treatments available to such patients (e.g. allogeneic peripheral blood stem cell transplantation as reported by Childs *et al.* [13]), the outlook in general remains poor, with an overall median survival of approximately 9 months. Moreover, the toxicity of IL-2 (with or without LAK cells) remains considerable. No advantage was found in a comparative study (128 patients) using tamoxifen alone or tamoxifen plus interferon alfa and IL-2 [14].

Over the past few years, innovative therapy with a variety of biological agents has shown great promise, and these are now becoming increasingly used as part of standard management in patients with advanced disease. For example, in a study of bevacizumab versus placebo in metastatic renal cell carcinoma, a highly significant prolongation of time to progression was reported in the treatment group [15]. This exciting result has been complemented by other studies suggesting activity for newer agents such as tyrosine kinase inhibitors, presumably via an antiangiogenic pathway. In general, in this fast-moving field, systemic treatment for these patients has largely shifted in recent years from cytokines to drugs targeting angiogenesis. These agents are discussed more fully in Chapter 6 – and also see Ref. [16] – an important on-line search of the Cochrane Collaboration Library to assess the value of targeted therapy for advanced renal cell cancer. In all, 28 studies met the inclusion criteria, and 10 were placebo-controlled. Two were too small to assess, and five more used nonspecific anti-angiogenic agents with poor activity. In all, 15 studies (5587 patients) tested anti-VEGF agents: bevacizumab (BEV), sorafenib, sunitinib, pazopanib, tivozanib, or axitinib. Three studies, in 1147 patients, tested the mammalian target of rapamycin (mTOR) inhibitors, temsirolimus or everolimus. Two studies included epidermal growth factor receptor (EGFR) inhibitors, and one tested the combination of temsirolimus plus BEV: in treatment-naive patients with mostly good-moderate prognostic risk; in separate trials, oral sunitinib (one trial) and intravenous BEV plus subcutaneous interferon-α (two trials) improved PFS compared with the previous standard of care interferon-α. Sorafenib did not appear to improve PFS over interferon-α in the first-line setting, and the addition of cytokines did not improve sorafenib efficacy. In poor-risk patients, the mTOR inhibitor temsirolimus improved PFS and overall survival. Several trials examined agents in the second-line setting. After cytokine therapy, sorafenib (one study) and pazopanib (one study) prolonged PFS over placebo. A preliminary report of the investigational VEGF receptor inhibitor axitinib gave superior PFS to sorafenib after either prior cytokine or prior sunitinib treatment. After cancer progression, 6 months of sunitinib and/or sorafenib therapy or everolimus prolonged PFS, with a marginal improvement in overall survival in several studies. In summary, agents showing useful activity in metastatic renal cell carcinoma include axitinib, sorafenib, sunitinib and temsirolimus, many of these newer agents sharing the obvious advantage of oral administration. See also Ref. [17]. Several important trials were reported in 2007, a breakthrough year for advanced or metastatic renal cell carcinoma [18–20]. In the first of these, oral sunitinib was compared with interferon alfa in 750 patients with previously untreated metastatic cancer. The median progression-free survival rate was significantly longer in the sunitinib group (11 months) compared with the interferon group (5 months), and on the whole treatment with oral sunitinib was better tolerated, these patients reporting a significantly better quality of life [18]. In the second [19], oral sorafenib was compared with placebo in an even larger study of over 900 patients who were resistant to standard therapy. The progression-free survival was 5.5 months for the surafenib group compared with 2.8 months for placebo patients, with a small increase in overall survival. More recently, over 600 patients with advanced poor-prognosis renal cell cancer were randomized in a three-arm phase III study to receive either interferon alfa or temsirolimus, or the combination; treatment was continued until progression of disease or withdrawal because of treatment-related side-effects [20]. In the group receiving only temsirolimus, a specific inhibitor of the mTOR kinase (see Chapter 6), overall survival was prolonged to 10.9 months, compared with 7.3 and 8.4 months in the other two arms. The improvement was reflected in a hazard ratio (for death) of 0.73 and a progression-free survival significant at the $P = 0.008$ level. Clearly, these newer agents, which act as inhibitors of both multi-kinase pathways and angiogenesis, have considerable promise in the management of this difficult condition, particularly since conventional cytotoxic chemotherapy has so little to offer in patients with metastatic renal cell cancer. Several studies have suggested that treatment failure after interferon or IL-2 can sometimes be salvaged by using a newer biologically targeted agent such as axitinib or everolimus, an orally administered inhibitor of mTOR, a component of an intracellular pathway that regulates cellular metabolism, growth, proliferation and angiogenesis (see Refs. [21,16] for a fuller discussion of recent evidence). An important large-scale, recent study coordinated from New York addressed the choice of two highly promising orally administered agents in a head-to-head study – pazopanib versus sunitinib – for patients with metastatic disease – see Ref. [22]. This was a study of 1110 patients randomly assigned to either of these two agents, and showed equivalence in efficacy but a side-effect profile in favour of pazopanib – less fatigue, hand-foot syndrome and thrombocytopenia.

Combination biological treatment has also become a clinical reality, with the publication of a large investigation from several European centres of a prospective study of bevacizumab plus interferon alfa-2a compared with interferon alone [23] in patients with metastatic disease. Among 649 patients included in the study, the number of progression events/deaths was 230/114 (of 325 patients in the combination group) versus 275/137 (of 316 patients in the interferon plus placebo group). The median duration of progression-free survival was significantly improved from 5.4 months to 10.2 months, a relative 37% improvement.

In addition to the emerging role for these newer agents in symptom palliation, treatment with radiotherapy may also be helpful, particularly in the relief of bone pain. Bone metastases are very common and in carefully selected patients, internal orthopaedic fixation of long bones is invaluable in prevention or treatment of pathological fractures, thereby allowing early mobility.

Prognosis

The prognosis in renal cell cancer depends on the stage and grade of the tumour, and the completeness of surgery (Figure 18.5). The 5-year survival is approximately 55%, most of the loss of life occurring in the first 2 years after diagnosis. Improvements in imaging techniques have probably been responsible for a slight rise in cure rates over the past 20 years. For stage I tumours, the 5-year survival is over 65%, whereas if the regional nodes are involved this falls to 30%. For stage IV tumours, there are very few 5-year survivors. With high-grade tumours only 30% of patients are alive at 5 years, while with low-grade tumours 80% of patients survive.

Carcinoma of the renal pelvis

Carcinomas of the renal pelvis [24] are uncommon (about 7% of all renal carcinomas) and are usually transitional cell carcinomas (TCCs) (80%) or squamous cell carcinomas, which may be more common in women. Clinical symptoms include haematuria (90%) and loin pain due to obstruction of the renal pelvis. On examination, in advanced cases, there may be a palpable loin mass.

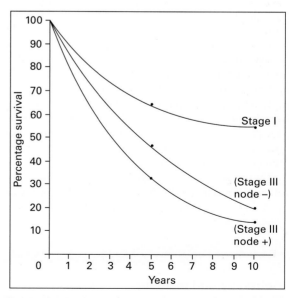

Figure 18.5 Prognosis of renal adenocarcinoma related to stage and lymph node involvement.

Investigation includes IVU, which usually shows a filling defect in the collecting system and occasionally demonstrates non-function where there has been long-standing postrenal obstruction by tumour. Half of all patients have malignant cells in the urine, so cytological examination of the urine is essential.

Surgery is again the most important method of treatment. Nephroureterectomy is usually required; for transitional tumours a part of the bladder wall is also usually removed, as a wide area of epithelium is at risk. As the histology of the renal pelvic tumour is not usually known preoperatively, the operation is the same for both TCCs and squamous carcinomas. However, local ureteric stump recurrence is reportedly less frequent with squamous carcinomas.

Radiotherapy may be worth considering for inoperable or recurrent cases but there is little evidence that it is ever curative. However, it may retard local progression of disease. In the follow-up period the possibility of a contralateral lesion must always be borne in mind. Repeated cystoscopy and cytological examination of the urine are both important since 50% of patients later develop a carcinoma of the bladder. About 10% of patients with TCC of the renal pelvis have a synchronous bladder carcinoma as well.

Carcinoma of the ureter

This rare tumour is usually a TCC, although sarcomas are occasionally encountered. Typically, the disease presents with frequency and dysuria. Ureteric colic is unusual. The diagnosis is usually made by IVU, which shows ureteric dilatation or distortion, or a non-functioning kidney. Retrograde pyelography demonstrates the site of the block. Urinary cytology may also be helpful.

Treatment is by nephroureterectomy, though occasionally the kidney may be preserved. In removing the ureter a cuff of bladder should be taken. Radiotherapy has occasionally been employed in patients with inoperable tumour, but with little success.

The prognosis depends largely on the cellular differentiation of the tumours. The 5-year survival rate is 80% with well-differentiated tumours, but only 10% with the most anaplastic forms.

Cancer of the urinary bladder

Aetiology and incidence

Bladder cancer is now the second commonest urological malignancy (the fourth commonest cancer in men in the western world, and ninth in women), with over 10 000 new cases annually in the UK and 45 000 new cases in the USA. Over three times as common in men as in women, it causes nearly 5000 deaths annually in the UK and as a result of occupational carcinogens identified in the 1950s, it remains an industrially prescribed disease. The incidence is rising, and global incidence rates are shown in Figure 18.6. At the end of the nineteenth century, it was recognized that workers in the aniline dye industry had a high incidence of bladder cancer, and the active carcinogen to which they were exposed was later identified as α-naphthylamine. Workers in the rubber industry form another important aetiological group. Chronic bladder infection or infestation also predisposes to malignant change; worldwide, the most important of these causes is schistosomiasis. Cigarette smokers are at greatly increased risk, which partly explains its much higher incidence in males. At least 50% of cases in males and 25% in females are causally related to cigarette smoking, particularly to duration of smoking, with the incidence decreasing comparatively rapidly in ex-smokers. In the USA, the disease is reportedly four times as common in white men as in black men and is commoner in urban areas. Other probable aetiological factors in bladder cancer include multiple urinary infections and previous exposure to cyclophosphamide [25].

Screening has increasingly been attempted; indeed, bladder cancer was probably the first solid tumour in males in which a systematic screening programme was seriously considered [26]. In low-risk groups (the general population), this has usually been done by dipstick testing for occult haematuria, a technique with high predictive accuracy but low yields (of the order of 2.5%) in unselected males aged 21–72 years. In higher-risk groups, the approach is clearly more logical although, even in men working in the rubber industry, it is nowadays difficult to confirm excess death rates, in contrast to studies performed in former years. At present, the cost and low yield argue against the wide introduction of screening programmes, although careful investigation of even a single episode of haematuria (or occult haematuria) is mandatory.

Recently, a number of associations have been reported between common genetic polymorphisms and bladder cancer risk [27]. These include deletion of one or two copies of the *GSTM1* gene and the *NAT2* acetylator genotype, particularly marked amongst cigarette smokers. As these polymorphisms are common in the population, they could account for up to 30% of bladder cancers,

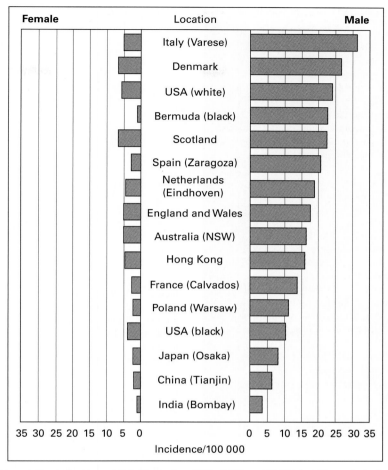

Female	Location	Male
	Italy (Varese)	
	Denmark	
	USA (white)	
	Bermuda (black)	
	Scotland	
	Spain (Zaragoza)	
	Netherlands (Eindhoven)	
	England and Wales	
	Australia (NSW)	
	Hong Kong	
	France (Calvados)	
	Poland (Warsaw)	
	USA (black)	
	Japan (Osaka)	
	China (Tianjin)	
	India (Bombay)	

35 30 25 20 15 10 5 0   0 5 10 15 20 25 30 35

Incidence/100 000

Figure 18.6 Geographic variation in incidence of bladder cancer, 1983–1987 per 100 000 (world population).

particularly important as previous industrial exposure cases are becoming less common.

Pathology and staging

Over 90% of bladder tumours are derived from transitional cell epithelium. In Western countries, TCC of the bladder is over five times as common as squamous cell carcinoma, although in Egypt, where schistosomal infestation is common, the squamous carcinoma is more frequent. Other histological types such as adenocarcinoma, leiomyosarcoma and rhabdomyosarcoma are rare. TCCs may be single or multiple, and are sometimes pedunculated, whereas squamous carcinomas are usually sessile and often necrotic in appearance. Multiple papillomatous tumours are often of low grade, but should be regarded as

premalignant. Fortunately, the majority of patients (70%) with bladder cancer present with superficial disease only.

In TCC, pathological grading is of considerable importance, and well-differentiated tumours carry a better prognosis independently of tumour stage. Pathological depth of infiltration of the bladder wall (P stage) directly correlates with survival. Very early lesions (papillary, grade 0) typically have a fine fibrovascular core, covered by normal mucosa. With grade I (well-differentiated) tumours, the urothelium is thickened, with a slight degree of pleomorphic change; grade II (moderately differentiated) and grade III (poorly differentiated) tumours are characterized by an increasing degree of nuclear pleomorphism and frequent mitotic activity easily observed with standard light microscopy.

Table 18.2 TNM and P staging for bladder cancer.

Tis	Preinvasive carcinoma (carcinoma *in situ*)
Ta	Papillary non-invasive carcinoma
T0	No evidence of primary tumour
T1	Tumour limited to the lamina propria (P1). Bimanual examination may reveal a mobile mass which cannot be felt after transurethral resection
T2	Tumour limited to superficial muscle (P2). Mobile induration of the bladder wall may be present, but should be impalpable following transurethral resection
T3	Invasion of deep muscle layer of the bladder wall (P3). On bimanual palpation a mobile mass is felt which persists after transurethral resection
T3a	Deep muscle invasion
T3b	Invasion through the muscle wall
T4	Invasion of prostate or other local structures (P4); tumour fixed or locally extensive
T4a	Tumour infiltrates prostate, uterus or vagina
T4b	Tumour fixed to pelvic and/or abdominal wall
N0	Regional lymph node involvement
N1	Involvement of a single ipsilateral regional node group
N2	Contralateral, bilateral or multiple regional node involvement
N3	Fixed regional lymphadenopathy (i.e. a fixed space between this and the tumour)
N4	Involvement of juxtaregional nodes
M0	No distant metastases
M1	Distant metastases

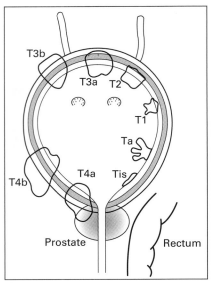

Figure 18.7 T staging of bladder cancer: Tis, carcinoma *in situ*; Ta, non-invasive papillary carcinoma; T1, limited to lamina propria; T2, superficial muscle involvement; T3a, deep muscle involvement; T3b, full thickness of bladder wall; T4a, invading neighbouring structures (prostate, vagina); T4b, involvement of rectum, fixed to pelvic wall.

The TNM staging notation (Table 18.2) allows a convenient shorthand description, based largely on the degree of local spread at presentation (Figure 18.7). The most important distinction lies between T2 and T3 tumours, since over 50% of all patients with T2 tumours will be alive at 3 years from diagnosis, whereas less than 25% of patients with T3 tumours (i.e. with invasion of the deep muscle of the bladder) will survive. The *Union Internationale Contre le Cancer* (UICC) staging criteria for bladder (and prostate) cancer now parallels the USA-based systems more closely. However, the resulting staging system takes far less account of clinical information; the above criteria, and TNM and P stage criteria, continue to be widely used, and important prognostic factors are included. In addition to TNM stage, pathological grade and histological type, and size, location and number of bladder tumours all influence clinical management. Multiple bladder tumours are so frequently encountered that the whole of the transitional cell epithelial surface must be considered at risk, and in some instances where tumours are widespread throughout the bladder, total cystectomy may be required even though the local invasiveness of each one may be unimpressive. The major sites of distant metastasis are lymph nodes, lung, liver and bone.

Patients with an abnormal chromosome complement have a poor prognosis. There appears to be a strong correlation between DNA content (ploidy) and level of invasion (pathological grade), depth of tumour invasiveness and response to certain types of therapy [24]. Tumours expressing A, B or H blood-group antigens have a better prognosis, though the reasons remain unclear. The development of a bladder cancer from normal or premalignant urothelial tissue may relate to the presence of transforming oncogenes, particularly those of the *ras* family which are known to be present on chromosomes 1, 11 and 12. There may be an association between *ras* expression and high histological grade. Additional adverse features such as amplification of the c-*erb*-B2 oncogene, the presence of tumour-associated antigen 138 or increased urinary excretion of fibronectin all appear to predispose to an increased likelihood of muscle invasion.

Clinical features

The majority of patients with bladder cancer complain of haematuria, usually painless, although other symptoms such as urgency of micturition, nocturia and frequency or reduction of the urinary stream may also be present. Loin or back pain may occur if tumour obstruction has led to hydronephrosis or if large intra-abdominal lymph node metastases are present. Even single episodes of haematuria should be fully investigated by cystoscopy. Fortunately, the majority of patients with superficial tumours do not develop invasive disease; indeed, it is probably true that superficial and deeply invasive bladder carcinomas are distinctly separate disorders [1].

Definitive diagnosis requires cystoscopy with biopsy, which gives a clear indication of the site, size, general appearance and multiplicity of tumours. This procedure is normally performed under general anaesthesia, permitting a full examination including thorough rectal and bimanual palpation, which is essential for accurate staging. Urinary exfoliative cytology is a valuable addition to diagnosis and is currently being evaluated as a means not only of diagnosis but also of monitoring response to treatment.

IVU should be performed, giving essential information regarding the anatomy and functioning of the kidneys and ureters, and often further information as to the site and extent of the primary tumour. Renal function should be assessed by measurement of blood urea and creatinine clearance, or other form of assessment such as diethylenetriaminepenta-acetic acid (DTPA) clearance. To evaluate the degree of extravesical spread MRI and CT are extremely valuable (Figure 18.8).

Management
Superficial bladder cancer

Management of superficial bladder tumours is almost entirely the province of the surgeon. Repeated cystoscopy may be required, together with biopsy of any suspicious site. Tumour mapping is an important preliminary and all visible tumours should be removed wherever possible. The aim of treatment is not only to eradicate the initial lesion but also to prevent a superficial relapse and, above all, prevent progression to muscle-invasive disease. Low-risk cases include those under 3 cm which are completed excised, of low pathological grade and favourable molecular marker staining (absent p53 antigen, normal ploidy). Other cases should be recognized as clearly carrying a higher risk of recurrence. A common management policy is to repeat cystoscopy in low-risk cases (with urine cytology) every 6 months for

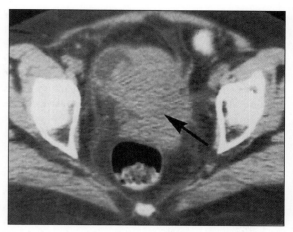

Figure 18.8 CT scan in advanced bladder cancer. The tumour (arrow) is shown extending posteriorly to the rectum and laterally to the side-walls of the pelvis. (Courtesy of Professor Dame Janet Husband.)

the first 2 years and yearly thereafter. For higher-risk superficial tumours, intravesical chemotherapy may be valuable (see below) and has been used for many years – long established in urological practice. More frequent follow-up will be required for high-risk groups: 3-monthly cystoscopy is often recommended, at least for the first year of follow-up. Small papillary tumours can be repeatedly treated by cystodiathermy, often for many years, although other methods such as cryosurgery and laser treatment are becoming more widely used. Intravesical chemotherapy using thiotepa, mitomycin C (probably the most commonly used agent), doxorubicin and other cytotoxic agents is sometimes able to prevent or treat small recurrences. Thiotepa is less used nowadays since it may cause considerable local discomfort. Although such tumours are rarely fatal, up to 10% of patients develop widespread intravesical recurrence after repeated cystodiathermy, necessitating further treatment either with radiotherapy or even total cystectomy. In these, intravesical chemotherapy may prove helpful in avoiding or delaying such treatment, thereby improving the quality of survival.

Because superficial bladder cancers can progress to more deeply penetrating lesions, both external radiotherapy and intravesical chemotherapy have now been tested as means of preventing this [28]. Bacille Calmette–Guérin (BCG) has been assessed in this way and also for recurrent carcinoma *in situ*. No clear-cut long-term benefit from these approaches has been shown and, in particular, radical irradiation appeared no better than more conservative treatment, in the largest trial yet reported. As Harland and colleagues pointed out, 'The prognosis for this group of patients (with pT1G3NxM0 disease) appears to be poor, irrespective of treatment'. Results of treatment are admittedly difficult to assess because although progression to muscle-invasive disease is common – up to 45% at 5 years – the follow-up time from many of the current studies is still rather short. BCG, first used when because post-mortem studies of patients dying from tuberculosis showed an unexpectedly low rate of malignant disease, is a fairly toxic form of treatment and an EORTC meta-analysis of several studies concluded that there was indeed a benefit, with rates of progression to muscle-invasive disease down from 13.8% to 9.8% at a 2.5 year median follow-up, much of the benefit coming from maintenance treatment see Ref. [29]. More recently, newer techniques such as intravesical interferon have shown promise. Photodynamic therapy has also been attempted, using haematoporphyrin derivatives (taken up by the malignant urothelium) followed by cystoscopy to reveal areas of fluorescence that correlate with areas of histologically proven tumour. The haematoporphyrin derivative can be used as a sensitizing agent for laser ablation.

A recent innovation showing considerable promise is the combination of intravesical BCG and mitomycin given via 'electromotive delivery' [30]. The rationale is based on the idea that BCG induces inflammation, which increases the permeability of the bladder mucosa, allowing more extensive penetration of mitomycin into the target tissues. A catheter electrode is retained in the bladder while a pulsed electric current is given externally over the lower abdomen during delivery of the drug. In the Italian study, over 200 patients were included, with a dramatically different disease-free survival (69 months vs. only 21 months for BCG alone), at a median follow-up of over 7 years.

Muscle-invasive disease

These cases account for about 15% of the total. Treatment for invasive (T2–T3) bladder carcinoma has been considerably refined in recent years, with increasing emphasis on multimodal approaches including transurethral surgery, systemic chemotherapy, improved techniques for radiation therapy and advanced reconstructive techniques following surgical cystectomy. As Kaufman *et al.* [31] have pointed out, 'all have the potential to improve the quality of life and cure the disease' – also see Ref. [32]. Choice of management for most patients usually

lies between a surgical procedure and radiation therapy (increasingly given with neoadjuvant and/or concomitant chemotherapy) or a combination of all modalities. The increasingly important role of chemotherapy is discussed more fully below. In some patients with small lesions located in a mobile portion of the bladder, a successful partial cystectomy may be possible. An adequate cuff of normal bladder should be removed, and the procedure is only recommended where the initial capacity of the remaining bladder is likely to be greater than 300–400 mL. Scrupulous surgical technique is important in order to avoid implantation tumour nodules developing at the anastomosis, and the operation is less widely used than formerly. Interstitial irradiation is an alternative to partial cystectomy in patients with T2 and early T3 lesions. A large study by van der Werf-Messing [33] gave a 5-year survival rate of 40% (T2) and 25% (T3), using interstitial (intravesical) irradiation with radium implants (sometimes with low-dose external irradiation), though her excellent results have proven difficult to replicate elsewhere.

The introduction of a satisfactory method of total cystectomy led in the past to rapid acceptance of this operation as the treatment of choice for many patients with deeply invasive (T3) tumours without extravesical or distant spread. However this procedure involves complete removal of the bladder, prostate and seminal vesicles (or bladder and urethra in the female), although some surgeons, even now, prefer a still more radical approach that combines total cystectomy with a pelvic lymph node dissection. Urinary diversion is usually achieved by fashioning a conduit from a section of resected ileum into which the ureters are implanted and which opens on to the abdominal wall (ileostomy), or by implanting the ureters directly into the sigmoid colon or rectum (Figure 18.9). Unfortunately, complication rates are substantial and reoperation is often necessary. Furthermore, the quality of life in patients undergoing different types of bladder diversion has not been fully investigated [34], and retention of a normal bladder is clearly desirable whenever possible.

Combinations of surgery and chemo-radiotherapy offer superior results to the use of total or radical cystectomy alone, though adverse side-effects have to be carefully considered, particularly in older patients. Recent surgical advances have included more acceptable methods of urinary diversion, including 'continent' types of stoma in which the patient can control the emptying of the urinary conduit by self-catheterization or other techniques, allowing more normal urinary function.

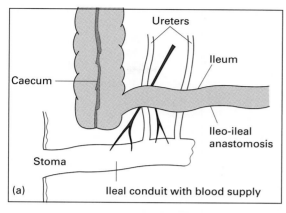

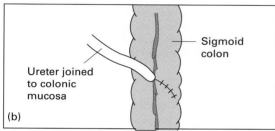

Figure 18.9 Common procedures for ureteric diversion following total cystectomy: (a) formation of an ileal conduit; (b) implantation into sigmoid colon.

A further important advance has been the possibility for the first time of continued sexual potency through careful sparing of critical neurovascular structures [35].

Radiotherapy or surgery?

In view of the effectiveness of radical radiotherapy for carcinoma of the bladder, it seems reasonable to ask whether cystectomy as primary management can be avoided altogether: the controversy rumbles on, though over 30 years ago, a large UK-based cooperative study attempted to answer this question, admittedly before the advent of modern conservative surgical or highly focussed radiotherapy techniques. In this landmark study, nearly 200 patients were allocated to receive either radical radiotherapy alone (60 Gy over 6 weeks) or preoperative irradiation (40 Gy over 4 weeks), followed by radical cystectomy a month later [36]. At 5 years, there was a trend in favour of the group undergoing both radiotherapy and surgery, with a survival rate of 38% compared with 29% for radical radiotherapy. Although the overall result did not achieve statistical significance, the combination

of preoperative irradiation and surgery seemed more effective in younger patients and in males. The difference between the two groups may have been exaggerated because 20% of patients randomized to radiotherapy and surgery could not complete the treatment. After local recurrence with radiotherapy alone, it was possible to perform salvage cystectomy with the impressive result of 52% 5-year survival after cystectomy. Similar results were later reported from centres in the USA and Denmark. More recently, several large groups have reported the results of treatment with radical radiotherapy alone, which increasingly seems closely comparable to those achieved by surgery.

The biological effectiveness of radiotherapy for bladder cancer is also shown by the phenomenon of post-irradiation tumour 'downstaging'. Several studies have shown that the P stage of the excised surgical specimen is frequently lower after radiotherapy than the initial tumour (T) staging would suggest. For example, in the Royal Marsden study, almost half (47%) of the bladder specimens excised after radiotherapy demonstrated this effect [36]. Sterilization of locally involved lymph nodes can also be achieved by radiotherapy, the same study showing an incidence of node metastasis of 23% (the expected proportion would be 40–50% with unirradiated T3 tumours). Only 8% of patients judged to be good responders to radiotherapy had histologically positive local nodes and required cystectomy, suggesting that preoperative irradiation may be particularly useful for those with limited or microscopic regional lymph node deposits. Perhaps the most important result of all was that where downstaging occurred the 5-year survival rate was 51%, whereas in patients who showed no such change the survival at 5 years was only 22%.

Although cystectomy remains a widely practised treatment for T3 tumours, these and other data suggest that radiotherapy (or perhaps, better still, chemo-radiation) may be its equal, with considerable advantages in terms of morbidity [37]. The quality of life for patients with an ileal conduit is clearly less satisfactory than for those who micturate normally. Common additional difficulties include odour, leakage, psychological adjustment to the stoma, and feelings of loss of sexual attractiveness. Many of these problems can be reduced by careful surgical technique but these patients naturally require a great deal of explanation and support preoperatively and postoperatively.

Radical external beam irradiation of bladder cancer requires supervoltage equipment and a multifield preferably conformal technique employing at least three or

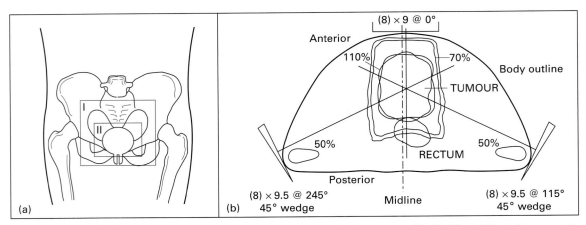

Figure 18.10 Classical external irradiation treatment technique for invasive (T3) carcinoma of the bladder. (a) Vertical representation of treatment volume: (I) for first phase of treatment, bladder and pelvic nodes are treated; (II) for second phase of treatment, the bladder is boosted to radical dose. Phase I is treated with the bladder full to minimize radiation damage to the small bowel. (b) Typical treatment plan in phase II of radical treatment (field sizes in cm). See text for detailed discussion as recent practice has altered.

four fields (Figure 18.10) and expert planning. Newer technologies, including three-dimensional conformal radiotherapy and intensity-modulated radiotherapy, improve the precision of radiotherapy delivery, directing high-dose radiation to the tumour itself rather than the whole bladder. One large UK-wide study (supported by Cancer Research UK) is currently assessing the role of chemo-radiotherapy and whole-bladder radiotherapy with a tumour boost. There is considerable debate as to whether it is essential to treat the local pelvic nodes as well as the bladder itself. Although it is difficult to show improved survival when the pelvic nodes are treated, the demonstration of downstaging as described above certainly strengthens the case. Treatment-related morbidity is greater when the pelvis is treated, even to the relatively modest dose of 40 Gy. With nodal involvement, overall 5-year survival is below 10%, suggesting that the disease is usually disseminated at diagnosis in node-positive cases. There may be a benefit in selected cases for recommending radical cystectomy followed by postoperative radiotherapy [38]. Current studies, including from the Medical Research Council (MRC) and the European Organization for Research and Treatment of Cancer (EORTC), mostly favour the use of neoadjuvant chemotherapy programmes with small-volume irradiation, probably a more logical approach. Chemoresponders may well be the same type of patients who downstaged with pelvic irradiation. Chemotherapy is discussed more fully below.

Apart from the importance of radiation treatment with curative intent, symptoms such as pain, haematuria and frequency usually respond well, and radiotherapy is the most valuable palliative treatment even in advanced (stage IV) tumours where there is virtually no prospect of cure [39].

Role of chemotherapy

The value of systemic chemotherapy for metastatic or advanced bladder cancer has become increasingly recognized over recent years. For example, important work from a large UK-based group has demonstrated a key benefit for the use of concomitant chemo-radiotherapy in muscle-invasive cancer – see Ref. [32]. In this study, the use of a mitomycin-fluorouracil combination significantly improved locoregional control, compared with radiotherapy alone (hazard ratio 0.68, with 5-year survival rates of 48% compared to 35%) – and without significant additional adverse events. It is also widely used for recurrent disease and also as an adjuvant to surgical or radiotherapeutic treatment, but its precise role still remains unclear. In studies from the USA, patients with muscle-invasive bladder cancer have often been treated with bladder-conserving transurethral surgery, combination chemotherapy and radiation therapy with concurrent cisplatin administration. In the Radiation Therapy Oncology Group (RTOG) study [40], 45% of the patients were alive and free of disease, the majority with functioning, tumour-free bladders (4 years follow-up data). Chemotherapy clearly increases complete remission rates in the adjuvant setting, but so far with only minimal detectable benefit in survival [41,42]. However, for many patients, conservative combination treatment will prove a more acceptable alternative to immediate cystectomy. Cisplatin, gemcitabine, cyclophosphamide, doxorubicin, mitomycin C, 5-fluorouracil (5-FU) and methotrexate all produce responses of the order of 20–30%. Many groups have attempted to improve the results still further with combination regimens, but no clear-cut survival advantage has yet been demonstrated although there are recent encouraging early reports. Cisplatin is often regarded as the most active agent, yet the long-term survival results of combination regimens including cisplatin seem to be almost identical with those of cisplatin therapy alone. M-VAC (methotrexate, vinblastine, doxorubicin and cisplatin) was until recently the most popular combination regimen in common use in Europe, but the combination of gemcitabine and cisplatin is almost certainly as effective and has lesser toxicity – see Ref. [43].

There is considerable interest in the concept of neoadjuvant chemotherapy in carcinoma of the bladder. In one of the largest studies so far reported, 376 patients were treated by radiotherapy or cystectomy, with or without neoadjuvant and adjuvant methotrexate [41]. No benefit was seen; indeed the chemotherapy, though relatively simple, proved too toxic for many patients to tolerate. A further British study in patients prospectively randomized to receive neoadjuvant cisplatin (as opposed to no chemotherapy) was also disappointing [42]. However, the results of multimodal therapy (including concomitant cisplatin-based chemotherapy) for muscle-invasive disease are clearly encouraging. For example, in an important study from Canada assessing the value of concomitant chemo-radiation, improved local control was seen in a cohort of 99 patients treated by concurrent cisplatin with preoperative or definitive radiation therapy [44]. With a mean follow-up of 6.5 years, the pelvic relapse rate was 25/48 (no chemotherapy) compared with 15/51 patients with chemotherapy; 3-year survival was 33% and 47%, respectively. However, the largest neoadjuvant chemotherapy randomized trial, with almost 1000 patients recruited internationally, showed a 3-year survival benefit of 5.5% when first published. Updated data with a 7.4-year median follow-up, and a more recently published meta-analysis, both showed a slightly greater effect [45]. The overall survival advantage appears to be of the order of 10–15% with modern neoadjuvant chemotherapy. The doublet combination of gemcitabine and cisplatin is increasingly regarded as the 'gold standard' for neoadjuvant chemotherapy for muscle-invasive bladder cancer – three courses given prior to surgery is a common recommendation though further studies will be required to determine which groups of patients really benefit from such intensive treatment. In less fit patients, carboplatin can be used instead of cisplatin, though it is generally felt that the response rate is slightly lower. At present, chemotherapy for advanced bladder tumours cannot be recommended in every case, particularly since these patients tend to be in poor health and often have impaired renal function. At our own centre, about 50% of potentially suitable patients are treated with chemotherapy, mostly because of frequent morbidity that limits more widespread use.

Prognosis

The likelihood of progression from early-stage superficial low-risk cases to the life-threatening muscle-invasive high-risk situation has been widely studied, and the EORTC have made a major contribution to our understanding – see, for example, Ref. [46]. A nomogram scoring system has been devised, depending on a variety of clinical and pathological factors. Important prognostic determinants include number of tumours identified, tumour size, prior recurrence rate, histological grade, presence of carcinoma *in situ* and so on. T1 tumours have a 5-year survival of about 75% with surgery alone, and it is becoming clear that smokers do less well, tending to present at a younger age and with more advanced and higher-grade tumours – see Ref. [47]. About 50% of all patients with invasive bladder cancer survive for 5 years, clearly stage-related. In T2 and early T3 lesions, the 5-year survival is 35%, while with more advanced disease, particularly where there is nodal involvement at diagnosis, only 10–15% will survive. There are virtually no long-term survivors when distant metastases are present at diagnosis. Adjuvant chemotherapy had not until recently contributed to a significant improvement in these long-term results, although chemotherapy is clearly more valuable if used concomitantly in a combined concurrent chemo-radiation programme [44,48], as is the case with so many other solid tumours treated with this approach. We await with interest the results of trials of more powerful chemotherapy regimens together with higher-dose radiotherapy, based on better precision and technical planning now routinely possible with equipment advances.

Table 18.3 World age-standardized incidence and mortality rates per 100 000 male population, world regions. 2008 estimates.

World region	Incidence rate	World region	Mortality rate
Australia/ New Zealand	104.2	Australia/ New Zealand	15.4
Western Europe	93.1	Western Europe	12.4
Northern America	85.6	Northern America	9.9
Northern Europe	73.1	Northern Europe	15.4
Caribbean	71.1	Caribbean	26.3
Southern Africa	53.9	Southern Africa	19.3
South America	50.2	South America	16.2
Southern Europe	50	Southern Europe	10.4
Central America	34.8	Central America	12.6
Central and Eastern Europe	29.1	Central and Eastern Europe	10.9
World	28	World	7.5
Western Africa	22.2	Western Africa	18.3
Middle Africa	16.4	Middle Africa	13.4
Eastern Africa	14.5	Eastern Africa	11.7
Western Asia	13.8	Western Asia	7.5
South-Eastern Asia	8.3	South-Eastern Asia	5.1
Eastern Asia	8.2	Eastern Asia	2.5
Northern Africa	8.1	Northern Africa	6.2
South-Central Asia	4.1	South-Central Asia	2.8

Carcinoma of the prostate

Incidence and aetiology

There are substantial worldwide variations in the incidence of carcinoma of the prostate (Table 18.3), which is among the commonest of all cancers in men (see Figure 18.1). In the UK, it accounts for about a quarter of all male cancer; almost 41 000 new cases were diagnosed in 2010, and it is the third largest cause of death from cancer in males, exceeded only by deaths from cancer of the lung and large bowel. In 2001, there were an estimated 198 000 new cases in the USA; in the UK, 20 000 new cases were recorded in 1997 (European Union 134 000 new cases), so the rise over the past 15 years

has been remarkable though largely of course due to 'ascertainment bias' following an increase over that same period of screening and prompt biopsy in men whose PSA is outside the normal range. A similar picture holds true in the USA, where the current incidence is up a total of 240 000 men in the USA (2011 figures), and with almost 34 000 deaths that same year. From the USA statistics, both incidence and mortality are considerably higher in black men than in white men [49]. In the USA, England, Australia and Japan there is strong evidence to suggest an increasing incidence and mortality during the past 50 years [50] and the current death rate is 1520 per 100 000 men. The positive autopsy rate for unexpected prostatic cancer is of the order of 30% in men over 50 years.

We are gradually learning more about the aetiology of prostatic carcinoma [51]. Its incidence increases in first-generation males after migration from a less prevalent to a more prevalent (and usually more socially affluent) area. This might suggest that change of diet could be an important potential culprit, particularly the intake of animal fats and red meat. Alternatively, there have been suggestions that the specifics of food components may be less important than the obesity which a Western diet so often produces. Other potential aetiological factors such as smoking, alcohol intake, vasectomy and physical activity have now all been excluded. Finally, the possible role of non-steroidal anti-inflammatory drugs has suggested a possible protective effect. A report from Canada, using a case-control design with over 2000 prostate cancer cases, showed a clear negative trend between cumulative duration of aspirin use and prostate cancer risk, with an 18% reduction over 8 years [52]. Growth of prostate cancer is stimulated by androgens and the cancer does not occur in castrated men. It is also thought to be less common in hepatic cirrhosis which is accompanied by impaired oestrogen degradation. Susceptible families occur, with a substantial inherited component in 5–10% of cases. It has also been suggested that factors operating in prenatal life may have an important aetiological influence, both prematurity and pre-eclampsia being inversely associated with incidence [53].

Somatic gene defects in prostatic cancer

At the time of diagnosis, prostate cancer cells contain many somatic mutations, gene deletions, gene amplifications, chromosomal rearrangements and changes in DNA methylation [51]. These alterations probably accumulate over a period of several decades. The most commonly reported chromosomal abnormalities appear to be gains at 7p, 7q, 8q and Xq, and losses at 8p, 10q, 13q and 16q. A striking heterogeneity in chromosomal abnormalities has been seen in different cases, in different lesions in the same case, and in different areas within the same lesion, and seven loci have been identified associated with prostate cancer on chromosomes 3, 6, 7, 10, 11, 19 and X ($P = 2.7 \times 10^{-8}$ to $P = 8.7 \times 10^{-29}$). Previous reports have confirmed common loci associated with prostate cancer at 8q24 and 17q (see Refs. [54,55]). Additional somatic genomic alterations appear to arise in association with the progression of prostate cancer. Mutations in the *TP53* gene, which are present in a minority of primary prostate cancers, may undergo clonal selection in the process of progression to metastatic prostate cancer.

Screening

Because of the frequency of prostatic carcinoma and its clear age relation, screening among unselected elderly males has increasingly been attempted, generally employing regular prostate-specific antigen (PSA) testing (see below) and clinical examination by digital rectal prostatic palpation [56,57]. The detection rate is of the order of 1%, but the majority of cases are confined to the prostate, strengthening the rationale. Regular testing for PSA clearly increases the sensitivity but an important study from the USA has provided data suggesting that screening and early detection are difficult to justify at present [58]. Data from the Surveillance, Epidemiology and End Results (SEER) Program of the National Cancer Institute were analysed, particularly with respect to assessment of national and regional trends. The incidence of prostate cancer rose dramatically during the two decades 1973–1994, but at a far greater rate than mortality, suggesting that earlier detection is now routinely taking place. However, because of lead-time bias and other factors, the benefits of screening and early detection remain unproven. The drawbacks are unequivocal, since the risk and harms of screening and resultant treatment are definite [59,60]. In the Cochrane database meta-analysis and review published in 2013, over 340 000 men were included in study. The conclusion was sobering to say the least: 'Prostate cancer screening did not significantly decrease prostate cancer-specific mortality in a combined meta-analysis of five RCTs. Only one study reported a 21% significant reduction of prostate cancer-specific mortality in a pre-specified subgroup of men aged 55 to 69 years. Pooled data currently demonstrates no significant reduction in prostate cancer-specific and overall mortality. Harms associated with PSA-based screening and subsequent diagnostic

evaluations are frequent, and moderate in severity. Overdiagnosis and overtreatment are common and are associated with treatment-related harms. Men should be informed of this and the demonstrated adverse effects when they are deciding whether or not to undertake screening for prostate cancer. Any reduction in prostate cancer-specific mortality may take up to 10 years to accrue; therefore, men who have a life expectancy less than 10 to 15 years should be informed that screening for prostate cancer is unlikely to be beneficial'. Nonetheless, an important study from Scandinavia confirmed that at 10 years, the routine use of biennial PSA screening reduced the risk of diagnosis of metastatic carcinoma of the prostate 1.8-fold, an impressive result that would be expected to lead to a genuine survival advantage [61]. On the other hand, this was balanced by a rise in the diagnosis of earlier-stage cancer which might never have required intervention if not diagnosed in the first place. It is important to remember, as pointed out, for example, by Hoffman [62], that 'The great majority of men with a diagnosis of prostate cancer die from other causes. Autopsy series suggest that 30% of men older than 50 years of age and 70% of those older than 70 years of age have occult prostate cancer' – a sobering thought, and in principle, profoundly challenging news for enthusiastic proponents of screening and early surgical intervention in fit healthy men with no symptoms. Without doubt, screening for prostate cancer remains one of the most controversial areas in cancer healthcare economics; many prominent organizations in the USA have developed active screening policies, often leading to early intervention, even though many men have a low risk of death even during 20 years of follow-up, provided the prostatic cancer is of low pathological grade. Despite this general point, information from SEER and Medicare claims suggests that in men already diagnosed with prostate cancer, the 10-year risk of death from competing causes are consistently higher, almost 60%, regardless of the tumour grade. It has been estimated, for example, that over 1900 prostatic biopsies are required to save a single life in men with a PSA level below 3 ng/mL (see Refs. [63,64]). Nonetheless, in the future it will doubtless become possible through testing for genetic susceptibility to identify high-risk individuals and offer the prospect of secondary prevention through regular screening and earlier treatment – see, for example, Eeles *et al.* [54,55] (whose recent study demonstrated 23 new prostate cancer susceptibility loci, taking us several steps further forward). An enticing alternative is to consider pharmacological prevention using a bioactive but well-tolerated agent in susceptible patients (i.e. beyond a certain age and also undergoing regular PSA screening through personal preference. One such agent is finasteride, a 5-alpha-reductase inhibitor; however, although this has been demonstrated as active in reducing the relative risk of developing prostate cancer, probably by at least one-quarter, no convincing long-term therapeutic benefit has yet been established – see, for example, Ref. [65].

Pathology and staging

Adenocarcinoma is overwhelmingly the most common cell type, although TCC may arise in the large prostatic ducts. Other unusual types include squamous, mucinous, carcinoid and small-cell carcinomas. Three-quarters of all prostatic cancers arise in the posterior or peripheral part of the prostate, and about 10% are discovered during prostatectomy for apparently benign prostatic hypertrophy. These tend to be more localized than when the diagnosis of carcinoma is suspected clinically.

Histological grading is of considerable importance, though the majority of prostatic cancers are moderately well differentiated. The incidence of lymph node metastases increases with the degree of anaplasia and there is no doubt that patients with low-grade lesions survive substantially longer (60% 5-year survival compared with 5% 5-year survival for patients with high-grade lesions).

No clinical or surgical staging system has yet found universal acceptance. The pattern of local invasion is shown schematically in Figure 18.11. The TNM system is increasingly employed (Table 18.4), but can be difficult in practice, particularly in determination of the T stage of the tumour. For this and other reasons, the UICC TNM staging criteria were revised in 1987. Even the more recent TNM system has not found wide acceptance. The widely used American system is simpler and correlates fairly closely with the TNM staging. Increasing attention is now paid to the pathological details of the prostatic specimen. The most widely used system is that

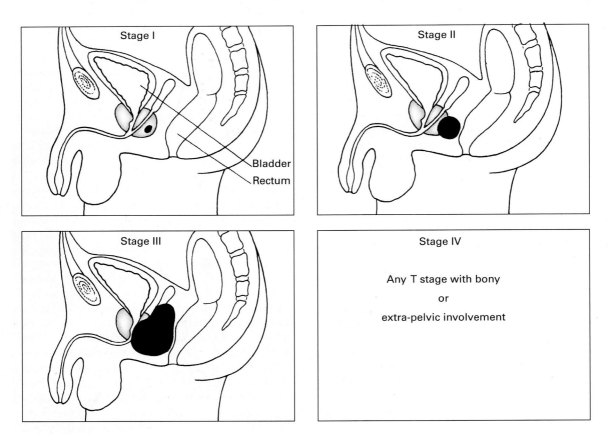

Figure 18.11 Local extension and clinical staging in carcinoma of the prostate.

Table 18.4 Staging systems for carcinoma of the prostate.

UICC 1978/1982	AUS stage	UICC 1987
T0 Occult carcinoma	A Ocullat carcinoma A1 One lobe A2 Multifocal or diffuse	T1 Incidental T1a Three foci or less T1b More than three foci
T1 Intracapsular tumour		
	B Confined to prostate B1 One lobe B2 Diffuse	T2 Clinically or grossly limited to gland T1a 1.5 cm T2b > 1.5 cm/more than one lobe
T2 The tumour can be felt (palpated) on examination, but has not spread outside the prostate		
T3 Extraprostatic extension	C Extracapsular extension	T3 Invades prostatic apex/beyond capsule/bladder neck/seminal vesical, not fixed
T4 Fixed invading adjacent organs		
T4 Fixed or invades other adjacent structures		
N1 Single regional node involved	D1 Pelvic node metastasis	N1 Single = 2 cm
N2 Multiregional nodes	N2 Single, 2–5 cm; multiple, 5 cm	
N3 Fixed node mass		
N4 Juxtaregional nodes		
M1 Distant metastasis	D2 Distant metastasis	M1 Distant metastasis

Stage grouping

Stage I	T1, T2a	N0	M0
Stage II	T2b, T2c	N0	M0
Stage III	T3	N0	M0
Stage IV	T4	N0	M0
	Any T	N1	M0
	Any	Any N	M1

Summary

Prostate

T1	Not palpable or visible
T1a	≤ 5%
T1b	< 5%
T1c	Needle biopsy
T2	Confined within prostate
T2a	≤One-half of one lobe
T2b	More than one-half of one lobe
T2c	Both lobes
T3	Through prostatic capsule
T3a	Extracapsular
T3b	Seminal vesicle(s)
T4	Fixed or invades adjacent structures: external sphincter, rectum, levator muscles, pelvic wall
N1	Regional lymph node(s)
M1a	Non-regional lymph node(s)
M1b	Bone(s)
M1c	Other site(s)

Table 18.4 (*continued*)

Prognostic grouping					
Group I	T1a–c	N0	M0	PSA < 10	Gleason ≤ 6
	T2a	N0	M0	PSA < 10	Gleason ≤ 6
Group IIA	T1a–c	N0	M0	PSA < 20	Gleason 7
	T1a–c	N0	M0	PSA ≥ 0 < 20	Gleason ≤ 6
	T2a	N0	M0	PSA ≥ 0 < 20	Gleason ≤ 6
	T2a	N0	M0	PSA < 20	Gleason 7
	T2b	N0	M0	PSA < 20	Gleason ≤ 7
Group IIB	T2c	N0	M0	Any PSA	Any Gleason
	T1–2	N0	M0	PSA ≥ 20	Any Gleason
	T1–2	N0	M0	Any PSA	Gleason ≥ 8
Group II	T3a, b	N0	M0	Any PSA	Any Gleason
Group IV	T4	N0	M0	Any PSA	Any Gleason
	Any T	N1	M0	Any PSA	Any Gleason
	Any T	Any N	M1	Any PSA	Any Gleason

Note: When either PSA or Gleason is not available, grouping should be determined by T category and whichever of either PSA or Gleason is available. When neither is available and prognostic grouping is not possible, use stage grouping.
AUS, American Urological Society; UICC, *Union International Contre le Cancer.*

of Gleason which was devised over 20 years ago for the USA-based Veterans' Administration Cooperative Urological Research Group (VACURG) [66]. The grades are shown below.

Grade 1: well-differentiated carcinoma with uniform gland pattern.

Grade 2: well-differentiated carcinoma with glands varying in size and shape.

Grade 3: moderately differentiated carcinoma with either (a) irregular acini often widely separated; or (b) well-defined papillary/cribriform structures. This is the commonest pattern seen in carcinoma of the prostate.

Grade 4: poorly differentiated carcinoma with fused glands widely infiltrating the prostatic stroma. Neoplastic cells may grow in cords or sheets and the cytoplasm is clear.

Grade 5: very poorly differentiated carcinoma with no or minimal gland formation. Tumour cell masses may have central necrosis.

About half of all tumours exhibit more than a single pattern. The commonest pattern (the primary) and the less common pattern (the secondary) can be recorded separately or can be summed to produce an average pattern called the pattern score (often simply termed the *Gleason score* or *index*) which correlates well with mortality [67].

Clinical and pathological characteristics have proven to be a fairly accurate reflection of the true degree of spread. Where radical prostatectomy has been performed and the specimen carefully analysed, close agreement between surgical and clinical findings is discovered in about three-quarters of all cases, although sometimes with unsuspected local invasion, usually of the seminal vesicles. Invasion of pelvic lymph nodes may be clinically silent but is increasingly likely with advanced stages of disease as the prostate has an unusually rich lymph node network. Drainage is most commonly to the obturator/hypogastric group and then to the external and common iliac nodes. Distant metastases are predominantly osseous, particularly to the pelvic and lower lumbar vertebrae, though ribs, dorsal spine and skull are not uncommonly involved. The bone metastases are typically osteosclerotic, as a result of the relatively slow clinical evolution of disease, although the pattern may be chiefly lytic or mixed.

Clinical features and investigation

Prostatic carcinoma is often asymptomatic, and is increasingly diagnosed at routine rectal examination. The typical finding is a firm, indurated or craggy gland which is usually enlarged. There may be obliteration of the median sulcus or spread to the lateral pelvic walls.

Many patients present with bone pain from secondary deposits, particularly in the back and pelvis.

In patients with local prostatic symptoms, the commonest complaints are urinary infection or obstruction, with changes in the urinary stream including hesitancy or urgency of micturition.

Histological diagnosis is always required and transrectal biopsy is widely favoured. If fragments from a transurethral resection of a hypertrophic gland show evidence of malignancy, further confirmation is not usually necessary. Other methods of biopsy include the perineal or retropubic routes. The PSA level is likely to be elevated (see below).

It is important to assess the local extent of disease as well as the presence of distant metastases in order to decide on the correct treatment, and to identify cases in which a local approach to treatment could be curative. An isotope bone scan should always be done since bone metastases are often asymptomatic, particularly in the skull, ribs and upper part of the vertebral column, and particularly if radical surgery is under consideration. Skeletal radiographs give further details of these deposits. Routine tests of renal function are often revealing, and IVU may show prostatic irregularity and back-pressure on the kidneys.

For patients who are candidates for surgery or radiotherapy of the primary tumour (with curative intent), it is essential to determine the full extent of local disease. Despite initial enthusiasm, routine lymphography has not become an established part of pretreatment investigation, since false-positive and false-negative results are not uncommon. CT scanning is more useful for detecting unsuspected nodal metastases, and also gives more detailed information regarding local extent of disease, particularly with respect to the degree of periprostatic invasion. However, it is not generally considered to be as valuable an investigation as it is with bladder cancer.

PSA has increasingly been employed as a valuable tumour marker, with a fairly good correlation between PSA level and extent of disease. If patients with localized disease are treated by radical prostatectomy, the concentration of PSA should fall to zero, the PSA level then proving extremely valuable if serially measured. An interesting new marker with potential clinical value, insulin-like growth factor (IGF)-1, has recently been reported by Chan *et al.* [68]. In this case-control study of men aged 40–82 years, the important finding was that those in the top quartile level for IGF-1 were over four times more likely to develop prostate cancer than those in the lowest quartile. The quartile correlation persisted with both low- and high-grade cancers, and was especially marked in patients over the age of 60. Since IGF-1 is a hormone that both stimulates cell growth and inhibits

natural cell death (apoptosis), high concentrations might act by encouraging rapid cell turnover, increasing the risk of random malignant transformation in the epithelial cells of the prostate. Other studies have now validated this initial observation.

The most important prognostic factors include initial performance status using standard scales (Karnofsky or ECOG), initial PSA level, Gleason score and T category. Some of these factors apply even in patients with evidence of advanced disease at diagnosis. The likelihood of local progression of disease is 25%, 50% and 75% (10 years) for well-differentiated (Gleason score < 4), moderately differentiated (Gleason score 5–7) and poorly differentiated (Gleason score > 7) tumours, respectively. The rapidity of reduction in PSA levels after therapy is also relevant. In patients with extensive disease, soft-tissue secondary sites may possibly be more responsive than bony sites to some types of hormone manipulation.

Management and results of radical treatment

There are a few areas in clinical cancer management where such diversity of opinion exists, even among experts [69–74]. Most would agree that with clinically localized prostatic cancer, without evidence of bone or extrapelvic metastases, an attempt at curative therapy should be made [69]. However, some experts take the view that the true incidence of early (T1) disease is so low that a localized approach is never really justifiable, preferring palliative methods of treatment in many such cases [70]. More aggressive surgeons are prepared to consider radical prostatectomy even in patients with local periprostatic extension (up to stage III disease), sometimes using hormonal treatment to produce tumour shrinkage preoperatively.

There are two possible approaches to treatment with curative intent: radical prostatectomy or radical radiotherapy. The radical surgical approach has evolved since the turn of the century, and currently consists of *en bloc* resection of the prostate, prostatic urethra and seminal vesicles with part of the surrounding connective tissue (Denonvillier's fascia). Only patients with the disease confined within the prostatic capsule and without lymph node metastasis are considered suitable, and the operation has always been more popular in the USA than in the UK. The surgical approach can be either retropubic or perineal. The suprapubic approach also allows for pelvic lymphadenectomy, if appropriate. Complications are discussed below. Over the past few years, surgical techniques have evolved rapidly, with the increasing use of laparoscopic operative approaches, and even robotic surgery. This fascinating methodology has the advantages of less perioperative pain and other complications, faster recovery and hospital discharge, less internal scarring and reduced postoperative sexual dysfunction. Over 40 000 such procedures have now been performed worldwide. Traditionally, following radical surgery, additional or adjuvant approaches such as hormonal therapy or radiotherapy have only been used in patients with evidence of disease recurrence. In support of this, for example, the large Early Prostate Cancer (EPC) study of 4400 men following radical prostatectomy, involving randomization to bicalutamide 150 mg daily or no treatment, showed no evidence at over 7 years' follow-up of any difference in survival, though admittedly this was a very low-risk group [71].

Radical radiation therapy, though more recently introduced, is certainly more widely applicable than surgery since minimal extracapsular extension or periprostatic invasion do not present major technical problems. Radical surgery demands a greater general level of medical fitness than radiotherapy. The normal prostate tolerates a high dosage of radiation, although excessive irradiation of surrounding tissues (bladder, prostatic urethra or large bowel) can cause serious problems (see Chapter 5).

In patients suitable for radical radiotherapy, a high dosage has to be given to the whole of the gland and periprostatic area. Although interstitial approaches using radium implants into the gland were initially employed by early workers, external beam irradiation is now usually preferred (but see below). There is a general agreement that a total dose of at least 70 Gy over 7 weeks (or equivalent over a shorter period) is required for eradication of prostatic cancer and even higher doses have been increasingly recommended. Some radiation oncologists (though far fewer than, say, 25 years ago) recommend irradiation to the pelvis as well as the prostate bed, because of the possibility of unsuspected periprostatic or lymphatic spread. As with bladder cancer, the appropriate choice of volume for treatment of prostatic cancer remains contentious [72]. Radiotherapists who prefer to avoid treatment of the pelvic contents, apart from the tumour bed itself, point to the lack of survival advantage in patients in whom prophylactic pelvic node irradiation has been undertaken. Avoiding irradiation of the whole pelvic contents often has the advantage of allowing a safer high dose to the main area of concern, the primary tumour itself. A variety of techniques have been used to achieve these high dosages. Multifield arrangements are invariably required, often

by preference using super-voltage equipment. Radical treatment using conformal or intensity-modulated radiation therapy is increasingly employed in order to reduce rectal side-effects (proctitis and rectal bleeding) [72–75]. Recent work from the MRC urology trials group in the UK showed that dose-escalated conformal radiotherapy with neoadjuvant androgen suppression provides considerably better prostate cancer control than conventional standard-dose conformal therapy but, perhaps not surprisingly, at a cost of greater side-effects [75]. This was a large randomized trial (843 men, all with localized disease), which confirmed a 5-year biochemical progression-free survival rate of 71% in the higher-dose group, compared with 60% in the standard-dose group. Significant additional side-effects included bowel dysfunction, together with late gastrointestinal and genitourinary toxicity, which was felt by the authors to offset the clinical advantage in terms of tumour control. With results now emerging for the important Anglo-Canadian PR3/PR07 trial of radiotherapy, it has become increasingly clear that for men with locally advanced or organ-confined prostate cancer, radical radiotherapy treatment + androgen deprivation reduces the risk of death by about half (as compared with treatment by androgen deprivation alone), a most important and encouraging result – see Ref. [76]; this study was fully updated at an ASCO presentation in 2012. At this update presentation it became clear that the risk of dying (measured at the 10 year point) from prostatic cancer (cause-specific deaths only) was reduced from 25% to 15%.

An alternative approach, receiving increasing attention, is the use of permanent interstitial implants, usually employing ^{125}I seeds, to the prostate (and periprostatic area if necessary) (Figure 18.12). This treatment delivers a very high local dose (in excess of 160 Gy) with remarkably low morbidity, and has become popular over the past 5 years [77]. A summary of treatment results is given in Table 18.5. Other promising new approaches include the use of temporary, high-dose rate intraprostatic brachytherapy, generally with ^{192}Ir line sources; and photodynamic therapy, again using intraprostatic implantation under direct vision.

The point has repeatedly been made that it is exceptionally difficult to assess the results of radical treatment for carcinoma of the prostate, because of its uncertain and often indolent natural history and the high death rate in any group of elderly men [78,79]. However, an important recent study from the MRC strongly supported the concept of early rather than delayed intervention,

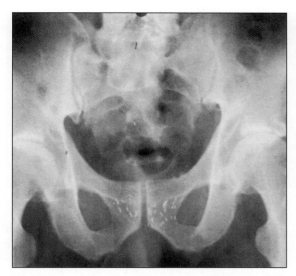

Figure 18.12 Transperineal interstitial implantation of the prostate. [125]I seeds are used to obtain a high local dose (in excess of 160 Gy). Intrarectal ultrasound is used for localization of the gland, avoiding the need for open operation.

Table 18.5 Results for early-stage prostate cancer. Each of these three methods of treatment is widely used but in the absence of formal randomized prospective studies the patient groups are unlikely to be strictly comparable.

	Patients	End-point	10-year result (%)
Radical retropubic prostatectomy			
Mayo Clinic	3170	PSA < 2 µg/L	52
Washington University	925	PSA < 6 µg/L	61
Johns Hopkins	2404	PSA < 2 µg/L	74
South Carolina/Baylor	1000	PSA < 4 µg/L	75
External beam radiotherapy			
Massachusetts General Hospital	1396	PSA control*	42
M.D. Anderson	643	PSA control*	61[†]
Fox Chase	408	PSA control‡	59[†]
Pooled institution analysis	1218	PSA control‡	68
Low-dose brachytherapy			
Northwest Prostate Institute	229	PSA control§	70
Arizona	695	PSA control§	71¶
Seattle (palladium-103 sources)	233	PSA control‡	83**
Seattle (iodine-125 sources)	125	PSA control‡	85

*Defined as prostate-specific antigen (PSA) < 10 µg/L and absence of two consecutive rises in PSA after nadir.
[†]Eight-year results.
‡Defined as absence of two consecutive rises in PSA after nadir.
§Using consensus definition of biochemical failure as three consecutive PSA rises after nadir.
¶Five-year results.
**Nine-year results.
Source: Jani and Hellman [73]. Reproduced with permission from Elsevier.

even for patients with advanced disease [80]. Following radical surgery, a disease-free survival rate comparable to the expected survival for men of similar ages has been claimed, although generally these series have been unrandomized and/or historically controlled [78–81].

Several centres have reported large series of patients treated by radiotherapy, in whom a proportion appear to have been controlled for lengthy periods, or even cured although 'cure' is difficult to define in the elderly population. One substantial study of 145 patients with localized cancers treated by surgical staging (lymphadenectomy, but without radical resection of the prostate) and radical radiation therapy reported as follows: at 15 and 20 years' follow-up, the actuarial survival was 46% and 25%; the cause-specific survival was 64.5% and 38% [82]. In following up these patients, it is important to realize that, in the irradiated prostate, subsequent biopsy may show evidence of persistent malignant cells for up to a year, without any supportive clinical suggestion that the treatment has failed. Up to 60% of patients with locally advanced disease may have positive biopsies up to 9 months after treatment, falling to only 24% at 12–30 months, without further treatment. Attempts at producing guidelines for treatment of clinically localized prostatic carcinoma have concluded that outcomes from both surgery and radiotherapy are essentially similar, or at least that current data are inadequate to make a clear

recommendation [83]. Patient preference is extremely important. Interestingly, and unlike the MRC report [80], surveillance for low- or intermediate-grade localized tumours resulted in 'only a marginal compromise of disease-specific survival at 5–10 years of follow-up'.

Treatment side-effects are summarized in Table 18.6. Complications of radical surgical treatment include

Table 18.6 Relative complication rates from local control treatments for prostate cancer.

Site	Prostatectomy	External beam radiotherapy	Brachytherapy	External beam radiotherapy and brachytherapy
Rectal	+	+++	+	++
Sexual (impotence)	+++	++	+	++
Urinary incontinence	+++	+	+	+
Urinary retention	+	+	+++	+++

Source: Jani and Hellman [73]. Reproduced with permission from Elsevier.

an operative mortality rate of 1.5–5%, permanent impotence in a large majority of patients (unless treated by nerve-sparing procedures, see below), frequency of micturition and urinary incontinence of about 10–15%. Rectovesical fistula and ureteric damage may also occur. Important complications of radical radiotherapy include diarrhoea, dysuria and perineal skin reaction (sometimes severe), and long-term sequelae include subcutaneous fibrosis, urethral stricture and fibrotic reduction of bladder capacity. Treatment with a full bladder may help to keep the small bowel out of the irradiated volume. The relatively lower level of impotence as a side-effect of radical radiotherapy is a valuable advantage, since this is almost certain to occur with radical surgery or hormonal treatment for prostatic cancer unless specific nerve-sparing surgical techniques are used. However, even with radical prostatic irradiation, impotence rates of up to 50% have been reported. The introduction of the nerve-sparing radical prostatectomy has led during the past decade to an enormous increase in the popularity of surgical treatment for localized carcinoma of the prostate, at least in the USA [84]. Additional surgical approaches for attempting to reduce side-effects include laparoscopic surgery and/or intraoperative nerve stimulation. Cryoablation and high-intensity focused ultrasound are also under assessment. Quality-of-life issues are now being recognized as increasingly important in assessing outcomes (see, for example, Ref. [85]). An important recent report from the Prostate Cancer Outcomes Study showed that functional outcomes – urinary incontinence and erectile dysfunction – after radical radiotherapy were superior at 2 and 5 years, but the rates at 15 years were equal – see Ref. [86].

Despite the wealth of data relating to aggressive management of early prostatic carcinoma, a policy of watchful waiting still has many advocates, particularly in patients with a low Gleason score (< 6) and low PSA (< 10 ng/mL, with a doubling time of more than 3 years). However, recent evidence from a 20-year Swedish study suggests that this may be unwise, because local progression and aggressive metastatic disease may develop even after 15 years [87]. The study followed 223 patients with early-stage localized prostate cancer. They received no initial treatment if the cancer was localized to the prostate. If the cancer progressed to symptomatic disease, patients were treated with oestrogens or orchidectomy. During the first 15 years, most cancers followed an indolent course: 25 (11%) of patients died of prostate cancer; 10 more died during follow-up. However, follow-up from 15 to 20 years showed a substantial decrease in cumulative progression-free survival (from 45% to 36%), survival without metastases (from 76.9% to 51.2%), and prostate-cancer-specific survival (from 78.7% to 54.4%). Mortality from prostate cancer increased from 15 (95% CI 10–21) per 1000 person-years during the first 15 years to 44 (95% CI 22–88) per 1000 person-years beyond 15 years of follow-up ($P = 0.01$). At least one recent study has shown that the rate of rise of preoperative PSA levels provides a useful prediction of outcome following radical prostatectomy [88]. And finally, greatly adding fuel to the controversy regarding the wisdom of early radical treatment with its many potential life-quality diminishing side-effects, the Prostate Cancer Intervention versus Observation Trial (PIVOT) study (PIVOT, 731 patients enrolled) has now reported its long-term follow-up results – see Ref. [89]. In this important trial, for men with localized cancer, and with the stated primary and secondary outcomes of all-cause and prostate-cancer-specific mortality, neither of these metrics was significantly reduced by radical prostatectomy as compared with observation, although those with a high PSA at presentation (above 10 ng/ml) comprising a group of 251 men (i.e. about a third of the total) did appear to benefit from radical surgery – with a prostate cancer-specific mortality of 5.6% compared with 12.8% in the surveillance group. Put another way, however, even this more adverse subset had about an 87% chance of remaining alive free of cancer at 12 years following diagnosis, with no radical treatment and no side-effects: more food for thought – and see also an excellent brief summary of the current position, at least as viewed from the UK, by Parker [90]. Needless to say, the controversy continues, but the tide seems to have turned against routine annual PSA testing, which seemed so popular just a decade ago, particularly in the USA – see, for example, Ref. [91]. More consideration is now being given to risk categorization: as Parker [90] points out, 'Using PSA testing alone to select men for biopsy has led to an epidemic of low-risk prostate cancer. Patient selection for biopsy using a risk calculator to estimate individual risk of serious cancer reduces unnecessary biopsies and the detection of low risk disease'.

Hormonal therapy and chemotherapy

In 1941, Huggins and Hodges discovered that prostatic cancers were almost always hormonally dependent [92]. Both oestrogen therapy and orchidectomy were found to be useful for palliation, particularly for bone metastases. Since the majority of patients are unsuitable for radical surgery, the use of oestrogen derivatives or orchidectomy was widely employed as a standard therapy for both early and advanced cases. Other oestrogen-related agents such as estramustine (an oestrogen with a nitrogen mustard moiety at position C-17) became briefly popular but are probably no better than diethylstilbestrol. We now know of course far more about the role of the androgen receptor, which is primarily responsible for mediating the effects of the hypothalamo-pituitary-gonadal axis on prostate growth. This is a cytoplasmic steroid receptor which forms a circulating complex with heat-shock protein-90 and on androgen binding, undergoes conformational change to allow nuclear transformation, thus driving gene transcription (see Ref. [93]).

Hormonal manipulation is used as definitive treatment for advanced disease (stages III and IV), although many oncologists offer local irradiation to patients with stage III disease who have no evidence of metastases elsewhere, if the clinical condition warrants an attempt at radical treatment.

The increasing availability of newer forms of androgen-ablating hormone therapy has widened the options, but their side-effects and acceptability differ.

However, it remains unclear whether the type of hormone therapy critically influences overall outcome, and also whether combined antiandrogen therapy is superior to single-agent or sequential treatment. Analogues of gonadotrophin-releasing hormone, called luteinizing hormone releasing hormone agonists, interfere with gonadotrophin release, leading to a fall in circulating testosterone. They initially produce an increase in luteinizing hormone and follicle-stimulating hormone levels, followed over a 1–2 week period by down regulation of surface receptors leading to chemically mediated castrate levels of testosterone. Hormonal agents include goserelin (Zoladex), a depot form of gonadotrophin-releasing hormone analogue, and flutamide [94], a pure antiandrogen that interferes with testosterone binding to the androgen receptor. Both of these, together with more traditional forms of hormone therapy (oestrogen derivatives, orchidectomy), appear to have similar response rates, though the analogue agents have fewer cardiovascular complications and are superior to diethylstilbestrol. Flutamide is probably similar in its mechanism of action to cyproterone acetate, which was introduced earlier (1973) and is also widely used. One advantage of treatment with flutamide and other non-steroidal pure antiandrogens over diethylstilbestrol is the potential for preservation of potency, but side-effects can be troublesome and include gynaecomastia, disturbances of hepatic function and gastrointestinal toxicity; half-life is short so multiple daily doses are necessary. Unlike the progesterone-like cyproterone acetate, these agents do not lead to central inhibition of luteinizing hormone release. Since they block negative testosterone feedback, increased serum levels of testosterone occur. Newer agents also include degarelix, an LHRH antagonist which binds competitively to pituitary LHRH receptors, reducing the level of luteinizing hormone without the initial testosterone flare – see Ref. [95].

Total androgen blockade, using combinations of hormonal agents in an attempt to block both testicular and adrenal output, has also been tested in several randomized controlled studies [96,97]. In patients with advanced disease, there appears to be a very small benefit: combinations of a gonadotrophin-releasing hormone analogue and an antiandrogen such as flutamide are generally employed. A large EORTC study confirmed an improved disease-free and overall survival with total androgen blockade during (and for 3 years after) external irradiation in patients with locally advanced disease [97]. More recently, work in this area has largely centred on the important question of whether intermittent androgen suppression for patients with a post-treatment rising PSA level, indicative of relapse, is a safe approach – as compared with the more demanding continuous therapy – see, for example, Ref. [98]. This issue is of course of profound importance for maintaining the patient's quality of life, a key objective in this group, and the current prevailing view is that intermittent androgen deprivation appears to be safe for a large proportion of those who prefer to be treated this way. Recent work has also suggested that more abbreviated courses of androgen blockade, perhaps of the order of 18 months, may somewhat unexpectedly be sufficient, and equal in efficacy to more extended programmes – perhaps yet another example of 'the law of diminishing returns'.

In palliative treatment of metastatic prostatic cancer, radiotherapy has an important role for painful bone metastases. These generally respond well to moderate doses of radiotherapy. In recent years, single-fraction hemibody irradiation has been increasingly used since widespread metastases in the lower spine are so common. Treatment of the lower half of the body to a single fraction dose of 7.5 – 10 Gy is well tolerated and often dramatically effective for pain relief.

In patients with widespread metastatic problems unresponsive to oestrogens or palliative irradiation, bilateral orchidectomy should be considered since worthwhile responses often occur. Patients with hormone-resistant prostatic carcinoma have particular problems [99] and long-term survival is unlikely, though it does seem important to keep the patient androgen-depleted. If antiandrogen treatment is withdrawn, testosterone levels may rise and survival may be shortened, especially in patients receiving gonadotrophin-releasing hormone analogues.

Chemotherapy for prostatic carcinoma has in the past been disappointing although a number of agents show modest levels of activity, including methotrexate, 5-FU, mitoxantrone, the taxanes (notably docetaxel and cabazitaxel), and cisplatin. Docetaxel is the first cytotoxic drug to have shown a survival advantage in patients with hormone-resistant prostatic cancer, admittedly short (2.4 months additional lifespan), in a well-controlled randomized trial that compared docetaxel plus prednisolone with mitoxantrone [100]. Using the 'numbers needed to treat' approach, treatment with this agent would produce an additional 12 months of life in 1 of 10 patients treated, with additional benefits in respect of quality of life. Cabazitaxel, a more recently introduced semi-synthetic taxane, has shown slightly better therapeutic efficacy compared with mitoxantrone, in a recent European trial (the TROPIC trial), particularly in patients with a higher Gleason score. Newer agents (or indications) also include vinorelbine [101], satraplatin (an oral platinum derivative) and, most importantly, abiraterone, a potent small-molecule agent that blocks the formation of testosterone by inhibiting cytochrome CYP17A1, an enzyme involved in the formation of both dehydroepiandrosterone and androstenedione, which may ultimately be metabolized into testosterone. This oral agent, given at a dose of 1000 mg daily together with prednisolone 10 mg daily, is associated with a remarkably high biochemical response rate, lowering PSA and improving the quality of life and even overall survival time in men with advanced hormone-resistant prostatic cancer [102]. See also the important studies from de Bono *et al.* [103] and Ryan *et al.* [104]. A large double-blind randomized study of over 1000 patients treated with or without abiraterone, published in 2013, confirmed an improved radiographic progression-free survival, showed a trend toward improved overall survival, and significantly delayed clinical decline and initiation of chemotherapy in patients with metastatic castration-resistant prostate cancer. Abiraterone has clearly added significantly to the powerful armamentarium of agents now in routine use for metastatic prostate cancer. Another agent of great interest, enzalutamide, has also shown impressive activity in the setting of castration-resistant post-chemotherapy relapse (see Ref. [105]). This is an oral androgen-receptor-antagonist agent which appears to target several steps in the androgen-receptor–signalling pathway, thereby inhibiting the major driver of prostate-cancer growth. Indeed this study was closed early because at the point of interim analysis, the median survival was 18.4 months versus 13.6 months – a relative reduction of 37% in risk of death though admittedly at the cost of side-effects such as fatigue, diarrhoea and vasomotor symptoms. In the UK, about 15% of patients receive chemotherapy at any point in their cancer journey; in the USA the figure is somewhat higher.

In patients with unresponsive widespread bone pain, treatment with radioactive phosphorus may be of value. Up to 75% of patients have been reported to benefit, though remissions tend to be short. ^{89}Sr has recently been marketed as a superior radionuclide for use in this way [99], and may possibly be preferentially taken up in metastases rather than treating the whole bone marrow. Many other newer therapies (including radiopharmaceuticals such as radium-223) are emerging as promising agents for advanced prostate cancer – see, for example, Mitka [106] and Parker *et al.* [107].

Overall, it has been estimated that patients with carcinoma of the prostate lose, on average, almost a decade of life; the disease is now claiming around 10 000 lives annually in the UK. In the USA, about 240 000 cases were diagnosed in 2012, with 28 000 deaths from this disease – second only to lung cancer. Prostate cancer is responsible for about 26% of all deaths from malignant disease in men over the age of 85. Nonetheless, with early diagnosis and improving outcomes, survivorship figures are high – for example, there are now over 250 000 men alive post-diagnosis in the UK alone.

Cancer of the urethra

Male urethra

This very rare tumour may arise in the prostatic, bulbar or penile urethra, and is thought to be commoner in patients with a history of chronic inflammation or stricture. In the prostatic urethra the tumour is a TCC, but in the penile urethra squamous carcinomas are more common. The tumour spreads by direct invasion into the perineum and penile tissues. The penile urethra drains to inguinal lymph nodes, and the prostatic urethra to pelvic nodes.

Urethral carcinomas present with a urethral mass, obstruction, fistula, pain and haematuria. The age range is 50–80 years. Prostatic urethral tumours are treated by radical prostatectomy or cystoprostatectomy, or by radical radiotherapy. This latter method is increasingly employed, using doses of the order of 60–70 Gy to the prostate. Radiation technique is similar to that employed for carcinoma of the prostate. Distal carcinomas are usually treated by amputation of the distal part of the penis. Lesions of the bulbomembranous urethra are generally treated by radical excision.

Female urethra

The tumour is twice as common in females, and the histological pattern is more varied (squamous carcinoma in the distal two-thirds and TCC in the proximal third). Adenocarcinoma may arise from the periurethral glands, and melanoma and sarcoma occasionally occur. Leucoplakia of the urethra is regarded as a premalignant change, as are urethral papillomas and polyps.

Presentation is usually with a mass, bleeding and offensive discharge. Lymphatic involvement occurs late, distal tumours draining to the inguinal nodes and those of the proximal urethra to the iliac nodes.

Tumours of the anterior urethra are sometimes treated by partial urethrectomy but there is a high risk of local recurrence, and nodal spread frequently occurs. Radical radiation therapy is increasingly used since surgical control of the more extensive tumours is hard to achieve and the results are very poor. Interstitial radioactive implants may be suitable for small tumours, and external beam radiation therapy for larger lesions. The usual tumour dose is of the order of 60 Gy, carefully fractionated to avoid stricture formation.

Cancer of the penis

Incidence and aetiology

Carcinoma of the penis is uncommon in Western countries, accounting for less than 0.2% of male cancer deaths. However, it is much more frequent in South-east Asia, and in parts of India and Africa. General hygiene is thought to affect the incidence, and early circumcision is associated with a very low risk. Men with phimosis also appear to be at higher risk. At present, a viral origin seems likely to explain at least a proportion of cases. At least one married couple has been described with coexistent penile and vulval carcinoma, and the viral hypothesis is strengthened by the observation that many patients with penile cancer also harbour condylomata acuminata. There is slight concordance between the incidence of penile and cervical carcinomas in sexual partners. In addition, there are several premalignant conditions that predispose to the development of the tumour. These include Bowen's disease (intraepithelial carcinoma), erythroplasia of Queyrat, leucoplakia, lichen sclerosus, balanitis xerotica obliterans and Paget's disease. Leucoplakia may coexist with an invasive carcinoma. These premalignant lesions should be treated by local excision. The carcinoma is almost always a squamous cell carcinoma, although melanoma, basal cell carcinoma and Kaposi's sarcoma have all been described.

Clinical features [108]

Presentation is usually with an exophytic, or occasionally an excavating, ulcerated lesion, most commonly arising in the glans or the inner surface of the prepuce – see also an excellent recent review by Arya *et al.* [109]. There is often wide surface extension before deeper invasion to the urethra and corpora cavernosa. Some carcinomas of the penis are clinically obvious with a circumferential exophytic necrotic tumour, whereas in other cases careful inspection with retraction of the prepuce is necessary to allow the tumour to be visualized. Local invasion to the inguinal nodes is common, and ulceration of inguinal node metastases often occurs. The superficial inguinal nodes drain the prepuce and most of the penile skin, whereas the glans and corpora cavernosa drain chiefly to the deep inguinal nodes. A biopsy should always be performed since non-malignant conditions such as lymphogranuloma venereum, trauma, local infection, penile warts (condylomata) or leucoplakia can all cause diagnostic confusion.

A TNM staging classification has been proposed (Table 18.7), but can be difficult to apply in practice, particularly since palpable inguinal lymph nodes may sometimes be due to local infection. Although relatively unlikely to disseminate widely, the commonest sites of blood-borne metastases (M1) are the skin (chiefly abdominal wall), lungs and bone, and chest radiography should always be performed as part of the investigation.

Treatment and prognosis

For very localized lesions, cryosurgery or laser excision may be adequate; for more extensive tumours wider excision has traditionally been considered the treatment of choice, although amputation of the penis has never been a popular method of treatment and radical local irradiation has increasingly been used as an alternative [108]. As the tumour is uncommon, few surgeons or radiotherapists have a large experience. Treatment is often individualized: a small non-infiltrating tumour, which can be surgically excised without amputation, is probably best treated by surgery, with local irradiation given wherever there is doubt about the adequacy of the resection edge of the specimen. Many oncologists are disinclined to offer radical irradiation in bulky lesions because of the probability of hypoxia within the necrotic part of the tumour, which limits the prospect of radio-curability; such tumours are probably best dealt with surgically, particularly if partial amputation will suffice. More proximal lesions would require total

Table 18.7 TNM staging for cancer of the penis. Data from Sobin *et al.* [112].

Stage grouping			
Stage 0	Tis	N0	M0
	Ta	N0	M0
Stage I	T1a	N0	M0
Stage II	T1b	N0	M0
	T2	N0	M0
	T3	N0	M0
Stage III A	T1, T2, T3	N1	M0
Stage III B	T1, T2, T3	N2	M0
Stage IV	T4	Any N	M0
	Any T	N3	M0
	Any T	Any N	M1

Penis			
Tis	Carcinoma *in situ*		
Ta	Non-invasive verrucous carcinoma		
T1	Subepithelial connective tissue		
T1a	Without lymphovascular invasion, not G3–4		
T1b	With lymphovascular invasion, or G3–4		
T2	Corpus spongiosum, cavernosum		
T3	Urethra		
T4	Other adjacent structures		
N1	Single palpable mobile unilateral inguinal	pN1	Single inguinal
N2	Palpable mobile multiple or bilateral inguinal	pN2	Multiple/bilateral inguinal
N3	Fixed inguinal or pelvic	pN3	Pelvic or extranodal

amputation, and radical irradiation is often preferred in the first instance, with surgery if there is local recurrence. Following surgery, attempts have been made to construct a predictive nomogram to assist further treatment decisions. In one large series (175 patients) from the Cleveland Clinic using data from 11 urology centres in Italy, the 2-year survival was a somewhat disappointing 58% (alive, disease-free) with 42% of patients already dead of disease [110].

A variety of radiotherapy techniques has been described, including superficial X-rays (with single or opposed direct fields), treatment by interstitial implantation or a radium mould, or by orthovoltage or supervoltage irradiation using photons or electrons. A wax block can be used to improve dose homogeneity. Interstitial implants often employ radioactive iridium. The total dose of external irradiation is usually 60 Gy in daily fractions over 6 weeks, or the equivalent over a shorter treatment period. With mould treatments using iridium wire or radium, the treatment can usually be completed within 1–10 days (the patient wearing the mould for 8–10 hours per day), to a total dose of the order of 60 Gy. The major complications of radiation therapy for carcinoma of the penis include urethral stricture (10–12% of patients), fibrosis, ulceration and local recurrence (10–40% depending on the size of the tumour). For larger and more infiltrating tumours, surgery is probably the treatment of choice, particularly where the inguinal nodes are obviously involved by tumour. Where the inguinal nodes are mobile, block dissection is generally preferable to local irradiation, although it is wise to perform aspiration cytology to confirm that the nodes are indeed metastatic. Where the inguinal nodes are clearly fixed and surgery is not possible, local irradiation can be useful as a palliative procedure. Although remissions have been documented in such cases, survival is poor. The majority of patients with stage I (T1 or T2 and N0) tumours are free of inguinal metastases but the incidence in stage II (T3, N0 or N1a) is well over 50%, and it is these patients who probably benefit most from block dissection.

Early carcinoma of the penis has an excellent cure rate with surgery and/or radiotherapy. Although few large series of patients have been reported, it seems probable that T1 or T2 and N0 cases are equally well treated by surgery or radiotherapy. Without treatment, patients with penile squamous cell carcinoma usually die within 2 years after diagnosis of the primary lesion, because of uncontrollable locoregional disease or from distant metastases. The spread of the tumour to locoregional lymph nodes (lymph-node positivity) is the most relevant prognostic factor. With currently available treatments, 5-year cancer-specific survival probabilities are 75–93% for patients with clinically node-negative disease, and progressively lower for those with increasingly extensive node-positive disease [108,110]. Patients with pathologically proven negative nodes have 5-year cancer-specific survival probabilities ranging from 85% to 100%.

In one recent series treated by ^{192}Ir, 25 of 31 patients had durable tumour control; most of the failures were successfully treated by salvage surgery [111]. Patients with deep involvement of penile structures or inguinal node involvement do far less well, and the survival rate is approximately 50%. Where there are inoperable inguinal metastases or distant involvement, the 5-year survival rate is well under 10%.

References

1 Cohen HT, McGovern FJ. Renal-cell carcinoma. *N Engl J Med* 2005; 353: 2477–90.

2 Chow WH, Gridley G, Fraumeni JF *et al.* Obesity, hypertension and the risk of kidney cancer in men. *N Engl J Med* 2000; 343: 1305–11.

3 George DJ, Kaelin WG. The Von Hippel–Lindau protein, vascular endothelial growth factor, and kidney cancer. *N Engl J Med* 2003; 349: 366–81.

4 Sobin LH, Wittekind Ch. *TNM Classification of Malignant Tumours*, 5th edn. New York: Wiley-Liss, 1997: 181.

5 Atkins MB, Bukowski RM, Escudier BJ *et al.* Innovations and challenges in renal cancer: summary statement from the Third Cambridge Conference. *Cancer* 2009; 115 (10 Suppl): 2247–51.

6 Vogelzang NJ, Priest ER, Borden L. Spontaneous regression of histologically proved pulmonary metastases from renal cell carcinoma: a case with 5-year follow-up. *J Urol* 1992; 148: 1247–8.

7 Young RC. Metastatic renal-cell carcinoma: what causes occasional dramatic regressions? *N Engl J Med* 1998; 338: 1305–6.

8 Kjaer M, Frederiksen MD, Engelholm SA. Postoperative radiotherapy in stage I and II renal adenocarcinoma. A randomized trial by the Copenhagen Renal Cancer Study Group. *Int J Radiat Oncol Biol Phys* 1987; 13: 665–72.

9 Ahmed T, Benedetto P, Yagoda A *et al.* Estrogen, progesterone and androgen-binding sites in renal cell carcinoma. *Cancer* 1984; 54: 477–81.

10 Yagoda A, Abi-Rached B, Petrylak D. Chemotherapy for advanced renal-cell carcinoma, 1983–93. *Semin Oncol* 1995; 22: 42–60.

11 Amato R. Modest effect of interferon-α on metastatic renal-cell carcinoma. *Lancet* 1999; 353: 6–7.

12 Rosenberg SA, Lotz MT, Muul LM *et al.* Observations on the systemic administration of autologous lymphokine-activated killer cells and recombinant interleukin-2 to patients with metastatic cancer. *N Engl J Med* 1985; 313: 1485–92.

13 Childs R, Chernoff A, Contentin N *et al.* Regression of metastatic renal-cell carcinoma after non-myeloblative allogeneic peripheral-blood-stem-cell transplantation. *N Engl J Med* 2000; 343: 750–8.

14 Henriksson R, Nilsson S, Colleen S *et al.* Survival in renal cell carcinoma: a randomised evaluation of tamoxifen vs. interleukin 2, alpha-interferon and tamoxifen. *Br J Cancer* 1998; 77: 1311–17.

15 Yang JC, Haworth L, Sherry RM *et al.* A randomized trial of bevacizumab, an anti-vascular endothelial growth factor antibody, for metastatic renal cancer. *N Engl J Med* 2003; 349: 427–34.

16 Coppin C, Kollmannsberger C, Le L *et al.* Targeted therapy for advanced renal cell cancer (RCC): a Cochrane systematic review of published randomized trials. *B J U Internat* 2011; 108: 1556–63.

17 Escudier B, Albiges L, Sonpavde G. Optimal management of metastatic renal cell carcinoma: current status. *Drugs* 2013; 73: 427–38.

18 Motzer RJ, Hutson TE, Tomczak P *et al.* Sunitinib versus interferon alfa in metastatic renal cell carcinoma. *N Engl J Med* 2007; 356: 115–24.

19 Escudier B, Eisen T, Stadler WM *et al.* Sorafenib in advanced clear-cell renal-cell carcinoma. *N Engl J Med* 2007; 356: 125–34.

20 Hudes G, Carducci M, Tomczac P *et al.* for the Global ARCC Trial. Temsirolimus, interferon alfa, or both for advanced renal-cell carcinoma. *N Engl J Med* 2007; 356: 2271–81.

21 Motzer RJ, Escudier B, Oudard S *et al.* for the RECORD-1 Study Group. Efficacy of everolimus in advanced renal call carcinoma: a double-blind, randomized, placebo-controlled phase III trial. *Lancet* 2008; 372: 449–56.

22 Motzer RJ, Hutson TE, Cella D *et al.* Pazopanib versus sunitinib in metastatic renal-cell carcinoma. *New Engl J Med* 2013; 369: 722–31.

23 Escudier B, Pluzanska A, Koralewski P *et al.* for the AVOREN Trial investigators. Bevacizumab plus interferon alfa-2a for treatment of metastatic renal cell carcinoma: a randomized, double-blind phase III trial. *Lancet* 2007; 370: 2103–11.

24 Hall MC, Womack S, Sagalowsky AI *et al.* Prognostic factors, recurrence, and survival in traditional cell carcinoma of the upper urinary tract: a 30-year experience in 252 patients. *Urology* 1998; 52: 594–601.

25 Wallace DMA. Occupational urothelial cancer. *Br J Urol* 1988; 61: 175–82.

26 Plail R. Detecting bladder cancer. *Br Med J* 1990; 301: 567–8.

27 Garcia-Closas M, Malats N, Silverman D *et al. NAT2* slow acetylation, *GSTM1* null genotype, and risk of bladder cancer: results from the Spanish bladder cancer study and meta-analyses. *Lancet* 2005; 366: 649–59.

28 Harland SJ, Kynaston H, Grigor K *et al.* on behalf of the National Cancer Research Institute Bladder Clinical Studies Group. A randomised trial of radical radiotherapy for the management of pT1G3NXM0 transitional cell carcinoma of the bladder. *J Urol* 2007; 178: 807–13.

29 Sylvester RJ, van der Meijden AP, Lamm DL. Intravesical Bacillus-Calmette-Guerin reduces the risk of progression in patients with superficial bladder cancer: a meta-analysis of the published results of randomized clinical trials. *J Urol* 2002; 168: 1964–70.

30 Di Stasi SM, Giannantoni A, Giurioli A *et al.* Sequential BCG and electromotive mitomycin versus BCG alone for high-risk superficial bladder cancer: a randomised controlled trial. *Lancet Oncol* 2006; 7: 43–51.

31 Kaufman DS, Shipley WU, Griffin PP *et al.* Selective bladder preservation by combination treatment of invasive bladder cancer. *N Engl J Med* 1993; 329: 1377–82.

32 James ND, Hussain S, Hall E *et al.* Radiotherapy with or without chemotherapy in muscle-invasive bladder cancer. *New Engl J Med* 2012; 366: 1477–88.

33 van der Werf-Messing B. Cancer of the urinary bladder treated by interstitial radium implant. *Int J Radiat Oncol Biol Phys* 1978; 4: 373–8.

34 Hautmann RE, Miller K, Steiner U *et al.* The ideal neobladder: 6 years of experience with more than 200 patients. *J Urol* 1993; 150: 40–5.

35 Brendler CB, Steinberg GD, Marshall FF *et al.* Local recurrence and survival following nerve sparing radical cystoprostatectomy. *J Urol* 1990; 144: 1137–41.

36 Bloom HJG, Hendry WF, Wallace DM, Skeet RG. Treatment of T3 bladder cancer: controlled trial of pre-operative radiotherapy and radical cystectomy vs. radical radiotherapy. Second report and review (for the Clinical Trials Group, Institute of Urology). *Br J Urol* 1982; 54: 136–51.

37 Dunst J, Sauer R, Schrott KM *et al.* Organ-sparing treatment of advanced bladder cancer: a 10-year experience. *Int J Radiat Oncol Biol Phys* 1994; 30: 261–6.

38 Shelley MD, Wilt TJ, Barber J, Mason MD. A meta-analysis of randomised trials suggests a survival benefit for combined radiotherapy and radical cystectomy compared with radical radiotherapy for invasive bladder cancer: are these data relevant to modern practice? *Clin Oncol* 2004; 16: 166–71.

39 Duchesne GM, Bolger JJ, Griffiths GO *et al.* A randomised trial of hypofractionated schedules of palliative radiotherapy in the management of bladder carcinoma: results of MRC trial BA 09. *Int J Radiat Oncol Biol Phys* 2000; 47: 379–88.

40 Tester W, Caplan R, Heaney J *et al.* Neoadjuvant combined modality program with selective organ preservation for

invasive bladder cancer: results of RTOG phase II trial 8802. *J Clin Oncol* 1996; 14: 119–26.

41 Shearer RJ, Chilvers CED, Bloom HJG *et al.* Adjuvant chemotherapy in T3 carcinoma of the bladder: a prospective trial. *Br J Urol* 1988; 62: 558–64.

42 Wallace DMA, Raghavan D, Kelly KA *et al.* Neoadjuvant (pre-emptive) cisplatin therapy in invasive transitional cell carcinoma of the bladder. *Br J Urol* 1991; 67: 608–15.

43 Roberts JT, von der Maase H, Sengelov L *et al.* Long-term survival results of a randomized trial comparing gemcitabine/cisplatin and methotrexate/vinblastine/ doxorubicin/cisplatin in patients with locally advanced and metastatic bladder cancer. *Ann Oncol* 2006; 17 (Suppl 5): v118–22.

44 Coppin CML, Gospodarowicz MK, James K *et al.* Improved local control of invasive bladder cancer by concurrent cisplatin and preoperative or definitive radiation. *J Clin Oncol* 1996; 14: 2901–7.

45 Advanced Bladder Cancer Meta-analysis Collaboration. Neoadjuvant chemotherapy in invasive bladder cancer: a systematic review and meta-analysis. *Lancet* 2003; 361: 1927–34.

46 Sylvester RJ, van der Meijden AP, Oosterlink W *et al.* Predicting recurrence and progression in patients with stage 1a T1 bladder cancer using EORTC risk tables: a combined analysis of 2596 patients from seven EORTC trials. *Eur Urol* 2006; 49: 466–75.

47 van Roekel EH, Cheng KK, James ND *et al.* Smoking is associated with lower age, higher grade, higher stage, and larger size of malignant bladder tumors at diagnosis. *Int J Cancer* 2013; 133: 446–54.

48 Sherwood BT, Jones GBD, Mellon JK *et al.* Concomitant chemo-radiotherapy for muscle-invasive bladder cancer: the way forward for bladder preservation? *Clin Oncol* 2005; 17: 160–6.

49 Greenlee RT, Hill-Hamon MB, Murray T *et al.* Cancer statistics 2001. *CA Cancer J Clin* 2001; 51: 15–36.

50 Grönberg H. Prostate cancer epidemiology. *Lancet* 2003; 361: 859–64.

51 Nelson WG, de Marzo AM, Isaacs WB. Mechanisms of disease: prostate cancer. *N Engl J Med* 2003; 349: 366–81.

52 Perron L, Bairah I, Moore L *et al.* Dosage, duration and timing of NSAID use and risk of prostate cancer. *Int J Cancer* 2003; 106: 409–15.

53 Ekbom A, Hsieh C-C, Lipworth L *et al.* Perinatal characteristics in relation to incidence of and mortality from prostate cancer. *Br Med J* 1996; 313: 337–41.

54 Eeles RA, Kote-Jarai Z, Giles GG *et al.* Multiple newly identified loci associated with prostate cancer susceptibility. *Nat Genet* 2008; 40: 316–21.

55 Eeles RA, Olama AA, Benlloch S *et al.* Identification of 23 new prostate cancer susceptibility loci using the iCOGS custom genotyping array. *Nat Genet* 2013; 45: 385–91.

56 Martin RM, Davey Smith G, Donovan J. Does current evidence justify prostate cancer screening in Europe? *Nat Clin Pract Oncol* 2005; 2: 538–9.

57 Albertsen PC. What is the value of screening for prostate cancer in the US? *Nat Clin Pract Oncol* 2005; 2: 536–7.

58 Albertsen PC, Hanley JA, Fine J. 20-year outcomes following conservative management of clinically localized prostate cancer. *JAMA* 2005; 293: 2095–101.

59 Ilic D, Neuberger MM, Djulbegovic M, Dahm P. Screening for prostate cancer. *Cochrane Database Syst Rev* 2013; Jan 31; 1: CD004720. doi: 10.1002/14651858.CD004720.pub3.

60 Schroder FH, Damhvis RA, Kirkels WJ *et al.* European randomized study of screening for prostate cancer: the Rotterdam pilot studies. *Int J Cancer* 1996; 65: 145–51.

61 Aus G, Bergdahl S, Lodding P *et al.* Prostate cancer screening reduces the absolute risk of being diagnosed with advanced prostate cancer: results from a prospective population-based randomized controlled trial. *Eur Urol* 2007; 51: 659–64.

62 Hoffman RM. Screening for prostate cancer. *New Engl J Med* 2011; 365: 2013–9.

63 Roobol M. Prostate specific antigen velocity in men with total prostate specific antigen less than 4 ng/ml. *Eur Urol* 2008; 53: 852–4; discussion 854–5.

64 Wilt TJ, Ahmed HU. Prostate cancer screening and the management of clinically localized disease. *Brit Med J* 2013; 346: f325.

65 Thompson IM, Goodman PJ, Tangen CM *et al.* Long-term survival of participants in the prostatic cancer prevention trial. *New Engl J Med* 2013; 369: 603–10.

66 Gleason DE, Mellinger GT, Veterans' Administration Co-operative Urological Research Group. Prediction of prognosis for prostatic adenocarcinoma by combined histological grading and clinical staging. *J Urol* 1974; 111: 58–64.

67 Andrén O, Fall K, Franzén L *et al.* How well does the Gleason score predict prostate cancer death? A 20-year follow-up of a population based cohort in Sweden. *J Urol* 2006; 175: 1337–40.

68 Chan JM, Stampfer MJ, Giovannucci E *et al.* Plasma insulin-like growth factor-I and prostate cancer risk: a prospective study. *Science* 1998; 279: 563–5.

69 Embleton M. What urologists say they do for men with prostate cancer. *Br Med J* 1999; 318: 276.

70 Dearnaley DP, Kirby RS *et al.* Diagnosis and management of early prostate cancer: report of a British Association of Urological Surgeons' working party. *Br J Urol* 1999; 83: 18–33.

71 McLeod DG, Iversen P, See WA *et al.* for the Casodex Early Prostate Trial Collaborative Group. Bicalutamide 150 mgm plus standard care vs standard care alone for early prostate cancer. *BJU Int* 2006; 97: 247–54.

72 Bayman NA, Wylie JP. When should the seminal vesicles be included in the target volume in prostate radiotherapy? *Clin Oncol* 2007; 19: 302–7.

73 Jani AB, Hellman S. Early prostate cancer: clinical decision-making. *Lancet* 2003; 361: 1045–53.

74 Chodak GW, Thisted RA, Gerber GS *et al.* Results of conservative management of clinically localised prostate cancer. *N Engl J Med* 1994; 330: 242–8.

75 Dearnaley DP, Sydes MR, Graham JD *et al.* Escalated-dose versus standard-dose conformal therapy in prostate cancer: first results from the MRC RT01 randomised controlled trial. *Lancet Oncol* 2007; 8: 475–87.

76 Warde P, Mason M, Ding K *et al.* Combined androgen deprivation therapy and radiation therapy for locally advanced prostate cancer: a randomized phase 3 trial. *Lancet* 2011; 378: 2104–11.

77 Duchesne GM. Radiation for prostate cancer. *Lancet Oncol* 2001; 2: 73–81.

78 Walsh PC, Partin AW, Epstein JI. Cancer control and quality of life following anatomical radical retropubic prostatectomy: results at 10 years. *J Urol* 1994; 152: 1831–6.

79 Johansson J-E, Holmberg L, Johansson S *et al.* Fifteen-year survival in prostate cancer: a prospective, population-based study in Sweden. *JAMA* 1997; 277: 467–71.

80 MRC Prostate Cancer Working Party Investigators' Report. Immediate and deferred treatment for advanced prostate cancer: initial results of the MRC. *Br J Urol* 1997; 79: 235–46.

81 Eustham JA, Kattan MW, Groshen S *et al.* Fifteen-year survival and recurrence rates after radiotherapy for localised prostate cancer. *J Clin Oncol* 1997; 15: 3214–22.

82 Gray CL, Powell CR, Riffenburgh RH *et al.* 20-year outcome of patients with T1–3 N0 surgically staged prostate cancer treated with external beam radiation therapy. *J Urol* 2001; 166: 116–18.

83 Middleton RG, Thompson IM, Austenfeld MS *et al.* Prostate cancer clinical guidelines panel summary report on the management of clinically localized prostate cancer. *J Urol* 1995; 154: 2144–8.

84 Walsh PC. The discovery of the cavernous nerves and development of nerve sparing radical retropubic prostatectomy. *J Urol* 2007; 177: 1632–5.

85 Sanda MG, Dunn RL, Michalski J *et al.* Quality of life and satisfaction with outcome among prostate-cancer survivors. *N Engl J Med* 2008; 358: 1250–61.

86 Resnick MJ, Koyama T, Fan K-H *et al.* Long-term functional outcomes after treatment for localized prostate cancer. *New Engl J Med* 2013; 368: 436–45.

87 Johansson JE, Andren O, Andersson SO *et al.* Natural history of early, localized prostate cancer. *JAMA* 2004; 291: 2713–19.

88 D'Amico AV, Chen M-H, Roehl KA, Catalona WJ. Preoperative PSA velocity and the risk of death from prostate cancer after radical prostatectomy. *N Engl J Med* 2004; 351: 125–35.

89 Wilt TJ, Brawer MK, Jones KS *et al.* Radical prostatectomy versus observation for localized prostate cancer. *New Engl J Med* 2012; 367: 203–13.

90 Parker C. Treating prostate cancer: no benefit from radical prostatectomy for men with low-risk disease. *Brit Med J* 2012; 345: e5122.

91 Kirby R, Patel U, Challacombe B, Dasgupta P. Changing paradigms in the investigation of an elevated PSA. *BJU Internat* 2013; 112: 283–5.

92 Huggins C, Hodges CE. Studies on prostatic cancer. I. The effect of castration, of estrogen and of androgen injection on serum acid phosphatase in metastatic carcinoma of the prostate. *Cancer Res* 1941; 1: 293–7.

93 Chen Y, Clegg NJ, Scher HI. Anti-androgens and androgen-depleting therapies in prostate cancer: new agents for an established target. *Lancet Oncol* 2009; 10: 981–91.

94 Crawford ED, Eisenberger MA, McLeod DG *et al.* A controlled trial of leuprolide with and without flutamide in prostatic carcinoma. *N Engl J Med* 1989; 321: 419–24.

95 Thomas BC, Neal DE. Androgen deprivation treatment in prostate cancer. *Brit Med J* 2013; 346: e8555.

96 Prostate Cancer Trialists' Collaborative Group. Maximum androgen blockade in advanced prostate cancer: an overview of the randomised trials. *Lancet* 2000; 355: 1491–8.

97 Bolla M, Collette L, Blank L *et al.* Long-term results with immediate androgen suppression and external irradiation in patients with locally advanced prostate cancer (an EORTC study): a phase III randomized trial. *Lancet* 2002; 360: 103–8.

98 Crook JM, O'Callaghan CJ, Duncan G, *et al.* Intermittent androgen suppression for rising PSA level after radiotherapy. *New Engl J Med* 2012; 367: 895–903.

99 Zlotta AR, Schulman CC. Can survival be prolonged for patients with hormone-resistant prostate cancer? *Lancet* 2001; 357: 326–7.

100 Tannock IF, de Wit R, Berry WR *et al.* Docetaxel plus prednisone or mitoxantrone for advanced prostate cancer. *N Engl J Med* 2004; 351: 1502–12.

101 Borden LS Jr, Clark PE, Lovato J *et al.* Vinorelbine, doxorubicin and prednisone in androgen-independent prostate cancer. *Cancer* 2006; 107: 1093–100.

102 Attard G, Reid AH, Yap TA *et al.* Phase I clinical trial of a selective inhibitor of CYP17, abiraterone acetate, confirms that castration-resistant prostate cancer commonly remains hormone driven. *J Clin Oncol* 2008; 26: 4563–71.

103 De Bono JS, Logothetis CJ, Molina A *et al.* Abiraterone and increased survival in metastatic prostate cancer. *New Engl J Med* 2011; 364: 1995–2005.

104 Ryan CJ, Smith MR, de Bono JS *et al.* Abiraterone in metastatic prostate cancer without previous chemotherapy. *New Engl J Med* 2013; 368: 138–48.

105 Scher HI, Fizazi K, Saad F *et al.* Increased survival with enzalutamide in prostate cancer after chemotherapy. *New Engl J Med* 2012; 357: 1187–97.

106 Mitka M. New research reveals positive therapies and methods for treating prostate cancer. *JAMA* 2012; 308: 441–2.

107 Parker C, Nilsson S, Heinrich D *et al.* Alpha emitter radium-223 and survival in metastatic prostate cancer. *New Engl J Med* 2013; 369: 213–23.

108 Novara G, Galfano A, De Marco V *et al.* Prognostic factors in squamous cell carcinoma of the penis. *Nat Clin Pract Oncol* 2007; 4: 140–6.

109 Arya M, Kalsi J, Kelly J, Muneer A. Malignant and premalignant lesions of the penis. *Brit Med J* 2013; 346: f1149. doi 10.1136/bmj.f1149.

110 Kattan MW, Ficarra V, Artibani W *et al.* Nomogram predictive of cancer specific survival in patients undergoing partial or total amputation for squamous cell carcinoma of the penis. *J Urol* 2006; 175: 2103–8.

111 Kiltie AE, Elwell C, Close HJ, Ash DV. Iridium-192 implantation for node-negative carcinoma of the penis: the Cookridge Hospital experience. *Clin Oncol* 2000; 12: 25–31.

112 Sobin LH, Gospodarowicz MK, Wittekind Ch, eds. *TNM Classification of Malignant Tumours*, 7th edn. Chichester: Wiley-Blackwell, 2009.

Further reading

Atkins MB, Avigan DE, Bukowski RM *et al.* Innovations and challenges in renal cancer: concensus statement from the First International Conference. *Clin Cancer Res* 2004; 10: 6277S–81S.

Badani KK, Kaul S, Menon M. Evolution of robotic radical prostatectomy: assessment after 2766 procedures. *Cancer* 2007; 110: 1951–8.

Barry MJ. Screening for prostate cancer among men 75 years of age or older. *N Engl J Med* 2008; 359: 2515–16.

Barry MJ. Screening for prostate cancer: the controversy that refuses to die. *N Engl J Med* 2009; 360: 1351–4.

Bill-Axelson A, Holmberg L, Ruutu M *et al.* Radical prostatectomy versus watchful waiting in early prostate cancer. *N Engl J Med* 2005; 352: 1977–84.

Brugarolas J. Renal-cell carcinoma: molecular pathways and therapies. *N Engl J Med* 2007; 356: 185–7.

Calabro F, Sternberg CN. State-of-the-art management of metastatic disease and initial presentation or recurrence. *World J Urol* 2006; 24: 543–56.

International Commission on Radiological Protection. *Radiation Aspects of Brachytherapy for Prostate Cancer.* ICRP Publication 98. Amsterdam: Elsevier, 2006.

Kaufman DS, McDougal WS, Zietman AL, Young RH. Case 18-2007: a 54-year-old man with early-stage prostate cancer. *N Engl J Med* 2007; 356: 2515–20.

Lee WR. What variables predict for metastasis in men with biochemical relapse following radiotherapy for prostate cancer? *Nat Clin Pract Oncol* 2005; 2: 340–1.

Mangar S, Khoo V. Radiotherapy for bladder cancer: improving outcomes. *Br J Cancer Management* 2005; 1: 4–7.

Michaelson MD, Iliopoulos O, McDermott DF *et al.* A 63-year-old man with metastatic renal-cell carcinoma. *N Engl J Med* 2008; 358: 2389–96.

National Institute for Clinical Excellence. *Guidance on Cancer Services. Improving Outcome in Urological Cancers.* Issued 2002. Available at www.nice.org.uk (No new publication of this comprehensive manual since 2002, at the time of writing).

National Institute for Clinical Excellence. *Quick Reference Guide: Prostate Cancer – Diagnosis and Treatment.* Issued 2008. Available at www.nice.org.uk.

Pelucchi C, Bosetti C, Negri E *et al.* Mechanisms of disease. The epidemiology of bladder cancer. *Nat Clin Pract Urol* 2006; 3: 327–40.

Pisansky TM. External-beam radiotherapy for localized prostate cancer. *N Engl J Med* 2006; 355: 1583–91.

Ray ME, Thames HD, Levy LB *et al.* PSA nadir predicts biochemical and distant failures after external beam radiotherapy for prostate cancer: a multi-institutional analysis. *Int J Radiat Oncol Biol Phys* 2006; 64: 1140–50.

Rixe O, Bukowski RM, Michaelson MD *et al.* Axitinib treatment in patients with cytokine-refractory metastatic renal-cell cancer: a phase II study. *Lancet Oncol* 2007; 8: 975–84.

Rosenberg SA. Interleukin-2 for patients with renal cancer. *Nat Clin Pract Oncol* 2007; 4: 497.

Schröder FH, Roach M, Scardino P. Management of prostate cancer. *N Engl J Med* 2008; 359: 2605–9.

Scottish Inter-Collegiate Guidelines Network (SIGN). Management of transitional cell carcinoma of the bladder (2005). Available at www.sign.ac.uk.

Sharifi N, Gulley JL, Dahut WL. Androgen deprivation therapy for prostate cancer. *JAMA* 2005; 294: 238–44.

Stamey TA *et al.* The prostate specific antigen era in the Unites States is over for prostate cancer: what happened in the last 20 years. *J Urol* 2004; 172: 1297–301.

von der Maase H. Current and future perspectives in advanced bladder cancer: is there a new standard? *Semin Oncol* 2002; 29 (1 Suppl. 3): 3–14.

Weiss RH, Lin PY. Kidney cancer: identification of novel targets for therapy. *Kidney Int* 2006; 69: 224–32.

Welch HG. Should I *Be Tested for Cancer? Maybe Not and Here's Why.* Berkeley, CA: University of California Press, 2004. [A brilliant critique of a number of screening controversies, most particularly the unsolved problem of screening for prostate cancer.]

19 Testicular cancer

Although testicular tumours are uncommon, with a frequency of just over 2 per 100 000 males per year, they have an importance well beyond this small number. First, they represent the most common malignant solid tumours in young men between the ages of 15 and 44, 85% of cases presenting during this period of adult life; second, they are exceptionally chemosensitive, with a high cure rate even with disseminated disease; and third, they often manufacture tumour markers that can be used to monitor treatment and predict recurrence before it is clinically evident. Furthermore, their incidence has risen considerably over the past decade, particularly in the 15–19 age group (Figure 19.1) [1]; in fact, in industrialized countries the incidence increased 10-fold during the twentieth century [2]. Worldwide incidence has doubled over the past 40 years (Figure 19.2), with a worldwide incidence overall of 6.3 cases per 100 000 each year. Some 1900 cases are now diagnosed annually in the UK (resulting in a lifetime risk for men of about one in 200), and over 7000 in the USA, with far lower prevalence rates in Asia and Africa. Consistently lower incidence rates are reported for black Americans compared with white, suggesting a genetic component to aetiology. Rates for Asian and Hispanic men are intermediate [3]. Surprising differences in prevalence have been noted, even between countries of Northern Europe in close geographic proximity, all of which have robust statistical reporting methods and reliable tumour registries (and where the incidence appears to be the highest in the

world) – such as Denmark and Finland [4]. During the same period there has been considerable progress in the management of these conditions, and death from testicular tumours is now extremely uncommon – see, for example, an excellent recent review by Horwich et al. [5], which also gives good practical advice regarding current treatment and follow-up, with emphasis on recognition of long-term consequences and side-effects.

Germ-cell tumours

Aetiology and incidence

About 95% of testicular tumours are *germ-cell tumours*, which are believed to arise in the pluripotent germ cell [3]. As elegantly stated by Boisen *et al.* [6], 'the resemblance of normal development and differentiation in testicular germ-cell tumours goes beyond morphology'. This cell, when malignant, can give rise to tumours which have either somatic or trophoblastic features or both. Somatic differentiation results in the mixture of tissues typically found in teratomas, while choriocarcinoma comes from trophoblastic differentiation. *Non-germ-cell tumours* are briefly described on page 403 and include lymphomas, metastatic deposits, and Leydig and Sertoli tumours. Although most male germ-cell tumours arise in the testis, they may occasionally be *extragonadal* in origin, and these are briefly outlined on page 403.

The presence of an undescended testis (cryptorchidism) is associated with a 10-fold increase in the incidence of

Cancer and its Management, Seventh Edition. Jeffrey Tobias and Daniel Hochhauser.
© 2015 John Wiley & Sons, Ltd. Published 2015 by John Wiley & Sons, Ltd.

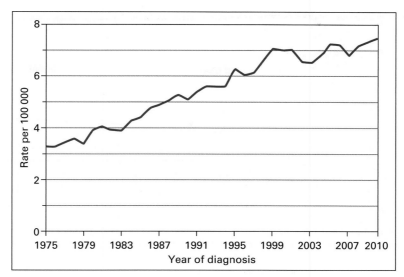

Figure 19.1 Testicular cancer (C62), European age-standardized incidence rates, Great Britain, 1975–2010. Source: http://info.cancerresearchuk.org/cancerstats/types/testis/incidence/?a=5441, accessed February 2014. © 2014 Cancer Research UK, Reproduced with permission.

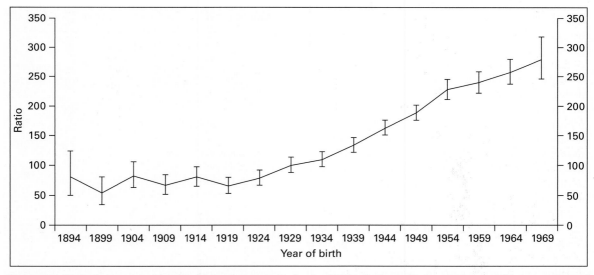

Figure 19.2 Testicular cancer incidence by birth cohort ratio, England and Wales ('reference' cohort is 1929 = 100) between 1894 and 1969. Note the sharp rise in incidence. Similar figures are available from other countries with reliable cancer registries.

testicular tumours [7]. About 10% of all patients with a testicular germ-cell tumour have a history of maldescent. Orchidopexy reduces, but does not abolish, this risk. Data from North America suggest that testicular tumours are rarer in black than in white Americans (approximately 1:5 in incidence). Teratomas of the testis (about 50% of all germ-cell tumours) present at an earlier age (peak age 20–30) than seminomas (peak age 30–50). The age-adjusted incidence in the UK is 3.8 per 100 000; incidence at different ages is shown in Figure 19.3. There is a trend towards higher prevalence in the wealthier social groups, and early onset of puberty and sexual activity are

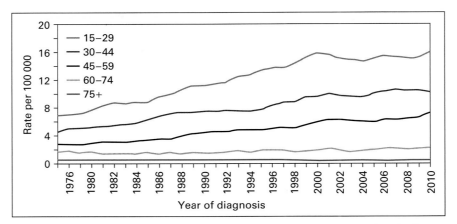

Figure 19.3 Testicular cancer incidence rates, by age, Great Britain, 1975–2010. Source: http://info.cancerresearchuk.org/cancerstats/types/testis/incidence/?a=5441, accessed February 2014. © 2014 Cancer Research UK, Reproduced with permission.

both thought to operate as important aetiological factors. Bilateral testicular tumours occur in about 5% of all cases. Teratoma and seminoma are the usual tumours at 10–40 years, but in older age groups lymphoma is much commoner. Familial instances of testicular germ-cell tumour have occasionally been described [2,8]. It is becoming clear that relatives of patients with testicular germ-cell tumours, though not themselves affected, carry certain abnormalities to a greater degree than expected: testicular microlithiasis, reduced sperm count, and perhaps a tendency towards relative infertility. In patients with an established and treated testicular cancer, a second primary testicular germ-cell tumour occurs in about 2% of cases. Risk factors are summarized in Table 19.1. The recommendation from the National Institute for Clinical Excellence (NICE), is that any patient with a mass or swelling in the body of the testis should be referred to a urologist urgently for investigation.

What could be the mechanism of carcinogenesis [2,7–9]? Both chemicals and viruses are possible candidates for inducing the final common pathway of tumour development and clonal evolution, that is, gonadotropin-driven mitosis in spermatogonia [10]. It seems likely that atrophy of the germinal epithelium with loss of feedback inhibition of the pituitary may result in an increase in pituitary-driven hormonal stimulation of the remaining testicular germ cells, resulting in neoplastic change. There may even be a higher risk of relapse with total aspermia (the greatest degree of atrophy), perhaps even accounting for the worrying possible association with vasectomy, in which the risk of testicular neoplasia may possibly be higher, particularly in patients whose

Table 19.1 Risk factors for testicular cancer.*

Demographic factorsAge 20–49 years
  High social class
  Caucasian
Medical characteristics
  Impaired fertility
  First born
  Undescended testis
  Carcinoma *in situ*
  Previous testicular tumour
  Inguinal hernia
  Testicular torsion
  Mumps orchitis
  Early puberty
Prenatal factors
Oestrogen exposure
Genetic factors
Close family relative with testicular cancer including certain
  rare familial syndromes
Other factors
Lack of exercise
  Sedentary lifestyle
  Maternal smoking

*Italics indicate factors under evaluation.
Data from http://www.cancerresearchuk.org/cancer-info/cancerstats/types/testis/riskfactors/

operation was complicated by haematoma or infection. Testicular atrophy following mumps orchitis may also result in neoplastic change via the same pathway. The role of testicular trauma has recently been more fully investigated and cannot confidently be excluded as a trivial factor [11], though it seems likely that genetic predisposition plays a far more important aetiological role, including both sibling and bilateral cases [2,10]. Germ-cell tumours are almost always hyperdiploid [12], often triploid or even tetraploid. A short arm isochromosome of chromosome 12 is the most frequent genetic marker in germ-cell tumours (even including *in situ* cases). Recent studies have suggested that an area on chromosome Xq27 may be responsible for about one-quarter of familial testicular cancer cases, and work is ongoing to identify the nature of this predisposing gene (now termed the *TGCT1* gene) and other genetic abnormalities that may predispose to testicular cancer [3,13]. It is already clear that the *TGCT1* locus at Xq27 is associated with a higher risk of bilateral tumours, and *TGCT1* may also predispose to undescended or cryptorchid testis.

Pathology

Several systems of classification are in current use (Table 19.2). In the UK, the commonest is the British Testicular Tumour Panel, while in the USA the Dixon and Moore classification is generally used [14]. Both are based on microscopic criteria, with an attempt to identify the predominant cell type. A major problem is that the tumours are often heterogeneous, the teratomas in particular displaying pleomorphism and a tendency to multiple cell types. Future classifications may depend increasingly on histochemical criteria, particularly in those which produce tumour markers.

Choriocarcinoma with any other cell type

Most testicular tumours are of germ-cell origin (Figure 19.4) and can usually be classified into seminomas (40%), teratomas (32%) or combined tumours with elements of both (14%). In the past 10 years there has been increased recognition that carcinoma *in situ* (also known as intratubular germ-cell neoplasia) may occur in the testis, and may, after about 5 years of apparent dormancy, develop into an invasive carcinoma. This specific histological change is found in almost every case as a precursor of invasive germ-cell tumours [15], and is particularly common in patients with a history of testicular maldescent [16]. The changes of carcinoma *in situ* are often widespread within the testis.

Table 19.2 Pathological classification of testicular tumours.

British Testicular Tumour PanelSeminoma
Malignant teratoma undifferentiated (MTU)
Malignant teratoma intermediate (MTI)
Malignant teratoma trophoblastic (MTT)
Teratoma differentiated

Dixon and Moore [14]
Pure seminoma
Embryonal carcinoma (pure or with seminoma)
Teratoma (pure or with seminoma)
Teratoma with embryonal carcinoma, choriocarcinoma or seminoma
Choriocarcinoma pure or with seminoma, embryonal carcinoma (or both)

World Health Organization
1. Tumours of single-cell type
    Seminoma
    Embryonal carcinoma
    Teratoma
    Choriocarcinoma
2. Mixed histological appearances
    Embryonal carcinoma with teratoma
    Embryonal carcinoma with teratoma and seminoma
    Embryonal carcinoma with choriocarcinoma
    Teratoma with seminoma

Source: Sobin and Wittekind (2006). Reproduced with permission from John Wiley and Sons.

Although the precise histological type of germ-cell tumour previously carried great prognostic significance, particularly in the distinction between seminoma and the teratomas (non-seminomas), dramatic improvements in treatment (particularly of teratomas) have reduced these disparities. Apart from the cell type, the most important prognostic feature, available from the operative specimen at orchidectomy, is the presence of tumour cells either at the cut end of the cord or within its vessels (intravascular invasion). Such tumours have an adverse prognosis. The initial concentrations of tumour markers (see below) also carry considerable prognostic significance.

The relationship between *in situ* carcinoma and invasive testicular cancer is now increasingly well recognized, although testicular biopsy remains unacceptable to many. Nevertheless, a high-risk group can be recognized by presence of *in situ* change – of practical importance because low-dose irradiation of an affected testis can prevent the later development of an invasive tumour without lowering testosterone levels or affecting sexuality.

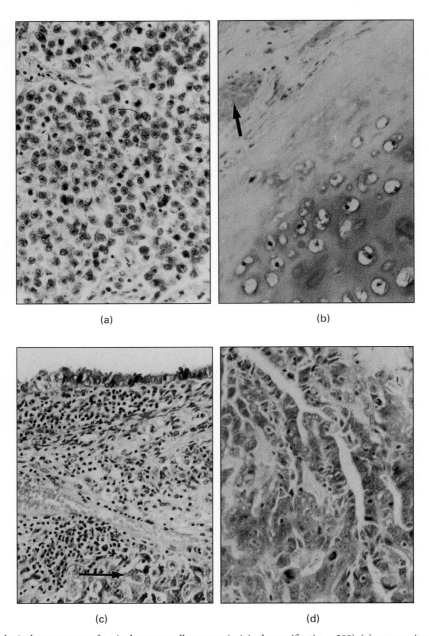

(a)

(b)

(c)

(d)

Figure 19.4 Histological appearances of testicular germ-cell tumours (original magnification ×200): (a) pure seminoma; (b) malignant teratoma differentiated, showing cartilage and smooth muscle (arrow); (c) MTI, showing differentiated epithelium and embryonal carcinoma (arrow); (d) MTU, showing embryonal carcinoma; (e) yolk sac tumour, showing a Schiller–Duval body (arrow); (f) chori-ocarcinoma, showing syncytiotrophoblast (arrow) and cytotrophoblast.

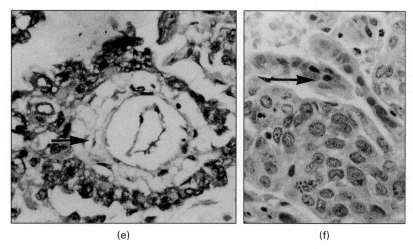

(e)   (f)

Figure 19.4 (*continued*)

Chromosomal analysis has identified a remarkably consistent single abnormality (isochrome 12p), which is almost as common in testicular tumours as the Philadelphia chromosome in chronic myeloid leukaemia. Other cytogenetic studies have suggested that seminomas may be an 'intermediate' step in the progression towards more malignant forms of testicular teratoma since the chromosome number for seminoma is intermediate between precursor *in situ* cell change and histologically more advanced disease [17].

Seminoma

Seminomas tend to be encapsulated and firm, with the cut surface pale grey and often featureless, and with little necrosis or haemorrhage. The microscopic appearance shows large round cells with distinct cell borders, clear cytoplasm, and large nuclei often with conspicuous nucleoli (Figure 19.4). Lymphocytic infiltration is frequently seen. When spread beyond the testis occurs, it is almost invariably to pelvic and para-aortic lymph nodes, later followed by involvement of mediastinal and supraclavicular nodes. Although chiefly testicular in origin, primary extragonadal seminomas are occasionally encountered in the retroperitoneal region, mediastinum, and suprasellar region or pineal area of the brain.

Teratoma (non-seminomatous germ-cell tumours)
Malignant teratoma undifferentiated (embryonal carcinoma)

Malignant teratoma undifferentiated (MTU) is the commonest non-seminomatous germ-cell tumour. It is often firm and nodular, showing areas of haemorrhage and necrosis. Microscopically, large anaplastic cells are usually seen, with less distinct cell borders and an eosinophilic cytoplasm containing nuclei of widely varying shapes. Some form of differentiation may occur, often with a glandular pattern (Figure 19.4).

Teratoma differentiated

Occasionally, a fully mature or differentiated testicular teratoma is encountered, in which mature bone, bone marrow and cartilage, and other tissues may be present. Even these tumours should be regarded as 'potentially malignant'.

Malignant teratoma intermediate (teratocarcinoma)

Malignant teratoma intermediate (MTI) usually shows characteristic differences from MTU, with a nodular appearance which, on sectioning, frequently feels gritty because of the presence of cartilage and/or bone. There is often a wide variety of germ-cell types, including cells derived from all three of the primitive germ-cell layers, including bone, cartilage, connective tissue and smooth muscle as well as cells suggestive of respiratory or gastrointestinal epithelium.

Malignant teratoma trophoblastic (MTT) (choriocarcinoma)

MTT is very much less common, and is histologically distinct because of the typical elements of cytotrophoblast and/or syncytiotrophoblast cells. It is highly malignant, metastasizing early and widely. It is extremely unusual to encounter a true trophoblastic testicular tumour confined to the testis. Typically these are bulky tumours at presentation and are more often associated with brain metastases than other types of teratoma. Drug resistance often develops early, and a prognostic distinction can be drawn between MTT and the commoner teratoma types (MTI and MTU). MTU probably has a more rapid doubling time than MTI, more commonly presents with lung deposits, seems more responsive to chemotherapy and carries a somewhat better prognosis.

Patterns of metastases

Clinical staging is based on a relatively predictable pattern of progression (Figure 19.5). The mode of spread is often lymphatic in the first instance, following the spermatic cord to the para-aortic nodes, thence to the retroperitoneal and retrocrural nodes, thoracic duct, posterior mediastinum and supraclavicular nodes (usually left-sided, although bifid or right-sided thoracic ducts occur in a small percentage of the population). Blood-borne spread frequently occurs, especially in MTT and MTU. In over 90% of cases this is associated with demonstrable nodal spread; in the remainder, metastases develop in the lungs in the absence of abdominal lymphatic disease. Liver involvement is unusual and exceptional in patients without lung deposits. Intracerebral and bone metastases are occasionally encountered. MTU is more commonly associated with locally invasive primary tumours and with haematogenous spread than MTI.

Clinical features

Patients typically present with a painless swelling of the testis, although pain occurs in about 25% of cases, particularly with rapidly growing tumours. Some young men present with a tumour of only 2–3 cm, while others are unaware of the change until the testis is well over twice its normal size. Some insist that a traumatic injury to the testis preceded its enlargement. Although small hydroceles are frequently present, invasion of the scrotal skin is extremely unusual and the tunica albuginea is rarely breached. Occasionally a spermatocele or varicocele may cause diagnostic difficulties.

The lymphatic drainage of the testis can be traced to the original embryonic site of origin in the abdomen (pelvic, common iliac and para-aortic nodes), rather than to adjacent nodes. Dissemination into these node groups is common and causes low back pain in about 10%. Patients may also notice lymphadenopathy in other sites, particularly the left supraclavicular nodes. If there is a history of inguinal or testicular surgery (usually herniorrhaphy or orchidopexy), inguinal node involvement may

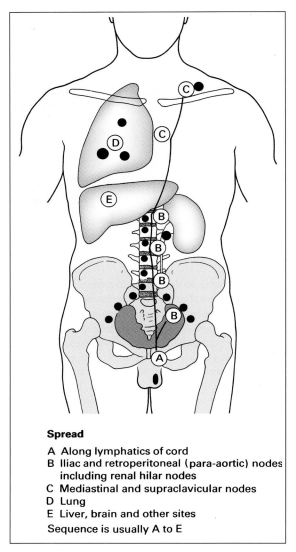

Spread

A Along lymphatics of cord
B Iliac and retroperitoneal (para-aortic) nodes including renal hilar nodes
C Mediastinal and supraclavicular nodes
D Lung
E Liver, brain and other sites
Sequence is usually A to E

Figure 19.5 Pathways of spread of testicular germ-cell tumours.

occur due to interference with the normal lymphatic pathways. Occasionally, abdominal swelling may occur from massive nodal deposits due to an unsuspected primary testicular tumour. The presenting symptoms will then be different: ureteric obstruction, acute abdominal pain or retrograde ejaculation as a result of pressure on the presacral plexus.

When patients present with obvious abdominal involvement, it is sometimes the case that the only sign of the primary tumour is testicular atrophy rather than a mass. Gynaecomastia may also occur (in up to

25% of patients with advanced disease), presumably due to ectopic hormone production by the tumour. Rarely, patients initially present with symptoms due to secondary spread in lung, brain or other sites. Infertility, due to azoospermia, may be the presenting complaint and clinical examination of the testes should be a routine procedure in the infertility clinic.

When considering the diagnosis, other causes of testicular swelling may cause difficulty, including cystic swellings (hydrocele if involving the testis, varicocele if clearly separate) and solid masses such as a testicular torsion, haematoma or scrotal inguinal hernia. The commonest mistake, however, is to confuse epididymo-orchitis in the young male, so often the cause of an important delay.

Tumour markers

These tumours often manufacture tumour markers, α-fetoprotein (AFP) and β-human chorionic gonadotrophin (β-HCG) being the best known (see also Chapter 4). AFP is synthesized by the fetal yolk sac, and plasma levels are elevated in about 70% of patients with MTU or MTI. It is never raised in patients with pure seminoma, and detection of AFP in such cases must be assumed to be due to foci of occult teratoma. Produced by trophoblastic elements in the tumour, β-HCG is detectable in the plasma of about 50% of patients with testicular teratoma and can also be modestly raised in patients with pure seminoma. With radioimmunoassay

techniques it is possible to measure these hormones at nanogram levels. The marker levels vary independently, reflecting their differing cell of origin. This may be confusing since treatment may lead to a fall in one marker without affecting the other. If raised, repeat measurements give a quantitative indication of tumour responsiveness and are an established part of management. At presentation, it is essential to obtain a preoperative sample for measurements of tumour markers.

The levels will fall after orchidectomy to within the normal range provided the patient has no metastases (Figure 19.5). If the preoperative levels of AFP and/or HCG are very high, the return of these values to normal may not be complete for several weeks since the half-life of AFP is 6–7 days and that of HCG is 16 hours. The level of both AFP and HCG at diagnosis gives an indication of prognosis: patients with AFP levels above 500 ng/mL and/or HCG above 10 000 ng/mL clearly do worse.

Tumour markers are also of great importance in the early diagnosis of relapse (Figure 19.6). Almost all patients with marker-producing tumours will develop elevated plasma levels as the first and most sensitive indication of relapse. Occasionally, patients with recurrent disease will develop a rise in only one marker even though both may previously have been elevated, due either to the differing sensitivity of components of the teratoma to chemotherapy or to the differential metastatic potential of the various elements of the primary. Tumour markers are particularly valuable in the diagnosis of extragonadal

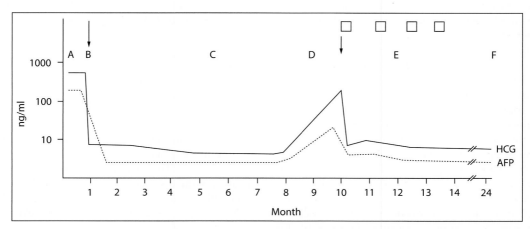

Figure 19.6 Serum markers in testicular teratoma. (A) Presentation with left testicular swelling: HCG 623 ng/mL, AFP 246 ng/mL. (B) Orchidectomy: HCG falls in 6 days to 10 ng/mL, AFP falls more slowly (half-life 6 days) to 4 ng/mL. (C) No rise in markers, clinical remission. (D) HCG and AFP rise, CT scan confirms enlargement of para-aortic nodes. (E) Cyclical intermittent combination chemotherapy produces rapid fall in HCG and slower fall in AFP, both to normal values. (F) Two years after presentation: normal markers, clinical remission, probable cure.

primaries since the differential diagnosis from other causes of a retroperitoneal, mediastinal or intracranial suprasellar mass is so wide.

Other tumour markers elaborated by testicular germ-cell tumours include placental alkaline phosphatase (PLAP) and lactate dehydrogenase (LDH). Although they are of far less value for disease monitoring than AFP and α-HCG, LDH in particular can provide useful information and is useful in patients who are otherwise marker-negative. Although about 90% of cases of pure seminoma have elevated PLAP levels, it is an unreliable marker since it is also raised in other conditions and in smokers. Glypican 3 (GPC3), a membrane-bound proteoglycan, has been recently reported to be positive as an immunohistochemical stain for yolk sac tumours and choriocarcinoma [18]. The oncofetal protein GPC3 may be useful in the diagnosis of non-seminomatous germ-cell tumours since embryonal carcinomas and immature teratomas express this less frequently.

Staging

Clinical staging systems vary widely, but all depend on the anatomical extent of spread at diagnosis (Table 19.3). In the UK, a simple system analogous to that used for Hodgkin's disease and other lymphomas (see Chapter 25) is often used. Greater detail can be incorporated in order to take account of the importance of tumour volume in the abdomen and lungs, characteristics recognized as crucial to the outcome. Radiological techniques such as lymphography, computed tomography (CT), magnetic resonance imaging (MRI) and positron emission tomography (PET) have helped our understanding. For example, the frequency of spread to the mediastinum was not appreciated until the advent of CT scanning; it is now recognized that nearly 30% of patients with testicular teratomas have evidence of involvement. Other investigations include intravenous urography and testicular ultrasonography, the latter particularly helpful in seminoma where irradiation of the para-aortic nodes may still be an important part of treatment at some centres, so care must be taken to avoid irradiation of the kidneys. The staging notation in Table 19.3 is based on investigations including CT and MRI.

In the USA, retroperitoneal lymph node dissection is still quite often performed, both for its value in staging and for possible therapeutic effect [19,20]. The tumour node metastasis (TNM) system is therefore partly surgically based (Table 19.3). In the UK, greater emphasis is placed on non-surgical approaches, and the accuracy of modern scanning methods is demonstrated by comparison with American data. These indicate that about 25% of lymph node dissection specimens in patients clinically thought to be free of extratesticular spread are indeed positive, a figure remarkably similar to British data from non-surgical series.

Management of testicular tumours

The last 25 years have seen major changes in management. Increased understanding of the importance of scrupulous staging, coupled with the advent of highly effective chemotherapy and routine use of tumour marker studies, has led to remarkable improvements and widespread acceptance that this is a tumour best treated by a multimodal approach. Expert surgeons, tumour pathologists, medical oncologists and radiation therapists all play an important and complementary role. Since these tumours are relatively uncommon and expert attention is so crucial, they are best treated in specialist units, or at the very least by study groups that will ensure uniformity of approach. For patients with a suspected testicular tumour, the correct surgical procedure is radical inguinal orchidectomy. Excision via the scrotal route, though still sometimes performed, should not generally be considered since trans-scrotal orchidectomy carries a real risk of scrotal recurrence or later development of inguinal node involvement. The spermatic cord should be excised as high as possible in order to provide information regarding the possibility of direct or intravascular spread of tumour, which has important implications for both management and prognosis. Before orchidectomy it is essential that the surgeon requests AFP and HCG levels, for the reasons described above.

Seminoma

If the tumour proves to be a pure seminoma, it is generally accepted that the surgeon has no further part to play, except perhaps for biopsy procedures if, for example, a supraclavicular node is discovered. Although American oncologists sometimes recommend surgery in seminomas with bulky abdominal lymph node metastases or where the HCG level is modestly raised, this is not usual practice in the UK. Radiotherapy alone will usually cure even bulky disease, and the addition of chemotherapy will increase this cure rate still further (see below).

Teratoma

For malignant teratomas, in the past, there has been an important difference of opinion between British and American authorities. For patients without abdominal

Table 19.3 Staging systems for testicular tumours.

UK notation

Stage I	Tumour confined to testis (tumour markers not elevated after orchidectomy, all investigations negative)
Stage II	Tumour in pelvic and abdominal (retroperitoneal) nodes (tumour markers may be persistently elevated. Positive lymphogram or CT scan of abdomen)
IIa	Nodes < 2 cm diameter
IIb	Nodes 2–5 cm diameter
IIc	Nodes > 5 cm diameter
Stage III	Mediastinal and/or supraclavicular nodes
Stage IV	Distant metastases*
	L1 less than three metastases, maximum diameter < 2 cm
	L2 more than three metastases, maximum diameter < 2 cm
	L3 maximum diameter > 2 cm

TNM staging notation

TX	Primary tumour cannot be assessed
T0	No evidence of primary tumour
Tis	Carcinoma *in situ* (non-invasive cancer cells)
T1	Tumour has not spread beyond the testicle and the narrow tubules next to the testicles where sperm undergo final maturation (epididymis). Cancer cells are not found inside blood vessels or lymph vessels next to the tumour. The cancer may have grown through the inner layer surrounding the testicle (tunica albuginea) but not the outer layer covering the testicle (tunica vaginalis)
T2	Similar to T1 except that the cancer has spread to blood vessels, lymphatic vessels, or the tunica vaginalis
T3	Tumour invades the spermatic cord (which contains blood vessels, lymphatic vessels, nerves, and the vas deferens)
T4	Tumour invades the skin surrounding the testicles (scrotum)
If the lymph nodes were taken out during surgery, there is a slightly different classification:	
pNX	Regional (nearby) lymph nodes cannot be assessed
pN0	There is no metastasis to regional lymph nodes
pN1	There is metastasis (spread) to one to five lymph nodes, with no lymph node larger than 2 cm across in greatest dimension
pN2	There is metastasis in at least one lymph node that is bigger than 2 cm but not larger than 5 cm; *or* metastasis to more than five lymph nodes that are not bigger than 5 cm across (in greatest dimension); *or* the cancer is growing out the side of the lymph node
pN3	There is metastasis to at least one lymph node that is bigger than 5 cm

*The number and size of lung metastases should be noted, in view of the prognostic importance of this observation.
Source: Sobin and Wittekind (2006). Reproduced with permission from John Wiley and Sons.

involvement, or evidence of only minimal nodal deposits (usually detected at CT or MRI), the standard British practice has been to recommend treatment by irradiation (or, more recently, by careful surveillance; see below).

In the USA, most of these patients would have been treated by extended retroperitoneal lymphadenectomy, removing all lymphatic and connective tissues along the great vessels from the diaphragm to the level of the iliac vessels, a formidable surgical procedure. Many American urologists claim that a lymph node metastatic rate of 25% fully justifies radical lymphadenectomy in all cases. In the UK, it is generally felt that combinations of radiotherapy and chemotherapy (or chemotherapy on relapse, if it

occurs) can effectively sterilize small-volume metastases in abdominal lymph nodes, and that the potential postoperative problems of aspermia (dry ejaculation) render such surgery unjustifiable.

Although it has been claimed that results of treatment by lymphadenectomy are superior to those in patients treated more conservatively, careful study of the literature does not bear this out. Comparisons are difficult since British patients are staged by clinical investigation, while most American urologists recommend lymphadenectomy as a staging as well as a potentially therapeutic procedure. It seems inescapable that many patients undergoing radical lymphadenectomy will have done so unnecessarily, in addition to having to face the undesirable sexual difficulties that the operation may bring. Reasonable comparison is possible between patients where lymphadenectomy confirms histologically positive para-aortic nodes and those from British series who have obviously positive CT or MRI appearances (stage II), where we see similar survival rates regardless of treatment. In stage I disease, a large series from Indiana University, following almost 400 patients treated surgically, showed a 99% survival [20]; conversely, an equally large British multicentre experience gave a similar (98%) outcome [21]. Chemotherapy proved necessary in 18.5% and 27%, respectively, but infertility was greater in the surgical group.

Over the past 10 years, this debate has largely become historic since the recognition that many patients with early disease, well staged and without adverse features, can be safely followed up by postorchidectomy surveillance. This requires serial marker studies and CT scanning, but does not include immediate postoperative treatment. Although approximately 20% of these patients relapse, close monitoring ensures that the relapse is almost always of small volume, and 99% of patients are curable by modern chemotherapy. Almost 80% of stage I surveillance cases require no postorchidectomy treatment whatever, that is, they are cured by this simple operation. However, surgery is recommended quite often after initial chemotherapy in order to reassess residual intra-abdominal disease (discussed further on page 401).

Radiotherapy
Seminoma

Although radiotherapy can be curative in pure seminoma, even in patients with advanced disease, the past few years have seen a marked shift in treatment approach, with a reduction in the use of radiotherapy. Historically, this treatment was given to almost all patients following orchidectomy, to both the para-aortic and pelvic nodes, an approach providing very good results, with overall cure rates of over 95%. However, alternative options are now available, including surveillance in well-staged patients [22] and also a single-dose treatment with single-agent carboplatin [23]. The biological benefit of adjuvant irradiation for patients with stage I disease was demonstrated in a large Canadian trial published in 1995 [24]. By 5 years, relapse had occurred in 18% of the patients undergoing close follow-up only, compared with only 5.5% after radiotherapy, the total series including over 170 patients. Following surveillance alone, relapse

is more likely with larger tumours. In general, the recommendation is that radiological surveillance should continue for 5 years as seminoma is a more indolent condition than other types of testicular germ-cell tumour. Well-tolerated single-agent carboplatin chemotherapy may prove to be as effective yet less toxic [23]. For patients with Stage 1 seminoma, a single dose of carboplatin will reduce the risk of relapse from about 1 in 6 to 1 in 25, and patients can be advised accordingly. About 99% of these patients are cured, regardless of the initial choice, as 'salvage' treatment is also effective for the small group who need it. In patients with more advanced (stage II) seminoma, an important study of 99 patients, mostly treated by orchidectomy and radiation alone (without chemotherapy), confirmed the excellent results achieved in patients with small-volume disease [25]. Those with stage IIa or IIb had a relapse-free survival rate of 89%, virtually all cured. For more bulky cases, the relapse-free survival dropped sharply, with chemotherapy clearly the preferred option. Infertility is not normally a problem following adjuvant radiation therapy, provided that the contralateral testis is protected from scattered irradiation by means of lead shielding. Where a scrotal operation such as orchidopexy, trans-scrotal biopsy or scrotal orchidectomy has been performed, the scrotal sac and ipsilateral inguinal nodes must also be treated. Although preservation of fertility cannot be guaranteed, an attempt at shielding the contralateral testis should certainly be made. One additional and crucial benefit for using chemotherapy routinely in patients with stage II disease, in comparison with adjuvant 'dog-leg' irradiation of abdominopelvic nodes, is the cumulative 12% absolute difference in risk of a second cancer during the subsequent 30 years following treatment with radiotherapy.

A report from the Royal Marsden Hospital in London has suggested that a single dose of neo-adjuvant carboplatin prior to radiotherapy can reduce the risk of relapse still further, in patients with Stage IIA and IIB seminoma – see Ref. [26]. In a single-arm study, 51 patients were treated between 1996 and 2011 with a single cycle of carboplatin followed by radiotherapy. The radiation field was reduced from an extended abdomino-pelvic field to just the para-aortic region alone and the radiation dose from 35 to 30 Gy in 39 patients – both features allowing for reduced late-stage radiation toxicity. After a median follow-up of 55 months, with 38 (74%) of the patients having been followed for over two years, there have been no relapses at all. Toxicity was low with grade 3 toxicity limited to four patients with grade 3 haematological toxicity (with no clinical sequelae) and one patient with grade 3 nausea (during radiotherapy). No patients experienced grade 4 toxicity. Patients with bulky abdominal disease are now routinely treated with chemotherapy prior to (or even instead of) irradiation.

For stages III and IV disease, chemotherapy gives much the best opportunity of cure, although some centres have reported encouraging results with whole-body irradiation. Occasionally, patients with 'pure' seminoma have an elevated serum β-HCG, and HCG can be demonstrated immunocytochemically. This does not appear to be associated with a worse prognosis. An elevated serum AFP is usually regarded as an indication for treatment as for non-seminomatous germ-cell tumours (see below).

Although seminoma is a highly curable tumour, many questions of management remain unanswered. Treatment of early-stage disease by orchidectomy alone (without adjuvant radiotherapy) is becoming increasingly popular since the surveillance results from major treatment centres are holding up well. Conversely, this approach is more difficult for seminoma than with non-seminomatous germ-cell tumours; useful marker elevations are generally unavailable. In the previously quoted Canadian study, however, only one of the 364 patients died of uncontrollable disease [24] despite the higher relapse rate in patients not given immediate adjuvant radiation therapy.

Teratoma

For non-seminomatous germ-cell tumours, chemotherapy has become the dominant form of treatment and radiotherapy is now much less widely employed. In the first place, surveillance of patients with stage I disease is associated with a high cure rate, at least 75%. Even more important, chemotherapy is almost always curative in the minority who do require treatment. With bulky stage II disease, the case for chemotherapy as the treatment of choice is totally established [27–29]. Patients with stages III and IV disease are usually cured with chemotherapy, although radiotherapy may still have a possible adjunctive role in the control of bulky abdominal disease (see below), though surgical resection of residual masses is generally preferred.

Chemotherapy

The emergence of highly effective chemotherapy for testicular teratoma has been one of the most exciting advances in cancer medicine over the past 30 years. In the early 1960s one or two agents were available with known but limited activity. The next important step was

the recognition of further agents of different classes, each with major activity. Vinblastine, bleomycin and cisplatin were all identified as independently effective.

These highly toxic regimens were a major advance, later replaced by a regimen that added cisplatin, a highly effective agent and the most powerful of all the cytotoxics for this condition, also relatively free from bone marrow toxicity, making it particularly suitable as part of a combination regimen. Over 20 years ago, Einhorn and colleagues at Indiana developed a combination of cisplatin, vinblastine and bleomycin (PVB) in patients with advanced disease [29]. This regimen is still sometimes used, although newer less toxic combinations, particularly bleomycin, etoposide and cisplatin (BEP), have now largely replaced it [27]. At major centres in both the USA and Europe, BEP is generally regarded as the 'gold standard' chemotherapy for testicular cancer.

Despite the remarkable results of modern therapy, the acute toxicity of all these regimens remains a serious problem, with gastrointestinal disturbance, granulocytopenia and infection, nephrotoxicity and pulmonary fibrosis as the major hazards. In Einhorn's earlier series (using PVB), four patients died in complete remission, two of these deaths being drug-related. Bleomycin is used in relatively large doses in these regimens and, as haematological toxicity has diminished, pulmonary toxicity from bleomycin has become increasingly recognized (see Chapter 6). However, an important study from the USA-based Eastern Cooperative Oncology Group confirmed that bleomycin remains an important component of therapy; both relapse-free survival and overall survival were better in the BEP group (86 and 95%) compared with the dual-agent etoposide/cisplatin group (69 and 86%) [30]. However, it was subsequently suggested that four cycles of EP are as valuable as three cycles of BEP, gaining an important toxicity advantage by avoiding the pulmonary symptoms and damage caused by bleomycin [31]. Although carboplatin is less toxic to the gastrointestinal tract than cisplatin, it is more myelotoxic and thus more difficult to use in combination with vinblastine and bleomycin. Later consequences of successful therapy are discussed in more detail below.

Some patients [32] are now recognized as having a particularly poor prognosis. Adverse features include presence of liver, bone or brain metastases; AFP at presentation of more than 1000 ng/mL; α-HCG more than 10 000 ng/mL; LDH above 10 times normal; mediastinal primary site; mediastinal node mass more than 5 cm; or more than 20 pulmonary metastases. Such cases are probably better treated by a still more

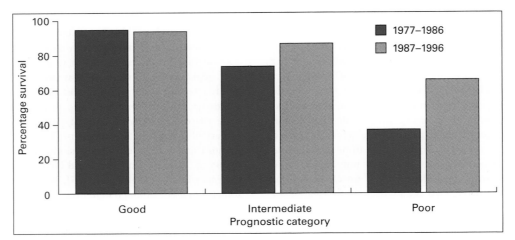

Figure 19.7 The 10-year actuarial survival for patients with disseminated non-seminomatous testicular germ-cell tumours (International Germ Cell Consensus Classification Group). Source: Sonneveld *et al.* [32]. Reproduced with permission from John Wiley and Sons.

intensive chemotherapy regimen, and about two-thirds of this group appear curable (see below) (Figure 19.7 and Table 19.4). It may be possible in patients with metastatic disease to increase the dose-intensity where necessary, by using pegfilgrastim support within a BEP-type regimen – see, for example, Ref. [33] – though it is not yet clear whether this offers superior results in these patients.

There is rarely any justification for giving more than four courses of similar chemotherapy. Although most patients are cured, it is important not to assume failure if after this time there is radiological evidence of residual disease, for example, visible lung metastases, which sometimes fade radiologically over several months. For treatment of late recurrence, or of truly refractory disease, the introduction of ifosfamide-based or other intensive regimens has for the first time given durable responses and a small proportion of cures. The VIP (vincristine, ifosfamide and cisplatin or carboplatin) regimen is one example of a logical combination; with BEP as the primary choice, patients treated with VIP will not previously have been exposed to vinblastine. High-dose stem-cell supported procedures have also been increasingly employed [34,35]. An important retrospective study from Einhorn's group in Indiana has confirmed the curative potential of this approach, even in patients who had relapsed or failed to respond to multiple previous lines of chemotherapy. Patients were treated with high doses of etoposide (750 mg/m^2) and carboplatin (700 mg/m^2), each for three consecutive

Table 19.4 Chemotherapy regimens commonly used for testicular cancer (see text).

Regimen	Drugs	Component Dosage	Days given
BEP: four cycles at 21-day intervals	Bleomycin	30 mg	1, 8, 15
	Etoposide	100 mg/m^2 per day	1–5
	Cisplatin	20 mg/m^2 per day	1–5
EP: same regimen without bleomycin			
VIP: day 1 = day 21	Vinblastine	0.11 mg/kg per day	1 and 2
	Ifosfamide	1200 mg/m^2 per day	1–5
	Cisplatin	20 mg/m^2 per day	1–5
VeIP: day 1 = day 21	Etoposide	75 mg/m^2 per day	1–5
	Ifosfamide	1200 mg/m^2 per day	1–5
	Cisplatin	20 mg/m^2 per day	1–5

Source: Oliver [27]. Reproduced with permission from Elsevier.

days and each followed by autologous peripheral-blood stem-cell transfusion; 173 patients received two such treatments, and a further 11 received one course. Most patients also received vinblastine and ifosfamide prior to the high-dose treatment. Overall, 116 had complete remission of disease, without relapse, over a median follow-up period of 48 months. The authors concluded that patients are potentially curable by this technique, even when used as third- or fourth-line therapy, an extremely encouraging result for this most drug-resistant group. The use of chemotherapy for patients with less advanced disease needs further exploration, particularly where there is only modest para-aortic involvement (stages IIa and IIb).

It is also clear that seminoma is a highly chemosensitive disease. Most cases present early, at a radiocurable stage, but for the few who have advanced disease or who later develop recurrence, there was little effective chemotherapy until the advent of cisplatin-based regimens. Current practice includes combinations of drugs similar to those used for teratoma, with radiotherapy sometimes still given to sites of bulk disease. However, single-agent cisplatin may be as effective for metastatic seminoma as the more complex combination regimens, and is still undergoing evaluation in this setting [27].

Long-term consequences of chemotherapy have been studied in considerable detail. The good news is that most patients will live a normal or near-normal life-span and enjoy good quality of life. However, some series especially those where treatment was intensive, have been more cautionary. For example, one report from Germany assessed a group of 90 patients (median follow-up 58 months) of whom only 19% were totally symptom-free [36]; 30% reported Raynaud's phenomenon, 21% had tinnitus or hearing loss, and two-thirds had elevation of follicle-stimulating hormone. Other abnormalities included persistent hypomagnesaemia, reduced Leydig cell functioning with borderline hypogonadism, arterial hypertension and peripheral neuropathy. Fortunately, second cancers are unusual [27,32], though the overall risk of both second cancers and cardiovascular disease are approximately similar to the risk from long-term smoking, that is, not inconsiderable.

Fertility following treatment for testicular cancer has of course become a major issue as a result of the increasing certainty of cure for the large majority of patients. In one important study assessing over 1400 men, the overall 15-year actuarial post-treatment paternity rate was 71% in the 554 men who attempted post-treatment conception, this figure being achieved without the use of cryopreserved semen [37]. This rate ranged from 48% in those receiving high-dose chemotherapy to 92% in the surveillance group; in addition, assisted reproductive technologies were used by 22% of the couples who attempted conception after treatment. Guidelines for fertility preservation have been issued by the American Society of Clinical Oncology [38].

Surgery after chemotherapy and radiotherapy
Surgery has an important role where there is residual disease after orchidectomy. Abdominal 'debulking' surgery, and even excision of pulmonary metastases by repeated thoracotomy, is frequently performed. Postponing surgery to the end of the chemotherapy programme gives an accurate histological picture of the effect of preceding treatment, as well as removing tumour in patients with residual disease. Ideally, it should be performed only after tumour markers have fallen to undetectable levels and at least one additional course of chemotherapy has been given beyond this point. Many cases show clear evidence of treatment-induced differentiation into mature teratoma; although this observation is encouraging, its significance and implications for long-term survival are not entirely clear. Most appear to be cured, without relapse after several years' follow-up.

Prognosis of testicular tumours (Table 19.5)
Mortality from germ-cell tumours continues to fall [31,32]. Stages I and II seminomas are nearly always curable by orchidectomy and radiotherapy (stage I, >95%; stage II, 85–90%). The prognoses of bulky stage II (stage IIc) and stages III and IV have greatly improved with chemotherapy (Figure 19.8a) and the majority are now cured even in these more advanced stages. It now seems clear that 80% of patients with stage I seminoma are cured by orchidectomy (surveillance alone), though adjuvant radiotherapy confers an even lower relapse rate [24,25].

In non-seminomatous germ-cell tumours the prognosis is excellent for stage I and early stage II disease. In addition, well over 70% of all patients with stage III disease will be cured, but bulky disease and stage IV patients are still at risk of incomplete drug response and relapse. Nevertheless, the last decade has seen great improvements even in this poor-prognosis group (Figure 19.8b). Patients treated at specialist centres have a better prognosis with strict adherence to current treatment protocols. Results from large centres in the

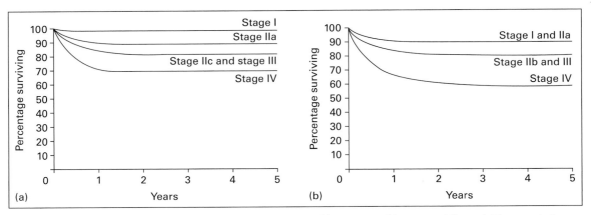

Figure 19.8 Prognosis of testicular germ-cell tumours related to stage: (a) seminoma; (b) teratoma (all types). These survival curves illustrate the dramatic improvement with advanced stages since the introduction of combination chemotherapy.

Table 19.5 Using tumour markers and other characteristics to assess risk in testicular germ-cell tumours.*

Risk status	Non-seminoma	Stages	Seminoma	Stages
Good outlook	No non-lung spread Good markers AFP < 1000 ng/mL HCG < 5000 ng/mL LDH < 1.5 IU/L	IS (S1) IIA (S1) IIB (S1) IIC (S1) IIIA	No non-lung spread AFP normal HCG and LDH can be any level	IIC IIIA IIIB IIIC

Intermediate outlook	No non-lung spread
	Intermediate markers
	  AFP 1000–10 000 ng/mL
	  HCG 5000–50 000 ng/mL
	  LDH 1.5–10
		IS (S2)
		IIC (S2)
		IIIB
			Non-lung spread
			AFP normal
			HCG and LDH can be
			any level
				IIIC with non-lung
				spread

Poor outlook	Non-lung spread[†]
	High markers
	  AFP > 10 000 ng/mL
	  HCG > 50 000 ng/mL
	  LDH > 10
		IS (S3)
		IIC (S3)
		All IIIC
			None (seminoma is
			never classified as
			poor outlook)	

*The 5-year survival rate for patients with a good prognosis is 91%, for intermediate prognosis 79%, and for poor prognosis 48%. These numbers are taken from a study of patients treated over 10 years ago. Survival is likely to be better today.
[†]Spread to sites such as the brain or liver (non-lung) generally indicates a poorer outlook.
AFP, alpha-fetoprotein; HCG, human chorionic gonadotrophin; LDH, lactate dehydrogenase.
Source: Data from American Cancer Society, Inc 2008.

UK are among the best reported, with overall survival of 80–90% following treatment with regimens containing cisplatin, bleomycin, vinblastine, etoposide and/or other drugs. Poor-prognosis patients clearly require special attention and specialist referral [34,35,39]. An international germ-cell consensus classification has been agreed, allowing metastatic cases to be reliably grouped as 'good', 'intermediate' or 'poor' prognosis [40]. The major effort in poor-prognosis patients lies in generating new chemotherapy programmes to improve on established regimens (see, for example, Ref. [35]), and to ensure through public education that late initial presentation occurs as infrequently as possible [41]. Overall, about 15% of men with metastatic testicular non-seminomatous germ-cell tumours will relapse, of whom about 30% are still curable with further intensive salvage treatment.

Late recurrences, though extremely unusual, do occur and vigilance needs to be maintained [42]. In this large series from Norway, the rates of relapse beyond 2 years were 1.4% and 3.2% for seminoma and non-seminoma respectively.

Extragonadal germ-cell tumours

Primary extragonadal germ-cell tumours are extremely uncommon, but have been described in a variety of sites including the retroperitoneum, anterior mediastinum, suprasellar or pineal area and the presacral region. Although the pathogenesis is not entirely clear, it is possible that these tumours result from malignant change in primordial germ cells that have migrated incompletely (cell 'rests') or in cells displaced during embryogenesis. There appears to be a genetic predisposition at least in some cases, since Klinefelter's syndrome is a well-described predisposing feature.

The commonest sites are the anterior mediastinum (1% of all mediastinal tumours) and retroperitoneum. In occasional cases, an associated congenital or developmental abnormality is present. The largest group are mixed tumours, but pure seminomas are more common than pure teratomas or choriocarcinomas. Since primary testicular tumours can be small and impalpable, one should always be wary when diagnosing a germ-cell tumour apparently arising from an extratesticular site, since metastases from an occult primary do occur. Acute leukaemia has been described in conjunction with mediastinal germ-cell tumours.

Both teratomas and seminomas show the same radiosensitivity and chemosensitivity as for primary testicular tumours. For mediastinal seminoma, surgery followed by radiotherapy appears effective, with long-term survival rates of about 50%. However, in bulky diseases, chemotherapy can be extremely effective at reducing tumour volume (eliminating the need for wide-field irradiation of the lungs) and is increasingly preferred. Similar regimens are used as for testicular primaries. For primary mediastinal non-seminomatous germ-cell tumours, some reports show good responses to modern chemotherapy, usually including cisplatin, vinblastine, etoposide, bleomycin and actinomycin D.

Primary germ-cell tumours of the brain are treated somewhat differently. Most of these are pineal or suprasellar tumours; both teratomas and seminomas occur. These latter can sometimes be cured by wide-field irradiation, including full irradiation of the whole central nervous system. The 5-year survival rate in children with radiosensitive pineal tumours (usually not biopsied but assumed to be seminoma or the less common pinealoblastoma) is 50%. With proven pineal teratomas (biopsy-proven or where AFP or β-HCG is clearly raised) the outlook is less good, although response to chemotherapy can be dramatic.

The apparent rarity of extragonadal germ-cell tumours may have to be revised in the light of reports describing patients originally thought to have undifferentiated carcinomas but with a clinical course and response to chemotherapy much more suggestive of extragonadal germ-cell tumour. This has been described as the *atypical teratoma syndrome* and in the majority of cases, serum markers (AFP and β-HCG) are raised, with subsequent staining of tissue sections by immunoperoxidase techniques showing intracellular AFP and β-HCG. Treatment with BEP or PVB is effective, with a high proportion of complete responders. In young men with mediastinal tumours which on biopsy prove to be 'poorly differentiated carcinoma', it is essential to consider this diagnosis and to measure plasma β-HCG and AFP. Even if these are negative, it is so important not to overlook this potentially curable tumour that response to platinum-based regimens should be fully assessed.

Management of non-germ-cell tumours of the testis

Orchidectomy alone is usually sufficient for Leydig and Sertoli cell tumours since these rarely metastasize. Lymphomas of the testis are usually large-cell centroblastic B-cell neoplasms. As they are frequently bilateral, irradiation of the contralateral testis is usually recommended even if the disease appears localized. These patients need careful staging as for other lymphomas (see Chapter 26). With paratesticular rhabdomyosarcomas, occult metastasis is so frequent that adjuvant combination chemotherapy is essential (see Chapter 24).

References

1 Møller H, Jørgensen N, Furman D. Trends in incidence of testicular cancer in boys and adolescent men. *Int J Cancer* 1995; 61: 761–4.
2 Harland SJ. Conundrum of the hereditary component of testicular cancer. *Lancet* 2000; 356: 1455–6.

3 Huddart R, Oliver RTD for Cancer Research UK. *Cancer-Stats – Testicular cancer, UK.* September 2002. Available at www.cancerresearchuk.org.

4 Looijenga LHJ, Oosterhuis JW. Clinical value of the X-chromosome in testicular germ-cell tumours. *Lancet* 2004; 363: 6–7.

5 Horwich A, Nicol D and Huddart R. Testicular germ cell tumours. *Brit Med J* 2013; 347: f5526.

6 Boisen KA, Kaleva M, Main KM et al. Difference in prevalence of congenital cryptorchidism in infants between two Nordic countries. *Lancet* 2004; 363: 1264–9.

7 Parker L. Causes of testicular cancer. *Lancet* 1997; 350: 827–8.

8 Oliver RTD. Testicular cancer. *Curr Opin Oncol* 1996; 8: 252–8.

9 Houldsworth J, Korkola JE, Bosl GJ et al. Biology and genetics of adult male germ cell tumors. *J Clin Oncol* 2006; 24: 5512–18.

10 Nicholson P, Harland SJ. Inheritance and testicular cancer. *Br J Cancer* 1995; 71: 421–6.

11 Swerdlow AJ, Huttly SRA, Smith PG. Testicular cancer and antecedent diseases. *Br J Cancer* 1987; 55: 97–103.

12 Chagant RSK, Rodriguez E, Bosl GJ. Cytogenetics of male germ-cell tumours. *Urol Clin North Am* 1993; 20: 55–66.

13 Rapley EA, Crockford GP, Teare D et al. Localization to Xq27 of a susceptibility gene for testicular germ-cell tumours. *Nat Genet* 2002; 24: 197–200.

14 Dixon FJ, Moore RA. Testicular tumours: a clinicopathological study. *Cancer* 1953; 6: 427.

15 Bosl GJ, Motzer RJ. Medical progress: testicular germ-cell cancer. *N Engl J Med* 1997; 337: 242–53.

16 Giwercman A, Grinsted J, Hansen B et al. Testicular cancer risk in boys with maldescended testis: a cohort study. *J Urol* 1987; 138: 1214–16.

17 Oliver RTD, Leahy M, Ong J. Combined seminoma/nonseminoma should be considered as intermediate grade germ cell cancer. *Eur J Cancer* 1995; 31A: 92–4.

18 Zynger DL, Dimov ND, Luan C et al. Glypican 3: a novel marker in testicular germ cell tumors. *Am J Surg Pathol* 2006; 30: 1570–5.

19 Sweeney CJ, Hermans BP, Heilman DK et al. Results and outcome of retroperitoneal lymph node dissection for clinical stage I embryonal carcinoma-predominant testis cancer. *J Clin Oncol* 2000; 18: 358–67.

20 Donohue JP, Thornhill JA, Foster RS et al. Primary retroperitoneal lymph node dissection in clinical stage A non-seminomatous germ cell testis cancer: review of the Indiana University experience 1965–89. *Br J Urol* 1993; 71: 326–35.

21 Read G, Stenning SP, Cullen MH et al. Medical Research Council prospective study of surveillance for stage I testicular teratoma. *J Clin Oncol* 1992; 10: 1762–8.

22 Choo R, Thomas G, Woo T et al. Long-term outcome of post orchidectomy surveillance for stage I testicular seminoma. *Int J Radiat Oncol Biol Phys* 2005; 61: 736–40.

23 Oliver RTD, Mason MD, van der Maase H. Radiotherapy versus single-dose carboplatin in adjuvant treatment of stage I testicular seminoma: a randomised trial. *Lancet* 2005; 366: 293–300.

24 Warde P, Gospodarowicz MK, Panzarella T et al. Stage I testicular seminoma: results of adjuvant irradiation and surveillance. *J Clin Oncol* 1995; 13: 2255–62.

25 Warde P, Gospodarowicz M, Panzarella T et al. Management of stage II seminoma. *J Clin Oncol* 1998; 16: 290–4.

26 Horwich A, Dearnaley DP, Sohaib A et al. Neoadjuvant carboplatin before radiotherapy in stage IIA and IIB seminoma. *Annals Oncol* 2013; 24: 2104–7.

27 Oliver RTD. Chemotherapy in testis cancer. In: Weiss RM, George NJR, O'Reilly PM, eds. *Comprehensive Urology.* London: Mosby, 2000: 673–8.

28 Kondagunta GV, Motzer RJ. Chemotherapy for advanced germ cell tumors. *J Clin Oncol* 2006; 24: 5493–502.

29 Einhorn LH, Donohue JP. *Cis*-diamine-chloroplatinum, vinblastine and bleomycin combination chemotherapy in disseminated testicular cancer. *Ann Intern Med* 1977; 87: 293–8.

30 Loehrer P, Johnson D, Elson P et al. Importance of bleomycin in favorable prognosis disseminated germ cell tumors: an Eastern Co-operative Oncology Group Trial. *J Clin Oncol* 1995; 13: 470–6.

31 Vasey P, Jones R. Testicular cancer: management of advanced disease. *Lancet Oncol* 2003; 4: 738–47. [Correspondence entitled BEP vs. EP for treatment of metastatic germ-cell tumours. *Lancet Oncol* 2004; 5: 146–7.]

32 Sonneveld DJA, Hoekstra HJ, van de Graaf WTA et al. Improved long term survival of patients with metastatic non-seminomatous testicular germ cell carcinoma in relation to classification systems during the cisplatin era. *Cancer* 2001; 91: 1304–15.

33 Grimison PS, Stockler MR, Chatfield M et al. Accelerated BEP for metastatic germ cell tumours: a multicenter phase II trial by the Australian and New Zealand Urogenital and Prostate Cancer Trials Group (ANZUP). *Annals Oncol* 2014; 25: 143–8.

34 Lotz J-P, Andre T, Donsimoni R et al. High-dose chemotherapy with ifosfamide, carboplatin and etoposide combined with autologous bone marrow transplantation for the treatment of poor-prognosis germ cell tumors and metabolic trophoblastic disease in adults. *Cancer* 1995; 75: 874–85.

35 Einhorn LH, Williams SD, Chamness A et al. High-dose chemotherapy and stem-cell rescue for metastatic germ-cell tumors. *N Engl J Med* 2007; 357: 340–8.

36 Bokemeyer C, Berger CC, Kuczyk MA, Schmoll H-J. Evaluation of long-term toxicity after chemotherapy for testicular cancer. *J Clin Oncol* 1996; 14: 2923–32.

37 Brydoy M, Fossa SD, Klepp O et al. Paternity following treatment for testicular cancer. *J Natl Cancer Inst* 2005; 97: 1580–8.

38 Lee SJ, Schover LR, Partridge AH *et al.* American Society of Clinical Oncology recommendations on fertility preservation in cancer patients. *J Clin Oncol* 2006; 24: 2917–31.

39 Stiller CA. Non-specialist units, clinical trials and survival from testicular cancer. *Eur J Cancer* 1995; 31A: 289–91.

40 International Germ Cell Collaborative Group. International germ cell consensus classification: a prognostic-factor based staging system for metastatic germ cell cancers. *J Clin Oncol* 1997; 15: 594–603.

41 Steele JPC, Oliver RTD. Testicular cancer: perils of very late presentation. *Lancet* 2002; 359: 1632–3.

42 Oldenburg J, Alfsen GC, Waehre H, Fossa SD. Late recurrences of germ cell malignancies: a population-based experience over three decades. *Br J Cancer* 2006; 94: 820–7.

Further reading

Alomary I, Samant R, Jenest P *et al.* The preferred treatment for stage I seminoma: a survey of Canadian radiation oncologists. *Clin Oncol* 2006; 18: 696–9.

Daufman DS, Saksena MA, Young RH *et al.* Case reports from the Massachussetts General Hospital: case 602007: a 28 year-old man with a mass in the testis. *N Engl J Med* 2007; 356: 842–9.

Ferry JA, Harris NL, Young RH *et al.* Malignant lymphoma of the testis, epididymis, and spermatic cord: a clinicopathological study of 69 cases with immunophenotypic analysis. *Am J Surg Pathol* 1994; 18: 376–90.

Lucia MH, Foster RS, Ulbright TM. Pathology of late recurrence of testicular germ cell tumors. *Am J Surg Pathol* 2000; 24: 257–73.

Sobin LH, Gospodarowicz MK, Wittekind Ch, eds. *TNM Classification of Malignant Tumours*, 7th edn. Chichester: Wiley-Blackwell, 2009.

Ulbright TM. Germ cell tumors of the gonads: a selective review emphasising problems in differential diagnosis, newly appreciated, and controversial issues. *Mod Pathol* 2005; 18: S61–79.

Ulbright TM, Amin MB, Young RH. *Tumors of the Testis, Adnexa, Spermatic Cord, and Scrotum*, 3rd Series, Fascicle 25. Washington, DC: Armed Forces Institute of Pathology, 1999.

Woodward PJ, Heidenreich A, Looijenga LH *et al.* Germ cell tumours. In: Eble JN, Sauter G, Epstein JI *et al.*, eds. *Pathology and Genetics of Tumours of the Urinary System and Male Genital Organs*. Lyon, France: IARC Press, 2004.

Young RH, Scully RE. *Testicular Tumors*. Chicago: ASCP Press, 1990.

20 Thyroid and adrenal cancer

Cancer of the thyroid

Thyroid cancer is exceptional in many ways. First of all, some thyroid cancers are very indolent with a long natural history, often over many decades, even where complete control of the tumour has not been achieved. Second, because most thyroid cancers take up iodine, the use of oral radioactive iodine – a highly specific therapy – can destroy both normal and neoplastic thyroid cells, with total ablation of the tumour and excellent 20-year survival rates. Third, in the majority of patients with metastases from well-differentiated thyroid carcinomas, the metastatic lesions retain their important characteristic radioiodine uptake, so that even patients with metastatic disease at presentation can be treated successfully. If necessary, these treatments can be repeated several times, using whole-body isotope scanning for assessment of progress and to determine whether further therapy is required [1].

There are important histological and behavioural differences between the major types of thyroid cancer which help to determine treatment strategy (Table 20.1). Although these tumour subgroups are well defined, several types of thyroid carcinoma have been recognized more recently, and further histopathological refinements seem likely [2]. The clinician needs a complete histopathological description of the tumour that should include not only the tumour type but also the degree of differentiation, since tumour grading is now known to have important prognostic significance [3]. The degree of local invasion into blood vessels, local structures and adjacent lymph nodes should also be described.

Thyroid lymphoma occurs rarely (1–3% of thyroid malignancies) and is discussed in Chapter 26.

Aetiology and incidence

There are about 14 000 new cases registered each year in the USA, and about 1100 deaths. In the UK the annual reported incidence is 2.3 (women) and 0.9 (men) per 100 000, leading to about 1000 new cases annually for England and Wales, i.e. about 1% of all newly diagnosed malignancies. The incidence of thyroid cancer, particularly the papillary subtype, has been increasing sharply for several years in a number of Western countries, though the factors responsible are not fully understood [4], and to some extent clearly represent a form of ascertainment bias (see below). In the USA, thyroid cancer is now the fifth most common cancer of women, the eighth overall – commoner than all the leukaemias put together (see Ref. [5]). In the Middle East, thyroid cancer is the second commonest cancer in women. As well as the importance of radiation carcinogenesis, such as following the Chernobyl accident (see below), an apparent increase in incidence may also reflect improved vigilance and advances in medical diagnosis. This resulted, for example, in the Colonna study, in a larger than expected incidence of small tumours (<1 cm in diameter), which were predominantly papillary in type. Recent attention has been drawn to the importance of increasingly sensitive investigations, often tantamount

Cancer and its Management, Seventh Edition. Jeffrey Tobias and Daniel Hochhauser.
© 2015 John Wiley & Sons, Ltd. Published 2015 by John Wiley & Sons, Ltd.

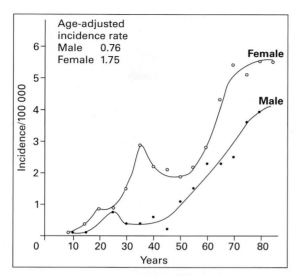

Figure 20.1 Age-specific incidence of thyroid cancer.

to screening of inappropriate patients – almost invariably asymptomatic – leading to diagnosis of very early relatively low-risk tumours ,and of course a corresponding increase in the *apparent* incidence of this disease – see, for example, Ref. [6]. These authors make a persuasive case, indeed they remind us forcefully that 'Unnecessary thyroidectomy is costly and harms patients'.

A number of aetiological factors have now been described. Like other thyroid diseases, thyroid cancer is commoner in women than in men (Figure 20.1), with a bimodal age distribution. The lower age peak of incidence is due to papillary and follicular tumours, and the rise in incidence in older patients is chiefly due to anaplastic cancers. Both thyrotoxicosis and Hashimoto's thyroiditis share a similar age distribution with well-differentiated thyroid carcinomas [7]. About 90% of all cases of thyroid cancer are differentiated (papillary and follicular, see below) with, potentially, an excellent prognosis. It is clearly one of the radiation-related cancers, more frequent both in survivors of the atom bomb and following childhood irradiation of the neck (the latter with a 50-fold increased incidence), usually with a latent period of 10–30 years. Recent evidence has confirmed a 12-fold increased incidence among women in Belarus following the explosion at the Chernobyl nuclear power plant near Kiev, Ukraine, in April 1986 [8]. In general, the risk of radiation carcinogenesis is higher in females, or where the radiation exposure occurred in very young children.

Medullary thyroid carcinoma has both a familial and a sporadic incidence and may form part of the syndromes of multiple endocrine neoplasia (MEN) (see Chapter 15).

Pathology
Papillary carcinoma

The commonest type of cancer is papillary carcinoma (Figure 20.2), comprising about 60% of all thyroid cancers, with a slightly greater proportion of those occurring in childhood. Together with well-differentiated follicular carcinoma, in at least 20% of cases the tumour appears to be multifocal in origin, and in older patients tends to have a more aggressive clinical course, with correspondingly poorer survival. Papillary carcinomas are almost three times commoner in women, with a peak incidence in the third and fourth decades. Any differentiated thyroid tumour that contains neoplastic papillae is by definition a papillary carcinoma, regardless of the presence of neoplastic follicles. The tumour is made up of cuboid cells and often contains psammoma bodies. A characteristic feature of papillary tumours is large empty nuclei, so-called orphan Annie nuclei. Over 90% of these tumours appear to be encapsulated, but lymph node invasion is common, though not necessarily prognostically important. Occasionally, papillary microcarcinomas (even up to 1 cm in size) are discovered in thyroidectomy specimens where a neoplasm was not suspected preoperatively. These small clinically undetected tumours can generally be ignored (from the point of view of further treatment) unless adjacent to one of the resection margins. A recent review of papillary microcarcinoma has recommended observation without immediate surgery as an appropriate initial strategy, provided the lesion is not situated close to the trachea or recurrent laryngeal nerve, and there are no nodal metastases demonstrable on ultrasonography [9]. Larger tumours, with evidence of extrathyroid invasion and/or invasion of the thyroid capsule, are associated with a worse prognosis, though in general this is a slow-growing and fully resectable tumour, with a low overall mortality [10]. For papillary cancer of the thyroid, the commonest genetic abnormalities are point mutations in BRAF and RAS, and rearrangement of the *RET* proto-oncogene, thus raising the prospect of useful targeted therapy with agents which act against RET, vascular endothelial growth factor receptor (VEGFR) and epidermal growth factor receptor (EGFR) tyrosine kinases, for patients with resistant or metastatic disease (see Ref. [11]).

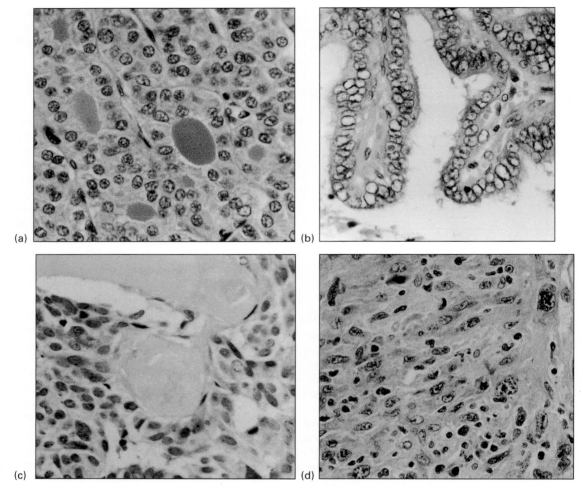

Figure 20.2 Histological appearances in thyroid cancer: (a) follicular carcinoma showing follicle formation (×200); (b) papillary carcinoma showing characteristic 'empty' nuclei (×200); (c) medullary carcinoma showing small cells with masses of amyloid (×200); (d) anaplastic carcinoma (×200).

Follicular tumours

Follicular tumours (Figure 20.2) are much less common (about 15% of all cases), often occurring in patients with a long history of goitre. They are unusual in children and are seen in a rather older age group than the papillary carcinomas, again with a slight female predominance. The mean age of diagnosis is about 10 years greater than for papillary cancer (52 compared with 41 years for patients with resectable disease [1]). Overall prognosis is good (Table 20.1). Lymph node involvement is uncommon, as the main route of dissemination is via the bloodstream with lung and bone as the commonest sites of metastasis.

Histologically, microangioinvasion is a common feature even though, as with papillary carcinomas, over 90% of these tumours appear macroscopically encapsulated. The presence of tumour within the capsular venous sinusoids or permeation of extrathyroidal veins are both important adverse prognostic features. The tumour can be difficult to distinguish from atypical adenomas, since the presence of nuclear pleomorphism and even bizarre nuclear forms is not necessarily tantamount to true malignancy, in the absence of evidence of microangioinvasion. In follicular carcinoma, the commonest genetic abnormalities include mutations in RAS and rearrangement of

Table 20.1 Clinical characteristics and survival in thyroid cancer.

Histological type	Response to radioiodine	Clinical behaviour	10-year survival (%)
Papillary	+++	Young patients. Often slow to evolve. Metastases usually lymphatic	95
Follicular	+++	Young middle-aged patients. Metastases often haematogenous (bone, lung)	90
Medullary	−	Young patients. Often familial. A key marker lesion in patients with multiple endocrine neoplasia type II. Non-MEN cases typically more indolent in behaviour Produces calcitonin as marker. C cell tumour. Often rapid clinical evolution. Surgery very important as radioresponsiveness variable	40
Anaplastic	−	Elderly patients. Predominantly local invasion with pressure symptoms	5
Small cell	−	Rapid but very radiosensitive. Usually localized	5
Lymphoma	−	Middle-aged group (highly radiosensitive)	40

the *PPAR-gamma* and *PAX8* genes, to create the *PPFP* fusion gene.

Medullary thyroid tumours

Remarkable progress has been made in our understanding of this rare genetic cancer over the past decade [12]. During this period, germline genetic testing has become the basis for important therapeutic decisions in patients affected by the syndrome characterized by medullary thyroid carcinoma and hyperparathyroidism, namely, MEN-2.

Medullary thyroid tumours (Figure 20.2) have a quite different derivation and are thought to arise from the parafollicular or C cells. The disease is often familial (see below). Typically, the stroma of the tumour has an amyloid appearance and the tumour itself may be bilateral. Medullary thyroid tumours have a high metastatic potential both to lymph nodes and to the bloodstream, and the extent of lymph node involvement is an important guide to prognosis [13]. The large majority secrete calcitonin, a particularly important tumour marker in view of the familial incidence of the disease and the obvious importance of identifying affected family members as early as possible [14]. Equally important is the use of the calcitonin assay for monitoring results of therapy. Familial medullary carcinoma of the thyroid is defined by the presence of the disease in four or more family members with no other evidence of MEN syndromes (see below) after careful screening. These cases tend to

have a later onset than in MEN-2-associated cases, often behaving clinically in a more indolent fashion. DNA testing can be particularly valuable in apparently familial cases, especially if the patient is under 40 years of age or has C-cell hyperplasia or multifocal tumours. If the test reveals no mutations in exons 10, 11, 13, 14 and 16 of the *RET* proto-oncogene, then the probability of the patient having MEN-2 is extremely low [15]. In patients with the codon 634 genotype, malignant transformation can occur as early as 1 year of age, though progression to lymph node involvement was not seen in a single case under the age of 14 years in a large European study of 207 patients from 145 families.

In the past, most patients reached the age of 30 years by the time of diagnosis. The mean age at diagnosis is expected to drop in the future, since the familial nature of the tumour is well understood and use of the calcitonin assay has now become widespread. Moreover, since age-related progression from C-cell hyperplasia to medullary thyroid carcinoma is associated with various germline mutations in the *RET* proto-oncogene, guidelines have become available for assessment of the optimal time for prophylactic thyroidectomy [16].

Multiple endocrine neoplasia

Other abnormalities are sometimes present in familial cases, particularly phaeochromocytoma and hyperparathyroidism, the so-called MEN syndromes, which can occur with both sporadic or familial forms of medullary thyroid cancer. They are inherited as autosomal dominant disorders with a high degree of penetrance but variable expression. The commonest variant of MEN, *Wermer's syndrome*, can involve the thyroid and parathyroid glands, pancreatic islets, pituitary or adrenal cortex (see Chapter 15). Two-thirds of patients have tumours of at least two of these endocrine glands. The second type of MEN, *Sipple's syndrome*, includes more patients with medullary thyroid carcinoma; approximately 95% of patients with MEN-2 will develop medullary carcinoma of the thyroid; 50% also have parathyroid hyperplasia and/or phaeochromocytoma. Mutations in the *RET* proto-oncogene, which codes for a tyrosine kinase receptor, have been implicated in over 90% of families with MEN-2, and predictive DNA testing of at-risk family members can now be performed [15]. Medullary thyroid cancer may be associated with ectopic hormone production from the thyroid tumour itself, and may produce adrenocorticotrophic hormone (ACTH), vasoactive intestinal peptide and also prostaglandins and serotonin.

The gene for MEN-2a (medullary thyroid cancer, phaeochromocytoma and parathyroid hyperplasia) is inherited as an autosomal dominant trait with incomplete penetrance so that 40% of carriers do not present with symptoms until 70 years of age [16,17]. About 90% of patients with MEN-2 have type 2a disease; the less common 2b variety is usually clinically apparent at an earlier age because of a characteristic facial appearance. Detection of presymptomatic carriers by provocation of calcitonin release identifies 90% by the age of 25 years, but DNA analysis is more reliable still [18]. The gene is located in the pericentromeric region of chromosome 10, and studies using DNA restriction fragment polymorphism provide accurate identification of the carrier state. A consensus statement from the European Community Medullary Thyroid Carcinoma Group has offered guidelines for combined biochemical and genetic MEN-2 screening, which should lead to rapid improvement in early detection and cure [19]. In patients at risk for MEN-2a and medullary carcinoma, prophylactic thyroidectomy is increasingly performed [20].

Anaplastic carcinoma

Anaplastic carcinoma of the thyroid (Figure 20.2) is the predominant form in elderly people, with 75% of patients beyond 60 years of age at diagnosis. They form only about 10% of all thyroid cancers, frequently occurring in women [21], but account for over half of thyroid cancer-related deaths [22]. Unlike well-differentiated thyroid cancer, they are generally rapidly growing tumours, often painful

and with pressure symptoms as an early feature, apparently arising in a long-standing goitre. The course of these tumours is quite different from that of the more slow-growing varieties commoner in younger patients, and several histological subtypes have been recognized, including spindle and giant-cell carcinomas in which there may be areas of well-differentiated carcinoma, supporting the suggestion that they sometimes arise from transformation of pre-existing well-differentiated thyroid cancer. For poorly differentiated cancer, the commonest genetic abnormalities include mutations in RAS and *PIK3CA*, together with overexpression of EGFR.

A very small number of 'anaplastic' carcinomas are characterized by infiltration with small lymphocyte-like cells, and are generally known as *small-cell* carcinomas of the thyroid. These are typically found in elderly patients and are rapidly growing and locally invasive. *Thyroid lymphomas* [23] are discussed in Chapter 26.

Diagnosis and investigation

Patients usually present with a firm mass in the neck, due to either the primary thyroid mass or an involved cervical lymph node. It is sometimes possible to classify the thyroid mass on clinical grounds as obviously benign, suspicious of cancer or 'probable' [24,25], although only a minority of thyroid cancers present with symptoms or signs of real prognostic value, and most cases have a benign cause. In making these distinctions, useful clinical criteria include the size and position of the mass, its mobility and the presence of signs of compression of vital structures in the neck. Findings that suggest the possibility of a locally advanced or more aggressive cancer include fixity of the thyroid nodule, recent hoarseness of the voice (which might indicate recurrent laryngeal involvement or vocal cord paralysis), fullness of the jugular vein or cervical lymphadenopathy.

Non-malignant conditions can simulate thyroid cancer; these include benign adenomas and multinodular goitres, as well as less common causes such as thyroglossal or colloid retention cysts. These may cause particular difficulty since they also produce the 'cold' nodule on thyroid isotope scanning so characteristic of malignant neoplasms (Figure 20.3). Ultrasound scanning will distinguish between cystic and solid lesions and is useful for monitoring and follow-up, for example, for a colloid nodule. The circulating thyroglobulin level may be elevated, but the test is still regarded by many as an unreliable marker of malignancy. New techniques for measuring thyroglobulin have been proposed [26]. Evidence of microcalcification in a soft-tissue radiograph, although

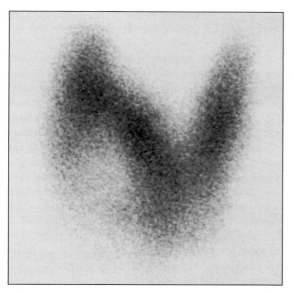

Figure 20.3 ^{123}I scan of thyroid, showing a cold nodule in the enlarged right node.

rarely seen, is strongly suggestive of papillary carcinoma, and is due to psammoma bodies. Apart from the mass itself, and the pressure effects such as stridor or recurrent laryngeal nerve involvement, patients with medullary carcinoma occasionally present with systemic endocrine symptoms from an associated MEN syndrome [14]. Most patients with thyroid cancer are clinically euthyroid. Autoimmune thyroiditis is associated with high levels of antithyroglobulin antibodies, low ^{131}I uptake and diffuse glandular enlargement, a syndrome quite different from de Quervain's subacute thyroiditis in which the thyroid is often painful or tender.

In general, thyroid scans suggestive of a 'cold' nodule (i.e. one which fails to take up radioiodine) should be regarded as potentially malignant. Fine-needle aspiration cytology (rather than open surgical biopsy) is usually adequate as the initial investigation. In the first place, this will immediately identify a thyroid cyst, to the great relief of the patient. Furthermore, cytological testing generally reveals the nature of the malignant lesion, with accurate prediction of the neoplastic cell type, although one limitation is that with follicular carcinoma the distinction between benign and malignant may be impossible, in which case surgical biopsy is essential. At most, only 20% of these patients will prove to have a malignant neoplasm. Radionuclide scanning may be useful when the fine-needle aspiration specimen is 'suspicious' or

indeterminate rather than clearly diagnostic, identifying 'hot' nodules that can be observed or treated medically [27]. In order to make an unequivocal diagnosis, hemithyroidectomy may sometimes be necessary or, in the case of larger lesions, partial or subtotal removal. For papillary (the largest single subtype), medullary and anaplastic cancers, needle aspiration may be sufficient, whereas in follicular carcinoma important histological features may not be recognizable in such small specimens. With routine fine-needle biopsy, only about half as many patients require diagnostic thyroidectomy for thyroid nodules, and a far higher proportion of surgically treated patients do indeed have cancer [28].

Papillary and follicular cancers are characteristically well differentiated and slow-growing, with a usually excellent prognosis [29].

Management
Surgical
A substantial thyroid resection may have been undertaken for diagnostic confirmation, consisting of unilateral thyroid lobectomy (hemithyroidectomy) with resection of the isthmus. However, there is no clear agreement, once the diagnosis has been established, as to whether the surgeon must then undertake a further operation to complete a total or near-total thyroidectomy. The risk of surgically induced hypoparathyroidism is low, probably about 3% in experienced hands. Repeat operations by inexperienced surgeons undoubtedly increase this hazard. In small cancers, completely enclosed by normal tissues, it may seem unjustifiable to advocate further surgery in view of the surgical risks. Nevertheless, routine total thyroidectomy is often recommended, even for *well-differentiated papillary tumours*, because of the high incidence of microscopic foci in the contralateral lobe [1,24]. A common recommendation in the UK is that a near-total or subtotal thyroidectomy be performed, though the use of serum thyroglobulin for follow-up has in recent years tended to modify this view. Younger patients under 40 years of age, with histopathology confirming a well-differentiated tumour, apparently completely removed, can be given suppressive thyroxine (T_4) to reduce thyroidstimulating hormone (TSH) to an undetectable level (0.2 mU/L) on current highly sensitive immunoradiometric assays, with follow-up using serum thyroglobulin as a marker (see below). The availability of thyroglobulin testing, coupled with a move towards more conservative surgery, has led to a controversy in selection of treatment options that has yet to be resolved.

For *follicular carcinomas* total thyroidectomy is usually best even in cases where metastases are present at the time of diagnosis, though this carries a risk of permanent hypoparathyroidism. In cases of papillary and follicular carcinomas, any obviously enlarged lymph nodes should be removed at the initial operation. *En bloc* resection of the thyroid gland and pathological nodes should be attempted even if bilateral lymph nodes are present. Despite the high incidence of histologically confirmed malignancies in clinically impalpable lymph nodes (probably of the order of 50%), prophylactic lymph node dissection is not usually recommended since recurrence after subsequent postoperative treatment with radioiodine will occur in less than 30% of patients.

In *papillary carcinoma*, the presence of palpable lymph nodes at diagnosis does not appear to affect the prognosis. There is no difference in outcome between patients treated by prophylactic neck dissection in whom lymph node involvement is confirmed histologically, and those with a later nodal recurrence who are then treated by therapeutic lymph node dissection (and possibly other methods as well). This is particularly true of the largest group of low-risk patients – women under 40 years of age with well-differentiated tumours. The classic large studies from Mazzaferri and Tubiana, assessing the long-term results in patients undergoing thyroidectomy for differentiated thyroid cancers, concluded that the completeness of surgical removal was still the most important prognostic factor [30,31].

With *medullary carcinomas*, routine neck node dissection is sometimes recommended, in addition to total thyroidectomy [19], a view substantiated by the high local recurrence rate of the order of 25%. For *anaplastic carcinomas* surgical removal of the tumour should be attempted wherever possible, although this is often technically difficult since early direct extension is the rule and tissue planes may be hopelessly destroyed. These tumours are only partly responsive to external beam irradiation so surgical removal of as much tumour as possible is important, even where this involves cutting directly across tumour. Because of the frequency of compression of the oesophagus, pharynx and trachea, maintenance of the airway by tracheostomy is often required.

For true *small-cell carcinomas* and *lymphomas* of the thyroid, thyroidectomy is unnecessary although it is occasionally performed for biopsy purposes. Where these tumours are suspected, 'Tru-cut' or other needle biopsy procedures are more often employed in order to avoid thyroidectomy wherever possible. They are highly radiosensitive, and surgery plays a correspondingly small part in the management.

Role of radiotherapy
Radioiodine therapy (^{131}I)

Use of ^{131}I has been an integral part of treatment for well-differentiated thyroid carcinoma for over 50 years [32–36]. Postoperative management depends on histological findings, extent of disease and completeness of surgery. In most cases of *well-differentiated thyroid cancer* (both papillary and follicular), ablation of residual thyroid tissue, together with neck and whole-body scanning, should be carried out postoperatively, using oral radioactive iodine, particularly if there is any doubt as to the completeness of surgery. About half of all follicular carcinomas fall into this category, rather fewer in the papillary group. Treatment with ^{131}I is not always necessary for well-differentiated tumours since occult and intrathyroid carcinomas have an excellent prognosis following surgery alone, and high doses of radioactive iodine can generally be avoided with safety in these predominantly young patients for whom radiation dose is an important consideration.

For patients in whom ^{131}I treatment is required, a moderately large dose has traditionally been given, of the order of 3 GBq (the becquerel has now replaced the curie; 1 Ci = 37 GBq), to ablate the residual thyroid tissue which always takes up iodine more avidly than the tumour, making therapeutic use of ^{131}I impossible in the presence of a significant volume of active residual thyroid tissue (Figure 20.4). However, recent large-scale studies have shown that for relatively low-risk cases, some of which have probably been surgically cured, a lower dose of radioiodine, of the order of 1.1 GBq, is quite sufficient, with lower risks to the patient [35,36]. If thyroxine (T_4) has been administered postoperatively, this must be discontinued one month before the radioiodine treatment in order to ensure that TSH rises. It is the rise in TSH rather than the hormone withdrawal that is important. After ^{131}I radioablation has been performed, a short 6-week course of triiodothyronine (T_3) is then given (in preference to T_4 which has a much longer duration of action and is therefore less flexible). After withdrawal of T_3 for 10 days, neck and whole-body scanning is again performed; residual uptake in the neck or elsewhere provides evidence of metastatic or unresected primary cancer. If this is demonstrated a therapeutic dose of ^{131}I (5.5–7.0 GBq) is indicated. It is the most highly targeted type of radiation therapy in common use for human cancer treatment and can be repeated at approximately

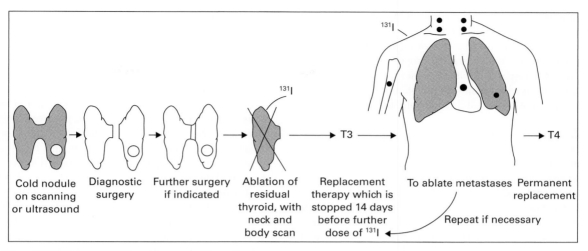

Figure 20.4 The use of ^{131}I in management of thyroid cancer.

3-monthly intervals (discontinuing exogenous T_3 10 days beforehand) for as long as the repeat scans confirm residual active disease, i.e. until the metastases are totally eradicated or treatment fails. An alternative to withdrawal of thyroid hormone therapy is the use of recombinant human thyrotropin [35].

Despite the dangers of significant radiation doses to the neck, marrow, gonads and other sites, it is important to realize that this specific and cytotoxic form of irradiation has produced many cures even in patients with widely metastatic disease. These patients (indeed most patients with thyroid cancer) need lifelong T_4 replacement since all thyroid tissue will have been ablated long before the final therapeutic dose. In a proportion of patients no longer responsive to radioiodine, hormone replacement with T_4 may produce further regression of disease (particularly in younger patients) because of the partial tumour dependency on TSH, which is suppressed by exogenous T_4. Occasionally, it is necessary to give therapeutic doses of ^{131}I when the patient has only just discontinued taking T_3 or T_4. In these cases TSH should be given for 2–3 days (by injection) before the ^{131}I is administered.

Although routine use of postoperative ^{131}I ablation is now regarded as over-treatment of many surgically treated cases of papillary carcinoma, the indications for use of radioiodine in selected patients were well demonstrated in classic studies by Mazzaferri and coworkers in Italy [30] and by Tubiana and coworkers in France [31]. Adverse features include age 40 years or over, a large primary tumour, poorly differentiated histological features and extracapsular extension. Local recurrence is more than twice as common after subtotal as after total thyroidectomy and may result in increased mortality. Radioiodine ablation is indicated where adequate uptake can be demonstrated in patients with multiple, locally invasive or large primary tumours, as well as those with distant metastases. New approaches to patient-specific dosimetry may offer better and more precise treatment and better radionuclide distribution [36]. Finally, the routine use of T_4 is valuable even in patients who have not undergone total thyroidectomy and who do not require it for physiological replacement.

Follow-up investigation and examinations are particularly important as patients may develop recurrences many years after apparent cure. Follow-up should include careful clinical palpation of the thyroid and regular chest radiography (about once every 3 years since pulmonary metastases and mediastinal nodes are relatively common sites), together with serum thyroglobulin measurements. Radioiodine tests are now much less used, and serum thyroglobulin can and should be measured when the patient is taking T_4 [26], yearly for the first 5 years after the patient is regarded as disease-free, and every second year of follow-up thereafter. Radioiodine testing (185 MBq is accepted as a safe outpatient dosage), with scanning 3–5 days afterwards, is increasingly used only in patients with an abnormal thyroglobulin level or in those known to have residual tumour postoperatively.

For patients with differentiated thyroid cancer who are unresponsive to radioiodine, an exciting advance has been reported recently, namely, the use of the MAP kinase inhibitor selumetenib, a well-tolerated oral agent with the potential to reverse the refractoriness to radioiodine even in patients with metastatic disease (see Ref. [37]). In an important study, a substantial proportion – 12 out of 20 patients – responded, with the majority then reaching the threshold for treatment with radioiodine and a reduction in their post-treatment thyroglobulin levels.

External irradiation and chemotherapy

In patients without adequate uptake of radioiodine, and particularly in those whose cancers are locally unresectable (including almost all cases of anaplastic carcinoma and many medullary carcinomas), external irradiation has an important role. A radical dose is required, typically of the order of 65 Gy in 7 weeks [38], in order to delay local recurrence and prevent troublesome symptoms from local obstruction. It can be curative, though rarely in patients with anaplastic carcinoma. In patients with *thyroid lymphomas* and *small-cell tumours*, both of which are highly radiosensitive, external beam irradiation is the definitive treatment [39]. For these tumours a lower dose is adequate, of the order of 40–50 Gy in 4–5 weeks. Since the total volume treated can be very substantial and at a site where spinal cord damage is a real threat, radical irradiation of the thyroid is technically difficult, and several groups have developed sophisticated techniques using wedged field arrangements or arc rotation planning. Others prefer a more straightforward approach with a single anterior direct field, shaped by lead blocks in order to protect the larynx and, if necessary, the lungs. The radiation fields should cover the whole thyroid gland, and if possible the first-stage supraclavicular or cervical lymph nodes. The field may have to be extended inferiorly to include the upper mediastinal area if there is evidence of disease at this level. Intratracheal deposits, for example, are well described and can lead to haemoptysis. Chemotherapy has a very limited role in the management of thyroid carcinomas but molecular targeted therapy appears to hold promise (see above) and both selumetenib, vandetanib and cabozantinib are increasingly used (see Refs. [40,11]).

Results of treatment

For well-differentiated tumours the results of treatment are remarkably good. One substantial subgroup of patients, those below 40 years of age with well-differentiated papillary carcinoma, have a normal survival pattern equal to that of a comparable population. The prognosis is affected by the age at diagnosis (the lower the better) and by the sex of the patient. One large American series, for example, confirmed a 10-year survival rate of 93% (papillary cancer) and 84% (follicular cancer) despite some patients developing local or even distant metastases [38,41,42]. Histological type also correlates with survival and, in general, the more well-differentiated the tumour, the better the prognosis. Features indicating a worse prognosis include male gender, positive family history, age above 40 years, tumour diameter above 4 cm, a poorly differentiated histology and lymph node or distant metastases. For papillary carcinoma, evidence of extrathyroid disease reduces the 10-year survival to about 50%. For medullary carcinomas the long-term survival is only about 40% [38,41], a reflection of its early metastatic potential and the ineffectiveness of ^{131}I therapy, itself a reflection of its different histogenesis. These figures are likely to improve as a result of genotype testing and prophylactic thyroidectomy [14,16,20], although over-treatment will doubtless occur in a proportion of *RET* mutation carriers owing to variation in expression and penetrance of the mutations, such as those affecting codons 611, 790, 791 and 804 [43].

Worst of all, anaplastic carcinoma has a very poor prognosis with about 5% of patients surviving 5 years and essentially no 10-year survivors; median survival for these tumours is only about 6 months [38]. It is important to distinguish small-cell carcinomas and thyroid lymphomas from the truly anaplastic group since their prognosis is undoubtedly better, and thyroid lymphoma, though uncommon, has an extremely good prognosis. For anaplastic carcinoma even highly aggressive treatments including surgery and external irradiation (and sometimes chemotherapy) have failed to improve the outlook [41].

It is difficult to assess the separate contributions of surgery and radiation therapy since they are used in a complementary fashion, with radiotherapy offered only to patients with incompletely resected tumours – those with a higher risk of local recurrence and poorer ultimate survival. Nevertheless, Tubiana and coworkers [31] achieved a 10-year survival rate of over 70% in patients with papillary carcinoma who had undergone incomplete surgery. In follicular and medullary carcinoma, the 10-year survival rates were 51 and 60%, respectively. For patients presenting with metastases, treatment with radioiodine (sometimes in combination with external irradiation to the primary tumour) may be very successful, with an overall survival rate of about 22% at 12 years. This reflects not only the effectiveness of ^{131}I therapy but also the indolent nature of this tumour, even when metastatic.

Chemotherapy for recurrent or metastatic thyroid cancer has been disappointing. The most active single agent is doxorubicin, with a response rate of about 30%, and with proven activity in all cell types. In addition, bleomycin has produced well-documented responses, and combinations of these and other agents have now been employed by several groups, reportedly with better response rates than with single agents alone. Duration of response is on the whole very short, quite apart from the fact that many of these patients are elderly and have rapidly advancing disease. Chemotherapy has only a limited role in the management of metastatic carcinoma of the thyroid, and treatment with external irradiation, radioiodine and exogenous T_4 should always be considered first. However, the recent availability of molecular targeted treatments has already made an impact and led to new ideas in the treatment of metastatic thyroid carcinoma. For example, vandetanib (ZD 6474) is a novel multi-targeted kinase inhibitor with potent activity against VEGFR II and other sites, making it an attractive agent for clinical trials in advanced disease, with particular relevance to medullary carcinoma, particularly since it is given as a once-daily oral dose. Its mechanism of action involves inhibition of VEGFR (antiangiogenesis) and also inhibition of the growth and survival of the tumour itself through inhibition of EGFR. It also inhibits RET kinase, an important growth factor in certain types of thyroid cancer. Vandetanib has shown encouraging early data in hereditary medullary thyroid cancer and has been awarded Food and Drug Administration (FDA) and European Union 'orphan drug' status, and FDA fast-track designation for this indication. It is currently undergoing clinical development in a range of tumours. Exciting results have also been reported with the VEGFR inhibitor motesanib diphosphate (AMG 706), an oral agent that also inhibits platelet-derived growth factor receptor and KIT. In an important international study from the USA and Europe, 93 patients with progressive, locally advanced or metastatic papillary, Hurthle cell or follicular cancer were treated with AMG 706 at a dose of 125 mg daily; stable disease or better was achieved in over 70% of cases, maintained for 24 weeks or longer in 35% [44]. Over 80% of patients had a fall in their circulating thyroglobulin during treatment.

Overall, about 8–10% of patients with thyroid cancer die of their disease [42]. Despite the excellent overall result in many patients with well-differentiated cancers, follow-up should be lifelong because of the lengthy natural history.

Cancer of the adrenal gland

These rare tumours arise from either the adrenal cortex or the adrenal medulla, and in adults the ratio of adreno-cortical carcinoma to malignant medullary tumours (malignant phaeochromocytoma) is approximately 2:1. Neuroblastoma, a common childhood tumour chiefly arising from the medulla, is discussed in Chapter 24.

Adrenocortical carcinoma

This very rare tumour represents only about 0.2% of all cases of cancer. About one-quarter of patients with adult Cushing's syndrome who have no obvious source of ectopic hormone production have an adrenal tumour, of which 30% are malignant [45]. Fewer than 40 cases are diagnosed in the UK per annum, most of which are hormonally active, presenting with features of Cushing's syndrome. In adrenal carcinoma patients, virilization, feminization or hyperaldosteronism (Conn's syndrome) are more common than in benign adenomas, although 30% of adrenocortical carcinomas are non-functional. The mean age at presentation is 45 years, with a female to male ratio of 2.5:1. Symptoms are usually present for 6–12 months before diagnosis, including glucocorticoid excess (45%), androgen excess (15%), both glucocorticoids and androgens (35%) and mineralocorticoids or estrogens (5%). Other symptoms include abdominal pain or discomfort, weight loss and extreme fatigue or weakness. Diabetes can also develop, as part of the presenting symptomatology. Benign adrenocortical tumours are typically yellowish in appearance and are adenomas often with lipid-laden large-cell or giant-cell patterns. Malignancy is likely if the mass is greater than 6 cm in diameter, characteristically with a more obviously necrotic or haemorrhagic appearance, with pleomorphic morphology and frequent mitoses. The distinction between adenoma and low-grade carcinoma can be difficult to make. Vascular invasion and distant dissemination (chiefly to bone, lung and liver) can occur.

At presentation, 70% have locoregional disease and 30% have metastases. The diagnosis is usually made biochemically (persistent hypercortisolaemia with absent dexamethasone suppression and low plasma ACTH), by computed tomography (CT) or magnetic resonance imaging (MRI) (Figure 20.5) and, ultimately, tissue diagnosis following laparotomy or CT-guided biopsy. In a large USA-based study using data from the Surveillance, Epidemiology and End Results (SEER) Program and the University of California [46], the size of the lesion proved to be a useful guide to the likelihood of malignancy. For instance lesions of over 4 cm had a 10% risk, i.e. about double that of the whole group studies; for lesions greater than 8 cm the risk increased ninefold. Adrenal hyperplasia is usually bilateral, and so unilateral adrenal enlargement is strongly suspicious of a benign or malignant tumour. Other imaging techniques include ultrasound and selective angiography with venous sampling. Non-functional tumours are more difficult to diagnose preoperatively and generally occur in patients under 20 years of age. Clinical features include a palpable abdominal mass (often of substantial size because of the 'silent' nature of the tumour), weight loss or fever.

A clinically useful staging system (McFarlane–Sullivan staging) has been developed, based largely on MRI and/or CT scanning, as follows.

Stage I   tumour size under 5 cm, no spread into adjacent tissues.

Stage II   tumour size above 5 cm but no adjacent local spread.

Stage III local or lymphatic invasion, adjacent to primary site.

Stage IV   further dissemination either locally or more widespread.

Treatment is primarily surgical, with wide resection usually via a substantial thoracoabdominal incision, and preoperative steroid therapy with metastatic disease. Systemic treatment with o,p'-DDD (a derivative of the insecticide DDT and generally known as mitotane) can

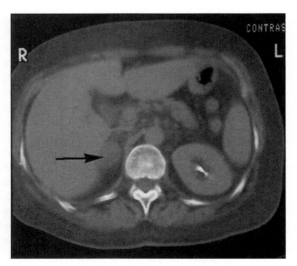

Figure 20.5 CT scan of abdomen showing adrenal tumour (arrow). Normal anatomy of other structures is also clearly shown.

be beneficial, although side-effects can be extremely troublesome, often necessitating a reduction in dosage. Mitotane is an agent that requires metabolic transformation for its therapeutic action [47], and individual cancers probably have differing characteristics in respect of the completeness of this process. In the majority of patients both a reduction in corticosteroid production and tumour regression can occur. Mitotane can often be given with little adverse effect, but the full daily dosage of 8–10 g may produce side-effects of anorexia, nausea, diarrhoea, confusion and lethargy, limiting treatment acceptability. These effects are largely due to contamination with DDT, and the pure drug is much better tolerated. Steroid replacement is usually necessary. Where there is failure of response to o,p'-DDD (or if side-effects are intolerable), palliation of Cushing's syndrome may be achieved by agents such as metyrapone, aminoglutethimide or ketoconazole, which interfere with steroid synthesis. An important recent study from Italy and Germany assessed the value of mitotane given as an adjuvant following radical resection of the primary cancer [48]. This was a retrospective analysis of 177 patients: the mitotane group were treated at Italian centres and the controls (surgery only) chiefly in Germany. Recurrence-free survival was significantly improved in the mitotane group (42 months compared with 10 months for Italian control patients and 25 months for German control patients). The relatively new agent gossypol is also under investigation, and has been shown to produce responses [49]. It is a derivative of the cotton plant, a polyphenolic aldehyde given by mouth that inhibits a variety of dehydrogenase enzymes (and has also been studied as a potential male contraceptive). Chemotherapy using cisplatin and etoposide occasionally produces responses. Surgical resection or embolization should also be considered, as well as palliative radiotherapy for patients with painful bone metastases. In fact radiation therapy to the tumour bed has been advocated as a potentially useful treatment, following initial surgery [50]; this recently published retrospective analysis from Germany suggested that adjuvant radiation therapy reduces local recurrence, and concluded that a randomized study would be worth pursuing. Overall, the prognosis is poor, with a median survival of 15 months, and only 20% of patients alive at 5 years. Adverse prognostic factors include age over 40 and metastases at presentation. Despite many advances in imaging and surgery, these results seem not to have improved during recent years [51].

Table 20.2 Symptoms caused by phaeochromocytoma.

Skin: attacks of sweating, flushing, blanching
Cardiovascular: hypertension, tachycardia, paroxysmal
   rhythm change, slow forceful beating chest pain, postural
   hypotension
Central nervous system: headache, tremor, irritability, mood
   change, psychosis, anorexia
Metabolic: weight loss, increased metabolic rate, glycosuria

Adrenal medulla

The cells of the adrenal medulla [52] have a different derivation from those of the cortex, developing from neuroectodermal tissue and giving rise to both benign and malignant tumours. In adult life these include *phaeochromocytoma* (benign in 90% of cases), *ganglioneuroma* or *neuroblastoma*. In childhood, neuroblastoma is much the commonest of the adrenal medullary tumours (see Chapter 24).

Phaeochromocytomas can arise from the adrenal medulla (90%), organ of Zuckerkandl or adrenal medullary cell rests in the pelvis; 10% are bilateral. They can occur sporadically or as part of a familial syndrome of MEN-2 (see Chapter 15). Other associated diseases include neurofibromatosis, von Hippel–Lindau and Sturge–Weber syndromes, cerebellar ataxia and tuberous sclerosis/astrocytoma. About 10% are histologically malignant, although conventional microscopic appearances are an unreliable guide to clinical behaviour and the diagnosis of malignancy must be made with caution.

Phaeochromocytoma can occur at any age but is commonest at 40–60 years. The annual incidence is 1 per 100 000 but it accounts for 0.1% of hypertension. Most patients are diagnosed as a result of investigation for sustained hypertension, but the secretion of catecholamines by the tumour may also cause paroxysmal symptoms (Table 20.2) (similar for both benign and malignant tumours) and include intermittent or paroxysmal headache, severe sweating attacks, postural hypotension, dysrhythmias and chest pain. Attacks may be precipitated by certain foods, posture and micturition. Pregnancy may provoke attacks due to pressure. Some patients present primarily with an abdominal or pelvic mass. Patients may be thin and agitated (resembling thyrotoxicosis).

Confirmation of the diagnosis is made by demonstration of excess catecholamines (adrenaline, noradrenaline and metabolites) in both urine and blood. The paroxysmal

nature of the disorder may lead to false-negative plasma catecholamine measurement, so 24-hour urine collections are essential. Measurement of vanillylmandelic acid (VMA) in the urine will provide the diagnosis in 85% of patients. False positives may occur on diets high in vanillin (bananas, nuts, coffee).

In others it may be necessary to resort to provocative tests using pharmacological agents. Phentolamine in *very small doses* (0.5–1.0 mg) will produce a fall in blood pressure of 25 mmHg lasting from 5 min to 4 hours. Histamine and tyramine provoke hypertension in these patients by liberating the excess catecholamines stored in nerve endings (but not in the tumour). The use of these drugs requires extremely careful monitoring. Provocative tests are now seldom necessary since the introduction of more sensitive tests. Indeed, the greater area of difficulty lies in distinguishing physiological hypersecretion.

Selective angiography and venous sampling may be necessary to localize the tumour, though CT or MRI generally give excellent visualization of the adrenal. In most cases the diagnosis of malignancy can be made only when the resected specimen is examined histologically, but occasionally a patient may have clinically obvious metastases. Despite the increasing availability of molecular diagnostic and prognostic markers, it remains impossible to predict the subsequent development of malignant disease, based on the initial histological findings in a resected tumour. Unfortunately, only the presence of metastases of chromaffin tissue at sites where no chromaffin tissue should be present will establish a definite diagnosis of a malignant phaeochromocytoma, the commonest site being bone, lungs, liver and nodal sites.

Treatment of these tumours is by surgical resection, with careful dissection and microscopic inspection of excision margins to ensure adequate clearance. Surgical excision of single metastatic deposits has also been recommended. Several recent reports have suggested that these tumours can be safely resected laparoscopically, provided that meticulous medical preparation is undertaken [53]. Preoperatively the blood pressure is controlled by gradually increasing doses of phenoxybenzamine (to produce α-adrenergic receptor blockade). In patients with arrhythmia, a beta-blocker is added after the blood pressure is brought under control (Figure 20.6). Used alone they can precipitate severe hypertension. After good blood pressure control has been achieved for 10 days the resection is performed, with continuous intraoperative intra-arterial blood pressure monitoring, and careful use of phentolamine and beta-blockers.

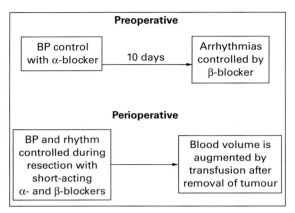

Preoperative

BP control with α-blocker → 10 days → Arrhythmias controlled by β-blocker

Perioperative

BP and rhythm controlled during resection with short-acting α- and β-blockers → Blood volume is augmented by transfusion after removal of tumour

Figure 20.6 Preoperative and perioperative management of phaeochromocytoma. BP, blood pressure.

A fall in blood pressure following removal can usually be controlled by blood transfusion.

The use of chemotherapy for metastatic disease is purely anecdotal but alkylating agents and doxorubicin have been reportedly effective. High-dose ^{131}I-meta-iodobenzylguanidine has also been used therapeutically [54] and has a symptom improvement rate of over 60%. In patients with symptomatic inoperable phaeochromocytoma, both alpha- and beta-blockers are valuable in controlling symptoms, and may have to be maintained for several years in patients with slow-growing tumours. Although long-term survival has been recorded, the majority of patients with malignant phaeochromocytoma die of the disease; extra-adrenal primary sites are said to have a particularly poor prognosis.

Cancer of the parathyroid glands

This tumour is very rare, with fewer than 300 cases in the world literature. Under 5% of all parathyroid tumours are malignant. The disease has been reported following irradiation of the neck. Most parathyroid carcinomas secrete parathyroid hormone, causing a very severe form of primary hyperparathyroidism, sometimes with a florid variety of osteitis fibrosa cystica. The tumour tends to be slow-growing, and long-term survival frequently occurs if complete surgical removal is performed. Local recurrence can lead to severe pressure symptoms in the neck, but can be surgically resectable. Distant metastases occasionally occur, chiefly to the lung and liver.

If a parathyroid carcinoma spreads to different sites, it can cause relentless hypercalcaemia and severe metabolic complications that are notoriously difficult to control and often result in death. Affected patients may require repeated palliative surgical extirpation of the metastatic nodules. Early *en bloc* resection of the primary tumour is the only curative treatment. Because the histopathological features of parathyroid carcinoma and adenoma may overlap, a definitive diagnosis of malignant potential or 'invasiveness' may depend on other criteria, such as the radiological features of the tumour, development of unexpected local recurrence or distant metastasis. An understanding of the molecular pathogenesis of parathyroid carcinoma could have considerable value with respect to early diagnosis, prognosis and new approaches to treatment.

No specific gene has been established as a direct contributor to the pathogenesis of sporadic parathyroid carcinoma, although several important molecular clues have been uncovered. Recent work has drawn attention to the possible importance of mutations in the *HRPT2* gene which are likely to have pathogenetic importance [55,40].

References

1 Schlumberger MJ. Medical progress: papillary and follicular thyroid carcinoma. *N Engl J Med* 1998; 338: 297–306.
2 LiVolsi VA. Well differentiated thyroid carcinoma. *Clin Oncol* 1996; 8: 281–8.
3 Akslen LA, LiVolsi VA. Prognostic significance of histologic grading compared with subclassification of papillary thyroid carcinoma. *Cancer* 2000; 88: 1902–8.
4 Colonna M, Guizard AV, Schvartz B *et al*. A time trend analysis of papillary and follicular cancers as a function of tumour size: a study of data from six cancer registries in France (1983–2000). *Eur J Cancer* 2007; 43: 891–900.
5 Bible, K C. Treating advanced radioresistant differentiated thyroid cancer. *Lancet Oncol* 2012, 13: 854–5.
6 Morris JC, Montori VM. Thyroid cancer: zealous imaging has increased detection and treatment of low risk tumours. *Brit Med J* 2013; 347: f4706.
7 Gasbarri A, Sciacchiatano S, Marasco A *et al*. Detection and molecular characterization of thyroid cancer precursor lesions in a specific subset of Hashimoto's thyroiditis. *Br J Cancer* 2004; 10: 1038.
8 Dobson R. Thyroid cancer has increased 12-fold in women since Chernobyl. *Br Med J* 2004; 328: 1394.
9 Ito Y, Miyauchi A. Therapeutic strategies for papillary microcarcinoma of the thyroid. *Curr Cancer Ther Rev* 2005; 1: 19–25.
10 Pellegriti G, Scollo C, Lumera G *et al*. Clinical behavior and outcome of papillary thyroid cancers smaller than 1.5 cm in

diameter: study of 299 cases. *Clin Endocrinol Metab* 2004; 89: 3713–20.

11 Leboulleux S, Bastholt L, Krause T *et al.* Vandetanib in locally advanced or metastatic differentiated thyroid cancer: a randomized, double-blind, phase 2 trial. *Lancet Oncol* 2012; 13: 897–905.

12 Cote GJ, Gagel RF. Lessons learned from the management of a rare genetic cancer. *N Engl J Med* 2003; 349: 1566–8.

13 Machens A, Gimm O, Ukkat J *et al.* Improved prediction of calcitonin normalisation in medullary thyroid carcinoma patients by quantitative lymph node analysis. *Cancer* 2000; 88: 1909–15.

14 Saad ME, Ordonez MG, Rashid RK *et al.* Medullary carcinoma of the thyroid: a study of the clinical features and prognostic factors in 161 patients. *Medicine* 1984; 63: 319–42.

15 Eng C. The RET proto-oncogene in multiple endocrine neoplasia type 2 and Hirschsprung's disease. *N Engl J Med* 1996; 335: 943–51.

16 Machens A, Niccoli-Sire P, Hoegel J *et al.* Early malignant progression of hereditary medullary thyroid cancer. *N Engl J Med* 2003; 349: 1517–25.

17 Mathew CGP, Easton DF, Nakamura Y *et al.* Presymptomatic screening for multiple endocrine neoplasia type 2A with linked DNA markers. *Lancet* 1991; 337: 7–11.

18 Lips CJM, Landsvater RM, Hoppener JWM *et al.* Clinical screening as compared with DNA analysis in families with multiple endocrine neoplasia type 2A. *N Engl J Med* 1994; 331: 828–35.

19 Calmettes C, Ponder BAJ, Fischer JA *et al.* Early diagnosis of the multiple endocrine neoplasia type 2 syndrome: consensus statement. *Eur J Clin Invest* 1992; 22: 755–60.

20 Wells SA Jr, Chi DD, Toshima K *et al.* Predictive DNA testing and prophylactic thyroidectomy in patients at risk for multiple endocrine neoplasia type IIa. *Ann Surg* 1994; 220: 237–50.

21 Cornett WR, Sharma AK, Day TA *et al.* Anaplastic thyroid carcinoma: an overview. *Curr Oncol Rep* 2007; 9: 152–8.

22 Wilson PC, Millar BM, Brierley JD. The management of advanced thyroid cancer. *Clin Oncol* 2004; 16: 561–8.

23 Mack LA, Pasieka JL. An evidence-based approach to the treatment of thyroid lymphoma. *World J Surg* 2007; 31: 978–86.

24 Sherman SI. Thyroid carcinoma. *Lancet* 2003; 361: 501–11.

25 Kebebew E, Clark OH. Differentiated thyroid cancer: 'complete' rational approach. *World J Surg* 2000; 24: 942–51.

26 Iervasi A, Iervasi G, Bottoni A *et al.* Diagnostic performance of a new highly sensitive thyroglobulin immunoassay. *J Endocrinol* 2004; 182: 287–94.

27 Fernandes JK, Day TA, Richardson MS, Sharma AK. Overview of the management of differentiated thyroid cancer. *Curr Treat Options Oncol* 2005; 6: 47–57.

28 Gharib H, Goeliner JR. Fine-needle aspiration biopsy of the thyroid: an appraisal. *Ann Intern Med* 1993; 118: 282–9.

29 Keston Jones M. Management of papillary and follicular thyroid cancer. *J R Soc Med* 2002; 95: 325–6.

30 Mazzaferri EL, Young RL, Oertel JE *et al.* Papillary thyroid carcinoma: the impact of therapy on 576 patients. *Medicine (Baltimore)* 1977; 56: 171–96.

31 Tubiana M, Schlumberger M, Rougier P *et al.* Long-term results and prognostic factors in patients with differentiated thyroid carcinoma. *Cancer* 1985; 55: 794–804.

32 Chatal JF, Hoefnagel CA. Radionuclide therapy. *Lancet* 1999; 354: 931–5.

33 Sawka AM, Thephamongkhol K, Brouwers M *et al.* A systematic review and meta-analysis of effectiveness of radioactive iodine remnant ablation for well-differentiated thyroid cancer. *J Clin Endocrinol Metab* 2004; 89: 3668–76.

34 Sisson JC. Applying the radioactive eraser: I-131 to ablate normal thyroid tissue in patients from whom thyroid cancer has been resected. *J Nucl Med* 1983; 24: 743–5.

35 Schlumberger M D, Catargi B, Borget I *et al.* Strategies of radioiodine ablation in patients with low-risk thyroid cancer. *New Engl J Med* 2012; 366: 1663–73.

36 Alexander EK, Larsen PR. Radioiodine for thyroid cancer – is less more? *New Engl J Med* 2012; 366: 1732–3.

37 Ho AL, Grewal RK, Leboeuf R, *et al.* Selumetenib-enhanced radioiodine uptake an advanced thyroid cancer. *New Engl J Med* 2013; 368: 623–632.

38 Wartofsky L, ed. *Thyroid Cancer: A Comprehensive Guide to Clinical Management.* New York: Humana Press, 1999: 515.

39 Souhami L, Simpson WJ, Carruthers JS. Malignant lymphoma of the thyroid gland. *Int J Radiat Oncol Biol Phys* 1980; 6: 1143–8.

40 Lumachi F, Basso SM, Basso U. Parathyroid cancer: etiology, clinical presentation and treatment. *Anticancer Res* 2006; 26: 4803–7.

41 Hundahl SA, Fleming ID, Freugen AM, Menck HR. A National Cancer Data Base report on 53 856 cases of thyroid carcinoma treated in the US, 1985–1995. *Cancer* 1998; 83: 2638–48.

42 Utiger RD. Follow-up of patients with thyroid carcinoma. *N Engl J Med* 1997; 337: 928–30.

43 Fitze G, Schierz M, Bredow J *et al.* Various penetrance of familial medullary thyroid carcinoma in patients with RET proto-oncogene codon 790/791 germline mutations. *Ann Surg* 2002; 236: 570–5.

44 Sherman S, Wirth LJ, Droz J-P *et al.* Motesanib diphosphate in progressive differentiated thyroid cancer. *N Engl J Med* 2008; 359: 31–42.

45 Luton J-P, Cerdas S, Billaud L *et al.* Clinical features of adrenocortical carcinoma, prognostic factors, and the effect of mitotane therapy. *N Engl J Med* 1990; 322: 1195–201.

46 Sturgeon C, Shen WT, Clark OH *et al.* Risk assessment in 457 adrenal cortical carcinomas: how much does tumor size predict the likelihood of malignancy? *J Am Coll Surg* 2006; 202: 423–30.

47 Schteingart DE. Adjuvant mitotane therapy of adrenal cancer: use and controversy. *N Engl J Med* 2007; 356: 2415–18.

48 Terzolo M, Angeli A, Fassnacht M *et al.* Adjuvant mitotane treatment for adrenocortical carcinoma. *N Engl J Med* 2007; 356: 2372–80.

49 Flack MR, Pyle RG, Mullen NM *et al.* Oral gossypol in the treatment of metastatic adrenal cancer. *J Clin Endocrinol Metab* 1993; 76: 1019–24.

50 Fassnacht M, Hahner S, Polat B *et al.* Efficacy of adjuvant radiotherapy to the tumor bed on local recurrence in adrenocortical carcinoma. *J Clin Endocrinol Metab* 2006; 91: 4501–4.

51 Kebebew E, Reiff E, Duh QY *et al.* Extent of disease at presentation and outcome for adrenocortical carcinoma: have we made progress? *World J Surg* 2006; 30: 872–8.

52 Lenders JW, Isenhofer G, Mannelli M, Pacak K. Phaeochromocytoma. *Lancet* 2005; 366: 665–75.

53 Flavio Rocha M, Faramarzi-Roques R, Tauzin-Fin P *et al.* Laparoscopic surgery for pheochromocytoma. *Eur Urol* 2004; 45: 226–32.

54 Sisson JC. Radiopharmaceutical treatment of pheochromocytomas. *Ann NY Acad Sci* 2002; 970: 54–60.

55 Shattuck TM, Välimäki S, Obara T *et al.* Somatic and germ-line mutations of the *HRPT*-2 gene in sporadic parathyroid carcinoma. *N Engl J Med* 2003; 349: 1722–9.

Further reading

Baudin E, Schlumberger M. New therapeutic approaches for metastatic thyroid carcinoma. *Lancet Oncol* 2007; 8: 148–56.

Biondi B, Filetti S, Schlumberger M. Thyroid-hormone therapy and thyroid cancer: a reassessment. *Nat Clin Pract Endocrinol Metab* 2005; 1: P32–P40.

Cooper DS, Doherty GM, Haugen BR *et al.* Management guidelines for patients with thyroid nodules and differentiated thyroid cancer. *Thyroid* 2006; 16: 1–33.

Gill V, Gerrard G. How much thyroxine is needed for thyroid cancer patients? *Clin Oncol* 2008; 20: 316–17.

Mallick U, Harmer C, Yap B *et al.* Ablation with low-dose radioiodine and thyroptropin alfa in thyroid cancer. *New Engl J Med* 2012; 366: 1674–85.

Mehanna HM, Jain A, Morton RP *et al.* Investigating the thyroid nodule. *Br Med J* 2009; 338: 710.

Pacini P, Schlumberger M, Dralle H *et al.* European consensus for the management of patients with differentiated thyroid carcinoma of the follicular epithelium. *Eur J Endocrinol* 2006; 154: 787–803.

Royal College of Physicians. *British Thyroid Association Guidelines for the Management of Thyroid Cancer*, 2nd edn. London: Royal College of Physicians, 2007.

21 Cancer from an unknown primary site

About 3% of all cancers, and 6% of cancer deaths, are cancers where the primary site is unknown after initial examination and investigation. In these cases, the primary tumour is too small to be clinically apparent. Usually the histological diagnosis, obtained from a metastasis, is of an adenocarcinoma or poorly differentiated carcinoma.

Diagnosis and treatment requires fine clinical judgement. Multiple investigations may be undertaken designed to disclose the primary site, but these are frequently ineffective in disclosing the primary tumour or in changing management. A diagnosis is established only in 15% of cases. After post-mortem, a further 70% of diagnosis is attained.

Site of presentation

The extent and nature of preliminary investigation will depend on the site of the metastasis [1]. The common metastatic sites include lymph nodes, bone, brain, liver and skin. Table 21.1 shows the most frequent primary tumours presenting at these sites. With each metastatic site, investigation will have a different emphasis. For example, a squamous carcinoma in a cervical node indicates that the nasopharynx or lung is the likely primary site, and full examination, including the larynx, pharynx and postnasal space, will often give the diagnosis. A left supraclavicular node suggests an intra-abdominal primary. Multiple liver metastases suggest gastrointestinal cancer, lung cancer or melanoma as the primary site Metastasis in an inguinal node or malignant ascites will necessitate gynaecological examination. Osteoblastic bone metastases suggest a prostate or thyroid primary.

Management will then be as for the underlying malignancy. When initial investigation has failed to give any clue to the primary cancer, the physician must ask 'If I find the primary, will there be any treatment which offers a reasonable chance of cure or long-term palliation or cure?' It is of critical importance to ensure that germ cell tumours are correctly diagnosed as these may present as poorly differentiated carcinomas but are highly responsive to chemotherapy.

The sites of origin of metastasis from an unknown primary site

The distribution of cancers that present as metastases from an occult primary is not the same as the overall distribution of cancer. In Table 21.2 the frequency of presentation of metastasis from an unknown primary is shown compared with the frequency of cancers in general. The commonest tumours are pancreas, lung, liver, stomach and colorectal cancer. Common cancers such as breast and prostate are much less frequent

Cancer and its Management, Seventh Edition. Jeffrey Tobias and Daniel Hochhauser.
© 2015 John Wiley & Sons, Ltd. Published 2015 by John Wiley & Sons, Ltd.

Table 21.1 Sites of metastases from an unknown primary site.

Site of metastasis	Likely primary site
High cervical nodes	Head and neck sites
	Thyroid, lung
Lower cervical nodes	Head and neck
	Lung
	Breast
	Gut (especially L. supraclavicular node)
Axillary nodes	Lung
	Breast
Skin	Breast
	Lung
	Melanoma
Bone	Myeloma
	Breast
	Kidney
	Prostate
	Lung
Brain	Lung
	Breast
	Prostate
	Melanoma
Inguinal nodes	Vulva
	Anorectal
	Prostate
	Ovary
Disseminated intra-abdominal adenocarcinoma (including liver metastasis)	Ovary
	Stomach
	Pancreas
	Gut

Table 21.2 Sites of origin of carcinomas presenting as metastases from unknown site.

	All unknown primary cases (%)	All cancers (%)
Pancreas	20	2
Lung	20	10
Unknown	15	
Liver	10	2
Stomach	10	5
Colorectal	81	5
Breast	3	26
Thyroid	3	1
Renal	3	2
Prostate	3	18
Ovary	2	5
Other	3	14

Table 21.3 Treatable cancers which may present as metastases from an unknown primary.

Curable tumours which must not be missed
Germ cell and trophoblastic tumours
Lymphomas
Well-differentiated thyroid cancer

Tumours which can be palliated by chemotherapy
Breast
Ovary
Small-cell carcinoma of the bronchus

Tumours which can be palliated by hormone therapy
Breast
Prostate
Endometrial

causes of metastasis from an unknown primary. This is probably because primary tumours in the breast are relatively easily detected clinically, while prostatic cancer is associated with an elevation of the acid phosphatase or prostate-specific antigen (PSA).

Tumours where treatment may be curative, or where prolonged palliation is possible, are shown in Table 21.3. Investigation must therefore be directed towards the confident exclusion of these cancers.

Several studies have shown that the yield of investigation is low when applied routinely to all patients in this situation. In most cases, therefore, a primary will not be found at presentation and, even if it is, it is extremely unusual for a treatable disease to be discovered. A further problem in adopting an attitude of intensive investigation is that the studies may give false-positive results. The patient may be subjected to a number of further investigations, often invasive, invariably expensive and usually resulting in failure.

Investigation and management

The following is a guide to the management of this difficult problem [1,2]. It must be emphasized that the degree to which investigation will be pursued will vary greatly with individual patients. The patient's age, fitness and degree of anxiety will all influence the decision, as well as the possibility of finding a treatable tumour. The decision about further investigation is one which demands judgement and skill. In the main, the less experienced the physician, the greater the number of investigations performed. It requires considerable clinical authority and careful explanation to help the patient understand that further investigation for the primary site may not be needed (or is not likely to be helpful) after the metastasis has been discovered and treatable causes excluded.

Review of histology

The most important first step is to discuss the biopsy with an experienced pathologist. The pathologist may have an idea where the primary site might be, but because of lack of clinical information, has left the diagnosis open. The usual appearance is of a poorly differentiated adenocarcinoma or an undifferentiated tumour. Special stains may be useful in providing further information, for example, immunocytochemical staining for large-cell lymphomas. These tumours are often difficult to distinguish from anaplastic carcinoma, but are very responsive to chemotherapy. Mucin stains may demonstrate intracellular mucin and point to an origin in the gut, pancreas or stomach. Monoclonal antibodies reactive with membrane and cytoplasmic proteins may help to determine the cell of origin. It is important not to miss a large-cell lymphoma as a cause of an undifferentiated tumour, and antibodies to the common leucocyte antigen (see Chapter 26 and Figure 3.12) and to epithelial antigens such as cytokeratins can usually make this distinction.

Table 21.4 lists some of the more frequently used reagents. Some work on paraffin sections, while others require frozen tissue. Biopsy material should therefore not be placed entirely in formalin when cancer is a possible diagnosis. Antibodies to epithelial membrane antigens (EMAs) are available which help to define epithelial tumours such as breast cancer or other poorly differentiated adenocarcinomas. Antibodies to prekeratin may be helpful in determining whether or not the tumour is of squamous origin; others react with melanoma-associated antigens. In a woman, if the node is taken from an axillary or a supraclavicular site, oestrogen and progesterone receptor positivity may indicate breast origin for the tumour. Occasionally, electron microscopy may help, for example, in showing pre-melanosomes in malignant melanoma, or intercellular bridges in poorly differentiated squamous carcinoma. Undifferentiated germ cell tumours are curable cancers of young people which are easily overlooked. They may contain human chorionic gonadotrophin (HCG) and α-fetoprotein

Table 21.4 Further pathological investigation in diagnosis in metastasis from an unknown primary site.

Cellular structure	Investigation or reagent	Tumour types identified	
Cytokeratins	Cam 5.2	Carcinomas	
Oestrogen and progesterone receptor	Antibodies	Breast cancer and other gynaecological tumours	
Epithelial membrane antigen (EMA)	Antibodies to EMA	Carcinomas (especially breast, gut, ovary, pancreas)	
Prostate-specific antigen (PSA)	Anti-PSA	Prostate cancer	
Common leucocyte antigen (CLA)	Anti-CLA	Lymphomas (98% positive)	
Desmin intermediate Vimentin filaments	Antibodies	Some sarcomas	
S100Melanoma-associated antigen	HMB-45	Melanoma	
Thyroglobulin	Anti-thyroglobulin	Thyroid carcinoma	
HCG	Anti-HCGAFP	Anti-AFP	Germ cell tumours
PLAP	Anti-PLAPP-remelanosomes	EM	Melanoma
Dense core granules	EM	Neuroendocrine tumours (small-cell lung cancer)	
Intermediate filaments	EM	Carcinoma	

EM, electron microscopy.

(AFP) and can be stained for the intracellular presence of these peptides by immunocytochemical techniques.

Imaging

The use of imaging is to determine the extent of the primary tumour and, on occasions may reveal the primary site.

A chest radiograph is an essential examination and may disclose a carcinoma of the bronchus or enlarged mediastinal lymph nodes suggestive of a lymphoma.

Computed tomography (CT) scans of the abdomen show the site of the primary tumour in 25% of cases. This is often the pancreas if the metastasis is an adenocarcinoma. Treatment is unaffected by knowledge of the pancreatic primary. Metastasis in the adrenal gland suggests a lung primary. If pulmonary metastases are small and numerous cancer of the colon, prostate or thyroid are likely causes. A few large metastases are more common with sarcomas. Calcification in hepatic metastases suggests a colonic cause. Mammography is essential if carcinoma of the breast is a differential diagnosis, since the presentation with a supraclavicular or axillary node does not exclude effective treatment.

Biochemical and haematological investigation

Certain tests should be carried out as a routine. These include an acid phosphatase and/or PSA measurement in men over 40 years old, to detect carcinoma of the prostate; and HCG and AFP determinations in young patients in case the tumour is of germ cell type. Hepatomas also produce AFP. Immunoelectrophoresis of plasma and examination of the urine for Bence-Jones protein is essential if myeloma is a possibility. The blood film may show leucoerythroblastic anaemia, most commonly seen with breast cancer. Polycythaemia and thrombocytosis may occur with renal carcinoma and hepatoma. Biochemical evidence of hypokalaemia and hyperglycaemia suggests Cushing's syndrome which, in this situation, is likely to be due to a small-cell lung cancer.

Molecular profiling

There is increased evidence that molecular profiling can assist more precise diagnosis and assist in selection of appropriate treatment. Microarray technology quantitating gene expression patterns in tumours have been validated in several tumour types including leukaemias and breast cancer but their role in cancers of unknown primary is uncertain. Additionally analysis of metastases may not always reflect the profile of the primary tumour. Testing of first-generation gene expression-based classifier for several specific cancer types demonstrated that identifying a small subset of patients having a colorectal-like gene expression profile predicted responses to treatment similar to those of known colon cancer patients [3]. A recent study in which molecular profiling and immunohistochemistry of metastatic disease were used, and in which the primary cancer was discovered some time later, showed a high level of agreement between the molecular profiling result and the final diagnosis [4]. Whether this can be applied more widely remains a focus of investigation. Several commercial services are already available but no firm evidence to validate routine clinical use is as yet available. Other promising approaches include microRNA and epigenetic profiling.

Other investigations

Serum markers may be of some help, but are rarely diagnostic except in hepatocellular cancers (AFP) and may be of value in excluding germ cell tumours (HCG, AFP). They include CEA for gastrointestinal carcinomas, PSA for prostate cancer and CA-125 for ovarian cancer.

Treatment

The element of uncertainty in the situation, added to the serious nature and generally poor prognosis, makes management difficult for the patient and physician. If the diagnosis has been established as a germ cell tumour or other treatable condition as outlined in Table 21.3, then treatment is along the appropriate lines.

Approximately 80% of patients will have histological appearances of poorly differentiated adenocarcinoma or poorly differentiated carcinoma. Some of these patients may have a germ cell tumour and be curable by chemotherapy [4]. These patients often have a tumour located in the midline (in the mediastinum or para-aortic region), are usually less than 50 years old and sometimes have a rapidly growing tumour. In these cases, if the histology is poorly differentiated *adenocarcinoma*, the response rate to germ-cell chemotherapy is low (about 30%) and usually short-lived. If the histology is poorly differentiated *carcinoma* the response rate approaches 80% in some series and some patients are cured. These findings indicate that younger patients with poorly differentiated mediastinal carcinomas should receive platinum-based germ-cell chemotherapy.

If the diagnosis is adenocarcinoma in an axillary lymph node, treatment for breast cancer should be considered, even if the mammogram is normal. Although mastectomy will show an occult primary in 40–70% of cases, it is not clear that an immediate operation contributes to cure. A trial of hormone therapy as initial treatment is an appropriate step in postmenopausal women. Women with malignant ascites showing adenocarcinoma should be treated for ovarian cancer especially if CA-125 is elevated. Peritoneal carcinomatosis in a woman strongly suggests an ovarian cancer, especially if the CA-125 is elevated. This can occur even if the ovaries are normal (so-called primary extraovarian serous carcinoma). Treatment is as for ovarian cancer although breast and bowel cancer can uncommonly present in this way.

Some tumours may show neuroendocrine features (such as neurosecretory granules) on electron microscopy. If the features are of a low-grade tumour in the liver, treatment is as for a presumptive carcinoid tumour. If the histology is high-grade, chemotherapy should be considered for a small-cell lung cancer. In many cases, however, no diagnosis will be reached, and the decision will then need to be taken as to whether chemotherapy should be used in an attempt to delay the progress of the disease. This depends very much on the clinical state of the patient and on the intensity of the patient's wish for treatment. Clinical pointers to responsiveness to chemotherapy (usually platinum-based) are tumours which are mediastinal or retroperitoneal, young age and tumours confined to the lymph nodes. Regressions can be induced with the use of drugs such as doxorubicin, paclitaxel and 5-fluorouracil. Often there is a failure of response or only a short-lived response. Recent combinations variably using paclitaxel, gemcitabine and platinum appear to be among the most active with around 25% survival at 2 years but randomized comparisons are needed because of the variable prognostic features in this heterogeneous group. Palliative treatment using radiotherapy to sites of pain or local swelling, and supportive measures (see Chapter 7) is then the mainstay of treatment.

Exceptionally, an isolated cerebral metastasis can be removed surgically. Removal of solitary brain secondaries (even when the primary site is known) is associated with less likelihood of recurrence in the brain and better quality of life than control with radiation alone.

Survival

Median survival is 3–5 months with 5–10% survival at 2 years. Response to chemotherapy is better if the histology is poorly differentiated carcinoma, if there are less than three metastatic sites, if carcinoembryonic antigen is not elevated and if the main location is in retroperitoneal or peripheral nodes.

References

1 Greco FA, Oien K, Erlander M *et al.* Cancer of unknown primary: progress in the search for improved and rapid diagnosis leading toward superior patient outcomes. *Ann Oncol* 2012; 23: 298–304.

2 Pavlidis N, Pentheroudakis G. Cancer of unknown primary site. *Lancet* 2012; 379: 1428–35.

3 Varadhachary GR, Talantov D, Raber MN *et al.* Molecular profiling of carcinoma of unknown primary and correlation with clinical evaluation. *J Clin Oncol* 2008; 26: 4442–8.

4 Hainsworth JD, Rubin MS, Spigel DR *et al.* Molecular gene expression profiling to predict the tissue of origin and direct site-specific therapy in patients with carcinoma of unknown primary site: a prospective trial of the Sarah Cannon research institute. *J Clin Oncol* 2013; 3: 217–23.

22 Skin cancer

Aetiology and pathogenesis

Over 46 000 new cases of skin cancer are reported every year in the UK. It is no surprise that skin cancers are the commonest of all malignancies since the skin is the largest and most accessible of our organs, directly exposed to environmental carcinogens. The earliest described and perhaps best-known example of a carcinogen-induced skin cancer, noted by Percival Pott in 1775, is carcinoma of the scrotal skin affecting chimney sweeps who came into direct contact with soot in chimney flues. In the nineteenth century, an increase in incidence of skin cancers was reported following treatment with medicines containing arsenic: arsenical fumes had already been implicated in the causation of scrotal cancers of copper miners and smelters. Towards the end of the century [1] it was suggested that strong sunlight might be a promoter of skin cancer; and shortly after the discovery of radium, Becquerel proposed that ionizing radiation might be the component of sunlight responsible for malignant change. The carcinogenic roles of ultraviolet (UV) radiation, X-rays and chemicals have now been confirmed; most important of all was the work of Yamagiwa and Ichikawa who demonstrated the carcinogenic properties of coal tar applied directly to the skin of experimental animals [2], although it was Kennaway who isolated and identified the carcinogen as 3,4-benzpyrene. Over the past 40 years, the incidence of melanoma has doubled every decade, probably as a result of increased exposure to sunlight and the loss of our ozone layer, currently estimated to be decreasing by 0.2–0.8% annually.

Sunlight and occupational factors

Epidemiological studies have provided important clues to the aetiology of skin cancer, whose incidence varies directly in proportion to the intensity of sunlight, so that skin cancers are much more common in Australia (with the world's highest incidence rates) and South Africa than in more temperate areas [3]. The increasing numbers of people in the UK taking holidays abroad* has certainly contributed to the increase in skin cancer rates over the past 30 years. A high proportion of skin cancers (particularly basal cell carcinomas) occur in sun-exposed areas of the body, and certain races such as fair-skinned Celts are particularly prone to developing skin cancer, probably due to a relative lack of protection by melanin pigment. By contrast, skin cancers are relatively uncommon in black races, presumably as a result of effective shielding by pigment in the superficial skin layers. For melanoma, the risk ratio between white and black skin is reportedly

---

* Up from some 11 700 000 in 1980 to a peak of 45 500 000 by 2008. Data from www.cancerresearch.co.uk).

Cancer and its Management, Seventh Edition. Jeffrey Tobias and Daniel Hochhauser.
© 2015 John Wiley & Sons, Ltd. Published 2015 by John Wiley & Sons, Ltd.

as high as 40%. Recent research into the epidemiology and genetics of basal squamous cell carcinomas suggests that they should be separately considered rather than, as previously, regarded collectively as a contrasting condition to melanoma but otherwise essentially similar to each other [4,5]. Public information programmes rightly emphasize the importance of avoiding overexposure to sunlight [3,6,7]. In black people, the distribution of skin cancers is much less determined by sunlight exposure than in white people, and is almost as common in unexposed areas such as the trunk and lower limbs. The use of psoralens and UVA in psoriasis is associated with a risk of cutaneous malignancy, particularly on the male genitalia, and an association has been noted between skin carcinoma (predominantly squamous cell) and non-Hodgkin's lymphoma [8], with UV sunlight as the presumed aetiological linkage factor. Recent work has drawn attention to the serious hazard of sunbed use, particularly in young people, and there are even calls for such devices to be banned (see Ref. [9]).

Occupational carcinogens have been an important cause of skin cancer, although increasing risk awareness has substantially reduced the hazard. However, industrial carcinogens such as petroleum derivatives, arsenicals and coal tar remain in common use, and protective clothing is still important. Even more critical is the need to keep radiation exposure to an absolute minimum, particularly for those working with X-rays, including medical, nursing and radiographic personnel who require regular monitoring of radiation exposure throughout their working lives.

Immunosuppression and viral causes

Skin cancer is a serious and frequent problem in immunosuppressed patients. In these patients, cancers typically arise in areas of the skin exposed to the sun, and are more aggressive than in non-immunosuppressed patients, often requiring multiple surgical procedures. Although this increase is often attributed to decreased cancer surveillance as a result of drug therapy and exposure to UVB radiation, recent studies have suggested that azathioprine, the commonly used immunosuppressive agent, may sensitize DNA to UVA radiation.

Recipients of renal allografts certainly have an increased risk of cancer, possibly as high as 250 times that of the general population. The most common malignancies are those involving the skin, including squamous and basal cell carcinomas, melanoma and Bowen's disease.

Squamous carcinoma is more frequent than basal cell carcinoma (a reverse of the usual pattern), sometimes multifocal and running an aggressive course.

Considerable interest has been aroused by the role of the wart viruses, *human papillomavirus* (HPV), and a pattern is now emerging in which HPV appears associated with the development of cancer in particular clinical settings. The genome of HPV-5 has been found in squamous carcinoma of the skin in renal allograft recipients and also in the squamous cancers that occur in the rare inherited skin disorder *epidermodysplasia verruciformis*, in which patients develop multiple warts. Although HPV is now less widely regarded as the key aetiological agent, it seems extremely likely that it does indeed have carcinogenic properties.

Kaposi's sarcoma is discussed separately on page 442.

Premalignant lesions

A group of premalignant skin lesions has been recognized in which malignant change is sufficiently common to justify close surveillance. These include the following:

Inherited disorders
Xeroderma pigmentosum

This is an autosomal recessive disease characterized by increased sensitivity to UV light, with multiple solar keratoses, premalignant lesions and ultimately malignant skin lesions on exposed surfaces. Melanoma, squamous carcinoma or basal cell carcinoma all occur. The defect is due to UV-induced damage causing a deficiency in the excision repair mechanism for DNA.

Naevoid basal cell carcinoma syndrome (Gorlin's syndrome)

This is a syndrome characterized by multiple basal cell carcinomas, particularly on the face and trunk, associated with cleft lip and skeletal abnormalities that include frontal bossing, mandibular cysts and bifid ribs [10]. It is inherited through a single autosomal dominant gene with complete penetrance but variable expression. About 40% of patients do not appear to have an affected parent.

There is also an increased tendency for other neoplastic changes, notably ameloblastoma and squamous cell carcinoma of, or around, the jaw, meningioma, melanoma and others. Management can be exceptionally difficult in view of the hundreds of naevi or invasive tumours these patients may develop, often in young adult life.

Albinism

This is a group of congenital diseases associated with defective skin pigmentation and an increased tendency to solar keratosis and squamous carcinoma *in situ*.

Epidermodysplasia verruciformis

This is an autosomal recessive disease characterized by multiple flat warts. These and even non-affected skin may evolve into squamous carcinoma (see above).

Genetic predisposition to melanoma

A melanoma predisposition gene, *CDKN2*, has now been identified that maps to chromosome 9p21–22 [11]. *CDKN2* mutations have been found in the germ line of affected members of melanoma kindred and there seems no doubt that, in a minority of cases, familial melanoma genuinely occurs, such families having been reported from Europe, the USA and elsewhere.

Another gene known as *BRAF* has also been implicated [12]: in a recent study investigating gene-sequence information from 115 specimens, mutations were detected in 23 of 43 (54%) from skin that was not chronically exposed to sun, showing a high level of *BRAF* mutation, particularly in respect of trunk primaries in young persons.

Because of the wide range of penetrants, the possibility of additional high- and low-risk genes and the uncertain medical benefit of this genetic information, routine testing for genetic abnormalities is not currently recommended outside of defined research protocols.

Carcinogen-induced disorders
Arsenical keratoses

After exposure to inorganic arsenicals, keratotic lesions may develop 10 years or more later on the palms and soles. These lesions are premalignant, although overt cancer is uncommon. Bowen's disease (see below) is often present as well, together with superficial basal cell carcinomas at other sites.

Solar keratoses

Although histologically similar to arsenical keratoses, the incidence of malignant change is much greater and the distribution also different, since these lesions chiefly occur on the face and dorsal aspect of the hands. Other changes of prolonged exposure to sunlight are present: furrowed elastic leathery skin, with wrinkling, atrophy and hyperpigmented or depigmented patches.

Radiation dermatitis

Following exposure to modest doses of superficial radiation (often given many years before for benign conditions such as ringworm, acne or hirsutism), the skin may assume a characteristic appearance, with depigmentation, atrophy of the skin, hair and sweat glands, and telangiectasia. These areas are more susceptible to malignant change. Basal cell carcinomas on the scalp are usually related to previous irradiation and may arise in skin without evidence of radiation change.

Miscellaneous disorders
Bowen's disease [13]

Often regarded as a premalignant skin disorder, this disease is in fact a superficial intraepidermal squamous cell carcinoma *in situ*, usually found on the trunk or limbs. If untreated, 3–5% of these lesions progress to become invasive squamous cell carcinoma. Characteristically, it spreads laterally within the cutis, often at several sites, and evolving slowly from a small erythematous papule to a crusting lesion. Histologically, the basal layer is intact but the epidermis shows premature keratinization and is disrupted, characteristically infiltrated with homogeneous cells with basophilic cytoplasm, small nuclei and frequent mitoses. There is an important association with internal malignancies, as many as one-quarter of all patients with Bowen's disease developing a deep-seated carcinoma during the 10 years following diagnosis.

Leucoplakia

These are indurated whitish plaques, often fissured with sharply defined borders, found on mucous membranes of the mouth. They may result from local irritation: ill-fitting dentures and smoking are frequently associated. The histology shows hyperplasia, hyperkeratosis and dyskeratosis; carcinoma *in situ* may arise, sometimes progressing to squamous cell carcinoma.

Genital carcinoma *in situ*

This disorder is now regarded as a form of intraepithelial neoplasia, presenting as a persistent red papule or plaque on the penis (and previously known as erythroplasia of Queyrat). The relationship with HPV remains contentious. Pathologically, there is an abnormal epidermis with an absent granular layer and small densely packed cells similar to those in Bowen's disease. Intraepithelial neoplasia may also be found on the vulva (see also Chapter 17).

Basal cell carcinoma [14]

Basal cell carcinoma (rodent ulcer) accounts for over 75% of all cases of skin malignancy in the Western world. Its incidence in the UK has increased by well over 200% over the past 20 years. In parts of New England, USA, 40% of the population will have developed a basal cell carcinoma by the age of 85 [15]. Age-specific incidence is shown in Figure 22.1. They are epithelial tumours without histological evidence of maturation or tendency to keratinization, and arise from the undifferentiated basal cells of the skin, which normally differentiate into structures such as hair or sweat glands. The tumour consists of uniform cells with darkly stained nuclei and little cytoplasm, often forming a characteristic palisade (Figure 22.2). The tumour generally arises on exposed areas, particularly the skin of the face and most characteristically around the nose, forehead, cheeks and lower eyelid, although it may sometimes occur on the limbs. Macroscopically, the lesions are often described as either

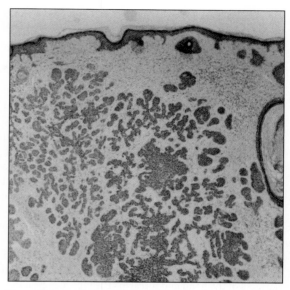

Figure 22.2 Basal cell carcinoma of the skin showing small nests of invading basal cells (×20).

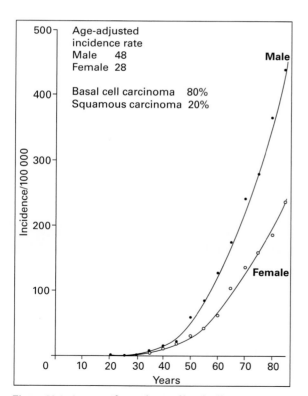

Figure 22.1 Age-specific incidence of basal cell carcinoma and squamous carcinoma of the skin.

nodular, pigmented, sclerosing (morphoeic), cicatrizing, infiltrating or ulcerative. There is usually a firm pink papule with a distinct raised edge, often serpiginous, with a pearly and telangiectatic appearance and with a depressed or frankly ulcerated centre with or without a central crust. Although non-inflammatory and typically painless, it may irritate and will often bleed repeatedly if scratched.

Untreated, these tumours invade laterally or deeply with local destruction of cartilage or even bone. In the sclerosing variety the typical features may be absent and the margin indistinct, making diagnosis more difficult. Superficial basal cell carcinomas, often multiple, also have an unusual appearance and are more common on the trunk with a more plaque-like scaling patch configuration or a fine pearly edge.

Despite the highly malignant microscopic appearance of basal cell carcinomas, metastasis to local lymph nodes or distant sites is exceptionally rare, a remarkable fact in view of the large size that many of these cancers can achieve, and an important contrast with the behaviour of squamous cell carcinomas. However, multiple primary tumours are not uncommon, with a reported incidence of second or subsequent tumours, from a recent large American prospective study, of 36% over the first 5 years of follow-up.

Squamous cell carcinoma

Squamous cell carcinomas of the skin are less common than basal cell carcinomas (Figure 22.1), though they share many characteristics. Sunlight or X-ray exposure, arsenic ingestion and occupational carcinogens are all aetiologically important. Multiple squamous cell carcinomas of the hand were common among radiation scientists in the early years of the twentieth century until the hazard was recognized and methods of dosimetry improved. Histologically, these are typical keratinizing squamous lesions (Figure 22.3), and to some extent the risk of local spread can be predicted from the histological appearance (more common with less well-differentiated tumours).

As with basal cell carcinomas, the commonest sites include sun-exposed areas of the head and neck, particularly the nose, temples, rim of the ear and lip, as well as the side and back of the neck, and the dorsal surfaces of the hand and forearm. The typical appearance is either a crusted scaly ulcer or a more nodular exophytic type that can fungate if untreated. The site of the tumour may be diagnostically helpful since squamous cell carcinomas, though commonest on the face, have a much more widespread distribution than basal cell carcinomas and a shorter history. A skin tumour of the hand or forearm is far more likely to be of squamous

cell origin. Squamous cell carcinoma may be difficult to distinguish macroscopically from the usually benign condition *keratoacanthoma*, characterized by a locally rapidly advancing, discrete and often bulky papule on the face or neck, and typically with a central plug of keratin filling the ulcerated central area.

Squamous cell carcinomas arising in areas of radiation dermatitis are both clinically and histologically more aggressive than other varieties, though the mean latent interval is about 20 years. In one large series of nearly 400 patients, the mortality was as high as 10%. These tumours are now less frequent because of higher-energy radiotherapy equipment, and the infrequent use of radiotherapy for benign skin disorders and arthritic conditions. This is also true of squamous carcinomas arising from chronic burn ulcers, known as *Marjolin's ulcer*, which in the past was a relatively common problem, typically characterized by a lengthy period of quiescence terminated by a highly aggressive phase with metastases to the lungs and other sites. A similar type of squamous cell carcinoma occasionally develops in chronic sinus tracts of osteomyelitis or other chronic infections and in the dysplastic or scar areas of chronic skin diseases such as lupus vulgaris or lupus erythematosus.

Squamous carcinomas arising at mucocutaneous junctions such as the anus and vulva tend to be aggressive, as do those developing in areas of radiation-damaged skin, patches of Bowen's disease, or against a background of carcinoma *in situ*. Sweat gland carcinoma, an uncommon condition, may also behave unpredictably. These tumours most commonly arise in the axilla and anogenital regions, and should be distinguished from the rare sebaceous gland cancers. Finally, squamous carcinomas are reportedly more common in areas of vitiligo, especially in black people.

Treatment of basal cell and squamous cell carcinoma

Because of their frequency and characteristic appearance, treatment without firm histological diagnosis is sometimes advocated. In general, this is unwise and can be dangerous since the lesions most likely to metastasize are those least likely to have been correctly diagnosed. Elderly patients may be too unwell for biopsy but in all other cases biopsy is essential. Benign conditions such as papillomas, sclerosing haemangiomas and keratoacanthomas can all be macroscopically confused with a basal or squamous cell carcinoma, and occasionally these two

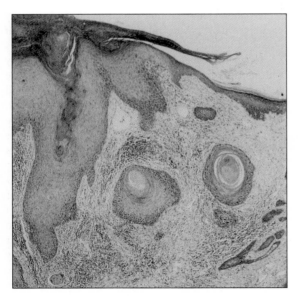

Figure 22.3 Squamous cell carcinoma of skin showing invading masses of squamous epithelium forming keratin pearls (×20).

major types of skin cancer can themselves be difficult to distinguish from each other.

There are several effective methods of treatment, including electrocautery and curettage, cryosurgery, excisional surgery, chemosurgery, radiotherapy and topical chemotherapy. Since all of these have their strong adherents and each method yields a very high success rate, formal comparisons are difficult. In addition, approaches such as electrocautery and cryosurgery are in general confined to such small lesions (usually under 5 mm diameter) that the very high success rate of over 95% is not representative of an unselected group. Cryosurgery, usually using liquid nitrogen, is effective for small lesions, particularly for superficial tumours such as Bowen's disease and the most superficial of basal cell carcinomas. It can be extremely useful in elderly or immobile patients. Chemosurgery, an interesting technique first described by Mohs [16], employs a zinc chloride paste fixative that is applied to the tumour, partly destroying it and allowing easy removal from the underlying skin while preserving its histological pattern. Further paste is then applied to any area of residual tumour, and the whole process repeated. This technique can be useful even for fairly large tumours and at sites where radiotherapy may be hazardous (see below), although it is time-consuming and laborious, and demands great expertise and care. Despite these potential drawbacks, this approach, often termed *micrographically controlled surgery*, has become a popular form of treatment, especially in the USA.

For basal cell and squamous cell carcinomas too large for electrocautery, most dermatologists would agree that the real choice lies between excisional surgery and radiotherapy. Each has its advantages. Surgery is quick, does not require multiple visits to hospital, and is the only way to produce a complete specimen for the pathologist. Conversely, for large tumours general anaesthesia is usually required, and skin grafting or flap rotation may well be necessary, with a less acceptable final cosmetic result as well as the risk of a higher postoperative complication rate. With tumours at difficult sites such as the inner canthus of the eye, surgery is probably best avoided since there is a risk of damage to the nasolacrimal duct, and surgical reconstruction can be very difficult. For squamous cell carcinomas, a wider excision is usually recommended because of the possibility of local lymphatic spread. There is no clear indication for routine lymph node dissection, although surgical excision is undoubtedly the treatment of choice for clinically involved regional nodes.

Radiotherapy is also highly effective, with a cure rate of over 90%. It is especially useful for tumours on the face, particularly around the eye, nose and nasolabial fold where tumours may infiltrate deeply and prove difficult to excise surgically without, in some cases, an unacceptable deformity. Both the columella of the nose and the ala nasae are difficult surgical sites, and radiotherapy is usually curative and gives excellent cosmesis. The radiation energy and effective depth-dose can be chosen to suit the individual tumour, and simple lead cut-outs can be tailor-made so that irregularly shaped tumours may be adequately treated without unnecessary treatment of large volumes of normal skin. For tumours of the lower eyelid and other sites where shielding of deeper structures is desirable (e.g. gums, teeth and tongue in treatment of cancer of the lip), simple shielding can be introduced for each treatment session. Figure 22.4 shows a lead shield inserted under local anaesthesia into the lower conjunctival sac, protecting the eye while the lower lid is treated. Direct electron beams are often employed. The major disadvantage of radiotherapy is that in order to produce the best cosmetic result, fractionated regimens of treatment of over 2–3 weeks are required. For the elderly or infirm, travelling may be tiring and a

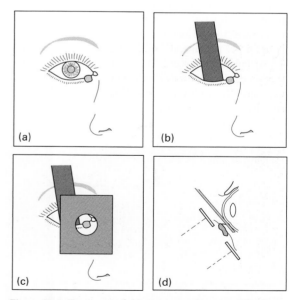

Figure 22.4 Treatment of skin cancer on lower eyelid: (a) typical position of tumour; (b) lead spatula inserted into lower lid before each treatment, shielding cornea and lens; (c) lead cut-out in position; (d) lateral view.

quick operation or treatment by a single large fraction of radiotherapy may be preferable.

A less highly fractionated course of radiotherapy (such as the Sambrook split course, in which two fractions of radiation are given some 6 weeks apart) has a very good cure rate but higher incidence of late skin changes: telangiectasia, atrophy and depigmentation. The aim of longer courses of radiotherapy is to reduce these late effects to a minimum, particularly important for facial skin cancers where a very high cure rate, coupled with a perfect cosmetic result, should be the aim. Acute skin changes consist of intense local erythema and inflammation, leading to early crusting, and resolution with healing which may take months to complete, particularly with larger lesions. Common fractionation regimens are shown in Table 22.1; they often reflect the capacity of the radiotherapy department to treat these common tumours, as much as the individual preference of the radiotherapist. Expressed in terms of the nominal standard dose (see Chapter 5), these treatments aim for a total of 1500–1900 ret. Squamous cell carcinomas require a wider treatment field than basal cell carcinomas, though most radiotherapists treat both lesions to the same doses and their radio-curability is probably identical. Radiotherapy is unsuitable for the naevoid basal cell carcinoma syndrome, as it gives poor results with marked skin damage.

In an important randomized study from France, patients with basal cell carcinoma of the face (less than four) were treated with either surgery or radiotherapy [17]. Of 347 patients, the surgical group ($N = 174$) had a 4-year failure rate of only 0.7% compared with a higher (7.5%) recurrence rate with radiotherapy ($N = 173$). Cosmetically, the surgical group also appeared to show an advantage. Both forms of treatment were conducted by highly experienced teams, although the radiotherapy technique did vary widely among the four participating hospitals.

Topical chemotherapy, usually using 5-fluorouracil, has been increasingly employed in recent years, particularly for recurrent lesions where surgery and/or radiation therapy have already been used. Although its precise role has not yet been determined, advantages include the possibility of repeated use where necessary, as well as its value in premalignant lesions and large areas of carcinoma in situ where other approaches might be difficult. It is valuable in treatment of multiple lesions, particularly superficial basal cell carcinomas, but is not usually recommended for thick or infiltrating lesions. Topical cytotoxic therapy produces acute inflammation which is a disadvantage, although steroids are usually helpful.

Recent work addressing the possibility of immunotherapy for treatment of non-melanoma skin cancers has been extremely encouraging [18]. Agents that can modulate the cutaneous immune response have now been developed, for example, the topical imidazoquinolines. These appear to work by stimulating both 'innate' and 'acquired' or 'adaptational' immunity, and by binding to receptors that recognize pathogens, activating host cells (including natural killer cells) to target the pathogen. One such agent, imiquimod, binds to the transmembrane receptor TLR7, with signalling through the TLR MyD88 pathway, stimulating a nuclear transcription factor cascade and enhancing the release of proinflammatory cytokines including tumour necrosis factor (TNF)-α and several of the interleukins (ILs). In recent years it has been used as a topical agent, with increasing success, particularly in squamous cell carcinoma of the skin and acquiring its formal acceptance from the Food and Drug Administration (FDA) in the USA in 2004 for basal cell carcinomas as well.

One further exciting new advance is the use of a new oral agent vismodegib, the first Hedgehog signalling-pathway-targeting agent to gain US FDA approval. This key pathway is a major regulator of cellular development. The substance acts as a cyclopamine-competitive antagonist of the smoothed receptor (SMO) which is part of the hedgehog-signalling-pathway. SMO inhibition causes the transcription factors GLI1 and GLI2 to remain inactive, thus preventing the expression of tumour mediating genes within the hedgehog pathway, which is known to be pathogenetically relevant in more than 90% of basal cell carcinomas. It is currently indicated for patients with basal cell carcinoma which has metastasized to other parts of the body, relapsed after surgery, or cannot

Table 22.1 Fractionation regimens in basal and squamous cell carcinoma.*

20–22 Gy × 1
14 Gy × 2 (6-week gap)
7.5 Gy × 5 (7–10 days)
6.75 Gy × 6 (alternate days)
6 Gy × 9 (over 3 weeks)
4.5 Gy × 10 (over 3 weeks)

*Single-fraction or two-fraction policies are generally adopted in elderly patients for whom repeated visits may be difficult. In general, however, better cosmetic results are achieved with more prolonged fractionation.

effectively be treated with surgery or radiation. In an important recent multi-centre study, 30% of patients ($n = 33$) with metastatic basal cell carcinoma had an objective response, and 43% of patients ($n = 63$) with locally advanced disease, with a median duration of remission of over 7 months in both groups – see Ref. [19]. Sadly, the adverse event rate was relatively high at 25%, with seven treatment-related deaths though this of course is a highly vulnerable group of heavily-pretreated patients with advanced disease and in some cases, poor skin coverage and a high risk of infection and other complications.

Overall results of treatment of both basal cell and squamous cell carcinoma are excellent [20]. Cure rates of 90–95% are regularly achieved by surgery or radiotherapy; for smaller tumours treated by curettage, cryosurgery or electrocautery the figures are claimed to be higher still. Sadly, the occasional tumour is encountered (particularly with basal cell carcinoma) which proves resistant to all methods of treatment, usually with multiple recurrences at the margins of the treated area, sometimes over a period of 10 years or more. These cases are characterized by relentless local invasion and destruction both laterally and deeply. Distant metastases to bone, lung or elsewhere are occasionally seen.

Malignant melanoma

Epidemiology and pathogenesis

Malignant melanoma is a far less common skin tumour than the cancers discussed above, but has a much worse prognosis. It accounts for about 4% of all skin cancers, with an annual incidence in the UK of about 6 per 100 000 population (Figure 22.5), but it has become more common during the last four decades [3,21], increasing at annual rates of 3–7% per year between the mid-1950s and the early 1980s. Broadly speaking, the incidence of melanoma appears to approximately double every decade, though fortunately survival rates are improving (see below). Despite the relatively low incidence of melanoma in relation to other far more common types of skin cancer, it is responsible for almost 80% of all deaths from skin cancer, both in the UK and Europe. There is wide international variation: the disease is almost 10 times as common in Australia and New Zealand as in Europe, occurring most frequently in patients between 40 and 70 years old, with a slight female preponderance. This is in contrast to basal cell and squamous carcinoma (Figure 22.1), implying a difference

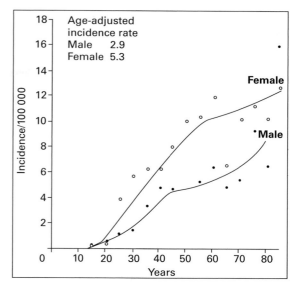

Figure 22.5 Age-specific incidence of melanoma in the United Kingdom.

in the relative importance of external factors such as sunlight in aetiology of these types of skin cancer.

Like other skin cancers, melanoma is commoner in the white population, presumably because pigmented skin is effective in screening solar UV light. The degree of sunburn, rather than sun exposure *per se*, may be an important aetiological feature [22]. About 75% of all malignant melanomas occur on an exposed site, chiefly affecting pale-complexioned white people, especially those with red hair and freckles [4]. The number of naevi on an individual's skin correlates quite closely with melanoma risk [23], and melanoma families have been widely reported [24]. The amount of received sunlight, as measured by distance from the equator, also correlates well with incidence. The earth's ozone layer has an important protective effect, filtering out carcinogenic UV light.

Much can be done to inform the public of the dangers of overexposure to the sun, and information about the value of early diagnosis is clearly worthwhile since the outcome is so dependent on stage (see below). Forceful advertising campaigns through public media and in medical waiting areas have become commonplace. As previously mentioned, the use of sunbeds for tanning is now known to be extremely hazardous, particularly in younger people, greatly increasing the risk of melanoma (including the rare but highly damaging ocular melanoma).

The major sites of melanoma in white people are the head and neck, trunk and limbs (Figure 22.6). In black people, the bodily distribution is different, with a greater likelihood of primary sites on the palms of the hands, soles of the feet and mucous membranes.

Clinical and pathological features

Although more than half of all melanotic lesions arise from a pre-existing benign naevus, some undoubtedly develop at sites of previously normal skin; in many cases the primary site is never discovered, the patient presenting either with lymphadenopathy or with more widespread involvement. Autopsy studies have shown that most of the organs of the body are capable of harbouring a primary melanotic focus: larynx, oesophagus, trachea, bronchus, gastrointestinal tract and leptomeninges have all been implicated. Certainly all these organs (and many more) contain clusters of melanocytes, but why these should undergo malignant change remains completely unknown.

Diagnosis of malignant melanoma is not always straightforward [25]. Almost all of us have pigmented melanocytic naevi (approximately 12 in the average white person), and many innocent pigmented naevi appear to enlarge slowly over the years. They are maximal in number in the third decade of life and then slowly disappear. Those undergoing any form of rapid change, particularly with ulceration or bleeding, must be regarded with suspicion: most dermatologists will advise excision biopsy. Important pointers for self-examination are summarized in Table 22.2. Other important skin conditions may be difficult to distinguish from malignant melanoma unless a biopsy is obtained; these include pigmented

Table 22.2 Signs for self-examination.

Major signs
Is an existing mole or dark patch getting larger or a new one growing?
Does it have a ragged outline?
Does it have a mixture of different shades of brown and black?

Minor signs
Is the mole inflamed or with a reddish edge?
Is it bleeding, oozing or crusting?
Is it bigger than all your other moles?
Is there also a change in sensation, like a mild itch?

Data from http://www.cancerresearchuk.org/cancer-info/ spotcancerearly/cancersymptomvideos/checkyourskin/ check-your-skin-for-signs-of-skin-cancer

basal cell carcinomas, solar keratoses, blue naevi, juvenile melanomas, pyogenic granulomas, sclerosing angiomas and benign pigmented melanocytic naevi.

Benign melanocytic naevi are derived from the intraepidermal melanocyte whose origin is from the neural crest. There are important differences between the various types of naevus, which may have a bearing on the pathogenesis of malignant melanoma. *Junctional naevi* are well-circumscribed, small, flat, pigmented lesions arising from clumps of pigmented cells at the junction of dermis and epidermis. The normal skin lines are not distorted. Their proliferation and penetration into the true dermis result in a *compound naevus*. These are larger than functional naevi and may be raised. Coarse hair may develop and, although the functional activity

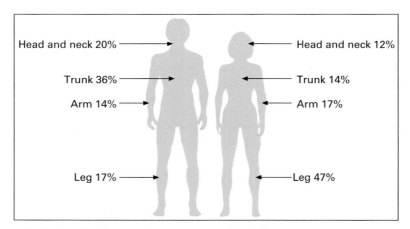

Figure 22.6 Percentage distribution of malignant melanoma on parts of the body.

may then abate, the pigmented cells deep in the dermis may then continue to multiply, resulting in an *intradermal naevus*. Here the melanocytes are no longer in contact with the epidermis. Clinically, the lesion has very little pigmentation, usually presenting as a raised papule, commoner in the older age groups. Although functional naevi are certainly capable of malignant change, this happens only rarely. It is not clear how frequently melanoma arises in a common melanocytic naevus.

In the past decade, there has been greater understanding of the importance of the *dysplastic naevus syndrome*, a condition originally recognized in familial melanoma but now regarded as more common in sporadic cases. The lesions tend to be larger than truly benign naevi, often irregular in outline and with more variable colour. The gene for familial dysplastic naevi has now been identified [26], located on chromosome 1. Despite the probable importance of the dysplastic naevus in the aetiology of malignant melanoma it should be recognized that the majority of these lesions appear stable or may even regress.

Enlargement of a pre-existing naevus occurs in 10–40% of patients with melanoma, though a more definite precursor, numerically less frequently encountered, is the *lentigo maligna* or Hutchinson's melanotic freckle. This epidermal lesion results from maturation of atypical melanocytes thought embryologically to result from neural crest tissue. It is one of three well-recognized macroscopic varieties of malignant melanoma, accounting for up to 10% of all cases and, if suspected, demanding immediate surgical excision. Occurring on sun-exposed areas in elderly patients, there is initially a flat pigmented area on the skin which represents a radial growth phase of the tumour, expanding slowly over many years. Later an invasive vertical growth develops, visible as nodules within the lesion. Surgical excision in the radial growth phase is often curative. *Superficial spreading melanomas* are usually larger, often 2–3 cm in diameter, chiefly occurring in middle age. They have an irregular edge, often with a pale central area. After 1–2 years the lesion may itch or ulcerate and may become nodular, due to vertical penetration of the lesion. In superficial spreading melanoma, about one-third of patients have evidence of pre-existing dysplastic naevi. *Nodular melanomas* develop more rapidly still, almost always characterized by deep dermal invasion by the time of diagnosis. There is no recognizable radial growth phase, and areas of skin not exposed to light are often affected. Typically there is a raised nodule on the skin surface and the normal skin markings are disturbed. Ulceration occurs

after 2–3 months and deep penetration occurs early. An association with a pre-existing naevus is less strong than in superficial spreading melanoma.

These three major types of melanoma account for almost 90% of all cases, the remainder arising from other types of naevus (congenital, blue, compound or intradermal), or from mucous membranes, meninges or other internal sites.

Stage of melanoma

The most important prognostic characteristics in malignant melanoma are the *level of invasion* (or microstage) and the *clinical stage of the tumour*. Clark *et al.* [27] described five separate levels of invasiveness (see Figure 4.1a), demonstrating that prognosis correlated well with depth of invasion. Subsequent work by Breslow [28] suggests that vertical tumour thickness in millimetres may be an even better guide and this method of pathological staging is now generally preferred. Tumours less than 0.75 mm in thickness very rarely metastasize. In addition, the *type* of primary may also influence the prognosis, nodular lesions in general having a worse prognosis stage than the more common superficial spreading variety, reflecting the increased probability of nodal involvement with nodular lesions. Thinner melanoma can usually be diagnosed on simple histological criteria including nuclear atypic asymmetry of the lesion, and the presence of single atypical melanocytes in the upper epidermis.

No single *clinical staging system* has been universally accepted, although patients with obvious lymphadenopathy undoubtedly do less well. A simple scheme is shown in Table 22.3. Involvement of regional nodes is usually judged clinically, but patients with palpable and histologically positive regional lymph nodes have a 5-year survival of less than 20%. Those with impalpable local lymph nodes but microscopical involvement have a 5-year survival of over 50%. In patients with melanomas up to 1.49 mm in depth, the survival rate is over 90%, reducing to 67% with tumours of 1.5–3.49 mm, and only 38% where the tumour is thicker still [21].

In reality, the problem of classification and case comparison is even more complex, since a surprising number of features are thought to have prognostic significance even in clinical stage I disease (Table 22.4). A diagnosis of regional lymphadenopathy or wider dissemination is of overriding prognostic significance. Important metastatic sites include liver, lung, spleen, bone, cardiac and central nervous system (particularly brain but also meningeal involvement). Clinical staging of melanoma naturally

Table 22.3 Clinical stage of malignant melanoma. Based on data from Sobin *et al.*, TNM Classification of Malignant Tumours 7e.

pTNM pathological classification

pT – primary tumour

pTX	Primary tumour cannot be assessed*
pT0	No evidence of primary tumour
pTis	Melanoma in situ (Clark Level I) (atypical melanocytic hyperplasia, severe melanocytic dysplasia, not an invasive malignant lesion)
pT1	Tumour 1 mm or less in thickness
	pT1a without ulceration and mitosis $< 1/mm^2$
	pT1b with ulceration or mitoses $\geq 1/mm^2$
pT2	Tumour more than 1 mm but not more than 2 mm in thickness
	pT2a without ulceration
	pT2b with ulceration
pT3	Tumour more than 2 mm but not more than 4 mm in thickness
	pT3a without ulceration
	pT3b with ulceration
pT4	Tumour more than 4 mm in thickness
	pT4a without ulceration
	pT4b with ulceration

pN – regional lymph nodes
The pN categories correspond to the N categories.

pN0	Histological examination of a regional lymphadenectomy specimen will ordinarily include 6 or more lymph nodes
	If the lymph nodes are negative, but the number ordinarily examined is not met, classify as pN0
	Classification based solely on sentinel node biopsy without subsequent lymph node dissection is designated (sn) for sentinel node, e.g. pN1 (sn).

Stage grouping

Stage 0	pTis	N0	M0
Stage I	pT1	N0	M0
Stage IA	pT1a	N0	M0
Stage IB	pT1b	N0	M0
	pT2a	N0	M0
Stage IIA	pT2b	N0	M0
	pT3a	N0	M0
Stage IIB	pT3b	N0	M0
	pT4a	N0	M0
Stage IIC	pT4b	N0	M0
Stage IIIA	pT1a–4a	N1a, 2a	M0
Stage IIIB	pT1a–4a	N1b, 2b, 2c	M0
	pT1b–4b	N1a, 2a, 2c	M0
Stage IIIC	pT1b–4b	N1b, 2b, 2c	M0
	Any pT	N3	M0
Stage IV	Any pT	Any N	M1

*pTX includes shave biopsies and regressed melanomas.

Table 22.4 Prognostic factors in clinical stage I malignant melanoma.

Low risk
Radial (lateral) growth phase
Thickness <0.76 mm or Clark's level 2

Intermediate risk
Level 3 invasion
Up to 1.5 mm thickness

High risk
Level 4 or 5
1.5–4.0 mm invasion
High mitotic rate
Satellite lesions
Ulceration
Axial location on hands or feet

takes account of the routes of spread, and a full blood count, chest radiography and liver function tests should be undertaken in all patients.

For those with small thin stage I lesions, further investigation is not generally necessary [21], though liver and brain scanning will undoubtedly reveal an occasional case of unsuspected occult disease. Abdominal computed tomography (CT), magnetic resonance imaging (MRI) or whole-body positron emission tomography (PET) may demonstrate unsuspected pelvic or para-aortic lymphadenopathy. Although these investigations are difficult (in terms of outcome) to justify as a routine, their increasing availability allows for better prognostic detail. Ultrasonography in skilled hands is a valuable, simple and non-invasive technique in melanoma since it provides reliable information for both hepatic and abdominopelvic staging. Recently, the use of radiolabelled monoclonal antibodies (generally using ^{111}In or ^{123}I) for whole-body scanning has occasionally provided additional information, identifying previously unrecognized metastatic sites.

Newer, more sensitive techniques have been used to analyse sentinel lymph nodes and detect melanoma cells not identified by standard histological methods [29,30]. The polymerase chain reaction (PCR) can be used to amplify RNA extracted from fresh tissue or paraffin-embedded specimens and detect one or more melanoma differentiation genes with a high degree of sensitivity [31]. Patients with sentinel lymph nodes that are positive for melanoma genes on PCR but negative on histological analysis have a risk of recurrence intermediate between that of patients whose sentinel nodes are

negative on both tests, and that of patients whose sentinel nodes are histologically positive. Patients whose sentinel nodes are negative on both histological analysis and PCR have a very low risk of recurrence.

Treatment
Surgery
Local excision

For localized (stage I) malignant melanoma confined to the primary site, surgical excision remains the cornerstone of management. Because of the propensity of local lymphatic invasion, most surgeons recommend wide excision of the primary lesion, with a particularly generous clearance proximally, although recent approaches have become more conservative [32]. A recent randomized study investigating the influence of width of margin of surgical excision (1 cm vs 3 cm) showed that the 1-cm margin was associated with a higher risk of loco-regional recurrence, but 3 years after surgical treatment overall survival was similar between the two groups [33]. Wide excision usually requires split-skin graft coverage, but in relatively good prognoses [Clark's level 1 or 2 (Figure 4.1a) and lentigo maligna lesions] less generous surgical excision with primary closure is probably adequate. A well-controlled study from the World Health Organization (WHO) Melanoma Group has shown that with tumours 1 mm or less in depth more conservative surgical excision is safe. The present view is that for each millimetre depth of tumour, a 1 cm margin is required, removing the need for surgical grafting in every case. Nodular lesions invade deeply usually as far as the papillary–reticular junction (Clark's level 3) or further and requiring deeper excision than primary lentigo maligna melanomas. Lesions of the hands and feet (e.g. subungual melanomas) are generally best dealt with by partial amputation of the digit.

Regional lymph node dissection

Is it necessary to undertake local lymphadenectomy in all cases of malignant melanoma? In patients with stage I disease, lymphadenectomy undoubtedly gives useful prognostic information. The presence of microscopic disease worsens the 5 year-survival from 70% of cases (true stage I, node-negative, lesions) to only 50% with occult regional lymph node involvement (proven only by surgery).

Whether regional lymphadenectomy makes a therapeutic contribution to prognosis remains hotly contested. In general, for patients with good-risk melanoma – a small lesion of a limb, not nodular in character and of Clark's level 1 – there is nothing to be gained by lymphadenectomy. For deeper lesions (e.g. nodular and spreading melanomas of Clark's level 3, 4 or 5), lymphadenectomy is often recommended. Removal of the first node into which the primary melanoma drains, sometimes referred to as the 'sentinel node', may be a reasonable compromise [32]. If negative for metastases, 'skip' lesions are unlikely. For melanoma of the trunk, early lymph node dissection does seem to carry a small survival advantage [34].

Dissection is normally performed if there are clinically involved lymph nodes in the primary nodal drainage area, though it is doubtful whether it genuinely adds to survival. Only 10% of patients with clinically detectable lymphadenopathy confirmed at lymphadenectomy are alive 5 years later. This unhappy situation is closely analogous to what we know from breast cancer studies, local node involvement generally reflecting disseminated but undetectable disease. In both of these illnesses, this prognostic information is gained by a procedure which is itself of doubtful benefit. Despite this dispiriting state of affairs, radical lymph node dissection for clinical stage II or III melanoma is the only practical means of therapy with any serious chance of success at present. For the highly selected group of patients with high-risk clinical stage II lesions of the distal portion of a limb, amputation may give the best chance of cure.

In the UK, few surgeons favour prophylactic lymph node dissection even in patients with high-risk lesions, even though it provides useful prognostic information. This view is borne out by careful analysis of a large group of Australian patients [35]. The extremely high incidence of this disease in Australia and New Zealand has led to special experience in the larger Australian centres, and the 5-year survival rates from Queensland appear better than anywhere else in the world (Queensland 81%, England 61%, USA 37%). Although this might suggest particular expertise, it is also true that a higher proportion of Australian patients have primary melanotic lesions confined to the epidermis, with a relatively good prognosis. Further results from Australia suggest a possible benefit of prophylactic lymph node dissection with melanomas of intermediate thickness, though the majority of patients suffer side-effects without any obvious advantage. However, a recent multicentre, randomized, controlled study showed no obvious benefit for prophylactic regional node dissection, at least in terms of survival [36]; these were melanomas of intermediate, 1–4 mm, thickness. Somewhat surprisingly, 5-year survival is only 20% better for patients with microscopic (non-palpable) nodal involvement than for patients who present with overt nodal disease (50% vs. 28%): there is clearly a limit to what can be achieved by surgical resection [28].

Increasingly over recent years, the role of sentinel node biopsy has been refined and clarified. To evaluate its contribution, Morton *et al.* [37] studied 1269 patients with an intermediate-thickness primary melanoma, using sentinel node biopsy to predict which patients had nodal metastases, whose survival could be prolonged by immediate lymphadenectomy. The incidence of sentinel node micrometastases was 16%; among those with node metastases, the 5-year survival rate was higher in those undergoing immediate lymphadenectomy, suggesting a valuable role for sentinel node biopsy as part of modern staging and management, in a disease in which appropriate surgical excision remains the cornerstone of success. Nonetheless it remains an open question as to whether sentinel node biopsy is genuinely beneficial from the point of view of overall survival, although it is now very widely used (see, for example, Ref. [38]).

Radiotherapy

There are few reports of the use of radiotherapy as an alternative to surgery for primary melanomas, although it is known that melanoma cells *in vitro* are not completely radio-resistant [39]. Despite the long-held clinical belief that radiation therapy is of no value, radiotherapy can in fact be quite useful for patients in whom surgery is unsuitable because the lesion is too advanced, particularly in lentigo maligna melanoma. Since many lesions are on the extremities, a high dose can usually be reached without danger to internal structures. Large infrequent fractions of treatment (>5 Gy) are often used in an attempt to overcome the shoulder effect thought to be largely responsible for resistance (see Chapter 5). An important recent study from Australia has finally confirmed that after many years of uncertainty regarding the role of radiotherapy as adjuvant therapy, it clearly does have a useful role in reducing the risk of loco-regional recurrence in high-risk cases – see Ref. [40]. The authors showed that with a median follow-up period of 40 months, risk of lymph node relapse was substantially reduced – 20 relapses in the treated group versus 34 cases in the untreated group, though the median overall survival versus unaltered. High-risk inclusion criteria included number of lymph nodes involved, extranodal spread and maximum size of the affected nodes.

Chemotherapy

Management of disseminated disease represents an almost insoluble problem. Median survival for patients

Table 22.5 Chemotherapy in melanoma.

Drug	Response rate* (%)
Single agents	
DTIC	22
Alkylating agents	10
Methotrexate	7
Cytosine arabinoside	10
Actinomycin D	13
Vindesine	15
Vincristine	10
Mitomycin C	14
Hydroxycarbamide	10
Nitrosoureas	14
Combination chemotherapy†	
DTIC + vinca	17
DTIC + nitrosourea	17
DTIC + vinca + nitrosourea	24
Vinca + nitrosourea	24
Vinca + nitrosourea + procarbazine	30

*Complete and partial response together. Most response rates refer to cutaneous lesions. Responses are uncommon in visceral lesions.
†Typical regimens.

with disease beyond the regional lymph node is only 6 months, though patients with predominantly skin involvement have a median survival of almost a year. Although malignant melanoma is often cited as a tumour in which spontaneous regression occurs, the actual incidence of the phenomenon is no more than 1%, and lengthy survival is exceptionally rare. Nevertheless, with the demonstration in the early 1970s of some degree of sensitivity to chemotherapy, the use of *cytotoxic drugs* for disseminated melanoma became widely adopted even though objective responses have been low (Table 22.5) and the overwhelming majority of these responses are less than complete. Furthermore, responses are usually seen in skin, but are very uncommon in liver, brain, bone and lung, sites that are the main cause of death. The most active agents are dacarbazine (DTIC) and vindesine, with response rates of 20–30%. It is not clear whether the use of drugs in combination offers genuinely superior results to treatment with single agents alone; other active agents include nitrosoureas (notably bis-chloroethyl nitrosourea and fotemustine) and cisplatin. Use of these, and also DTIC, has become more common with the

advent of new-generation 5-hydroxytryptamine (5-HT)$_3$ antagonists such as ondansetron, which offer superior control of nausea and vomiting; however, combinations such as bleomycin, lomustine, vincristine and DTIC have mostly failed to live up to their early promise. Another experimental approach has been the use of high-dose chemotherapy (generally with melphalan, ifosfamide or DTIC) supplemented by autologous marrow transplantation, though this has not as yet proven more beneficial than conventional chemotherapy and should not be used outside controlled clinical trials.

There is also evidence of occasional responses to tamoxifen, although reports are still scanty. Interestingly, there are well-documented historic cases of remission (or, conversely, sudden unexpected relapse) in melanoma patients who have become pregnant, clearly suggesting a degree of hormone-related tumour behaviour.

An alternative approach, for patients with primary melanoma of an extremity and with loco-regional or recurrent disease, is the use of regional cytotoxic perfusion. Although this was used in the 1960s and 1970s as an adjuvant to primary surgical treatment, there is no convincing evidence that it reduces the likelihood of metastatic disease. Melphalan and cisplatin are most commonly used, the latter particularly in hepatic metastases. Responses are relatively common (up to 40%) though generally partial and short-lived. Regional perfusion has mostly been used for unresectable limb lesions with recurrent disease, or for widespread skin metastases confined to a single limb.

Immunotherapy

Reports of occasional spontaneous regression of disease in melanoma, coupled with the demonstration of antigen and antimelanoma antibodies in the sera of a few patients with the disease, have led to the use of 'active immunotherapy' in this disease. Non-specific intralesional treatment with bacille Calmette–Guérin (BCG) produces local responses in patients with recurrent cutaneous or nodal disease, and interferon (IFN)-α has also been used in this way. Unfortunately, most responses are short-lived, and of little or no value for patients with recurrent visceral or bone metastases. However, a recent case report, widely discussed in the international media, has raised hopes once again for a successful form of immune-mediated treatment [41]. The patient was a 52-year-old male with recurrent melanoma, with pulmonary, inguinal and iliac node metastases. The tumour had failed to respond to high-dose IFN, IL-2 and local excision. Treatment was given with an experimental programme of cloned autologous CD4+ T cells with specificity for the melanoma-associated antigen NY-ESO-1, collected by leucopheresis, and cultured. Treatment was given by a single 2-hour infusion (approximately 5 billion T cells infused, without any form of preconditioning). The resulting remission proved durable over a 2-year period. By way of explanation, the authors felt that the treatment had somehow induced the patient's own T cells to respond to other antigens of his tumour. Perhaps more impressive was the publication of a recent report by the European Organization for Research and Treatment of Cancer (EORTC) Melanoma Group, assessing the value of adjuvant pegylated interferon alfa-2b in resected stage III disease [42]. This interferon is the best studied of the immune adjuvant therapies currently available, and pegylation, the process of covalent attachment of polyethylene glycol polymer chains, can be routinely achieved by their incubation with the target macromolecule. The covalent attachment of polyethylene glycol to an agent can mask it from the host's immune system and can induce hydrophobic drugs and proteins to become water-soluble. In this large-scale European study, 1256 patients were randomly assigned postoperatively to observation alone or weekly treatment with this interesting agent, over a 5-year period. Although there was no overall difference in survival between the two groups, the recurrence-free survival was certainly improved. At a median of 3.8 years' follow-up, the number of recurrences was 328 (interferon group) versus 368 (no adjuvant treatment), an interesting result, and statistically achieving a hazard ratio of 0.82.

Recently, the identification of peptides associated with melanoma has led to the development of new approaches towards vaccines, either for primary or secondary prevention. The best-known peptide, melanoma antigen (gene) family (MAGE), a recombinant peptide epitope, is able to produce an immune response which, it is hoped, will prove to be protective.

Biological response modifiers and hyperthermia

Following the interest in immunotherapy of melanoma in the 1970s, attention naturally turned to the use of IFN, a biological response modifier of established value in other neoplasms, notably B-cell lymphoid tumours (see Chapter 6). IFN-α, IFN-β and IFN-γ have all been shown to have activity, in about 10–20% of patients, though most responses are short-lived, generally in patients with a relatively small tumour burden. IFN-α is sometimes used for intralesional therapy and may occasionally result in complete disappearance of the injected lesion. Recent studies have attempted to assess IFN-α in combination with chemotherapy, or as a single agent at high doses, with varying success [43].

IL-2 has also been used over the past 5 years, either as a single agent or with cultured autologous lymphocytes, which then become cytolytic for the autologous tumour cells. These lymphokine-activated killer (LAK) cells have a response rate reportedly up to 25% with a few unmaintained long-term responses. Unfortunately, IL/LAK cell therapy has numerous dose-related side-effects, making it difficult to use (see Chapter 6).

More recently, the use of targeted therapy has made a profound impact on the management of melanoma – see, for example, Ref. [44]. Both vemurafenib, a BRAF enzyme inhibitor, and ipilimumab, an antibody that activates the body's immune system to fight melanoma by inhibiting the cytotoxic T lymphocyte-associated antigen 4 (CTLA-4) molecule have been shown to have marked activity in patients with metastatic melanoma [45, 46]. These new observations are of great importance, and both of these agents have extended survival in melanoma, a notoriously difficult end-point. In the case of vemurafenib, only patients whose tumour expresses the common V600E mutation (i.e. at amino acid position 600 on the BRAF protein, the normal valine is replaced by glutamic acid) or the less common V600K mutation will respond though this includes about 60% of all cases. In an important study from the Memorial Sloan Kettering group from New York, USA, 675 patients with previously untreated metastatic melanoma patients, all with the V600E mutation, were randomly assigned either vemurafenib (960 mg orally twice daily) or dacarbazine (1000 mg/m^2, intravenously every 3 weeks). At 6 months, overall survival was 84% in the vemurafenib group compared with 64% in the dacarbazine group [45]. Vemurafenib was associated with a relative reduction of 63% in the risk of death and of 74% in the risk of either death or disease progression, as compared with dacarbazine ($p < 0.001$ for both). Common adverse events included arthralgia, rash, fatigue, alopecia, development of keratoacanthoma or squamous cell carcinoma, photosensitivity, nausea, and diarrhoea; 38% of patients required dose modification because of toxic effects. Clearly, vemurafenib improved the rates of both overall and progression-free survival in patients with previously untreated melanoma with the BRAF V600E mutation. In the case of ipilimumab, a key study from the Harvard group was recently published, again to considerable media interest [46]. A total of 676 HLA-A*0201-positive patients with unresectable stage III or IV melanoma, whose disease had progressed while they were receiving therapy for metastatic disease, were randomly assigned to receive ipilimumab plus the specific glycoprotein peptide vaccine gp100, ipilimumab alone, or gp100 alone. The primary end point was overall survival, which was increased to 10.0 months for patients receiving ipilimumab plus gp100, as compared with 6.4 months among patients receiving gp100 alone ($p < 0.001$). The median overall survival with ipilimumab alone was 10.1 months. No difference in overall survival was detected between the two ipilimumab groups, and grade 3 or 4 immune-related adverse events occurred in 10–15% of patients treated with ipilimumab. Other BRAF inhibitors and monoclonal antibodies directed against CTLA-4, a co-inhibitory receptor that represses effector T-cell activity, are of course under study at present, notably dabrafenib and tremelimumab. In addition, recent work with nivolumab, which targets the programmed-death-1 [PD1] receptor, has shown good activity in combination with ipilimumab, for patients with advanced melanoma, raising the prospect of powerfully synergistic combinations of targeted therapies – see Ref. [47]. For good reviews of the current role of immunotherapy for melanoma and also recent ideas on vaccine therapy, see Refs. [48,49].

Hyperthermia, the use of heat treatment for cancer, has also been used with some success in melanoma, especially when combined with limb perfusion using melphalan chemotherapy. Although cell kill appears better at temperatures above 41–45 °C, toxic reactions at this level can be severe and milder hyperthermia (39–40 °C) is more commonly used. Studies of this approach continue, under the supervision of EORTC and WHO.

Palliative radiotherapy

Palliative irradiation is undoubtedly useful in selected patients with troublesome deposits, particularly in brain or bone. Although melanoma is not among the more radiosensitive of malignant diseases, resistance can partly be overcome by the use of large infrequent fractions of treatment. Long-term local control of both primary and metastatic lesions is achieved in about 25% of cases. Newer approaches, including neutron and charged particle therapy, radiosensitizers and hyperthermia, are all being investigated. A further interesting type of regional treatment using novel irradiation is the concept of boron neutron capture therapy [50], exploiting the uptake of phenylalanine (a molecule important in melanogenesis) into melanin-producing melanoma cells. The phenylalanine is coupled to boron to produce the boron-labelled melanin substrate analogue $^{10}B_1$-p-boronophenylalanine. If these cells are irradiated with non-toxic thermal neutrons, the ^{10}B nuclide

'captures' the neutrons, then disintegrates to produce a high-energy lithium atomic nucleus together with an α-particle. The energy is deposited locally, selectively destroying the melanin-synthesizing melanoma cells. This technique has been used in patients with melanoma, with encouraging early results [50].

Prognosis

Prognosis in melanoma is always difficult to determine, a reflection of the multitude of potentially important features (Table 22.4). The sharp increase in incidence of melanoma in wealthier social groups is reflected in a higher mortality rate in these same social classes. For both sexes, people in more affluent social classes are about 50% more likely to die of melanoma than the most economically deprived group, presumably related to access to foreign holidays and more time spent in the sun. The average length of life lost in patients with melanoma is greater than a decade. Several authors have made the point that cure of skin melanomas is only possible with earlier diagnosis.

Young patients seem to do better than older age groups. Overall, about 90% with melanoma are alive 5 years after diagnosis, whereas only 74% of young men survive that long. Taking all age groups together, a little over 50% of patients with stage I disease will survive 5 years free of recurrence (Figure 22.7), though it is important to recognize that late relapses occur, so that 5-year survival figures are not definitive. About one-quarter of patients with clinical stage I disease have lymph node involvement at diagnosis (pathological stage II), 75% of these later developing evidence of dissemination. A further 20% of patients with true stage I disease develop distant metastases without ever having had local lymph node enlargement. About 20% of all patients destined to develop recurrent disease will remain disease-free during the first 5 years from diagnosis. For this reason a 5-year survival rate of 60% for stage I melanoma signifies an overall cure rate of about 50% of all patients with early-stage disease. There is also a difference dependent on the primary site of the lesion. Analysis of over 12 000 cases from the Swedish Cancer Registry [51] demonstrated a worse prognosis for scalp and neck lesions, followed by those on the lower limbs and trunk.

Early detection of recurrence appears to give the best opportunity for effective secondary treatment, so patients who have had resection of thick primary lesions require close follow-up [52], for example, 2-monthly for the first year and 3-monthly in the second.

For patients with regional lymphadenopathy at diagnosis, the cure rate is probably no more than 15%,

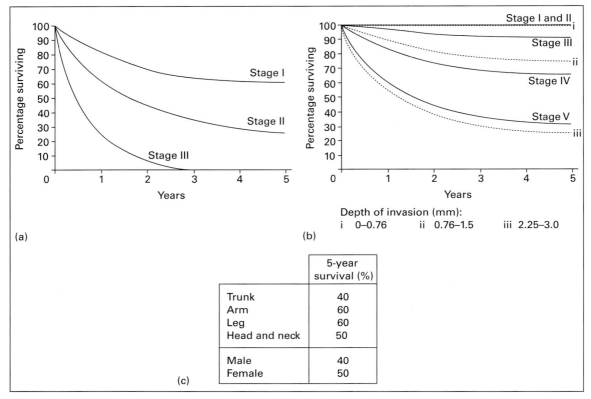

Figure 22.7 Prognosis in melanoma: (a) prognosis related to stage grouping; (b) prognosis related to stage (I–V) and depth of invasion (dashed lines); (c) prognosis related to site and sex.

while those with disseminated disease at presentation have a median survival of less than 6 months. These dreadful figures will only improve with increased public and professional awareness resulting in earlier diagnosis and treatment. Although both chemotherapy and 'immunotherapy' are at present relatively ineffective, it is at least now widely accepted that disseminated melanoma is not totally resistant to treatment.

Skin lymphomas

These are discussed separately in Chapter 26.

Miscellaneous rare tumours

Dermatofibrosarcoma protuberans

This is a soft-tissue sarcoma arising in the skin. It develops as firm nodules which grow slowly and may become large and be locally invasive. In general, it does not metastasize

but may recur after simple excision. Wide excision is the treatment of choice. Radiotherapy may be useful if major surgery (e.g. amputation) would otherwise be required.

Kaposi's sarcoma

Originally described by Moritz Kaposi in 1872, this sarcoma was rare in Europe until recently [53]. Kaposi initially described the tumour in elderly Ashkenazi Jewish men, and its incidence in Europe remained low at about 0.3 per million before the AIDS epidemic. However, it is common in Africa, accounting for 10% of all cancers in Kenya and Uganda. There is a much higher frequency in both renal allograft recipients and patients with AIDS; in fact, it is the commonest neoplasm among people with AIDS [54]. The tumour appears to be sustained by immunosuppression, which if discontinued may allow regression of the neoplasm. It is increasingly regarded as a sexually transmitted disease, six times more common, for example, in homosexual or bisexual men than in other AIDS risk groups in the United States – see, for example, the classic article by Levine [55]. It is clearly linked to infection with human herpesvirus 8 (see pages 28–29 and 30–31). Kaposi's sarcoma herpesvirus (KSHV) is linked to the pathogenesis of all forms of Kaposi's sarcoma – classic, endemic African and AIDS types – and is also a well-recognized complication in patients who have had organ transplants [54]. KSHV is also associated with lymphoproliferative disorders, including primary effusion lymphoma and multicentric Castleman's disease. KSHV is a gamma-2 herpesvirus, a family characterized by their ability to replicate in lymphoblastoid cells. Members of this family such as Epstein–Barr virus and herpesvirus saimiri cause lymphoid malignancy.

Pathologically, there is proliferation of endothelial vascular channels with numerous interweaving bands of spindle cells, consistent with proliferating endothelium. In the classic form of the disease a pigmented nodule appears on the leg or foot, often growing slowly. It may ulcerate, but lymph node spread is unusual until multiple new lesions have appeared and the disease is more advanced. The disease often results in brawny infiltration with diffuse swelling of the thigh or lower leg. This is a very indolent unresponsive type of tumour. In children, lymph nodes appear early with a clinical picture similar to lymphoma. In AIDS, the nodular and lymphadenopathic forms convey lesions also appearing on the mucous membranes. Speed of progression varies greatly with the presentation, often atypical by contrast to 'classical' Kaposi's sarcoma, with lesions at mucosal or inconspicuous sites. This form of disease seems more prevalent in homosexual males than in other groups with human immunodeficiency virus (HIV) positivity.

Nodular localized disease is treated with radiotherapy. It is a sensitive tumour and single fractions of 8 Gy using electrons are effective, with a complete response rate of 60–90%. In cases of 'classic' non-AIDS-related Kaposi's sarcoma, radiotherapy doses may need to be higher. The tumour is also sensitive to chemotherapy, effective agents (with response rates) including actinomycin D (90%), DTIC (60%), liposomal doxorubicin (70%), bleomycin (60%), paclitaxel and etoposide (35%), which has the advantage of oral administration. Combination chemotherapy gives a high proportion of complete responders. The usual combinations are actinomycin D and vinblastine, or actinomycin, vincristine and DTIC. IFN-α produces tumour responses in about 40% of patients who have AIDS, and is increasingly regarded as first-line therapy in selected patients with epidemic cutaneous Kaposi's sarcoma [53].

In the classic form of the disease, patients live for many years. In AIDS-related cases, the prognosis is much worse, patients dying of opportunistic infections in addition to the sarcoma. The introduction of highly active antiretroviral therapy (HAART) is an important component of long-term tumour control in persons with HIV positivity, and a proportion of patients with Kaposi's sarcoma do not require other additional treatment. At present, the treatment goal for patients with Kaposi's sarcoma is long-term palliation with minimal toxicity. Complete tumour response, even with long-term disease-free survival, does not necessarily imply that the tumour has been cured, even though HAART can certainly induce tumour responses in over one-quarter of all patients with AIDS/Kaposi's sarcoma, particularly those who were previously untreated for HIV. Nowadays, HAART is considered to be fundamental to the antitumour treatment of HIV/Kaposi's sarcoma, forming part of almost all treatment regimens currently in use.

Merkel cell (primary cutaneous neuroendocrine) tumours

These curious and unusual tumours, first described by Friedrich Merkel in 1875 and often presenting as a discrete nodular mass, have attracted increasing attention in recent years, particularly since the discovery of a 'Merkel Cell polyomavirus' (MCPyV). MCPyV-DNA has been found to be 'clonally integrated' in the majority of patients with this condition (around 75%), which may play a causative role. Histologically, they are round-cell tumours containing neurosecretory granules, and resemble small-cell carcinoma. Risk factors include age (generally over 65 years), fair skin and sun exposure. They are commoner in immunocompromised patients, for example, organ transplant recipients and HIV +ve persons. Although often running an aggressive course, they can be surprisingly radiosensitive, and response rates of over 90% have been documented, suggesting that the traditional approach (surgical resection) may be unnecessary – see, for example, Hruby et al. [56]. Use of intratumoral Interferon-B has also had some success. Nevertheless, 40% are locally recurrent and 55% give rise to regional node metastases, indeed these tumours have a frequency of nodal involvement around 20% at the time of initial presentation. The overall 2-year survival rate is 72% (slightly better in women). So far fewer than 2000 cases have been reported in the world literature.

Extramammary Paget's disease

These lesions are located near apocrine sweat glands, in the anogenital region, breast areola and axillae. They are probably a form of carcinoma *in situ*, and present as red scaly plaques, slowly increasing in size. They are usually removed surgically.

Metastatic carcinoma

Nodules of secondary carcinoma are not infrequently found in the skin, especially with cancer of the breast, penis, vulva and melanoma. If the diagnosis is in doubt, excision biopsy may be necessary. Treatment is generally directed toward the underlying disease if possible. Radiotherapy is often extremely useful for ulcerating or painful deposits.

References

1 Department of Health, Health Education Authority (UK). *Sun Conscious? Fashion and Beauty: the New Testament*. London: Health Education Authority, 1998.

2 Yamagiwa K, Ichikawa K. Experimental study of the pathogenesis of carcinoma. *Cancer Res* 1918; 3: 1–29.

3 Wakefield M, Bonett A. Preventing skin cancer in Australia. *Med J Aust* 1990; 152: 60–1.

4 Zanetti R, Rosso S, Martinez C *et al*. The Multicentre South European Study 'Helios' I. Skin characteristics and sunburns in basal cell and squamous cell carcinoma of the skin. *Br J Cancer* 1996; 73: 1440–6.

5 Rosso S, Zonetti R, Martinez C *et al*. The Multicentre South European Study 'Helios' II. Different sun exposure patterns in aetiology of basal cell and squamous cell carcinoma of the skin. *Br J Cancer* 1996; 73: 1447–54.

6 Rees JL. The melanoma epidemic: reality, and artefact. *Br Med J* 1996; 312: 137–8.

7 Anonymous. Do sunscreens prevent skin cancer? *Drug Ther Bull* 1998; 36: 49–51.

8 Adami J, Frisch M, Yuen J. Evidence of an association between non-Hodgkin's lymphoma and skin cancer. *Br Med J* 1995; 310: 1491–5.

9 el Ghissassi F, Baan R, Straif K *et al*. A review of human carcinogens. Part D. Radiation. *Lancet Oncol* 2009; 10: 751–2.

10 Gorlin RJ. Nevoid basal cell carcinoma syndrome. *Medicine (Baltimore)* 1987; 66: 98–113.

11 Rivers J. Is there more than one road to melanoma? *Lancet* 2004; 363: 728–30.

12 Kefford R, Bishop JN, Tucker M *et al*. Genetic testing for melanoma. *Lancet Oncol* 2002; 3: 653–4.

13 Cox NH. Guidelines for the management of Bowen's disease. *Br J Dermatol* 1999; 141: 633–41.

14 Rubin AI, Chen EH, Ratner D. Basal-cell carcinoma. *N Engl J Med* 2005; 353: 2262–9.

15 Goldberg LH. Basal cell carcinoma. *Lancet* 1996; 347: 663–7.

16 Neville JA, Welch E, Leffell DJ. Management of non-melanoma skin cancer in 2007. *Nat Clin Pract Oncol* 2007; 4: 462–9.

17 Avril M-F, Auperin A, Margulis A *et al*. Basal cell carcinoma of the face: surgery or radiotherapy? Results of a randomised study. *Br J Cancer* 1997; 76: 100–8.

18 Sauder DN. The emerging role of immunotherapy in the treatment of non-melanoma skin cancers. *Nat Clin Prac Oncol* 2005; 2: 326–7.

19 Sekulic A, Migden MR, Oro AE *et al*. Efficacy and safety of vismodegib in advanced basal-cell carcinoma. *New Engl J Med* 2012; 366: 2171–2179.

20 Bath-Hextall F, Bong J, Perkins W, Williams H. Interventions for basal cell carcinoma of the skin: systematic review. *Br Med J* 2004; 329: 705–8.

21 MacKie RM, Fruedenberger T, Aitchison TC. Personal risk-factor chart for cutaneous melanoma. *Lancet* 1989; ii: 487–90.

22 Mirror AJ, Mihm MC. Mechanisms of disease: melanoma. *N Engl J Med* 2006; 355: 51–65.

23 Green A, Swerdlow AJ. Epidemiology of melanocytic naevi. *Epidemiol Rev* 1989; 11: 204–21.

24 Anderson DE, Smith J, McBride CM. Hereditary aspects of malignant melanoma. *JAMA* 1967; 200: 741–6.

25 Tsao, H, Atkins MB, Sober AJ. Medical progress: management of cutaneous melanoma. *N Engl J Med* 2004; 351: 998–1012.

26 Bale SJ, Dracopoli NC, Tucker MA *et al*. Mapping the gene for hereditary cutaneous malignant melanoma-dysplastic nevus to chromosome 1p. *N Engl J Med* 1989; 320: 1367–72.

27 Clark WH, From L, Bernadino EA, Mihn NC. The histogenesis and biologic behaviour of primary human malignant melanomas of the skin. *Cancer Res* 1969; 29: 705–27.

28 Breslow A. Tumour thickness, level of invasion and node dissection in stage I cutaneous melanoma. *Ann Surg* 1975; 182: 572–5.

29 Busam KJ. Advances in molecular staging of melanoma patients: multimarker analysis of archival lymph node tissue. *J Clin Oncol* 2003; 21: 3550–1.

30 Krown SE, Chapman PB. Defining adequate surgery for primary melanoma. *N Engl J Med* 2004; 350: 823–5.

31 Kuo CT, Hoon DS, Takeuchi H *et al*. Prediction of disease outcome in melanoma patients by molecular analysis of paraffin-embedded sentinel lymph nodes. *J Clin Oncol* 2003; 21: 3566–72.

32 Rivers JK, Roof MI. Sentinel lymph-node biopsy in melanoma: is less surgery better? *Lancet* 1997; 350: 1336–7.

33 Thomas JM, Newton-Bishop J, A'Hern R *et al*. Excision margins in high-risk malignant melanoma. *N Engl J Med* 2004; 350: 757–66.

34 Cascinelli N, Mrabito A, Santinami M *et al*. Immediate or delayed dissection of regional nodes in patients with melanoma of the trunk: a randomised trial. *Lancet* 1998; 351: 793–6.

35 Davis NC, McLeod R, Beardmore G, Little J, Quinn R, Holt J. Melanoma is a word not a sentence. *Aust NZ J Surg* 1976; 46: 188–92.

36 Piepkorn M, Weinstock MA, Barnhill RL. Theoretical and empirical arguments in relation to elective lymph node dissection for melanoma. *Arch Dermatol* 1997; 133: 995–1002.

37 Morton DL, Thompson JF, Cochran AJ *et al.* Sentinel-node biopsy or nodal observation in melanoma. *N Engl J Med* 2006; 355: 1307–17.

38 Torjesen I. Sentinel node biopsy for melanoma: unnecessary treatment? *Brit Med J* 2013; 346: e8645.

39 Barranco SC, Romsdahl MM, Humphrey RM. Radiation response of human melanoma cells grown *in vitro. Cancer Res* 1971; 31: 830–3.

40 Burmeister BH, Henderson MA, Ainslie J *et al.* Adjuvant radiotherapy versus observation alone for patients at risk of lymph-node field relapse after therapeutic lymphadenectomy for melanoma: a randomised trial. *Lancet Oncol* 2012; 13: 589–597.

41 Hunder NN, Wallen H, Cao J *et al.* Treatment of metastatic melanoma with autologous CD4$^+$ T cells against NY-ESO-1. *N Engl J Med* 2008; 358: 2698–703.

42 Eggermont AM, Suciu S, Santinami M *et al.* for the EORTC Melanoma Group. Adjuvant therapy with pegylated interferon alfa-2b versus observation alone in resected stage III melanoma: final results of EORTC 18991, a randomized phase III trial. *Lancet* 2008; 372: 117–26.

43 Marabito A. Effect of long-term adjuvant therapy with interferon alpha-2a in patients with regional node metastases from cutaneous melanoma: a randomised trial. *Lancet* 2001; 358: 866–9.

44 Gibney GT, Sondak VK. Has targeted therapy for melanoma made chemotherapy obsolete? *Lancet Oncol* 2013; 14: 676–7.

45 Chapman PB, Hauschild A, Robert C, *et al.* Improved survival with vemurafenib in melanoma with BRAF V600E mutation. *N Engl J Med* 2011; 364: 2507–16.

46 41.Hodi FS, O'Day SJ, McDermott DF *et al.* Improved survival with ipilimumab in patients with metastatic melanoma. *N Engl J Med* 2010; 363: 711–23.

47 Wolchok JD, Kluger H, Callahan MK *et al.* Nivolumab plus ipilimumab in advanced melanoma. *New Engl J Med* 2013; 369: 122–133.

48 Zikich D, Schachter J, Besser MJ. Immunotherapy for the management of advanced melanoma: the next steps. *Am J Clin Dermatol* 2013; 14: 261–72.

49 Blanchard T, Srivastava PA, Duan F. Vaccines against advanced melanoma. *Clin Dermatol* 2013; 31: 179–190.

50 Mishima Y, Honda C, Ichihashi M *et al.* Treatment of malignant melanoma by single thermal neutron capture therapy with melanoma-seeking ^{10}B-compound. *Lancet* 1989; ii: 388–9.

51 Thörn M, Adami HO, Ringborg U *et al.* The association between anatomic site and survival in malignant melanoma: an analysis of 12 353 patients from the Swedish Cancer Registry. *Eur J Cancer* 1989; 25: 483–91.

52 Sylaidis P, Gordon D, Rigby H, Kennedy J. Follow-up requirements for thick cutaneous melanoma. *Br J Plast Surg* 1997; 50: 349–53.

53 Antman K, Chang Y. Medical progress: Kaposi's sarcoma. *N Engl J Med* 2000; 342: 1027–38.

54 Flore O. *Kaposi's sarcoma. Lancet* 2004; 364: 740–1.

55 Levine AM. AIDS-related malignancies: the emerging epidemic. *J Natl Cancer Inst* 1993; 85: 382–97.

56 Hruby G, Scolyer RA, Thompson JF. The important role of radiation treatment in the management of Merkel cell carcinoma. *Brit J Dermatol* 2013; 169: 975–82.

Further reading

Bharath AK, Turner RJ. Impact of climate change on skin cancer. *J R Soc Med* 2009; 102: 215–18.

Hwang ST, Janik JE, Jaffe ES, Wilson WH. Mycosis fungoides and Sézary syndrome. *Lancet* 2008; 371: 945–57.

Kong M-F, Jogia R, Jackson S *et al.* Malignant melanoma presenting as a foot ulcer. *Lancet* 2005; 366: 1750.

O'Donovan P, Perrett CM, Zhang X *et al.* Azathioprine and UVA light generate mutagenic oxidative DNA damage. *Science* 2005; 309: 1871–4.

Parrish JA. Immunosuppression, skin cancer and ultraviolet A radiation. *N Engl J Med* 2005; 353: 2712–13.

Sobin LH, Gospodarowicz MK, Wittekind Ch, eds. *TNM Classification of Malignant Tumours*, 7th edn. Chichester: Wiley-Blackwell, 2009

Thomas JM, Giblin V. Cure of cutaneous melanoma is only possible with earlier diagnosis. *Br Med J* 2006; 332: 987–8.

Yarchoan R, Tosato G, Little RF. Therapy insight. AIDS-related malignancies: the influence of antiretroviral therapy on pathogenesis and management. *Nat Clin Pract Oncol* 2005; 2: 406–15.

23 Bone and soft-tissue sarcomas

Sarcomas are cancers of mesenchymal tissues. Although they are uncommon there is great variety, and a working classification is given in Tables 23.1 and 23.2. They occur in both children and adults. Some types, such as osteosarcoma and Ewing's sarcoma, are most frequent in adolescence. There is a slight male preponderance. The age-specific incidence is shown in Figure 23.1.

Bone sarcomas

The best-understood aetiological factor in bone sarcoma is ionizing irradiation [2]. From 1917 to 1926 many factories were established in the USA and Canada in which there was large-scale production of watches and instruments coated with paint that was made luminous by the action of radium on zinc sulphide. The deplorable factory conditions and the technique taught to the young female employees of pointing their brushes in their mouths led to osteosarcoma of the jaw and also at sites remote from the skull as a result of the absorption of radium from the gut and its deposition in bone. The cumulative risk of developing osteosarcoma was as high as 70% over the ensuing 40 years.

External beam radiation produces a bone or soft-tissue sarcoma in 1 in 3000–5000 treated patients. The latent period is 5–30 years (median 10 years). Radiation-induced bone sarcoma is especially likely to occur in children and is one of the commonest second cancers complicating cancer treatment. The major risk of radiation-induced bone cancer is in children with heritable retinoblastoma, and with Ewing's sarcoma, where the relative risk is increased 350-fold. The absolute risk in Ewing's sarcoma is 7%. In other childhood cancers, the relative risk is 30-fold. The absolute rate is only 0.1–0.5% [3]. The frequency of osteosarcoma and other bone sarcomas is greatly increased in patients with Paget's disease, the tumour arising in the affected bone. This, and prior radiation, are the main causes of the increased frequency of bone sarcoma in the elderly.

Osteosarcoma occurs with a 500-fold increased incidence in patients who are cured of the familial form of retinoblastoma (see Chapter 24, pages 486–487 and also 489). In this disease, there is loss of both alleles at 13q14. Allele loss at this site has been found in sporadic cases of osteosarcoma. Loss of heterozygosity and mutation of the *p53* tumour-suppressor gene on chromosome 17p is a frequent finding in sporadic osteosarcoma. A familial

Cancer and its Management, Seventh Edition. Jeffrey Tobias and Daniel Hochhauser.
© 2015 John Wiley & Sons, Ltd. Published 2015 by John Wiley & Sons, Ltd.

Table 23.1 Primary malignant bone tumours.

Osteosarcoma: usually high-grade malignancy, most benign form is parosteal osteosarcoma; usually metaphyseal; can be in flat bones; peak ages 12–24 and 50–80

Ewing's sarcoma: high-grade malignancy; diaphyseal in long bones, often in flat bones; age 5–30

Chondrosarcoma: variable malignancy; usually metaphyseal; age 40–60

Other spindle cell tumours

Malignant fibrous histiocytoma

Fibrosarcoma: age 30–50; long bones; metaphyseal usually, similar distribution to osteosarcoma

Haemangiopericytoma

Haemangioendothelioma

Other round-cell tumours

Primary lymphoma of bone

Mesenchymal chondrosarcoma

Angiosarcoma

Giant-cell tumour: occasionally malignant; epiphyseal; age 30–40

Table 23.2 A simple staging system for bone sarcomas [simplified from Enneking *et al.* [1].

Stage	Histological grade	Site
IA	Low	Intracompartmental
IB	Low	Extracompartmental
IIA	High	Intracompartmental
IIB	High	Extracompartmental
III	Regional or distant metastases Any grade or local extent	

cancer syndrome, Li–Fraumeni syndrome, in which sarcomas in childhood are associated with an increased incidence of cancer at an early age in close relatives, is associated with a germline mutation in *p53*. Only 4% of

sporadic cases of osteosarcoma, with no suggestive family history, are associated with germline *p53* mutation [4].

In Ewing's sarcoma a characteristic translocation t(11;22) has been found both in cell lines and in primary tumours. The same translocation has been shown in neuroepithelioma and Askin's tumour, suggesting that all three round-cell tumours arise from a common lineage. The translocation leads to the expression of an aberrant protein that contains part of either the *FLIa* or *ERG* gene [5]. These transcripts occur in 95% of cases. Three other genes are occasionally partners. The detection of the

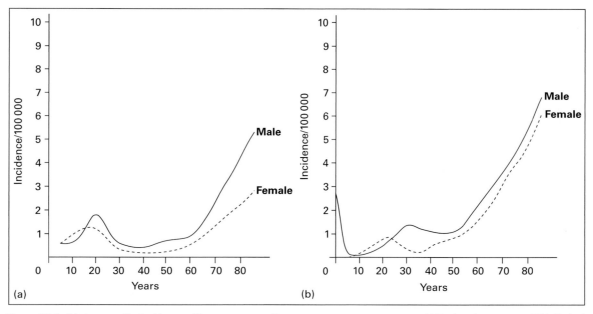

Figure 23.1 (a) Age-specific incidence of bone sarcomas. Commonest types: osteosarcoma, 31%; chondrosarcoma, 17%; Ewing's sarcoma, 8%. (b) Age-specific incidence of soft-tissue sarcomas. Commonest types: fibrosarcoma, 16.1%; liposarcoma, 12.4%; leiomyosarcoma, 10%.

transcript may be useful diagnostically in distinguishing other small round-cell tumours. The type of transcript does not appear to relate to clinical outcome.

Although rare, primary malignant bone tumours are very important and their management is changing. Until the late 1960s, the treatment was usually by amputation or radiotherapy alone, and the results were poor, with osteosarcoma and Ewing's tumour cured in only 10–20% of patients. In recent years, the management of malignant bone tumours has changed considerably. Local control of disease can often now be achieved without amputation by the use of internal prosthetic replacement. The use of intensive chemotherapy preoperatively and postoperatively has prolonged survival in both Ewing's tumour and osteosarcoma.

These changes have meant that the management of these uncommon tumours has become highly specialized. They are undoubtedly best managed in centres with special expertise in the complex pathology, radiology, surgery, chemotherapy, radiation therapy, prosthetics, nursing, psychology, and rehabilitation techniques that form such an essential and integrated part of the management.

Osteosarcoma

This is the commonest malignant tumour of bone (31% – approximately 3 cases per million) and accounts for 3–4% of all childhood malignancies. In the UK, there are approximately 150 new cases each year. The term 'osteosarcoma' is now preferred to 'osteogenic sarcoma', which is a confusing term because several of the bone tumours do show evidence of calcification or even apparent bone production as part of their evolutionary development. In the USA, the annual incidence is approximately 400 children and adolescents below the age of 20 with approximately 500 additional adult cases.

Pathology

The tumour usually arises in the epiphyseal region and consists of malignant osteoblasts, which make osteoid. Within the tumour there may be areas of chondroblastic or fibroblastic differentiation so that small biopsies may not be representative. The tumour cells produce alkaline phosphatase, which is a useful cytochemical marker. Typically, the tumour contains mixed fibroblastic, osteoblastic and chondroblastic elements, but other forms are the telangiectatic type, in which there are blood-filled spaces in the tumour, and the small-cell variant, which may be difficult to distinguish from Ewing's sarcoma.

The histological differential diagnosis includes other forms of primary malignant bone tumour or soft-tissue sarcoma, especially malignant fibrous histiocytoma of bone. Histological grading of the degree of malignancy gives a rough guide to prognosis and is one of a number of prognostic variables to be considered while assessing comparisons between treatments [6].

Local invasion occurs when the tumour breaks through the bone and the periosteal surroundings (Figure 23.2) and invades the soft tissue including the nerves and blood vessels around the joint. A staging system has been proposed, based on grade and compartmental extension (Table 23.2).

Juxtacortical (parosteal) osteosarcoma is an unusual variant in which new bone formation is especially dense and which presents as a large exostosis. The pathology and clinical behaviour are less malignant. A further variant, periosteal osteosarcoma, has an intermediate degree of malignancy. Osteosarcoma arising in Paget's disease occurs in an older age group and often develops in flat bones. The tumours are usually aggressive and metastases occur early.

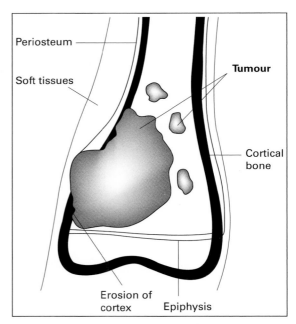

Figure 23.2 In this central osteosarcoma the tumour has arisen next to the epiphysis. It has eroded the cortical bone, broken through the periosteal barrier and spread into the soft tissues. The 'islands' of the central tumour are actually connected contiguously to the main tumour mass when seen in three dimensions.

Clinical features

The disease mostly affects adolescents, the peak incidence being in the age range 10–20 years during the adolescent growth spurt. There is also a second peak of incidence much later in life, around age 80 years. In the younger (and more numerous) age group, boys are affected more often than girls (1.5:1). Most of the tumours occur around the knee, and the lower femur and upper tibia account for 60% of all cases. The presentation is with pain and swelling, often brought to attention by minor trauma. The pain is typically worse at night and may be present for many weeks before swelling appears. (Nocturnal bone pain is always a serious symptom in oncology, often indicating bone involvement.) On examination there is usually a firm swelling, which may be warm and tender with limitation of movement of the joint.

Radiological appearances

Generally there is a destructive lesion in the metaphyseal region, usually but not always with new bone formation in spicules. There may be a Codman's triangle caused by elevation of the periosteum (Figure 23.3). The parosteal

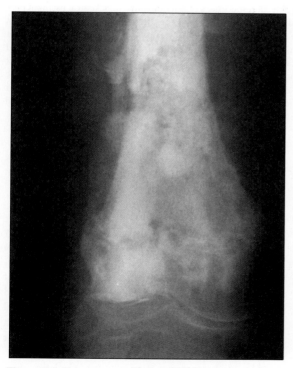

Figure 23.3 Osteosarcoma of the lower left femur. There is extensive bone destruction, with elevation of the periosteum (Codman's triangle) and new bone formation.

variety is associated with slow growth, exostosis and dense new bone, and the telangiectatic type with rapidly progressive destruction. The way in which the radiological appearances are produced by the tumour extension is clearly shown in radiographs of thin sections taken through the whole specimen (Figure 23.4).

Investigation

Routine investigation should include chest radiography, isotope bone scan (which may show skeletal metastases) and computed tomography (CT) of the thorax. This should be performed before surgery. CT scanning is the most sensitive method of detecting pulmonary metastases and these will be present in about 30% of cases. If local resection is contemplated (see below), magnetic resonance imaging (MRI) of the affected limb is essential to delineate tumour extent (Figures 23.5 and 23.6) including the extent of the soft-tissue component and the intramedullary extension. In interpreting MRI scans, care must be taken not to confuse oedema with soft-tissue infiltration. The serum alkaline phosphatase is frequently elevated.

Treatment
Surgery

Before 1980, amputation was the main surgical treatment for osteosarcomas of the limbs. For tumours around the knee, the amputation was generally at the mid-thigh level, and the 'received wisdom' was that to be of value, the stump must extend at least 10 cm from the ischial tuberosity. Higher tumours, or those which extend high up the femoral shaft, were (and occasionally still are) treated by disarticulation.

In recent years, conservative surgery has been used wherever possible, in fact in over 75% of cases treated in large and experienced centres with good multidisciplinary expertise – see, for example, Ref. [7]. A substantial internal prosthesis is inserted after removal of the tumour (Figure 23.7) and in some countries a bone allograft is used. The functional results of prostheses are usually excellent for the lower femur and upper tibia but somewhat less satisfactory in the upper humerus. Pathological fractures and/or extensive infiltration along the bone shaft or into soft tissue make prosthetic replacement less feasible. Conservative limb-preserving surgery is now increasingly performed for pelvic tumours, either with removal of part of the pelvic ring without reconstruction (for tumours of the pubis and ischium not involving the hip joint) or with insertion of a metallic prosthesis. Local recurrence of the tumour is becoming less common

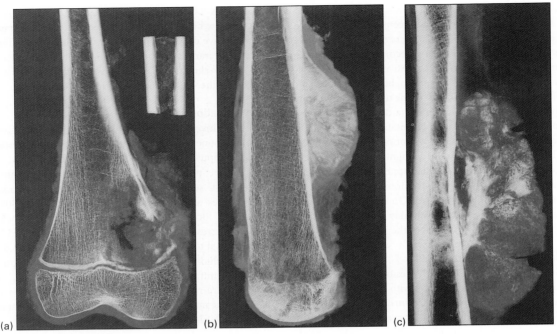

(a)   (b)   (c)

Figure 23.4 Fine-detail radiographs of sagittal longitudinal slabs of resection specimens of osteosarcoma. (a) Classical osteosarcoma of distal femur in a boy aged 14 years. The lesion stops at the unfused epiphysis. It is destroying the cortex and extends subperiosteally, lifting the periosteum and forming a Codman's triangle. There are spicules of new bone formation. This is the commonest site for osteosarcoma. The insert shows the normal intramedullary cavity higher in the femur. (b) Parosteal osteosarcoma in an 18-year-old male, arising from the posterior aspect of the distal femur (the typical site of this tumour). The tumour is confined to the outer aspect of the cortex and contains trabecular bone which is covered with fibrous tissue on the outer surface. The bone cortex is intact and the medulla is not involved. The fused epiphysis is visible. (c) Periosteal osteosarcoma of the mid-femur in a woman aged 50. The tumour is made up of radiolucent tumour cartilage and shows patchy calcification. In a few places there is a trabecular pattern with mineralized tumour osteoid. There is involvement of the subadjacent medulla.

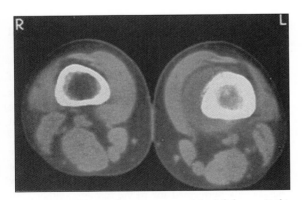

Figure 23.5 CT scan of osteosarcoma of the left femur. At this level the bone radiograph was only slightly abnormal. The scan shows erosion of the cortex, periosteal reaction and considerable soft-tissue swelling.

with skilful surgery and with the use of preoperative chemotherapy. Local recurrences in long bones can often be successfully treated by amputation.

Chemotherapy

The use of complex and intensive adjuvant chemotherapy has resulted in an increase in survival from 20–25% without chemotherapy to 45–80% with current treatment – see, for example, Ref. [8]. Because of the rarity of the tumour, international study groups have developed over recent years, with the aim of mounting substantial studies, with cooperation between European and North American trial groups a welcome development – see, for example, Ref. [9].

Adjuvant programmes typically use cisplatin, doxorubicin, ifosfamide and high-dose methotrexate, though details of chemotherapy programmes vary

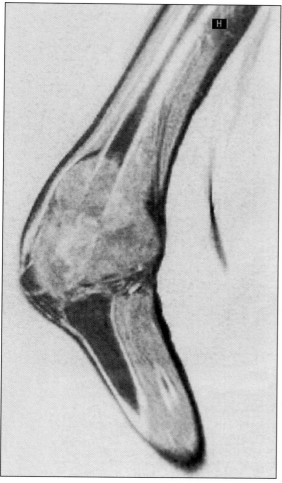

Figure 23.6 MRI scan of the lower femur in a 16-year-old girl with osteosarcoma. A large soft-tissue mass surrounds the lower femur, extending into the soft tissues.

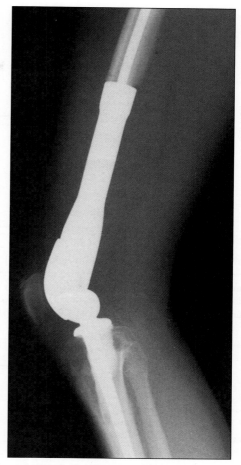

Figure 23.7 Endoprosthetic replacement of osteosarcoma of the distal femur. Following chemotherapy the tumour was resected and the lower femur and knee replaced by the prosthesis. Chemotherapy was then continued for 3 months. This patient now walks normally and can run and climb stairs.

internationally. The value of extremely high doses of methotrexate has still not been shown convincingly but the usual practice is to give high doses with folinic acid rescue. Ifosfamide is widely used in chemotherapy combinations. There is some evidence that response rates are higher when the drug is given in very high dose but the toxicity is greatly increased and the effect on survival is uncertain and has increasingly been questioned – see Ref. [10]. Although other agents such as cyclophosphamide, etoposide, bleomycin and actinomycin are sometimes used, there is little evidence to suggest they are more effective than the three-drug combination MAP (methotrexate, doxorubicin, cisplatin). In large-scale

studies about 60% of patients with no detectable metastases at presentation are cured (Figure 23.8a) [11,12].

It is now regarded as standard-of-care to employ chemotherapy both before surgery (induction or neoadjuvant chemotherapy) and also postoperatively (Figure 23.9). This has the advantages of starting systemic treatment early, of allowing time for the manufacture of an endoprosthesis, of facilitating surgery if the tumour reduces in size, and of allowing histological assessment of response when the tumour is resected. In an important large-scale study from France, children with localized high-grade osteosarcoma of a limb were randomized to

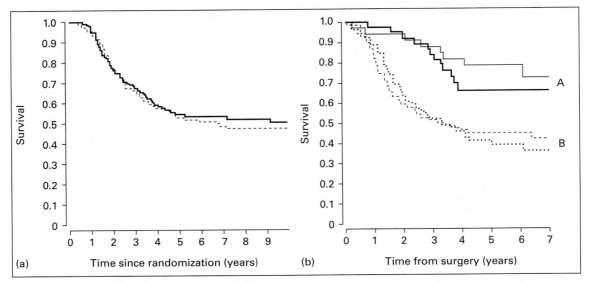

Figure 23.8 (a) A randomized trial of two chemotherapy regimens in osteosarcoma. Survival at 5 years is 55% with few recurrences after that time. (b) Survival in the two arms of the trial according to whether there was a good (A) or poor (B) histological response. (Source: Souhami *et al.* [11]. Reproduced with permission from Elsevier.)

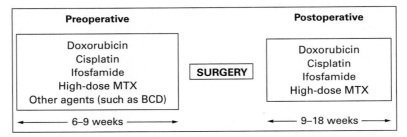

Figure 23.9 Schematic representation of a typical chemotherapy programme for osteosarcoma. BCD is a combination of bleomycin, cisplatin and actinomycin D. MTX is methotrexate. Limb preservation surgery is increasingly employed.

high-dose methotrexate, etoposide and ifosfamide or alternatively high-dose methotrexate and doxorubicin [13]. There were 56% good responders in the first arm compared with 39% for methotrexate/doxorubicin, and a slightly higher event-free survival at 77 months. The authors felt that avoidance of doxorubicin- or cisplatin-containing regimens was valuable since lower long-term cardiotoxicity and ototoxicity should be expected. The hope that non-responding or partially responding tumours would have a better prognosis if chemotherapy was intensified preoperatively has not been fulfilled, despite the observed improvement in histological response following dose-dense chemotherapy [14]. This important study has called into question the traditional view that survival is undoubtedly better

in patients whose tumours show a good histological response following preoperative chemotherapy (Figure 23.8b). For relapsing patients no longer effectively treatable by primary or conventional regimens, combinations of agents including gemcitabine and docetaxel have become widely used. More recently, the addition of mifamurtide has offered further hope for these mostly young patients and their families. Mifamurtide, an immune stimulator which activates both monocytes and macrophages, is a fully synthetic derivative of muramyl dipeptide (MDP), the smallest naturally occurring immune stimulatory component of cell walls from a *Mycobacterium* species, and is given as a one-hour liposomally enclosed infusion, generally well tolerated. In an impressive study from the US-base

Children's Oncology Group, 662 patients with localized non-metastatic osteosarcoma were treated with standard chemotherapy regimens (combining methotrexate, cisplatin and doxorubicin, with or without ifosfamide – a 2 × 2 factorial design), and randomized to mifamurtide or placebo control (see Ref. [15]). The results showed a 30% reduction in mortality and an overall 6 year absolute survival improvement of 7% – the first major advance in recent years.

Treatment of pulmonary metastases

Patients who develop pulmonary metastases [16] may still be curable by surgery. If a patient develops pulmonary metastases, CT and/or PET scanning should be used to determine if there is a possibility that they can be resected. Neoadjuvant and adjuvant chemotherapy may not only delay or prevent pulmonary metastases but also provide benefits to patients by reducing the number of pulmonary metastases when they do occur, increasing the chance of a potentially curative resection. The prognosis after removal of metastases is better if the lesions are unilateral, if there are less than six, if they appear late after chemotherapy has stopped, and if they can technically be totally resected. When a metastasis is detected, chemotherapy is often started, logically enough, using agents that have not previously been given. If no new metastases have appeared within 2–3 months, thoracotomy is undertaken. This approach helps to prevent needless thoracotomies in patients destined to develop further pulmonary metastases very soon and to die quickly of their disease. This topic is well surveyed by Treasure and Utley in a comprehensive, recent 2013 review [17].

Radiotherapy

Before modern chemotherapy was introduced, high-dose radiotherapy to the primary tumour was used in order to avoid amputation in those destined to die of metastases. If these did not occur within 6–12 months, a delayed amputation was performed. Unfortunately, local radiotherapy seldom provides long-lasting control of the primary and local recurrence and fractures often occur. Radiotherapy is still of value in palliation of an advanced tumour and in treatment of painful bone metastases.

Whole-lung irradiation (17.5 Gy in 20 fractions) has been used to prevent pulmonary metastases. Some studies have shown prevention, or delay in onset, of pulmonary metastases, while others have not and the value of this treatment remains uncertain. Its use has been superseded by chemotherapy.

Parosteal and periosteal osteosarcoma

Parosteal osteosarcoma is a rare slow-growing variant that arises from the surface of the bone, usually the distal posterior femur (see Figure 23.4b). It metastasizes late and adjuvant chemotherapy is not indicated. Treatment is by wide local excision. Periosteal osteosarcoma (see Figure 23.4c) is rare and is of a higher grade than parosteal lesions. There are usually areas of chondroblastic differentiation. Although less likely to metastasize than classical central tumours, chemotherapy may be indicated. For current guidelines in this rare tumour, see Ref. [18].

High-grade surface osteosarcomas

These are rare variants that can occur at any age. Histologically and clinically they are indistinguishable from central high-grade tumours and are treated in the same way. They should not be mistaken for periosteal tumours, which have a reduced tendency to metastasize.

Small-cell osteosarcoma

A rare variant of osteosarcoma, these tumours resemble Ewing's sarcoma and may contain cytoplasmic glycogen. The tumour cells produce alkaline phosphatase, indicating their osteoblast origins, as does the presence of tumour osteoid. They metastasize rapidly and although responsive to chemotherapy, the prognosis is less good than for other variants.

Chondrosarcoma

This is the second commonest bone tumour but occurs later in life than osteosarcoma, with a peak incidence at 40–60 years. It may arise *de novo* as a sarcomatous transformation of benign enchondromata, in multiple enchondromatosis (Ollier's disease) and, rarely, in Paget's disease. See Ref. [19], for a useful review.

Presentation

These tumours are usually slow-growing. The commonest site is the pelvis, followed by the femur, humerus, scapula and ribs. The most usual symptom is a painful swelling, but in slow-growing lesions, pain may not be a symptom at first. The disease tends to grow more rapidly in younger patients.

The radiograph typically shows a destructive bone lesion with areas of calcification normally as flecks (rather than spicules as in osteosarcoma) (Figure 23.10).

Pathology [20]

The low-grade tumour resembles cartilage but without tumour osteoid being formed and with a greater degree

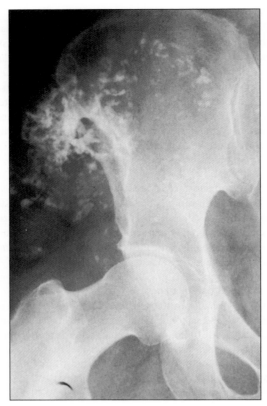

Figure 23.10 Chondrosarcoma of the ilium. The ilium is eroded by the tumour which shows patchy calcification. The tumour extends into the soft tissues laterally.

of cellular pleomorphism. Low-grade tumours tend to be locally invasive and not to metastasize, but pulmonary metastases are frequent in high-grade tumours. Sometimes low-grade tumours change to a more malignant variety after repeated local recurrence. At this stage a spindle cell component may dominate the histological appearance.

Treatment and prognosis

The mainstay of treatment is surgery, with complete removal of the tumour with associated soft tissues. In a long bone this can sometimes be accomplished, without amputation, by *en bloc* resection and insertion of an endoprosthesis. In the pelvis a surgical approach is often impossible. It is essential that the initial resection is radical with wide margins. Local recurrence will otherwise occur, requiring much more extensive surgery. Radiotherapy is used as a palliative treatment but the tumour is radioresistant and local control is usually short-lived.

From the little evidence available the tumour also appears to be resistant to cytotoxic drugs [21] unless the tumour is dedifferentiated, when responses may occur to drugs such as cisplatin, doxorubicin and ifosfamide.

Prognosis is largely determined by histological grade. The 10-year survival is 80% for grade I tumours and 25% for grade III.

Mesenchymal chondrosarcoma

This rare variant occurs in teenage children and young adults. The axial skeleton and skull bones are often affected. The tumour shows calcification on plain radiography. The tumour contains small-cell components, which may make distinction from a round-cell sarcoma difficult. It responds to chemotherapy but radical excision is essential for survival. Radiation may be used if the resection margins are not clear at operation. Chemotherapy regimens are usually based on cisplatin, doxorubicin and ifosfamide.

Ewing's sarcoma

This is a malignant round-cell tumour of bone whose aetiology is unknown. It is the second commonest primary bone tumour of children and adolescents after osteosarcoma, and this tumour and its related malignancies (see below) account for about 3% of childhood tumours. The characteristic chromosomal translocation is discussed on pages 447 and 456. In summary, these tumours are characterized by translocation of the EWS gene with a member of the ETS family genes (see an excellent review of the biology of Ewing's and related tumours by Ross *et al.* [22]). Ewing's sarcoma is characterized by EWS fusions with FLI1 in over 90% of cases, ERG in 5–10% of cases, with FEV, ETV1 and ETV4 fusions occurring in less than 1% of cases. Several studies report that a reciprocal translocation of band q24 on chromosome 11 and band q12 on chromosome 22 leads to an in-frame fusion, producing an EWS–FLI1 fusion gene in 85% of cases. EWS–ETS fusions can vary in chromosomal breakpoints, and differences in these breakpoints may be related to varying severities of prognosis. EWS and ETS family combinations are specific to ES, but combinations of EWS with other genes result in a number of other pathologies. The peak incidence is 10–20 years and, like osteosarcoma, it is slightly more common in males (1.5:1). It is very rare in Africans and black Americans.

Presentation

Pain and swelling are the usual symptoms and may be present for many months before diagnosis. Pulmonary

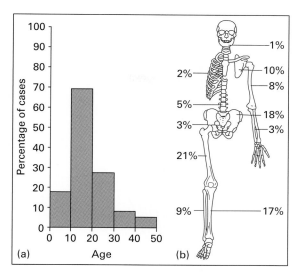

Figure 23.11 Ewing's sarcoma: (a) age at onset; (b) site of primary tumour.

symptoms, due to metastases, may first bring the patient to the doctor. The flat bones of the pelvis are the commonest site of involvement, although the femur is the commonest single bone to be involved, the tibia and humerus less frequently. The tumour can also arise in the vertebrae, skull and ribs (Figure 23.11b). Fever and weight loss are not infrequent, especially with large and metastatic tumours.

Pathology

The tumour usually arises in the diaphysis and occasionally in the metaphysis. Epiphyseal involvement is unusual. Histologically it consists of small round cells. It resembles, and must be distinguished from, non-Hodgkin's lymphoma, metastatic neuroblastoma and some types of rhabdomyosarcoma. On conventional histology it may be impossible to distinguish Ewing's sarcoma from primitive neuroectodermal tumours (PNETs) of other types (such as Askin's tumour). Indeed, it seems likely that classical Ewing's sarcoma and PNETs are part of a spectrum of round-cell tumours showing varying degrees of neural differentiation. Immunohistochemical techniques will show neural markers in PNETs (such as neurone-specific enolase and neural cell adhesion molecule). When PNET presents in bone, it seems that the prognosis is not substantially different from that for Ewing's sarcoma [23]. Differentiation from lymphoma can be made by use of antibodies to the common leucocyte antigen (which stain lymphoma) and by the lack of surface immunoglobulin

in Ewing's sarcoma. Ewing's tumour usually stains with antibodies to MIC2, an antigen almost always present in the tumour cells.

The tumour typically permeates the medullary and cortical bone, and for this reason wide margins are needed in planning radiotherapy or surgery. Glycogen can often be demonstrated in the cytoplasm by the periodic acid–Schiff (PAS) stain, and the distinction from these other tumours can usually be made on clinical, radiological and biochemical grounds. Metastases to lung and to the bones occur frequently.

Investigation

Diagnosis is by biopsy and expert opinion on the histology. The radiograph usually shows a diffuse erosion in a flat bone (Figure 23.12) or in the diaphyseal region of a long bone (Figure 23.13). There is a marked periosteal reaction, sometimes with an 'onion skin' appearance, usually with evidence of a soft-tissue mass that is often extensive.

Further investigation should include a full blood count, which may show anaemia and leucocytosis in advanced or rapidly progressive cases; chest radiography; CT scan of the primary site and of the thorax, which may show single or multiple metastases; isotope bone scan to detect bone metastases, which are common; plasma lactate dehydrogenase and liver function tests; and urine vanillylmandelic acid if there is a possibility that the diagnosis is neuroblastoma. MRI is invaluable in indicating the degree of intramedullary and soft-tissue extension of the tumour. About 20% of patients have radiologically detectable metastases at diagnosis. Sensitive molecular

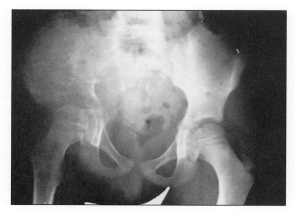

Figure 23.12 Ewing's sarcoma of the right ilium. The bone is diffusely expanded by a large radiolucent tumour.

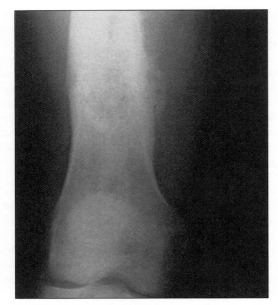

Figure 23.13 Radiograph of Ewing's tumour of the femur. Note the diaphyseal position, the periosteal elevation, and the new bone formation.

tests for the t(11;22) translocation (see above) can detect Ewing's tumour cells in the bone marrow of an even greater proportion (up to 50% in some series), associated with larger tumours and a worse prognosis.

Treatment

This must be both local and systemic. Local treatment alone is associated with cure in only 10–20% of cases, and the prognosis has been improved considerably by the use of chemotherapy – see Ref. [24] for an excellent review.

Local treatment

Unlike most primary bone sarcomas, Ewing's sarcoma is radiosensitive. Indeed the mainstay of local treatment used to be radical megavoltage radiotherapy. Doses of 55–65 Gy are given to the primary site in 2-Gy fractions over 6–7 weeks. Care must be taken not to irradiate all the soft tissues of a limb to this dose, or troublesome oedema will occur below the irradiated site. In practice, this involves careful avoidance of a strip of soft tissue the whole length of the treatment field (Figure 23.14). Additionally, the final 15–20 Gy are given to a smaller field around the residual tumour, that is, using a 'shrinking field' technique. This area of radiotherapy requires great skill and precision, with the use of modern conformal

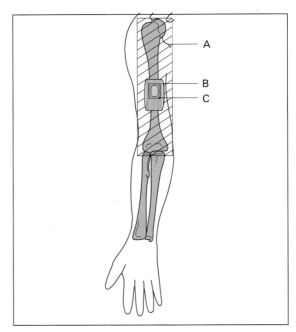

Figure 23.14 Radiation fields in Ewing's sarcoma. (A) The whole bone is irradiated to a modest diaphyseal humeral dose (30 Gy). (B) The field is shrunk down to the tumour and adjacent bone to 45 Gy. (C) The tumour itself is boosted to 60–70 Gy. If the tumour is well clear of the epiphyses these may not be included in the radiation field.

and IMRT techniques to ensure the best possible tumour localization and avoidance of sensitive surrounding tissues.

In recent years, troublesome late local recurrences have been seen in some patients after treatment with radiotherapy and chemotherapy. For this reason, there is increasing use of surgical excision and endoprosthetic replacement of bone as an adjuvant to chemotherapy and radiotherapy. Surgery alone may sometimes be sufficient to gain control, but because of the permeating nature of the tumour, a combination of surgery and radiation is sometimes necessary. Another reason for wishing to avoid radiation is the risk of later development of radiation sarcoma. The 20-year risk of induction of a radiation sarcoma after treatment of Ewing's tumour in childhood is 7%. The problem is that surgery for large tumours often proves to be histologically intralesional so that follow-up radiation cannot be avoided. The decision between surgery and radiation is therefore highly complex, especially in pelvic tumours [25]. Malignant round-cell bone tumours should be managed by those who are very familiar with these problems and not in hospitals with limited experience.

Chemotherapy

Adjuvant chemotherapy is an essential part of management and has been responsible for the improved prognosis in recent years [26]. The most useful agents are doxorubicin, cyclophosphamide, vincristine, actinomycin D and ifosfamide. Responses are also seen with etoposide, methotrexate and nitrosoureas. A variety of different combinations is in use, with none showing clear superiority. It is probable that all first-line agents should be used and that the dose of drugs should be kept as high as possible. In recent years, the tendency has been to use chemotherapy very intensively over a period of 9–12 months rather than to use lower doses for 1–2 years. A typical regimen begins with ifosfamide, doxorubicin, etoposide and vincristine (VIDE regimen) for 12 weeks followed by local treatment (with surgery and radiotherapy). Chemotherapy is continued postoperatively, with actinomycin substituted for doxorubicin when the maximum dose of doxorubicin has been reached. The patient must be kept under regular review during this time, with regular blood counts and chest radiography, plus bone scans when clinically indicated. The use of very high-dose chemotherapy with autologous peripheral blood stem-cell support is still experimental. It is being assessed in high-risk cases such as patients who have a small number of pulmonary metastases at presentation. Preliminary results suggest that a minority of these patients may be cured by this procedure, depending on their remission status at the time of high-dose therapy. A further new avenue of treatment with potential benefit is the molecular targeted approach, with insulin-like growth factor-1 receptor targeted monoclonal antibodies as one example that has shown promise in early phase human clinical trials (see Ref. [27]). As this author points out, 'With an improved understanding of the genome, transcriptome, proteome and other "-omic" events that promote and sustain Ewing pathogenesis, the use of nascent biologically targeted therapeutics is on the horizon. Understanding how and when to integrate such therapies into clinical practice, although challenging, may lead to a paradigm shift towards more personalized therapy'. At least one agent within this family, figitumumab (a fully human IgG2 monoclonal antibody targeting the insulin-like growth-factor-1 receptor), has emerged as being of potential benefit for relapsed chemo-refractory cases – see Ref. [28].

Prognosis

In localized disease, the use of radical local treatment with the most intensive chemotherapy regimens has now led to 5-year survival rates of up to 70%. Most of these children have probably been cured. Although many factors including a proper multidisciplinary team approach have contributed to this improved survival, there is little doubt that chemotherapy has been the major influence [26,29].

Pelvic lesions have a worse prognosis than limb tumours. Very small tumours (e.g. in the jaw and in the small bones of the hand and feet) have an excellent prognosis and it is not clear how much chemotherapy is necessary in these cases. The main determinants of prognosis are tumour volume and the presence of metastases. Large tumours are more likely both to recur locally and to metastasize.

Patients presenting with metastatic disease may frequently obtain a complete response of the tumour followed by later relapse. With conventional chemotherapy the outlook remains poor, although patients with only a few pulmonary metastases have a reasonable chance of cure. The value of high-dose chemotherapy is currently under investigation and molecularly targeted treatments also have the potential to improve outcomes still further – see, for example, Ref. [30].

Giant-cell tumour of bone (osteoclastoma)

This tumour occurs at age 20–40 and typically involves the epiphysis of a long bone. It causes a well-defined lytic lesion that eventually erodes the cortex of the bone, giving rise to soft-tissue extension. The presentation is with pain and swelling typically around the knee, the tumour occurring with equal frequency in the lower femur and upper tibia. Radiography shows a lytic lesion. Similar cystic changes can be caused by aneurysmal bone cysts or the cystic lesion of osteitis fibrosa cystica (primary hyperparathyroidism).

Pathologically the tumour consists of giant cells and spindle cells [31]. Occasionally, the appearances are frankly malignant and the tumour is then more locally invasive and metastases may occur. The tumours can be graded (I–III) according to the appearance of the stromal cells. It is possible, but not proven, that radiation treatment of giant-cell tumour might provoke malignant transformation. This is an uncommon development and usually it is the more aggressive (grade III) tumours that are irradiated, so the issue is not clear.

Treatment is usually by thorough curettage of the entire cavity of a localized lesion. The cavity can then be filled by bone chips. More extensive lesions can be treated by excision and endoprosthetic replacement of bone. Some tumours are not amenable to surgery, for example, those in vertebrae. In these cases radiotherapy, usually given at a dose of 40–50 Gy over 4–5 weeks, is the mainstay of treatment. There is no effective chemotherapy, although drugs used in osteosarcoma treatment have been used. Solitary pulmonary metastases can be excised, sometimes without recurrence.

Other malignant spindle cell tumours of bone (malignant fibrous histiocytoma, fibrosarcoma)

These tumours have a similar anatomical distribution to osteosarcoma but occur in the 30–50 age range, and in the diaphysis a little more commonly. The *fibrosarcomas* are often of low grade. Many of the tumours are associated with a long history of pain before the diagnosis is established by radiography followed by biopsy. Fibrosarcoma is treated by surgical excision. Although chemotherapy may be considered in high-grade lesions, there is little information on the chemosensitivity of this rare tumour.

Malignant fibrous histiocytoma consists of spindle cells with histiocytic-like cells. The radiological features are of bone lysis. The tumour is of high grade, with spindle-cell features (see page 461). Treatment is by overall excision, but there is clear evidence of chemosensitivity and the tumour is now treated with chemotherapy as well. It is sensitive to high-dose methotrexate, ifosfamide and doxorubicin. The prognosis is poor with surgery alone (30% overall survival at 3–4 years) but it seems that chemotherapy will improve this. As with osteosarcoma, these tumours tend to be resistant to radiotherapy, although radiotherapy may be helpful as an adjuvant to surgery, or for local recurrence.

Bone tumours of vascular origin

Haemangioendothelioma is a locally invasive tumour that does not usually metastasize. The lesion can occur at any age and is radiologically lytic. It may be multicentric. Treatment is by excision. Haemangiopericytoma is a vascular tumour, taking on a spindle cell appearance and of variable malignancy. Treatment is by surgery. Angiosarcoma is an exceedingly rare undifferentiated tumour that arises from vascular endothelium (demonstrated by staining for factor VIII). Although usually solitary, multiple contiguous bones may be involved. The tumour is excised if possible. Little is known of its chemosensitivity.

Non-Hodgkin's lymphoma of bone

Non-Hodgkin's lymphoma may occur in bone and be completely localized with no evidence of disease elsewhere. Nevertheless, the risk of spread is great. The tumours are lytic and destructive, typically having ill-defined margins. Both high-grade and low-grade tumours are described. In Europe, they are usually B-cell disorders, but T-cell lymphomas are possibly more common in Japan. An associated soft-tissue mass is often present. Full staging is essential (see Chapter 26) to determine if there is systemic spread and to ensure that the bone lesion is not a metastasis from a nodal lymphoma. Radiotherapy (30–40 Gy) controls the local disease, and systemic chemotherapy is now usually given, especially if there is any doubt about whether the tumour is localized, and in all high-grade tumours. In elderly patients with clinically localized disease it is permissible to follow an expectant policy and treat with cytotoxic agents only if metastasis occurs. Very rarely, the tumour may arise at a number of bone sites in a multifocal distribution.

Soft-tissue sarcomas

Progress in the management of adult sarcomas has been hampered by the relative rarity and heterogeneity of these tumours. In addition, they are relatively unresponsive to radiotherapy and chemotherapy (although the situation has improved over recent years – see below), and many tumours have a high incidence of local recurrence after surgery. In adults, the clinical behaviour of these tumours is becoming clearer, and some important points in management are now established. This important area of specialist oncology is well covered in a recent publication from the ESMO/European Sarcoma Network working party – see Ref. [32]. In childhood sarcomas, the picture is different, with some degree of responsiveness to chemotherapy proving the rule, leading in many instances to an improvement in survival rate (see Chapter 24).

Aetiology

The overall incidence in adults is low – about 2 per 100 000, accounting for 1% of all cancers. About 11 000 new cases are diagnosed annually in the USA, chiefly in adults though patients of any age can be affected. Overall, gastrointestinal stromal tumours – GISTs – account for less than 1% of all gastrointestinal tumours, but nonetheless they are the most common mesenchymal neoplasms of the gastrointestinal tract, though only about 25–35% are truly malignant. GISTs are usually found in the stomach or small intestine, but can occur anywhere along the GI tract, and rarely show evidence of involvement beyond the GI tract.

Most cases of soft-tissue sarcoma are sporadic. Soft-tissue sarcoma may also arise in a previously irradiated area. The latency and frequency are similar to those for bone sarcoma. Soft-tissue sarcoma is one of the tumours which occurs in Li–Fraumeni syndrome (see page 33). Patients with von Recklinghausen's disease have a tendency towards malignant change in fibromatous or neurofibromatous lesions (neurofibrosarcoma is the typical tumour type). Angiosarcoma of the liver occurs more frequently in workers chronically exposed to PVC. Patients with gross lymphoedema may rarely develop a lymphangiosarcoma of the oedematous limb (Stewart–Treves syndrome), most typically in the upper arm, following radiotherapy for breast carcinoma.

Pathology and molecular genetics

Soft-tissue sarcomas can arise wherever mesenchymal tissue is present (Table 23.3). The commonest varieties in adults result from malignant transformation of fibrous tissue (fibrosarcomas), striated muscle (rhabdomyosarcoma), smooth muscle (leiomyosarcoma), fat (liposarcoma) and blood vessels (haemangiopericytoma, angiosarcoma). GISTs are relatively uncommon tumours of the gastrointestinal tract (up to 3% of all gastrointestinal malignancies), occurring chiefly in the stomach (70%), small intestine (about 20%) and oesophagus (about 10%). They are thought to arise from interstitial cells that normally form part of the autonomic nervous system. Uterine carcinosarcoma, which appears to be a remarkable example of epithelial-to-mesenchymal transition in its pathogenesis (and therefore may respond differently to chemotherapy programmes, compared with most other types of soft-tissue sarcoma), is briefly discussed in Chapter 17. At the genetic level, this tumour is characterized by abnormalities in both the P13K and RAS pathways. Tumours of peripheral nerves (e.g. schwannoma, neurofibrosarcoma) are discussed in Chapter 11 and mesothelioma in Chapter 12. Other rarer tumours occur and are discussed below. The characteristic cytogenetic changes that accompany some sarcomas are described in the appropriate sections. See Refs. [33,34] for excellent and illuminating reviews of this important area.

It has become clear in recent years that histological features, particularly tumour grade, have an important bearing on outcome. Pathological grading according to the classification described by Trojani and colleagues is

recognized as both reproducible and predictive. Features such as tumour size larger than 10 cm, the presence of tumour necrosis, and obvious vascular invasion by tumour cells are all significant adverse risk factors [35].

Genetic mutations in soft-tissue sarcoma

The discovery that the molecular changes that occur in this diffuse group of tumours provide potential targets for therapy (and also aid classification) has led to a dramatic conceptual and practical advance.

GISTs are benign but may become malignant. When they do, they frequently overexpress a mutant, active, signal transduction receptor tyrosine kinase c-*KIT* (about 75–80% of cases) or platelet-derived growth factor (PDGF) receptor α (about 8%). These two mutations are mutually exclusive, and overall about 85–90% of GISTs have a mutation in one of these two kinase genes [36,37]. Dramatic responses to the tyrosine kinase inhibitor imatinib, initially used in chronic myeloid leukaemia (see chapter 28, page 579), have shown that tumour growth is at least partially stimulated by c-*KIT*. *Inflammatory myofibroblastic tumours* may become high-grade sarcomas and overexpress the mutant tyrosine kinase ALK.

Desmoplastic round-cell tumours are related to Ewing's sarcoma (see pages 454–457) and express the EWS–WTI fusion protein, a transcriptional regulator that induces PDGF-α, which is a mitogen. It is not yet known if inhibitors to this protein might result in tumour regression.

Other sarcomas overexpressing receptor tyrosine kinases are *congenital fibrosarcoma* and *mesoblastic nephroma* (N-TRK-3 in both) and *dermatofibrosarcoma protuberans* (PDGF-β). Over 95% of these tumours have the chromosomal translocation t(17;22), which appears to fuse the collagen gene *COL1A1* with the PDGF gene, resulting in an unlimited and self-stimulating signal for cellular division. The signal transduction protein Ras is overexpressed in neurofibrosarcomas. From the point of view of diagnostics and classification, characteristic translocations have been found in myeloid liposarcoma and synovial sarcoma (see below).

Gastrointestinal stromal tumour (GIST) [36]

These are the commonest mesenchymal neoplasms of the gastrointestinal tract, with up to 6000 new cases diagnosed annually in the USA. As pointed out above, we now know a good deal more about their pathogenesis and molecular genetics, with considerable implications for successful management with targeted therapy (see below). They occur within a wide age range, with a

Table 23.3 Soft-tissue sarcoma: a simplified classification.

Tissue of origin	Benign neoplasm	Sarcoma
Fibrous tissue	Fibroma (single or multiple, as in protuberans)	Fibrosarcoma (including dermatofibrosarcoma fibromatosis)
Muscle		

Striated	Rhabdomyoma	Rhabdomyosarcoma
		  Embryonal
		  Alveolar
		  Pleomorphic
		  Botryoidal

Smooth	Leiomyoma (including uterine 'fibroids')	Leiomyosarcoma
Mixed origin		Malignant fibrous histiocytoma (possibly a mixture of other pathologies)
Fat	Lipoma	Liposarcoma
Blood vessels	Angioma, haemangioma	Haemangiosarcoma, Kaposi's sarcoma, lymphangiosarcoma, haemangiopericytoma
Peripheral nerves	Neuroma, neurofibroma, neurilemmoma (including schwannoma)	Neurofibrosarcoma, malignant neurilemmoma (including malignant schwannoma and neuroepithelioma)
Pleura and peritoneum		Mesothelioma
Unknown		Synovial cell sarcoma
		Alveolar soft part sarcoma (malignant non-chromaffin paraganglioma)
		Perivascular epithelioid cell tumour, also known as PEComa

median age at diagnosis of 58 years; three-quarters of patients are over the age of 50 at diagnosis. They are usually sporadic but may be inherited in an autosomal dominant manner, and are more commonly diagnosed than expected in patients with type 1 neurofibromatosis. Germline mutations of genes encoding succinate dehydrogenase subunits have occasionally been identified. About half of all cases are located within the stomach, 25% in the small bowel, and 10% in the colon or rectum. The remainder occur as extraintestinal primaries. It is thought that they might arise from the interstitial cells of Cajal, or possibly that these share a common stem cell. Morphologically, they can be further classified into one of three types – epithelioid, spindle cell or mixed – with substantial histological variation. An approximate prediction of behaviour can be made from both tumour size and mitotic activity; site also has prognostic importance since small bowel tumours carry a higher risk of progression of disease than gastric tumours. Lymphatic spread is very uncommon.

The oncogenic kinase mutations are briefly outlined above. Of the large majority of cases expressing a KIT mutation, most involve the juxtamembrane domain (exon 11), though mutations can also occur in the extracellular domains (exons 8 and 9) and in the kinase I and II domains (exons 13 and 17). These mutations are found even in very small tumours (less than 1 cm), suggesting that the mutations characteristically occur early. The chromosomal changes associated with the common mutations include 14q deletion, 22q deletion, 1p deletion, 8p gain, 11p deletion, 9p deletion and 17q gain. Loss of the long arm of chromosome 22 is seen in about half of tumours, and losses on chromosomes 1p, 9p and 11p are clearly associated with malignant progression. Occasional familial clusters are encountered though the disease is rarely diagnosed in children.

Fibrosarcoma

These tumours are composed of fusiform fibroblasts that form collagen strands and reticulin. The histological definition of malignancy may be difficult, and well-differentiated tumours such as dermatofibrosarcoma protuberans seldom metastasize but may be locally invasive. Anaplastic tumours invade locally and also spread rapidly to the lungs.

The tumours usually arise on the limbs or trunk but may occur in any soft tissue. Typically, the patient notices a painless firm lump. In dermatofibrosarcoma protuberans the history is of a slowly enlarging skin nodule becoming violaceous and later ulcerating.

Malignant fibrous histiocytoma (high-grade spindle cell tumour)

In recent years, this term has become less widely used as a pathological entity. The term 'high-grade spindle-cell tumour' is often preferred. It is certainly not a new disease and cases previously diagnosed as poorly differentiated fibrosarcoma or pleomorphic rhabdomyosarcoma are now included in this category. The term does not describe a specific tumour but an appearance that can be found in sarcomas of many types. The typical histological pattern is one of malignant spindle cells often arranged in a 'storiform' or herringbone fashion. As with fibrosarcomas, the presentation is usually with a painless lump or nodule, though this tumour can also occur as a primary bone tumour.

Liposarcoma

These tumours present in middle age and occur in subcutaneous fat and in retroperitoneal tissues. They do not arise from pre-existing lipomas. There are four histological types:

1 well-differentiated (with mature fat);
2 myxoid, with a particularly characteristic t(12;16)(q13;p11) translocation;
3 round-cell type;
4 a pleomorphic variant.

The translocation in the myxoid tumour deregulates the *CHOP* gene, which is involved in adipocyte differentiation.

Rhabdomyosarcoma

This is a complex group of tumours with several distinct subtypes.

Embryonal rhabdomyosarcoma

These tumours occur in early childhood and young adult life. They consist of malignant spindle and round cells, and often occur in the head, neck and orbit (see Chapter 24).

Alveolar rhabdomyosarcoma

This tumour is composed of large, round and polygonal cells. It occurs in adolescents and young adults and has a wider anatomical distribution, often presenting in the trunk. These are highly malignant tumours and metastasize early.

Pleomorphic rhabdomyosarcoma

In these tumours the cells vary greatly in size and shape, and giant cells are often present. Many are now classified as malignant fibrous histiocytoma. They occur in adult life (over the age of 30), usually on the limbs, arising from deep muscle groups.

Botryoidal rhabdomyosarcoma ('sarcoma botryoides')

These tumours consist of polypoid growths in the urinary and genital tracts, usually in young children. Histologically the tumour consists of an area of cells with high mitotic activity surrounded by acellular oedematous tissue.

Leiomyosarcoma

The uterus is the commonest site of origin. The tumours probably occur as a result of malignant change in a uterine fibroid (leiomyoma). The histological diagnosis is usually made after hysterectomy for fibroids. Other leiomyosarcomas arise from smooth muscle at other sites such as subcutaneous tissue, stomach, bowel and retroperitoneum.

Synovial sarcoma

Synovial sarcomas [25] arise around joints, bursae and tendon sheaths. The cell of origin is not known but may not be the synovial lining cell. Pathologically, the monophasic form consists of sheets of spindle cells, whereas in the biphasic form there are 'glandular' spaces lined by cuboidal epithelial cells. The tumours may contain calcified areas. Tumours with few mitoses and a large 'glandular' component may have a better survival. A consistent chromosomal translocation is present: t(X;18)(p11.2;q11.2). There are two alternative chromosomal breakpoints, one associated with the monophasic appearance and the other with the biphasic. Synovial sarcomas occur in young adults, especially in the hands, feet and knees, but do not involve the joint lining. They present as hard lumps near a joint. Local spread and metastasis occur and local recurrence after excision is frequent. They are relatively chemosensitive tumours.

The prognosis is better for small tumours (greater than 7.5 cm) and if there is no neural or vascular invasion.

Angiosarcoma, lymphangiosarcoma and haemangiopericytoma

Angiosarcomas are rare, highly malignant neoplasms arising from the vascular endothelium itself. There are rare instances of their occurring in the liver (see Chapter 15). They usually arise in the skin, subcutaneous tissues and glandular sites such as breast and thyroid. Lymphangiosarcomas may arise in areas of chronic oedema (e.g. in the arm after mastectomy). Haemangiopericytoma (glomus tumour) is thought to arise from the contractile cells (pericytes) in small blood vessels. It usually occurs in the extremities and retroperitoneal spaces but is also found in the head and neck; benign and malignant variants occur.

Kaposi's sarcoma

This tumour of great significance is discussed in Chapter 22. It arises from endothelial cells and presents as pigmented skin lesions that grow slowly. Formerly, the tumour was commonest in Jewish and Italian men, and was much more frequent in West Africa than in Europe or the USA. This has changed with the recognition of AIDS, in which Kaposi's sarcoma occurs much more frequently and with a much more aggressive course. This tumour is associated with human herpesvirus 8 (see pages 28–30).

Alveolar soft part sarcoma

This rare neoplasm occurs in young adults, usually women. It is usually a slow-growing tumour, occurring typically in the extremities, and typically arising in the thigh in adults and in the head and neck in children. Although lung metastases usually occur, they grow slowly and may be compatible with long survival.

Epithelioid sarcoma

This is a rare tumour occurring on the extremities and with a tendency to spread to skin, bone and draining nodes. The cell of origin is unknown, but the histological appearances can be similar to a carcinoma or chronic inflammatory lesion. As with other tumours, the presence of an undiagnosed mass on a limb or intra-abdominally should raise the suspicion of a sarcoma. Diagnosis and staging should precede surgical excision whenever possible, and the operative procedure should be carefully planned.

Perivascular epithelioid cell tumour is also known as PEComa. This term is used to describe a family of mesenchymal tumours consisting of perivascular epithelioid cells (PECs). These are rare tumours, more common in women than men, that can occur in any part of the human body. The cell type from which they originate remains unknown, the name referring to the characteristic microscopical morphologic appearance. Histologically they consist of perivascular epithelioid cells with a clear or granular cytoplasm and central round nucleus, lacking prominent nucleoli. Some PEComas display malignant features, whereas others can cautiously be labeled as having 'uncertain malignant potential'. The most common tumours within this family are *renal angiomyolipoma* and *pulmonary lymphangioleiomyomatosis*, both of which are more common in patients with tuberous sclerosis complex. The genes responsible for this multi-system genetic disease have also been implicated in other PEComas.

'Clear-cell sarcoma' (soft part melanoma)

This tumour typically arises in the extremity, usually around the knee in a young adult. Ultrastructurally the tumour contains premelanosomes and is a form of undifferentiated melanoma.

Diagnosis, investigation and staging

Many sarcomas present clinically with a lump or mass, sometimes tender but not infrequently painless. With gastrointestinal tumours, notably GISTs, patients may present with dysphagia, gastrointestinal haemorrhage or even symptoms suggestive of intestinal obstruction. Up to 75% of GISTs are discovered when they are less than 4 cm in diameter and are either asymptomatic or associated with nonspecific symptoms. They are frequently diagnosed incidentally during radiologic studies or endoscopic or surgical procedures performed to investigate GI tract disease or to treat acute symptoms such as haemorrhage, obstruction, or occasionally a perforated viscus. Clinical manifestations of GISTs include vague, nonspecific abdominal pain or discomfort (probably the most common symptom), early satiety or a sensation of abdominal fullness. A palpable abdominal mass is rarely encountered. GISTs of the oesophagus may of course present as with any oesophageal mass or tumour, that is, with dysphagia and weight loss. Surgical biopsy generally leads to a rapid diagnosis, though the pathological variety of subtypes is extremely wide, and diagnostic 'incompleteness' is not unusual unless the biopsy material is referred to a major centre for sarcoma pathology. When a GIST is suspected, immunohistochemistry using the CD117 stain is generally diagnostic if positive. Tumours previously regarded as leiomyosarcoma of the stomach or small bowel would probably nowadays be reclassified as GISTs on the basis of CD117 positivity.

Clinical staging in soft-tissue sarcoma is important for management and also offers a guide to prognosis. Many of these tumours metastasize to the lungs. Lymph node metastases are frequent, particularly in alveolar rhabdomyosarcoma and Ewing's sarcoma. Other important distant sites include the liver, bone marrow and brain.

Staging investigation should therefore include chest radiography and CT scan of the thorax in order to detect pulmonary metastases. MRI of the primary is essential to determine the extent of the tumour and infiltration into local structures. Operability is better assessed by this means than by any other. Although there is no generally accepted staging system, the classification of the American Joint Committee on Cancer is useful prognostically (Table 23.4).

Management of the primary tumour

Biopsy is generally required for an accurate diagnosis, although increasingly it is not recommended for gastric lesions that are highly suspected of being a GIST [36]. Where necessary, the most satisfactory procedure is needle biopsy followed by a planned approach to local and systemic treatment in collaboration with medical and radiation oncologists and surgeons. For GISTs, the goal of surgery is complete gross resection with preservation of

an intact pseudocapsule. These tumours must be handled with great care to avoid tumour rupture and consequent intra-abdominal dissemination. Excellent guidelines for the management of soft-tissue sarcomas have recently been issued by a panel of UK-based sarcoma specialists (see Ref. [39] for an excellent review, in which they stress the key importance of a multidisciplinary approach at specialist centres for every patient: '*Any patient with a suspected soft tissue sarcoma should be referred to a diagnostic centre and managed by a specialist sarcoma multidisciplinary team*').

Regrettably, in the case of soft-tissue sarcomas, the patient with a lump on a limb is sometimes operated upon ('shelled out') by an inexperienced surgeon who has no prior knowledge of the diagnosis. Such operations are often marginal or intralesional resections that subsequently pose formidable problems in management. Where a sarcoma is suspected preoperatively and confirmed by frozen section, it is unwise to attempt an excision biopsy at the same procedure since such surgery is often inadequate and definitive surgery must then be undertaken at a second operation. This problem also arises when excision biopsy of a 'benign' mass has been attempted, and the diagnosis of malignancy was not suspected even at operation. Examples are leiomyosarcoma of the uterus, which is usually diagnosed after hysterectomy for fibroids, and soft-tissue sarcomas of the head and neck region, which frequently present with cervical lymphadenopathy rather than with the primary tumour itself.

Traditionally, radical surgery has usually been recommended for soft-tissue sarcomas arising in the extremities, and amputation has been widely used. For high lesions of the thigh, this may require disarticulation or even hemi-pelvectomy in an attempt to control the tumour. These radical operations were introduced because of the risk of local recurrence.

Removal of the tumour without a wide margin of normal tissue (so-called marginal excision) carries an average local failure rate of 80%. Wide local excisions are accompanied by failure rates of up to 45% with surgery alone. Radical excisions with a suitably wide margin (including compartmentectomy, a procedure which is far less often performed now than formerly – see below) or amputation, have local failure rates of less than 10%. These figures led to the adoption of radical surgery as the mainstay of treatment.

The management of GISTs has been revolutionized by the introduction of the c-*KIT* tyrosine kinase inhibitor (TKI) imatinib mesylate (Glivec) (see page 579), initially

---

Table 23.4 A simplified stage grouping of soft-tissue sarcomas. See current UICC/TNM classification [38] for further detail.

Stage I	Low-grade (1) tumour. No nodal or distant spread (G1 T1 – 2 N0 M0)
Stage II	Intermediate-grade (2) tumour. No nodal or distant spread (G2 T1 – 2 N0 M0)
Stage III	High-grade (3) tumour. No nodal or distant spread (G3 T1 – 2 N0 M0)
Stage IV	A Tumour of any grade with lymph node metastases only (G1 – 4 T1 – 2 N1 M0)
	B Distant metastases (G1 – 4 T1 – 2 N0 1 M1)
T1 tumours are less than 5 cm diameter (subgroup A)	
T2 tumours are more than 5 cm diameter (subgroup B)	

Grade is based on necrosis, pleomorphism and mitotic activity.

used for treatment of chronic myeloid leukaemia. This specific inhibitor of tyrosine kinase enzymes gives a response rate of over 50%, even in metastatic or inoperable cases. Patients who become resistant probably do so because of mutation of the binding site on the c-Kit protein, so that imatinib no longer 'fits' in the pocket. This then leads to uncontrolled inactivation of the signalling pathway, and hence renewed tumour growth. Fortunately, these tumours may then also respond to another of the multiple tyrosine kinase inhibitor agents, sunitinib (Sutent). This agent, also available as an oral preparation, is a multikinase inhibitor that targets several TKIs implicated in tumour growth, pathologic angiogenesis, and metastatic progression. It inhibits platelet-derived growth factor receptors (i.e. PDGFR-alpha, PDGFR-beta), vascular endothelial growth factor receptors (i.e. VEGFR1, VEGFR2, VEGFR3), stem cell factor receptor (KIT), Fms-like tyrosine kinase-3 (FLT3), colony-stimulating factor receptor type 1 (CSF-1R), and also the glial cell-line–derived neurotrophic factor receptor (RET). It was recently assessed in a large randomized study of 312 patients, all with an imatinib-resistant GIST [40]. The median time to tumour progression was over 27 weeks for the sunitinib group, compared with under 7 weeks for placebo, and treatment was reasonably well tolerated. The explanation for this relative lack of cross-resistance may well be due to the far higher level of binding affinity of sunitinib to c-Kit, as well as its effect in blocking the activity of the PDGF receptor as well as various vascular endothelial growth factor-derived angiogenic-mediated pathways. Other important tyrosine kinase inhibitors include sorafenib, dasatinib and nilotinib, all second-generation investigational agents, but still more important is the demonstration of clinically useful activity of regorafenib, which has now received FDA approval for locally advanced, unresectable GISTs no longer responsive to imatinib or sunitinib. The key phase III GRID trial of 199 patients with metastatic or unresectable GIST showed that regorafenib plus best supportive care (BSC) significantly improved progression-free survival compared to placebo plus BSC. Patients were treated with BSC and randomized to either regorafenib (160 mg daily, orally, for 3 weeks followed by a 1-week break), or placebo. Median PFS was considerably increased in these heavily pretreated patients 4.8 months for regorafenib compared with just 0.9 months for placebo + BSC – see Ref. [41].

The common problem of distant metastases, coupled with the realization that radiotherapy can play a useful part in local control [42], has led over the past 15 years or so to a modification of this assumption of the need for extensive surgery. Wide surgical excision, coupled with high-dose pre- or post-operative irradiation, is increasingly accepted as a satisfactory alternative, with a better functional and cosmetic outcome than can be achieved by amputation – see, for example, Ref. [43]. Myxoid liposarcomas respond particularly well to radiotherapy, a feature probably related to their intensely vascular internal structure. The radiation dose must be high (at least 60 Gy in 6 weeks) to minimize the risk of local recurrence. Many centres particularly in the USA recommend a higher dose of 66 Gy given in 6-and-a-half weeks. For tumours of the limbs, the dose can sometimes even be taken to 70 Gy. The affected compartment should be considered at risk and uniformly irradiated to this high dose. A strip of skin and subcutaneous tissue (a 'corridor') should be left unirradiated to allow adequate lymphatic drainage from the distal limb. A proportion of these patients develop local recurrence that may well require amputation, but wide local excision combined with radical radiotherapy offers a satisfactory method of local control in the majority (80–90%) of all patients with soft-tissue sarcomas of the extremities. Surgical removal of the whole of the affected compartment – 'compartmentectomy' – was until relatively recently generally recommended, though a wide local excision with an adequate margin is now considered absolutely acceptable by most experts; the only question being, as in several other areas in oncology – what constitutes an 'adequate margin'? A clearance with at least 2–3 mm all round is probably sufficient though opinions and therefore local practices vary and it may prove difficult or impossible to achieve this in every case. As pointed out by Swallow and Catton, 'Due to anatomical constraints, tumours of the head and neck and retroperitoneum are typically excised with close margins, providing a rationale for adjuvant radiation' – see Ref. [44]. These operations are often technically as difficult, if not more so, than amputation, in view of the important structures that must be preserved, as well as the need especially in larger tumours, to resect a substantial volume of tissue with primary closure wherever possible (Figure 23.15). When pre-operative radiotherapy is offered (a clinical decision to be made on a case-by-case basis), a dose of 50 Gy in 5 weeks is usually preferred, with surgical resection 6 weeks later, at which time the tumour may well have reduced in size, allowing for an easier surgical resection. Radiotherapy is not always recommended for grade 1 (very low grade) tumours treated with wide local excision since the risk of recurrence is low. It may also not be

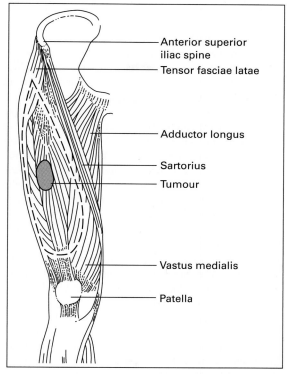

- Anterior superior iliac spine
- Tensor fasciae latae
- Adductor longus
- Sartorius
- Tumour
- Vastus medialis
- Patella

Figure 23.15 Compartmentectomy. The diagram illustrates the wide surgical excision of soft tissue situated, in this case, in the rectus femoris.

needed for higher-grade tumours of smaller size where the risk of local recurrence is judged to be low. Each case must be decided on its merits. The dose and timing of radiation and the use of both pre- and post-operative radiotherapy are issues requiring further study. One important UK-based trial (VORTEX – Randomized trial of *Vo*lume of Postoperative *R*adiotherapy given to Adult Pa*T*ients with *Ex*tremity Soft Tissue Sarcoma) is attempting to reduce functional impairment by reducing the radiotherapy volume, hopefully without compromise of the local control rate.

Radiotherapy treatment is particularly valuable in soft-tissue sarcomas with multiple or extensive primary sites, such as soft-tissue angiosarcomas or Kaposi's sarcoma, and in myxoid liposarcoma. It is essential in cases where there is doubt about surgical margins. For responsive tumours such as angiosarcoma, Kaposi's and myxoid liposarcoma, recent reports confirm a high degree of local control using wide-field irradiation, sometimes in combination with surgery, with durable remissions

(possibly cures) lasting 10 years and more even in patients with multifocal sites of primary disease, for example, on the scalp. Most recurrences in patients treated by limb-sparing surgery and post-operative high-dose radiotherapy will have occurred within 5 years, or not at all.

Hyperthermia has been used as an adjunct to radiation therapy, but there has not yet been a controlled comparison of this technique. Hyperfractionated and accelerated radiotherapy are also being assessed in current trials.

The management of soft-tissue sarcomas of childhood is further discussed in Chapter 24.

Chemotherapy [45–47]

A number of agents are effective in producing partial (or occasionally complete) remissions in patients with local recurrence and/or metastatic disease. A wide variety of agents has been shown to have activity, although in general the response rates to single agents are low and of brief duration. In the occasional patient, a complete and durable response to chemotherapy is obtained. Many

Table 23.5 Chemotherapy in soft-tissue sarcoma.

Drug regimen	Approximate response rate (%)
Single agents	
Ifosfamide	25
Doxorubicin	25
Dacarbazine (DTIC)	15
Cyclophosphamide	10
Vincristine	10
Methotrexate	10
Cisplatin	10
Actinomycin	10
Combination chemotherapy	
Doxorubicin, DTIC, ifosfamide	25–35
Vincristine, actinomycin, cyclosphosphamide (VAC)	20
Vincristine, doxorubicin, DTIC (VADIC)	35
Doxorubicin, cyclophosphamide methotrexate (ACM)	30
Cyclophosphamide, vincristine, doxorubicin, DTIC (CyVADIC)	40
Cyclophosphamide, vincristine, doxorubicin, actinomycin (CyVADACT)	35

classes of drug have activity (Table 23.5). Doxorubicin is one of the most active and widely used agents. It has been extensively used alone and in combination with ifosfamide, itself an active drug with a response rate of 25%. The combination of doxorubicin and ifosfamide is generally regarded as the standard combination most widely used, though in published studies of patients with advanced disease, this two-drug combination has not always appeared superior to doxorubicin alone. Other drugs with activity (although less clear-cut than for ifosfamide and doxorubicin, and far less commonly used) include dacarbazine (DTIC), methotrexate, gemcitabine, actinomycin D and vinca alkaloids.

Undoubtedly, the most responsive of these tumours are the embryonal rhabdomyosarcomas, in which the success of combination regimens (particularly employing vincristine, actinomycin D, doxorubicin and cyclophosphamide) for metastatic disease has led to their routine use as adjuvant treatment immediately following local radiotherapy and/or surgery. At least 60% of patients with embryonal rhabdomyosarcomas can be cured with current adjuvant chemotherapy, and cure is even possible in patients with evidence of residual disease postoperatively and in a proportion of patients with metastatic disease. The majority of these patients will be children or young adults, and these encouraging results have not so far been seen with other forms of soft-tissue sarcoma in adults.

A wide variety of single agents and combination regimens has been used in advanced soft-tissue sarcomas (Table 23.5). The highest response rates have been reported with doxorubicin, ifosfamide and dacarbazine, with a response rate of approximately 25%. A much smaller proportion of patients will achieve complete response. The addition of cyclophosphamide and vincristine or vinorelbine to these two drugs has increased the response rate only to about 40%, at the cost of considerable toxicity. Epirubicin is also active, with approximately similar response rates. Attempts at improving the poor response figures have mostly centred on the use of these drugs in combination. In respect of chemotherapy recommendations for the various histological sub-types of soft-tissue sarcoma, the recent ESMO publication [32] reported.

At the time of writing these Guidelines, there is no formal demonstration that multiagent chemotherapy is superior to single-agent chemotherapy with doxorubicin alone in terms of overall survival. However, a higher response rate may be expected, in particular in a number of sensitive histological types, according to several, although not all, randomized clinical trials.

Therefore, multiagent chemotherapy with adequate-dose anthracyclines plus ifosfamide may be the treatment of choice, particularly when a tumour response is felt to be able to give an advantage and patient performance status is good. In angiosarcoma, taxanes are an alternative option, given their high antitumour activity in this specific histological type. An alternative option is gemcitabine ± docetaxel. Doxorubicin plus dacarbazine is an option for multiagent first-line chemotherapy of leiomyosarcoma, where the activity of ifosfamide is far less convincing on available retrospective evidence. Imatinib is standard medical therapy for those rare patients with dermatofibrosarcoma protuberans who are not amenable to non-mutilating surgery, or with metastases deserving medical therapy.

A newer agent, brostallicin, has reportedly proven active in a proportion of patients with drug-resistant soft-tissue sarcomas [47]. This is a synthetic α-bromoacryloyl agent, a derivative of distamycin-A, initially derived from the culture mycelium *Streptomyces distallicus*, which acts as a DNA minor groove-binding agent.

The use of chemotherapy as an adjuvant to surgery with or without radiotherapy remains controversial 45 – and see also Ref. [48]. In general, the numbers of patients in the clinical trials have been too small to detect differences of less than 20% in survival, and improvements of this size are clearly implausible with present drugs. Although several years ago, a large meta-analysis suggested that doxorubicin-based chemotherapy prolongs progression-free survival in localized soft-tissue sarcoma with a small effect on overall survival (Figure 23.16), a recent large-scale study from the European Organization for Research and Treatment of Cancer (EORTC) (350 patients, mostly with high-grade tumours, using a combination of doxorubicin and moderate-dose ifosfamide) failed to show any worthwhile benefit [49]. See also Ref. [50].

The problem of defining the patients who will benefit from chemotherapy is made more difficult by the heterogeneity of histology, grade, stage and site [51]. At present adjuvant chemotherapy is best offered in the setting of a trial, or in younger adults with high-grade tumours where the risk of metastasis is very high. Adjuvant chemotherapy is regarded as 'standard of care' for adults who have the subtypes of soft-tissue sarcomas that typically occur in paediatric patients (Ewing's sarcoma, rhabdomyosarcoma), and adjuvant chemotherapy is not warranted in patients with low- and intermediate-risk disease (stages I and II). For patients with higher-risk disease (stage III), the available randomized trials still

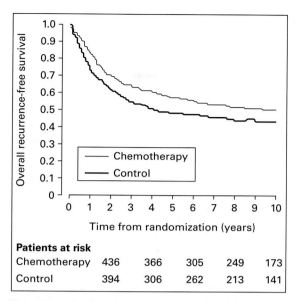

Figure 23.16 Kaplan–Meier curves of overall recurrence-free survival for adjuvant chemotherapy versus control. (Source: Casali and Blay [45]. Reproduced with permission from Oxford University Press.)

do not convincingly demonstrate a clinical benefit to adjuvant chemotherapy. A full account of potential risks and benefits is important when discussing adjuvant chemotherapy with patients who have stage III disease. The role of signal transduction inhibitors remains to be determined but drugs active against tyrosine kinases (and possibly other substrates) overexpressed in the different tumours offer possible opportunities for some progress. Current agents under active study include pazopanib, crizotinib, cediranib and sunitinib but reports detailing responses are still largely anecdotal though a recent randomized study did show useful activity for pazopanib, a selective orally-administered multi-targeted receptor tyrosine kinase inhibitor of VEGFR-1, VEGFR-2, VEGFR-3, PDGFR-a/β and c-kit that blocks tumour growth and appears to inhibit angiogenesis in previously treated patients.

For advanced metastatic disease other studies will be necessary to elucidate small but possibly important differences in chemotherapy effectiveness, and also to monitor toxicity. Interestingly, possible differences in responsiveness to chemotherapy are beginning to emerge, for example, from a recent study in patients with myxoid liposarcoma that demonstrated an unusually high response rate to trabectedin (ecteinascidin-743),

an antitumour agent extracted from the marine tunicate (sometimes known as unichordates or sea squirts) *Ecteinascidia turbinata*, which like brostallicin appears to act as a DNA minor groove-binding agent. In this study, a median progression-free survival of 14 months was noted, even in pretreated patients refractory to conventional therapy [52], with some of the tumours undergoing long-lasting local control. Trabectedin has emerged as an agent with real potential in the management of these difficult soft-tissue sarcomas and is now in regular use, for example, at our own centre; further trials are currently underway to refine its use in greater detail (see Refs. [53,54]). It has now been approved for use in uterine sarcoma and is also increasingly employed in relapsed ovarian carcinoma in conjunction with pegylated liposomal doxorubicin (see page 342). Current regimens for metastatic uterine carcinosarcoma include either an in-patient programme of ifosfamide or out-patient-based carboplatin/paclitaxel, currently being directly compared in a GOG study.

Survival

Overall survival correlates closely with stage, Trojani tumour grade, and site. The 5-year survival for stage I is approximately 80%, stage II 60%, stage III 30% and stage IV 10%. The more distal the tumour, the better the prognosis. Lymph node spread is important prognostically, and is commoner in rhabdomyosarcoma and synovial sarcoma. The prognosis for retroperitoneal tumours is poor, with 5-year survival of 15–35%. This figure is worse for higher-grade lesions and those where no surgical removal is possible. At present, the use of adjuvant chemotherapy as part of the initial treatment strategy is uncertain, and the most recent studies do not support its routine use, at least with the standard ifosfamide/doxorubicin regimen.

References

1 Enneking WF, Spannier SS, Goodman MA. A system for the surgical staging of musculoskeletal sarcoma. *Clin Orthop Relat Res* 1980; 153: 106–20.

2 Lagrange J-L, Ramaioli A, Chateau M-C, for the Radiation Therapist and Pathologist Groups of the Fédération Nationale des Centres de Lutte Contre le Cancer. Sarcoma after radiation therapy: retrospective multiinstitutional study of 80 histologically confirmed cases. *Radiology* 2000; 216: 197–205.

3 Hawkins M, Kinnier-Wilson M, Burton HS *et al.* Radiotherapy, alkylating agents, and risk of bone cancer after childhood cancer. *J Natl Cancer Inst* 1996; 88: 270–3.

4   Brugieres L, Gardes M, Moutou C. Screening for germ line p53 mutations in children with malignant tumors and a family history of cancer. *Cancer Res* 1993; 53: 452–5.

5   Delattre O, Zucman J, Melot T *et al*. The Ewing family of tumors: a sub-group of small round-cell tumours defined by specific chimeric transcripts. *N Engl J Med* 1994; 331: 294–9.

6   Bielack SS, Kempf-Bielack B, Delling G *et al*. Prognostic factors in high-grade osteosarcoma of the extremities or trunk: an analysis of 1,702 patients treated on neoadjuvant co-operative osteosarcoma study group protocols. *J Clin Oncol* 2002; 20: 776–90.

7   Grimer RJ. Surgical options for children with osteosarcoma. *Lancet Oncol* 2005; 6: 85–92.

8   Anninga JK, Gelderblom H, Fiocco M *et al*. Chemotherapeutic adjuvant treatment for osteosarcoma: where do we stand? *Eur J Cancer* 2011; 47: 2431–45.

9   Whelan JS, Jinks RC, McTiernan A *et al*. Survival from high-grade localised extremity osteosarcoma: combined results and prognostic factors from three European osteosarcoma intergroup randomised controlled trials. *Ann Oncol* 2012; 23: 1607–16.

10 Maki RG. Ifosfamide in the neoadjuvant treatment of osteogenic sarcoma. *J Clin Oncol* 2012; 30: 2033–5.

11 Souhami RL, Craft AW, Van den Eijken JW *et al*. Randomised trial of two regimens of chemotherapy in operable osteosarcoma: a study of the European Osteosarcoma Intergroup. *Lancet* 1997; 350: 911–17.

12 Whelan J, Seddon B, Perisoglou M. Management of osteosarcoma. *Curr Treat Options Oncol* 2006; 7: 444–55.

13 Le Deley M-C, Guinebretiere J-M, Gentet J-C *et al*. SFOP OS94: a randomised trial comparing preoperative high-dose methotrexate plus doxorubicin to high-dose methotrexate plus etoposide and ifosfamide in osteosarcoma patients. *Eur J Cancer* 2007; 43: 752–61.

14 Lewis IJ, Nooij MA, Whelan J *et al*. Improvement in histologic response but not survival in osteosarcoma patients treated with intensified chemotherapy: a randomised phase III trial of the European Osteosarcoma Intergroup. *J Natl Cancer Inst* 2007; 99: 112–28.

15 Meyers, PA, Schwartz, CL, Krailo MD *et al*. Osteosarcoma: the addition of muramyl tripeptide to chemotherapy improves overall survival--a report from the Children's Oncology Group. *J Clin Oncol* 2008; 26: 633–8.

16 Saeter G, Hole J, Stenwig AE *et al*. Systemic relapse of patients with osteogenic sarcoma: prognostic factors for long-term survival. *Cancer* 1995; 75: 1084–93.

17 Treasure T, Utley M. Surgical removal of asymptomatic pulmonary metastases: time for better evidence. *Brit Med J* 2013; 346: f824.

18 Grimer RJ, Bielack S, Fleger S *et al*. Periosteal osteosarcoma – a European review of outcome. *Eur J Cancer* 2005; 41: 2806–11.

19 Mavrogenis AF, Gambarotti M, Angelini A *et al*. Chondrosarcomas revisited. *Orthopedics* 2012; 35: e379–90.

20 Mankin HJ, Cantlay KD, Lipielo L *et al*. The biology of human chondrosarcoma. 1. Description of the case, grading and biochemical analyses. *J Bone Joint Surg A* 1980; 62: 160–76.

21 Earl HM. Chemotherapy of rare malignant bone tumours. *Baillière's Clin Oncol* 1987; 1: 223–41.

22 Ross KA, Smyth NA, Murawski CD, Kennedy JG. The biology of Ewing Sarcoma. *ISRN Oncol* 2013; 2013: 759725.

23 Terrier P, Henry-Amar M, Tricke TJ *et al*. Is neuroectodermal differentiation of Ewing's sarcoma of bone associated with an unfavourable prognosis? *Eur J Cancer* 1995; 31A: 307–14.

24 Subbiah V, Anderson P, Lazar AJ *et al*. Ewing's Sarcoma: standard and experimental treatment option. *Curr Treat Options Oncol* 2009; 10: 126–40.

25 Scully SP, Temple HT, O'Keefe RJ *et al*. Role of surgical resection in pelvic Ewing's sarcoma. *J Clin Oncol* 1995; 13: 2336–41.

26 Lessnick SL, Dei Tos AP, Sorensen PH *et al*. Small round cell sarcomas. *Semin Oncol* 2009; 36: 338–46.

27 Ludwig JA. Ewing sarcoma: historical perspectives, current state-of-the-art, and opportunities for targeted therapy in the future. *Curr Opin Oncol* 2008; 20: 412–8.

28 Olmos D, Postel-Vinay S, Molife LR *et al*. Safety, pharmacokinetics, and preliminary activity of the anti-IGF-1R antibody figitumumab (CP-751,871) in patients with sarcoma and Ewing's sarcoma: a phase 1 expansion cohort study. *Lancet Oncol* 2010; 11: 129–35.

29 Lin PP, Jaffe N, Herzog CE *et al*. Chemotherapy response is an important predictor of local recurrence in Ewing sarcoma. *Cancer* 2007; 109: 603–11.

30 Kelleher FC, Thomas DM. Molecular pathogenesis and targeted therapeutics in Ewing Sarcoma/primitive neuroectodermal tumours. *Clin Sarcoma Res* 2012; 2 (1): 6. doi: 10.1186/2045-3329-2-6.

31 Mendenhall WM, Zlotecki RA, Scarborough MT *et al*. Giant cell tumor of bone. *Am J Clin Oncol* 2006; 29: 96–9.

32 The ESMO / European Sarcoma Network Working Group. Soft tissue and visceral sarcomas: ESMO Clinical Practice Guidelines for diagnosis, treatment and follow-up. *Ann Oncol* 2012; 23 (Supplement 7): vii192–99.

33 Thway, K. Pathology of soft tissue sarcomas. *Clin Oncol* 2009; 21: 695–705.

34 Verweij J, Baker LH. Future treatment of soft tissue sarcomas will be driven by histological subtype and molecular aberrations. *Eur J Cancer* 2010; 46: 863–8.

35 Trojani M, Contesso G, Coindre JM *et al*. Soft-tissue sarcomas of adults: study of pathological prognostic variables and definition of a histopathological grading system. *Int J Cancer* 1984; 33: 37–42.

36 Rubin BP, Heinrich MC, Corless CL. Gastrointestinal stromal tumour. *Lancet* 2007; 369: 1731–41.

37 Joenssu H, Roberts P, Sarlomo-Rikala M *et al*. Clinical response induced by the tyrosine-kinase inhibitor STI571 in metastatic gastrointestinal stromal tumor expressing

a mutant c-kit proto-oncogene. *N Engl J Med* 2001; 344: 1052–6.

38 Sobin LH, Gospodarowicz MK, Wittekind Ch, eds. *TNM Classification of Malignant Tumours*, 7th edn. Chichester: Wiley-Blackwell, 2009.

39 Grimer RJ, Judson I, Peake D. Seddon B. Guidelines for the management of soft tissue sarcomas. *Sarcoma* 2010; 2010: 506182. doi: 10.1155/**2010**/506182.

40 Demetri GD, Van Oosterom AT, Garrett CR *et al.* Efficacy and safety of sunitinib in patients with advanced gastrointestinal stromal tumour after failure of imatinib: a randomised controlled trial. *Lancet* 2006; 368: 1329–38.

41 Demetri GD, Reichardt P, Kang YK, *et al.* Efficacy and safety of regorafenib for advanced gastrointestinal stromal tumours after failure of imatinib and sunitinib (GRID): an international, multicentre, randomised, placebo-controlled, phase 3 trial. *Lancet* 2013; 381: 295–302.

42 O'Sullivan B, Ward I, Haycocks T, Sharpe M. Techniques to modulate radiotherapy toxicity and outcome in soft tissue sarcoma. *Curr Treat Options Oncol* 2003; 4: 453–64.

43 Nystrom LM, Rymer NB, Reith JD *et al.* Multidisciplinary management of soft tissue sarcoma. *ScientificWorldJournal* 2013; 2013: 852462. Published online 2013 July 28.

44 Swallow CJ, Catton CN. Local management of adult soft tissue sarcomas. *Semin Oncol* 2007; 34: 256–69.

45 Casali PG, Blay JY; ESMO/CONTICANET/EUROBONET Consensus Panel of experts. Soft tissue sarcomas: ESMO Clinical Practice Guidelines for diagnosis, treatment and follow-up. *Ann Oncol* 2010; 21Suppl 5: v198–203.

46 Gronchi A, Frustaci S, Mercuri M *et al.* Short, full-dose adjuvant chemotherapy in high-risk adult soft tissue sarcomas: a randomized clinical trial from the Italian Sarcoma Group and the Spanish Sarcoma Group. *J Clin Oncol* 2012; 30: 850–6.

47 Leahy M, Ray-Coquard I, Verweij J *et al.* Brostallicin, an agent with potential activity in metastatic soft tissue sarcoma: a phase II study from the EORTC soft tissue and bone sarcoma group. *Eur J Cancer* 2007; 43: 308–15.

48 Blay JY, Le Cesne A. Adjuvant chemotherapy in localized soft tissue sarcomas: still not proven. *Oncologist* 2009; 14: 1013–20.

49 Woll PJ, van Glabbeke M, Hohenberger P *et al.* for the EORTC Soft Tissue and Bone Sarcoma Group. Adjuvant chemotherapy with doxorubicin and ifosfamide for resected soft tissue sarcoma: interim analysis of a randomised phase III trial. *J Clin Oncol, 2007 ASCO Annual Meeting Proceedings Part I* 2007; 25 (18S): 10008.

50 Patrikidou A, Domont J, Cioffi A, Le Cesne A. Treating soft-tissue sarcomas with adjuvant chemotherapy. *Curr Treat Options Oncol* 2011; 12: 21–31.

51 Pisters PW, O'Sullivan D, Maki RG. Evidence-based recommendations for local therapy for soft tissue sarcomas. *J Clin Oncol* 2007; 25: 1003–8.

52 Grosso F, Jones RL, Demetri GD *et al.* Efficacy of trabectedin (ecteinascidin-743) in advanced pretreated myxoid liposarcomas: a retrospective study. *Lancet Oncol* 2007; 8: 595–602.

53 Demetri GD, Chawla SP, von Mehren M *et al.* Efficacy and safety of trabectedin in patients with advanced or metastatic liposarcoma or leiomyosarcoma after failure of prior anthracyclines and ifosfamide: Results of a randomized phase II study of two different schedules. *J Clin Oncol* 2009; 27: 4188–96.

54 Trabectedin for the treatment of advanced soft tissue sarcoma. 2010. National Institute for Health and Clinical Excellence (NICE-UK report).

Further reading

Beal K, Allen L, Yahalom J. Primary bone lymphoma: treatment results and prognostic factors with long-term follow-up of 82 patients. *Cancer* 2006; 106: 2652–6.

Ferrari S, Smeland S, Mercuri M *et al.* Neoadjuvant chemotherapy with high-dose ifosfamide, high-dose methotrexate, cisplatin, and doxorubicin for patients with localised osteosarcoma of the extremity: a joint study by the Italian and Scandinavian Sarcoma Groups. *J Clin Oncol* 2005; 23: 8845–52.

Hameed M. Small round cell tumors of bone. *Arch Pathol Lab Med* 2007; 131: 192–204.

Marina N, Gebhardt M, Teot L, Gorlick R. Biology and therapeutic advances for pediatric osteosarcoma. *Oncologist* 2004; 9: 422–41.

Miettinen M, Lasota J. Gastrointestinal stromal tumors: review on morphology, molecular pathology, prognosis, and differential diagnosis. *Arch Pathol Lab Med* 2006; 130: 1466–78.

Roylance R, Seddon B, McTiernan A *et al.* Experience in the use of trabectedin (ET-743, Yondelis) in 21 patients with pre-treated advanced sarcoma from a single centre. *Clin Oncol* 2007; 19: 572–6.

Sinkovics JG. Adult human sarcomas I. Basic science. *Expert Rev Anticancer Ther* 2007; 7: 31–6.

Sinkovics JG. Adult human sarcomas II. Medical oncology. *Expert Rev Anticancer Ther* 2007; 7: 183–210.

Smeland S, Muller C, Alvegard A *et al.* Scandinavian Study Group Osteosarcoma study SSG VIII: prognostic factors for outcome and the role of replacement salvage chemotherapy for poor histological responders. *Eur J Cancer* 2003; 39: 488–94.

24 Paediatric malignancies

An approach to cancer in children

As we stated in previous editions, the diagnosis of cancer in a child is an exceptional and painful test of the strength of family life. Happy families usually cope better with the shock, grief and disruption. When the diagnosis has been made, the physician must take time to be alone with the parents, explaining the diagnosis, prognosis and approach to investigation and treatment. The majority of children with cancer are cured, so for many tumours a cautiously optimistic account can be given. The parents will feel extreme anxiety about the diagnosis and this anxiety may show itself as demanding behaviour towards the staff. Sometimes parents feel that they have been responsible in some way – that there is a genetic factor to which they have contributed or that the cancer has arisen as a result of avoidable physical or mental trauma or faulty diet. Parents are justifiably concerned about avoidable delays in diagnosis and investigation. They need to express these feelings and must be reassured that they are not responsible for the illness. Above all, they must feel confident in the hospital and its staff.

Talking to children and their parents requires tact, humanity, patience and a clear head. Every new case will prove an additional test of these qualities, and the doctor will have to deal with the anguish of the parents as well as the physical and emotional suffering of the child. All children, except for the very youngest, need some account of why they are in hospital and what is likely to happen, and with older children and adolescents these explanations will need to be accurate and complete. It is impossible to generalize about how much to tell. Children of 6–8 years will understand that they are ill, and grasp the elements of treatment. At 10–11 years they will know more, and teenagers will know about cancer and leukaemia. The physician must talk to the child and try to gauge his or her feelings and understanding. For children of about 11 years or more, a personal and private relationship with the doctor is important. They often want to ask questions directly and may be anxious to avoid upsetting their parents. At other times they may feel that the truth is being filtered by their parents. The doctor should try to encourage the family to be open with each other with respect to the illness. Honesty and frankness are important in gaining the parents' trust and in helping them to participate in treatment.

The complexity of treatment makes it difficult for any doctor to provide detailed answers to all the questions which a parent or the child might ask, but it is essential that a single experienced clinician should be seen to be in charge of the team, so that both the patient and the parents can identify with an individual.

With most childhood cancers, the disease is quickly brought under control and the child feels and looks well,

Cancer and its Management, Seventh Edition. Jeffrey Tobias and Daniel Hochhauser.
© 2015 John Wiley & Sons, Ltd. Published 2015 by John Wiley & Sons, Ltd.

except for the side-effects of treatment. These side-effects come to dominate the illness, since the acute anxiety about the diagnosis fades with time and with the induction of a remission or disappearance of the tumour. The nausea, vomiting and hair loss, and the disruption of school and family life because of frequent hospital trips, all place a great strain on the child and family, who will need support and reassurance from the medical team. A skilled multidisciplinary team is an essential part of management. Case discussion with nursing staff, counsellors, psychologists and medical staff is a useful way of ensuring that treatment and support are made as effective as possible. In teenagers, the disruption to school work, the blow to body image and development, and the possible loss of contact with friends mean that family and school will need to act in harmony with the hospital staff to try to minimize the stress of the illness and the disruption to the child's education.

After successful treatment the long-term sequelae of treatment may bring problems, for example, intellectual and neurological impairment following brain tumours such as medulloblastoma (see Chapter 11), growth defects after extensive radiation (see Chapter 5) and infertility after chemotherapy.

If the disease recurs, the implications for prognosis are usually grave. If there is still a chance of cure, intensive treatment may be needed again and the depression of morale in the child and family will make extra support necessary. If the chance of cure is slim or non-existent, the parents must be told and the aims of palliative treatment explained and agreed upon. Many parents still hope that a cure will be found, yet they must at the same time begin to accept the likelihood of the child's death. The conflict may be great and there must be an opportunity for the family to express their feelings. Parents should know that freedom from pain or discomfort is usually possible.

Parents will be desolate that relapse has occurred and may sometimes feel that they were wrong to allow aggressive treatment with its attendant side-effects, and all to no avail. These feelings may be directed at the medical team. At this difficult stage, sympathetic discussion and explanation are essential. Senior staff must remember that those members of the team who are less experienced may themselves need to be reassured and supported.

Very young children do not have a clear idea of death but may express their fears of separation in play or in conversation. Adolescents will usually have an adult perception of death, but the huge psychological impact of a cancer diagnosis at this most critical and sensitive time in a young adult's life cannot be overestimated. In dealing with a dying child, the doctors should allow the patient and family to indicate how far and fast they wish to go in discussion and should not force unpalatable facts upon them [1]. Many families need to retain some hope of recovery in dealing with the situation. At the same time the doctor must listen to, and understand, expressions of anger and grief as part of the process of acceptance that the child will die.

Tumours of childhood

Although all childhood tumours are uncommon, cancer is the commonest natural cause of death in childhood (of all causes, second only to accidents). The incidence figures for the UK are shown in Figure 24.1 and Table 24.1. About 1600 children are diagnosed in the UK with cancer each year, and in teenagers cancer is the leading cause of death after accidents (unintentional injury, including road traffic incidents). Extraordinary advances have been made in the management of almost all the common childhood tumours, such that the 5-year survival rate has improved over recent decades from 30% to about 80%. An estimated 33 000 childhood cancer survivors are now alive in the UK, an astonishing statistic. With a better understanding of the diseases and far more effective treatments, cure is frequently achieved. As treatment policies become more sophisticated, paediatric oncology has become a specialized branch of cancer treatment. Childhood cancer is undoubtedly best treated in a specialized paediatric oncology centre. With some tumours, the chances of survival are possibly improved by 10–15%. Conversely, in cancers such as Wilms' tumour, where results may be equal in survival to those in non-specialist centres, this may be at the expense of overtreatment in the non-specialist hospitals [2]. In recent years, units for the care of adolescents with cancer have been established in some cancer centres. These units are based on the principles of paediatric cancer units, but with special expertise in managing the cancers found in this age group and the particular emotional consequences of cancer at this age.

Aetiology and incidence

Little is known of the aetiology of childhood tumours. Ionizing radiation may be a predisposing cause, either when given during pregnancy or as a result of deliberate irradiation, for example, to the thymus for thymic hyperplasia, which has been responsible for an increased risk of thyroid carcinoma. Transplacental carcinogens have long

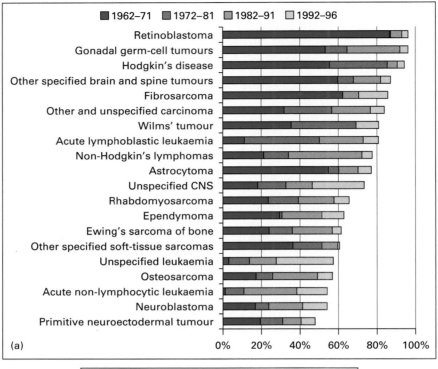

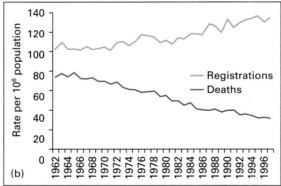

Figure 24.1 (a and b) Registration rates for successive calendar periods (expressed as proportions of the rate for 1963–1967) for children aged 0–14, UK, 1962–1996, showing the increasing incidence for all major childhood tumour types since the 1960s. The considerable reduction in childhood cancer mortality in the UK since the 1960s (despite stable or increasing incidence rates) reflects dramatic improvements in survival. Only about 25% of children with cancer diagnosed in the UK during the decade 1962–1971 survived for more than 5 years. Nearly 75% of those diagnosed during 1992–1996 survived for more than 5 years. Data from Cancer Research UK.

been thought to be a possible cause of childhood cancer. The clearest demonstration of the potential importance of this mechanism was shown by the association of adenocarcinoma of the vagina in teenage girls with treatment of the mother 20 years previously with diethylstilbestrol for early threatened abortion.

Genetic factors are frequently involved [3]. Several tumours of childhood are now known to be associated with chromosomal abnormalities. Some of these are acquired and are discussed in the sections on the tumours concerned. Others are heritable (constitutive) abnormalities, and these are listed in Table 3.5 (see

Table 24.1 Average annual registrations and incidence rates per million population in the UK, 1978–1987.

Diagnostic group	Cases per year	Age 0–1	Age 1–4	Age 5–9	Age 10–14
Leukaemia					
Acute lymphoblastic	323	16.3	58.6	26.6	14.9
Acute non-lymphocytic	64	9.5	7.3	4.1	5.6
Lymphomas					
Hodgkin's disease	58	–	1.4	4.3	9.8
Non-Hodgkin's lymphoma	70	2.2	5.0	7.1	7.5
Brain and spinal cancer	290	27.3	30.9	27.2	22.7
Neuroblastoma	74	32.1	14.9	2.7	0.4
Wilms' tumour	70	12.9	16.6	4.0	0.5
Bone					
Osteosarcoma	32	–	0.2	1.7	6.3
Ewing's sarcoma	28	–	0.6	2.7	4.2
Soft-tissue sarcoma	80	11.9	8.9	6.1	6.3
Germ-cell and gonadal cancer	39	6.9	4.7	1.4	3.9
All cancers	**1240**	**153.6**	**161.1**	**92.8**	**91.7**

page 35). Some congenital malformations appear to be associated with paediatric tumours. There is an increased risk of tumours (usually neurogenic sarcomas) developing in children with von Recklinghausen's disease. The rare syndrome of hemihypertrophy may be associated with both Wilms' tumour and hepatoblastoma. Wilms' tumour can be associated with aniridia and a wide variety of congenital abnormalities.

In addition to inherited non-malignant diseases in which there is an increased risk of cancer, there are inherited gene mutations that give rise to a high risk of cancer without any other manifestations. An example is retinoblastoma, which has a marked familial incidence particularly in the bilateral form of the disease, where half the offspring of affected children will themselves develop the disease. Li–Fraumeni syndrome, due to *p53* mutation, is another example where there is a high risk of cancer in families of children with sarcoma (see pages 32–34). In alveolar rhabdomyosarcoma, clinically more aggressive than the embryonal sub-type, the majority of cases exhibit one or more characteristic chromosomal translocations, such as t(2;13)(q35;q14), which results in the expression of a PAX3–FOXO1 fusion transcription factor. Certain genes are now known to cooperate with PAX3–FOXO1, as well as the target genes of the fusion transcription factor that contribute to various aspects of clinical behaviour – N-MYC, IGF2, MET, CXCR4, CNR1, TFAP2B, FGFR4 and P-cadherin, and PAX3/7–FOXO1 cooperating factors such as the abrogation of the *p53* pathway, IGF2 deregulation, N-MYC and miR17-92 amplification, are among the bewildering array of factors potentially involved. Hopefully, the characterization of these pathways will lead to a better understanding and allow the design of novel targeted therapies – see Ref. [4].

Other genetic influences remain to be elucidated. If a child with an identical twin develops acute leukaemia, then the risk of the twin also developing this disease is high. The overall risk of cancer in childhood is 1 in 600, but in siblings 1 in 300.

Geographical and racial variations also exist, which may eventually throw further light on aetiology. In the UK, children from affluent backgrounds who live in rural or isolated areas are more likely than others to develop cancer, according to the 11th report from the Committee on Medical Aspects of Radiation in the Environment (COMARE), an independent expert advisory committee (see Ref. [5]). This group looked at more than 32 000 cases of childhood cancer diagnosed under the age of 15 years, finding that the prevalence was very unevenly distributed. In particular, childhood leukaemia, central nervous system (CNS) tumours and bone tumours were more common in affluent areas and areas of low population density. There was certainly an excessive number of cases in the top socioeconomic groupings. A recent report has suggested a possible link between risk of childhood neuroblastoma (the second commonest childhood solid tumour) and marijuana use in early pregnancy [6].

Liver cancer is commoner in the Far East, retinoblastoma in India, intestinal lymphoma in Israel and Burkitt's lymphoma in Uganda. Ewing's sarcoma is exceptionally rare in Africans. In the UK and the USA, the proportion of various groups of tumours is reasonably constant: 20–25% consists of tumours of the CNS and eye, 33% are leukaemias and 35% are solid tumours (chiefly Wilms' tumour and neuroblastoma). Most of these tumours have their maximal incidence at ages 0–4 years, although some, such as bone tumours and lymphomas, have a later peak between 6 and 14 years. In general, younger children appear to have a better survival than older groups, particularly with neuroblastoma and retinoblastoma. With the relative improvement in treatments of other paediatric illnesses, cancer has assumed an increased importance as a cause of death despite the many advances in management.

Childhood tumours of the CNS are common, and are discussed with adult brain tumours in Chapter 11; leukaemia is discussed in Chapter 28 and paediatric lymphomas in Chapter 26.

With respect to clinical management, the reader should be aware that paediatric oncology is a highly specialized and rapidly moving branch of oncology, increasingly managed only by acknowledged experts in the field who have undergone specialist training. The following account of the major specific tumours should be understood as a brief summary of current thinking rather than a precise text for specific case management. The good news of course is that with modern multi-disciplinary management, almost 80% of children and young adolescents can now be cured – one of the most outstanding achievements in the field of oncology.

Neuroblastoma

After brain tumours, leukaemia and lymphoma, neuroblastoma is the commonest of paediatric tumours, accounting for some 7% of the total and about 15% of all deaths from cancer in the paediatric age group [7]. About 1 in 6000 children will develop neuroblastoma by the age of 5 years, and over 80% of cases occur below the age of 4 years. About one-quarter of all cases occur under the age of 1 year, a group in which a very high rate of survival (approaching 90%) is regularly achieved with modern treatment. Most cases are sporadic but there are reports of twins with both affected, as well as families with two or more affected siblings. Overall, the survival has undoubtedly improved in recent years (Figure 24.2).

Pathology

Neuroblastomas are embryonal tumours that arise from neural crest tissue, which normally develops into the adrenal medulla and sympathetic ganglia. The common primary sites are therefore the adrenal medulla and the sympathetic nervous tissue in the retroperitoneum. About 65% of primary tumours develop within the abdomen, over half of these from the adrenal medulla [7]. However, tumours may also arise in the posterior mediastinum and spine, predominantly extradurally from paravertebral sympathetic ganglia (Figure 24.3). Because of their derivation from the adrenal medulla, elaboration and secretion of adrenal medullary hormones or metabolites are characteristic of these tumours (see below).

Neuroblastomas sometimes undergo spontaneous regression and differentiation. Small neuroblastomas are not infrequently found in the adrenals in fetal autopsies. In infancy there is a widely disseminated form of the disease (stage 4S) that undergoes spontaneous regression. In other cases the tumour shows pathological features indicating varying degrees of differentiation, from small round undifferentiated cells to ganglion cells and Schwann cell-like stroma. The degree of neural differentiation is related to improved prognosis as is lower mitotic rate and absence of necrosis. Neuroblastomas are often positive on periodic acid–Schiff (PAS) staining, and express a variety of neuroendocrine markers (chromogranin-A, synaptophysin, neurone-specific

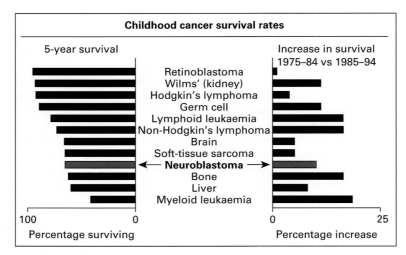

Figure 24.2 Improvement in survival of infants and children diagnosed with neuroblastoma. Source: Linet *et al.* (1999).

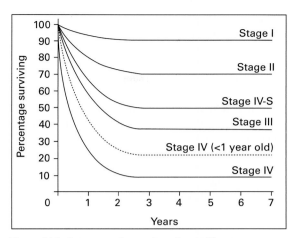

Figure 24.3 Common primary sites of neuroblastoma.

enolase). Electron microscopy may show dense neurose-cretory granules.

The N-*myc* gene, found on chromosome 2p24, is frequently amplified. It is thought to exert its tumorigenic effect, at least in part, by directly or indirectly regulating the expression of micro-RNAs which are involved with neural cell differentiation and/or apoptosis. More than 10 copies of this gene per cell confers a strong indication of poor prognosis, and this is now widely used to help tailor intensity of treatment. Assessment of gene amplification is now a routine part of pathological examination. Deletion of chromosome 1p is present in 40%. This region of chromosome 1 may contain a tumour-suppressor gene, and loss of heterozygosity at this site may predict early relapse. A significant gain of genetic material at 17q is frequently confirmed, and is associated with poor prognosis. Recent work has also strongly implicated the chromosomal locus 6p22 as being associated with susceptibility to neuroblastoma and also to a particularly aggressive clinical course (see Ref. [8]).

Neuroblastomas tend to spread very widely, by local, lymphatic and haematogenous routes, and important sites of blood-borne dissemination include bone marrow (often forming clusters of large, poorly differentiated cells), liver (sometimes resulting in enormous hepatomegaly) and bone (a single destructive lesion being a typical neuroblastoma metastasis). Unlike other paediatric soft-tissue tumours, the lungs are seldom the site of metastases. Skin and periorbital metastases are common, and overall about half of all cases present with evidence of haematogenous spread of disease [7].

Clinical features

Clinical presentation is unusually varied, due to the variety of primary sites, the early wide dissemination and the secretion of pharmacologically active metabolites (Table 24.2). As the recent authors of an authoritative review point out, 'the clinical hallmark of neuroblastoma is heterogeneity, with the likelihood of cure varying widely according to age at diagnosis, extent of disease, and tumour biology' [7]. The commonest presentation is of an abdominal mass, sometimes painless but often accompanied by mild or recurrent abdominal pain. Other common symptoms include irritability, fever, lethargy, anaemia or bone pain from a metastasis. Occasionally, lymph node or skin metastases, hepatomegaly or proptosis are the first clinical signs. Subcutaneous metastases often have a blue/black colour. Liver metastases may be painful. Other primary sites of presentation include presacral neuroblastoma causing urinary frequency or obstruction; posterior mediastinal tumours causing dyspnoea; intraspinal tumours causing spinal cord compression; cervical sympathetic tumours causing Horner's syndrome; and olfactory bulb tumours (aesthesioneuroblastoma) causing nasal obstruction and epistaxis. There is an association between neuroblastoma and myoclonic or opsoclonic movements, though the mechanism is unclear. Rarely, secretion of large amounts of catecholamines and intestinal peptides can cause sweating, pallor and

Table 24.2 Presenting symptoms of neuroblastoma.

Constitutional
Fever, malaise, weight loss, anaemia

Primary site
Adrenal: pain and abdominal mass
Presacral: loss of bladder control, frequency of micturition
Paravertebral: spinal cord compression
Cervical sympathetic: Horner's syndrome
Olfactory bulb: unilateral nasal block and epistaxis

Metastases
Liver: pain, weight loss, fever
Bone: pain (preceding X-ray change), anaemia, pathological fractures
Orbit: proptosis
Central nervous system: malignant meningitis

Remote effects
Diarrhoea: due to secretion of vasoactive intestinal polypeptide
Myoclonus or opsoclonus
Hypertension

diarrhoea. Some authorities advocate the wide-scale use of mass population-based screening at 6 months of age using analysis of urinary catecholamine metabolites (see below) but others argue against, as a significant number of tumours regress spontaneously (see Ref. [9]).

Diagnosis and investigation

The definitive diagnosis is by biopsy of the affected site but a confident diagnosis may already have been made biochemically. Catecholamine metabolites are produced in about 90% of all children with neuroblastomas, and screening for urinary metabolites should be undertaken if the diagnosis is suspected. Homovanillic acid (HVA) or vanillylmandelic acid (VMA) are the most reliable and widely used measurements. The diagnosis can often be made on a random urine sample. Both HVA and VMA should be measured since either metabolite may be increased.

Plain radiography of the abdomen will frequently demonstrate calcification in the primary tumour, typically with a diffuse pattern. Liver metastases may also calcify. The chest radiograph is often normal, though abnormal mediastinal shadowing often occurs with primary intrathoracic tumours (typically in the posterior mediastinum). Parenchymal lung metastases are very unusual. Skeletal survey and isotope bone scanning are useful in detecting osseous metastases. Bone marrow aspiration is mandatory in all cases of neuroblastoma. Over 40% of children have marrow involvement even when bone radiographs are normal, so marrow aspiration is generally recommended. Computed tomography (CT) and/or magnetic resonance imaging (MRI) and abdominal ultrasonography give excellent delineation of tumour as well as providing accurate imaging of the liver.

Meta-iodobenzylguanidine (MIBG) is taken up by adrenergic nervous tissue and can be used to identify both primary and metastatic neuroblastoma; 10% of cases show no uptake. Because over 90% of neuroblastomas show avidity or selective concentration of MIBG, scanning by means of MIBG scintigraphy has become an important part of tumour staging, demonstrating both primary site and metastatic disease. It is now the imaging isotope of choice as it has better image resolution than the ^{131}I isotope previously employed [7]. Early diagnosis by screening the urine of all 6-month-old babies has been attempted in Japan, but population-based studies from Germany and North America suggest that screening does not reduce overall mortality. Some small tumours may be detected early but these may regress spontaneously.

Differential diagnosis

The clinical diagnosis of neuroblastoma is not always straightforward, particularly if the child presents with failure to thrive and without other obvious abnormalities to suggest a diagnosis of malignancy. The differential diagnosis in children presenting with an abdominal mass often lies between neuroblastoma and Wilms' tumour. Other abdominal tumours which may cause diagnostic difficulty include hepatoblastoma and intestinal lymphoma. If the child presents with bone metastases, these may be difficult to distinguish radiologically from a primary Ewing's tumour, bone lymphoma or even a non-malignant cause such as osteomyelitis or tuberculosis.

Difficulty may also occur when the child presents with spinal cord compression, when a variety of malignant and non-malignant causes must be considered. These include intraspinal cysts, neurofibroma, spinal tuberculosis, primary intraspinal tumours, medulloblastoma and other tumours which spread within the CNS (see Chapter 11), and other rare causes of extradural compression such as Hodgkin's disease.

Clinical staging

Clinical staging of neuroblastoma is important as a means of selecting the most appropriate treatment and to give an assessment of prognosis [10]. Several classifications have been proposed and all are based on an accurate assessment of the extent of spread. This International Neuroblastoma Staging System (INSS) classification has on the whole proved extremely valuable for both consistency of treatment and case-to-case cross-centre comparison. The degree of histological differentiation (i.e. tumour grade) influences prognosis, but this information is difficult to fit into a simple staging classification. The same is true for catecholamine excretion and age, though age at diagnosis is probably the single most important prognostic factor. A new classification has been proposed that for the first time includes information obtained from cytogenetic analysis in addition to the more traditional methods outlined above; this International Neuroblastoma Risk Group (INRG) stratification is likely to replace the previous INSS approach. In the new system, extent of disease will be defined preoperatively by imaging studies and bone marrow morphology. Stages M and MS are proposed in order to categorize tumours that are widely metastatic or have an INSS 4S pattern of disease, respectively [7]. Traditionally, the cut-off for age-related risk assessment has been 1 year, but recent work suggests that this may be too low [7].

Up to 70% of children have disseminated tumour at diagnosis, often in the bone marrow. The prognosis worsens with increasing stage. However, the IV-S (S indicates special) category has been defined because these children have a surprisingly good prognosis, with a survival rate similar to patients with stage I tumours. Most IV-S patients are under the age of 1 year, and stage IV-S comprises about 5% of the total. These children have small primary tumours, with metastases typically to the liver, skin or bone marrow. Children below the age of 1 year also have a much better prognosis even with stage III and IV disease. Within this group those with stage IV and without tumour N-*myc* amplification have a very good outcome. A high mitotic rate, hypodiploidy and karyotypic abnormalities of chromosome 1 are also associated with a poor prognosis.

In addition to age and disease extent, the primary site is also prognostically important. Tumours arising in the mediastinum and the neck have a better prognosis than those in the abdomen, probably since more are localized at the time of diagnosis. This is particularly the case with thoracospinal lesions that produce early spinal cord compression. Curiously, pelvic tumours also appear to have a better prognosis, and more frequently undergo differentiation to ganglioneuroma or even spontaneous remission; again this may relate to the fact that most of these children are under the age of 15 months. These various biological features are increasingly employed as an important part of the treatment decision strategy, helping influence the type of chemotherapy and its intensity. For this disease, the concept of 'molecular staging' has become a reality.

Clinical management

Current clinical management of neuroblastoma is unsatisfactory and refinements in treatment are continuously being suggested – see, for example, Ref. [11], for a thoughtful analysis of critical current problems and obstacles to further progress. Unlike many of the paediatric malignancies, chemotherapy has not yet made a dramatic improvement in the survival of these children, although the initial chemosensitivity of this tumour is not in doubt. The intensity of treatment is based on assessment of risk, using the known prognostic features described above. As well as the INSS stage, age at diagnosis, histopathology, N-*myc* gene status, and DNA mitotic index are all useful for assigning each patient into a low-, intermediate- or high-risk group. This will in turn be used to determine the treatment programme, in particular the need for intensive treatment, which is necessary for the highest-risk stages – see Ref. [12] for a

useful discussion of treatment risks and benefits. When the tumour is localized, it is generally curable. However, long-term survival for children with advanced disease is poor, despite aggressive multimodal therapy. High-risk neuroblastoma is treated with intensive chemotherapy, surgery, radiation therapy, bone marrow/autologous stem-cell transplants, and biological-based therapy that may include *cis*-retinoic acid. With current treatments, patients with low- and intermediate-risk disease have an excellent prognosis with cure rates above 90%. In contrast, therapy for high-risk neuroblastoma results in cures only about 30% of patients.

Local treatments with surgery and/or radiation therapy are therefore very important, and may be curative in children with localized disease. A 2-year survival rate of 80% has been achieved by the use of surgery alone in apparently localized cases. Radiotherapy is usually recommended after incomplete excision, but probably best avoided where surgery appears complete. Long-term survivors have certainly been documented where surgery was incomplete, but supplemented by postoperative radiotherapy, although the contribution of radiotherapy is difficult to quantify. Most children with clinical stage II and III disease will be in this category. Even in children with stage IV disease, in whom chemotherapy may be the most important part of treatment, attention must be paid to controlling the primary disease.

In stage IV cases chemotherapy is usually the first treatment, but radiotherapy and surgery will often be required at a later stage in order to achieve control of the bulky primary tumour. Some surgeons feel that, in this situation, preoperative irradiation makes surgery technically easier. In these more advanced cases, the local treatment is usually withheld until at least two cycles of chemotherapy have been given.

Guidelines for treatment of neuroblastoma are given in Table 24.3. Combinations of vincristine, cyclophosphamide, actinomycin D and doxorubicin are usually used. Agents such as cisplatin, etoposide and ifosfamide are increasingly used in combination therapy. All these drugs have been shown to be active as single agents in neuroblastoma (Table 24.4). With these more intensive regimens (such as OPEC, Table 24.4) the response rates are 60–70% but only 25–30% of advanced disease is cured though useful additional responses can sometimes be secured after failure of first-line therapy – see, for example, Ref. [13]. The use of high-dose chemotherapy and autologous bone marrow transplantation may improve survival in high-risk cases [14]. Patients who receive high-dose therapy with a stem-cell or bone

Table 24.3 Guidelines for treatment of neuroblastoma.

Stage I	Surgery alone
Stage II	Surgery with postoperative irradiation is considered if surgery incomplete
	Chemotherapy sometimes used for stage IIB after incomplete excision unless the child is less than 6 months old
Stage III	Chemotherapy followed by 'debulking' surgery with local irradiation and further chemotherapy
Stage IV	As for stage III, but intensive chemotherapy is the mainstay of treatment
Stage IV-S	If possible no treatment is given. If the child has symptoms because of tumour size, surgery ± minimal chemotherapy is justified

Table 24.4 Chemotherapy for neuroblastoma.

Single agents
Vincristine
Actinomycin D
Doxorubicin
Cyclophosphamide
Ifosfamide
Cisplatin/carboplatin
Etoposide/teniposide
High-dose melphalan

Combination chemotherapy
VAC I: vincristine, actinomycin and cyclophosphamide
VAC II: vincristine, doxorubicin and cyclophosphamide
OPEC: vincristine, cisplatin, etoposide and cyclophosphamide
VECI: vincristine, carboplatin, teniposide and ifosfamide

marrow transplant after complete or partial chemotherapy response are more likely to be long survivors: the toxicity of these treatments is diminishing and further trials are in progress. Controversy continues as to whether the marrow or peripheral blood for transplantation support needs to be purged of supposedly malignant cells – see, for example, Ref. [15] – but the question remains unanswered. Targeted radiotherapy also holds considerable promise, using ^{131}I-MIBG either as primary therapy or at relapse. Low-dose radioiodine-tagged MIBG has been shown to be useful for disease palliation but higher doses will be more myelotoxic and possibly even require stem-cell support. Other newer treatments include novel combinations of cytotoxic drugs,

derivatives of vitamin A (e.g. fenretinide), treatment intensification with bone marrow transplantation and of particular interest at the present time, the use of therapeutic vaccines that attempt to boost or initiate a better immune response using interleukins such as IL-2 and chimeric Monoclonal Antibody14.18 (Ch14.18) for children with high-risk neuroblastoma. This is an antibody showing real potential in the treatment of certain types of cancer by targeting GD2, a glycolipid on the surface of tumour cells and is a chimera, composed of a combination of mouse and human DNA – a monoclonal antibody that induces antibody dependent cell-mediated cytotoxicity, a mechanism of cell-mediated immunity, whereby the immune system actively targets a cell that has been bound by specific antibodies.

Results from the landmark US-based NCI's phase III study were published in 2010 (see Ref. [16]). In that important study, immunotherapy with Ch14.18 significantly improved patient outcome compared with standard therapy in patients with high-risk neuroblastoma, with a two-year estimate for event-free survival at 66% in the Ch14.18 immunotherapy group and 46% in the standard therapy group. Side effects of Ch14.18 included nerve pain (which can be severe), systemic oedema sometimes leading to hypotension, dyspnoea and tachycardia, and allergic reactions.

Finally, at least one large randomized study has suggested that 13-*cis*-retinoic acid, a vitamin A derivative, has improved the event-free survival, even in late-stage cases. For high-risk cases, almost all patients treated in major centres over the past decade have undergone stem-cell transplantation and the use of 13 *cis*-retinoic acid post-transplant became widely accepted.

Although overall results remain disappointing, survival has improved in recent years as a result of better diagnosis, treatment strategy, biochemical monitoring and possibly chemotherapy. Survival is clearly related to age, N-*myc* gene amplification status, presence of bone-marrow metastases, and stage (Figure 24.2). Children living beyond 3 years from diagnosis are usually considered cured. See also the comprehensive recent global statistical report published by the International Neuroblastoma Risk Project Group [17], which gives a good quantitative account of the overall survival improvement following treatment in the modern era.

Wilms' tumour
Incidence and aetiology
Named after Max Wilms, a German surgeon (1867–1918) who first described this condition, Wilms' tumour

(nephroblastoma) accounts for about 8% of all paediatric tumours, with a peak incidence below the age of 4 years. Inherited cases account for less than 1%. With neuroblastoma it forms much the largest group of intra-abdominal malignancies of childhood. However, there are pronounced behavioural differences between these two tumours, particularly in their response to treatment. In the USA, about 500 new cases are diagnosed annually, and there is a slight male preponderance.

Although most cases (about 75%) are sporadic, there is also a familial form. Aniridia, gonadal dysplasia and mental retardation may be associated with Wilms' tumour (sometimes termed the WAGR complex), as may musculoskeletal deformity. It can also be associated with Beckwith–Wiedemann syndrome, which comprises hemihypertrophy, macroglossia and omphalocele. Chromosomal analysis shows deletion at the level of band 13 of the short arm of chromosome 11 (11p13) (Figure 24.4). Cases with small deletions do not show mental retardation. The tumour-suppressor *WT1* gene is a transcription factor, inactivated in about 10% of cases, and recent work suggests that the *WTX* gene on the X chromosome is inactivated in up to 30% of cases [18]. Other described germline abnormalities are XX/XY mosaicism and trisomy 8 or 18. The peak age of incidence is 3–5 years, though it has on rare occasions been discovered at birth.

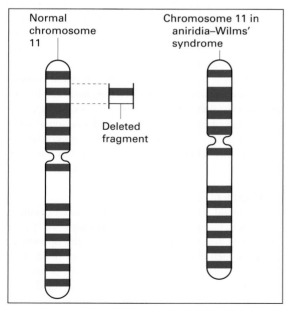

Figure 24.4 Deletion of part of the short arm of chromosome 11 in aniridia–Wilms' syndrome.

Pathology

Almost the whole kidney can be replaced by either a centrally or peripherally placed tumour, often exhibiting areas of patchy haemorrhage or degeneration, and sometimes with a lobulated appearance. Necrosis and cystic change are both common, and although a very large size may be attained without obvious extrarenal involvement, extension of solid cores of tumour cells along the renal vein and inferior vena cava are common. Other direct sites of spread may include the perinephric fat, colon, adrenal gland or liver as well as the renal pelvis itself, and the local draining lymph nodes. Occasionally, the tumour may be extrarenal in origin, presumably arising in ectopic cell rests remaining at the time of mesonephric crest migration.

Histologically, Wilms' tumour contains both mesenchymal and epithelial elements, often admixed and with differing stages of maturity. Within the epithelial element, there is usually evidence of a renal origin, with embryonic tubular or glomerular structures sometimes lined by recognizable epithelium and occasionally arranged in rosettes. The most favourable histological group usually contains all three elements. A monomorphic epithelial form is particularly favourable. Undifferentiated stroma may form a large proportion of the tumour though this too may show areas of differentiation to form smooth muscle, bone or cartilage. A variety of histological types have been described, which probably represent differing degrees of differentiation. Some tumours are so undifferentiated as to defy unequivocal histological diagnosis. About 5% of tumours are anaplastic. Nuclear enlargement and hyperploidy are associated adverse features. Tumours with these features have a great propensity to metastasis. There is a particular form of bone-metastasizing tumour that is probably a distinct entity. More highly differentiated forms also occur, and a specific group of 'mesoblastic nephromas' has only minimal nuclear pleomorphism, mitotic activity and metastatic potential, and is often surgically curable. Loss of heterozygosity on the short arm of chromosome 11 has been widely reported as the most consistent karyotypic abnormality in the tumour.

Clinical features

The common presentation is with a symptomless, painless abdominal mass more commonly on the left and often discovered by the parent or during a routine examination [19]. There may be recurrent abdominal pain of moderate severity. Abdominal distension is common although, unlike neuroblastoma, these tumours tend not to cross the midline. Haematuria occurs in 30% of cases. Hypertension is unusual but is occasionally severe and sometimes accompanied by complications such as retinopathy or encephalopathy. It is thought to be due to excess renin production by the tumour or to renal ischaemia from renal artery stenosis. Fever, anorexia and lethargy may also be presenting symptoms.

About one-fifth of children with Wilms' tumour have evidence of distant metastases at presentation, though figures from central referral hospitals suggest a much higher incidence (up to 60–70%), representing a preponderance of advanced and complicated cases. Direct spread to extrarenal fat and other local organs is common, and local nodal spread occurs predominantly to the para-aortic and other intra-abdominal lymph node groups. Haematogenous spread occurs typically to the lung parenchyma, brain and bone, although liver, mediastinum, vagina and testis are well-known secondary sites (Figure 24.5). Bilateral presentation occurs in 5% of cases, which are usually regarded as being bilateral primary tumours rather than secondary spread. Bilateral Wilms' tumour can also be metachronous. Children with bilateral tumours are younger and have 10 times the incidence of associated congenital anomalies.

Investigation and staging

Plain chest and abdominal radiographs will help to define the extent of the primary tumour and demonstrate obvious pulmonary metastases. CT scanning of the chest is

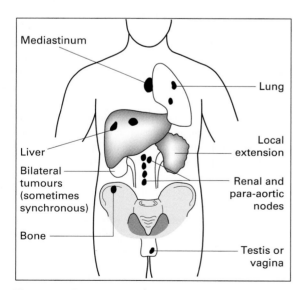

Figure 24.5 Common sites of metastasis in Wilms' tumour.

more sensitive but may not alter management since small metastases (not visible on chest radiography) respond to chemotherapy. Abdominopelvic ultrasonography will give accurate preoperative information as to the size and extent of disease. Visualization of the inferior vena cava is important prior to surgery and can be achieved with ultrasound or contrast venography. The most precise definition of tumour size is achieved with CT or MRI of the abdomen.

Routine urine examination often reveals microscopic haematuria, and measurement of catecholamine excretion will be necessary in cases that are difficult to distinguish clinically from neuroblastoma, especially if there is hypertension. Isotope bone scanning is usually recommended since symptomless bone secondaries may be present. These investigations should help distinguish the true Wilms' tumour from a variety of malignant and non-malignant conditions that it may clinically resemble.

Although neuroblastoma is the most important differential diagnosis, other intra-abdominal childhood tumours may cause difficulty, such as retroperitoneal sarcoma and hepatoblastoma. Important non-malignant causes of childhood abdominal masses include renal haematomas, hydronephrosis, multilocular cystic kidney, horseshoe kidney, perirenal haematoma and splenomegaly.

Staging systems have become more logical with increased understanding of the natural history of these tumours and of the importance of complete surgical removal. At present, the National Wilms' Tumour Study Staging System (Table 24.5) is most widely used. This staging system has now been successfully used for 10 years, and data are accumulating to suggest that extent of disease at operation and the presence of lymph node involvement are the most influential prognostic factors. Large referral centres have better results than smaller hospitals where the occasional case is treated, with the implication that non-specialist clinicians should be strongly dissuaded from treating a child with a curable cancer.

Management

There should be close co-operation between paediatric surgeon, radiotherapist, paediatric oncologist and pathologist to ensure that all clinicians have the opportunity to assess each child before surgery is performed. There has been some controversy over the use of preoperative biopsy because of the risk of intra-abdominal dissemination of tumour. If this is done it should be a fine-needle biopsy to minimize this risk. Even in the presence of obvious metastatic disease, careful assessment

Table 24.5 Staging and guidelines for the management of Wilms' tumour.

Stage I	Tumour limited to the kidney, and completely resected. Renal capsule intact, tumour removed without rupture, no residual disease	Surgery and vincristine
Stage II	Tumour extends beyond kidney but is completely resected. Penetration is into the perirenal soft tissue or fat; infiltration of renal vessels outside the kidney, or para-ortic lymph node involvement. No residual tumour	Surgery; adjuvant combination chemotherapy using vincristine and actinomycin D
Stage III	Residual tumour confined to the abdomen, or tumour biopsied or ruptured before or during surgery. Involved lymph nodes beyond para-aortic chains. Tumour not completely resected	As for stage II but whole-abdominal irradiation for diffuse spread, and chemotherapy includes doxorubicin
Stage IV	Distant blood-borne metastases (usually to lung, liver, bone and/or brain). Lymph node metastases beyond the abdomen	Surgery and more intensive combination chemotherapy
Stage V	Bilateral tumours at presentation	Individual treatment often including bilateral renal surgery with low-dose postoperative radiotherapy and adjuvant combination chemotherapy

of operability should be made because control of the primary tumour without surgery is difficult. The advent of effective irradiation and chemotherapy has allowed surgeons to reconsider operating on children whose tumours are inoperable at first presentation – see, for example, Ref. [20].

Guidelines for the management of Wilms' tumour are set out in Table 24.5. Surgical removal should be performed in order both to remove the tumour in its entirety, without biopsy or other disturbance of the capsule, and to assess the extent of intra-abdominal disease with careful delineation of any area of residual tumour. Before resection it must be confirmed that the contralateral kidney is intact. Enlarged lymph nodes should generally be resected or at least biopsied. There is no substitute for surgical experience and the planning of the surgery must be meticulous. Surgery should not be attempted if the tumour is fixed and if there is hepatic infiltration. Under these circumstances chemotherapy is usually given first, as it is if there are metastases.

Postoperative chemotherapy with combinations of vincristine, actinomycin D and/or doxorubicin should be used (Table 24.6). However, the possible roles of preoperative chemotherapy and routine postoperative irradiation of the tumour bed remain controversial. There

is evidence that preoperative chemotherapy is valuable in the management of doubtfully resectable tumours.

Although postoperative radiotherapy has been employed routinely for many years as an adjuvant to surgery, the development of effective chemotherapeutic regimens has led to a reappraisal of the role of radiotherapy [21]. In stage I disease, postoperative radiotherapy confers no benefit and 10 weeks' treatment with doxorubicin and vincristine are as effective as longer periods.

Children with stage II disease should be treated postoperatively with combination chemotherapy. Combination chemotherapy using vincristine and actinomycin D, if intensive, gives as good a result as regimens using doxorubicin (with its attendant cardiotoxicity).

Stage III disease has presented a bigger challenge. Evidence from European trials has indicated that preoperative chemotherapy reduces the stage of tumour at surgery and may allow radiotherapy to be omitted from the programme. If radiotherapy is omitted it is probable that three-drug regimens are necessary.

Stage IV disease should be treated with intensive combination chemotherapy. The successful treatment of disseminated Wilms' tumour demands an aggressive approach, often requiring surgical resection of residual pulmonary

Table 24.6 Chemotherapy in Wilms' tumour.

	Response rate (complete and partial) (%)
Single agents	
Vincristine	70
Doxorubicin	60
Actinomycin D	40
Cyclophosphamide	35
Etoposide	30
Cisplatin	30
Combination therapy*	
Actinomycin D and vincristine	95
Vincristine and doxorubicin	90
Vincristine, doxorubicin, cyclophosphamide	90

*Response rates are approximate as these combinations have not been thoroughly tested in metastatic disease, and different combinations are used in different stages of the disease.

and hepatic metastases with additional use of both radiotherapy and chemotherapy.

In patients with bilateral (stage V) disease, surgery is attempted only after initial chemotherapy has reduced the tumour mass as far as possible. The aim of surgery is then to preserve as much of both kidneys as possible. Chemotherapy is usually continued postoperatively. If surgical clearance is impossible, and the disease cannot be eradicated, bilateral nephrectomy and transplantation is a last resort.

The routine use of chemotherapy has radically altered the outlook in this disease, and now forms part of the initial management. Avoidance of radiotherapy whenever possible has reduced the long-term complications such as growth retardation within the irradiated area, scoliosis and radiation-induced second tumours, often an unresectable and rapidly fatal sarcoma. Trials are in progress to clarify further the details of postoperative treatment. At present, important chemotherapy-induced complications include nausea and vomiting, peripheral neuropathy, alopecia and skin reactions (including recall phenomena in previously irradiated areas, following actinomycin D treatment).

Treatment of recurrent disease is always difficult because of the previous administration of chemotherapy and radiotherapy. The same agents may again be effective, particularly in cases where recurrence is late, well after discontinuation of the initial adjuvant chemotherapy. Other drugs such as cisplatin, ifosfamide, vinblastine, bleomycin and etoposide may be of value in children resistant to first-line treatment. High-dose chemotherapy with stem-cell transplantation has also been used in selected recurrent cases resistant to conventional relapse chemotherapy. Palliative irradiation (sometimes in combination with surgery) may also be useful for brain, lung, extradural, bony and hepatic metastases.

Prognosis

The prognosis in Wilms' tumour has improved greatly as a result of routine adjuvant chemotherapy, although a better understanding of the role of surgery, radiotherapy and supportive care has also contributed – see, for example, Ref. [22]. At present, the prognosis in this disease is better than for any other childhood malignancy and the overall survival rate is now 80–90% (Figure 24.6). Several prognostic factors are known to be important including age at diagnosis (the younger the better), histological findings such as degree of differentiation (with a better prognosis in well-differentiated tumours) and tumour stage. Prognosis for stage I disease is excellent with 5-year survival rates of at least 90%; with stage IV disease this falls to 54%.

Clear-cell sarcoma of the kidney

This rare tumour, which has a peak incidence at ages 1–4 years with a male preponderance, is characterized by early bone metastasis. After primary treatment it may relapse at an interval of several years. Treatment is with surgery and chemotherapy. The regimens have generally followed those used for Wilms' tumour, but there is some

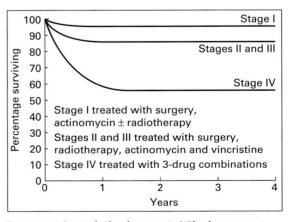

Figure 24.6 Survival related to stage in Wilms' tumour.

evidence that longer periods of treatment are associated with better survival [23].

Other malignant renal tumours in childhood, all uncommon and some extremely rare, have been well reviewed by an expert group from University College London and Great Ormond Street Hospital in London [24].

Malignant mesenchymal tumours (soft-tissue sarcoma)

Incidence, aetiology and classification

This very heterogeneous group of tumours account for 7% of childhood tumours, with an incidence of 0.8 per 100 000 children. The tumours become much less common after 14 years of age. Little is known of their cause, although genetic factors are important in Li–Fraumeni syndrome and most certainly in the aggressive alveolar rhabdomyosarcoma (see above for a fuller discussion).

The histological types of soft-tissue sarcoma in children are similar to those found in adults (see Chapter 23), but the relative frequency is different, with rhabdomyosarcoma and fibrosarcoma predominating (Table 24.7). Histological diagnosis may be difficult. Advances in molecular genetics may help in classification.

Rhabdomyosarcoma

This tumour is the commonest soft-tissue sarcoma of childhood. *Embryonal rhabdomyosarcoma* is the most frequent histological type, with a peak incidence at 2–5 years. *Alveolar rhabdomyosarcoma* is commoner in adolescence. The tumours can arise at a variety of sites: in the head and neck (chiefly the orbit, nasopharynx, oropharynx or palate), the pelvis (particularly bladder, uterus and vagina) or, less commonly, the extremities or trunk.

Pathology

There are four main histological subtypes of rhabdomyosarcoma: embryonal, alveolar, pleomorphic and mixed types [25]. The first two account for more than 90% of all cases. Macroscopically, the tumours are usually nodular, often with a surrounding inflammatory and oedematous reaction. Although they may appear to be circumscribed, true encapsulation is very uncommon. Sarcoma botryoides has a characteristic macroscopic appearance, described as resembling bunches of grapes, which consist of mucinous polyps of tumour.

Microscopically, these tumours are highly malignant. Pathological diagnosis can be difficult, particularly if cross-striation is regarded as an essential part of the histological diagnosis (Figure 24.7). Differentiation from other small round-cell tumours can be made by showing positivity for desmin and vimentin, and lack of staining with markers for Ewing's tumour or lymphoma. *Embryonal rhabdomyosarcoma* is often poorly differentiated, with long, slender, spindle-shaped cells with a single central nucleolus and eosinophilic cytoplasm, often without obvious cross-striations. The cells usually have an irregular pattern without the cellular arrangements

Table 24.7 Childhood soft-tissue sarcoma.

	Relative frequency (%)
Rhabdomyosarcoma	52
Fibrosarcoma (including histiocytoma)	10
Mesenchymoma	6
Synovial sarcoma	6
Liposarcoma	4
Leiomyosarcoma	2
Vascular sarcomas	5
Others	15

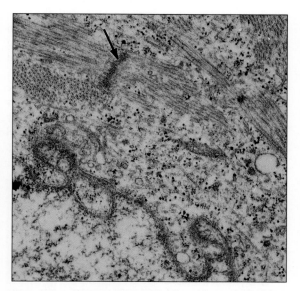

Figure 24.7 Electron micrograph of a portion of rhabdomyoblast. Thick and thin filaments are shown, and there is formation of Z bands (arrow) (×26 600).

that are characteristic of alveolar rhabdomyosarcoma. *Sarcoma botryoides* is a polypoid form of embryonal rhabdomyosarcoma. The embryonal group is the commonest form of paediatric rhabdomyosarcoma and accounts for the majority of head, neck and genitourinary cases.

Alveolar rhabdomyosarcoma arises more commonly on the limbs and trunk. Microscopically, these tumours have a more organized pattern and the cells tend to be separated by connective tissue bands. The typical cell is round with scanty eosinophilic cytoplasm, which is sometimes vacuolated and may contain glycogen. Cross-striations are often seen, and giant multinucleate cells are common. Pleomorphic rhabdomyosarcomas are rare in childhood, and almost always arise in skeletal muscle.

All varieties are highly malignant and exhibit rapid growth with early dissemination. Early lymph node involvement is common, producing obvious lymphadenopathy, which may be the initial presenting feature particularly in head and neck tumours. Blood-borne metastases are also frequent, particularly to lung and marrow, though other sites such as brain, liver and other soft-tissue sites may also be involved. However, there are prognostic implications of the pathology as shown by the international classification (Tables 24.8 and 24.9).

Clinical features

Clinically, the commonest presentation is with a painless mass either clearly visible in the case of extremity and trunk lesions, or causing displacement as with the characteristic proptosis of orbital rhabdomyosarcoma, which accounts for 30% of all head and neck cases. A grouping of major sites has been summarized by an international workshop as shown in Table 24.10.

In the pelvis, the commonest primary sites are the genitourinary tract and perianal area. Bladder tumours are more common in boys and present with urinary symptoms. There may be hydronephrosis. Vaginal tumours present with a vaginal mass or bleeding.

Table 24.8 Pathology and prognosis in rhabdomyosarcoma.

Prognosis	Pathology
Good	Botryoid, spindle cell
Intermediate	Embryonal
Poor	Alveolar undifferentiated
Uncertain	Rhabdoid

Source: Newton *et al.* [25]. Reproduced with permission from John Wiley and Sons.

Table 24.9 Preclinical staging of childhood rhabdomyosarcoma.

T	T1	Confined to organ of origin (subgroup according to size <5 or >5 cm)
	T2	Spread to adjacent structures (subgroup according to size <5 or >5 cm)
N	N0	No involved nodes
	N1	Regional nodes involved
	NX	Uncertain
M	M0	No distant metastases
	M1	Distant metastases

Stage grouping (and 5-year survival rates)

Stage I	T1	N0 or NX	M0	78%
Stage II	T2	N0 or NX	M0	65%
Stage III	Any T	N1	M0	67%
Stage IV	Any T	Any N	M1	26%

Table 24.10 Major sites of rhabdomyosarcoma.

Orbit (non-parameningeal)
Head and neck (non-parameningeal)
Head and neck (parameningeal), nasopharynx, nasal cavity, paranasal sinuses, middle ear, pterygoid fossa
Genitourinary
Limbs
Other

Deep-seated parameningeal tumours may cause indirect symptoms such as facial and other cranial nerve palsies and discharge from the ear with tumours in the middle ear, or airway obstruction and nasal discharge from nasopharyngeal primaries. Dysphagia may occur with tumours in the oropharynx. Lymph node metastasis is common with testicular and genitourinary sites and may be the presenting sign, but is very unusual with head and neck (particularly orbital) primaries.

Investigation and staging

Important investigations include chest radiography and thoracic CT scan, bone scan, ultrasonography of the liver, and CT and/or MRI of the abdomen (in patients with abdominopelvic primary tumours). In head, neck and orbital cases, detailed plain radiographs, CT and/or MRI are essential for determining the local extent of the primary site. In the orbit, scanning may show extension into the nasal or maxillary sinus when it is then considered parameningeal. Intracranial extension is uncommon.

For parameningeal sites, MRI will frequently reveal invasion of the skull base and intracranial extension. An ear, nose and throat examination is necessary. In other head and neck sites, an examination under anaesthesia may be necessary to delineate the tumour. In genitourinary sites, CT has largely rendered urography unnecessary. CT scanning of the abdomen is also necessary in paratesticular tumours to identify enlarged para-aortic lymph nodes. Numerous staging systems have been proposed, but these have now been consolidated to form a widely accepted system of pretreatment staging based on the tumour node metastasis (TNM) system (Table 24.9).

Management

As with most paediatric tumours, current management [26,27] is complex and, for the majority of patients, includes surgery, radiotherapy and chemotherapy since none of these modalities alone gives satisfactory results. This integrated multimodal approach to treatment has led to a substantial improvement in prognosis – see, for example, Ref. [28] for an update on current treatment protocols and results from the US-based Children's Oncology Group. Until recently, radical surgical removal of the primary was always felt to be mandatory, a view which has undergone revision in recent years. Combination chemotherapy should now be used as the initial treatment, followed by local treatment with surgery and radiotherapy. Although surgery should be as complete as possible, careful judgement is required in order to avoid the risk of long-term mutilation. This has led, for example, to an increasing preference for wide excision (including compartmentectomy) rather than amputation for children with tumours of the extremities. When coupled with radical postoperative irradiation and early (adjuvant) chemotherapy this approach gives acceptably low local recurrence rates and allows for later amputation in the small number of cases where local recurrence occurs in the absence of more generalized disease.

With more deeply situated primary tumours such as those in the nasopharynx, primary surgery plays no part other than to establish the histological diagnosis. In some of the deeply situated but more accessible abdominopelvic primaries, the role of surgery is more uncertain, though it is increasingly accepted that major procedures such as total cystectomy or exenteration should not be performed in the first instance since effective irradiation and chemotherapy may result in cure with far less long-term damage. Combinations of chemotherapy and irradiation are increasingly used to achieve local control in orbital rhabdomyosarcoma, and it is sometimes possible to save

the eye. Embryonal and alveolar rhabdomyosarcoma are relatively sensitive to irradiation (particularly embryonal rhabdomyosarcoma), though high doses are required for effective control (50–60 Gy over 5–6 weeks).

Chemotherapy has now been established as an important part of treatment in both metastatic and recurrent cases, and also as an adjuvant to local treatment. Many agents are known to produce objective responses in significant numbers of patients, including vinca alkaloids, alkylating agents, actinomycin D, doxorubicin, methotrexate, ifosfamide, cisplatin, carboplatin and etoposide (Table 24.11). Chemotherapy of metastatic disease usually produces only temporary remission. Treatment with combination chemotherapy is preferable using, for example, vincristine, actinomycin D and cyclophosphamide, although actinomycin D should not be given synchronously with radiation because of radiation recall phenomena that are sometimes dangerous, and cyclophosphamide is usually deferred until after radiotherapy because of the danger of myelosuppression. Adjuvant chemotherapy is usually continued for 9 months. Localized tumours require only 6 months' therapy. Tumours in special sites may require particular treatment strategies; for example, in parameningeal tumours prophylactic treatment with intrathecal chemotherapy and cranial irradiation may be needed.

At present, multicentre studies in both Europe and the USA are attempting to provide answers to several unresolved issues such as the need for radiotherapy, the most

---

Table 24.11 Chemotherapy in rhabdomyosarcoma in childhood.

Single agents
Vincristine
Actinomycin D
Doxorubicin
Cyclophosphamide
Mitomycin C
Cisplatin
Ifosfamide
Etoposide

Combination chemotherapy regimens
Vincristine, actinomycin D, cyclophosphamide
Vincristine, actinomycin D, cyclophosphamide, doxorubicin
Other regimens including cisplatin, ifosfamide and etoposide
as part of study protocols especially in poor-prognosis
disease

acceptable and effective form of adjuvant chemotherapy, and the duration of adjuvant treatment.

Prognosis

The stage of disease is the most important prognostic factor; both the extensiveness of the primary lesion (which will govern the likelihood of resectability) and the presence of metastases affect survival. Overall 5-year survival rates according to pretreatment stage are given in Table 24.9. As with other paediatric tumours, age at presentation also affects prognosis. The median survival is better for children under 7 years. Younger children have less extensive disease at the time of diagnosis, and in general a more favourable tumour type (predominantly embryonal rhabdomyosarcoma) than older children. Site may also be important, and orbital tumours in general have a better prognosis though other head and neck tumours, particularly nasopharynx, have a poor prognosis presumably due to their inaccessibility, late presentation and unsuitability for surgical resection as well as propensity for spread to the CNS.

Recurrence tends to occur early, usually (90%) within the first 2 years.

Retinoblastoma
Incidence and inheritance

Retinoblastoma is a rare but important tumour with a familial incidence. The rate appears to have doubled over the past 40 years and retinoblastoma now has a frequency of 1 per 15 000 live births, accounting for about 3% of all childhood malignancies. This lifetime cumulative incidence rate results in an estimated 18 000–30 000 live births worldwide. A higher incidence is noted in developing countries, very likely due to lower socioeconomic status and also the presence of human papilloma virus sequences within the retinoblastoma tissue. Its increasing incidence is also partly due to the fact that it is an inherited disease in which survival is increasing, which in turn leads to an increase in the number of children born to previously affected parents.

There are two forms of the disease, namely, the inherited or non-inherited types (all cancers are considered genetic in that mutations of the genome are required for their development, but this does not imply that they are heritable, or transmitted to offspring). About 55% of children with retinoblastoma have the non-heritable variety; when there is no history of the disease within the family, the disease is labeled 'sporadic', though this does not necessarily indicate that the particular case is of the non-heritable form. Bilateral cases (the minority, about one-third of all patients) are commonly heritable, while unilateral cases are more commonly non-heritable. The number (and size) of tumours in each eye may vary and in certain rare cases, groups of patients have been reported in which bilateral retinoblastoma is associated with pinealoblastoma – alternatively termed 'trilateral retinoblastoma'.

Genetic Abnormalities, Testing and Counselling

Genetic testing should be performed in all cases as identifying the *Rb1* gene mutation that led to a child's retinoblastoma is important in both the clinical care of the affected individual and also in the potential approach to the care of present and future siblings and even, later in life any offspring of treated patients. As mentioned above, many cases are of the heritable form though most children with retinoblastoma have a normal karyotype. In those with associated mental retardation (see below), a deletion on the long arm of chromosome 13 is present (13q14). Chromosome loss and loss of heterozygosity at this site can be shown in all patients. Tumour formation occurs only when both genes are lost.

The *Rb1* gene codes for a nuclear phosphoprotein which is DNA-binding. The introduction of the normal *Rb1* gene product suppresses tumorigenicity. The *Rb1* gene may be inactivated in other tumours, for example, small-cell carcinoma of the lung and breast cancer. The gene product appears to have a general cell-cycle suppressor function.

Patients with retinoblastoma have a greatly increased likelihood of developing a second tumour. Those with bilateral (inherited) disease have a 20% risk of a monocular cancer, of which the commonest is osteosarcoma, and occasionally Ewing's sarcoma, Wilms' tumour and soft-tissue sarcoma.

Most cases of retinoblastoma are sporadic (non-familial). When familial, it is inherited by an autosomal dominant gene, though some individuals can apparently carry this defective gene without developing the tumour. Sporadic non-familial cases are mostly unilateral, with only a small risk that the offspring of these patients will subsequently develop the disease (Figure 24.8). However, in sporadic bilateral cases, there is a 50% chance of the offspring developing the disease. In retinoblastoma families, most affected children will themselves develop bilateral disease so that in apparently unilateral familial cases, a close watch must be kept on the contralateral eye. In genetic counselling (Table 24.12) it is also important to recognize that about 4% of normal parents of an affected child will produce more than one child with the disease. Retinoblastoma can on rare occasions be associated with

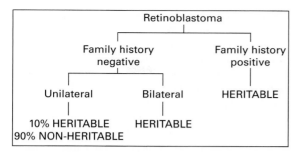

Figure 24.8 Inheritance of retinoblastoma.

Table 24.12 Genetic counselling in retinoblastoma.

Bilateral disease is almost always familial

Offspring of survivors of hereditary retinoblastoma, or of bilateral sporadic cases, will have a 50% chance of developing the tumour

Unaffected parents with a child with unilateral disease have a 1–4% chance of having another affected child

Survivors of unilateral sporadic disease have a 7–10% chance of having an affected child, and are therefore presumed to be silent carriers

If two or more siblings are affected, there is a 50% chance that subsequent siblings will have the tumour

Unaffected children from retinoblastoma families may occasionally (5%) carry the gene, but if they have an affected child the risk in subsequent children is 50% since the parent is then identified as a silent carrier

---

mental retardation, microcephaly and skeletal deformity, in which cases a deletion at 13q14 may be observed. If the *RB1* mutation of an affected individual is identified, amniotic cells in any later at-risk pregnancy can also be tested for the potential family mutation and any foetus carrying the mutation can be delivered early, allowing earlier treatment of any eye tumours, with better visual outcomes and preservation of sight.

Pathology

Retinoblastoma is thought to arise from a retinal neuroepithelial progenitor. Microscopically, the tumour typically consists of an admixture of undifferentiated and small cells with deeply staining nuclei and scant cytoplasm, though larger cells are often found, sometimes with a tendency to rosette formation around the central cavity.

Retinoblastoma is typically multifocal. This is presumably due to spread of tumour within the retinal layers, as well as to synchronous tumour development within

different parts of the retina in cases of bilateral disease, since spread via the optic nerves and chiasm does not generally occur. The commonest route of spread, the so-called 'endophytic type' of tumour, is forward into the vitreous humour, and this growth within the globe tends to occur before other involvement of periglobal structures. The 'exophytic' growth pattern is when the tumour arises from the outer retinal layers and grows outwards. Retinal detachment may occur during this process, but extension of growth into the choroid does not usually occur other than with very large tumours. Seeds of tumour may break off and implant themselves in the eye. Invasion of the choroid increases the risk of haematogenous spread. Invasion of the sclera may also occur, carrying a poor prognosis; the optic nerve itself may be directly invaded by the tumour via the lamina cribrosa, and the tumour may thence spread to the subarachnoid space with dissemination of tumour cells into the cerebrospinal fluid, with consequent seeding along the base of the brain.

Blood-borne metastases occur, most commonly to the bone marrow, liver, lymph nodes and lungs.

Clinical features

Most children present under the age of 2, usually with a white pupil (leucocoria) or, less commonly, with strabismus, glaucoma, defects in visual fixation, or inflammatory changes within the eye. Any family history of retinoblastoma should immediately raise suspicion, and the most important investigation is a careful ophthalmological examination by an experienced ophthalmic surgeon. This gives an assessment of tumour site, extent, involvement of the contralateral eye and evidence of multicentricity. The corneal light reflex or Hirschberg test is valuable as a means of checking for symmetrical reflection of beam of light in the same spot on each eye, when a light is shined into each corne – to assist in determining whether the eyes have a significant but subtle strabismus. Only the ophthalmologist can reliably exclude important non-malignant diseases such as *Toxocara* infection or retinal dysplasia; biopsy is considered unwise since this may provide a pathway for tumour dissemination.

Investigation

Tumour calcification may also be present radiologically. Chest radiography, full blood count and isotope bone scanning should be performed in all cases, with cerebrospinal fluid examination whenever there is suspicion of CNS involvement. CT and MRI are now used to assess disease extent.

Table 24.13 A simplified staging system with prognosis (percentage 3-year survival) in retinoblastoma. For a more detailed assessment, see Ref. [29].

Stage I	Single or multiple tumours of size less than 4 disc diameters at or behind the equator (90–100%)
Stage II	Single or multiple tumours of size 4–10 disc diameters at or behind the equator (90–100%)
Stage III	Tumours anterior to the equator or a single tumour larger than 10 disc diameters at or behind the equator (70–85%)
Stage IV	Multiple lesions, some greater than 10 disc diameters. This group includes any lesion extending anteriorly to the ora serrata (70–75%)
Stage V	Massive tumours involving over half the retina, or tumours with vitreous seeding (33–70%)
Stage VI	Residual orbital disease. Extension into the optic nerve and through the sclera (30%)

Staging

Size, site and multicentricity of tumour have led to the widely accepted clinical staging system that has now been in clinical use for over 25 years (Table 24.13). This simple system depends on ophthalmoscopic examination with accurate diagrammatic representation of the retinal lesion in relation to standard reference landmarks such as the optic nerve head, ora serrata (junction of the retina and ciliary body) and so on. A new international classification has recently been introduced based more on response characteristics to chemotherapy (see Further reading). The new system addresses more closely the twin objectives of treatment: overall survival of the patient, and preservation of the eye and its functioning.

Treatment

Treatment [30] depends on the presenting stage. In recent years, treatment philosophy has moved away from immediate or early enucleation of the more severely affected eye to a more conservative policy with a much greater reliance on chemotherapy and radiotherapy as the preferred local technique. The excellent results of this approach (see below) are highly dependent on careful ophthalmological assessment in every case. Eradication of tumour with preservation of vision has in most cases become a realistic aim. An outstanding recent review from the multidisciplinary team from Toronto makes

several powerful points: 'Parents are now leading the effort for widespread awareness of the danger of leucocoria. Genome-level technologies could make genetic testing a reality for every family affected by retinoblastoma. Most importantly, active participation of survivors and families will ensure that the whole wellbeing of the child is prioritised in any treatment plan' – see Ref. [31].

With very small tumours (<7 mm diameter), cryosurgery and photocoagulation are both effective, though with tumours near the optic disc or macula external beam irradiation is preferable because light coagulation close to these critical parts of the eye carries a risk of permanent visual damage. For these tumours, external irradiation using a single lateral field is both simple and effective.

For larger tumours (3–10 mm) brachytherapy (see Chapter 5) with radioactive cobalt plaques is frequently used, but smaller tumours near the optic disc or macula are better treated with external beam irradiation. With single tumours above 10 mm, external beam irradiation of the whole eye is frequently used and usually requires multifield treatment to ensure homogeneous irradiation of the whole globe, particularly where there is vitreous seeding. Use of an anterior field allows for more adequate sparing of the contralateral eye even though the lens and cornea are unavoidably treated. This technique is also suitable where there are multiple tumours confined to one eye. A dose of 35 Gy in 3–4 weeks is sufficient to control most intraocular retinoblastomas. With posteriorly situated tumours, a lens-sparing approach is preferable, using contact lenses to locate the cornea.

With obvious infiltration of the optic nerve, enucleation is preferable.

Chemotherapy has become the preferred initial treatment for many children with retinoblastoma, particularly infants with bilateral tumours and older children with extensive bilateral disease (when chemotherapy is frequently combined with external beam radiation). The main indications for chemotherapy for intraocular retinoblastoma include tumours that are large and/or those that cannot be treated with local therapies alone in children with bilateral disease. It is also quite often used in patients with unilateral disease when the tumours are small but cannot be controlled with local therapies alone. This approach has avoided some of the bony deformity that is the inevitable consequence of external beam radiation to the developing skull. With bilateral tumours, preservation of sight is more difficult, and it is best to treat each eye individually, on its own merits, rather than assuming that enucleation of the worse eye will invariably be required. Where there is residual tumour in the orbit after removal of the eye, postoperative irradiation should be given to include the whole orbit and optic foramen. A dose of 50 Gy in 5 weeks is both effective and well tolerated in children requiring postoperative irradiation of the orbit, in whom the radiation tolerance of the eye is no longer a consideration. Particular care is required to ensure immobilization either by means of a head cast or with sand bags.

In all cases of retinoblastoma, treatment planning must be precise, aiming to cover all areas of disease without unnecessarily jeopardizing the lens of both the affected and the contralateral eye. Unfortunately, and even with modern beam-shaping and intensity-modulated radiotherapy approaches, with the radiation dose required to control most retinoblastomas (35–40 Gy in 3.5–4 weeks) significant complications are still common, particularly when the child is very young. The commonest complication, cataract formation, is unavoidable when anterior beams are used, though not all cataracts are clinically significant and, if necessary, lens extraction is fairly simple and effective. Vascular injury from irradiation, though easily visible to the ophthalmologist, rarely impairs vision, but occasionally retinal haemorrhage may result in secondary glaucoma that can be troublesome. Irreversible damage to the orbital bones is a frequent complication preventing normal growth and impairing the long-term cosmetic outcome. Following radiation, there is a greatly increased risk of second cancers, especially bone sarcoma. Overall, during a 20-year period follow-up, the relative risk is increased 350-fold, with 12% of patients developing a second malignant neoplasm, particularly in inherited-retinoblastoma genetically affected patients, in whom the second-cancer rate is reportedly as high as 35%. The use of anthracyclines and alkylating agents almost certainly adds to this risk. These late-onset cancers are most likely to occur within the irradiated site, although the risk of malignancy elsewhere is also greatly increased. Sadly, after highly effective treatment of the primary or first tumour, enucleation of the affected eye is often necessary when cure seemed to have been initially achieved.

Cytotoxic chemotherapy is increasingly used. It has a clear role in bilateral disease, in poor-risk tumours with optic nerve invasion (detected following enucleation) or choroidal invasion, in relapsed disease (in the orbit or metastatic) and when disease recurs in a sole remaining eye. Vincristine, carboplatin and etoposide are the drugs most usually employed in combination chemotherapy. The results of treatment for advanced and extraocular retinoblastoma are poor. Adjuvant chemotherapy for

these high-risk tumours has improved the chances of cure. Surgical or radiation cure is rare in patients with massive orbital disease or extensive optic nerve involvement at presentation. In these very advanced cases, death is as likely to result from intracranial involvement as from distant metastases, and although combination chemotherapy, whole-brain irradiation and intrathecal chemotherapy have undoubtedly produced worthwhile responses, no cures have yet been reported. Cooperative paediatric groups in the UK, USA, Australia and elsewhere are currently conducting new clinical trials to assess these many issues further.

Prognosis [32]

The results of treatment are very good (Table 24.13), particularly in early cases and where specialized facilities and experienced clinicians are available. Cure rates of 90% have been achieved in the UK as a whole. In one large series, children with stage I and II disease had a cure rate of 100%, and even those with stage IV and V disease had a cure rate of 75%. When conservative measures have failed, enucleation of the eye can be curative, though there is still a 10–15% overall mortality rate due to intracranial spread or distant metastases. A few children, successfully treated, will later die from a second radiation-induced tumour (usually osteosarcoma).

Histiocytoses

This group of disorders, comprising 3–4% of paediatric tumours, originates from the macrophage/monocyte series of cells. These cells arise in the bone marrow, circulate briefly as blood monocytes and then migrate to tissues where they become fixed macrophages in the liver, spleen, lung, bone marrow and tissues (histiocytes) or antigen-presenting (dendritic) cells This subject is well covered in a recent review from pathologists at Harvard – see Ref. [33]. As they point out, 'Langerhans cell histiocytosis (LCH) combines in one nosological category a group of diseases that have widely disparate clinical manifestations but are all characterized by accumulation of proliferating cells with surface markers and ultrastructural features similar to cutaneous Langerhans cells (LCs) ... Important questions about LCH remain unanswered. First, despite having phenotypic features of LCs, LCH cell gene-expression patterns differ from those in LCs. ... Second, LCH's prominent inflammatory component and occasional benign clinical course suggest that LCH may not be a neoplasm. However, the demonstration that LCH cells are clonal, along with the recent discovery of activating BRAF mutations in

LCH cells, *strongly suggests that LCH is a neoplastic disease.* [our italics]. These new observations point the way to rationally targeted therapies'. The disorders described below in class 1 are often multifocal, sensitive to cytotoxic agents and irradiation, but nevertheless can be fatal.

The classification of histiocytoses has recently been altered and is now based on the nature of the histiocytic infiltrate.

• Class 1 histiocytosis is characterized by the presence of the Langerhans' cell. These cells may not be malignant and may respond to immunological mediators. Under electron microscopy, the cells show typical Birbeck granules. Opinion is still divided as to whether this is a malignant disease. In some cases, however, monoclonality of cells has been demonstrated [34].

• Class 2 lesions are characterized by a reactive macrophage infiltrate. The two disorders in this category are the rare and rapidly fatal familial erythrophagocytic lymphohistiocytosis, and infection-associated haemophagocyte syndrome.

• Class 3 comprises malignant histiocytic tumours, including monocytic leukaemia (see Chapter 28).

Langerhans' cell histiocytosis (class 1 histiocytosis)

Langerhans' cell histiocytosis [34] was previously termed histiocytosis X, a now outdated term that encompasses a spectrum of disease comprising Letterer–Siwe disease, eosinophilic granuloma and Hand–Schüller–Christian disease. Letterer–Siwe disease, an acute disorder with onset in infancy, is characterized by hepatosplenomegaly, lymph node enlargement, thrombocytopenia and skin rash. A greasy scaly scalp or nappy (diaper) rash is usually the presenting feature. Widespread infiltration of the skin, liver, lungs, spleen and bone marrow gives rise to hepatic dysfunction, dyspnoea and marrow failure. Lytic lesions in bone are common. The form of the disease previously called eosinophilic granuloma has a presentation that ranges from a single isolated bone lesion, typically in older children, to multiple punched-out bone lesions. The prognosis is worse below the age of 3 years. Presentation is usually with bone pain or lymphadenopathy. The disease may regress spontaneously. Other patients present with multiple eosinophilic granulomas. Occasionally, diabetes insipidus may occur due to pituitary involvement, as well as exophthalmos from orbital deposits (Hand–Schüller–Christian disease). Enlargement of liver and spleen occurs, as does skin infiltration, but the disease is less aggressive than Letterer–Siwe disease. As with eosinophilic granuloma, the disease may become quiescent and does not usually relapse if the activity ceases for 3–4 years. Diabetes insipidus is permanent, and chronic neurological disability may occur as a result of cirrhosis with prolonged portal hypertension.

Prognosis and treatment

Mortality is highest in infants and in children with organ infiltration (lung, liver, bone marrow). Single bone lesions can be treated by curettage and local steroid injection. Radiation in low dosage is often dramatically effective but carries the risk of bone sarcoma in later life. More generalized disease can be treated with cytotoxic drugs of which the most useful are prednisolone, vinblastine, etoposide, chlorambucil and methotrexate. However, the disease may follow a very indolent course and may even remit completely even without treatment, and it is important to avoid toxicity. In many cases (especially those where the disease is confined to the bone or skin), treatment can be withheld for long periods of time.

Rare paediatric tumours

The tumours described above, the intracranial tumours of childhood, and the leukaemias and lymphomas constitute 92% of all childhood malignancies; the remaining 8% are made up of a variety of uncommon diseases seen only sporadically even in large paediatric centres. Some, such as hepatoblastoma and orchioblastoma, are true paediatric tumours whereas others, such as adenocarcinoma of the kidney or transitional cell carcinoma of the bladder, are essentially adult tumours seen very rarely in the paediatric age group. The principles of management of some of these rare paediatric malignancies are not yet clearly established. The importance of a joint approach, with full pretreatment assessment by paediatric surgeon, radiotherapist and paediatric oncologist (working closely with a histopathologist with special experience in these tumours), cannot be emphasized too strongly. A good outline of these rare conditions is provided in a recent text – see Ref. [35].

Hepatoblastoma

This rare tumour (though the commonest of primary paediatric liver cancers) occurs in children below the age of 5 – usually below the age of 3. It is occasionally associated with Wilms' tumour. It can be associated with anomalies such as hemihypertrophy as well as with familial adenomatous polyposis coli (FAP) and Fanconi's syndrome. In cases associated with FAP there is germline mutation of the *APC* gene on chromosome 5q. Cytogenetic abnormalities in tumours are deletions in 1p, 1q and 11p (a site commonly involved in Beckwith–Wiedemann syndrome in which hepatoblastoma may occur).

The pathological features are immature hepatic epithelial cells or a mixture of these cells with mesenchymal elements [36]. It usually arises in the right lobe and presents with a visible asymptomatic mass which later causes pain and weight loss. Like hepatocellular carcinoma (which occurs in children over the age of 5), the tumour produces α-fetoprotein (AFP), which may be elevated above the normal infantile range. The tumour can be delineated by ultrasound and CT scanning. Arteriography is essential if an unusual resection is to be attempted. Occasionally, the tumour is associated with thrombocytosis (thrombocytopenia is more likely to indicate a vascular tumour).

The tissue diagnosis is usually made by biopsy to exclude other liver tumours. It does not appear possible to cure these children without complete surgical excision. Up to 75% of the liver can be removed but haemorrhage can be severe and great skill is necessary. Preoperative chemotherapy is now given to most cases of hepatoblastoma. The tumour shrinks and surgical excision is facilitated. As pointed out in a useful recent review, '… even in patients with advanced local disease, complete resection is now a possibility because of improvements in liver transplantation techniques' – see Ref. [37].

Cisplatin and doxorubicin are the most effective agents. Responses are also reported to alkylating agents such as ifosfamide. Recent studies have also suggested a possible role for dose-dense cisplatin since this is clearly the most active agent presently available – see Ref. [38]. Of 62 high-risk patients, the 3-year event-free survival was 67%, a remarkable achievement. Serum AFP can be used to assess response to treatment. Prognosis is worse the more sections of the liver that are involved, if there is diffuse invasion, and if there are metastases. A very high AFP and node involvement are adverse indicators.

Germ-cell tumours

All the adult germ-cell tumours (see Chapters 17 and 19) are occasionally seen in childhood. In addition, specific childhood forms occur though none is common.

Sacrococcygeal germ-cell tumours

These are the most common germ-cell tumours of childhood and the commonest tumour of the newborn. The female to male ratio is 4:1. The tumour arises on the inner margin of the distal part of the coccyx. The tumour is often external with variable internal components between the coccyx and the rectum. Approximately 10% of tumours in the newborn are malignant, but above 3 months of age 50% are malignant. Where possible, tumour should be surgically excised. When this is not possible, and if there are malignant elements (embryonal carcinoma, choriocarcinoma), chemotherapy should be given. If a good response is obtained, surgical excision may then be possible.

Head and neck germ-cell tumours

Of childhood teratomas, 10% arise in the head and neck. The sites are very variable (orbit, soft tissue, nasopharynx), and they may cause respiratory obstruction. Treatment is with surgery and chemotherapy (if malignant). Pineal teratomas are discussed in Chapter 11.

Testicular germ-cell tumours

The main histological variants are the yolk sac tumour (endodermal sinus tumour, Teilum tumour, orchioblastoma), embryonal carcinoma and differentiated tumour. Below the age of 2, yolk sac tumours are probably less likely to metastasize than in older children. The differentiated tumours are benign. Before effective chemotherapy was available, 9% of children under 2 years old were alive 2 years after treatment, while only 25% of older children survived. This difference may be less marked since the advent of platinum-based chemotherapy. The management follows the guidelines outlined for adult testicular tumours (see Chapter 19).

Sex cord and stromal tumours of the testis

Leydig cell tumours and Sertoli cell tumours occur rarely, the Leydig cell tumour at age 4–5 years and the Sertoli cell tumour below the age of 2 years. Leydig cell tumours, which may be accompanied by testicular virilization, are slow-growing and cured by orchidectomy. Sertoli cell tumours may cause feminization, and orchidectomy is adequate treatment.

Gonadoblastomas are very rare tumours, chiefly found in patients with testicular feminization (XY or XY/X0 karyotype with dysgenetic gonads and feminine phenotypes). The tumour develops in an abnormal gonad, which is frequently indeterminate or no more than a rudimentary streak. The testes may be maldescended, in which case they are present in the inguinal canals or abdomen.

Ovarian germ-cell tumours

The classification of these tumours is discussed in Chapter 17. Dysgerminomas, embryonal carcinoma and teratoma are managed as outlined in that chapter; as in adults, surgery and combination chemotherapy are the major modalities.

Late sequelae of treatment of cancer in childhood

As more children and adolescents survive cancer, we are becoming increasingly aware of late effects of treatment – see, for example, an excellent recent summary Editorial [39]. The importance of these problems has in turn led to re-examination of the primary treatment in some stages of some tumours, if the same survival can be achieved at less long-term cost. There are three areas of particular concern: effects on growth [40], gonadal function [41], quality of life [42] and the occurrence of second cancers [43,44]. All these important issues are well discussed in a recent guidance document from Scotland – see Ref. [45] – which offers several new recommendations, for example, in fertility, cardiac health, bone health, metabolic syndromes and even dental health: an extremely valuable and practical set of guidelines.

Growth

Studies in acute lymphoblastic leukaemia where both chemotherapy and prophylactic cranial irradiation were administered have shown significant decreases in height during treatment, which is regained to a varying degree when treatment stops. The site of damage is not definitely known but growth hormone deficiency and a lack of responsiveness of the epiphysis to growth hormone, induced by chemotherapy, certainly play a part. In children treated with radiation for brain tumours, growth retardation is greater in those who are also given chemotherapy. It is not known which cytotoxic agents are most likely to produce growth impairment.

Radiation of a growing epiphysis results in arrest of bone growth at that site. The dose required to produce permanent closure of the epiphysis is not known with certainty, but most schedules of treatment for cancer will do so. In a young child this may lead to a gross disparity in limb length, failure of development of the spine (after mantle treatment for Hodgkin's disease, for example) or asymmetry of the chest wall or head and neck.

Gonadal function

Children treated with nitrosoureas and procarbazine for brain tumours have a high incidence of gonadal dysfunction [41,42]. Although puberty progresses

normally, follicle-stimulating hormone levels are high (and luteinizing hormone to a lesser degree). In later life, the boys have small testes and severe oligospermia. In girls, ovarian function appears to return to normal and prospects for fertility are often good though recent studies have given more information regarding the risk factors for infertility than were previously available – see, for example, Ref. [46]. The outcome following successful treatment for childhood cancer depends on a variety of factors including exposure to alkylating agents, and in particular, the use of pelvic or total-body irradiation – all of course adverse factors, and well summarized by Anderson [47] and studied in detail by the Childhood Cancer Survival Study (CCSS) of 3531 female survivors of childhood cancer treatment who reported having ever been sexually active (excluding those with known ovarian failure). The effects of pelvic irradiation are particularly striking though the separate effects of uterine and ovarian irradiation were not separable in this study. It is suggested that even low-level irradiation of the uterus may have a more damaging outcome than previously thought. The majority of female cancer survivors will have normal reproductive function and would be expected to have a successful pregnancy [48], though there remains an additional risk of preterm delivery and/or a low-birthweight baby. For some women with apparently normal menstrual periods and thought likely to be fully fertile, a reduced level of antimullerian hormone, itself known to be a marker of ovarian reserve, will give a useful clue in doubtful cases or patients where gonadal function needs assessing because of primary infertility in an apparently normal clinical setting. It is not known if the menopause will be premature in patients who have had treatment, but it is wise to assume that this is likely, and counsel patients accordingly. In some acute lymphoblastic leukaemia protocols, spinal irradiation may of course affect either the ovaries or even the testes.

In boys who do not receive alkylating agents there is much less germinal epithelial damage. If mustine, vincristine (Oncovin), prednisone and procarbazine therapy has been given for Hodgkin's disease, severe oligospermia and high follicle-stimulating hormone levels are the rule. Damage appears to be less long-lasting if treatment is given prepubertally.

Second cancers and other chronic conditions

The possibility of inducing a second cancer by treatment is particularly important in childhood cancers because of the long period of risk. For example, it now

Table 24.14 Relative risk of bone cancer according to primary diagnosis.

Diagnosis	Relative risk
Retinoblastoma	350
Ewing's sarcoma	250
Rhabdomyosarcoma	30
Wilms' tumour	30
Hodgkin's disease	30

appears that about one in every 180 survivors of a childhood CNS cancer will develop a non-neurological second malignancy within 15 years, according to a very large recent international population-based study of over 8400 survivors [49]. Most of these occurred within 10 years from the initial diagnosis, and the risk was particularly marked in patients surviving a glioma or primitive embryonal tumour. One of the commonest types of radiation-induced second cancer is bone sarcoma [43], the relative risk depending on the primary diagnosis (Table 24.14). The secondary cancer is usually osteosarcoma, and it typically develops within the initial radiation field (though often not, in the case of the inherited form of retinoblastoma; see Figure 24.8).

Acute non-lymphoblastic leukaemia may develop after treatment with chemotherapy: alkylating agents, etoposide and nitrosoureas appear to be the drugs most likely to be associated. The risk seems higher after treatment for Hodgkin's disease (where radiation is often also given). Leukaemia is also more common after successful treatment for childhood brain tumours. Overall, the relative risk of leukaemia determined by the Late Effects Study Group was 14 times greater [44]. A recent report from the same group has confirmed an even higher incidence of solid tumours, particularly breast cancer, two-thirds occurring in patients who received both chemotherapy and radiation [50]. The scale of these risks has been clearly demonstrated in a large study from the Sloan-Kettering Cancer Centre in New York [51]. These investigators calculated the frequencies of cancer and chronic conditions in over 10 300 survivors, comparing these with their siblings and demonstrating that long-term survivors of childhood cancer are more likely to have a reduced health status, and indeed to die prematurely than other adults. As well as the second cancers noted above, other problems included a higher

rate of cardiovascular disease, renal dysfunction, severe musculoskeletal problems and endocrinopathies. Sadly, the incidence of these chronic conditions increased over time and did not appear to plateau during the course of observations, underscoring the necessity of continued follow-up of survivors of childhood cancer, with emphasis on surveillance for second cancers (e.g. breast, colorectal, melanoma and other skin cancers), coronary artery disease, late-onset anthracycline-related cardiomyopathy, pulmonary fibrosis and so on. As a group, the cancer survivors were eight times as likely as their siblings to have severe or life-threatening chronic health conditions, particularly survivors of bone tumours, CNS tumours and Hodgkin's disease.

Cancer in children of survivors

Apart from an increased risk of cancer in children of survivors of hereditary cancer such as retinoblastoma, there does not appear to be an excess incidence of cancer in offspring of survivors of paediatric cancer [52].

References

1 Kreicbergs U, Valdimarsdottir U, Onelöv E et al. Talking about death with children who have severe malignant disease. *N Engl J Med* 2004; 351: 1175–86. [Correspondence *N Engl J Med* 2005; 352: 91–2.]

2 Pritchard J, Stiller CA, Lennox EL. Overtreatment of children with Wilms' tumour outside paediatric oncology centres. *Br Med J* 1989; 299: 835–6.

3 Stiller CA. Epidemiology and genetics of childhood cancer. *Oncogene* 2004; 23: 6429–44.

4 Marshall AD, Grosveld GC. Alveolar rhabdomyosarcoma – The molecular drivers of PAX3/7-FOXO1-induced tumorigenesis. *Skelet Muscle* 2012; 2: 25. Doi: 10.1186/2044-5040-2-25.

5 Elliott A (Chairman). *The Distribution of Childhood Leukaemia and Other Childhood Cancers in Great Britain, 1969–1993*. Committee on Medical Aspects of Radiation in the Environment (COMARE), 11th report. Available from www.comare.org.uk.

6 Bluhm EC, Daniels J, Pollock BH et al. Maternal use of recreational drugs and neuroblastoma in offspring: a report from the Children's Oncology Group (United States). *Cancer Causes Control* 2006; 17: 663–9.

7 Maris JM, Hogarty MD, Bagatell R, Cohn SL. Neuroblastoma. *Lancet* 2007; 369: 2106–20.

8 Maris JM, Mosse YP, Bradfield JP et al. Chromosome 6p22 locus associated with clinically aggressive neuroblastoma. *N Engl J Med* 2008; 358: 2585–93.

9 Hiyama E, Iehara T, Sugimoto T et al. Effectiveness of screening for neuroblastoma at 6 months of age: a retrospective

population-based cohort study. *Lancet* 2008; 371: 1173–80. [Correspondence *Lancet* 2008; 372: 372–3].

10 Brodeur GM, Pritchard J, Berthold F *et al.* Revisions of the International Criteria for neuroblastoma diagnosis, staging, and response to treatment. *J Clin Oncol* 1993; 11: 1466–77.

11 Gains J, Mandeville H, Cork N *et al.* Ten challenges in the management of neuroblastoma. *Future Oncol* 2012; 8: 839–58.

12 Navarro S, Piqueras M, Villamon E *et al.* New prognostic markers in neuroblastoma. *Expert Opin Med Diagn* 2012; 6: 555–67.

13 Kushner BH, Modak S, Kramer K *et al.* Ifosfamide, cisplatin, and etoposide for neuroblastoma: a high-dose salvage regiment and review of the literature. *Cancer* 2013; 119: 665–71.

14 Matthay KK, Villablanca JG, Seeger RC *et al.* Treatment of high-risk neuroblastoma with intensive chemotherapy, radiotherapy autologous bone marrow transplantation and 13-cis-retinoic acid. *N Engl J Med* 1999; 341: 1165–73.

15 Klingebiel T. Role of purging in PBSC transplantation for neuroblastoma. *Lancet Oncol* 2013; 14: 919.

16 Yu AL, Gilman AL, Ozkaynak MF, *et al.* for the Children's Oncology Group. Anti-GD2aAntibody with GM-CSF, interleukin-2, and isotretinoin for neuroblastoma. *New Engl J Med* 2010; 363: 1324–34.

17 Moroz V, Machin D, Faldum A *et al.* for the International Neuroblastoma Risk Group Project. Changes over three decades in outcome and the prognostic influence of age-at-diagnosis in young patients with neuroblastoma: a report from the International Neuroblastoma Risk Group Project. *Eur J Cancer* 2011; 47: 561–71.

18 Rivera M, Kim W, Wells J *et al.* An X chromosome gene, WTX, is commonly inactivated in Wilms' tumor. *Science* 2007; 315: 642–5.

19 Ahmed HU, Arya M, Tsiouris A *et al.* An update on the management of Wilms' tumour. *Eur J Surg Oncol* 2007; 33: 824–31.

20 Pietras W. Advances and changes in the management of children with nephroblastoma. *Adv Clin Exp Med* 2012; 21: 809–20.

21 D'Angio GJ, Breslow N, Beckwith JB *et al.* Treatment of Wilms' tumour: results of the third National Wilms' Tumour Study. *Cancer* 1989; 64: 349–60.

22 Davidoff AM. Wilms Tumor. *Adv Pediatr* 2012; 59: 247–67.

23 Seibel NL, Li S, Breslow NE *et al.* Effect of duration of treatment on treatment outcome for patients with clear cell sarcoma of the kidney: a report from the National Wilms' Tumour Study Group. *J Clin Oncol* 2004; 22: 468–73.

24 Uddin Ahmed H, Arya M, Levitt G *et al.* Review Part 1: primary malignant non-Wilms' renal tumours in children. *Lancet Oncol* 2007; 8: 730–7.

25 Newton WA, Gehan EA, Webber BL *et al.* Classification of rhabdomyosarcomas and related sarcomas. Pathological aspects and proposal for a new classification: an Intergroup Rhabdomyosarcoma Study. *Cancer* 1995; 76: 1073–85.

26 Maurer HM, Beltangady M, Gehan EA *et al.* The Intergroup Rhabdomyosarcoma Study 1. A final report. *Cancer* 1988; 61: 209–20.

27 Flamant F, Rodary C, Voute PA, Otten J. Primary chemotherapy in the treatment of rhabdomyosarcoma in children: trial of the International Society of Paediatric Oncology preliminary results. *Radiother Oncol* 1985; 3: 227–36.

28 Raney RB, Waterhouse DO, Meza JL *et al.* Results of the Intergroup Rhabdomyosarcoma Study Group D9602 protocol, using vincristine and dactinomycin with or without cyclophosphamide and radiation therapy, for newly diagnosed patients with low-risk embryonal rhabddabdomyosarcoma: a report from the Soft Tissue Sarcoma Committee of the Children's Oncology Group. *J Clin Oncol* 2011; 29: 1312–8.

29 Sobin LH, Gospodarowicz MK, Wittekind Ch, eds. *TNM Classification of Malignant Tumours*, 7th edn. Chichester: Wiley-Blackwell, 2009.

30 Harnett AN, Hungerford J, Lambert G *et al.* Modern lateral external beam (lens sparing) radiotherapy for retinoblastoma. *Ophthalmic Paediatr Genet* 1987; 8: 53–61.

31 Dimaras H, Kimani K, Dimba EA *et al.* Retinoblastoma. *Lancet* 2012; 379: 1436–46.

32 Sanders B, Draper GJ, Kingston JE. Retinoblastoma in Great Britain 1969–80, incidence, treatment and survival. *Br J Ophthalmol* 1988; 72: 576–83.

33 Badalian-Very G, Vergilio JA, Fleming M, Rollins BJ. Pathogenesis of Langerhans cell histiocytosis. *Annu Rev Pathol* 2013; 8: 1–20.

34 Willman CL, Busque L, Griffith BB *et al.* Langerhans cell histiocytosis (histiocytosis X): a clonal proliferative disease. *N Engl J Med* 1994; 331: 154.

35 Schneider DT, Brecht IB, Olson TA, Ferrari A. *Rare Tumors in Children and Adolescents*. Springer, 2012. ISBN 9783642041969.

36 Haas JE, Muczynski KA, Krailo M *et al.* Histopathology and prognosis in childhood hepatoblastoma and hepatocarcinoma. *Cancer* 1989; 64: 1082.

37 Honeyman JN, La Quaglia MP. Malignant liver tumors. *Semin Pediatr Surg* 2012; 21: 245–54.

38 Zsiros J, Brugieres L, Brock P *et al.* Dose-dense cisplatin-based chemotherapy and surgery for children with high-risk hepatoblastoma (SIOPEL-4): a prospective, single-arm feasibility study. *Lancet Oncol* 2013; 14: 834–42.

39 Lancet Oncology Editorial. It doesn't stop at cure: monitoring childhood cancer survivors. *Lancet Oncol* 2013; 14: 671.

40 Clayton PE, Shalet SM, Morris-Jones P *et al.* Growth in children treated for acute lymphoblastic leukaemia. *Lancet* 1988; i: 460–2.

41 Livesey EA, Brook CGD. Gonadal dysfunction after treatment of intracranial tumours. *Arch Dis Child* 1988; 63: 495–500.

42 Jenney ME, Levitt GA. The quality of survival after childhood cancer. *Eur J Cancer* 2002; 38: 1241–50.

43 Hawkins MM, Kinnier-Wilson M, Burton HS *et al.* Radiotherapy, alkylating agents and the risk of bone cancer after childhood cancer. *J Natl Cancer Inst* 1996; 88: 270–8.

44 Jenkinson HC, Hawkins MM, Stiller CA *et al.* Long-term population-based risks of second malignant neoplasms after childhood cancer in Britain. *Br J Cancer* 2004; 91: 1905–10.

45 Wallace WHB, Thompson T, Anderson A. Long term follow-up of survivors of childhood cancer: summary of updated SIGN guidance. *Brit Med J* 2013; 346: f1190.

46 Barton SE, Najita JS, Ginsburg ES *et al.* Infertility, infertility treatment, and achievement of pregnancy in female survivors of childhood cancer: a report from the Childhood Cancer Survivor Study cohort. *Lancet Oncol* 2013; 14: 873–81.

47 Anderson RA. Infertility in women after childhood cancer. *Lancet Oncol* 2013; 14: 797–8.

48 Edgar AB, Wallace WH. Pregnancy in women who had cancer in childhood. *Eur J Cancer* 2007; 43: 1890–4.

49 Maule M, Scélo G, Pastore G *et al.* Risk of second malignant neoplasms after childhood central nervous system malignant tumours: an international study. *Eur J Cancer* 2008; 44: 830–9.

50 Bhatia S, Robinson LL, Oberlin O *et al.* Breast cancer and other second neoplasms after childhood Hodgkin's disease. *N Engl J Med* 1996; 334: 745–51.

51 Oeffinger KC, Mertens AC, Sklar CA *et al.* Chronic health conditions in adult survivors of childhood cancer. *N Engl J Med* 2006; 355: 1572–82.

52 Sankila R, Olsen JH, Anderson H *et al.* Risk of cancer among offspring of childhood-cancer survivors. *N Engl J Med* 1998; 338: 1339–44.

Further reading

Alston RD, Rowan S, Eden TOB *et al.* Cancer incidence patterns by region and socioeconomic deprivation in teenagers and young adults in England. *Br J Cancer* 2007; 96: 1760–6.

Anon. Clinical trials in children, for children [Editorial]. *Lancet* 2006; 367: 1953.

Aslett H, Levitt G, Richardson A, Gibson F. A review of long-term follow-up for survivors of childhood cancer. *Eur J Cancer* 2007; 42: 1781–90.

Bhatia S. What is the risk of second malignant neoplasms after childhood cancer? *Nat Clin Pract Oncol* 2005; 2: 182–3.

Birch JM, Pang D, Alston RD *et al.* Survival from cancer in teenagers and young adults in England, 1979–2003. *Br J Cancer* 2008; 99: 830–5.

Bleyer A, Viny A, Barr R. Cancer in 15- to 29-year olds by primary site. *Oncologist* 2006; 11: 590–601.

Burton A. The UICC My Child Matters Initiative Awards: Combating cancer in children in the developing world. *Lancet Oncol* 2006; 7: 13–14.

Ellis CN, ed. *Inherited Cancer Syndromes: Current Clinical Management.* Berlin: Springer Verlag, 2004.

Ellison LF, Pogany L, Mery LS. Childhood and adolescent cancer survival: a period analysis of data from the Canadian Cancer Registry. *Eur J Cancer* 2007; 43: 1967–75.

Ferrari A, Bisogno G, de Salvo P *et al.* The challenge of very rare tumours in childhood: the Italian TREP project. *Eur J Cancer* 2007; 43: 654–9.

Gommersall LM, Arya M, Mushtaq I, Duffy P. Current challenges in Wilms' tumor management. *Nat Clin Pract Oncol* 2005; 2: 298–304.

Gupta N, Banerjee A, Haas-Kogan D, eds. *Pediatric CNS Tumors.* Berlin: Springer Verlag, 2004.

Hart R. Preservation of fertility in adults and children diagnosed with cancer. *Br Med J* 2008; 337: 1045–8.

Haupt R, Spinetta JJ, Ban I *et al.* Long term survivors of childhood cancer: cure and care. The Erice Statement. *Eur J Cancer* 2007; 43: 1778–80.

Hewitt M, Weiner SL, Simone JV. *Childhood Cancer Survivorship: Improving Care and Quality of Life.* Washington, DC: National Academy Press, 2003.

Kreitler S, Arush MWB, eds. *Psychosocial Aspects of Pediatric Oncology.* Hoboken, NJ: Wiley, 2004.

Lacey EKF, Clarke NMP. The big idea. Paediatric oncological pathology: a new phenomenon. *J R Soc Med* 2008; 101: 324–6.

Liben S, Papadatou D, Wolfe J. Paediatric palliative care: challenges and emerging ideas. *Lancet* 2008; 371: 852–64.

Linet MS, Ries LA, Smith MA, Tarone RE, Devesa SS. Cancer surveillance series: recent trends in childhood cancer incidence and mortality in the United States. *J Natl Cancer Inst.* 1999; 91: 1051–1058.

Linn Murphree A. Intraocular retinoblastoma: the case for a new group classification. *Ophthalmol Clin North Am* 2005; 18: 41–53.

Martinez-Monge R, Cambeiro M, San-Julian M *et al.* Use of brachytherapy in children with cancer: the search for an uncomplicated cure. *Lancet Oncol* 2006; 7; 157–66.

Metzger ML, Billett A, Link MP. The impact of drug shortages on children with cancer – the example of mechlorethamine. *New Engl J Med* 2012: 367: 2641–3.

Mitchell W, Clarke S, Soper P. Survey of psychosocial support provided by UK paediatric oncology centres. *Arch Dis Child* 2005; 90: 796–800.

Neglia JP, Friedman DL, Yasui Y, *et al.* Second malignant neoplasms in five year survivors of childhood cancers: childhood cancer survivor study. *J Natl Cancer Inst* 2001; 93: 618–29.

Pearson AD, Pinkerton CR, Lewis IJ *et al.* High-dose rapid and standard induction chemotherapy for patients aged over 1 year with stage 4 neuroblastoma: a randomised trial. *Lancet Oncol* 2008; 9: 247–56.

Pinkerton R, Shankar AG, Matthey K. *Evidence-based Pediatric Oncology*, 2nd edn. Oxford: Blackwell Publishing, 2007.

Ribeiro RC, Pui CH. Saving the children – improving childhood cancer treatment in developing countries. *N Engl J Med* 2005; 352: 2158–60.

Senior K. Teenagers with cancer: an improving picture. *Lancet Oncol* 2006; 7: 366.

Wawszczyk R. A teenager's experience of cancer. *J R Soc Med* 2005; 98: 370–1.

Whelan J, Dolbear C, Mak V *et al*. Where do teenagers and young adults receive treatment for cancer? *J Public Health (Oxf)* 2007; 29: 178–82.

Wilne SH, Dineen RA, Dommett RM, Walker DA. Identifying brain tumours in children and young adults. *Brit Med J* 2013; 347: f5844.

World Health Organization. The 58th World Health Assembly adopts resolution on cancer prevention and control. Available at www.who.int/mediacentre/news/release//2005/pr_wha05/en/index.html, accessed 18 August 2006.

25   Hodgkin's lymphoma

The prognosis of Hodgkin's Lymphoma (this term is now preferred to 'Hodgkin's Disease') has greatly improved, both for patients with localized disease, who are often curable by radiotherapy, and for those with disseminated disease treated with cytotoxic drugs. The overall cure rate is now of the order of 80–90%, and modern approaches are increasingly geared towards a reduction of treatment-related complications (sometimes fatal in the long-term – see below), since these tragic risks can be considerably reduced by proper treatment individualization and entry of the patient into a well-conducted clinical trial. These points are further discussed below. Success has been achieved not only because of the introduction of new methods of treatment, but also because it has become apparent how radiotherapy and chemotherapy can be employed to best advantage. There have also been improvements in staging techniques and a better understanding of the patterns of spread, which have led to more rational treatment.

Incidence and epidemiology

The incidence of Hodgkin's Lymphoma rises steeply from the age of 10–20 years. There is a slight fall in middle age, followed by a rise after 50 years to reach a maximum at age 70 years and over (Figure 25.1). The male-to-female ratio in Western countries is about 1.5:1. Although the relative age incidence varies in different parts of the world, the male predominance usually holds (Table 25.1).

The reported variation in incidence appears to reflect genuine differences in the frequency of the disease rather than in the accuracy of diagnosis. In some countries such as Colombia and Nigeria the incidence in childhood (age 5–14) is five times that in the UK, but in adult life it is four times less common. In these countries the history also tends to be less favourable compared with western Europe and North America. In Japan and possibly other Far Eastern countries, the incidence appears to be substantially lower than in the West.

Cancer and its Management, Seventh Edition. Jeffrey Tobias and Daniel Hochhauser.
© 2015 John Wiley & Sons, Ltd. Published 2015 by John Wiley & Sons, Ltd.

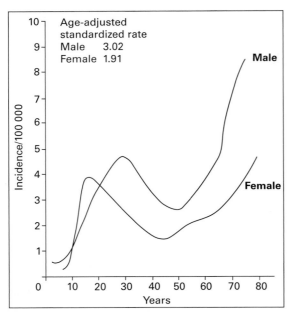

Figure 25.1 Hodgkin's disease: age-specific incidence.

Table 25.1 Hodgkin's lymphoma: annual incidence rates (per 100 000) in various countries.

	Male	Female
England	2.2	1.3
USA		
Whites	2.3	1.4
African-Americans	1.3	0.7
Japan	0.6	0.3
Sri Lanka	0.1	0.1

Aetiology

Genetic, family and social factors

There is an excess of human histocompatibility antigen identity in affected siblings. In the family of a patient the risk of siblings having the disease is greater than normal, possibly about six times that of the normal population, with siblings of the same sex most likely to be affected. The disease is slightly more frequent in higher socioeconomic groups. The meaning of rare, but dramatic, clusters of cases is unknown but may suggest an environmental rather than (or as well as) a genetic cause [1].

Infections

Epstein–Barr virus (EBV) is the infectious agent that has the strongest claim to an association with Hodgkin's Lymphoma. This virus infects B cells, the acute infection, infectious mononucleosis, being controlled by a cytotoxic T-cell response. A history of infectious mononucleosis in the previous 3 years is associated with a four-fold risk of Hodgkin's lymphoma [2]. EBV is a widely ubiquitous herpes virus, spread mainly through saliva. The majority of primary EBV infections throughout the world are subclinical and antibodies to EBV have been demonstrated in all population groups with a worldwide distribution – approximately 90–95% of adults are EBV-seropositive. Cells similar to Reed–Sternberg (RS) cells have been found in lymph node biopsies from patients with infectious mononucleosis. The EBV genome can be detected in RS cells in 75% of cases of mixed cellularity histology, 40% of the nodular sclerosing variety, but not in lymphocyte-predominant disease.

The role of EBV remains open, since the finding of viral genome and latent membrane protein does not prove that it is a cause of transformation – the same findings are present in non-neoplastic proliferation.

Pathology

The Hodgkin Reed–Sternberg cell

Lymph nodes from patients with Hodgkin's Lymphoma contain two categories of cells. The first is the cell that is the hallmark of the disease and which is thought to be the malignant component, the RS cell or its mononuclear counterpart (Figure 25.2). The second consists of a pleomorphic cellular infiltrate, the composition of which varies considerably in different patients.

The malignant cells are large, often with slightly basophilic cytoplasm. The nuclei are usually lobulated and there may be two or more in a single cell. The classical RS cell has two or more nuclei, usually with large nucleoli which are acidophilic. The mononuclear variety of cell is sometimes seen in reactive inflammatory nodes, and cells with a similar appearance to RS cells may occasionally be found in infective lesions (infectious mononucleosis) and other lymphoproliferative disorders such as phenytoin-induced lymph node enlargement and non-Hodgkin's lymphoma. The Hodgkin RS cell is a B lymphocyte derived from the germinal centre of lymph nodes [3]. The mechanism provoking the infiltrate of normal cells that make up the bulk of the nodal enlargement in the disorder is unclear. Their function is unknown.

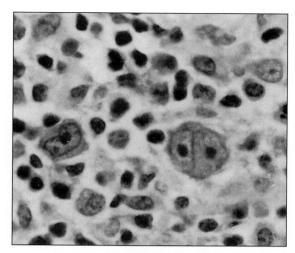

Figure 25.2 Section of a lymph node in Hodgkin's disease, showing typical binucleate Reed–Sternberg cell and mononuclear Hodgkin's cell (×400).

The techniques of immunohistochemistry and molecular genetics have been used in Hodgkin's Lymphoma to characterize the RS cell. Immunophenotyping shows B-cell characteristics in RS cells. CD20 and CD15 are usually expressed. CD30, an activation antigen on lymphoid cells, is strongly expressed on RS cells (and on other lymphomas and so-called Ki-1-positive lymphomas). Soluble CD30 is found in the serum of untreated patients. No consistent karyotypic abnormality has been found in Hodgkin's disease although a variety of chromosomal translocations have been detected.

Classification

The histological classification that is widely used is based on the revised American–European classification [4], which divides the microscopic appearance into five categories.

1 *Lymphocyte rich.* The appearances are of small lymphocytes with scarce RS cells and mononuclear variants. These are sparse within B-lymphocyte-rich node.

2 *Nodular lymphocyte predominant.* The tumour has a nodular appearance with mononuclear Hodgkin's cells that have a B-cell phenotype that differs from typical RS cells. The disease usually presents as stage 1 disease. There is a risk of development of a B-cell non-Hodgkin's lymphoma, usually after an interval of 10 years.

3 *Nodular sclerosis.* There are broad bands of collagen separating cellular nodules of Hodgkin's disease. The tumour contains mononuclear 'lacunar' cells that are

typical of this form. Nodular sclerosing disease has been subcategorized into two groups, where group 1 has a lymphocyte-predominant infiltrate in the nodules and group 2 has a more pleomorphic appearance with numerous RS cells. Patients in group 1 have been reported to have a better prognosis [5].

4 *Mixed cellularity.* The infiltrate is pleomorphic with lymphocytes, macrophages, eosinophils and polymorphs.

5 *Lymphocyte depleted.* There is either diffuse fibrosis with fewer RS cells, or a reticular type with numerous RS cells or their mononuclear variant.

The nodular sclerosing and mixed cellularity categories make up 80–90% of all cases. Prognostically, lymphocyte-predominant histology is most favourable and lymphocyte-depleted histology least so. Most of the relationship between prognosis and histology relates to disease stage. In patients of similar tumour stage, histology has little influence on outcome.

Sometimes the pathologist has difficulty in deciding if the patient has Hodgkin's disease or not, and mistakes can occur. The clinician should be very careful in cases which have atypical histology obtained from non-nodal sites, and with clinically odd presentations such as isolated disease presenting in the gut or skin. The differential histological diagnosis includes the following:

- reactive nodes with immunoblasts, which may be seen in infectious mononucleosis, other herpes virus infections or toxoplasmosis;
- hypersensitivity to drugs such as phenytoin;
- angioimmunoblastic lymphadenopathy (see Chapter 26);
- T-cell lymphoma (see Chapter 26);
- metastatic melanoma;
- non-Hodgkin's lymphoma, particularly the distinction from sclerosing B-cell mediastinal lymphoma and Ki-1 lymphoma (see Chapter 26).

In patients with proven Hodgkin's disease, other histological abnormalities may be found. The spleen or liver may show granulomatous infiltration of unknown cause. After intensive chemotherapy the lymph nodes may show an unusual appearance, with vascular invasion and atypical lymphocyte-depleted histology with few inflammatory elements, appearances similar to a non-Hodgkin's lymphoma.

Abnormal immunity in Hodgkin's Lymphoma

Host defence against infection is abnormal in advanced Hodgkin's Lymphoma even before treatment.

Radiotherapy and chemotherapy can impair these defence mechanisms still further. In advanced disease, there are depressed delayed hypersensitivity reactions to a variety of antigens including tuberculin, *Candida*, mumps and histoplasmin.

Patients with Hodgkin's lymphoma are susceptible to opportunistic infections. These include infections with bacteria such as *Pseudomonas* and tuberculosis, fungi such as *Candida* and *Aspergillus*, and viruses such as herpes zoster and herpes simplex. In all these diseases, susceptibility is probably due to depressed cell-mediated immunity (CMI).

The more advanced the disease, the greater the likelihood of anergy, but there is little clinical value in tests of immune competence as part of the routine investigation of a newly diagnosed case. The degree of spread of the disease is better assessed by more straightforward investigations.

The treatment of patients with advanced disease with cytotoxic drugs is hazardous for many reasons, one of the most important being the additional depression of immunity, which can even occasionally result in overwhelming or fatal infection. Fortunately, this is now uncommon but as ever, vigilance and attention to clinical detail is essential to avoid this tragic consequence.

Clinical features

In the majority of cases the clinical presentation is straightforward [6]. The patient will have accidentally noticed an enlarged painless lymph node in the neck or elsewhere, and a biopsy gives the diagnosis. The initial site of presentation (Figure 25.3) includes cervical nodes (70% of all cases), axilla (25%) and inguinal area (10%). The lymph nodes usually grow slowly and are sometimes visible on photographs months or years before being noticed by a patient. Occasionally, the nodes are described as growing very rapidly and sometimes they are tender if there has been a recent upper respiratory infection. The nodes may fluctuate in size with such infections and may mislead the physician into believing that the node enlargement is only inflammatory.

About a quarter of all patients have constitutional symptoms at presentation. Fever is the commonest of these and is generally of low grade but may occasionally be hectic, up to 40°C, which usually occurs in the evening and falls to normal in the morning. In advanced disease, bouts of fever lasting 1 or 2 weeks may occur (Pel–Ebstein fever) but this is unusual and not specific

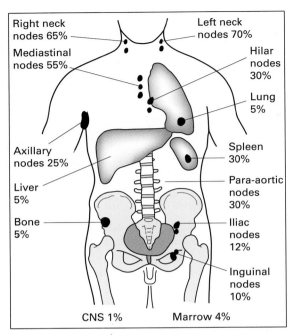

Figure 25.3 Frequency of sites of involvement at presentation in patients with Hodgkin's disease.

for Hodgkin's Lymphoma. Drenching sweats may occur at night, waking the patient from sleep. Lesser degrees of sweating occur in many normal individuals and are hard to evaluate. Weight loss is especially associated with advanced or bulky disease. The triad of constitutional symptoms (fever, sweats and more than 10% loss of body weight) is clinically important because cases with one or more of these features have a poorer prognosis.

Generalized pruritus occurs in 5–10% of patients at the time of presentation, but more patients will develop this symptom during the course of the disease when it relapses. If severe, it can be very disabling, the skin becoming excoriated from scratching, especially at night. The cause is not understood. The symptom abates with successful treatment. Alcohol-induced pain is felt in involved lymph nodes in a very small number of patients (2–5%). It is aching or stabbing in nature, comes on within minutes of drinking, and lasts from a few minutes to an hour. It is associated with mediastinal disease of nodular sclerosing histology.

Other rare systemic features of Hodgkin's Lymphoma include autoimmune haemolytic anaemia (although a positive antiglobulin test in the absence of haemolysis is more common) and immune thrombocytopenia.

A variety of erythematous skin rashes may occur, including erythroderma, erythema multiforme, psoriasiform lesions and bullous eruptions.

Enlarged nodes may produce symptoms due to compression. Examples include limb oedema and pain due to nerve entrapment; cough, stridor or superior vena caval obstruction from mediastinal disease; obstruction of the inferior vena cava or the ureters by para-aortic nodes; and obstructive jaundice due to nodes in the porta hepatis. Internal mammary node enlargement may give rise to a chest wall mass in the parasternal region. In contrast to non-Hodgkin's lymphoma, the tonsil and Waldeyer's ring are rarely involved. When this does occur it is usually associated with upper cervical node involvement.

Hodgkin's Lymphoma occasionally presents as a pulmonary lesion and then must be distinguished from infection or other bronchial tumours by sputum cytology, culture and biopsy. Endobronchial Hodgkin's Lymphoma is very rare, the clinical features being wheezing and haemoptysis. Much more commonly, pulmonary infiltration occurs from direct spread from enlarged hilar or mediastinal nodes. Pulmonary nodules of Hodgkin's Lymphoma are easily missed on chest radiographs, and computed tomography (CT) is very useful when the diagnosis is in doubt. Pleural infiltration usually presents as an effusion, and is nearly always associated with mediastinal and pulmonary disease. If the mediastinal disease is massive, the pleural effusion may be due to lymphatic obstruction rather than direct invasion by tumour. The same is true for chylous effusions. A diagnosis of pleural infiltration can be made reliably only by biopsy or by CT scan showing nodules of tumour in the pleura or subpleural lung. Cytological examination is usually unrewarding since RS cells are rarely found.

Bone marrow involvement occurs at presentation in approximately 5% of patients and is nearly always associated with widespread disease elsewhere, and with constitutional symptoms. The diagnosis is by marrow biopsy. The number of positive routine marrow biopsies in patients with early-stage disease is very small, but a normal blood count does not preclude involvement in those with advanced disease. However, marrow involvement is more likely if there is anaemia, thrombocytopenia or leucopenia. The disease is focal within the marrow, so false-negative biopsies are frequent.

Occasionally, the bones are involved in a more localized way by Hodgkin's Lymphoma, either by direct spread from adjacent nodes or by metastatic spread (in which case there is usually widespread disease elsewhere). The commonest histology is nodular sclerosis.

The presentation is with pain, the serum alkaline phosphatase is elevated, radiographs may show either osteoblastic or osteolytic lesions, and an isotope bone scan is positive. A solitary bone deposit does not necessarily indicate stage IV disease (i.e. diffuse involvement of an extranodal tissue; see Table 25.2) and may respond to local treatment, with a good prognosis.

Skin and subcutaneous infiltrations are uncommon as presenting features but may occur over lymph node masses or in their drainage areas, usually in the context of aggressive disease. The nodules of tumour are often painless but may ulcerate. Subcutaneous lesions may occur in the breasts. Primary cutaneous Hodgkin's Lymphoma is a great rarity.

Table 25.2 Ann Arbor staging classification for Hodgkin's Lymphoma, still in wide use after 30 years.

Stage I	Involvement of a single lymph node region or of a single extralymphatic site or organ
Stage II	Involvement of two or more node regions on the same side of the diaphragm, or of a localized extranodal involvement and one or more lymph node regions on the same side of the diaphragm (IIE)
Stage III	Involvement of lymph nodes on both sides of the diaphragm which may also include the spleen (IIIS) or a localized extranodal site (IIIE), or both (IIISE)
Stage IV	Diffuse involvement of one or more extralymphatic organs

Notes

1 Suffix A: no constitutional symptoms. Suffix B: constitutional symptoms present. These include fevers, night sweats and/or loss of 10% or more of body weight over 6 months. Pruritus is not included.

2 Localized extranodal involvement can at times be difficult to distinguish from stage IV disease. A good working rule is that localized spread means that the lesion in question could still be treated with radiotherapy.

3 Stage III disease can be usefully subdivided according to the extent of intra-abdominal node involvement. Stage III1 means involvement of spleen and splenic, coeliac or portal nodes or any combination of these. Stage III2 means involvement of para-aortic, iliac or mesenteric nodes with or without upper abdominal disease.

4 In the case of the marrow or liver, diffuse involvement means the demonstration of any amount of unequivocal Hodgkin's disease since localized spread at these sites is not recognized and radiotherapy is not regarded as a treatment option.

When Hodgkin's Lymphoma involves the central nervous system (CNS), it is usually spinal rather than cerebral. This is a rare presentation and usually occurs by extension through the intervertebral foramina from adjacent lymph nodes to cause epidural compression. The clinical features are of root pain, paraesthesiae or spinal cord compression. All are medical emergencies because there is a serious risk of paraplegia (see Chapter 8). When this occurs as the presenting symptom, laminectomy and radiotherapy are the usual methods of histological diagnosis and treatment. If the diagnosis is already established, prompt treatment with radiotherapy and steroids is usually adequate. Compression of the spinal cord may be localized and does not necessarily constitute an indication for chemotherapy. Hodgkin's Lymphoma may on rare occasions present with leptomeningeal spread, with a clinical syndrome of basal malignant meningitis causing cranial nerve palsies, or symptoms and signs of raised intracranial pressure.

The gut is rarely the primary site of Hodgkin's Lymphoma and the diagnosis should be viewed with suspicion, since gastrointestinal non-Hodgkin's lymphomas are so much more common. Nevertheless, there are isolated cases of the disease arising in the oesophagus, stomach, and small and large bowel. The presentation is usually indistinguishable from other tumours at these sites. When the disease occurs in the small bowel it usually affects the terminal ileum and may cause malabsorption syndrome.

The urinary tract is seldom clinically involved, and the commonest manifestation is ureteric compression with hydronephrosis. It is very unusual for direct renal infiltration to be clinically apparent. Rarely, cases of nephrotic syndrome occur which are due either to an immune complex glomerulonephritis or to compression of the renal veins by tumour masses.

Hodgkin's Lymphoma may be accompanied by paraneoplastic syndromes (see Chapter 9). In the CNS, patients may rarely develop progressive multifocal leucoencephalopathy. This is a relentless, fatal, demyelinating disorder, now known to be caused by a papovavirus. It is characterized by dementia, disorientation and focal signs leading to coma and death. Subacute cerebellar degeneration may occur with progressive ataxia, especially truncal ataxia, due to degeneration of Purkinje cells in the vermis. It usually does not improve with treatment of the disease. Guillain–Barré syndrome occurs in the disease more commonly than would be expected by chance. Segmental granulomatous angiitis may occur in the brain, which may respond to treatment of Hodgkin's Lymphoma and which is possibly related to varicella-zoster infection.

Patterns of spread

In early Hodgkin's Lymphoma, lymph node groups are much more commonly involved than others (Figure 25.3). By far the commonest site of presentation is the neck, while involvement of mesenteric nodes is rare. Following localized treatment, adjacent lymph nodes are the most frequent sites of relapse, a finding which led to the introduction of extended-field radiotherapy. In more detailed analyses, certain patterns of spread have been found. Bilateral cervical node enlargement is unusual unless there is also mediastinal disease; mediastinal disease is itself frequently associated with involved neck nodes. Unilateral upper cervical nodes involved with nodular sclerosing disease are seldom associated with disease at other sites. Nodular sclerosing Hodgkin's disease in the mediastinum is more frequently found in women and is not usually associated with subdiaphragmatic disease. Splenic involvement is uncommon when the presentation is with isolated inguinal node enlargement. Splenic disease, as the sole intra-abdominal site, occurs in only 10% of patients. In the abdomen the coeliac plexus is the commonest site of node involvement.

When the disease involves the liver or bone marrow, splenic disease is nearly always present. Involvement of the liver with sparing of the spleen is so unusual that the pathological findings should be questioned. It is not clear if splenic involvement is a source of dissemination, although vascular invasion in splenic Hodgkin's Lymphoma may signify a worse prognosis.

Staging classification [7,8]

The Ann Arbor classification is widely used as a description of clinical or pathological stage and is outlined in Table 25.2. This staging notation (with explanatory notes) is used throughout this chapter. The original Ann Arbor scheme did not take account of bulk of disease, number of sites of involvement or laboratory findings such as erythrocyte sedimentation rate (ESR) and lactate dehydrogenase, which influence prognosis. The scheme has been revised to take account both of these changes and of modern imaging methods.

Clinical stage refers to the anatomical description of the extent of the disease on the basis of clinical examination, chest radiography, CT and isotope scans. *Pathological stage* is based on information obtained by biopsy and other surgical procedures. The stage refers to staging based on histological identification of additional sites of spread.

When comparison was made between the results of clinical and pathological staging (based on laparotomy) it was found that for each clinical stage there was a 25–30% chance of error as judged by pathological stage. Although modern scanning techniques have reduced the falsenegative rate of clinical staging, occult intra-abdominal disease in normal-sized para-aortic nodes and spleen is impossible to detect reliably.

Investigation

Clinical examination

The presence of constitutional symptoms should be noted. The sites of clinically apparent disease should be carefully documented, and a diagram made of the major nodal masses.

Haematology and biochemistry

Full blood counts are normal in most patients with localized nodal disease without constitutional symptoms (stages IA and IIA). Mild anaemia, polymorphonuclear leucocytosis and a high ESR are more common with advanced disease. The anaemia is usually normochromic or slightly hypochromic and is typical of the anaemia of chronic disease. Autoimmune haemolytic anaemia may rarely occur at presentation. Lymphopenia usually signifies advanced disease but eosinophilia, which occurs in a few patients, has no prognostic significance. The ESR is a somewhat unreliable guide to extent and activity of disease but a high ESR (>40 mm/hour) is usually associated with more widespread disease.

Liver enzymes and plasma bilirubin are often abnormal with hepatic involvement, but an isolated modest elevation in aspartate aminotransferase or γ-glutamyltransferase sometimes occurs in the absence of proven involvement. The plasma alkaline phosphatase is often elevated, particularly in patients with advanced disease. Usually it is the liver isoenzyme which is responsible, but bone phosphatase may sometimes be contributory. An elevated alkaline phosphatase is not conclusive evidence of extensive disease if it is an isolated finding.

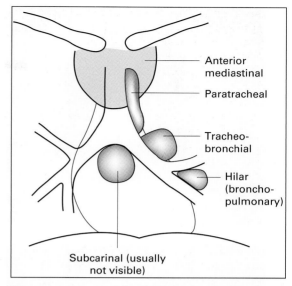

Figure 25.4 Anatomical distribution of the major lymph node groups that may be involved in Hodgkin's disease.

Routine radiography
Chest radiography

Chest radiography is essential. Enlargement of mediastinal and bronchopulmonary lymph nodes is very common, and the anatomical distribution of the lymph node groups is shown in Figure 25.4. Mediastinal adenopathy is particularly common in women with nodular sclerosing disease. Massive mediastinal node enlargement may occur, leading to superior vena caval obstruction (Figure 25.5). The thymus may be involved and often the mass projects laterally to the right and is seen anteriorly on lateral films. The bronchopulmonary lymph nodes may be enlarged with more subtle radiological changes. Usually there is associated mediastinal node enlargement.

The pulmonary changes may be due to compression of a bronchus, to direct intrapulmonary extension from a lymph node mass or, less commonly, to localized intrapulmonary Hodgkin's disease. Bronchial compression may cause atelectasis of a whole lobe with associated consolidation within the collapsed area. Direct extension from lymph nodes (Figure 25.6) is not infrequent. In patients who have been previously treated with radiation to mediastinal nodes, extension of the disease into the lung may be very difficult to distinguish radiologically from radiation pneumonitis and fibrosis.

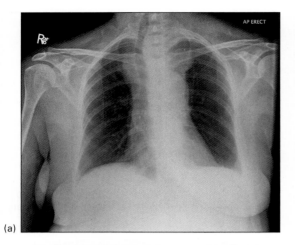

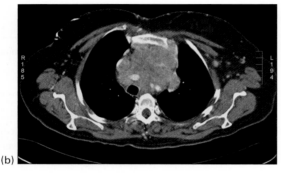

Figure 25.5 Chest radiograph showing a large well-defined mediastinal mass. The patient was a woman of 22, with nodular sclerosing Hodgkin's disease. (a) Anteroposterior chest radiograph. (b) Transaxial CT scan, same patient.

Tuberculosis and other infections may produce similar radiological appearances. A chest radiograph may also show enlargement of the cardiac shadow due to a pericardial effusion, or erosion of a rib or sternum due to local extension from lymph nodes.

Other imaging techniques

Thoracic CT scan will determine whether there is intrapulmonary spread of disease and will demonstrate small pulmonary and subpleural nodules of tumour. Involvement of mediastinal nodes is demonstrated. The additional information may lead to a change in treatment policy and the scans are of value in the planning of involved field (IF) radiotherapy.

Abdominal CT scanning of the abdomen is especially important in its capacity to show widespread disease in asymptomatic patients, because the management

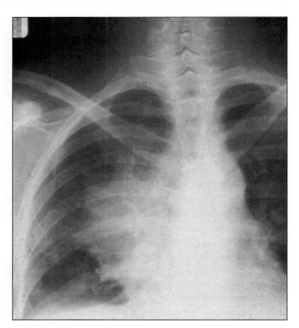

Figure 25.6 Involvement of hilar nodes with extension into the lung on the right.

will then of course be altered. MRI scanning may give additional useful information, and CT/PET fusion (see Chapter 4) is increasingly regarded as the "gold standard" with its excellent combination of anatomic detail with functional activity – especially valuable in disease monitoring, where over-treatment (e.g. with unnecessary radiation therapy following highly successful chemotherapy) can be damaging. It has for the first time permitted a more logical use of shrinking-field radiotherapy techniques during the treatment, as it may allow a safe reduction in radiation volume, tailoring the therapy to the individual requirement – see, for example, the important Swiss-German study from Engert *et al.* [9].

Bone scanning may sometimes be useful in demonstrating isolated areas of involvement. The information obtained from routine use is limited, but if there is bone pain it is an important investigation as a positive scan may change treatment policy. The areas revealed on the scan should also be examined radiologically because increased uptake on a bone scan has many possible causes – an important diagnostic pitfall.

In lymphography (now very rarely used), lymphatic channels are cannulated and low-viscosity contrast material is injected slowly. Radiographs of the pelvis and abdomen are taken at the time of injection and the next

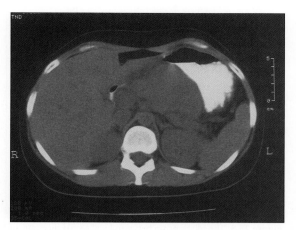

Figure 25.7 CT scan of the abdomen in a patient with stage III Hodgkin's disease. A large mass of lymph nodes is displacing the barium-filled stomach to the left.

day. Although the technique provides information about the involvement of lymph nodes that may not be enlarged on CT scan, it has largely been abandoned because it is technically difficult, uncomfortable and hypersensitivity reactions can occur.

Barium studies of the stomach and bowel are unnecessary unless there are clear symptoms requiring investigation. In the stomach, the usual radiological appearance of Hodgkin's disease is of a mass indenting the barium, occasionally with appearances suggesting ulceration (Figure 25.7). In the small and large bowel, the typical appearance is of a long segment of infiltration with a coarse and distorted mucosal pattern and thickening of the bowel wall. The involvement may be patchy and discontinuous.

Percutaneous biopsy

Some of the indications for percutaneous biopsy have already been discussed. Marrow trephine is a worthwhile investigation in patients for whom treatment may be with radiotherapy alone, since an involved marrow will indicate the need for chemotherapy. However, in localized Hodgkin's disease without constitutional symptoms only 5% of patients will have a positive trephine biopsy. Diagnosis may be difficult because typical RS cells may not be present. The mononuclear Hodgkin's cell may be found and may be sufficient for diagnosis. The involvement is usually focal so there are considerable sampling errors.

Percutaneous liver biopsy is not a reliable investigation because Hodgkin's Lymphoma may be focal within the liver. It can be useful in selected cases with abnormal liver function tests, constitutional symptoms or hepatomegaly, and if positive may remove the need for further staging procedures. There may be a considerable problem in interpreting liver biopsy material. Focal mononuclear infiltrates are frequently found, and pathologists are usually reluctant to diagnose the disease on the basis of occasional malignant-looking mononuclear cells. In both liver and marrow, non-caseating granulomata may be found, the cause of which is unknown, and these should not be confused with Hodgkin's Lymphoma.

Staging laparotomy and splenectomy

The introduction of laparotomy and splenectomy in the 1960s, now largely historic, showed that even in patients with clinical, localized (stage I or II) supradiaphragmatic disease there was a significant chance of finding disease below the diaphragm. Although this led to a greater understanding of the mode of spread of Hodgkin's Lymphoma, the advent of modern imaging techniques and the increased efficacy of chemotherapy have meant that the procedure rarely has a role in staging or subsequent investigation.

No purpose is served by a staging laparotomy and splenectomy if no change in the proposed treatment will follow – it has to have genuine discriminant value and there is no known therapeutic benefit from removing a diseased spleen. In clinically and radiologically localized disease above the diaphragm, a laparotomy might disclose subdiaphragmatic disease in 40% of patients. However, a policy of limited assessment followed by radiotherapy, with chemotherapy if there are adverse prognostic features or if relapse occurs, does not lead to reduced survival. Patients who are known beyond doubt to have stage IIIB, IVA or IVB disease, on the basis of clinical evidence and preliminary investigations, should not be subjected to laparotomy since drug treatment will be used (see below). In centres where it is routine practice to use chemotherapy for massive mediastinal disease and stage IIIA disease (Table 25.2), a laparotomy is also unnecessary.

Nowadays, treatment policy is therefore very seldom changed by laparotomy. Furthermore, splenectomy carries additional roles in patients who are already immunosuppressed by the disease and its treatment. Splenectomy adds to this susceptibility, with increased risk of infection with *Haemophilus influenzae* and

Streptococcus pneumoniae. Because staging laparotomy is now used only in unusual and specific circumstances, patients who have been treated for supradiaphragmatic disease with radiotherapy alone must be carefully watched for early symptoms of subdiaphragmatic relapse, which will occur in a substantial minority.

Treatment

There is now a good-to-excellent chance of cure for all patients, even when they present with extensive disease. Traditionally, the mainstay of treatment of localized disease has been radiotherapy, though this approach is increasingly being questioned in view of recent research showing results at least as good, with less overall hazard, with chemotherapy – see, for example, Ref. [10]. Chemotherapy is always used for advanced disease, and combined- chemo-radiation in selected particularly challenging clinical situations. The best chance of cure is when the patient first presents. Careful assessment of the treatment strategy is critical at this stage. While many patients can still be cured after relapse, recurrence of disease usually worsens the outlook.

The methods of using radiotherapy and drugs are changing fast and as ever, an understanding of the principles of these treatments is important in planning the correct approach in each individual patient.

Principles of radiotherapy

Like all lymphomas, Hodgkin's Lymphoma is highly sensitive to radiotherapy. The probability of long-term control (Figure 25.8) at the irradiated site is dependent on dose. The dose that is needed to eradicate clinically inapparent disease in adjacent nodes, or in nodal areas in remission after chemotherapy, is less than that required for greatly enlarged nodes and bulky tumour masses. The usual practice has been to treat both the involved and adjacent fields to the same dose level, usually in the region of 40 Gy in 25 daily fractions.

There has been considerable debate over many years as to whether it is preferable to treat only the sites of clinical involvement (involved field, IF) or whether to extend the field to adjacent nodes (extended field, EF). Because Hodgkin's Lymphoma spreads from the site of clinical involvement to adjacent lymph nodes, the contiguous, clinically uninvolved, nodes were included in the field when radiotherapy was the only curative treatment. Now that chemotherapy for relapse after radiation failure is so much more successful than it was at the time when

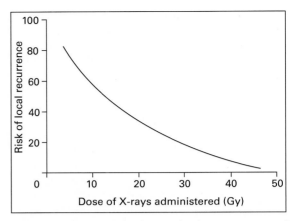

Figure 25.8 The relationship between local recurrence rate and dose of radiation administered.

EF radiation was first introduced, the long-term survival advantage for EF rather than IF is not apparent (see below).

Extended radiation fields commonly employed are the mantle field for treating disease in the neck, mediastinum and axillae, and the inverted-Y field for nodes in the para-aortic and iliac regions (Figure 25.9). The lungs, larynx and humeral heads are shielded. When large mediastinal masses are irradiated the field is often

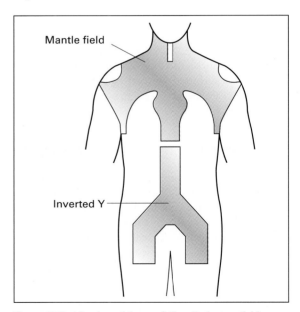

Figure 25.9 Mantle and inverted Y radiotherapy fields commonly employed for supradiaphragmatic and infradiaphragmatic nodal involvement in Hodgkin's disease.

progressively contracted as resolution occurs in order to avoid irradiating large volumes of lung (see Chapter 5). Recently, there has been an increasing tendency to reduce the size of the radiation fields in localized disease, especially when chemotherapy is given additionally (see below). The long-term effects of radiation are of increasing concern, particularly secondary fibrosis and cardiac toxicity.

Increasingly, patients with limited-stage disease are treated not with traditional radiotherapy at all, but with conventional combination chemotherapy, for example, using the 4-drug ABVD, which is generally associated with an equal response and disease-specific survival rate but a lower mortality from other causes – see Ref. [10] – and more fully described below.

Principles of chemotherapy [1]

Many classes of cytotoxic agents show activity against Hodgkin's Lymphoma. The approximate response rates obtained with the different drugs, when used as single agents in advanced disease, are shown in Table 25.3.

When cytotoxic drugs are used as single agents, the likelihood of a complete response is small and, if obtained, the response is not usually sustained for more than a few months. The major step forward was the development of combination chemotherapy. The first combination drug

regimen, and one that set the standard against which newer schedules have been judged, was MOPP (mustine, vincristine, prednisone and procarbazine). The details of this and other commonly employed regimens are given in Table 25.4. Current policies typically use either six cycles in total or two further cycles after achieving complete remission. Regimens have been developed in which seven or eight drugs have been combined into a single cycle usually over 10–14 days. Response rates are high but the regimens have not yet been shown to be more effective than standard combinations, of which the current benchmark is ABVD (doxorubicin, bleomycin, vinblastine and dacarbazine) introduced in the 1980s. The response to chemotherapy is usually rapid, with disappearance of fever and reduction in tumour masses. Previously untreated patients have a 40–50% chance of long-term relapse-free survival with these regimens and may be cured. The likelihood of achieving sustained complete response seems to be somewhat less in men, in patients over the age of 40 years, in those with marked constitutional symptoms and in patients with multiple sites of disease, especially if bulky. In these patients, alternating regimens of different drugs may improve response and survival. There are several other alternating combinations in common use such as LOPP (chlorambucil, vincristine,

Table 25.3 Approximate response rates to some of the commonly used agents in Hodgkin's Lymphoma (of historical interest only, but the basis of highly successful combination chemotherapy regimens).

	Complete response (%)	Partial response (%)	Total
Alkylating agents			
Nitrogen mustard	10	50	60
Cyclophosphamide	10	45	55
Chlorambucil	15	45	60
Vinca alkaloids			
Vincristine	30	30	60
Vinblastine	30	30	60
Other agents			
Prednisolone	0	60	60
Procarbazine	20	35	55
Doxorubicin	10	45	55
Bleomycin	5	40	45
DTIC	5	40	45

Table 25.4 Commonly used combination chemotherapy regimens in Hodgkin's Lymphoma.

ChlVPP (28-day cycle; for LOPP substitute vincristine for vinblastine)
Chlorambucil 6 mg/m² days 1–14 p.o.
Vinblastine 6 mg/m² days 1, 8 i.v.
Procarbazine 100 mg/m² days 1–14 p.o.
Prednisolone 40 mg days 1–14 p.o.
ABVD (28-day cycle)
Doxorubicin 25 mg/m² days 1, 15 i.v.
Bleomycin 10 mg/m² days 1, 15 i.v.
Vinblastine 10 mg/m² days 1, 15 i.v.
DTIC 375 mg/m² days 1, 15 i.v.
EVAP (alternates with LOPP every 28 days)
Etoposide 150 mg/m² days 1, 2, 3; max. 200 mg
Vinblastine 6 mg/m² days 1, 8; max. 10 mg
Doxorubicin 25 mg/m² days 1, 8
Prednisolone 25 mg/m² days 1–14; max. 200 mg
MOPP (28-day cycle)
Mustine 6 mg/m² days 1, 8 i.v.
Vincristine 2 mg (max.) or 1.4 mg/m² days 1, 8 i.v.
Procarbazine 100 mg/m² days 1–19 p.o.
Prednisolone 40 mg/m² days 1–14 p.o.

procarbazine and prednisolone) with EVAP (etoposide, vinblastine, doxorubicin and prednisolone). Response rate, duration and survival are much worse if the patient has previously been treated with single- or multiple-drug therapy. Previous radiotherapy does not seem to jeopardize response, although the toxicity may be greater (see below). The general principles of administration of the drugs are discussed in Chapter 6.

Risk-adapted treatment

Some patients with apparently localized disease treated with radiotherapy may relapse at distant sites. This is because there is more widespread microscopic disease than is detected at diagnosis (a fact confirmed by past experience with staging laparotomy). Most of these patients can receive chemotherapy on relapse and some may be cured. Other patients have clinical and biochemical features indicating a poor prognosis even if the disease appears localized.

These considerations, and the increasing evidence that radiation therapy is an important cause of later second cancer, has led to attempts to define patients who should receive chemotherapy as part of initial treatment, and to reduce the extent of radiation by adding chemotherapy as an adjuvant or associated initial treatment.

A simple prognostic score has been devised by an international collaborative group [8] based on biochemical and clinical factors for patients with advanced disease treated with chemotherapy, allowing identification of patients in whom more intensive treatments might be considered as initial treatment [12].

Management as determined by stage

In the following discussion, guidelines are given as to the management of Hodgkin's Lymphoma at presentation according to clinical and pathological stage. Clinical practice varies, so a consensus view is presented.

Clinical stage IA, IIA

In this category, patients without constitutional symptoms have one or more groups of nodes involved on one side of the diaphragm, and investigation has failed to show disease elsewhere. For this group of patients radiotherapy produces good results. The usual practice for patients with cervical and mediastinal disease has traditionally been to irradiate the mantle field (Figure 25.9) to a dose of 40–44 Gy in 20–25 fractions. For those presenting with inguinal node disease, the inverted-Y

radiation field is generally used. The use of chemotherapy in localized disease and the treatment of massive mediastinal disease are discussed separately, but in recent years there has certainly been a tendency, even in early-stage patients with favourable prognostic factors, towards a 'less radiotherapy, more chemotherapy' approach [12]. The overall likelihood of undiagnosed intra-abdominal disease (usually high para-aortic or splenic) is 35%. Two treatment strategies have been advocated.

1 To treat with either mantle field or IF irradiation only, and to rely on salvage irradiation or chemotherapy on relapse. The advantage of this approach is that it avoids over-treatment of a large number of patients, especially those with good histology, low risk scores and below 40 years of age in whom the risk of occult intra-abdominal disease is low (20%). About 70% of all patients will be cured by this approach. However, the question of whether treatment on relapse is as effective as early treatment is still somewhat controversial. More recent trials have shown that in those patients with 'poor' prognostic factors, combined radiation and chemotherapy offers better survival than radiation alone. In the 'good' prognosis group survival is not worse if chemotherapy treatment is delayed, although relapse is, as expected, more frequent in those treated with radiotherapy alone.

2 To treat with mantle or EF radiotherapy followed by six cycles of, or with, chemotherapy followed by irradiation. Again many patients will be over-treated and long-term sequelae of radiotherapy and chemotherapy are worrying (see below). Excellent long-term disease-free survival is usually obtained and this approach may be safest if the histology and other prognostic factors (such as ESR) are adverse. A meta-analysis using individual patient data has shown that the 10-year risk of disease relapse is greater (by 12%) in patients receiving reduced radiation fields, but survival is unchanged because of the efficacy of chemotherapy on relapse [13]. Similarly, the use of chemotherapy with radiotherapy is associated with a 17% reduction of relapse at 10 years but no definite effect on mortality.

The policy for this group of patients will, therefore, vary in different institutions. In the UK, most major centres adopt strategy 1 for patients without adverse features, reserving chemotherapy for relapse. Patients with adverse factors (poor histology, large tumour bulk, adverse prognostic score [8]) would usually be treated by chemotherapy and IF radiotherapy to sites of disease. A recent large multicentre study from the European Organization for Research and Treatment of Cancer (EORTC) has helped refine these recommendations further [14]. The aim of this large study (over 700 patients) was to reduce the toxicity of treatment using a combination of low-intensity chemotherapy and IF radiotherapy. Patients were stratified into 'favourable' and 'unfavourable' groups, based on the prognostic factors of age, number of involved areas, symptoms and mediastinal width. Chemotherapy (in the experimental arm of the study) consisted of six cycles of epirubicin, bleomycin, vinblastine and prednisone (EBVP) followed by IF radiotherapy. It was randomly compared in the favourable group to subtotal nodal irradiation, and in the unfavourable group to six cycles of MOP[P]/ABV (doxorubicin, bleomycin and vinblastine) hybrid, also together with IF radiotherapy. In favourable patients, the combination of EBVP and IF radiotherapy was superior to conventional radiotherapy (88% vs 78% event-free survival at 10 years). In the unfavourable group, the 'classical' MOPP/ABVD together with IF radiotherapy was substantially better than the experimental group: again, 88% event-free survival, compared with only 68% in the IF radiotherapy group, and leading to 10-year overall survival rates of 87% and 79%, respectively ($P = 0.0175$). In a further important study from the European cooperative group, chemotherapy (using MOPP plus ABV) and IF radiotherapy were compared with subtotal nodal radiotherapy without chemotherapy, for patients with early-stage disease with favourable prognostic features [12]. Again this was a large randomized study of over 1500 patients. The results showed a clear advantage for the combined-modality group, with an estimated 5-year survival rate of 98% versus 74% ($P < 0.001$). The authors made the bold statement that in contrast to previous recommendations for treatment, 'chemotherapy plus involved-field radiotherapy should [now] be the standard treatment for Hodgkin's disease with favorable prognostic features'. However, more recently, as mentioned above, the use of combination chemotherapy using ABVD has begun to replace routine radiotherapy even for early-stage patients: the ground appears to be shifting yet again. For example, in an important study from the North American-based NCIC and ECOG groups, 405 patients with excellent-prognosis non-bulky stages IA and IIA disease were randomized between treatment with this chemotherapy regimen alone (4–6 courses), or with subtotal nodal radiation therapy – see Ref. [10]. At 12 years following treatment (the study – HD.6 – was commenced in 1994), the overall survival figures were 94% (chemo-alone group) and 87% (with radiotherapy – a difference of $p = 0.04$), with 6 "deaths from other causes" in the ABVD group and 20 in the radiotherapy group.

Clinical stage IIIA

In this category, patients have presented with localized disease but scanning has demonstrated spread to lymph nodes in the abdomen (or, uncommonly, the spleen). The distinction between IIIA1 and IIIA2 is useful in deciding on treatment within the IIIA category as a whole. Although stage IIIA1 patients (see Table 25.2) can be treated with total nodal irradiation (TNI), with chemotherapy reserved for relapse, stage IIIA2 patients do not do well with this approach and the prognosis is improved by adding chemotherapy to the TNI. However, the evidence suggests that, provided an effective regimen is used, chemotherapy alone is as effective as TNI and chemotherapy in stage IIIA. In most centres current policy would be treatment with chemotherapy, with radiation reserved for sites of residual or initially bulky disease and given at the completion of the chemotherapy programme. A meta-analysis of trials where chemotherapy for advanced disease has been compared with chemotherapy plus radiation has shown no difference in survival but, as expected, a reduction in relapse rate if radiation is given in addition. In trials that compared additional radiation to additional chemotherapy, failure-free survival was the same, but overall survival was superior for the chemotherapy alone treatment because of the late sequelae attributable to radiotherapy – an echo of the results of the NCIC-ECOG HD.6 study for lower-risk patients, quoted above in more detail [15], and see Ref. [10].

Clinical stage IIB, IIIB, IVB

These patients present with constitutional symptoms and widespread disease, or more localized disease (IIB) on scanning with the pathological stage unknown. The mainstay of treatment is chemotherapy with ABVD, or a more complex chemotherapy regimen especially in poorer-prognosis patients (see Principles of chemotherapy, above). In many European centres, the combination known as BEACOPP is widely used – bleomycin, etoposide, doxorubicin, cyclophosphamide, vincristine, procarbazine and prednisone, supported by G-CSF, with excellent results – see, for example, the current ESMO guidelines from Eichenauer et al. [16]. Although pathological stage IIB disease (an unusual category) can be treated with EF or IF radiotherapy alone, the risk of relapse is high and this approach is now very uncommon, though an important study from Holland published a few years ago suggested that even in patients with advanced disease, the use of IF radiotherapy in patients who have achieved a partial remission with chemotherapy can be valuable [17]. In this large study of over 700 patients, the 8-year event-free and overall survival in patients who had only achieved a partial remission following chemotherapy were extremely close to those achieving a complete remission from chemotherapy, suggesting a definite role for 'adjuvant' radiotherapy in this group. Recent work from Germany, using a meta-analysis of all available trials comparing ABVD-type regimens with escalated-BEACOPP (i.e. at an intensified dose), suggests that the latter regimen is more effective and wherever possible, should replace ABVD in this setting – see Ref. [18].

Massive mediastinal disease

It is not uncommon to find a huge mediastinal mass in a relatively asymptomatic patient, in which the mass, on chest radiography, occupies more than one-third of the transverse diameter of the chest or is greater than 10 cm across (see Figure 25.5). Several studies have suggested that it is difficult to control the disease by radiation alone and that early chemotherapy improves both relapse-free survival and overall survival. The usual practice is to give chemotherapy first, allowing a smaller volume to be irradiated.

Treatment on relapse including high-dose chemotherapy

Relapse after a standard chemotherapy regimen [19] is self-evidently an adverse prognostic feature. Local relapse in a previously unirradiated nodal area can be treated by irradiation which, if the original disease was localized (e.g. to the mediastinum), should be with curative intent. Frequently, the relapse will be more generalized, often of a higher or more unfavourable tumour grade, and further chemotherapy will be the treatment of choice. A new biopsy for confirmation is essential. If a single chemotherapy regimen has been previously used (e.g. ChlVPP), then a different regimen should be employed (e.g. ABVD).

Although durable remissions can be obtained with conventional chemotherapy on relapse, increasing interest is being shown in the results of high-dose chemotherapy with peripheral blood stem cells as support. These procedures are becoming less difficult. Although now well established as a successful form of salvage therapy for many patients with non-Hodgkin's lymphoma (see Chapter 26), high-dose therapy for Hodgkin's disease took longer to become established. However, it has now become one of the standard indications for patients with chemosensitive first relapse [20]. The most commonly used drug combination in the UK is probably a regimen containing bis-chloroethyl nitrosourea

(BCNU), etoposide, cytosine arabinoside and melphalan. Depending on selection criteria, about half of all patients who receive high-dose chemotherapy in complete or partial second remission will have long-term (5 years or more) freedom from progression. In Europe, a combination of IGEV (ifosfamide, gemcitabine, vinorelbine and dexamethasone) or ICE (ifosfamide, carboplatin, etoposide) is often used. Bulky disease and/or initial remission of under a year are known adverse features and often influence patient selection. At present, high-dose chemotherapy with stem-cell autologous transplantation should be considered for patients with extensive (stage III or IV) disease who are not in complete remission after initial chemotherapy; for patients who have relapsed quickly after remission; for patients who have relapsed after two different chemotherapy regimens; and for patients who are not responding completely to a salvage chemotherapy regimen. Allogeneic transplantation, ideally from a well-matched related (sibling) donor, is also increasingly undertaken, though still remains controversial and, of course, far more hazardous. As patients with primary refractory Hodgkin's disease have a poor outcome even following high-dose chemotherapy and autologous stem-cell transplantation, this group are potentially important candidates for allogeneic transplantation, particularly now that reduced-dose conditioning regimens are becoming more widely used. In palliative situations, gemcitabine-based therapy often offers the best compromise between finding an active programme with potential benefit, without too great a hazard from treatment toxicity.

Hodgkin's Lymphoma in childhood

Hodgkin's Lymphoma is uncommon in childhood, accounting for 5% of paediatric cancer. The disease is often localized and appears particularly sensitive to chemotherapy. The histological subtypes are the same as in adults. However, there are several problems in management of the disease in young children. First, high-dose radiation profoundly affects bone growth in children where the epiphyses are not yet fused. Second, the long-term consequences of chemotherapy in childhood are now being seen (see below). Because of these complications and the excellent results of treatment, current efforts are directed to reduction of long-term treatment toxicity while maintaining the excellent cure rates.

Children with clinical stage I, with minimal disease, can be treated by IF irradiation with good results.

For children with clinical stage II and III disease and with bulky stage I disease, EF irradiation produces relapse-free survival of about 50% at 5 years. However, there is a strong argument for treatment with low-dose (20–25 Gy) EF irradiation, in order to avoid radiation sequelae, together with six cycles of chemotherapy, often given as three cycles before and after radiotherapy. Etoposide-containing regimens should not be given because of the risk of chemotherapy-induced leukaemia. Relapse-free 5-year survival of about 80% is achieved by this means. Chemotherapy alone may be as effective as the combined-modality treatment and it is clearly preferable to avoid EF irradiation wherever possible. As Schellong [21] has pointed out:

> For two decades now, combined chemo-radiotherapy has been preferred in most of the studies on childhood Hodgkin's disease (HD), because combined modality is the precondition for (1) reducing the radiation dose, (2) reducing the radiation fields, (3) shortening chemotherapy, (4) omitting splenectomy and laparotomy, and thus, for optimizing the benefit/risk ratio between cure rates and late effects. Recently, the rationale for this approach has been strengthened by worrying data about the increasing incidence of secondary breast cancer in women treated for Hodgkin's Disease in childhood, adolescence or [early] adult life. Nearly all breast cancers were localized in the former radiation field, and the relative risk was much higher after doses >40 Gy than after lower doses.

As in adults, chemotherapy is now the mainstay of treatment of stage IIIB and IV disease, with high rates of prolonged relapse-free survival, presumably equating to cure in most cases. In an important study from Canada, the overall and event-free survival rates at 8.5 years were 94% and 88%, respectively [22], though some of the patients in this series had a more favourable initial clinical stage (123 children, clinical stages I–IIIB). In a somewhat larger long-term follow-up study from the UK, following 358 children over 20 years, the overall survival rates were 89.3% at 10 years and 89% at 20 years [23]. Most of these children had been treated with ChlVPP chemotherapy alone, with only a relatively small proportion undergoing radiotherapy as well, usually because of bulky mediastinal disease. For stage I disease (111 patients), the treatment was initially by preference, with IF radiotherapy alone.

High-dose radiation in children who have not reached skeletal maturity produces cessation of growth with distortion of limbs and pelvis, failure of chest wall growth and small stature due to impaired vertebral development. Almost all boys treated with chemotherapy will develop long-term irreversible azoospermia [24]. Girls fare better, with over 80% recovering normal menstruation. The risk of second cancer is 18 times that of the general population, with most being radiation-related. There is an excess of cancer of the breast and thyroid, and of bone and soft-tissue sarcoma [25].

Hodgkin's Lymphoma during pregnancy (see also Chapter 8, page 137).

Occasionally, Hodgkin's Lymphoma is diagnosed for the first time during pregnancy. If this occurs during the first 20 weeks, it is probably best to advise termination and then to proceed to the usual evaluation and treatment. During the last trimester, provided the patient is not ill, it is possible to wait until delivery before investigation and treatment. More difficult problems arise if the pregnancy is advanced (20 weeks or more) and the disease is progressing and/or the patient is constitutionally unwell, or if the pregnancy is early but termination is refused.

In a woman in advanced pregnancy in whom treatment cannot be delayed until delivery because the disease is advanced or growing rapidly, it is probably best to treat with combination chemotherapy. There are several reports of normal full-term children born to women who have received combination chemotherapy during pregnancy but clearly it is prudent to postpone such treatment for as long as possible. Single-agent chemotherapy was used in the past, but this is not good practice since there is little to suggest that the adverse effects on the fetus are less and there is a grave problem of worsening the long-term prognosis by this treatment. If a woman refuses termination early in pregnancy and has progressive disease, chemotherapy should be delayed as long as possible to allow the early, crucial stages of fetal development to proceed. If the patient has apparently localized supradiaphragmatic disease but it is felt inadvisable to wait until after delivery, localized radiotherapy is given and full investigation is deferred. In this situation, where a decision has to be made between chemotherapy and irradiation, abbreviated staging using ultrasound can be helpful.

If a woman with previously diagnosed, investigated and treated Hodgkin's Lymphoma relapses during pregnancy, then similar considerations apply. In women who have been successfully treated for Hodgkin's Lymphoma there is no evidence that pregnancy will provoke recurrence or adversely affect prognosis.

Toxicity of treatment

The potential toxicities of radiotherapy and chemotherapy have been dealt with in general terms in Chapters 5 and 6. The following brief account specifically concerns Hodgkin's Lymphoma [26].

Acute toxicity of chemotherapy
Bone marrow suppression

This is a common accompaniment of all standard chemotherapeutic regimens in Hodgkin's Lymphoma. Most centres make dosage reductions in response to depressed blood counts, rather than delay the cycle, although delay may be necessary on occasions. The toxicity tends to be cumulative and particular care should be taken as treatment progresses, especially in the elderly, in those who have received EF radiotherapy in the past and in ill patients with extensive disease. After TNI the problem is particularly severe since over 50% of the adult haemopoietic marrow is within the irradiation field. Recovery of the marrow after TNI takes years and is often incomplete, so chemotherapy should be introduced with caution in these patients.

Immunosuppression

Treatment adds to the depression of CMI that is commonly present in advanced disease. Lymphopenia is an invariable consequence of EF irradiation and persists for several months after treatment. Depression of CMI is induced by most cytotoxic agents, especially alkylating agents and steroids. For this reason, herpes zoster and herpes simplex are very common in heavily treated patients and may be life-threatening. Less common nowadays is reactivation of tuberculosis, but other opportunistic infections such as *Pneumocystis*, cytomegalovirus and *Aspergillus* are occasionally seen.

Long-term complications of radiation

Radiation pneumonitis, leading to fibrosis, is a relatively common complication if the radiation dose is above 40 Gy. For this reason very large mediastinal masses require special consideration. Chemotherapy is often used to produce tumour shrinkage before irradiation, though it is not clear whether it is sufficient to irradiate the residual volume only. For smaller nodal areas complications are exceptionally rare.

With earlier radiation techniques there was an increased risk of myocardial infarction and cardiac death, which was greater with higher total dose and larger mediastinal radiation fields. The relative risk has

fallen from about sixfold to two-fold using modern techniques. Nonetheless, a recent large British study of over 7000 Hodgkin's Lymphoma survivors (treated in the UK between 1967 and 2000) showed that the risk was real and most marked in patients who had been treated with supradiaphragmatic radiotherapy, anthracyclines or vincristine [27], and that the risk remains high for at least 25 years after treatment. Occasionally, mediastinal irradiation may cause pericarditis with a pericardial effusion that usually resolves. This may cause pain but is usually asymptomatic. Constrictive pericarditis is an extremely uncommon complication of mediastinal irradiation using modern techniques.

Clinical hypothyroidism is an infrequent (5%) complication of mantle field irradiation, although transiently elevated thyroid-stimulating hormone levels are more frequent (30%). This complication is of insidious onset and thyroid function should be checked yearly in patients at risk. Radiation damage to the bowel following infradiaphragmatic irradiation may uncommonly occur, giving rise to diarrhoea (sometimes bloody), steatorrhoea and intestinal obstruction. It is related to both the volume and the total dose administered, and is more likely to occur if the bowel has been tethered in one site by previous inflammation or surgery.

In the CNS the commonest symptom of radiation damage is Lhermitte's syndrome of tingling and paraesthesiae in the legs, often provoked by neck flexion. This usually passes off with no sequelae. Transverse myelitis should not occur with modern planning techniques. Very high repeated doses over peripheral nerves can rarely lead to peripheral neuropathy, usually within 1–5 years.

Impaired spermatogenesis occurs with doses of irradiation to the testes as low as 50 cGy and is more rapid, complete and long-lasting with higher doses, being invariable and often permanent at doses above 5 Gy (see Chapter 5). During pelvic irradiation, with effective shielding, the dose should be below 100 cGy. The dose that causes permanent cessation of ovarian function is higher than for the testis. Oophoropexy is sometimes performed in order to move the ovaries outside a possible pelvic irradiation field (see above), with somewhat inconsistent results.

Long-term complications of chemotherapy (see also Chapter 6)

As pointed out by Meyer and colleagues [10], recent results show that 'improving long-term survival is less dependent than previously assumed on further reducing deaths due to progressive Hodgkin's lymphoma and instead emphasize a need for treatments that will not lead to deaths from late treatment effects'. This is a remarkable testament to the enormous advances made in the management of often previously fatal condition, over the past 30 years.

Female fertility may be depressed after chemotherapy, but the effect is variable. In most women the period of reproductive life may be shortened. This complication must be discussed carefully with each patient, especially if the decision to have children might otherwise be deferred. Persistent amenorrhoea and the onset of the menopause are likely to occur in older premenopausal women. Amenorrhoea frequently occurs during treatment but normal menstruation usually returns. Many patients have had normal children after treatment. On the other hand, the hazard of teratogenicity during chemotherapy is usually regarded as an indication for termination (see above).

In men azoospermia is almost inevitable after chemotherapy, especially with regimens containing alkylating agents and procarbazine. Recovery from sterility is rare. Sperm storage before chemotherapy is strongly advised – in fact should be regarded as mandatory – for men who are concerned about the effects on fertility. In advanced Hodgkin's Lymphoma, oligospermia is common before treatment begins. There is little doubt that ABVD has a lower risk of gonadal toxicity than the MOPP or similar regimens chiefly used for Hodgkin's Lymphoma.

During the first 5 years after MOPP chemotherapy, the cumulative risk of herpes zoster is approximately 15%, and after MOPP with TNI is 50%. Disseminated zoster (9%) is more common in those receiving combined-modality treatment than in those receiving chemotherapy or radiation alone (2%). Bacterial infections, especially pneumococcal, also occur more often, particularly in children, in patients over 50 years and probably in those who have undergone splenectomy.

Second malignancies

In recent years, it has become apparent that following chemotherapy for Hodgkin's Lymphoma, there is an increased risk of the patient developing a second malignancy [25,26,28,29]. The association was first documented for acute non-lymphocytic leukaemia (ANL). At present, the risk of developing ANL in the 7 years after chemotherapy alone, or after combined-modality

treatment, is approximately 2%. However, in patients over the age of 40 years, the risk of ANL may be higher. It is now apparent that the risk of solid tumours is greater than that of leukaemia and occurs with a relative risk of approximately 4 for lung cancer, 17 for non-Hodgkin's lymphoma and 2 for all other tumours combined (all patients and all treatments). Lung cancers, breast cancer and bone sarcomas are especially likely to occur within the radiation field; the increased risk becomes apparent after a delay of 10–15 years, and seems to continue well beyond that period. If treatment is given early in life, the overall cumulative risk after 30 years is about 15%, a far from trivial figure, and for many cancers the risk seems greatest when treatment was given at a young age. The risk is lower if chemotherapy has induced an early menopause, presumably because of its protective effect in relation to breast cancer, one of the commoner post-treatment malignancies. However, the overall relative risk for all cancers is greatest for combined-modality treatment. In the large long-term follow-up from the UK Children's Cancer Study Group, the 20-year cumulative incidence of malignancy was 7.3% [29]. This was felt to be a relatively low figure, which might well be due to the relatively small number of patients who had undergone combined chemoirradiation treatment, coupled with the modest dose of radiotherapy (35 Gy, IF only, by preference). The haematological second malignancy rate was 1.6%. The cumulative probability is shown in Figure 25.10.

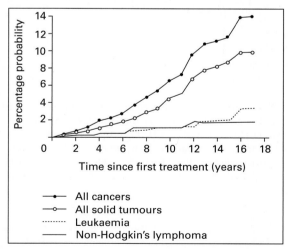

Figure 25.10 Second malignancies after treatment for Hodgkin's disease. (Source: Swerdlow *et al.* [30] Reproduced with permission from BMJ Publishing Group Ltd.)

Both alkylating agents and procarbazine are potential carcinogens, but the cause of the increased incidence of ANL is not known. It may be less common after ABVD; however, this regimen was introduced into clinical practice more recently than MOPP, and since the leukaemia risk is highest more than 5 years after chemotherapy, it may be a little soon to assume that ABVD is not as leukaemogenic though this is widely held – probably correctly – to be the case. The risk of leukaemia relates to survivors rather than to those treated. It is important to appreciate that despite the many potential long-term consequences of treatment, the risk posed by recurrent Hodgkin's Lymphoma is considerably greater than the hazard from a second malignancy.

References

1 Cartwright RA, Watkins G. Epidemiology of Hodgkin's disease: a review. *Haematol Oncol* 2004; 22: 11 – 26.

2 Hjalgrim H, Askling J, Rostgaard K *et al.* Characteristics of Hodgkin's Lymphoma after infectious mononucleosis. *New Engl J Med* 2003; 349: 1324–32.

3 Küppers R, Rajewsky K. The origin of Hodgkin and Reed–Sternberg cells in Hodgkin's disease. *Annu Rev Immunol* 1998; 16: 471–93.

4 Harris NL. A revised European–American classification of lymphoid neoplasms: a proposal from the International Lymphoma Study Group. *Blood* 1994; 84: 1361–92.

5 MacLennan KA, Bennett MH, Tu A *et al.* Relationship of histopathological features to survival and relapse in nodular sclerosing Hodgkin's disease: a study of 1659 patients. *Cancer* 1989; 64: 1686–93.

6 Urba WJ, Longo DL. Hodgkin's disease: review article. *N Engl J Med* 1992; 326: 678–87.

7 Lister TA, Crowther D, Sutcliffe SB *et al.* Report of a committee convened to discuss the evaluation and staging of patients with Hodgkin's disease: Cotswolds Meeting. *J Clin Oncol* 1989; 7: 1630–6.

8 Hasenclever D, Diehl V. A prognostic score for advanced Hodgkin's disease. *N Engl J Med* 1998; 339: 1506–14.

9 Engert A, Haverkamp H, Kobe C *et al* for the German and Swiss Hodgkin's study groups. Reduced-intensity chemotherapy and PET-guided radiotherapy in patients with advanced stage Hodgkin's lymphoma (HD15 trial): a randomized, open-label, phase 3 non-inferiority trial. *Lancet* 2012; 379: 1791–99.

10 Meyer RM, Gospodarowicz MK, Connors JM *et al.*, for the NCIC and ECOG collaborative groups. ABVD alone versus radiation-based therapy in limited-stage Hodgkin's Lymphoma. *New Engl J Med* 2012; 366: 399–408.

11 Canellos GP, Anderson JP, Propert KJ *et al.* Chemotherapy of advanced Hodgkin's disease with MOPP, ABVD and MOPP alternating with ABVD. *N Engl J Med* 1992; 327: 1478–84.

12 Fermé C, Eghbali H, Meerwald JH *et al.* for the European EORTC-GELA group. Chemotherapy plus involved-field radiation in early-stage Hodgkin's disease. *N Engl J Med* 2007; 357: 1916–27.

13 Specht L, Gray RG, Clarke MJ, Peto R. Influence of more extensive radiotherapy and adjuvant chemotherapy on long-term outcome of early-stage Hodgkin's disease: a meta-analysis of 23 randomized trials involving 3888 patients. *J Clin Oncol* 1998; 16: 830–40.

14 Noordijk EM, Carde P, Dupouy N *et al.* Combined-modality therapy for clinical stage I or II Hodgkin's lymphoma: long-term results of the European Organisation for Research and Treatment of Cancer H7 randomized controlled trials. *J Clin Oncol* 2006; 24: 3128–35.

15 Loeffler M, Bronsteanu O, Hasenclever D *et al.* Meta-analysis of chemotherapy versus combined modality treatment trials in Hodgkin's disease. *J Clin Oncol* 1998; 16: 818–29.

16 Eichenauer DA, Engert A and Dreyling M, for the ESMO Guidelines Working Group. Hodgkin's lymphoma: ESMO clinical practice guidelines for diagnosis, treatment and follow-up. *Ann Oncol* 2011; 22 (Suppl 6): vi 55–58.

17 Aleman BM, Raemaekers JM, Tomisic R *et al.* for the EORTC Lymphoma Group. Involved-field radiotherapy for patients in partial remission after chemotherapy for advanced Hodgkin's lymphoma. *Int J Radiat Oncol Biol Phys* 2007; 67: 19–30.

18 Skoetz N, Trelle S, Rancea M *et al.* Effect of initial treatment strategy on survival of patients with advanced-stage Hodgkin's lymphoma: a systematic review and network meta-analysis. *Lancet Oncol* 2013; 14: 943–52.

19 Hoppe RT. Development of effective salvage treatment programs for Hodgkin's disease: an ongoing clinical challenge. *Blood* 1991; 77: 2093–5.

20 Schmitz N, Buske C, Gisselbrecht C. Autologous stem cell transplantation in lymphoma. *Semin Hematol* 2007; 44: 234–45.

21 Schellong G. Paediatric Hodgkin's disease: treatment in the late 1990s. *Ann Oncol* 1998; 9 (Suppl. 5): 115–19.

22 Chow LM, Nathan PC, Hodgson DC *et al.* Survival and late effects in children with Hodgkin's lymphoma treated with MOPP/ABV and low-dose, extended-field irradiation. *J Clin Oncol* 2006; 24: 5735–41.

23 Capra M, Hewitt M, Radford M *et al.* for the Children's Cancer and Leukaemia group (formerly UKCCSG). Long-term outcome in children with Hodgkin's lymphoma: the United Kingdom Children's Cancer Study Group HD 82 trial. *Eur J Cancer* 2007; 43: 1171–9.

24 Shafford EA, Kingston JE, Malpas JS *et al.* Testicular function following the treatment of Hodgkin's disease in childhood. *Br J Cancer* 1993; 68: 1199–204.

25 Batia S, Robison LL, Oberlin O *et al.* Breast cancer and other second neoplasms after childhood Hodgkin's disease. *N Engl J Med* 1996; 334: 745–51.

26 Hancock SL, Hoppe RT. Long-term complications of treatment and causes of mortality after Hodgkin's disease. *Semin Radiat Oncol* 1996; 6: 225–42.

27 Swerdlow AJ, Higgins CD, Smith P *et al*. Myocardial infarction mortality risk after treatment for Hodgkin disease: a collaborative British cohort study. *J Natl Cancer Inst* 2007; 99: 206–14.

28 Tucker MA, Coleman CN, Varghese A, Rosenberg SA. Risk of second cancers after treatment for Hodgkin's disease. *N Engl J Med* 1988; 318: 76–81.

29 Swerdlow AJ, Barber JA, Hudson GV *et al*. Risk of second malignancy after Hodgkin's disease in a collaborative British cohort: the relation of age at treatment. *J Clin Oncol* 2000; 18: 498–509.

30 Swerdlow AJ, Douglas AJ, Vaughan-Hudson G *et al*. Risk of second primary cancers after Hodgkin's disease by type of treatment: analysis of 2846 patients in the British National Lymphoma Investigation. *Br Med J* 1992; 304: 1137–43.

Further reading

Brice P, Bouabdallah R, Moreau P *et al*. Prognostic factors for survival after high-dose therapy and autologous stem cell transplantation for patients with relapsing Hodgkin's disease: analysis of 280 patients from the French registry. *Bone Marrow Transplant* 1997; 20: 21–6.

Cheson BD, Pfistner B, Juweid ME *et al*. Revised response criteria for malignant lymphoma. *J Clin Oncol* 2007; 25: 579–86.

Diehl V. Hodgkin's disease: from pathology specimen to cure. *N Engl J Med* 2007; 357: 1968–71.

Diehl V, *et al*. Hodgkin lymphoma: clinical manifestations, staging and therapy. In: Hoffman R *et al*. eds. *Hematology: Basic Principles and Practice*, 5th edn. Philadelphia, Pa.: Churchill Livingstone Elsevier, 2009.

Fuchs M, Diehl V, Re D. Current strategies and new approaches in the treatment of Hodgkin's lymphoma. *Pathobiology* 2006; 73: 126–40.

Newland A, Provan D, Myint S. Preventing severe infection after splenectomy. *Br Med J* 2005; 331: 417–18.

Re D, Thomas RK, Behringer K, Diehl V. From Hodgkin disease to Hodgkin lymphoma: biologic insights and therapeutic potential. *Blood* 2005; 105: 4553–60.

Sureda A. Autologous and allogeneic stem cell transplantation in Hodgkin's lymphoma. *Hematol Clin North Am* 2007; 21: 943–60.

26 Non-Hodgkin's lymphomas

Incidence and aetiology

Recent years have seen a considerable growth in our knowledge of the aetiology and pathogenesis of non-Hodgkin's lymphomas (NHLs). They are a heterogeneous group of neoplasms which, in Western countries, occur predominantly in the elderly. The overall age-specific incidence is shown in Figure 26.1, but this obscures markedly different age incidences with some rarer forms of NHL (which occur in childhood or early adult life) – see, for example, Ref. [1]. It seems clear that the incidence of NHL is rising quite rapidly, but the causes are not fully known. For example, the incidence of follicular lymphoma, the second commonest variety of nodal lymphoid malignancies in Western Europe, has risen sharply from 2 – 3/100 000 in the 1950s to 5 – 7 in recent years – see, for example, Ref. [2]. The AIDS epidemic has contributed to the rising incidence of B-cell lymphomas – see, for example, Ref. [3].

Cancer and its Management, Seventh Edition. Jeffrey Tobias and Daniel Hochhauser.
© 2015 John Wiley & Sons, Ltd. Published 2015 by John Wiley & Sons, Ltd.

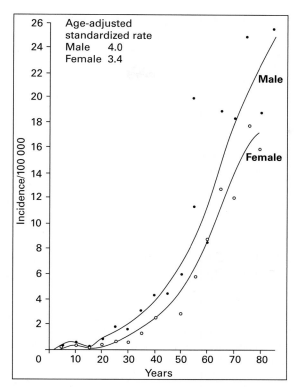

Figure 26.1 Age-specific incidence of non-Hodgkin's lymphoma.

Geographical distribution

In the late 1950s, in a landmark study, the surgeon Denis Burkitt reported cases of a lymphoma occurring in the jaw and abdomen of Ugandan children [4], diagnosed predominantly at 3 years of age. Burkitt showed that the tumour appeared in regions of high humidity – the wet tropical areas. The tumour was then reported in Papua New Guinea in the same climatic regions. Cases are now reported in the Western countries, but with an incidence of only 1% of that in Africa. Western cases have few jaw tumours and in Middle Eastern cases the ileocaecal region is more usually involved. Epstein–Barr virus (EBV) was identified in cultured tumour cells from African cases, and almost all African cases have high serum titres of anti-EBV. Since almost all the normal population has been infected, a cofactor has been postulated, possibly falciparum malaria. This is also suggested by the lower incidence of the tumour in cities and in regions where malaria has been controlled. The age of onset is higher in children who have migrated to areas of high malaria prevalence.

Lymphomas are a common Middle Eastern cancer (10% of all cancer cases), but they differ from European cases in that many are intestinal, often arising in a background of diffuse small-intestinal thickening generally termed immunoproliferative small-intestine disease. Current hypotheses favour the view that this is an early stage of lymphoma.

A lymphoma characterized by skin rash, hepatosplenomegaly and hypercalcaemia was reported in 1977 in patients from the southern Japanese island of Kyushu. Later, cases were described in the UK in patients from the Caribbean and in the USA. T-lymphotrophic viruses isolated in Japan and in the USA were shown to be identical. This retrovirus is designated human T-cell lymphotropic virus (HTLV)-1. The virus is transmitted in breast milk and possibly in semen. It seems that HTLV-1 lymphoma may also be endemic in eastern China. It is not clear what environmental stimulus causes activation of an infection acquired in infancy, since the age of onset of the overt disease is 40–60 years. The overall incidence in Japan is 5 per 100 000 and 3 per 100 000 in the Caribbean. HTLV-1 also causes spastic paraparesis in Jamaica.

Viral causes

There is strong evidence that *HTLV-1* is the cause of adult acute T-cell leukaemia/lymphoma. The virus appears to act early in oncogenesis, causing transformation that leads to further genetic alteration. This results in malignant clonal proliferation that is no longer dependent on the virus. Transformation depends on a protein (Tax) that interacts with other cellular activators leading to production of factors causing lymphoid proliferation, such as interleukin (IL)-2, and deregulation of cell cycle control.

EBV is implicated in the pathogenesis of endemic Burkitt's lymphoma, AIDS-related lymphomas, angiocentric T/natural killer (NK) lymphoma and possibly Hodgkin's disease. EBV can transform lymphoid cells, but it is not clear how it might maintain this state. The full expression of transforming proteins is only possible in conditions of profound immunosuppression, such as after bone marrow transplantation, and this is probably the way in which post-transplant lymphoid proliferations are caused. In chronic latent infection other transforming events must occur, such as c-*myc* mutation and overexpression of *bcl*-6.

Kaposi's sarcoma herpesvirus (human herpesvirus type 8, HHV8) has been found in a rare lymphoid malignancy known as primary effusion lymphoma (PEL) often in patients with AIDS. Infection with HHV8 is far more common in AIDS than in PEL. A cofactor is presumably needed for transformation, possibly EBV infection. HHV8 codes for a variety of proteins that might interfere with B-lymphoid and endothelial cell function including a viral cyclin, a viral IL-6 and a viral G protein-coupled receptor.

An important recent report from the USA (Baylor College of Medicine) has demonstrated that patients with hepatitis C have a 20–30% additional risk of developing an NHL and also a three-fold risk above normal of developing Waldenström's macroglobulinemia [5]. This was a large retrospective cohort study, in human immunodeficiency virus (HIV)-negative US veterans (97% men), of almost 150 000 hepatitis C-infected patients who were compared for risk with a panel of almost four times this number of uninfected people, matched for age and sex.

Lymphomas in other immunodeficiency states

Table 26.1 indicates the wide range of disorders predisposing to NHL, with the majority clearly suggesting states of immune deficiency. Patients with AIDS are at high risk of developing NHL [6]. The clinical features of these lymphomas are discussed on page 531. Almost all are B-cell tumours. In organ transplant recipients, lymphomas account for one-third of all the associated malignancies. The tumours are usually immunoblastic and often intracranial. If the immunosuppression has included ciclosporin in high dose, the lymphomas are more frequent and often arise in lymph nodes or the intestinal tract. With other immunosuppressive

---

Table 26.1 Disorders predisposing to development of lymphoma.

Congenital
Chédiak–Higashi syndrome
Ataxia telangiectasia
Wiskott–Aldrich syndrome
Swiss-type agammaglobulinaemia
Klinefelter's syndrome
Coeliac disease
Bloom's syndrome
X-linked lymphoproliferative disease

Acquired
AIDS
Chronic immune suppression (e.g. renal allograft recipients)
Sjögren's syndrome
Rheumatoid arthritis
Common variable hypogammaglobulinaemia

---

treatments, intracerebral lymphoma is more common. In ataxia telangiectasia and Wiskott–Aldrich syndrome there is a high incidence of lymphoma. In these cases, and in transplant recipients, there is sometimes a clinical association with EBV infection.

In the X-linked lymphoproliferative syndrome (discussed above) immune deficiency in young boys is associated with overwhelming EBV infection.

Coeliac disease

Patients with this disease have a 200-fold increase in incidence of lymphoma of the intestine. The tumours are T cell in origin and have distinct clinical features (see pages 535–536).

Pathology and molecular genetics of lymphoma

Genetic abnormalities occur in many types of NHL [7]. A reciprocal translocation of chromosomal material between chromosomes 8 and 14, t(8;14)(q24;q32), occurs in tumour cells in Burkitt's lymphoma. More than 80% of tumours have this translocation. Interestingly, translocations between chromosomes 14 and 18 can be detected in a remarkably high proportion (possibly 50%) of healthy people, which clearly suggests that the translocation is by itself insufficient for the development of an immediate clinical syndrome of follicular lymphoma [6].

Translocations between 8 and 22 t(8;22) and from 2 to 8 t(2;8) occur in the remaining 20%. The immunoglobulin heavy-chain locus is located at 14q32 and the light chain at 2p11 and 22q11. Each of these sites is the site of gene rearrangement in the normal B lymphocyte. The break on chromosome 8 is always at band 8q24 which is the c-myc proto-oncogene site. There is heterogeneity at the site of the immunoglobulin locus break. The c-myc is abnormally expressed for B cells, although it is at a level appropriate for proliferating cells. The African, endemic, cases do not show c-myc rearrangement, but the sporadic cases do.

Follicle centre cell lymphomas of the follicular type and some diffuse large-cell lymphomas show a characteristic chromosomal translocation in 85% of cases. This is between 14q32 (the heavy-chain locus) and 18q21. The breakpoint on chromosome 18 is rearranged in the majority of follicular lymphomas. The gene is bcl-2 (B-cell leukaemia and lymphoma 2), which codes for a mitochondrial protein that inhibits apoptosis. The expression of *bcl*-2 is associated with worse prognosis in large-cell lymphomas.

T-cell malignancies also show non-random chromosomal abnormalities. The most common site is at 14q11, the site of the T-cell receptor gene (α and β chains).

It is still not clear what role these lympho-specific translocations play in oncogenesis. They are sometimes related to control of proliferation. For example, a t(2;5) translocation occurs in anaplastic large-cell lymphoma, producing a tyrosine kinase (ALK) that may prove to be a drug target. In mucosa-associated lymphoid tissue lymphomas, a t(1;14) translocation activates *bcl*-10, which may protect the cell from apoptosis. In small-lymphocyte lymphomas, a t(9;14) translocation is often present that activates *PAX*-5, a transcription factor that may stimulate B-cell proliferation in some lymphomas.

An important clinical application of molecular techniques has been the detection of rearrangement of antigen-receptor genes as a manifestation of clonality. These genes (T-cell receptor genes and immunoglobulin genes) rearrange during normal development of the cells, producing an antigen-specific clone. Neoplastic expansion of a clone is accompanied by a specific rearrangement which can be detected at low levels using molecular and immunological techniques.

The classification of lymphomas has been in a state of constant change for many years [6–9]. The problem has been that lymphomas derived from different cells, or at different stages of lymphoid differentiation, may nonetheless have very similar prognoses and require similar treatments. A purely clinical classification, ignoring biology, lacks a rational scientific basis, while a classification based on biology alone risks becoming a list of entities, providing little help to the clinician. A consensus has emerged in which modern methods of determining the cell of origin and the characteristic genetic abnormalities have been linked to practical clinical considerations concerning treatment and prognosis. This is summarized in the World Health Organization (WHO) classification, which is closely aligned to others (such as Revised European–American lymphoma, REAL) that have had wide acceptance (Table 26.2). The Kiel classification (Table 26.3) is similar but also groups according to clinical behaviour.

During fetal life precursors of T lymphocytes are formed and migrate to the thymus, and then to the developing lymph nodes and spleen. Maturation into mature T cells takes place at various stages, especially in the thymus. The sequence of maturation can be defined by their surface antigen structure. Monoclonal antibodies

Table 26.2 The WHO classification of non-Hodgkin's lymphomas.

B-cell neoplasms
B-cell chronic lymphocytic leukaemia/lymphocytic lymphoma
B-cell prolymphocytic leukaemia
Mantle cell lymphoma
Follicular lymphoma
Splenic marginal zone lymphoma
Marginal zone B-cell lymphoma (MALT type)
Nodal marginal zone lymphoma ± monocytoid cells
Hairy cell leukaemia
Diffuse large-cell lymphoma subtypes: mediastinal (thymic), intravascular, primary effusion
Burkitt's lymphoma
Plasmacytoma
Plasma cell myeloma

T and putative natural killer cell neoplasms
T-cell prolymphocytic leukaemia
T-cell large granular lymphocyte leukaemia
Natural killer cell leukaemia
Natural killer cell lymphoma, nasal and nasal-type
Mycosis fungoides
Sézary syndrome
Angioimmunoblastic T-cell lymphoma
Peripheral T-cell lymphoma, unspecified
Subcutaneous panniculitis T-cell lymphoma
Adult T-cell leukaemia/lymphoma (HTLV-1 positive)
Anaplastic large-cell lymphoma (T- and null-cell types)
Primary cutaneous anaplastic large-cell lymphoma
Subcutaneous panniculitis-like T-cell lymphoma
Enteropathy-type T-cell lymphoma
Hepatosplenic γδ T-cell lymphoma

to T-cell surface antigens have been especially helpful in this respect. The sequence of maturation is shown in Figure 26.2. By the time the T cell leaves the thymus its function as a helper cell or cytotoxic/suppressor cell is established.

In the lymph nodes the T cells lodge in the paracortical region (Figure 26.3) and around the central arterioles in the spleen. Some T cells recirculate from the lymphatic system to the blood and then back to the lymph nodes where they enter the paracortical region through postcapillary venules.

Early B lymphocytes are formed in the fetal liver and subsequently in the bone marrow. From there they migrate to the lymph nodes. They are found in the follicles, which consist of an outer mantle zone of small

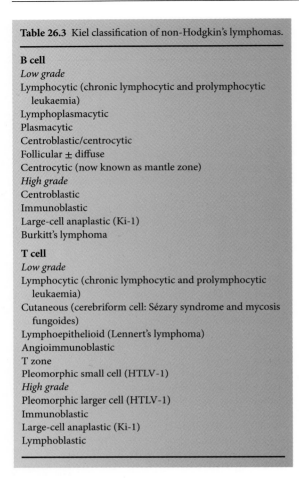

Table 26.3 Kiel classification of non-Hodgkin's lymphomas.

B cell
Low grade
Lymphocytic (chronic lymphocytic and prolymphocytic
    leukaemia)
Lymphoplasmacytic
Plasmacytic
Centroblastic/centrocytic
Follicular ± diffuse
Centrocytic (now known as mantle zone)
High grade
Centroblastic
Immunoblastic
Large-cell anaplastic (Ki-1)
Burkitt's lymphoma

T cell
Low grade
Lymphocytic (chronic lymphocytic and prolymphocytic
    leukaemia)
Cutaneous (cerebriform cell: Sézary syndrome and mycosis
    fungoides)
Lymphoepithelioid (Lennert's lymphoma)
Angioimmunoblastic
T zone
Pleomorphic small cell (HTLV-1)
High grade
Pleomorphic larger cell (HTLV-1)
Immunoblastic
Large-cell anaplastic (Ki-1)
Lymphoblastic

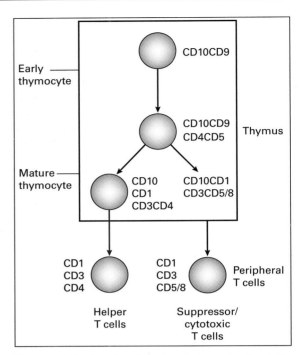

Figure 26.2 T-cell surface phenotype during maturation in the thymus. The T-cell antigens are identified by monoclonal antibodies and are helpful in categorizing the various forms of T-cell lymphoma and leukaemia.

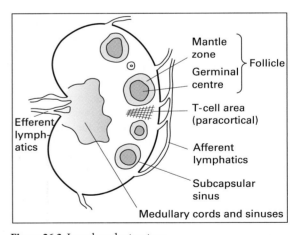

Figure 26.3 Lymph node structure.

lymphocytes and a germinal centre composed of cells where the nucleus is either irregular in shape or large and round. In lymphoma, the cells with a nucleus of irregular outline are called cleaved cells or *centrocytes* and those with a large round non-cleaved nucleus are *centroblasts*. Some B lymphocytes recirculate between nodes and blood. After contact with antigen, B cells transform into antibody-secreting plasma cells.

As B cells terminally differentiate, the genes which code for the enormous variety of potential immunoglobulin molecules rearrange to code for one immunoglobulin molecule only. At this point the 'clonal' nature of the cell is established. Similarly, rearrangement of the genes which code for the four components of the T-cell antigen receptor occurs during T-cell clonal development in the thymus. This rearrangement can be detected relatively simply using molecular biological techniques. In a cell suspension that may contain lymphoma cells (which are

clonal), clonal rearrangement can be detected if as few as 5% of the cells comprise the tumour population. Gene rearrangement is therefore a useful technique for determining, for example, marrow contamination. Detection of a chromosomal abnormality, such as the t(14;18) translocation in follicular lymphoma, by polymerase chain reaction (PCR) is even more sensitive but is not possible in tumours that do not have such an abnormality.

Macrophages, or mononuclear phagocytes, are formed from pluripotent haemopoietic stem cells in the marrow. They are liberated into the bloodstream as monocytes and lodge in tissues at sites of inflammation (histiocytes). They also play a part in repopulating the 'fixed' tissue phagocytic cells: Kupffer cells and splenic, alveolar and peritoneal macrophages. The antigen-presenting cells (dendritic cells) in lymph nodes and spleen may also be part of the mononuclear phagocyte system.

A simplified guide to the stage of differentiation of lymphocytes to which various NHLs and leukaemias correspond is shown in Figure 26.4 and a synopsis of the immunological classification of lymphoreticular neoplasms is shown in Table 26.2.

The pathological classification of the NHL has a long and tortuous history, from Rappaport's early recognition over half a century ago (1956) that there was a critical and indeed essential difference between the behaviour of 'nodular' and 'diffuse' lymphomas, to the Lukes–Collins (USA) and Kiel (European) approach, both depending fundamentally on the separation between B-cell- and T-cell-derived lymphomas (both published in 1975); and finally to the current New Working Formulation (NWF) now widely used throughout the world. Our current understanding is dominated by an immuno-logical and molecular perspective, based on a series of crucial insights gained over many decades of work. Even more recently we have the REAL classification (1994, a modification of the NWF) and the WHO classification published in 2001 (see below). The following cell types have been identified: small lymphocytes (B and T), lymphoplasmacytic cells, plasma cells, centrocytes (small and large), centroblasts (small and large), immunoblasts (B and T) and lymphoblasts (B and T).

B-cell neoplasms make up the majority of NHLs (Table 26.2). The most common are the follicular lym-phomas, which are derived from the B cell of the follicle centre. However, the tumour cells do not always form follicles and may also give rise to a diffuse lymphoma.

T-cell lymphomas probably constitute about 10% of NHLs (Table 26.2). The T-cell lymphomas can be divided into three broad categories: cutaneous lymphomas, thymic lymphomas and peripheral T-cell lymphomas. Morphologically they are diffuse, with a wide variety of cellular morphology.

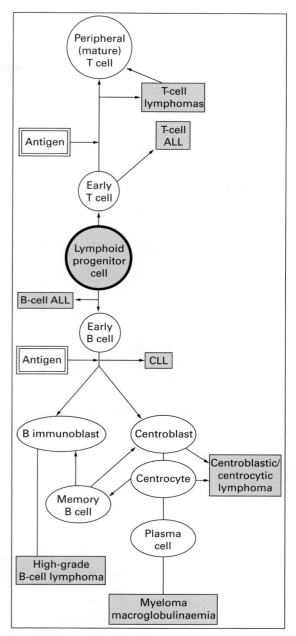

Figure 26.4 Simplified scheme of cell origin of non-Hodgkin's lymphomas: origin of B-cell and T-cell lymphomas, and origin of macrophage tumours. ALL, acute lymphoblastic leukaemia; CLL, chronic lymphocytic leukaemia.

It is not yet clear how many lymphomas are neoplasms of malignant macrophages or NK cells. Those that are should not, strictly speaking, be called lymphomas. Histochemical evidence has suggested that they may account for 5% of diffuse large-cell lymphomas. This part of the classification remains contentious because of the lack of a clonal marker for macrophages.

Although the immunological classification of lymphoma is logical and in many respects superior, for most cases the pathological diagnosis rests on conventional light microscopical appearances (Figure 26.5). The WHO classification currently divides NHLs into B-cell, T-cell and NK-cell lymphomas [8–10], which are of course distinct and separate in epidemiology, histopathology and outcome. Traditional clinical prognostic indices rely only on patient factors and staging, but molecular prognostic markers reflect the intrinsic lymphoma biology and measure tumour load, providing an opportunity for novel therapeutic targets. Lymphomagenesis involves mutations, deletions or dysregulations of genes critical in the control of cell cycle and apoptosis, which are in turn prognostically important. Genome-wide gene expression

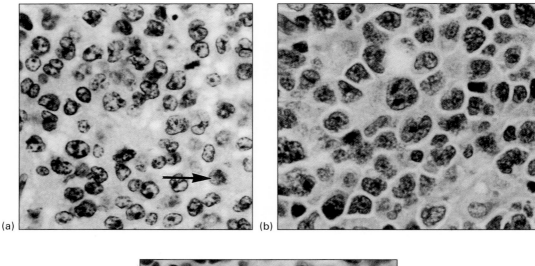

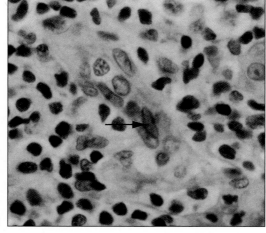

Figure 26.5 Histological appearance in non-Hodgkin's lymphoma (original magnification ×400). (a) Follicle centre cell lymphoma predominantly containing centrocytes but with scattered centroblasts (arrow). (b) Follicle centre cell lymphoma composed principally of centroblasts. (c) Peripheral T-cell lymphoma showing proliferating high endothelial venules (arrow) and a mixture of small and large lymphocytes, some with clear cytoplasm, others showing an irregular nuclear outline.

profiling, either by allowing lymphomas to be classified according to different stages of lymphoid maturation or by defining specific gene expression signatures, is also of prognostic significance. In lymphomas where viral infections of the neoplastic cells occur, quantification of viral copies is a valuable surrogate marker for tumour load and prognosis. Molecular markers, together with patient and clinicopathological features, will in the future provide more accurate prognostic models for risk stratification, helping refine treatment intensity and improving treatment outcomes.

Clinical features

NHLs usually arise in peripheral lymph nodes, but may also develop at a wide variety of extranodal sites. The clinical features of extranodal lymphomas are described later (see page 534 et seq.).

Nodal lymphomas

Presentation

Painless enlargement of a lymph node is the most frequent presentation of NHL, and the commonest site is the neck. Sometimes the nodes fluctuate in size, which can lead to delay in diagnosis. NHLs tend to be more widespread at presentation than Hodgkin's disease and to be present at more unusual lymph node sites, for example, Waldeyer's ring. Although the presentation is usually straightforward, the enlarging lymph node mass may cause initial symptoms due to compression, for example, swelling of the arm or leg, simulating deep venous thrombosis or superior vena caval obstruction (SVCO).

Retroperitoneal lymph node enlargement can result in backache and obstructive renal failure, and nodes in the aorta hepatis may cause obstructive jaundice.

Widespread infiltration of the liver is usually accompanied by weight loss, anorexia and fever. Even without liver involvement, constitutional symptoms are not infrequent, with weight loss, night sweats and fever. Intra-abdominal lymphoma may present with fever of unknown origin, especially if there is hepatic or bone marrow involvement.

Clinical examination must be meticulous. The neck should be carefully examined, and it is often easier to determine the extent of disease if the examination is carried out from behind the patient. Node enlargement should be sought in the preauricular and postauricular regions, in the occipital, supraclavicular and infraclavicular areas, and deep behind the sternomastoid. The axilla should be carefully examined in both the apex and the walls. Epitrochlear nodes are often missed. In the abdomen the size of the liver and spleen should be noted and an attempt made to examine abdominal and retroperitoneal nodes by deep palpation. The inguinal nodes are often slightly enlarged in normal individuals, but pathological inguino-femoral nodes may extend downwards into the medial aspect of the thigh. Examination of the oropharynx and nasopharynx should be routine, as should rectal examination which may lead to detection of large masses of pelvic nodes.

Diagnosis and investigation

The diagnosis is by node or tissue biopsy. Although there is usually little difficulty about the diagnosis, other conditions may simulate lymphoma (Table 26.4), especially at extranodal sites, and precise immunological classification is becoming increasingly important in management. For these reasons, a lymph node biopsy should be regarded as an important clinical investigation and not as a trivial affair.

Inexperienced surgeons sometimes biopsy a superficial node, which frequently shows reactive hyperplasia, or a node in the neck or groin which may not be obviously abnormal. If there is a deeper, clearly pathological, node this should be removed. Immunohistochemistry helps a great deal in diagnosis, particularly in distinguishing large-cell lymphomas from anaplastic carcinoma, and in the diagnosis of T-cell tumours. Some of these investigations can be done only on fresh or frozen tissue, so the biopsy should not all be placed in formaldehyde and

Table 26.4 Lymph node enlargement simulating lymphoma.

Follicular histology
Reactive hyperplasia
Rheumatoid arthritis and related arthritides
Angiofollicular hyperplasia
Toxoplasmosis

Diffuse histology
Phenytoin sensitivity
Dermatopathic lymphadenopathy
Metastatic carcinoma and melanoma

Other histologies
Sinus histiocytosis with massive lymph node enlargement
Infectious mononucleosis
Cat scratch fever
Metastatic carcinoma (especially melanoma)

the pathologist will advise as required. If the node shows reactive hyperplasia, or an equivocal result, one should not hesitate to biopsy another node if clinical suspicion is high. If the nodes are in an inaccessible site, it may be necessary to proceed to laparotomy or mediastinotomy. It is often better to do this than repeatedly biopsy equivocally enlarged peripheral nodes.

In the investigation of NHL there are certain routine tests that are inexpensive, harmless and sometimes rewarding, and these should be performed. A chest radiograph may show hilar, mediastinal or paratracheal node enlargement. Parenchymal lung lesions are less common, as are pleural effusions, but the latter occur not infrequently when there is massive mediastinal disease. Occasionally the effusion is chylous due to rupture of lymphatics in the mediastinum. Lung infiltrates and effusions which contain lymphoma cells usually occur when there is associated mediastinal or hilar disease.

The blood count may show anaemia, which is usually normochromic and typical of the anaemia of chronic disease (with a low serum iron and iron-binding capacity). Occasionally it is due to autoimmune haemolysis, and a Coombs' test and reticulocyte count should be performed if this is suspected. The blood film may show circulating lymphoma cells. However, immunological methods may detect a malignant population that is not apparent on the blood smear, and the proportion of patients with blood involvement will certainly prove to be higher than the present 10% of cases identified by the blood film. Recent methods of demonstrating monoclonality in B cells have been applied to bone marrow and have suggested a high level (30–50%) of involvement in both follicular and diffuse lymphomas. An abnormal blood film implies marrow disease, but this may not always be detected on aspiration and biopsy. Conversely, marrow involvement on biopsy is not always associated with an abnormal peripheral blood picture. The blood urea and electrolytes should be measured to exclude renal failure. The liver enzymes should also be measured since a rise in alkaline phosphatase and aminotransferases may indicate liver infiltration, and the alkaline phosphatase and bilirubin may be elevated if there are nodes in the aorta hepatis causing compression.

Other investigations include computed tomography (CT) of the abdomen or pelvis to demonstrate intra-abdominal or pelvic disease, an intravenous urogram if there is evidence of renal impairment, and bone radiography and scan if there is bone pain or tenderness at a particular site. Before the advent of CT, lymphography was widely used to demonstrate pelvic and para-aortic nodes. CT is a less troublesome alternative to lymphography and has about the same sensitivity. It has the advantage of being able to demonstrate nodal masses in the mesentery and in the upper abdomen, sites poorly demonstrated by lymphography.

How far should these tests be done as a routine and combined with more invasive tests such as liver or marrow biopsy? This depends on what the treatment strategy is to be. If there is a prospect that the disease is localized and the patient might be cured by radiotherapy, extensive investigation is needed to define the true extent of the disease. However, if treatment is to be with palliative local radiotherapy, for example, in an elderly patient with clinically localized disease, then invasive investigations are meddlesome. If the histology and clinical features indicate widespread poor-prognosis disease, then intensive chemotherapy will be used and it becomes irrelevant to persist with unpleasant investigations such as liver biopsy.

Staging notation

The staging notation is the same as that employed for Hodgkin's disease (see Table 25.2). Unlike Hodgkin's disease the great majority of patients will have stage III or IV disease at presentation.

Most cases of NHL presenting as nodal disease should be regarded as widespread, irrespective of histology [8]. In both nodular and diffuse lymphomas it is likely that there will be evidence on mediastinal and abdominal CT, and a not inconsiderable chance of detecting disease in the marrow or liver. While 30% of patients have clinically localized disease (stages I and II) at presentation, after sequential investigation the proportion falls to about 15%. Laparotomy makes little contribution to assessment of spread.

Follicular lymphoma

Centroblastic and centrocytic follicular lymphomas constitute up to 30% of all cases of NHL (figures from Europe; possibly a lower proportion, about 20%, in the USA). At present, the current incidence of follicular lymphoma is approximately 1 per 24 000 persons per year (figures from the USA), and rising. These are tumours of the follicle centre (B cell), a mixture of small cleaved centrocytes and large centroblasts. Depending on the proportion of these cells they are referred to as follicular small cleaved (centrocytic) mixed or large-cell (centroblastic) lymphoma. The distinction from diffuse lymphomas of the follicular centre cell is occasionally arbitrary since a single node may show follicular and diffuse changes, especially in the large-cell (centroblastic) types. Spontaneous fluctuations in lymph node size and even regressions occur.

An unusual form of lymphoma with a nodular appearance is the lymphoma derived from small B cells surrounding the follicle. This has a different phenotype from the follicular centre cell.

The tumours always express CD20 and CD22 and frequently CD19. The translocation from 18q21 to 14q32 at the site of the heavy-chain enhancer has been previously discussed (see pages 518–519 et seq.). The resulting overexpression of *bcl*-2 may block programmed cell death, contributing to expansion of the tumour. The large-cell variants appear to have the highest growth fraction and small-cell variants the lowest, and this may account for the greatest likelihood of cure of the large-cell variant by chemotherapy.

The tumours occur in middle or old age with painless (often prolonged) enlargement of nodes. Involvement of marrow and blood is frequent, especially in the centrocytic types. Clinical stage I and II disease occurs in 40% of cases, but only 20% have stage I and II after investigation.

Treatment: stages I and II

Many studies have suggested that a watch-and-wait policy confers no disadvantage, and may be the preferred option. In practice, patients may find this hard to accept, especially if the nodes are highly visible.

In this group localized or extended-field irradiation produces impressive results, with 60–80% of patients free of the disease at 10 years. Recurrence is frequent at adjacent lymph node sites, but further radiation can be given. Current data suggest that about 50% of patients will be cured by treatment of involved and adjacent lymph nodes [11]. Additional chemotherapy has not yet been shown to be unequivocally beneficial when radiation is used. However, in stage II disease in an infirm elderly patient, excellent symptomatic control can be obtained with the use of intermittent oral chlorambucil, sometimes combined with prednisolone.

Treatment: stages III and IV

Some of these patients with low-grade follicular lymphomas will live for several years without symptoms from their disease (Figure 26.6). There has been considerable debate about how soon treatment (with chemotherapy) should begin. The median period before symptoms develop is 4 years. It seemed that, until recently, no advantage in survival was achievable with an immediate treatment policy using conventional chemotherapy compared

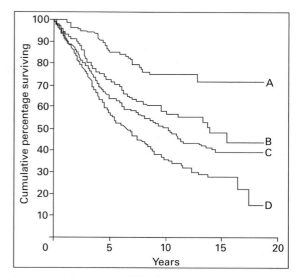

Figure 26.6 Prognosis in follicular non-Hodgkin's lymphoma. The curves indicate the death rate from lymphoma according to stage at presentation. A, stage I/IE ($N = 2441$); B, stage II/IIE ($N = 186$); C, stage III/IIIE ($N = 397$); D, stage IV/IVE ($N = 423$). The relationship between prognosis and clinical stage is clearly shown. The 15-year overall cause-specific survival is 37%. Data from the British National Lymphoma Investigation.

with the traditional watch-and-wait approach that was the standard of care for many patients a decade ago [11].

With low-dose oral chemotherapy, symptoms can usually be brought under control. However, with this approach, relapse will occur relatively quickly and the interval between treatments will shorten.

The purine analogue fludarabine is one of the most effective of the newer agents [12]. It is relatively free of immediate side-effects, and 50% of patients relapsing after chlorambucil have a remission. Myelosuppression and immunosuppression are cumulative and limit dose and duration. Interferon-α has been shown to prolong progression-free survival in some trials, and there is some suggestion of improved overall survival. It is used after or with chemotherapy and may justify the increased toxicity. Rituximab (an anti-CD20 monoclonal antibody) produces responses in drug-insensitive relapse [13] and is established as an important component of treatment in selected cases – see Ref. [2]. Often recommended as a 2-year maintenance programme, it clearly contributes to an extension of progression-free survival. One of the mechanisms by which it appears to eradicate CD20-positive lymphoma cells is via antibody-dependent cellular cytotoxicity, binding rituximab to the tumour cells, with further downstream effects via IgG receptors. Its role in early treatment is being further defined in a variety of studies – see, for example, Ref. [14]. These results indicate that response rate and progression-free survival are undoubtedly improved by its use in combination with chemotherapy. There is accumulating evidence that overall survival may also be improved though this is far less clear. If confirmed, this will clearly require a revision of the traditional watch-and-wait policy, at least in selected patients [15]. In patients who have achieved only a partial remission after chemotherapy, the use of radiolabelled (yttrium-90) ibritumomab has been associated with a significant conversion rate to complete remission, though its use after treatment with rituximab has not been established. This agent is a recombinant murine IgG1 κ monoclonal antibody specific for the B-cell antigen CD20. It is also sometimes used in the management of diffuse high-grade lymphoma (see below).

Poor prognosis is indicated by systemic symptoms, high serum lactate dehydrogenase and poor performance status. A high response rate can be achieved with more intensive chemotherapy. However, early studies with cyclophosphamide, vincristine and prednisolone did not show any advantage to this approach. Subsequently, even more intensive doxorubicin-containing therapy has been shown to produce a high rate of complete response. Nevertheless, longer-term follow-up has failed to show a convincing benefit for more intensive therapy. The role of high-dose chemotherapy (with bone marrow or blood stem-cell support) is under evaluation in young and high-risk patients. Prolonged remissions can be obtained but there is as yet no convincing demonstration of improved survival.

Mantle cell lymphoma

The term 'mantle cell lymphoma' [16] is that used in the REAL classification. Previous terms were *centrocytic*, *intermediate lymphocytic* or *diffuse small cleaved cell lymphoma*. It is a relatively infrequent lymphoma (5–10% of cases). It affects men more than women, usually aged about 60 years or over – see, for example, Ref. [17]. It presents as widespread nodal disease, often with marrow and spleen involvement. It may present as a primary disorder in the spleen, or as a generalized nodular infiltrate in the gastrointestinal tract [18]; the bowel disease in this disorder is particularly difficult to treat as it is characteristically diffuse, unresectable and responds poorly.

The malignant B cells appear as small cleaved cells occasionally admixed with larger blastic cells. They express CD20, CD19 and CD22 and surface immunoglobulin and IgD. There is a t(11;14) translocation which moves *bcl*-1 next to the immunoglobulin heavy-chain enhancer. This results in overexpression of cyclin D1. This overexpression is associated with an aggressive clinical course and a worse prognosis but probably plays a role in pathogenesis and is a target for new agents – see below, for example, in work using targeted therapy against Bruton's Tyrosine Kinase (BTK), a cytoplasmic protein expressed in B-cells and myeloid cells and clearly essential for the regulation of B-cell proliferation and survival. Activation of B-cell receptor signalling appears to be essential for the proliferation of the malignant B-cell – hence the recent concentration on designing inhibitors of B-cell receptor-associated kinases such as BTK. The presence of blastic cells is also adverse prognostically.

Treatment is currently unsatisfactory though recent improvements have been made, notably in the newer approach with BTK inhibition. Initially the tumour responds to COP (cyclophosphamide, vincristine and prednisolone), CHOP (cyclophosphamide, doxorubicin, vincristine and prednisolone) and other regimens such as ESHAP, but often only for a short time. Responses to fludarabine are also short-lived. Encouraging results have been reported using rituximab in combination with chemotherapy [19], and also with the use of both bortezomib and temsirolimus. The important study from Holland comparing a large group of older patients (560 enrolled, 532 included in the analysis) treated either with rituximab, cyclophosphamide and fludarabine or R-CHOP as per younger patients demonstrated that the latter was the more effective regimen; maintenance treatment afterwards, with rituximab, added still further to the benefit [17]. High-dose chemotherapy is also being evaluated and more effective supportive care has meant that patients over the age of 60 can now increasingly be considered for more intensive regimens, justified in selected cases by the better outcome. An important recent study of over 100 patients recruited from the MD Anderson group has identified Ibrutinib, an oral BTK inhibitor, as a useful salvage agent for patients with relapsed or refractory mantle cell lymphoma, with some durable responses – see Ref. [20]. In this difficult group, the overall response rate was 68%, including some patients who had previously received targeted therapy with bortozemib. Estimated median duration was an impressive 17.5 months. Current studies include a formal comparison of ibrutinib versus temsirolimus, and also phase III studies of ibrutinib in combination with bendamustine and rituximab – both known to be active agents in this extremely challenging cohort of patients – as well as the potential of incorporating it into the 'standard' approach with R-CHOP.

Stage I and II follicular large-cell (centroblastic) lymphoma

This is a much less common form of NHL and has a more rapid course. In true stage I disease radiation therapy may cure some patients. Relapse-free survival is prolonged if chemotherapy (such as CHOP) is added (see page 528 for chemotherapy details). Chemotherapy alone with CHOP or ProMACE (prednisone, methotrexate, doxorubicin, cyclophosphamide and etoposide) – MOPP (mustine, vincristine, prednisone and procarbazine) produces excellent results. At present the weight of evidence favours intensive chemotherapy as the mainstay of treatment, and the role of radiation is less clear.

Adult diffuse intermediate- and high-grade lymphoma

Included in this category are the diffuse tumours called centrocytic/centroblastic, large-cell, immunoblastic, undifferentiated and pleomorphic peripheral T-cell lymphomas and follicular large-cell lymphoma (see below). The largest group is the diffuse large-cell type. Diffuse large-cell lymphoma is the commonest form of NHL. Most of the tumours are B cell in origin, many of them having the immunophenotype and genetic abnormalities associated with follicular cell lymphoma (CD10, *bcl*-2 rearrangement, *bcl*-6 expression). T-cell tumours can appear identical clinically and it is not clear if there is any prognostic significance to the cell type. Immunoblastic tumours are usually of B-cell origin, and lymphoblastic tumours may be B or T cell. The justification for grouping them all therapeutically is that there is no clear reason for adopting different treatment strategies in each type.

The patients are usually middle-aged or older. Most cases are stage III or IV but large-cell types are localized (stage I or II) in 25% of cases. Routine investigation includes chest and abdominal CT scanning and bone marrow aspiration and biopsy. An international prognostic index [18] used age, performance status, serum lactate dehydrogenase, stage and extranodal spread to define four risk groups depending on age (Table 26.5 and Figure 26.7).

As far as treatment is concerned, radiotherapy alone is not adequate treatment for stage II disease, and the relapse rate in stage I disease is 40%. Treatment for stage I and II cases therefore now includes combination chemotherapy. Radiotherapy to the involved field with

Table 26.5 International Diagnostic Index for non-Hodgkin's lymphomas.*

Factor†	Score	
	0	1
Age	<60	≥60
Performance status	0, 1	2, 3, 4
Stage	I, II	III, IV
Extranodal disease	<2 sites	>2 sites
LDH	Normal	High
Low-risk score 0, 1		
Low intermediate-risk score 2		
Higher intermediate-risk score 3		
High-risk score 4, 5		

*Originally defined for diffuse lymphomas, it applied to follicular lymphomas as well.
†To these factors may be added β_2-microglobulin in plasma (lower score when normal) and obesity (higher score). LDH, lactate dehydrogenase.

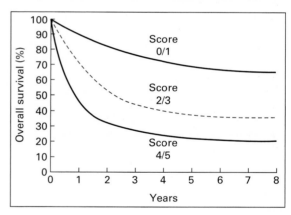

Figure 26.7 The 5-year survival rates for aggressive non-Hodgkin's lymphoma according to the International Prognostic Index Score (see Table 26.5).

three cycles of CHOP has been shown to be superior to eight cycles of CHOP without radiation both with respect to progression-free survival and overall survival [21]. However, stages I and II include patients with widely differing prognoses. CHOP and radiotherapy are excellent treatment for stage I with no adverse prognostic factors according to the international index. For patients with bulky stage II more intensive chemotherapy gives improved survival [22]. The optimum treatment for the intermediate groups of stage I and II is not yet defined.

Table 26.6 Combination chemotherapy regimens in advanced diffuse nodal non-Hodgkin's lymphoma.

CHOP (21 days)
Cyclophosphamide (1 m² day 1)
H-doxorubicin (70 mg/m² day 1)
O-vincristine (2 mg i.v. day 1)
Prednisolone (100 mg p.o. days 1–5)

M-BACOD (21 days)
Methotrexate (200 mg/m² days 1, 8, 15; with folinic acid)
Bleomycin (15 mg/m² day 1)
A-doxorubicin (45 mg/m² day 1)
Cyclophosphamide (600 mg/m² day 1)
O-vincristine (2 mg/m² day 1)
Dexamethasone (6 mg/m² p.o. days 1–5)

Pro(M)ACE-CytaBOM (21 days)
Prednisolone (60 mg/m² days 1–14)
A-doxorubicin (25 mg/m² day 1)
Cyclophosphamide (650 mg/m² day 1)
Etoposide (120 mg/m² day 1)
Cytarabine (300 mg/m² day 1)
Bleomycin (15 mg/m² day 8)
O-vincristine (2 mg/m² day 8)
Methotrexate (120 mg/m² day 8; with folinic acid)

MACOP-B
Methotrexate (400 mg/m² days 8, 36, 64)
A-doxorubicin (50 mg/m² days 1, 15, 29, 43, 57, 17)
Cyclophosphamide (350 mg/m² days 1, 15, 29, 43, 57, 71)
O-vincristine (2 mg/m² days 8, 22, 36, 50, 64, 78)
Prednisolone (75 mg/m² p.o. days 1–84, reducing)
Bleomycin (20 mg/m² days 22, 50, 78)

For stage III and IV disease, treatment is with intensive combination chemotherapy. The CHOP regimen has been widely used (Table 26.6) but several more intensive combinations have been used. These regimens have incorporated the following features: additional agents such as methotrexate, cytosine arabinoside and etoposide, treatment at closer intervals to avoid the problem of relapse between cycles, and the use of multidrug combinations such as ProMACE–CytaBOM (cytarabine, bleomycin, O-vincristine and methotrexate) (Table 26.6). Typically, treatment durations of about 4–6 months are used, but the MACOP-B (methotrexate, A-doxorubicin, cyclophosphamide, O-vincristine, prednisolone and bleomycin) regimen lasts only 12 weeks, with chemotherapy cycles being given weekly. These regimens are very myelosuppressive, and mucositis is common especially with MACOP-B. However, a randomized comparison of three of these regimens with CHOP has failed to show any survival advantage and CHOP remains the standard chemotherapy approach [22]. The best results require the maximum dosage and the risks of toxicity are constantly present. The more intensive programmes are not suitable for elderly or infirm patients, and considerable care is needed in all patients regardless of age. Several novel agents are currently under study, including pixantrone, an aza-anthracenedione compound that acts as an inhibitor of topoisomerase II and has less cardiotoxicity than doxorubicin. It has shown activity in several clinical trials and has achieved fast-track approval by the Food and Drug Administration (FDA) for use in relapsed aggressive NHL.

With many of these CHOP or CHOP-like regimens, complete response rates (in single-institution selected series) are 80% or greater. Relapse is uncommon after 3 years, and cure rates of 60% can be achieved, depending on the composition of the patient groups included, with respect to the prognostic index. If a complete response is not attained, the outlook is poor, most patients dying within 2 years. Failure to attain early complete response may be an indication for autologous or allogeneic stem-cell transplantation (see below).

The anti CD-20 monoclonal antibody rituximab has rapidly become an established part of treatment of these conditions [23,24], increasing the complete response rate and prolonging event-free and overall survival, even in elderly patients in whom toxicity is always an important issue. A number of other biological targeted therapies are also under investigation, including complexes of antibodies tagged with radioactive molecules such as ibritumomab tiuxetan (Zevalin; rituximab tagged with radioactive yttrium) and tositumomab (Bexxar), an antibody with radioactive iodine attached. Their major disadvantage is that they cannot be used with chemotherapy because they lower blood counts. Generally they are used when chemotherapy is no longer proving effective.

Adult lymphoblastic lymphoma

Adult lymphoblastic lymphomas [25] are diffuse high-grade lymphomas characterized by cells with scant cytoplasm, small nucleoli and nuclei which may be of a convoluted or non-convoluted form. The mitotic rate is high. There is often strong phosphatase activity. The immunophenotype is variable but many are T-cell tumours. Both T-cell and B-cell forms express terminal deoxyribonucleotidyltransferase. The cells show T-cell markers (see Figure 26.2), some having a 'thymic' pattern of antigen expression. B-cell types may show common acute lymphoblastic leukaemia antigen (CALLA). Chromosomal breaks at the location of the T-cell receptor α and δ chains are frequent (14q11).

The disease is most frequent in adolescence and in young adults, and in males more than females. A mediastinal mass and SVCO are frequent. There is widespread nodal involvement. Bone marrow involvement is frequent and the distinction between this and lymphoblastic leukaemia is sometimes a matter of definition. Many haematologists will call this leukaemia if there are more than 25% of lymphoblasts in the marrow. Although involvement of the central nervous system (CNS) at diagnosis is unusual, it may occur during the course of the disease, especially if there is marrow involvement.

Treatment has depended to some degree on whether these patients have been regarded as having leukaemia or lymphoma and on whether they are children or adults. There is no clear clinical basis for this distinction. Children have usually been treated with either acute lymphoblastic leukaemia protocols or those based on the LSA2L2 regimen (see pages 533–534). Both these regimens are relatively successful but LSA2L2 probably cures only half of the patients; other regimens such as COMP (cyclophosphamide, vincristine, methotrexate and prednisolone) or A-COP (A-doxorubicin, cyclophosphamide, O-vincristine and prednisolone) appear to be at least as effective. All employ intrathecal treatment as prophylaxis for CNS disease. Established CNS disease is treated as described on page 538. With the introduction of intensive chemotherapy regimens the prognosis has improved, with a 3-year relapse-free survival rate of 60%. Poor prognostic features are age greater than 30 years, high initial white cell count and failure to obtain complete response. The role of high-dose chemotherapy (and peripheral blood stem-cell support) is under investigation for these patients.

Small non-cleaved cell lymphomas (SNCC lymphomas, Burkitt's lymphoma, lymphoblastic lymphoma Burkitt's type)

These tumours are characterized by diffuse infiltration of lymph nodes with cells with a round nucleus with multiple nucleoli, and scanty cytoplasm containing lipid and macrophages. The distinction between Burkitt's and non-Burkitt's type is somewhat arbitrary. The cells are B cells with surface IgM. They express HLA-DR, CALLA, CD19, CD20 and CD21, all B-cell markers. The chromosomal translocations are described on pages 518–519.

In Western countries about 30% of childhood NHL and 1–2% of adult cases are of Burkitt type. In so-called endemic areas (equatorial Africa, New Guinea) the incidence is 40 times higher than in the West, where the incidence is 2 per million below the age of 20.

Recent work on the use of gene-expression microarray technology has helped improve the accuracy of both diagnosis and prognosis [26]. Since the distinction between Burkitt's lymphoma and diffuse large-B-cell lymphoma is still unclear, these authors used transcriptional and genomic profiling, and generated a molecular signature for Burkitt's, aiding identification of previously unclassifiable cases. Over 20% of these patients had a chromosomal breakpoint at the *myc* locus, associated with complex chromosomal changes and a dramatically less favourable clinical course.

The presentation and management of Burkitt's lymphoma in childhood is discussed below (pages 532–533). Adult patients have in the past been treated with one of the regimens outlined in Table 26.6. This may not be the correct policy, and outcomes are probably better if protocols based on the childhood regimens are adopted. Recent results are comparable with those obtained in children. The regimen consisted of CHOP with intermediate-dose methotrexate, and cytosine arabinoside and methotrexate given intrathecally. However, a more recent study from the NCI, addressing the possibility of a less intensive therapy option for patients with this histology showed surprisingly good results, although the trial was admittedly an uncontrolled prospective study rather than a randomized methodology – see Ref. [27]. A total of thirty consecutive patients (including some who were HIV-positive) were treated with a regimen including infused etoposide, doxorubicin, cyclophosphamide, vincristine, prednisolone and rituximab (EPOCH-R). Almost every patient responded well, with a free-from-progressive – disease rate of over 95% at a follow-up period greater than 6 years. None of the patients died during the study period from Burkitt's lymphoma.

Primary mediastinal B-cell lymphoma

Primary mediastinal B-cell lymphoma (PMBL) [28] is a recently defined entity. It occurs in young adults with a female preponderance. It presents with the typical symptoms of an anterior mediastinal mass: cough, dysphagia, hoarse voice, chest pain and SVCO. The tumour remains localized to the mediastinum where it may invade locally into adjacent lung and pleura. It consists of medium to large B cells often with marked fibrosis. The tumour expresses CD20 and other B-cell markers. It is not distinguishable histologically from other diffuse large-cell B-cell tumours. The likely origin is in thymic B cells. Various chromosomal abnormalities have been described. Mutation of the *bcl*-6 gene, common in other large-cell lymphomas, is absent in PMBL.

The differential diagnosis includes other mediastinal lymphomas and tumours. PMBL is the commonest mediastinal lymphoma in adults. Immediate chemotherapy is the first step in management. SVCO responds rapidly and emergency radiation is not usually needed. The regimens contain anthracyclines and there is no clear superiority for any. Mediastinal radiation is often given after chemotherapy, especially if response is incomplete (although the presence of fibrosis makes this difficult to assess). There is no certain evidence that it is necessary. Extensive masses and invasion are associated with worse outcomes. In these patients, and those with a poor response to initial therapy, high-dose chemotherapy with stem-cell support has been used. Approximately 60% of patients appear to be cured with current approaches.

Ki-positive lymphomas

The Ki-positive lymphoma [29] is a rather distinctive lymphoma that expresses CD30 (Ki-1) from the outset (other lymphomas may express CD30 later in their clinical course). The cells are large and may contain phagocytosed red cells. Breaks in chromosome 5 are often present. Seventy per cent are of T-cell origin.

The tumours often occur in children or young adults. Skin rash may be present at presentation. The treatment is as for high-grade lymphoma. Approximately 50% of patients will be long-term survivors.

Lymphoplasmacytic lymphoma and Waldenström's macroglobulinaemia

Lymphoplasmacytic lymphoma and Waldenström's macroglobulinaemia [30] occur in the elderly. They are tumours of small lymphocytes mixed with plasma cells, which often produce IgM in large quantities. Typically they present with lymph node enlargement, anaemia and symptoms of hyperviscosity: bleeding, retinal haemorrhages, mental confusion and renal impairment. On examination there may be hepatomegaly, splenomegaly (which may be massive but is often not present) and lymph node enlargement. Patients may have distal sensorimotor peripheral neuropathy and cranial nerve palsies (in these patients the IgM is often directed to a myelin-associated protein). Rarely, there may be urticarial red skin lesions due to dermal infiltration (Schnitzler's syndrome).

Investigation reveals anaemia, high erythrocyte sedimentation rate (ESR), monoclonal immunoglobulin that may be a cryoglobulin, and abnormal platelet function. The bone marrow shows focal infiltration with small lymphocytes with occasional plasma cells. There is involvement of spleen, liver and lymph nodes. Pulmonary infiltration may be due to tumour or opportunistic infection.

Treatment is with plasmapheresis if hyperviscosity is life-threatening. Alkylating agents, fludarabine and 2-deoxychloroadenosine are effective treatments, but relapse occurs. The therapeutic role of anti-CD20 antibody is currently being assessed.

Angioimmunoblastic T-cell lymphoma

This disease, which for several years was not thought to be malignant, is a T-cell lymphoma characterized by proliferating vascular endothelium replacing the paracortical region, interspersed with T cells and plasma cells. It presents with lymph node enlargement, rash, hepatosplenomegaly, fever and dysproteinaemia with polyclonal hyperglobulinaemia. Initial response to treatment is not sustained and a progressive lymphoma supervenes.

Stem-cell transplantation in non-Hodgkin's lymphomas

Although modern combination regimens will cure 50–60% of patients with high-grade NHL, those who relapse are seldom, if ever, curable by conventional chemotherapy. High-dose chemotherapy with autologous bone marrow transplantation [31] or peripheral blood stem-cell support can achieve a five- to seven-fold increase in drug dosage. The procedure is based on the proposition that this increase is adequate to cure a patient who has disease resistant to lower drug doses. Above these doses non-haematological toxicity is likely to be fatal. Major improvements in supportive care, the use of autologous peripheral blood stem-cell support and haemopoietic growth factors have all reduced the morbidity and mortality from the procedure.

Evidence from uncontrolled trials shows that in relapsed patients about 30–40% will live beyond 3 years after high-dose stem-cell-supported treatment, and 60–75% of patients will have a major response [32].

Prognostic factors include general health, tumour mass, the responsiveness of the tumour to previous chemotherapy, and the number and variety of previous regimens. These encouraging results have led to use of the procedure in first remission in high-risk patients, or in patients failing to achieve complete response with the first treatment. The problem is that in both these categories there is considerable heterogeneity of prognosis and this means that randomized comparison of the treatment is essential.

The first randomized trial has been reported [31] in which patients who had relapsed after chemotherapy, but who still had chemosensitive disease, were treated either with chemotherapy and irradiation alone or with the addition of high-dose therapy. A clear relapse-free survival and overall survival advantage was found in those receiving the high-dose treatment, although the numbers of patients randomized was small. High-dose therapy should therefore be considered in patients who fail to achieve complete response with initial treatment, in selected patients with poor-prognosis tumours (e.g. high-grade T-cell lymphomas, adult lymphoblastic lymphoma, poor-prognosis high-grade nodal lymphoma of follicular centre cells) even in first complete response, and in patients who, after first relapse, achieve a second complete response.

One problem with autologous stem-cell or marrow transplantation is the potential contamination of the transfused cells by tumour. A wide variety of 'purging' procedures has been adopted to eliminate residual tumour cells, but there is no convincing evidence that these are necessary or effective. The problem therapeutically is mainly the residual disease in the patient rather than in the transfused cells. One possible way forward is to use concurrent administration of high-dose rituximab both before and after autologous stem-cell transplantation for these patients, and a number of studies have offered encouraging results [33]. Despite decades of work in this exciting area, the precise role and achievements of high-dose chemotherapy supported by autologous stem-cell transplantation remain controversial, particularly perhaps the role of this approach as part of the first-line treatment of aggressive NHL [32]. The authors of this meta-analysis felt that its use was not warranted in patients with 'good-risk' disease. A recent large-scale US and Canadian-based study concluded that in the current era of effective treatment both in the first instance and as salvage for relapse, early autologous transplantation as consolidation in aggressive NHL certainly increased the progression-free survival time but not the patient's overall survival – see Ref. [34].

HIV- and AIDS-related non-Hodgkin's lymphomas [35,36]

The occurrence of NHL in patients infected with human immunodeficiency virus (HIV) is now regarded as part of the definition of AIDS. The introduction of highly active antiretroviral therapy has diminished the frequency of AIDS and the diseases that complicate it, including some of the HIV-related lymphomas. Previously the risk of lymphoma was 60 times that of the non-infected population. The diminished frequency appears to be directly related to the recovery of immune competence.

The lymphomas include Hodgkin's disease, nodal lymphomas, primary CNS lymphoma and PEL. These are usually diffuse large-cell immunoblastic or SNCC lymphomas (Burkitt's-like) and other diffuse large-cell types. Ki-1 anaplastic large-cell lymphoma may occur, of B-cell type. The immunoblastic lymphomas are now much less common, while the Burkitt's type and Hodgkin's disease have not become less frequent at present. EBV infection is closely associated with primary CNS lymphoma and with PEL. The latter is always associated with HHV8 genome in the tumour cells.

Typically, the NHL occurs in a patient who has had AIDS for 1–2 years and whose CD4 cell count is very low. Most patients present with widespread disease, and extranodal sites are often involved (CNS 40%, bone marrow 35%, gastrointestinal 25% and numerous other sites less frequently). SNCC lymphomas commonly involve the CNS and bone marrow, and large-cell types the gastrointestinal tract. Tumours where EBV is detected are especially likely to involve the meninges as are those presenting in the marrow, nasal sinuses and testes. In these cases CNS prophylaxis should be considered. It is estimated that as more patients with established AIDS live longer (due to antibiotic therapy) one-third or more will develop NHL. Coincident infection with HTLV-1 is increasingly recognized, especially in intravenous drug abusers. Chemotherapy appears to improve survival. Haematological toxicity may be ameliorated by granulocyte colony-stimulating factor but immunosuppression is a serious problem. In patients with established AIDS the complete response rates are relatively low and median survival is about 6 months. Poor prognostic features are AIDS present before diagnosis of NHL, poor performance status, low CD4 count and extranodal disease. However, when the lymphomas arise in patients without AIDS and with good immune function, full-dose chemotherapy can be delivered and appears to produce more durable remission. Treatment of CNS disease is discussed on pages 537–538.

Non-Hodgkin's lymphoma in childhood

Incidence and aetiology

NHLs are more common in children than Hodgkin's disease (1.5:1) and are the third most frequent childhood cancer [37,38]. The annual incidence is 0.6 per 100 000 children below 15 years of age, with a peak onset at age 6–10 years (see Figure 26.1). A variety of inherited diseases predispose to childhood NHL (see Table 26.1). Other aetiological factors are discussed on pages 535–536.

Pathology

The distinction between childhood NHL and leukaemia is to some extent semantic. Many childhood lymphomas spread to the bone marrow and the frequency of diagnosis of marrow involvement is increasing as techniques for the demonstration of monoclonal B-cell populations improve. A convention is to regard more than 25% infiltration as compatible with lymphoma. The lymph nodes almost always show diffuse involvement, and follicular patterns are very rare. The main categories are shown in Table 26.7. Diffuse lymphoblastic lymphoma is the commonest type. Some of these tumours show a convoluted nuclear morphology and show positivity with T-cell markers – these are T-cell tumours. Others show surface immunoglobulin and are thus B-cell tumours. Other tumours have neither T nor B markers.

Approximately 20% of cases are large-cell lymphomas of diverse lineage. Some appear to be tumours of the follicle centre cell, others are B-cell immunoblastic tumours, while yet others express T-cell markers. Many of these tumours express the CD30 antigen (Ki-1, Ber-h2) which characterizes activated B and T cells. The majority of these appear to be peripheral T-cell tumours.

Childhood NHL has a greater tendency to involve extranodal sites such as the gut, bone marrow and CNS.

Table 26.7 Pathology of childhood non-Hodgkin's lymphoma.

Diffuse lymphoblastic lymphoma: B cell, T cell
Diffuse large-cell lymphoma
Burkitt's lymphoma

Table 26.8 Distribution (%) of main primary site of disease in children with non-Hodgkin's lymphoma.

Intra-abdominal	30
Peripheral nodes	25
Mediastinal	22
Skeleton	7
Nasopharynx	10
Subcutaneous and skin	3.5
Epidural	1
Thyroid	0.5
Testis	0.5
Breast	0.5

The lymph nodes of Waldeyer's ring and the mediastinum are frequently involved. The distribution of the main mass of disease at presentation is shown in Table 26.8, and a staging system in Table 26.9. About 50% of the tumours arising in the mediastinum are of T-cell origin.

Childhood B-cell lymphomas

The majority of NHLs in childhood are B-cell tumours. These diffuse lymphomas consist of either large-cell type or SNCCs. The large-cell lymphomas are usually found in boys and are often extranodal, occurring in the nasopharynx, lung, mediastinum, bone, soft tissues and tonsils.

Table 26.9 A simple staging system for childhood non-Hodgkin's lymphoma and small non-cleaved cell (Burkitt's) lymphoma.

Stage	Description
IA	Single nodal area, or single extranodal site excluding the mediastinum
IIA	Single extranodal tumour with involved regional nodes. Two or more nodal areas on one side of the diaphragm. Primary gut lymphoma and mesenteric nodes
III	Two or more nodal sites above and below the diaphragm. All primary intrathoracic tumours. Extensive primary intra-abdominal disease. All paraspinal or epidural tumours
IV	Involvement of CNS or marrow
Burkitt's lymphoma	
I	Single extra-abdominal site
II	Multiple extra-abdominal sites
III	Intra-abdominal tumour
V	Intra-abdominal tumour with extra-abdominal sites

The SNCC lymphomas are either Burkitt's lymphoma, or a form in which the cells are more pleomorphic. Endemic Burkitt's lymphoma occurs predominantly in Africa but the tumour is sporadic in Western countries. In Africa, the presentation is usually with jaw or orbital tumours that grow rapidly. Other sites of involvement include the ovaries, retroperitoneal tissues, kidneys and glandular tissues such as breast and thyroid. Invasion of the lymph node and marrow is infrequent.

Spread to the CNS is common and occurs early, often with paraplegia and cranial nerve palsy. A staging system which relates to prognosis is shown in Table 26.9. In Western countries SNCC lymphoma is more likely to present with an abdominal mass, or with enlarged cervical nodes. Marrow involvement is more frequent than in African cases.

Many childhood B-cell lymphomas are generalized diseases with a risk of marrow and CNS involvement. However, some cases have a lower risk of meningeal spread. These cases include localized tumours of the gut, and patients with localized nodal disease. With localized gut lymphoma it is not clear if any treatment should be given after complete resection, but it is usual practice to treat with chemotherapy. CNS prophylaxis does not appear to be necessary in these cases.

Childhood T-cell lymphomas

These tumours often present with anterior mediastinal or cervical node enlargement. They disseminate rapidly to the bone marrow, CNS and testes. The cells may have convoluted nuclei and focal acid phosphatase activity in the cytoplasm. They usually exhibit T-cell markers, reacting with T-cell monoclonal antibodies, and also express CD30 (see above). In childhood, Ki-1 (CD30-positive) lymphomas may be accompanied by a skin rash (lymphomatoid papulosis), which may be the presenting feature on which a rapidly evolving lymphoma develops.

Histologically, the mediastinal tumours are described as lymphoblastic. The distinction between the childhood and adult forms of lymphoblastic lymphoma is arbitrary, and this and the treatment are more based on historical patterns of care rather than on clear evidence that such distinctions are important.

The patients are usually male. SVCO may be present from the outset, which might need urgent treatment (usually with steroids and vincristine) before the diagnostic biopsy can be taken. This therapy can make subsequent diagnosis difficult, but the situation may be life-threatening and aggravated by biopsy under anaesthesia. Marrow failure from infiltration, or CNS symptoms, may be the presenting feature.

In some large treatment series these childhood tumours have not been characterized by modern methods. It appears that many pleomorphic large-cell lymphomas of childhood are T-cell tumours even when there is no mediastinal mass present.

Diagnosis and investigation

Diagnosis is by lymph node or tissue biopsy. Initial staging investigations should be performed quickly since progress of the disease may be rapid. A marrow aspiration and biopsy should be performed and the cerebrospinal fluid (CSF) examined for cells. Biochemical tests of liver and kidney function are necessary with measurement of plasma calcium and urate since tumour lysis syndrome (see Chapter 8) may occur when treatment starts.

Precise immunohistochemical definition of the tumour is now often possible. Although at present the relationship to prognosis is not clear, in the next few years the application of these techniques may allow a more precise definition of risk and therefore lead to greater precision in selecting treatment.

Treatment
Large-cell non-Hodgkin's lymphoma

During the 1960s the prognosis of acute lymphoblastic leukaemia in childhood was improving rapidly with the use of more intensive drug regimens and prophylactic treatment of the CNS. However, childhood lymphomas were still rapidly fatal, 85% of children dying within 1 year and only 10–15% surviving 5 years.

Many modern protocols of intensive treatment are derived from the LSA2L2 programme introduced by Wollner in 1971. The 5-year survival of 70–80% is now regularly obtained, with few children relapsing beyond this time. The protocols have the following components:
1 an intensive induction regimen using cyclophosphamide, vincristine, doxorubicin, prednisolone and intrathecal methotrexate;
2 a consolidation phase using antimetabolites (cytosine arabinoside, thioguanine, asparaginase);
3 a maintenance phase lasting 1 year, using sequential alternating pairs of drugs.

The results of protocols of this type are shown in Figure 26.8. Survival is better in stage I and II disease.

In a randomized study in paediatric NHL of all stages that compared the LSA2L2 protocol with the slightly less aggressive COMP regimen, the Children's Cancer Study Group in the USA found the COMP regimen

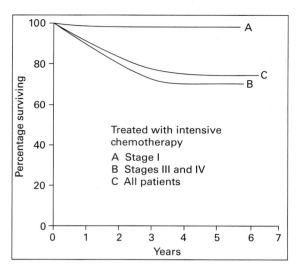

Figure 26.8 Results of intensive chemotherapy of large-cell non-Hodgkin's lymphoma in childhood.

to be slightly less effective [37]. Other regimens have been based on German protocols for acute leukaemia, and on high-dose cyclophosphamide [38], which are as successful as LSA2L2. There is better disease-free survival at 2 years for localized disease (81%) than for generalized disease (46%). In non-localized disease the LSA2L2 protocol proved better than the COMP regimen for patients with lymphoblastic disease.

Lymphoblastic lymphoma in childhood tends to present with mediastinal disease and includes many cases of T-cell lymphoma. Non-lymphoblastic disease tends to be more localized and have an intra-abdominal presentation. In cases with a better prognosis (stage I and II disease, Table 26.9) a randomized trial has shown that radiotherapy can be omitted from the treatment and that treatment of moderate intensity combined with intrathecal methotrexate is associated with a 4-year survival of nearly 90% [39]. There are considerable potential long-term advantages in reducing the amount of chemotherapy and radiation which these children receive [40]. Failure of bone growth, bone cancers, leukaemia and sterility are sequelae of childhood treatment that may be avoided if less intensive treatment can be given without diminished survival. As with adults, the anti-CD20 monoclonal antibody rituximab is increasingly used in the paediatric age group, as an adjunct to 'conventional' chemotherapy and also following high-dose stem-cell transplantation [24].

The optimum treatment for tumours expressing CD30 has not yet been defined, but regimens based on COMP or the LSA2L2 programme have generally been employed.

Other regimens have been used, some of which include cranial irradiation as prophylactic CNS treatment. With the LSA2L2 protocol, using intrathecal methotrexate only, the incidence of CNS relapse is about 16%. The incidence is probably lower when cranial irradiation is used in addition. The risk of CNS disease appears to be low for those with stage I nodal disease and for those whose intra-abdominal lymphoma has been resected.

Small non-cleaved cell lymphoma (including Burkitt's lymphoma)

For SNCC lymphoma (including Burkitt's lymphoma) the chemotherapy approach is rather different from that for lymphoblastic lymphoma, with greater emphasis on high doses of alkylating agents. Treatment does not need to be prolonged beyond 10 weeks, but should be very intensive during this time. Radiation therapy has no part to play in initial treatment. Almost all children will have a complete remission but 50% will relapse. Cure is still possible if CNS relapse occurs, but many regimens now include some form of CNS prophylaxis.

Children who survive 2 years are cured. The 2-year disease-free survival figures for each stage (Table 26.9) are as follows: I and II, 80%; III, 65%; and IV, 40%. In stage III it is advisable to remove as much bulk as possible before treatment. With 90% removed the results approach those for stage I. More aggressive regimens are being developed for stage IV cases. Very high-dose chemotherapy with autologous peripheral stem-cell support is being assessed, and newer agents such as ifosfamide and etoposide are being introduced into protocols.

Extranodal presentation of non-Hodgkin's lymphoma

NHLs may present at a variety of extranodal sites, and when they do they often pose particular problems in diagnosis and management. In addition to presentation at an extranodal site, there may be involvement of these sites later in the course of the disease, at a time when a nodal lymphoma relapses and disseminates. In this latter circumstance, this is usually part of a generalized spread of the disease. Treatment will usually be palliative, particularly if the patient has already undergone intensive previous chemotherapy. There are of course exceptions to this general rule.

Table 26.10 Staging systems for gastric lymphoma.

	TNM	Ann Arbor
Limited to stomach wall	I	I
Mucosa alone	IA	
Submucosa	IB	
Serosal	IC	
Adjacent (perigastric) nodes	II	II$_1$
Non-adjacent intra-abdominal	III	II$_2$
Nodes outside abdomen	III	III
Disseminated, non-nodal disease	IV	IV

The account which follows concerns the management of NHLs presenting at an extranodal site, in the absence of clinically overt disease elsewhere.

Gastrointestinal lymphoma

Lymphomas may occur at any site in the gastrointestinal tract [41], but the stomach and the small intestine are most frequently involved. The aetiology and pathogenesis are not well understood. The gut-associated lymphoid tissue in a normal individual shows a well-defined pattern of lymphocyte traffic. Immunoglobulin-bearing cells in the follicle centre of small-intestinal lymphoid nodules (Peyer's patches) migrate into the bloodstream and return to the lamina propria of the small bowel, where they differentiate to plasma cells. A similar 'homing' mechanism may take place with gastric and large-bowel lymphocytes and with lymphocytes bearing immunoglobulin of other classes.

Non-Hodgkin's lymphoma of the stomach
Pathology and clinical features
Lymphoma of the stomach is an uncommon tumour, comprising less than 0.5% of all gastric neoplasms. The patient is usually middle-aged or elderly, but the disease can affect young adults. In many cases the tumour begins as a low-grade lesion in the mucosa with destruction of the glandular tissue, so-called lymphoepithelial lesions. This low-grade tumour may occur diffusely in the stomach and remain localized to the stomach wall for several years. Some tumours are of large-cell type and spread early to adjacent lymph nodes. The two most widely used staging systems are given in Table 26.10.

The presentation of gastric lymphoma is similar to that of adenocarcinoma of the stomach, with nausea, anorexia and upper abdominal discomfort as the chief symptoms and occasionally haematemesis or chronic iron-deficiency anaemia as associated features. Barium meal shows a large gastric ulcer or appearances similar to adenocarcinoma of the stomach. On endoscopy, a malignant ulcer is usually seen, but occasionally the appearance can simulate a benign gastric ulcer. Biopsy evidence can be misleading since the specimen may show small lymphocytes which are hard to distinguish from an inflammatory infiltrate. There is a close association between the low-grade gastric lymphoma of mucosa-associated lymphoid tissue and infection with *Helicobacter pylori* [42].

Treatment
In the past, treatment of gastric lymphoma has usually been by surgical resection if possible. The lack of randomized trials means that clear-cut guidance concerning non-surgical treatment is difficult.

If the diagnosis of a low-grade lymphoma has been made on biopsy and *H. pylori* infection is present, it is usual to treat the infection with antibiotics and a proton-pump inhibitor. About 60% of patients will show a complete histological response of the tumour, which will be at the molecular level in half of these. The remission may last several years. If relapse occurs, or if there is failure to achieve complete response, many physicians would use chemotherapy as the next step, keeping surgery in reserve. It is usual to use combination chemotherapy in fit patients. When chemotherapy is started in an unresected or recurrent gastric lymphoma, there is a risk of gastric perforation. The first treatment must be given under close medical supervision.

For higher-grade stage I tumours and those not associated with *H. pylori*, surgery is often the first treatment, but chemotherapy is generally employed [43]. For localized high-grade tumours and all tumours of stage II or worse there is a higher risk of relapse. These relapses may be outside the abdomen (in 50% of cases of stage II$_1$ or III disease). Stage II$_2$ low-grade tumours were formerly often treated by gastric and upper abdominal radiotherapy, but increasingly the preference is to use chemotherapy. Stage III high-grade tumours should be treated with combination chemotherapy, assuming that the patient's performance status is adequate. For stage II$_2$ or III, chemotherapy also seems the most appropriate treatment; it is clearly indicated for stage IV disease.

Small-bowel lymphoma [44]
Pathology
Lymphoma of the small intestine represents the most common bowel tumour of children below the age of

10 years and there is a rise in incidence in adults above the age of 50 years. There is a male preponderance (male to female ratio 5:1) and there are two predisposing conditions. In long-standing untreated coeliac disease there is an increased incidence of intestinal lymphoma, and in this situation the lymphoma has now been shown to be of T-cell type and the bowel is usually widely involved. In the Middle East, there is a high incidence of an intestinal lymphoma that is usually preceded by a diffuse plasma cell and lymphocytic proliferation in the small bowel, known as immunoproliferative disease of the small intestine. In this early phase there is excess production of the heavy chain of IgA (α-chain disease). At this early stage, the disease may respond to treatment with antibiotics, but it subsequently progresses and a B-cell lymphoma develops that may be rapidly evolving. The secretion of heavy chains in the blood may disappear with the onset of lymphoma.

In the typical case of intestinal lymphoma in Europeans, no predisposing cause can be detected. The neoplasm arises in the lymphoid tissues of the mucosa of the bowel, invades and ulcerates the mucosa, and penetrates the bowel wall to the serosal surface. Histologically, many small-bowel lymphomas are of the diffuse large-cell type, but in adults some of the lymphomas are of lower grade [44].

Clinical features

The presentation is usually with subacute or acute intestinal obstruction with colicky abdominal pain, vomiting and constipation. There may be diarrhoea or even malabsorption, but this is unusual. Gastrointestinal haemorrhage occurs, usually of a chronic type leading to iron-deficiency anaemia. When perforation occurs the clinical picture is typical of perforation of the bowel at any site. Occasionally, patients may present with ascites, usually chylous in nature, but sometimes due to widespread dissemination of intraperitoneal lymphoma. With more extensive abdominal disease there may be fever and anaemia.

The diagnosis is usually made at laparotomy or by a barium follow-through examination, which may show infiltration of the bowel wall with ulceration and segments of narrowing, above which are areas of bowel dilatation.

The management of NHL of the small intestine is often difficult. This is in part due to the fact that the disease often presents as an acute surgical emergency. The prognosis is dependent on adequate surgical excision of the tumour. A simple system of staging, which relates quite well to prognosis, is shown in Table 26.11.

Table 26.11 Staging of intestinal lymphoma.

IA	Single tumour confined to gut
IB	Two or more tumours confined to gut
IIA	Local node involvement
IIB	Local extension to adjacent structures
IIC	Local tumour with perforation and peritonitis
III	Widespread lymph node enlargement
IV	Disseminated tumour (to liver, spleen and elsewhere)

All cases should be further staged with chest radiography and bone marrow aspiration. A liver biopsy should be performed during the laparotomy. Complete local excision of the tumour with the resection margins free of disease, and without involvement of mesenteric nodes, will frequently result in a cure, and the role of radiation therapy and adjuvant chemotherapy is still to be determined in this type of case. If the lymphoma is of low-grade histology and complete excision has been carried out, then it is probable that no further treatment is needed. If, as is more likely, there is local node involvement and the histology is of a diffuse large-cell type, most oncologists would treat the patient further, and in recent years the tendency has been to use combination chemotherapy. There is a particular danger in the use of combination chemotherapy in patients in whom the tumour has not been resected completely, with perforation of the bowel wall occurring as a result of tumour lysis. This has a high mortality. In unresectable tumours it is therefore prudent to begin chemotherapy in lower doses, both to allow healing of the bowel wall as the tumour regresses more slowly, and to avoid neutropenia which will add to mortality if perforation should occur. Without combination chemotherapy the 5-year survival of diffuse lymphomas of the gut is about 20% and of follicular lymphomas about 50%, but this clearly depends on the stage.

The combination of drugs usually employed will include cyclophosphamide, vincristine, doxorubicin and prednisolone in various regimens as for diffuse NHLs at other sites (see Table 26.6). In children, the likelihood of CNS involvement is small and it does not appear that prophylactic treatment of the CNS is an essential part of management.

The lymphoma complicating coeliac disease presents particular problems. The preferred designation is *enteropathy-associated T-cell lymphoma*. The mean time of onset is 7 years after the diagnosis of coeliac disease but may be many years later. The lymphoma does not regress on a gluten-free diet and, typically, patients do not show anti-gliadin antibody in the blood. Cutaneous and pulmonary spread of the lymphoma is characteristic. The small bowel is frequently involved, with an ulcerative lesion that may be the harbinger of the malignant change. Resection of the lymphoma is carried out where possible. Although chemotherapy is usually given postoperatively, the prognosis is poor due to the inadequate nutritional state of the patient and the risks of perforation and haemorrhage.

α-Chain disease [45]

The lymphoma which follows immune proliferative smallintestine disease (IPSID) is characterized by transformation of the nodular mucosal infiltrate into a high-grade B-cell lymphoma where there is secretion of α-heavy chain (subclass 1). Recent studies have suggested that IPSID is a neoplasm from the beginning. Although in the early stage IPSID may regress with antibiotics, when it transforms to a high-grade tumour treatment with chemotherapy is difficult and usually unsuccessful.

Lymphomatous polyposis

In this extremely unusual disease, polyps develop in the ileocaecal region, characteristically in patients over 50 years of age. The polyps consist of a centrocytic tumour and the mesenteric nodes are usually involved. The tumour disseminates widely early on. Treatment with chemotherapy produces regression but the prognosis is poor (see also Mantle cell lymphoma, pages 526–527).

Non-Hodgkin's lymphoma of bone (see also Chapter 23, page 458) [46]

NHL frequently invades the marrow and may sometimes cause localized bone lesions with pain, vertebral collapse and pathological fractures. Occasionally, NHL presents as a primary bone lesion, and most of these cases are of large-cell lymphoma. Sometimes the lesion is localized with no evidence of NHL at other sites, even after extensive investigations. In children, isolated lymphoma of bone may be mistaken for Ewing's sarcoma [47]. Immunohistochemical studies will usually resolve any diagnostic difficulty. In most cases of NHL of bone the lesion is confined to one bone, and a long bone is usually affected. The antecedent history is often very long and the lesions are often very large with extensive soft-tissue infiltration.

The diagnosis is based on the finding of a bone lesion in the absence of widespread lymphoma at other sites including the bone marrow. Pretreatment staging therefore includes CT scanning of the abdomen and mediastinum and a bone marrow examination.

Although radiotherapy (40–45 Gy) produces local control in over 90% of cases, and should encompass a generous margin of normal bone and soft tissue, dissemination to lymph nodes occurs in approximately 50% of cases. It is usual practice therefore to give combination chemotherapy before radiotherapy. It is not known whether, in the era of intensive chemotherapy, radiation treatment can be dropped, and at present local treatment is given even if the chemotherapy response is excellent. In general the prognosis of primary bone lymphoma is extremely good, particularly in patients treated, as is customary nowadays, with combined-modality therapy [46]. In the very elderly it may be reasonable to treat with radiation alone in the first instance.

Central nervous system involvement with lymphoma

Primary lymphomas of the brain and spinal cord occur but are rare. Usually the CNS is involved as part of the pattern of spread of generalized disease and there is a particular tendency for the CNS to be involved in diffuse lymphomas, especially of childhood, of T-cell type and when there is marrow involvement.

Primary lymphoma of the brain

Primary lymphoma of the brain [48–50] is an uncommon tumour occurring more frequently in AIDS, in renal allograft recipients and in those on long-term immunosuppressive therapy. The histological appearances are usually of a high-grade lymphoma with centrocytic, centroblastic and lymphoplasmacytic forms. They arise in the cerebrum (70% of cases), cerebellum and brainstem (25% of cases) and rarely in the spinal cord. They tend to be multicentric, and perivascular infiltration is common. Presentation is with the signs and symptoms of a brain tumour (see Chapter 11). Although rare in the spinal cord, seeding into the CSF occasionally occurs late in the disease. An unusual complication is migration of lymphoma cells into the vitreous of the eyes causing visual loss. Patients do not usually show lymphoma elsewhere at presentation or later in the disease. Bone marrow and CSF examination are essential staging investigations.

In non-AIDS-related cases, treatment was traditionally with radiotherapy but the disease was difficult to control, local relapse being common even after doses as high as 45–50 Gy. Chemotherapy is now usually given either alone or before irradiation. As recently pointed out by

Bessell and colleagues [50], 'there is an unconfirmed consensus that combined chemo-radiotherapy is superior to radiotherapy alone'. Combinations are based on high-dose methotrexate, cytosine arabinoside and alkylating agents that can penetrate the blood–brain barrier such as nitrosoureas, procarbazine and temozolomide. The role of radiation is now well defined. Patients over 60 years of age have a worse prognosis. For fit patients, response rates of 60–80% (depending on criteria) are achieved with median survival of 50 months. Treatment is often toxic, especially if radiation is included. If CSF seeding has occurred, it is very difficult to cure the disease even with chemotherapy, neuraxis radiation and intrathecal treatment. Treatment with dose intensification using autologous stem-cell support has been employed by several groups but its role remains undefined.

At the start of the AIDS epidemic CNS lymphoma was recognized as an associated tumour. Typically, the lymphoma is a high-grade B-cell neoplasm, generally occurring in patients already gravely ill with AIDS (many cases being diagnosed at autopsy). The presentation is with focal neurological signs, cranial nerve palsies, fits and mental confusion. On CT scan the tumour mass may be difficult to delineate and ring-enhancing lesions may make distinction from toxoplasmosis difficult. Treatment is often challenging for many patients, and usually unsuccessful even in the short term, since these patients are ill and immunocompromised. Radiation may help localized disease. Chemotherapy is associated with a high risk of opportunistic infection, and must be given with great care.

Secondary lymphoma of the central nervous system

Involvement of the CNS occurs in about 9% of all cases of NHL. The clinical presentation is either with lymphomatous meningitis (55%) or with extradural compression (45%) (Figure 26.9). The great majority of patients have diffuse large-cell (centroblastic) lymphoma or diffuse centrocytic lymphoma as the primary disease. Light microscope evidence of involvement of the bone marrow at diagnosis is present in 70% of cases, probably an underestimate if more sensitive tests of involvement are undertaken. Patients usually have advanced nodal spread at diagnosis, and involvement of retroperitoneal nodes is common. Other risk factors for the development of secondary CNS lymphoma include a raised serum lactate dehydrogenase level, advanced stage, a high age-adjusted International Prognostic Index score at presentation, and special anatomic sites of documented involvement, for example, the testis [51]. Lymphomatous involvement of

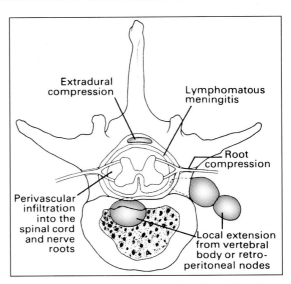

Figure 26.9 Involvement of the spinal cord with lymphoma. Extradural compression may result from lymphomatous involvement of the vertebral body or by extension from para-aortic nodes. Leptomeningeal infiltration is probably haematogenous and is particularly common when bone marrow is involved.

the CNS is particularly frequent in childhood lymphomas and in lymphomas of T-cell type.

The clinical presentation of lymphomatous meningitis is with cranial nerve palsies, mental confusion and raised intracranial pressure. Root lesions frequently occur due to compression and perivascular infiltration. The CSF is examined cytologically and, if possible, surface markers (light chain restriction, T-cell markers) should be identified in an attempt to distinguish the cells from reactive lymphocytes that might be found in tuberculous or fungal meningitis and which may be part of the differential diagnosis. In recent years, both PCR and flow cytometry assays have become available to aid diagnosis.

Epidural compression usually occurs in the thoracic spine, but nerve roots may be compressed, including the cauda equina. These patients usually have retroperitoneal lymphoma and sometimes intravertebral deposits. The clinical syndrome is with a paraparesis and is a medical emergency whose management is discussed in Chapter 8.

Lymphomatous meningitis is a serious complication and very few patients in whom it has developed will be cured. Management is with intrathecal chemotherapy using methotrexate in combination with cytosine arabinoside and craniospinal irradiation. Patients at high risk (e.g. many childhood lymphomas, diffuse large B-cell lymphoma, and T-cell lymphomas in childhood and adolescence) should receive prophylactic treatment of the CNS with intrathecal methotrexate and cranial irradiation in an attempt to avoid this complication [52]. Regimens for systemic treatment often include drugs that penetrate the CSF and these may confer adequate protection. Alternatively, the risk of CNS disease in adults may be lower than had been predicted. Newer approaches that have become increasingly used in clinical practice include stem-cell transplantation, intrathecal administration of rituximab, and liposomal cytarabine.

Non-Hodgkin's lymphoma of the nasopharynx and Waldeyer's ring [53]

NHL may present in the lymphoid tissue of the oropharynx and nasopharynx, in the absence of clinical evidence of disease elsewhere. Primary sites include tonsil (about 50% of cases), nasopharynx (about 30%) and base of tongue. Nasal and nasopharyngeal tumours are much more common in China and South America. These tumours often have the phenotype of NK cells, characteristically with a distinct pathology of vascular destruction. Others are T-cell or B-cell tumours. The tumours in Waldeyer's ring are usually B-cell tumours and histology may be follicular or diffuse, centroblastic or centrocytic. The presentation is with difficulty in swallowing and nasal congestion. There may be enlargement of cervical lymph nodes, or evidence of disease elsewhere.

Approximately 20% of patients have localized disease (stage I) and 40% have involvement of cervical nodes (stage II). Lymphangiography – though now almost entirely an obsolete investigation – demonstrated during the 1970s that almost all patients with stage III disease have involved abdominal nodes. Approximately 50% of patients have stage III disease at presentation, and 10% of patients stage IV disease (in bone marrow or liver). Patients who present with stage I disease do not usually prove to have more extensive disease on investigation.

The gastrointestinal tract may be involved, and a barium meal and follow-through should be performed as part of the initial investigations.

For patients with disease localized to Waldeyer's ring and cervical nodes, treatment is usually with radiotherapy. Many patients (possibly 60%) will be free of disease at 5–10 years. For patients with stage III and IV disease, treatment is with chemotherapy, but it is not clear if the prognosis has been greatly improved by modern regimens. Survival depends on stage and cell type, NK cell tumours having a good prognosis. For all groups 2-year survival is only 60%.

Ocular non-Hodgkin's lymphoma

Uncommonly the conjunctiva, orbit and globe of the eye can be the site of NHL. Orbital lymphomas present with unilateral proptosis, external ocular palsy and intraocular lymphoma with visual disturbance. Conjunctival lymphoma presents with swelling of the lid and visible tumour.

These tumours are uncommon, and their prognosis is not known with certainty. They must be distinguished from the more frequent benign lymphoid proliferations that affect the eye, especially pseudolymphoma of the orbit. They are usually treated with local radiotherapy, but systemic spread probably occurs in about half the cases.

Non-Hodgkin's lymphoma of the lung

NHL may spread to the lung either directly from mediastinal nodes or as part of a more widespread dissemination (usually in advanced and drug-resistant cases). Both Hodgkin's lymphoma and NHL may involve the lung and cause considerable diagnostic difficulty.

Lymphomatoid granulomatosis

This disease usually arises in the lung. It consists of a pleomorphic infiltrate, often involving vessel walls with areas of necrosis and atypical lymphoid cells. The disease is indolent, often over many years. Malignant invasive lymphoma occurs in up to 50% of cases, even if the disease is not considered malignant at the onset. In some cases T-cell monoclonal proliferation has been demonstrated (by T-cell receptor gene rearrangement). Cases have been described in AIDS. Spread to the skin and CNS occurs. Local resection may be curative. More widespread disease has a worse prognosis but long-term remissions may be obtained by steroids and chemotherapy. The EBV genome has occasionally been demonstrated.

Cutaneous non-Hodgkin's lymphoma

The skin is a frequent site of secondary spread of NHL of all types. It is usually involved in the context of disseminated and often drug-resistant disease. Clinically, there are subcutaneous lumps or papular infiltrates in the dermis. Treatment is of the underlying disease where possible. Superficial X-rays are very helpful in controlling troublesome lesions, and electron therapy is useful for widespread cutaneous infiltrates.

The skin may also be the site of a *primary cutaneous lymphoma (PCL)*, defined as NHL disorders presenting in the skin without evidence of extracutaneous disease at the time of diagnosis. These tumours are of many types and are often indolent, and represent the second commonest group of extranodal NHL after the gastrointestinal lymphomas with an annual incidence of about 1/100 000. They can be broadly classified into those of T-cell and B-cell origin, of which the T-cell variants (primary cutaneous T-cell lymphomas) are the commonest in Europe and the USA (about 75% of the total), though different proportions are found elsewhere, for example, most parts of Africa and Asia. This specialist topic is well covered by Willemze and Dreyling [54].

Primary cutaneous T-cell lymphoma

The two major syndromes of primary cutaneous T-cell lymphoma [55–57] are mycosis fungoides (MF), the commonest cutaneous T-cell lymphoma, accounting for over 50% of all cases, and Sézary syndrome. Others also occur, and the current WHO/EORTC (European Organization for Research and Treatment of Cancer) classification can be found in Willemze *et al.* [58].

This disease is uncommon. The onset is usually at 50–70 years of age, though many cases may have a long history with an origin much earlier in life. Men are slightly more affected than women, and there are some curious occupational links, for example, glassworkers, pottery and ceramics workers. Occasional family clustering has been recorded. There are stages in the clinical evolution, although in individual cases they are often not easily separable.

The lesions of MF typically occur as patches in the first instance, characteristically on the trunk and buttocks, often very itchy. In the *erythematous* or *pretumour stage* there is a rash that may resemble psoriasis with fine red scaly patches, sometimes up to 15 cm in diameter. Alopecia is common if the disease affects the scalp.

There are often poikilodermatous changes that suggest the diagnosis. This phase may last for many years with numerous diagnoses offered. The diagnosis can only be substantiated by biopsy and by showing monoclonality of T cells by molecular methods. There is acanthosis, parakeratosis and clusters of histiocytes (Darier–Pautrier abscesses). When the lesion progresses to the *infiltrative* or *plaque stage*, indurated plaques are usually present. Microscopically, these show infiltration of the upper dermis and epidermis with lymphoma cells, which are helper T-cells. There is usually no significant lymph node enlargement. If the nodes do enlarge, they may show 'dermatopathic lymphadenopathy' and, later, clear evidence of tumour infiltration. In the *tumour stage* the lesions enlarge and ulcerate. Involvement of internal organs may occur. MF is usually a lymphoma of the helper/inducer cell-surface phenotype (CD4) and should

be distinguished from other more aggressive T-cell lymphomas that also involve the skin, for example, peripheral T-cell lymphomas, which require more aggressive treatment, generally with chemotherapy. Typically, the lesions stain for CD4, though occasionally they may stain for CD8 (often a marker for a more aggressive disease process) or are negative for both antigens.

In the erythrodermic phase (Sézary syndrome), the skin shows infiltration with T cells. Lymph node enlargement and hepatomegaly may be present. The patient complains of intense itching, the skin becomes red and thickened and may be swollen. Hair is lost and palmar hyperkeratosis occurs with dystrophy and loss of nails. The circulating cells were called *cellules monstreuses* by Sézary. They do not infiltrate the marrow until late in the disease. Hepatosplenomegaly may occur and there may be lymph node enlargement. In general, Sézary syndrome is increasingly regarded as a form of leukaemia and therefore requires systemic treatment, though skin-directed therapies such as PUVA and/or topical steroids are often useful as an adjunct.

The most important prognostic factor for Primary Cutaneous T-cell Lymphoma is the extent of disease. A staging system is shown in Table 26.12.

Treatment in the first stage is with steroid creams and topical nitrogen mustard or nitrosoureas, avoiding

Table 26.12 Staging system for primary cutaneous T-cell lymphoma.

T1	Plaques occupying less than 10% of body surface
T2	Plaques over more than 10%
T3	Tumours
T4	Generalized erythroderma (Sézary syndrome)
N0	No clinically or pathologically involved nodes
N1	Nodes enlarged, pathology negative
N2	Pathologically involved
N3	Clinically and pathologically involved
M0	No visceral involvement
M1	Visceral involvement

Stage group

1A	T1	N0	M0
1B	T2	N0	M0
2A	T1–2	N1	M0
2B	T3	N0,1	M0
3	T4	N0,1	M0
4A	T1–4	N2,3	M0
4B	T1–4	N0–3	M1

over-aggressive approaches wherever possible as early use of chemotherapy is on the whole unlikely to lead to an improved survival. As Willemze and Dreyling point out, 'a stage-adapted conservative therapeutic approach is recommended for MF and its variants'. Cutaneous hypersensitivity to nitrogen mustard can be troublesome. Local radiation can be used for unsightly lesions. More widespread disease responds to psoralens and ultraviolet light A (PUVA) and whole-body electron beam therapy; PUVA is complicated by secondary skin cancers in a few patients. Narrow-band UVB can be used for patients with patches or only very thin plaques. Whole-body electrons cause depilation and loss of sweating. Neither appear to change prognosis. Wide-field irradiation is the treatment usually used in the mycotic stage.

Chemotherapy is increasingly used, and although responses frequently occur, there is no benefit from aggressive early treatment using combination chemotherapy of the type used for other lymphomas. Responses to alkylating agents and anthracyclines are variable and usually short-lived, even if responses have been reported to fludarabine and 2-chlorodeoxyadenosine. Interferon also produces responses, some of which are long-lasting. New approaches that have shown some clinical effectiveness include the oral histone deacetylase inhibitor vorinostat (suberoylanilide hydroxamic acid), which at a dose of 400 mg daily has reportedly reduced the troublesome symptom of pruritus in about half of all cases, as well as producing significant partial responses even in heavily pretreated patients [59]. Other newer agents include the retinoid bexarotene, anti-CD5 and anti-CD6 monoclonal antibodies, and the use of toxin-coupled antibodies to the IL-2 receptor. The monoclonal antibody alemtuzumab (Campath) is increasingly used for cutaneous T-cell lymphoma.

Prognosis is related to stage. Patients with stage 1A disease probably have a normal lifespan with few of them progressing to tumour stage. For stage 2 disease, survival is 85% at 5 years and 70% at 10 years. More extensive skin disease, nodal involvement, tumour stage and visceral involvement are all poor prognostic factors.

Primary cutaneous B-cell lymphoma

Primary cutaneous B-cell lymphoma [57] represents a group of disorders of which the commonest form is probably derived from germinal centre B cells. It presents as a single red patch or nodule, without ulceration, occurring at any site. The diagnosis may present difficulty both clinically and pathologically, and the EORTC-WHO classification currently recognizes three main sub-types.

These are: primary cutaneous marginal zone lymphoma, primary cutaneous follicle centre lymphoma (both of these typically behave in a relatively indolent fashion with 10-years survival around 90%), and primary cutaneous diffuse large B-cell, leg type lymphoma, which is more common in women, has a more aggressive natural history and a worse survival of about 50% at 5 years. Radiation is used for localized lesions, but the disease responds to chemotherapy using a conventional combination of drugs. Patients with localized disease generally have an excellent prognosis.

Malignant angioendotheliomatosis

This disorder is characterized by widespread skin lesions, fever, dementia, neurological signs and organ failure. There is intravascular proliferation of atypical mononuclear cells within small blood vessels. Recent studies have shown this to be a lymphoid tumour with positive B-cell markers and numerous karyotypic abnormalities.

Non-Hodgkin's lymphoma of the thyroid [60]

These tumours usually present as a rapidly enlarging thyroid mass in middle-aged or elderly women. They are associated with Hashimoto's thyroiditis, and areas of thyroiditis may be found in the gland on biopsy. Histologically, they are usually diffuse large-cell tumours that are generally of B-cell type. Follicular and plasmacytoid forms are unusual, and T-cell tumours are rare. The evolution of the disease in a gland affected by autoimmune disease is reminiscent of the development of lymphomas in Sjögren's syndrome. The mass does not take up radioactive iodine and cannot be distinguished clinically from other thyroid cancers. Diagnosis is made by biopsy or thyroidectomy. However, radical surgery has little role in management since the tumours are sensitive to radiotherapy.

Staging investigations are necessary since the prognosis is excellent with local treatment if the disease is confined to the gland. These investigations should include chest radiography, abdominal CT scan and/or lymphography, and marrow aspiration and biopsy. Relapse in the gut is relatively frequent and a small-bowel barium examination may be useful.

If there is no local extension of the tumour from the gland and no evidence of involvement of adjacent nodes, radiotherapy (40 Gy in 4 weeks) to the gland and adjacent nodes will cure 90% of patients. Only 50% of patients with local and nodal extension will be cured, and the prognosis is also worse over the age of 65 years.

Adjuvant chemotherapy should therefore be considered in these cases, and is clearly necessary for patients with more widespread disease. It seems likely that T-cell tumours will also require chemotherapy. There are, as yet, few data to show whether chemotherapy will improve the prognosis.

Non-Hodgkin's lymphoma of the testis [61,62]

NHL of the testis is usually a diffuse large-cell (centroblastic) lymphoma. The patients are generally over the age of 50 years, an age when seminoma and teratoma are uncommon. The tumours are mostly unilateral but there is a considerable risk of contralateral involvement. Presentation is with painless enlargement of the testis. After investigation most patients are found to have stage I or II disease (Ann Arbor system, see Table 25.2). The disease has a tendency to spread to abdominal nodes and to Waldeyer's ring. Occasionally, CNS relapse occurs.

Staging investigations should include lymphangiography and/or CT scan of the abdomen, and bone marrow examination. Localized disease (IE and IIE) can be treated with radiotherapy to the pelvic and para-aortic lymph nodes. Bilateral or advanced (stage III and IV) disease carries a poor prognosis and systemic chemotherapy is required. The prognosis is not good. Overall 60% of patients will have died at 3 years.

References

1   Armitage JO, Coiffier BM.D,, Dalla-Favera R, eds. *Non-Hodgkin's Lymphomas,* 2nd edn. Philadelphia: Lippincott Williams & Wilkins, 2009.

2   Dreyling M, Ghielmini M, Marcus R et al. Newly diagnosed and relapsed follicular lymphoma: ESMO clinical practice guidelines for diagnosis, treatment and follow-up. *Ann Oncol* 2011; 22 (Suppl. 6): vi59–63.

3   Boshoff C, Weiss R. AIDS-related malignancies. *Nat Rev Cancer* 2002; 2: 373–82.

4   Burkitt D. Determining the climatic limitations of a children's cancer common in Africa. *Br Med J* 1962; ii: 1019–23.

5   Giordano TP, Henderson L, Landgren O et al. Risk of non-Hodgkin lymphoma and precursor proliferative diseases in US veterans with hepatitis C virus. *JAMA* 2007; 297: 2010–17.

6   Staudt LM. A closer look at follicular lymphoma. *N Engl J Med* 2007; 356: 741–2.

7   Sarris A, Ford R. Recent advances in the molecular pathogenesis of lymphomas. *Curr Opin Oncol* 1999; 11: 351–63.

8   Harris NL, Jaffe ES, Stein H et al. A revised European–American classification of lymphoid neoplasms: a proposal from the International Lymphoma Study Group. *Blood* 1994; 84: 1361–92.

9   Aisenberg AC. Coherent view of non-Hodgkin's lymphomas. *J Clin Oncol* 1995; 13: 2656–75.

10 Kwong YL. Predicting the outcome in non-Hodgkin lymphoma with molecular markers. *Br J Haematol* 2007; 137: 273–87.

11 MacManus MP, Hoppe RT. Is radiotherapy curative for stage I and II low grade follicular lymphoma? Results of long-term follow-up study of patients treated at Stanford University. *J Clin Oncol* 1996; 14: 128–290.

12 Tallman MS, Hakimian D. Purine nucleoside analogs: emerging roles in indolent proliferative disorders. *Blood* 1995; 86: 2463–74.

13 McLaughlin P, Grillo-Lopez AJ, Link BK et al. Rituximab chimeric anti-CD20 monoclonal antibody therapy for relapsed indolent lymphoma: half of patients respond to a four-dose treatment program. *J Clin Oncol* 1998; 16: 2825–33.

14 van Oers M H, Van Glabbeke M, Giurgea L et al. Rituximab maintenance treatment of relapsed/resistant follicular non-Hodgkin's lymphoma: long-term outcome of the EORTC 20981 phase III randomized intergroup study. *J Clin Oncol*. 2010; 28: 2853–2858.

15 Marcus R. Use of rituximab in patients with follicular lymphoma. *Clin Oncol* 2007; 19: 38–49.

16 Leonard JP, Schattner EJ, Coleman M. Biology and management of mantle cell lymphoma. *Curr Opin Oncol* 2001; 13: 342–7.

17 Kluin-Nelemans E, Hoster E, Hermine O, et al. Treatment of older patients with mantle-cell lymphoma. *New Engl J Med* 2012; 367: 520–31.

18 International NHL Prognostic Factors Project. A predictive model for aggressive non-Hodgkin's lymphoma. *N Engl J Med* 1993; 329: 987–94.

19 Forstpointner R, Unterhalt M, Dreyling M et al. Maintenance therapy with rituximab leads to a significant prolongation of response duration after salvage therapy with a combination of rituximab, fludarabine, cyclophosphamide, and mitoxantrone (R-FCM) in patients with recurring and refractory follicular and mantle cell lymphomas: results of a prospective randomized study of the German Low Grade Lymphoma Study Group (GLSG). *Blood* 2006; 108: 4003–8.

20 Wang ML, Rule S, Martin P et al. Targeting BTK with ibrutinib in relapsed or refractory mantle-cell lymphoma. *New Engl J Med* 2013; 369: 507–16.

21 Miller TP, Dahlberg MS, Cassady JR et al. Chemotherapy alone compared with chemotherapy plus radiotherapy for localised intermediate and high-grade non Hodgkin's lymphoma. *N Engl J Med* 1998; 339: 21–6.

22 Fisher RI, Gaynor ER, Dahlberg S et al. Comparison of a standard regimen (CHOP) with three intensive

chemotherapy regimens for advanced non-Hodgkin's lymphoma. *N Engl J Med* 1993; 328: 1002–6.

23 Feugier P, Van Hoof A, Sebban C *et al.* Long term results of the R-CHOP study in the treatment of elderly patients with diffuse large B cell lymphoma. *J Clin Oncol* 2005; 23: 4117–26.

24 Jetsrisuparb A, Waingnon S, Komvilaisak P. Rituximab combined with CHOP for successful treatment of aggressive, recurrent, paediatric B-cell large cell non Hodgkin's lymphoma. *J Pediatr Haematol Oncol* 2005; 27: 223–6.

25 Piccozi VJ, Coleman CN. Lymphoblastic lymphoma. *Semin Oncol* 1990; 17: 960–1104.

26 Hummel M, Bentink S, Berger H *et al.* A biologic definition of Burkitt's lymphoma from transcriptional and genomic profiling. *N Engl J Med* 2006; 354: 2419–30.

27 Dunleavy K, Pittaluga S, Shovlin M *et al.* Low-intensity therapy in adults with Burkitt's lymphoma. *New Engl J Med* 2013; 369: 1915–25.

28 van Besien K, Kelta M, Bahaguna P. Primary mediastinal B-cell lymphoma: a review of the pathology and management. *J Clin Oncol* 2001; 19: 1855–64.

29 Kadin ME, Sakko K, Berliner N *et al.* Childhood Ki-1 lymphoma presenting with skin lesions and peripheral lymphadenopathy. *Blood* 1986; 68: 1042–9.

30 Treon SP, Girtz NA, Dimopoulos M *et al.* Update on treatment recommendations from the Third International Workshop on Waldenstrom's Macroglobulinemia. *Blood* 2006; 107: 3442–6.

31 Philip T, Guglielmi C, Hagenbeek A *et al.* Autologous bone marrow transplantation as compared with salvage chemotherapy in relapses of chemotherapy-sensitive non-Hodgkin's lymphoma. *N Engl J Med* 1995; 333: 1540–5.

32 Greb A, Bohlius J, Trelle S *et al.* High-dose chemotherapy with autologous stem-cell support in first-line treatment of aggressive non-Hodgkin lymphoma: results of a comprehensive meta-analysis. *Cancer Treat Rev* 2007; 33: 338–46.

33 Khouri IF, Saliba RM, Hosing C *et al.* Concurrent administration of high dose rituximab before and after autologous stem-cell transplantation for relapsed aggressive B-cell non-Hodgkin's lymphomas. *J Clin Oncol* 2005; 23: 2240–7.

34 Stiff PJ, Unger JM, Cook JR. Autologous transplantation as consolidation for aggressive non-Hodgkin's lymphoma. *New Engl J Med* 2013; 369: 1681–90.

35 Kirk O, Pederson C, Cozzi-Lepri A *et al.* Non-Hodgkin's lymphoma in HIV-infected patients in the era of highly active antiretroviral therapy. *Blood* 2001; 98: 3406–12.

36 Sander AS, Kaplan L. AIDS lymphoma. *Curr Opin Oncol* 1996; 8: 377–85.

37 Anderson JR, Wilson JF, Jenkin DT *et al.* Childhood non-Hodgkin's lymphoma: the results of a randomized therapeutic trial comparing a 4-drug regimen (COMP) with a 10-drug regimen (LSA2-L2). *N Engl J Med* 1983; 308: 559–65.

38 Hvizdala EV, Berard C, Callihan T *et al.* Lymphoblastic lymphoma in children: a randomized trial comparing LSA2L2

with the A-COP therapeutic regimen: a Paediatric Oncology Group Study. *J Clin Oncol* 1988; 6: 26–33.

39 Philip T, Pinkerton R, Biron P *et al.* Effective multiagent chemotherapy in children with advanced B-cell lymphoma: who remains the high-risk patient? *Br J Haematol* 1987; 65: 159–64.

40 Murphy SB, Magrath IT. Workshop on paediatric lymphomas: current results and prospects. *Ann Oncol* 1991; 2 (Suppl. 2): 219–23.

41 Isaacson PG, Spencer J. Malignant lymphoma of mucosa associated lymphoid tissue. *Histopathology* 1987; 11: 445–62.

42 Wotherspoon AC, Doglioni C, Diss TC *et al.* Regression of primary low grade B-cell gastric lymphoma of the mucosa-associated lymphoid tissue type after eradication of *Helicobacter pylori. Lancet* 1993; 342: 575–7.

43 Liu HT, Hsu C, Chen CL *et al.* Chemotherapy alone versus surgery followed by chemotherapy for stage I/IIE large cell lymphoma of the stomach. *Am J Hematol* 2000; 64: 175–9.

44 List AF, Greer JP, Cousa JC *et al.* Non-Hodgkin's lymphoma of the gastrointestinal tract: an analysis of clinical and pathological features affecting outcome. *J Clin Oncol* 1988; 6: 1125–33.

45 Ben-Ayed F, Halphen M, Najjar T *et al.* Treatment of alpha chain disease: results of a prospective study in 21 Tunisian patients by the Tunisian-French Intestinal Lymphoma Study Group. *Cancer* 1989; 63: 1251–6.

46 Beal K, Allen L, Yahalom J. Primary bone lymphoma: treatment results and prognostic factors with long-term follow-up of 82 patients. *Cancer* 2006; 106: 2652–6.

47 Hameed M. Small round tumors of bone. *Arch Pathol Lab Med* 2007; 131: 192–204.

48 Eichler AF, Batchelor TT. Primary central nervous system lymphoma: presentation, diagnosis and staging. *Neurosurg Focus* 2006; 21: E15.

49 Poortmans MPP, Kluin-Nelemans HC, Haaxma-Reiche H *et al.* High-dose methotrexate-based chemotherapy followed by consolidating radiotherapy in non-AIDS related primary central nervous system lymphoma: EORTC Lymphoma Group phase II trial 20962. *J Clin Oncol* 2003; 21: 4483–8.

50 Bessell EM, Hoang-Xuan K, Ferreri A, Reni M. Primary central nervous system lymphoma: biological aspects and controversies in management. *Eur J Cancer* 2007; 43: 1141–52.

51 Tomita N, Kodama F, Kanamori H *et al.* Secondary central nervous system lymphoma. *Int J Hematol* 2006; 84: 128–35.

52 Arkenau HT, Chong G, Cunningham D *et al.* The role of intrathecal chemotherapy prophylaxis in patients with diffuse large B-cell lymphoma. *Ann Oncol* 2007; 18: 541–5.

53 Gurkaynak M, Cengiz M, Akyurek S *et al.* Waldeyer's ring lymphomas: treatment results and prognostic factors. *Am J Clin Oncol* 2003; 26: 437–40.

54 Willemze R, Dreyling M. Primary cutaneous lymphomas: ESMO clinical practice guidelines for diagnosis, treatment and follow-up. *Ann Oncol* 2010; 21: v177–80.

55 Willemze R, Meijer CJL. EORTC classification for primary cutaneous lymphoma: a comparison of the REAL classification and the proposed WHO classification. *Ann Oncol* 2000; II (Suppl. I): 11–5.

56 Koh HK, Foss FM , eds. *Cutaneous T Cell Lymphoma. Haematology/Oncology Clinics of North America Series.* Philadelphia: WB Saunders, 1995, 2000.

57 Pandolfino TL, Siegel RS, Kuzel TM *et al.* Primary cutaneous B-cell lymphoma: review and current concepts. *J Clin Oncol* 2000; 18: 2151–68.

58 Willemze R, Jaffe ES, Burg G *et al.* WHO–EORTC classification for cutaneous lymphomas. *Blood* 2005; 105: 3768–85.

59 Duvik M, Talpur R, Ni X *et al.* Phase 2 trial of oral vorinostat (suberoylanilide hydroxamic acid, SAHA) for refractory cutaneous T-cell lymphoma (CTCL). *Blood* 2007; 109: 31–9.

60 Mack LA, Pasieka JL. An evidence-based approach to the treatment of thyroid lymphoma. *World J Surg* 2007; 31: 978–86.

61 Zouhair A, Weber D, Belkacemi Y *et al.* Outcome and patterns of failure in testicular lymphoma: a multicenter rare cancer network study. *Int J Radiat Oncol Biol Phys* 2002; 52: 652–6.

62 Al-Abbadi MA, Hattab EM, Tarawneh MS *et al.* Primary testicular diffuse large B-cell lymphoma belongs to the nongerminal center B-cell-like subgroup: a study of 18 cases. *Mod Pathol* 2006; 19: 1521–7.

Further reading

Canellos GP, Lister TA, Young B, eds. *The Lymphomas*, 2nd edn. Philadelphia: Saunders Elsevier, 2006.

Cheson BD, Leonard JP. Monoclonal antibody therapy for B-cell non-Hodgkin's lymphoma. *N Engl J Med* 2008; 359: 613–26.

Copelan EA. Medical Progress: Hematopoietic stem-cell transplantation. *N Engl J Med* 2006; 354: 1813–26.

Freedman J. *Lymphoma: Current and Emerging Trends in Detection and Treatment.* New York: Rosen Publishing, 2006.

Goedert JJ, Coté TR, Virgo P *et al.* Spectrum of AIDS-associated malignant disorders. *Lancet* 1998; 351: 1833–9.

Gross TG, Termuhlen A. Pediatric non-Hodgkin's lymphoma. *Curr Oncol Rep* 2007; 9: 459–65.

Gupta RK, Lister TA. Management of follicular lymphoma. *Curr Opin Oncol* 1996; 8: 360–5.

Hwang ST, Janik JE, Jaffe ES, Wilson WH. Mycosis fungoides and Sézary syndrome. *Lancet* 2008; 371: 945–57.

Leonard JP, Coleman M, eds. *Hodgkin's and Non-Hodgkin's Lymphoma.* New York: Springer, 2006.

Levine AM, Gill PS, Meyer PR *et al.* Retrovirus and malignant lymphoma in homosexual men. *JAMA* 1985; 254: 1921–5.

Liu V, Cutler CS, Young AZ. A 44-year-old woman with generalized, painful, ulcerated skin lesions. *N Engl J Med* 2007; 357: 2496–505.

Solal-Celigny P, Roy P, Colombat P *et al.* Follicular lymphoma. International prognostic index. *Blood* 2004; 104: 1258–65.

Weinstein HJ, Hudson MM, Link MP, eds. *Pediatric Lymphomas.* Berlin: Springer, 2007.

27 Myeloma and other paraproteinaemias

Myeloma

Incidence and aetiology

Myeloma (multiple myeloma, myelomatosis, plasma cell myeloma) is chiefly a disease of the elderly (Figure 27.1), and is almost twice as common in males as in females. Annual incidence is approximately 4 per 100 000 and is twice as frequent in American black as in white people. The incidence has increased over the past 40 years [1], and it now accounts for about 10% of all haemotological malignancy. Family clusters have been reported, with an increased incidence in first-degree relatives [2], suggesting a cancer-susceptibility locus. An increased risk of developing myeloma has also been reported in relatives of carriers of the *BRCA1* and *BRCA2* mutations. Use of serum electrophoresis in screening programmes reveals a far higher incidence of paraproteinaemia (a monoclonal immunoglobulin band) and up to 3% of an asymptomatic population over the age of 70 have a monoclonal gammopathy. Most of these have a form of 'benign' paraproteinaemia (see pages 556–557) but a minority subsequently develop symptomatic myeloma. As with other B-cell neoplasms, there appears to be an unequivocal relationship between radiation exposure and subsequent development of myeloma [3]. An increased incidence has been reported in a group of American radiologists, presumably due to lifelong radiation exposure, and also in survivors of Nagasaki and Hiroshima with a delay of 20 years. The past few years have seen many important changes in management, with the introduction of a number of important new agents, and the increasing use of both autologous and allogeneic stem-cell transplantation. As a result, the prognosis for patients with myeloma, stagnant for so long, at last appears to be improving.

Pathogenesis
Immunoglobulin abnormalities

Multiple myeloma is one of a number of B-lymphocyte neoplasms [4] characterized by continued synthesis and release of immunoglobulins (Table 27.1), with neoplastic proliferation of a clone of B lymphocytes resulting in large numbers of immature plasma cells that infiltrate the bone marrow and which can occasionally be found in the blood. The oncogenic event may occur earlier in the B-cell differentiation pathway but clonal expansion occurs at the plasma cell stage (Figure 27.2). Production of large amounts of a monoclonal immunoglobulin is therefore characteristic of multiple myeloma.

Cancer and its Management, Seventh Edition. Jeffrey Tobias and Daniel Hochhauser.
© 2015 John Wiley & Sons, Ltd. Published 2015 by John Wiley & Sons, Ltd.

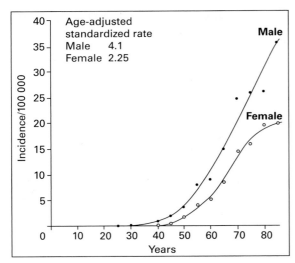

Figure 27.1 Age-specific incidence of myeloma in the UK.

Table 27.1 Immunoglobulin-producing neoplasms.

Benign (but see text)
Monoclonal gammopathy of unknown significance
Cold agglutinin disease

Malignant
Myeloma
Waldenström's macroglobulinaemia
Primary amyloidosis
Non-Hodgkin's lymphomas
Heavy-chain diseases (γ, α or μ)

The basic structure of normal immunoglobulins consists of two pairs of polypeptide chains, one pair of light chains (each 22 kDa) and one pair of heavy chains (each 55–70 kDa), held by covalent (disulphide) and non-covalent bonds. There is variability in heavy-chain structure, with five separate types of heavy chain, γ, α, μ, δ and ϵ, these differences forming the basis of the five classes of immunoglobulin: IgG, IgA, IgM, IgD and IgE. Furthermore, there are altogether 10 different heavy-chain sequences, four γ, two α, two μ and only one each of δ and ϵ. Of the γ immunoglobulins, IgG3 is particularly prone to polymerize, as are IgA and IgM. However, there are only two types of light chain, κ and λ. IgG, IgD and IgE are found in the plasma as single molecules of molecular mass 160–200 kDa. IgM is a macroglobulin (molecular mass 900 kDa) synthesized as a pentamer of IgG structure. IgA is formed by plasma cells

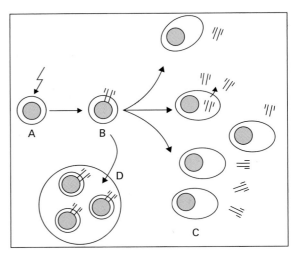

Figure 27.2 Pathogenesis of myeloma: (A) oncogenic event in a B cell; (B) expansion of a clone of malignant B cells; (C) proliferation of plasma cells leading to bone lesions and production of paraprotein; (D) suppression of normal B cells leads to hypogammaglobulinaemia.

in the gut and respiratory tract, and is therefore found in external secretions such as saliva, tears, bronchial and gastrointestinal mucosa, as well as in the blood. It has an important role in primary defence against invading pathogens.

Normal immunoglobulins are diverse in their detailed structure, synthesized in response to a variety of antigenic stimuli. Each immunoglobulin molecule recognizes one antigenic structure only, and the portion of the molecule which confers this specificity is known as the idiotypic determinant. In contrast, in myeloma the product of the neoplastic plasma cell clone is an immunoglobulin of a single homogeneous structure (i.e. a single idiotype), the myeloma or M protein (not to be confused with IgM), or paraprotein. There is always light-chain restriction, that is, to either κ or λ type.

In most patients, whole immunoglobulin molecules are often synthesized, but in about one-quarter, there may be a disproportionate production of one component so that free light chains are produced. In approximately 1% of patients (often termed non-secretors), no monoclonal protein can be detected in the plasma or urine.

When free light chains are secreted into the blood, they cross the glomerular membrane and are detectable in the urine. They have the unusual property of producing a cloudy precipitate (Bence Jones protein) when the urine is heated to 50–60 °C, with dissociation of the precipitate as the temperature is raised near boiling point. Excretion of free light chains occurs in 40–50% of all cases of myeloma, and is detected nowadays by immunoelectrophoresis of the urine.

The major classes of immunoglobulin have differing physical properties, which may be clinically relevant since many aspects of the disease are attributable to the physical characteristics or deposition of the immunoglobulin itself. For example, IgM has a high molecular weight, and hyperviscosity syndrome is not uncommon (see below). IgA molecules polymerize in the plasma and will also cause hyperviscosity. Excess light chains may be deposited in the renal tubule and contribute to renal failure (see pages 548–549). Polymerization of light chains is one component of amyloid, which also contributes to renal disease. The incidence of the different types of myeloma roughly parallels the concentrations of normal serum immunoglobulins and reflects the number of plasma cells normally found in each group. IgG myeloma is the commonest type, followed by IgA. IgM production is rarely due to a true myeloma but is usually part of Waldenström's macroglobulinaemia or non-Hodgkin's lymphoma (see page 530). IgD myeloma is very uncommon, and IgE exceedingly rare. More than 5×10^9 plasma cells must be present for the paraprotein to be detectable as a discrete immunoglobulin band.

In myeloma an assessment of tumour mass can be made using a formula that includes haemoglobin, calcium, presence of multiple bone lesions, paraprotein concentration and blood urea. Patients with a large tumour mass (in excess of 0.5×10^{12} cells) have a worse prognosis and respond less frequently to chemotherapy. Some of the important prognostic features are shown in Table 27.2. One of the more successful attempts to determine likely prognosis has used only serum β_2-microglobulin and initial haemoglobin levels. In this formula, larger values imply a worse prognosis [5].

Depression of production of normal immunoglobulin is a characteristic feature of the disease and one which helps to differentiate it from benign varieties of monoclonal gammopathy, though the mechanism of suppression of normal immunoglobulin production is not clear. This depression affects all classes of normal immunoglobulin and contributes greatly to susceptibility to bacterial infection.

Other causes of monoclonal immunoglobulin production (Table 27.1) include monoclonal gammopathy of unknown significance (MGUS), previously erroneously termed 'benign monoclonal gammopathy'. This is common in the elderly and may cause diagnostic difficulty,

Table 27.2 Prognostic features in myeloma.

Good	Poor
Low serum β_2-microglobulin (<2 mg/L)	High serum β_2-microglobulin (>2 mg/L)
Haemoglobin > 10 g/dL	Haemoglobin < 8.5 g/dL
Serum calcium normal	Serum calcium > 2.9 mmol/L
No lytic bone lesions	More than three bone lesions
Low paraprotein level	High paraprotein level
IgG < 50 g/L	IgG > 70 g/L
IgA < 30 g/L	IgA > 50 g/L
Urine light chains < 2 g/day	Light chains > 5 g/day
Plasma urea < 8 mmol/L	Urea > 8 mmol/L

particularly as it may later progress to myeloma. The current understanding of the MGUS–myeloma relationship is that a spectrum exists from the relatively benign disorder to the frankly malignant. Although MGUS shares certain features with myeloma (excess immunoglobulin synthesis and occasional Bence Jones proteinuria), the marrow plasma cell infiltrate is modest (<10%) and there are no bone lesions. Progression of MGUS to myeloma is well described and may occur slowly, with a period of 'smouldering' disease that can cause difficulty for the clinician.

It is not yet clear which oncogenes or other DNA sequences are the most critical for myeloma development, either *de novo* or within an existing background of MGUS. Initial studies suggest that both the *myc* and *ras* oncogene series may be implicated. It is also known that of the cytokines, interleukin (IL)-6 is an important agent capable of stimulating plasma cell growth and differentiation, and lymphotoxin, or tumour necrosis factor (TNF)-β, is a known mediator of osteoclast activation and therefore of myeloma bone destruction [6]. It is now clear that myeloma develops as a 'multistep transformation process', with cellular proliferation regulated through several different pathways [7].

Pathological features

Both the bone and the bone marrow are infiltrated by malignant plasma cells, typically round or oval, often with an eccentrically placed nucleus like their normal counterpart. The cytoplasm is densely basophilic due to the RNA-producing paraprotein, with a clear perinuclear zone where the Golgi apparatus is situated.

Abnormal forms are often present, sometimes large and binucleate or trinucleate, with the nucleus eccentrically placed. The marrow infiltration is often patchy, unlike leukaemia – hence the name multiple myeloma – but the histological diagnosis is highly probable when the level of infiltration exceeds 20% of all nucleated marrow cells, though the diagnosis is not excluded by lesser degrees of involvement. The bone gets destroyed by the tumour.

Typically the lesions are lytic and fractures are common (Figure 27.3). The mechanism of lysis is not fully understood but osteoclastic-activating factors produced by the myeloma or mature B cells have been described. Any bone can be affected and common sites include vertebrae, pelvis, skull, ribs and proximal long bones.

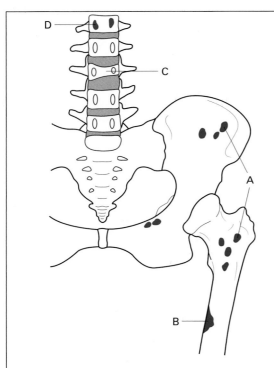

A The typical lesion is of multiple rounded translucencies without sclerosis
B Some lesions may be very large and fractures of long bones are frequent
C Vertebral osteoporosis and collapse is very common
D Loss of the vertebral pedicle is an easily missed sign of infiltration

Figure 27.3 Diagrammatic representation of bone lesions in myeloma.

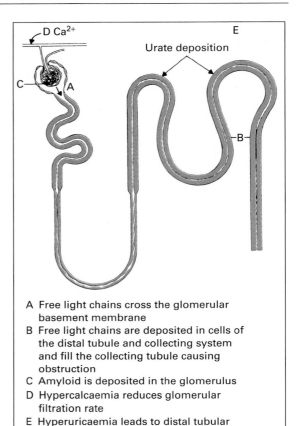

A Free light chains cross the glomerular basement membrane
B Free light chains are deposited in cells of the distal tubule and collecting system and fill the collecting tubule causing obstruction
C Amyloid is deposited in the glomerulus
D Hypercalcaemia reduces glomerular filtration rate
E Hyperuricaemia leads to distal tubular and interstitial urate deposition

Figure 27.4 Renal damage in myeloma.

The kidney is affected in several ways (Figure 27.4). First, light chains are taken up by distal renal tubular cells, a major site of catabolism of normal light chains. The massive load of light chains results in tubular damage and large casts of light chains and albumin fill and obstruct the tubule, imposing a further load on the remaining nephrons. Specific defects in tubular reabsorption occur, due to protein aggregation in renal tubule cells, and leading to tubular reabsorptive defects with leakage of amino acids, glucose, potassium and phosphate (acquired Fanconi's syndrome).

Second, amyloid deposition in glomerular blood vessels occurs in 10% of patients, particularly in cases where light chains alone are produced. In myeloma this protein consists in part of polymerized light-chain fragments; λ light chains are much more likely to lead to amyloid formation. Other features contributing to renal impairment include recurrent hypercalcaemia with dehydration, hypercalciuria and nephrocalcinosis, urate deposition and renal tubular leakage. Urinary tract infection is common and pyelonephritis may develop. Together, these processes constitute 'myeloma kidney'. There may even be renal deposition of malignant plasma cells, typically late in the disease when there is a large tumour mass.

Clinical features

Patients with myeloma may be asymptomatic for many years before presenting with weakness, bone pain, anorexia and other symptoms due to abnormal proliferation of the malignant plasma cells, direct effects of the abnormal immunoglobulin, or hypercalcaemia.

Diffuse bone pain is often the major complaint, with skeletal abnormalities present in about two-thirds of patients. The pain is typically dull or aching, often felt in the spine, ribs or pelvis. Pathological fractures are common, and acute back pain from a vertebral crush fracture is a frequent first presentation of myeloma. This may lead to acute cord compression (see Chapter 8). In its later stages, multiple myeloma may be among the most painful of all cancers, with multiple sites of vertebral and long bone fracture from widespread malignant infiltration.

Typical radiological appearances include generalized osteopenia or osteoporosis (particularly evident in the dorsal and lumbar spine and sacroiliac area), and punched-out osteolytic lesions, with little or no sclerosis. Full radiological skeletal survey often reveals unsuspected bone lesions and should always be performed at diagnosis. In addition to the ribs, vertebrae and hips, these lesions are characteristically found in the skull, usually remaining asymptomatic until they reach a large size. Biopsy of any of these sites reveals heavy infiltration with abnormal plasma cells.

Many patients present with fatigue and lassitude due to anaemia, and recurrent bacterial infection due to immunoparesis. Nausea, anorexia and dehydration may be due to hypercalcaemia and lead to deteriorating renal function.

Hyperviscosity syndrome may develop in patients in whom the type and level of abnormal immunoglobulin contributes to an increase in plasma viscosity. This is most commonly seen in patients with Waldenström's macroglobulinaemia (see below) but also occurs in patients with myeloma, especially with IgA, IgM and IgG3 paraproteins. Clinically, this syndrome consists of neurological symptoms, chiefly vertigo, confusion and transient ischaemic episodes; retinopathy with distended retinal veins, haemorrhages and papilloedema; and hypervolaemia with increased vascular resistance. A bleeding tendency is frequently due to both thrombocytopenia and clotting disturbances due to interference of the coagulation system by paraprotein, leading to reduced platelet aggregation. Clinically, this may cause purpura, epistaxis, mucosal bleeding and retinal haemorrhage. A positive Hess test, reduced thromboplastin generation time and defective clot retraction may all occur.

In addition to cord compression from direct involvement of the vertebrae by myeloma, patients often suffer other neurological complications. Direct extradural involvement may occur through involvement of nerve roots via the intervertebral foramina. Soft-tissue deposits may occur in the orbit or base of skull, leading to proptosis or cranial nerve palsies. Carpal tunnel syndrome may develop, due to amyloid infiltration. Megaloblastic anaemia can occur, possibly due to defective folate metabolism, although many patients have some degree of macrocytosis with no megaloblastic change and of uncertain cause. Recurrent infection is also a common feature of the disease and is frequently one of the presenting complaints. Leucopenia predisposes to infection, as does the generalized depression of normal immunoglobulins. This immunoglobulin abnormality usually fails to become normal even with 'successful' treatment that may suppress the monoclonal immunoglobulin band. Some patients also have impairment of phagocytosis and cellular immune responses.

The plasma volume may be high as a result of the increase in total plasma protein, contributing to the anaemia even when the total red cell mass is near normal. The M band is also responsible, by direct coating of erythrocytes, for the raised erythrocyte sedimentation rate (ESR) and erythrocyte rouleaux formation that are so characteristic of myeloma. Typically, the ESR is more than 80 mm/hour. Bone marrow involvement is almost invariable, though for diagnostic purposes direct biopsy of a tender area is more likely to be positive. Abnormal plasma cells can account for up to 95% of the nucleated cell population. A practical point: many haematologists advise against sternal marrow puncture in patients with myeloma, in view of the extreme fragility of bone and the danger of inadvertently entering the mediastinum.

Hypercalcaemia is common, chiefly attributable to bone destruction from abnormal plasma cell proliferation, although other factors which activate osteoclasts have been described [8]. In many patients, a highly potent osteoclast-activating factor has been identified [6,9]. Approximately one-third of patients have an abnormally elevated plasma calcium at diagnosis, and the majority develop hypercalcaemia during the course of the illness. Indeed, myeloma is the diagnosis par excellence that may result in profound and treatment-resistant hypercalcaemia, often of sufficient severity to require emergency treatment (see Chapter 8). The symptoms include polyuria, polydipsia, constipation, nausea, vomiting, dehydration and mental confusion. Hypercalciuria is even more frequent.

Impaired renal function is extremely common. Once hypercalcaemia and renal impairment have developed, a vicious circle becomes established in which there is worsening renal function, increasing hypercalcaemia, further dehydration with falling glomerular filtration rate, and increasing tubular obstruction and dysfunction from light-chain deposition. This is a medical emergency and its management is described below.

Diagnosis

In a typical case when there are bone lesions, anaemia, paraproteinaemia, hypercalcaemia, Bence Jones proteinuria and marrow involvement, there is no diagnostic difficulty. In less florid cases, the differential diagnosis can be extensive and may include the following:

1 Other causes of anaemia, bone pain and hypercalcaemia such as metastatic cancer.

2 Other causes of paraproteinaemia such as MGUS, occult primary tumours (Table 27.3), Waldenström's macroglobulinaemia or lymphomas (Table 27.4).

3 Other causes of lytic lesions in bone such as breast, renal, thyroid or bronchial carcinoma.

4 Other causes of spinal cord compression such as metastatic cancer.

5 Other causes of anaemia and raised ESR such as connective tissue diseases, malignancy and infection especially where cold agglutinins are formed as in *Mycoplasma* infections and infectious mononucleosis, although these patients are generally younger.

6 Solitary plasmacytomas (see below).

7 Primary amyloidosis, which may be accompanied by plasmacytosis in the marrow and also by a proteinuria.

The diagnosis may be difficult if there is minimal marrow involvement, no detectable paraprotein, or a solitary bone lesion on skeletal radiography. In doubtful cases, the marrow examination may have to be repeated. However, if there is no pressing indication for treatment, a period of observation may allow the diagnosis to be established more easily (Table 27.4). Occasionally, immunological testing using light and heavy chain antibodies to establish monoclonality may be necessary to exclude a 'reactive'

Table 27.3 Causes of monoclonal gammaglobulinaemia other than myeloma.

Monoclonal gammopathy of unknown significance
Non-lymphoid and lymphoid malignancy
Carcinoma of breast, gastrointestinal tract, ovary, bladder, prostate and others
Soft-tissue sarcomas
Melanoma
Non-Hodgkin's lymphoma
Waldenström's macroglobulinaemia
Autoimmune diseases
Rheumatoid arthritis
Polyarteritis nodosa

Table 27.4 Causes of macroglobulinaemia.

Benign
Benign macroglobulinaemia
Cold agglutinin disease
Neoplasms
Waldenström's macroglobulinaemia
IgM myeloma
Non-Hodgkin's lymphomas
Chronic lymphatic leukaemia

plasmacytosis. In patients with 'smouldering myeloma' there is usually a paraprotein level of 3 Gm/dL or greater, a plasma-cell infiltration of at least 10%, and/or Bence Jones proteinuria of at least 1 Gm/24 hour. Until recently, the diagnosis of this low-level type of myeloma was followed by a period of observation or surveillance, but the recent demonstration of benefit – including the key yardstick of improved overall survival (OS) – from early treatment with lenalidomide and dexamethasone, has called into question this traditional view – see Ref. [10]. In this important randomized study from Spain, the OS-surrogate 3-year progression-free survival using these simple oral agents was even more impressive, shifting from 30% (no treatment) to 77% (active treatment), with acceptable side-effects.

Treatment

As mentioned in the introduction to this chapter, the past few years have seen a number of important, even dramatic, changes in management – see, for example, Ref. [11], for an excellent and up-to-date review. After a long sequence of disappointments, the outlook has now improved significantly, with an increased number of patients treated by multiple-agent chemo and targeted therapy, and enjoying more prolonged durable remissions and an improved quality of life. Advances in bone marrow transplantation and peripheral blood stem-cell enrichment techniques, together with exciting advances in biological therapy, have substantially widened the treatment opportunities.

When patients, just diagnosed with myeloma, present with dangerous manifestations such as dehydration, hypercalcaemia or spinal cord compression, the first treatment should be to correct the metabolic disturbance or serious local problem (see Chapter 8). Intravenous fluid replacement, correction of hypercalcaemia, local irradiation and occasionally decompressive laminectomy should, in these circumstances, take precedence. In the majority of patients, however, the presenting clinical syndrome is more slowly evolving and, in contrast to these clinical emergencies, there will be time to confirm the diagnosis before instituting treatment.

Chemotherapy, intensive treatment approaches and targeted therapy

Despite remarkable and rapid recent advances in chemotherapy for myeloma (see below), the traditional approach, using oral melphalan, is still sometimes used, especially with more elderly or unfit patients – though much less often than in former years. This form of medication improved survival from a median of 6–12 months (untreated) to 2–3 years [9,12] in the earliest attempts towards active and partially effective therapy for myeloma. Usually given by mouth, doses vary from 6 to $10\,mg/m^2$ over 4–7 days every 46 weeks. The addition of oral prednisolone has slightly improved the remission rate. Typical doses range from 60 to $80\,mg/m^2$ (with melphalan) in divided doses and accompanied by a histamine H_2-receptor antagonist such as ranitidine $150\,mg$ twice daily. Combined melphalan–prednisolone oral therapy is generally well tolerated, although in long survivors there is undoubtedly a small risk of development of acute myeloblastic leukaemia related to chronic melphalan therapy. High-dose intravenous melphalan is, however, still widely used as part of high-dose stem-cell supported treatment, often in younger fitter patients during their first remission (see below).

The introduction of more complex induction chemotherapy regimens and more active maintenance programs, often incorporating targeted as well as cytotoxic therapy, seems clearly to have led at last to a higher survival rate, even in older patients who cannot necessarily be expected to tolerate the most intensive treatment regimens [13,14].

Most patients with myeloma (over 80%) will respond to chemotherapy, with prompt improvement in symptoms, particularly pain, tenderness and hypercalcaemia. The paraprotein level generally falls within the first three cycles, although the immunoparesis of the unaffected immunoglobulins usually takes longer to recover, and may never do so. Other parameters such as haemoglobin, albumin and blood urea may return to normal limits and can be useful for monitoring progress. In patients who respond to chemotherapy, it is rarely necessary to continue the initial treatment beyond six to nine courses, since little further is to be gained. By this time many will have entered a 'plateau' phase, in which no further reduction of the paraprotein occurs, and treatment can reasonably be discontinued; alternatively, disease will be progressing and further strategies will be necessary.

Over the past 15 years many more complex regimens including intensive-dose regimens and targeted therapies have been tested, in an attempt to raise remission rates and duration, and ultimately to improve survival [9,15]. Increasingly, agents used 'upfront' including bortozemib, thalidomide and high-dose steroid therapy as well as a vinca alkaloid, multiple alkylating agents and doxorubicin. An alternative approach, to improve convenience of intensive treatment, is to use oral regimens including high-dose dexamethasone and idarubicin, sometimes also incorporating thalidomide (see below). One typical oral anthracylene regimen, known as Z-Dex, includes idarubicin $10\,mg/m^2$ daily for 4 days together with dexamethasone $40\,mg$ daily for 4 days, on a 3-week cycle. This is generally easier for patients than the well-known combination of vincristine, infused doxorubicin and high-dose dexamethasone (VAD), which requires insertion of a Hickman line, and often considerable periods of inpatient care, also making it less widely acceptable.

Intensive treatment should be offered to younger fitter patients, although there is no absolute consensus as to which combination of agents is most effective. Commonly used agents include vinca alkaloids, multiple alkylating agents, bortozemib, thalidomide, lenalidomide and doxorubicin together with high-dose dexamethasone. Regimens such as ABCM (doxorubicin, BCNU, cyclophosphamide and melphalan), VAD or VMCP–VBAP (vincristine, melphalan, cyclophosphamide and prednisolone alternating with vincristine, BCNU, doxorubicin and prednisolone) are widely used. In this younger group, the initial results of high-dose melphalan therapy, with or without autologous bone marrow transplantation (BMT) during first remission as initially described by McElwain and colleagues, have been extremely promising [16]. With an intensive single-exposure treatment, complete remission is seen in about one-third of patients, with elimination of malignant plasma cells in the marrow, reduction of paraprotein to undetectable levels and return of normal marrow function. In many cases, the immunoparesis has resolved as well, an impressive feature and unusual with conventional treatment.

An important and now classic study from France, comparing results of conventional with high-dose treatment (including autologous BMT), confirmed response rates of 81% with high-dose therapy (including complete responses in 22%) compared with 57% (complete responders 5%) in the conventionally treated arm [17]. Event-free 5-year survival was 52% compared with 12%. These are substantial differences that have altered current treatment recommendations in myeloma, particularly since stem-cell autotransplantation is widely applicable to reasonably fit patients up to age 65. Autologous stem-cell transplantation is now routinely offered during first remission to a substantial group of patients. A further group of highly selected younger patients may alternatively derive great benefit from allogeneic BMT if a donor is available, although the use of allogeneic transplantation still remains contentious. In a large recent study from Italy and the USA, patients with closely matched donors (HLA-identical siblings) were offered an allogeneic graft procedure as well as the standard chemotherapy (vincristine, doxorubicin, dexamethasone) together with melphalan with autologous stem-cell rescue [18]. Patients without a donor were treated with the same three-drug regimen in the first instance, followed by two myeloablative courses of melphalan, each followed by an autologous graft. Overall survival clearly favoured the first group: 80 months versus 54 months at a median 45-month follow-up. This important study is likely to prove highly influential in directing therapy for patients with an HLA-matched sibling, since the survival advantage was clear-cut, even compared with an intensive double-transplant of autologous stem cells in the comparator group of patients. Additional studies from other co-operative groups in the USA and Europe have amplified these initial findings more securely – see, for example, Refs. [19,20].

The main areas of controversy in the use of BMT for multiple myeloma are summarized in Table 27.5. It is clear that autologous bone marrow or stem-cell transplantation has now become the central basis of management for younger fit patients with myeloma, particularly where the tumour burden has initially been reduced by conventional multiagent chemotherapy as described above. Further useful remissions can sometimes be achieved by a second autologous transplantation procedure, if sufficient stem cells have been collected, preferably at the first harvest. Allogeneic stem-cell transplantation clearly offers a further alternative for suitable, generally younger, patients with a matched donor, with the additional potential benefit of a graft versus host effect coupled with the certainty of 'clean' or uncontaminated marrow, though with considerably greater morbidity than with the autologous approach.

After discontinuation of first-line chemotherapy, patients should be carefully monitored since further treatment will always be required, although sometimes only after many months or years. If treatment is discontinued following a well-documented response, it may be worth reinstituting the same therapy at the point of relapse since a second response is often seen. Relapse is usually detectable by a rise in the monoclonal immunoglobulin band, although some patients become symptomatic again without such a rise. Further supportive therapy with blood transfusion, antibiotics or palliative radiotherapy is often required if the patient becomes anaemic, or develops infections or painful bony lesions. Erythropoietin has become more widely used as a means of avoiding anaemia without frequent transfusion [22].

Second-line chemotherapy in myeloma remains unsatisfactory; likewise, treatment for the 25% of patients who are unresponsive when first treated ('primary chemoresistance'). Responses to secondary chemotherapy are usually of short duration, at the cost of inflicting more undesirable side-effects than seen with first-line agents. In an elderly population, careful judgement is always required before considering such treatment and it is important to establish that no further response can be obtained with first-line chemotherapy. The increasing use of thalidomide as a second-line treatment in relapsed myeloma has given this controversial agent a new role, even in newly diagnosed patients, that is, as first-line therapy [23]. It is capable of reducing serum and urine paraprotein levels, and can be taken orally at a daily dose of 200 mg but increasing to 800 mg in tolerant patients. It is also sometimes used as part of a combination programme with such agents as cyclophosphamide

Table 27.5 Summary of the evidence for key questions in the management of multiple myeloma by chemotherapy.

Question	Conclusion	Evidence
Is chemotherapy better than placebo?	Urethane is not better than placebo; cyclophosphamide is superior to placebo	2 randomized controlled trials enrolling 137 patients
Is melphalan the best single-agent therapy?	No survival advantage for patients treated with single-agent melphalan	5 randomized controlled trials enrolling 1651 patients
Is melphalan plus prednisone more effective than single-agent melphalan?	The study authors favoured the doublet, but the available data do not support a clear-cut survival advantage	1 randomized controlled trial enrolling 183 patients
Is combination chemotherapy better than melphalan plus prednisone?	No difference in survival between the groups; response rates were significantly higher with chemotherapy	Collaborative meta-analysis of data from individual patients, including 6633 patients from 27 randomized trials
Is interferon beneficial in management of multiple myeloma?	Progression-free survival was improved with interferon, but the survival benefit was small	Meta-analysis of individual patient data from 4012 patients who participated in 24 randomized trials
Does early treatment offer benefit over deferred treatment in early-stage myeloma?	Treatment just after diagnosis does not improve survival or response rate, compared with deferring therapy until disease progression	3 randomized controlled trials enrolling 365 patients
Is there an effective salvage therapy after first-line therapy has failed?	No experimental treatment has produced good results in any of the studies	10 randomized controlled trials enrolling 808 patients
Can high-dose chemotherapy be used in patients with impaired renal function?	Actuarial 3-year survival rates were comparable in both groups; melphalan $140\,mg/m^2$ is the optimum dose for patients with impaired renal function	Matched pair analysis of 126 patients with renal failure and controls

Source: Kumar *et al.* [21]. Management of multiple Reproduced with permission from Elsevier.

and dexamethasone (CDT). Toxicity is mostly mild, at least at lower doses (<600 mg). This antiangiogenic agent may possibly have a place as maintenance oral therapy in myeloma and several studies are currently in progress. For example, in elderly patients, a recent large randomized multicentre trial from Italy confirmed the superiority of an oral regimen using melphalan, prednisolone and thalidomide (compared with oral melphalan and prednisone together), at least from the point of view of higher response rates and longer event-free survival [24]. The combined complete or partial response rates were 76% for the three-drug regimen and 48% for melphalan and prednisone alone; the 3-year survival rates were 80% and 64% respectively, though at the cost of increased side-effects. A further large French study has strongly supported these findings. A proposed mechanism for the cytotoxic activity of thalidomide is outlined in Figure 27.5. A further related oral agent, lenalidomide,

has also emerged as an extremely active drug, with a better toxicity profile than thalidomide (less sedation and peripheral neuropathy) though with more associated myelosuppression. This simple piperidinedione agent, a structural analogue of thalidomide introduced in 2004, is clearly more powerful (reportedly well over 200 times more potent as an immunomodulator) than thalidomide, in respect of TNF inhibition and increased stimulation of T-cell proliferation and IL-2 production. It seems likely to emerge as an extremely important agent in myeloma, probably for first-line therapy in the immediate future (see below), and has recently been compared in a large European study with high-dose dexamethasone in relapsed or refractory myeloma [26]. This group assessed the benefits of these two treatments in over 350 patients, who received oral lenalidomide (25 mg daily on days 1–21 every 4 weeks), with or without dexamethasone 40 mg orally given according to a standard protocol.

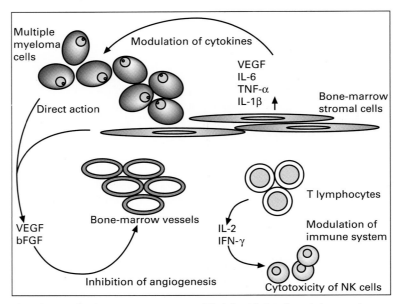

Figure 27.5 A proposed mechanism for the antitumour activity of thalidomide in relapsed chemoresistant multiple myeloma. FGF, fibroblast growth factor; IFN, interferon; IL, interleukin; NK, natural killer; TNF, tumour necrosis factor; VEGF, vascular endothelial growth factor. (Based upon Kumar *et al.* [21] and Singhal *et al.* [25].)

Time to progression of disease was clearly better in the lenalidomide group (11.3 months vs 4.7 months). A complete or partial response was noted in 106 patients in the lenalidomide group but only 42 in the comparator arm. Overall survival was also significantly improved. It is also highly active for patients with smouldering myeloma. In addition, a large number of studies have now been reported using targeted biological therapy with borte-zomib, a first-in-class proteasome inhibitor, mostly in patients with late-stage relapsed myeloma. In one recent study comparing treatment with standard dexametha-sone [27], bortezomib led to a dramatic improvement, with 89% of patients alive after a year, resulting in fast-track approval by the Food and Drug Administration (FDA) for use of bortezomib after progression following at least two different types of myeloma chemotherapy. For a more recent update on this agent, see Ref. [28].

With the advent of increasingly active immunomodu-lators, such as lenalidomide, pomalidomide (and others), and various targeted therapies, it is becoming increasingly difficult to assess the competing claims of all the newer anti-myeloma agents (and the associated complex regi-mens) advocated by scattered research groups in a logical and coherent series of clinical trials. Additional agents now increasingly used in second, third or fourth-line treatment include bendamustine, an alkylating agent

causing intra-strand and inter-strand cross-links between DNA bases, and carfilzomib, a tetrapeptide epoxy-ketone, which binds and inhibits the chymotrypsin-like activity of the 20S proteasome, an enzyme that appears to act by degrading unwanted cellular proteins.

The proper sequencing of treatments for myeloma is becoming highly challenging. Treatment decisions are increasingly governed by our understanding of the pathogenesis of myeloma, for example, with patients exhibiting interstitial deletion of chromosome 13q generally regarded as having a poor prognosis [29]. This abnormality appears to occur in about 40% of cases, though virtually all these have translocation t(4;14) as well. For this group, it may be sensible to avoid the use of autologous transplantation entirely, since they appear to do poorly with this approach.

Radiotherapy

Radiotherapy is of great value in multiple myeloma and is often required as part of the initial treatment, particularly for patients who present with painful bone deposits in the vertebrae or long bones, especially if there is a likelihood of pathological fracture or cord compres-sion [13]. Occasionally, surgical vertebral stabilization is required for large tumours with cord compression (Figure 27.6). Radiotherapy is the most important

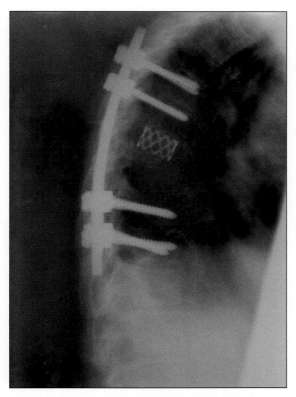

Figure 27.6 Lateral view of thoracic spine to show orthopaedic stabilization following vertebrectomy in a case of myeloma with spinal cord compression.

modality in myelomatous spinal cord compression, either alone or in combination with surgical decompression. Magnetic resonance imaging (MRI) should be performed to define the extent of the compression, and treatment should be started early at the onset of radicular pain. Radiotherapy is often combined with internal fixation, particularly where a weight-bearing long bone is affected by lytic deposits. Since myeloma deposits are relatively radiosensitive, large doses are rarely required [13].

Objective success and considerable clinical relief of symptoms have been claimed with systemic or hemibody irradiation (HBI) in myeloma [30], particularly in patients with symptomatic relapses unresponsive to standard chemotherapy. With HBI, pulmonary complications are unusual if the dose to the upper half of the body is kept below 8 Gy. Overall median survival with this technique is 12 months in drug-resistant cases (with many surviving beyond 2 years), comparable with second-line chemotherapy regimens but generally more acceptable. However, HBI cannot be recommended as first-line

therapy to consolidate a chemotherapy remission. Total body irradiation is widely used in many centres as part of the marrow-ablative protocol for patients undergoing allogeneic transplantation, often in conjunction with high-dose melphalan.

A further recent advance has been the use of pamidronate, clodronate and other bisphosphonate agents (e.g. ibandronate and zoledronic acid) to protect against skeletal complications and improve the quality of life in patients with advanced stages of disease [31]. In an MRC study of over 500 patients assessing the potential of oral clodronate as part of primary management, several benefits were noted [32]. Fewer patients developed vertebral or other pathological fractures, height loss was reduced, and hypercalcaemia was also less frequent. The authors recommended that treatment with clodronate should be instigated early in the course of the disease.

Prognosis

Patients with myeloma experience remissions and relapses requiring careful judgement for optimal choice and timing of therapy. Some survive over 5 years, requiring little in the way of chemotherapy, but repeated courses of radiotherapy and general support measures. Such patients usually have a low tumour burden based on simple criteria (Table 27.2). Retrospective analyses have shown that tumour burden is a good predictor of response and survival [13,14]. As pointed out above, cytogenetics can to some extent be used to identify differing prognostic groups, requiring different tailored approaches to management. For patients with a better prognosis, the paradigm of aiming to manage myeloma as a relatively indolent chronic disorder is gradually being realized, particularly since the advent of a much wider spectrum of effective treatments. Median survival in the best prognostic groups is approximately 5 years, compared with only 6 months in the worst (Figure 27.7). However, there is no longer any serious doubt that patients are surviving longer with modern treatments, as evidenced by a recent longitudinal study assessing outcomes with patients treated before and after 2000 [33]. In this study, survival after relapse was twice as long (24 months vs 12 months) in the more recently treated group. In addition, patients treated with one or more of the newer drugs (thalidomide, lenalidomide and/or bortezomib) had longer survival from relapse (30.9 months vs 14.8 months; $P < 0.001$). Patients treated aggressively for smouldering myeloma, as in the Mateos study noted above, have a reasonably good prognosis with an overall survival of over 90% at 3 years.

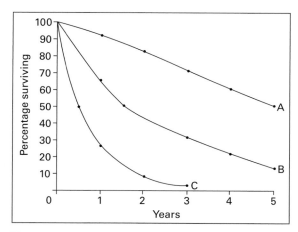

Figure 27.7 Prognosis in myeloma related to tumour mass: A, low; B, moderate; C, high (see also Table 27.2, page 547).

Since patients with myeloma often develop renal failure, it is not surprising that simple renal function is generally regarded as the most important prognostic criterion at diagnosis, although in recent years more weight has been given to total tumour mass, initial β_2-microglobulin level and number of bone lesions. Apart from disease recurrence and renal dysfunction, other myeloma complications are due to progressive pancytopenia as a result of therapy and crowding of normal marrow elements by abnormal plasma cells. Anaemia (often requiring repeated transfusion), infection and thrombocytopenia with bleeding are all common. Occasionally, infection, renal failure and hypercalcaemia may become totally resistant to treatment.

Solitary plasmacytoma

Solitary plasmacytoma [13,34,35] is a single-site plasma cell lesion occurring in either bone (common sites including vertebrae, clavicles, sternum or skull) or soft tissue (particularly nasal or oral cavity, bowel or bronchus). The typical histological picture is of malignant plasma cell infiltration, as in myeloma. In many patients no other evidence of myeloma develops, provided adequate local treatment with radiotherapy is given. However, solitary plasmacytoma can be the initial manifestation of myeloma; all patients must be carefully investigated since a proportion with apparently solitary lesions actually have multiple myeloma at the outset, and many others will undoubtedly develop myeloma later, although latent periods of several years are not

unusual. Progression is more common in those who present with a plasmacytoma in bone than in those where the site is extramedullary. Although we lack unequivocal evidence that aggressive chemotherapy for solitary plasmacytomas will *prevent* the development of generalized myeloma, younger and fitter patients are often treated with chemotherapy prior to local irradiation of the lesion. One-third of patients remain disease-free for 10 years or more, the remainder developing myeloma within a median time period of 2–3 years. Non-secretory disease and persistence of myeloma-specific protein after local treatment are both important adverse prognostic features.

Monoclonal gammopathy of unknown significance

There are many diseases in which a monoclonal immunoglobulin band is found but without evidence of a plasma cell neoplasm [36] (see Table 27.4). The commonest cause, and the one which creates greatest diagnostic confusion, is MGUS, which is a disease of the elderly. It is common, with a prevalence of 0.5% in adults over 40 years and at least 5% in those over 70 years; it accounts for 40% of all paraproteinaemias. The monoclonal immunoglobulin concentration is usually less than 30 g/L. A large majority (85%) have an IgG paraprotein without other abnormalities in plasma proteins or symptoms of the kind found in patients with multiple myeloma. Bence Jones protein is occasionally found. The ESR is usually raised. MGUS requires no treatment, although it clearly predisposes to myeloma. In one series, for example, 22 patients with MGUS went on to develop multiple myeloma at a median time interval of just under 10 years after initial recognition of the M protein. Long-term (30-year) follow-up has confirmed that myeloma develops in up to 16% of those with MGUS, with an annual actuarial rate of 0.8% [9]. Although the cause of MGUS is unknown, these gammopathies are often characterized by a rearrangement of immunoglobulin genes that results in the production of a monoclonal protein, typically with a plasma-cell clone and its associated monoclonal protein remaining stable over many years. As with myeloma, common phenotypic profiles occur, including CD38+, CD56+ and CD19−, although the proportion of phenotypically normal plasma cells is higher in patients with MGUS than in those with myeloma. In general, patients with MGUS have two populations of plasma cells, one normal and polyclonal and the other clonal with the abnormal immunophenotype.

Macroglobulinaemia

This group of conditions is characterized by the production of monoclonal IgM (see Table 27.4). The correct diagnosis may prove elusive and require months or years of careful assessment as the disease process gradually develops and becomes more clear-cut, particularly in patients with slowly evolving IgM-producing non-Hodgkin's lymphoma, in whom the paraprotein elevation may precede lymphadenopathy or other lymphoma-related symptoms, or may even masquerade as a genuine case of myeloma.

Benign macroglobulinaemia follows a similar course to other forms of MGUS (see above).

Cold agglutinin disease is a disorder of the elderly in which patients suffer vascular disturbances in the extremities due to intracapillary red-cell agglutination in parts of the body exposed to cold. A deep blue–violet discoloration may occur (acrocyanosis) that may lead to gangrene. A moderate haemolysis is usually present, but physical examination is usually normal. The disease is due to a monoclonal IgM, which has the property of being a cold agglutinin. If simple measures (gloves or mittens and warm boots) are inadequate, treatment with alkylating agents can be helpful.

Waldenström's macroglobulinaemia (see also page 530) [37]

This condition, typically occurring in the elderly, is characterized by marrow infiltration with lymphoid cells that have an appearance intermediate between lymphocytes and plasma cells (lymphoplasmacytoid). Monoclonal lymphocytes are present in both blood and marrow, and the morphology is suggestive of a differentiating B-cell neoplasm. There is often enlargement of lymph nodes, liver and spleen. Unlike IgM myeloma, bone lesions are very uncommon, although diffuse osteoporosis may occur. Monoclonal IgM is often produced in very large amounts, sometimes producing hyperviscosity.

The patient typically presents with ill-health and weakness, often with night sweats. Symptoms of hyperviscosity may predominate, with headache, mental confusion, retinal haemorrhages and renal impairment. The macroglobulin may produce haemolytic anaemia or act as a cold agglutinin, producing haemorrhage by interaction with platelets and clotting factors. Purpura and bleeding are not infrequent. Investigations reveal anaemia, variable thrombocytopenia, a raised serum IgM and occasionally immunoparesis.

The disease is usually only slowly progressive and, in the absence of symptoms, treatment can be withheld. Chlorambucil or cyclophosphamide usually produce regression of lymphadenopathy and a fall in IgM levels. Fludarabine is also effective but immunosuppressive. Steroids are of little value, but plasmapheresis will produce reduction of viscosity and may be essential if clinical hyperviscosity is present, until chemotherapy has reduced IgM production. Prognosis is variable, but average survival is 3–4 years. In aggressive cases, combination chemotherapy as for myeloma may be valuable.

POEMS syndrome

This rare multisystem disease, still poorly understood, was first described in the mid-1950s and later given the acronym POEMS because of the five main features usually present; namely, *p*olyneuropathy, *o*rganomegaly, *e*ndocrinopathy, *m*onoclonal gammopathy and *s*kin changes. Most patients have at least three, although not necessarily all, of the above features. At least one site of plasmacytoma is always present. Characteristically, the polyneuropathy, which probably represents the commonest presentation of POEMS, is bilateral, symmetrical and progressive, often to a startling degree, and accompanied by clear-cut changes in the electromyogram. The commonest sites of soft-tissue swelling or enlargement include liver, spleen and lymph nodes, with changes, at least in the enlarged lymph nodes, often reminiscent of Castleman's disease (giant angiofollicular hyperplasia, the multicentric plasma cell variant). In the enlarged liver the histological changes are less specific. Common endocrinopathies include diabetes or glucose intolerance, hypothyroidism and elevated oestrogen levels. Typically, the plasma cell abnormality appears to be a variant of osteosclerotic myeloma, or MGUS (see pages 556–557). The commonest immunoglobulin abnormalities are IgA and IgG-γ. Elevations in vascular endothelial growth factor (VEGF) levels are usually present, a feature often now regarded as essentially pathognomonic of the POEMS syndrome. Treatment is generally by local radiotherapy if only a single plasmacytoma is present, or with more intensive myeloma-specific chemotherapy (including autotransplantation and high-dose chemotherapy) for more extensive disease. Targeted therapy, particularly with bevacizumab, seems logical in view of the raised VEGF levels, and is increasingly used, although it is not regarded as first-line therapy. Prognosis of the neuropathy and other changes appears on the whole remarkably good (see Refs. [38,39]).

Heavy-chain diseases

These diseases are lymphocyte neoplasms in which there is production of incomplete heavy chains of immunoglobulin, without light chains. The first patient was described by Franklin and coworkers in 1964 [40]. So far, only γ, α and μ heavy-chain diseases have been described. Interestingly, each has distinct clinical features.

γ Heavy-chain disease

γ Heavy-chain disease usually affects elderly patients, producing lymphadenopathy, tonsillar enlargement, palatal oedema and hepatosplenomegaly. Bone lesions are unusual. Occasionally there are associated autoimmune diseases such as systemic lupus erythematosus or Sjögren's syndrome. Anaemia is common but marrow biopsy is not always diagnostic. The lymph nodes are sometimes replaced with lymphoplasmacytoid cells; the γ heavy-chain fragment is found in serum or urine, and there may also be immunoparesis. Chemotherapy is usually minimally effective. Although this disease may occasionally regress without treatment, survival is usually for less than 3 years.

α Heavy-chain disease (see also Chapter 26, page 537)

This is the commonest of the heavy-chain diseases, chiefly found in young Mediterranean adults aged 20–30, predominantly in the Middle East and South America. It is a disease of the small bowel although occasionally the stomach, large bowel and postnasal space are affected. There is often a lengthy history of gastrointestinal disturbance, and some patients have been previously diagnosed as having immunoproliferative disease of the small intestine. Because of massive lymphoid infiltration of the bowel, severe malabsorption and diarrhoea occur and although the histological appearances may initially not appear to be malignant, a true lymphoma usually develops.

α Heavy chains are present in the blood but their detection is difficult. The marrow is not involved and liver, spleen and lymph nodes are not enlarged. The diagnosis is made by small-bowel biopsy. Treatment with chemotherapy at the stage of frank lymphoma is only temporarily effective, and whole-abdominal irradiation has sometimes been used. Before this stage, treatment with oral tetracycline may produce lengthy remissions.

μ Heavy-chain disease

In this very rare disease, μ heavy chains are found in the plasma. The clinical disease mimics long-standing chronic lymphatic leukaemia, or a non-Hodgkin's lymphoma, usually with marked visceral organomegaly, and treatment is similar to that used for these diseases.

References

1 Velez R, Beral V, Cuzick J. Increasing trends of multiple myeloma mortality in England and Wales 1950–79: are the changes real? *J Natl Cancer Inst* 1982; 69: 387–92.

2 Lynch HT, Ferrara K, Barlogie B *et al.* Familial myeloma. *N Engl J Med* 2008; 359: 152–7.

3 Sirohi B, Powles R. Multiple myeloma. *Lancet* 2004; 363: 875–87.

4 Cuzick J. Radiation-induced myelomatosis. *N Engl J Med* 1981; 304: 204–10.

5 Cuzick J, Cooper EH, MacLennan ICM. The prognostic value of serum β$_2$ microglobulin compared with other presentation features in myelomatosis. *Br J Cancer* 1985; 52: 1–6.

6 Tricot G. New insights into the role of microenvironment in multiple myeloma. *Lancet* 2000; 355: 248–50.

7 Hallek M, Bergsagel DL, Anderson KC. Multiple myeloma: increasing evidence for a multistep transformation process. *Blood* 1998; 91: 3–21.

8 Mundy GR, Raisz LG, Cooper RA *et al.* Evidence for the secretion of an osteoclast stimulating factor in myeloma. *N Engl J Med* 1974; 291: 1041–6.

9 Gahrton G. Treatment of multiple myeloma. *Lancet* 1999; 353: 85–6.

10 Mateos M-V, Hernandez M-T, Giraldo P *et al.* Lenalidomide plus dexamethasone for high-risk smoldering multiple myeloma. *New Engl J Med* 2013; 369: 438–47.

11 Usmani S Z, Crowley J, Hoering A *et al.* Improvement in long-term outcomes with successive total therapy trials for multiple myeloma: are patients now being cured? *Leukemia* 2013; 27: 226–32.

12 Niesvisky R, Siegel D, Michaeli J. Biology and treatment of multiple myeloma. *Blood Rev* 1993; 7: 24–33.

13 Pulte D, Gondos A, Brenner H. Improvement in survival of older adults with multiple myeloma: results of an updated period analysis of SEER data. *Oncologist* 2011; 16: 1600–3.

14 Bladé J, Rosiñol L. Changing paradigms in the treatment of multiple myeloma. *Haematologica* 2009; 94: 163–6.

15 Bataille R, Harousseau J-L. Medical progress: multiple myeloma. *N Engl J Med* 1997; 336: 1657–64.

16 Selby PJ, McElwain TJ, Nandi AC *et al.* Multiple myeloma treated with high dose intravenous melphalan. *Br J Haematol* 1987; 66: 55–62.

17 Attal M, Harousseau J-L, Stoppa A-M *et al.* A prospective randomized trial of autologous bone marrow transplantation and chemotherapy in multiple myeloma. *N Engl J Med* 1996; 335: 91–7.

18 Bruno B, Rotta M, Patriarca F *et al.* A comparison of allografting with autografting for newly diagnosed myeloma. *N Engl J Med* 2007; 356: 1110–20.

19 Shimoni A, Hardan I, Ayuk F *et al.* Allogenic hematopoietic stem-cell transplantation with reduced-intensity conditioning in patients with refractory and recurrent multiple myeloma: long-term follow-up. *Cancer* 2010; 116: 3621.

20 Harousseau J-L, Moreau P. Autologous hematopoietic stem-cell transplantation for multiple myeloma. *N Engl J Med* 2009; 360: 2645–54.

21 Kumar A, Loughran T, Alsina M *et al.* Management of multiple myeloma: a systematic review and critical appraisal of published studies. *Lancet Oncol* 2003; 4: 293–304.

22 Rizzo DJ, Lichtin AE, Woolf SH *et al.* Use of epoietin in patients with cancer: evidence-based clinical practice guidelines of the American Society of Clinical Oncology and American Society of Hematology. *Blood* 2002; 100: 2302–20.

23 Rajkumar SV, Blood E, Vesole D *et al.* Phase III clinical trial of thalidomide plus dexamethasone compared with dexamethasone alone in newly diagnosed multiple myeloma: a clinical trial coordinated by the Eastern Cooperative Oncology Group. *J Clin Oncol* 2006; 24: 431–6.

24 Palumbo A, Brighaen S, Caravita T *et al.* For the Italian Multiple Myeloma Network. Oral melphalan and prednisone chemotherapy plus thalidomide compared with melphalan and prednisolone alone in elderly patients with multiple myeloma: a randomized controlled trial. *Lancet* 2006; 367: 825–31.

25 Singhal S, Mehta J, Desikan R *et al.* Antitumour activity of thalidomide in refractory multiple myeloma. *N Engl J Med* 1999; 341: 156–7.

26 Dimopoulos M, Spencer A, Attal M *et al.* Lenalidomide plus dexamethasone for relapsed or refractory myeloma. *N Engl J Med* 2007; 357: 2123–32.

27 Richardson PG, Barlogie B, Berenson J *et al.* A phase 2 study of bortezomib (Velcade) in relapsed, refractory myeloma. *N Engl J Med* 2003; 348: 2609–17.

28 Picot J, Cooper K, Bryant J, Clegg AJ. The clinical effectiveness and cost-effectiveness of bortezomib and thalidomide in combination regimens with an alkylating agent and a corticosteroid for the first-line treatment of multiple myeloma: a systematic review and economic evaluation. *Health Technol Assess.* 2011; 15(41): 1–204.

29 Fonseca R, Barlogie B, Bataille R *et al.* Genetics and cytogenetics of multiple myeloma: a workshop report. *Cancer Res* 2004; 64: 1546–58.

30 McSweeny EN, Tobias JS, Blackman G *et al.* Double hemibody irradiation in the management of relapsed and primary chemoresistant myeloma. *Clin Oncol* 1993; 5: 378–83.

31 Terpos E, Sezer O, Croucher PI, *et al.* The use of bisphosphonates in multiple myeloma: recommendations of an expert panel on behalf of the European Myeloma Network. *Ann Oncol* 2009; 20: 1303–17.

32 McCloskey EV, MacLennan ICM, Drayson MT *et al.* For the MRC Working Party for Leukaemia in Adults. A randomized trial of the effect of clodronate on skeletal morbidity in multiple myeloma. *Br J Haematol* 1998; 100: 317–25.

33 Kumar SK, Rajkumar SV, Dispenzieri A *et al.* Improved survival in multiple myeloma and the impact of novel therapies. *Blood* 2008; 111: 2516–20.

34 Frassica DA, Frassica FJ, Schray MF *et al.* Solitary plasmacytoma of bone: the Mayo Clinic experience. *Int J Radiat Oncol Biol Phys* 1989; 16: 43–8.

35 Dimopoulos MA, Goldstein J, Fuller L *et al.* Curability of solitary bone plasmacytoma. *J Clin Oncol* 1992; 10: 587–90.

36 Bladé J. Monoclonal gammopathy of undetermined significance. *N Engl J Med* 2006; 355: 2765–70.

37 Ghobrial IM, Gertz MA, Fonseca R. Waldenström's macroglobulinaemia. *Lancet Oncol* 2003; 4: 679–85.

38 Miralles GD, O'Fallon JR, Talley NJ. Plasma-cell dyscrasia with polyneuropathy. The spectrum of POEMS syndrome. *N Engl J Med* 1992; 327: 1919–23.

39 Dispenzieri A, Kyle RA, Lacy MQ *et al.* POEMS syndrome: definitions and long-term outcome. *Blood* 2003; 101: 2496–506.

40 Franklin EC, Lowenstein J, Bigelow B, Meltzer M. Heavy chain disease: a new disorder of serum gammaglobulin. *Am J Med* 1964; 37: 332–50.

41 Brenner H, Gondos A, Pulte D. Recent major improvement in long-term survival of younger patients with multiple myeloma. *Blood* 2008; 111: 2521–6.

Further reading

McCarthy PL. Second transplant as a standard for multiple myeloma. *Lancet Oncol* 2014; 15: 786–8.

Palumbo A, Boccadoro M. A new standard of care for elderly patients with myeloma. *Lancet* 2007; 370: 1191–2.

San Miguel JF, Schlag R, Khuageva NK *et al.* Bortezomib plus melphalan and prednisone for initial treatment of multiple myeloma. *N Engl J Med* 2008; 359: 906–17.

28 Leukaemia

Leukaemias are neoplastic proliferations of white blood cells (WBCs). Although relatively uncommon, they have been the subject of intensive investigation because of the insights they give into aetiology and pathogenesis of the malignant process. The chemotherapy that has been responsible for the increasing cure rate in acute leukaemia has served as an example for the treatment of other malignancies. Allogeneic bone marrow transplantation (BMT) was developed as a treatment for acute leukaemia. Autologous BMT has also been widely used in treatment and some of the findings have been of great importance in designing studies of autologous BMT in solid tumours. For these reasons, the principles of management are described in this chapter, but more detailed discussion and guidance is given in the references listed at the end of the chapter.

Incidence and aetiology

The incidence and mortality of leukaemia is shown in Figure 28.1. In childhood (below 15 years of age), acute lymphoblastic leukaemia (ALL) accounts for 80% of all cases, acute myeloblastic leukaemia (AML) and its variants for 17%, and chronic granulocytic leukaemia (CGL) for approximately 3% [1]. Three-quarters of cases of ALL occur below the age of 6 years. In the USA, about 3000–5000 new cases of ALL are diagnosed annually. In adults, the outlook for ALL is far worse than in children, as many more have unfavourable cytogenetic characteristics such as the t(9;22) translocation, and patients over the age of 60 years may have a lowered tolerance of the intensive chemotherapy essential for cure. The death rate from acute leukaemia in the population is approximately 7 per 100 000. As a whole, leukaemia is slightly more common in males (male to female ratio of 3:2), and its incidence over the last decade appears to have been constant. Acute leukaemia is most common in the elderly (Figure 28.1), and over 15 years of age 85% of cases are AML. In adults, AML and ALL have a very similar prognosis, but childhood ALL has different clinical features and a much better prognosis than adult ALL, or AML at any age.

A variety of aetiological factors have been implicated. Ionizing irradiation is known to be leukaemogenic. Survivors of the Hiroshima and Nagasaki atom bombs have an increased risk of leukaemia, and the risk is greater for those who were near the centre of the explosions. The most frequent types were AML and CGL and the increased incidence began 2 years after the explosion and then declined after 6 years. Exposure to ionizing irradiation in pregnancy doubles the risk of childhood leukaemia, as does therapeutic irradiation which, in the past, was used for the treatment of ankylosing spondylitis.

Cancer and its Management, Seventh Edition. Jeffrey Tobias and Daniel Hochhauser.
© 2015 John Wiley & Sons, Ltd. Published 2015 by John Wiley & Sons, Ltd.

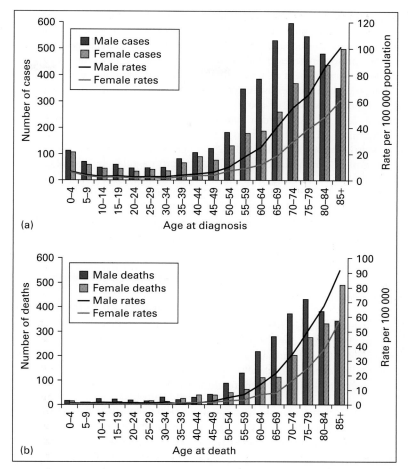

Figure 28.1 (a) Leukaemia (C91–C95), average number of new cases per year and age-specific incidence rates by sex, UK, 2008–2010. (b) Leukaemia (C91–C95), average number of deaths per year and age-specific mortality rates by sex, UK, 2009–2011. (Source: http://info.cancerresearchuk.org/cancerstats/types/leukaemia/mortality/?a=5441 accessed February 2014. © 2014 Cancer Research UK, Reproduced with permission.)

Viruses are not well-established causes except for the family of human T-cell leukaemia viruses (HTLVs) prevalent in Japan and other Asian countries.

Benzene and some of its derivatives predispose to the development of both leukaemia and aplastic anaemia. An excess of leukaemia (predominantly AML) has been reported in refinery workers. Other occupations with increased risk appear to be welders and workers in industries using DDT.

An important cause of leukaemia is anticancer treatment itself. There is an increased risk of leukaemia after treatment for Hodgkin's Lymphoma (see also Chapter 25, pages 513–514) and ovarian cancer [2]. The risk increases with time from treatment and depends on the nature of the drugs used, alkylating agents and etoposide being particularly implicated. There is a higher relative risk for young patients. A large study of over 420 000 patients in the USA showed that patients who have received chemotherapy for any reason are 4.7 times more likely to develop acute myeloid leukaemia than the general population – see Ref. [3]. In treatment-related leukaemia, typical chromosomal abnormalities occur, of which the most consistent is translocation involving chromosome 11. This also occurs following benzene exposure. The chromosome 11 band 23–32 appears to be consistently involved, and the functional effect is to alter cell signalling and growth. In childhood leukaemia, recent studies have suggested that deletions, amplifications, point mutations and/or structural rearrangements are frequently present in genes encoding the regulators of B-lymphocyte development in up to 40% of all cases. Chromosome 11 abnormalities in leukaemic bone marrow cells have been observed in about 15% of cases of ALL, almost 20% of AML, and a similar number in refractory anaemia (RA) cases. Bands 11p13, 11p14 and 11p15 on the short arm and 11q14, 11q21 and 11q23 on the long arm of chromosome 11 are the most likely to be involved in these rearrangements, with rearrangements of band 11q23 detected most frequently. The main target appears to be the *PAX*-5 gene, which is altered in over 30% of patients. Smoking increases the risk of leukaemia by 50%. The risk is mainly for AML and acute myelomonocytic leukaemia (AMML) (see below). The risk of childhood leukaemia is also probably increased in children whose mothers smoked marijuana or who were exposed to benzene and other solvents in pregnancy.

Certain constitutive abnormalities predispose to leukaemia. In Down's syndrome (trisomy 21) there is a substantially increased risk of acute leukaemia, up to 10–15 times the expected incidence, and usually ALL, at least in the younger age group [4]. Bloom's syndrome, Fanconi's anaemia and ataxia telangiectasia are all autosomal recessive diseases characterized by chromosome breakage and an increased risk of leukaemia. A defective DNA repair mechanism may be responsible. AML is the usual leukaemia in Fanconi's anaemia, and ALL in ataxia telangiectasia. It is also widely accepted that certain syndromes of myelodysplasia or myelofibrosis can be genuinely 'pre-leukaemic'.

Pathogenesis

The clonal nature of leukaemia proliferation has been elegantly established by studies on patients who are heterozygous for glucose 6-phosphate dehydrogenase (G6PD). In patients with chronic myeloblastic leukaemia (CML) who are heterozygous for G6PD, leukaemic cells have been shown to express only one G6PD isozyme. Similar clonality has been shown in AML [5].

The oncogenic event endows the clone with a proliferative advantage, because it is not subject to growth regulation. The leukaemic mass increases, but this does not appear to be the sole reason for the suppression of normal haemopoiesis. In the process of clonal expansion somatic genetic instability gives rise to subclones with diverse features within the tumour.

These genetic changes *consequent* to the early events inducing the leukaemic process may themselves confer a growth stimulus. Early in the development of CML, and also in some cases of ALL particularly in adults, there is a translocation between chromosomes 9 and 22 (t9;22)(q34;q11). This juxtaposes the *bcr* gene and the *abl* gene: the fusion protein results in a tyrosine kinase that gives rise to phosphorylation of substrates involved in growth regulation. Several of the translocations in acute leukaemia result in expression of transcription factors which themselves regulate expression of other genes (see below). The sum of these changes is an uncontrolled capacity for self-renewal and an unresponsiveness to apoptotic signals.

The acute leukaemias

Pathology and classification

Acute leukaemias often retain many of the cytoplasmic and membrane characteristics of their normal counterparts, so it is possible to relate the various types of acute leukaemia to a particular stage of myeloid or lymphoid maturation [6]. A simplified scheme is shown in Figure 28.2.

The diagnosis is made from blood and marrow films. In the typical case there are leukaemic blasts in the blood and the marrow is packed with uniform-looking blast cells. Cases of ALL almost always show these appearances, but in adult AML the leukaemic process may be much more subtle, with few blasts in the blood. The marrow must show over 30% of blasts for the diagnosis to be made with confidence. When there are less than 20% blasts the diagnosis of myelodysplastic state is usually made.

The acute leukaemias have been subdivided on morphological grounds using a scheme devised by a French–American–British (FAB) study group [6]. An outline is given in Table 28.1.

In AML, the myeloblasts may contain Auer rods, which are pink-staining, rod-like inclusions that are probably aberrant forms of the cytoplasmic granules found in normal granulocyte precursors. These granules are often prominent in the cytoplasm in AML and are particularly frequent and often large in the M3 variety (hypergranular promyelocytic leukaemia). In monocytic leukaemia (M5) the blasts are large with abundant cytoplasm, and in erythroleukaemia (M6) there are erythroblasts and myeloblasts in the marrow. The World

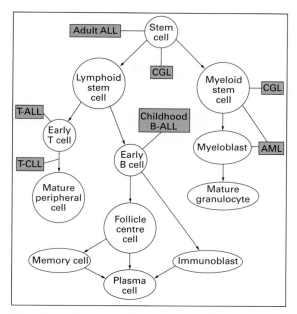

Figure 28.2 Maturation of haemopoietic and lymphoid cells in relation to types of leukaemia.

Health Organization (WHO) has classified acute myeloid leukaemia as follows.

• *AML with characteristic genetic abnormalities*: includes AML with cytogenetic abnormalities including translocations between chromosomes 8 and 21 t(8;21), inversions in chromosome 16, or translocations between chromosomes 15 and 17 t(15;17). Patients in this category generally have a high rate of remission and a better prognosis than other types of AML.

• *AML with multilineage dysplasia*: includes patients who have had a pre-leukaemic myelodysplastic syndrome (MDS) or myeloproliferative disease that then transforms into AML. This type of AML often occurs in elderly patients, with a worse prognosis.

• *AML and MDS, therapy-related*: includes patients who have had previous chemotherapy and/or radiation, and subsequently develop AML or MDS. These leukaemias may also be characterized by specific chromosomal abnormalities, and often carry a worse prognosis.

• *AML not otherwise categorized*: includes subtypes of AML that do not fall into the above categories.

• *Acute leukaemias of ambiguous lineage*: these occur when the leukaemic cells cannot be classified as either myeloid or lymphoid cells, or where both types of cells are present together.

In ALL, cytogenetic characterization has also been increasingly recognized as an important predictor of

Table 28.1 Morphological classification of acute leukaemia. The percentages indicate the proportions of the subtypes of acute leukaemia of myeloid and monocytic origins.

Myeloblastic leukaemia (55%)
M0: almost no differentiation, antimyeloperoxidase staining (5% of cases), ?worse prognosis
M1: poorly differentiated, stains for myeloperoxidase, Auer rods (20% of cases)
M2: differentiated beyond promyelocyte, may show t(8;21) and B-cell antigens (30% of cases)

Promyelocytic leukaemia (10%)
M3: hypergranular, Auer rods; t(15;17)
M3 (variant): granules absent but myeloperoxidase present

Myelomonocytic leukaemia (20%)
M4: granulocyte features but monocyte esterase present, urine lysozyme present, monocytosis, E0 variant shows eosinophilia

Monocytic leukaemia (15%)
M5: monocytic features (less in children), esterase positive, high white cell count, gum hypertrophy, urine lysozyme present

Erythroleukaemia
M6: rare

Megakaryoblastic
M7: rare

Acute lymphoblastic leukaemia
L1: small monomorphic cells
L2: large heterogeneous cells
L3: Burkitt-like

outcome. Some of the commoner abnormalities are summarized in Table 28.2. At present, the subclassification of ALL remains highly contentious. Until recently, subtyping of the various forms of ALL was made according to the FAB classification, used for all acute leukaemias (including acute myelogenous leukaemia). The FAB classification was essentially morphological, as follows.

• ALL-L1: small uniform cells.

• ALL-L2: large varied cells.

• ALL-L3: large varied cells with vacuoles (bubble-like features).

However, the recent WHO International Panel on ALL now recommends that this should be discontinued, as the morphological classification seems to have little if any clinical or prognostic relevance. Instead it advocates the use of an immunophenotypic classification, taking account of more fundamental cytogenetic

Table 28.2 Some of the commoner cytogenetic abnormalities in acute lymphoblastic leukaemia.

Cytogenetic change	Risk category
Presence of Philadelphia chromosome	Poor prognosis
t(4;11)(q21;q23)	Poor prognosis
t(8;14)(q24.1;q32)	Poor prognosis
Complex karyotype (more than four abnormalities)	Poor prognosis
Low hypodiploidy or near triploidy	Poor prognosis
High hyperdiploidy	Good prognosis
Deletion of 9p	Good prognosis

Table 28.3 Cytochemistry and lineage characteristics of acute leukaemia.

Phenotypic feature	Leukaemia
Sudan black	+ AML –ALL
Myeloperoxidase	+ AML –ALL
α-Naphthylbutyrate esterase	+ AML –ALL
Tdt expression	ALL (T and B)
Immunoglobulin gene heavy-chain rearrangement	B-ALL
TCR gene arrangement	T-ALL
Cytoplasmic or surface immunoglobulin	B-ALL
TCR expression	T-ALL

TCR, T-cell receptor; Tdt, terminal deoxynucleotidyltransferase, a DNA polymerase measured by fluorescence or biochemically.

characteristics. Subtypes are classified by determining the surface markers of the abnormal lymphocytes, with two main immunological types: pre-B cell and pre-T cell. The mature B-cell ALL-L3 is now classified as Burkitt leukaemia/lymphoma. In contrast to the older system, this approach to subtyping clearly helps determine the prognosis and most appropriate treatment for ALL.

As noted in Table 28.2, some cytogenetic subtypes have a worse prognosis than others.

• A translocation between chromosomes 9 and 22, known as the Philadelphia chromosome, occurs in about 20% of adult and 5% of pediatric cases of ALL.

• A translocation between chromosomes 4 and 11 occurs in about 4% of cases and is most common in infants under 12 months.

• Not all translocations of chromosomes carry a poorer prognosis. Some translocations are relatively favourable, for example hyperdiploidy (>50 chromosomes) is, perhaps unexpectedly, a good prognostic factor.

In ALL, the commonest variety (previously termed L1) is characterized by scanty cytoplasm and fewer nucleoli. In the less common form (previously termed L2) the blasts are larger, with a larger nucleolus. This form, which is more common in adults, is more easily mistaken for AML and may account for some cases designated as undifferentiated leukaemia. The L3 form is of large homogeneous cells with prominent nucleoli and basophilic cytoplasm resembling Burkitt's lymphoma cells. The commonly used immunocytochemical stains, often of great value in diagnostically difficult or doubtful cases, are shown in Table 28.3. In occasional instances of undifferentiated acute leukaemia, the cytochemical stains may be unhelpful. In ALL in particular, these markers

may help to distinguish common ALL from T-cell ALL and Burkitt's lymphoma.

Immunological phenotype in leukaemia

The normal maturation sequence of lymphoid and myeloid cells is accompanied by expression of cell surface and cytoplasmic proteins that can be detected by antibodies. In the leukaemias, this antigen expression can be used to 'phenotype' tumours, reflecting different stages of maturation [7]. Some of these subdivisions have little prognostic or therapeutic importance, but they help in understanding the pathogenesis of leukaemia. An abbreviated summary is given in Table 28.4.

Table 28.4 Useful cellular markers in acute leukaemia.*

Stem cells: Tdt, HLA-DR, CD34
Myeloid: CD11, CD13, CD14, CD33
Monocytic: CD11, CD14
Megakaryocytic: CD17, AN51, J15
B cell: C10, CD19, CD20, CD24, Tdt, SIg
T cell: CD2, cyCD3, CDS, CD7

*Several other markers may be used, and the panel of markers shown is an indication of those in wide use. The markers are, in any case, used in conjunction with morphological and clinical features.
cy, cytoplasmic; SIg, surface immunoglobulin; Tdt, terminal deoxynucleotidyltransferase.

Table 28.5 Common chromosomal abnormalities in leukaemia.

Leukaemia	Abnormality
CML	t(9;22). Demonstrable karyotypically in 80% of cases. More restricted translocation in many of the remainder
AML	
M2 (M1 less frequently)	t(8;21), good prognosis
M3	t(15;17), good prognosis
M4	Various translocations involving 11q23, inv16 (good prognosis)
M5	t(9;11), other translocations of 11q23, poor prognosis
ALL	t(12;21) TEL–AML1 fusion product, good prognosis
	Ph[1] chromosome, poor prognosis
T-cell ALL	t(11;14), poor prognosis; t(8;14), poor prognosis
B-cell ALL	t(8;14), poor prognosis
Undifferentiated or AUL	t(4;11), very poor prognosis
CLL	Trisomy 12, bad prognosis; deletion 13q14, bad prognosis

AUL, acute undifferentiated leukaemia.

Genetic and chromosomal abnormalities in leukaemia

A wide range of acquired karyotypic abnormalities have now been found in leukaemia (Table 28.5) and in recent years a more precise definition of the genes involved has become possible – see, for example, the recent work on genetic and epigenetic landscapes of adult AML from the Cancer Genome Atlas Research Network [8]. This new knowledge has been profoundly valuable in both classification and treatment, which increasingly is directed by the genetic basis of the individual case. Furthermore, considerable progress has now been made in understanding how these genetic changes lead to the development of leukaemia. It seems likely that, as in other cancers, several sequential changes are necessary for the development of the full malignant characteristics.

In CML, the Philadelphia (Ph[1]) chromosome is usually present. This is at chromosome 22q, which bears a reciprocal translocation from chromosome 9q. This moves the C-*abl* (tyrosine kinase) proto-oncogene from 9 to 22 and fuses it to a gene at the breakpoint cluster region (*bcr*). Production of fusion protein results in a 210-kDa protein in CML (and another, 185 kDa, in ALL). When CML undergoes blastic transformation (see below) further chromosomal abnormalities occur. Cases of CML which are Ph[1]-negative sometimes have a more restricted *abl–bcr* translocation that is not detected cytogenetically.

In AML and AMML there are specific chromosomal abnormalities associated with the different categories (M1–M7) described in Table 28.1. These are outlined in Table 28.5. This represents a very simplified summary of many different abnormalities in a rapidly changing field. In these leukaemias the leukaemic event occurs at the stem-cell level and is followed by defective maturation. In older patients, there seems to be a particular association with cytogenetic abnormalities involving chromosomes 5 and 7. Recent progress has identified the *FLT3* gene as the most frequently mutated gene in cases of acute myelogenous leukaemia. In AML, the myeloid cells of the blood and bone marrow grow uncontrollably, crowding out and destroying normal haemopoietic precursors. In the leukaemic cells of *FLT3*-positive AML, acquisition of the gene promotes relentless growth. About 30–35% of patients have either internal tandem duplications in the juxtamembrane domain, or mutations in the activating loop of FLT3. *FLT3* mutations occur in a broad spectrum of subtypes in adult and paediatric AML, and are particularly common in acute promyelocytic leukaemia (APL). Overall, about 30% of adult AML patients carry the *FLT3* gene, and it is clear that *FLT3* mutations confer an additional risk of extreme leucocytosis, with leucostasis, increased relapse rate and a poor overall prognosis. Other relatively common abnormalities include mutations in the nucleophosmin gene (*NPM*), the CCAAT/enhancer-binding protein α gene (*CEBPA*), the myeloid-lymphoid or mixed lineage leukaemia gene (*MLL*) and the neuroblastoma RAS viral oncogene homologue (*NRAS*). All these genotypic abnormalities are now known to carry prognostic significance, in cytogenetically normal AML (see Schlenk *et al.* in Further reading). In T-cell ALL, breakpoints occur at 14q11, which is the site of the T-cell receptor genes α and β, and 7q33–36 (β T-cell receptor). The translocation t(8;14)(q24;q11) involving oncogenes such as C-*myc*, similar to that found for immunoglobulin genes in Burkitt's lymphoma, may result in disordered cell growth. Another T-cell-specific translocation is t(11;14). Chromosome 9p is frequently deleted or translocated in ALL and is especially associated with lymphomatous clinical features. About 5% of children and 25% of adults with ALL are Ph[1]-positive, associated with a poor prognosis.

In leukaemia some of the gene translocations and deletions described above involve oncogenes, which may thereby be inappropriately activated or mutated leading to disordered growth. Thus, the receptor for colony-stimulating factor (CSF)-1 is the product of the C-*fms* gene and is expressed in acute non-lymphocyte leukaemia. The intracytoplasmic domain has protein tyrosine kinase activity. CD20 (Table 28.4) is a B-cell protein with signal transduction properties. Both of the fusion proteins resulting from the *abl–bcr* translocation in CML and ALL (above) have tyrosine kinase activity and are leukaemogenic in mice. *p53* is frequently mutated in CML and the resultant protein has defective function, being unable to serve as a check to entry into cell cycle. The AML associated translocation t(8;21) blocks the action of a protein complex (CBFB–AML1) that activates several genes. This repression is also achieved by the inv(16) mutation found in AML. Both are associated with a better prognosis. In ALL, the genetic translocations give rise to transcription factors many of which act through the HOX system of transcriptional control. An example is the translocation t(12;21) that creates the TEL–AML1 fusion protein which represses transcription. Some of these genetic changes confer increased susceptibility or resistance to the action of cytotoxic drugs [9].

These examples indicate that the result of the genetic instability is the formation of proteins that alter growth and differentiation in the cell.

Clinical features and management
Acute leukaemia in childhood

The disease usually presents at the age of 4–5 years. The symptoms are due to marrow infiltration causing anaemia, thrombocytopenia, infection and bone pain, especially in long bones. As with other forms of acute leukaemia, the history is of a few weeks of malaise, sometimes with fever even in the absence of obvious infection. Oral and pharyngeal ulceration may occur. Although petechiae are often found on examination, presentation with other haemorrhagic phenomena is less common.

On examination the child is usually pale. There may be lymph node enlargement, splenomegaly and slight hepatic enlargement. The bones may be tender on pressure, particularly over the sternum. Skin petechiae are common (and may also be seen on the palate), as are haemorrhages in the eye, present either in the retina or as larger sub-hyaloid haemorrhages. Skin infiltration with leukaemia is uncommon and takes the form of plaques of tumour of purple colour. In the mouth there may be mucosal ulceration and gingivitis.

Occasionally the patient has symptoms of meningeal involvement at presentation. This usually manifests itself as headache, vomiting and neck stiffness. Papilloedema may be present. Cranial nerve palsies may occur as in other forms of malignant meningitis.

Investigation usually reveals anaemia, thrombocytopenia and an elevated total WBC count with numerous lymphoblasts. In 40% of cases, the total WBC is not elevated but blasts are usually present. 'Aleukaemic leukaemia' is a term used to describe those cases where blasts are not present in the blood film (approximately 5% of cases). In all cases, a bone marrow examination is essential, with cytochemical and immunological studies when possible (as outlined above). A chest radiograph is usually normal, but in T-cell ALL may show a mediastinal mass due to thymic enlargement. This form of ALL is common in adolescent boys. Bone radiographs are not infrequently abnormal and the typical abnormality is of radiolucent bands in the metaphyseal region. Diffuse demineralization also occurs, and discrete osteolytic lesions.

Biochemical investigation may show a raised uric acid due to rapid proliferation and death of leukaemic cells. A lumbar puncture may show leukaemic cells even if there is no clinical evidence of disease in the central nervous system (CNS).

For further details, see the excellent recent review by Mitchell *et al.* (see Further reading).

Treatment
Remission induction and consolidation (Figure 28.3)

There is a significant risk of death in the first few weeks during induction therapy, which can be minimized by supportive measures at, or before, the start of chemotherapy. Anaemia must be corrected. If the kidneys are enlarged or the creatinine raised, the risk of tumour lysis syndrome is greatly increased and steps must be taken to prevent and treat this complication (see Chapter 8, pages 137–139). With more intensive regimens, such as those used for B-cell ALL and AML, platelet support will be necessary. Infections must be detected early and treated vigorously (see also section on supportive measures in adult acute leukaemia). In common ALL, haematological and clinical remission is induced with vincristine, prednisolone and L-asparaginase. Vigorous hydration, allopurinol and urinary alkalinization are necessary in the induction period. With this regimen, over 95% of patients will remit within 3 weeks. Children with B-cell ALL and other bad prognostic features do not do well with this standard therapy and more intensive protocols are needed using cyclophosphamide, cytosine

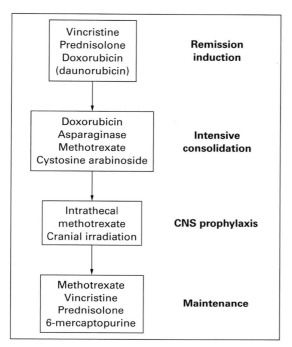

Figure 28.3 Outline of management of acute lymphoblastic leukaemia in childhood.

arabinoside, anthracyclines and methotrexate. This has been investigated in more detail in an extremely important global study of over 44 000 patients with childhood ALL, of whom just over 1000 failed the initial attempt at remission-induction – see Ref. [10]. Children in this small group had several characteristics in common – older age at diagnosis, higher white-cell count, a T-cell phenotype, presence of Philadelphia chromosome, and 11q23 rearrangement. High hyperdiploidy was on the other hand a relatively favourable feature. Ten-year survival was only 32%, much lower than for the total group, but allogeneic transplantation was valuable especially in the T-cell leukaemia group.

In AML, remission is induced with cytosine and daunorubicin. Recent trials are assessing the value of using additional drugs such as thioguanine and etoposide. Myelosuppression is much more severe with these regimens and skilled supportive care is needed.

In ALL, following the induction of complete or partial remission, the treatment is intensified by using drugs such as asparaginase, an anthracycline (daunorubicin or doxorubicin), cytosine arabinoside and cyclophosphamide [11]. Methotrexate in high dose may add to the durability of remission. These drugs are myelosuppressive, but

at this stage the bone marrow has recovered following the elimination of most of the leukaemic population. Intensification for AML has posed great problems in management. The results for intensive conventional chemotherapy have improved at the time when allogeneic transplantation has been introduced, with impressive current results. Many children will not have a donor, which leaves only the alternatives of a matched unrelated donor for patients at high risk of relapse after obtaining remission (such as those with monosomy 7), or autologous BMT (usually given after several cycles of intensive consolidation therapy). Trials of these different approaches are in progress. For very young children (infants under the age of 1 year), a 'hybrid' protocol designed to treat elements of both ALL and AML may be the most effective way forward [12].

Maintenance therapy in childhood acute lymphoblastic leukaemia

The duration of 'maintenance' chemotherapy has not been defined. With more intensive induction and consolidation regimens, it seems probable that prolonged maintenance therapy will be less necessary. 6-Mercaptopurine and methotrexate are the most widely used drugs, often in conjunction with vincristine and prednisolone. In cases with poor prognostic features (Table 28.6), more aggressive regimens have been used as intermittent pulsed therapy. At the end of treatment a testicular biopsy is sometimes performed, if prophylactic irradiation has not been given, in order to detect occult disease. Relapse at any site is unusual beyond a year after treatment has stopped. Thioguanine is not used in maintenance because prolonged use carries a risk of splenomegaly and portal hypertension due to obstruction of liver sinusoids without cirrhosis.

Table 28.6 Adverse prognostic features in childhood ALL.

Adverse cytogenetic markers
CNS disease at presentation
Early marrow relapse
Testicular relapse
T-cell phenotype
Ph[1] chromosome present
Potential new adverse features: still to be evaluated
    Slow initial response
    Persistent minimal residual disease on remission
    Adverse gene expression profiles

Prophylaxis of central nervous system disease

The importance of CNS prophylaxis was demonstrated in the early 1970s. Before that time, infiltration of the meninges by leukaemic cells was responsible for relapse in half of all cases. The lymphoblasts infiltrate the meninges diffusely and extend to the spinal meninges and sheaths of cranial nerves. Clinical presentation is with symptoms of raised intracranial pressure: headache, nausea and vomiting, with a stiff neck and papilloedema. Convulsions may occur and palsies of cranial nerves (particularly VII, VI and III) often develop, and may be the first sign. The diagnosis is made on lumbar puncture when leukaemic blasts are found. The risk of coning from the lumbar puncture is small.

Prophylactic treatment greatly diminishes the frequency of CNS relapse. Nowadays the usual regimen is cranial irradiation (18 Gy in 8–10 fractions over 2 weeks) together with intrathecal methotrexate (10 mg/m^2 × 4 over the same period). However, the long-term consequences of CNS radiation have been of sufficient concern to lead to attempts to dispense with prophylactic irradiation [13; see also Pui *et al.* in Further reading]. The results are not easy to interpret. It seems that for 'standard-risk' ALL (WBC <50 × 10^9/L) intrathecal methotrexate is adequate prophylaxis, but for all the higher-risk cases CNS radiation is necessary. It is not clear if additional drugs (such as cytosine arabinoside) confer additional advantage. Established CNS disease (which now occurs in 5–10% of cases) is treated by intrathecal methotrexate twice weekly with cranial irradiation to a higher dose (often 24 Gy over 2–3 weeks), together with, or followed by, spinal irradiation. However, lasting control of CNS disease is unusual. Intrathecal cytosine arabinoside is also used in patients who are thought to be resistant to methotrexate. Additional measures are generally felt to be necessary for children who fall into the poor-prognosis category [14], with early consideration of treatment intensification and allogeneic BMT during first remission. Very-high-risk ALL in first complete remission has been defined by the presence of at least one of the following criteria: (i) failure to achieve complete remission after the first four-drug induction phase; (ii) cytogenetic t(9;22) or t(4;11) clonal abnormalities; and (iii) poor response to prednisone, associated with a T immunophenotype, or WBC of 100 × 10^9/L or greater, or both.

Treatment and prophylaxis of testicular disease

Relapse in the testis is common and is one reason for the worse prognosis of ALL in boys. Testicular relapse may be less frequent in regimens including high-dose methotrexate. It occurs in about 25% of prepubertal boys but is less common in older children. Relapse may not be clinically apparent at first, swelling and hardness being late signs. It is usually bilateral, and testicular biopsy shows peritubular leukaemic infiltration. Treatment is by testicular irradiation, generally to a dose of the order of 24 Gy in 2–3 weeks. The role of prophylactic testicular irradiation is still undecided.

Treatment on relapse

If children relapse during initial or maintenance treatment or up to 1 year after cessation of therapy, the outlook is poor and BMT is considered (see below). Following later relapses, remission can usually be reinduced by intensive therapy and may be durable. This may not be the case with relapse following more intensive regimens, which would then imply that BMT will need to be considered for this group as well.

Allogeneic BMT has been used in an attempt to improve results in childhood ALL when the prognosis is poor. The procedure does not have a proven survival advantage over chemotherapy on relapse in standard-risk ALL. The following clinical situations have been regarded as indications for consideration of allogeneic BMT in childhood ALL: second or third remission, especially if relapse occurred while on maintenance therapy; and poor-prognosis cases such as those with t(4;11) acute undifferentiated leukaemia, t(8;14) B-cell ALL, and Ph^1-positive ALL. These children may benefit from BMT in first remission.

Results of BMT in first remission in high-risk cases have been promising [14], with 60% 3-year relapse-free survival. In standard-risk cases in second remission, 65% 5-year relapse-free survival is reported. The results depend greatly on the factors used to select patients. Autologous BMT or stem-cell transplantation has generally been rather less impressive than allogeneic transplantation, possibly because of marrow contamination but also because some high-dose regimens have not included total-body irradiation (TBI). Newer treatment regimens of combined chemotherapy and TBI may improve results of autologous BMT [15]. Allogeneic BMT has a greater mortality than autologous transplantation, partly because of graft-versus-host disease. Conversely, the graft-versus-leukaemia effect may improve overall results. Some of the problems and adverse consequences associated with BMT are discussed further in Chapter 8.

If relapse occurs in the CNS despite prophylaxis, a further remission may be obtained with more intrathecal methotrexate or craniospinal irradiation. Methotrexate can also be given through an Ommaya or Rickham reservoir, which allows direct delivery of the drug into the cerebral ventricular system. Systemic relapse is inevitable, and further systemic treatment is usually given.

A relapse of ALL is a very serious event. With conventional reinduction chemotherapy only 20% of children will be alive at 2 years. For this reason attempts have been made to intensify the remission induction treatment after first relapse, using allogeneic or autologous BMT. It seems possible that about one-third of children with relapsed AML may be curable by this means.

Prognosis

Overall, about 80% of children with ALL are cured with modern treatment, a truly remarkable achievement over the past 40 years with estimates "that contemporary treatment may further increase the cure rate to near 90%" – see Refs. [16] and [17]. The important prognostic features are given in Table 28.6. Survival is better in girls than in boys and is shown in Figure 28.4. Since so many children are now surviving as long-term cured patients, the late effects of treatment are a major and indeed increasing concern. In brief, they include a potential for multiple organ damage such as neuropathy, cardiomyopathy, hypothyroidism, subfertility and of course, significant psychological damage – these points are dealt with more fully in Chapter 24. The relatively common neurological sequelae of CNS and spinal irradiation have led to a reduction in dosage and even usage in low-risk cases. The late onset of brain tumours induced by CNS irradiation appears to be more frequent in children who carry a polymorphism for the mercaptopurine detoxifying enzyme (thiopurine methyltransferase) that also makes them more liable to acute toxicity and for development of secondary AML [9]. These concerns

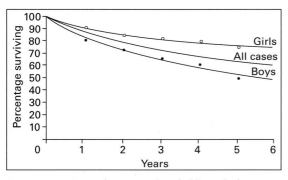

Figure 28.4 Survival in acute lymphoblastic leukaemia in children.

have led to the introduction of more sophisticated and risk-adapted strategies of treatment that take into account the known prognostic factors, to which are added the rapidity of response and the much-improved detection of minimal residual disease. The use of microarray technology may allow further refinement of treatment decisions [18]. Important issues relating to support of these patients in the community, both during and also after treatment completion, have recently been well reviewed by Grigoropoulos *et al.* [19].

Acute lymphoblastic leukaemia in adults

The clinical features are similar to those in children except for the greater percentage of patients with a mediastinal mass. Above the age of 12 years, ALL has a significantly worse prognosis. More cases (20%) are Ph[1]-positive and at least some cases represent CGL presenting in the acute phase. Only 30% are common ALL, 12% are B-cell ALL, 8% T-cell ALL and 30% of cases are unclassifiable (null cell ALL). Although the long-term prognosis appears to be as poor as in adult AML, adult ALL is usually regarded separately because CNS relapse is common.

The treatment of adult ALL is similar to the childhood disease with the following general modifications.

1 Induction treatment is more intense, with regimens that include vincristine, prenisolone, anthracyclines and asparaginase.

2 More intensive 'consolidation' therapy with regimens that include cytosine arabinoside and anthracyclines, high dose methotrexate and teniposide.

3 Testicular relapse is less frequent and prophylactic treatment is not given.

Currently, intensive induction regimens in unselected cases produce complete remission in 80% of cases, with about 40% remaining in remission at 3 years [20]. Poor prognostic factors include age over 60, WBC above 30×10^9/L, late achievement of complete response, Ph[1]-positivity, mature or precursor B-cell phenotype, and abnormal cytogenetics. Prophylaxis of the CNS may in future be avoided for some patients, since the high risk of CNS relapse is mostly confined to patients with B-cell ALL, elevated lactate dehydrogenase or alkaline phosphatase, and a high proliferative fraction [18]. Treatment strategies adapted to the *prognostic category* have increasingly been recommended [21], for example, very intensive induction regimens for patients with mature B-cell ALL, including high-dose chemotherapy with peripheral blood stem-cell transplantation during first remission. Current studies are addressing the importance of minimal residual disease, since assessments using more sensitive genetic technology have shown that the amount of residual leukaemia, in patients whose leukaemia appears to be in remission, varies considerably. There are a variety of such techniques to determine whether very small burdens of leukaemia cells are present in individual patients.

Allogeneic BMT is the preferred treatment in first remission in the high-risk groups defined above. Some centres would consider all first-remission ALL over the age of 21 as an indication for BMT on the grounds that the prognosis is worse in adults than in children. Ph[1]-positive leukaemias show a high rate of remission in first relapse with the use of the signal transduction tyrosine kinase inhibitor imatinib mesylate (ST 1571 - see pages 579–580).

Following second remission the results of allogeneic BMT are clearly superior since survival rates of 30–40% are obtained. Results with autologous BMT are also clearly superior to chemotherapy alone in second relapse, but not proven to be so in first relapse. However, peripheral blood stem-cell-supported transplant may prove to be the preferred treatment in this situation. Molecular techniques for the detection of minimal residual disease can certainly identify patients at high risk of relapse. These methods have led to the assessment of intensification of treatment in patients where residual disease can be detected.

Acute myeloid leukaemia in adults

Although a rare disorder, with about 10 000–12 000 new cases diagnosed annually in the whole of the USA, AML is the most common type of myeloid leukaemia, with a prevalence of 3.8 per 100 000, rising to almost 18 per 100 000 in adults over the age of 65 years. About 2000 new cases occur in the UK each year, with a median age at presentation of 67 years. It accounts for about 1.5% of all deaths from malignant disease. Risk factors include exposure to ionizing radiation, benzene and previous cytotoxic chemotherapy, as well as survival of nuclear bombing (Hiroshima and Nagasaki). A possible occupational risk has been noted in male members of airline crews who have flown for more than 500 000 hours. Since very few people exposed to these various environmental causes develop AML, a possible explanation might be genetic variation in enzymes that detoxify carcinogens such as benzene or cytotoxic drugs [22].

In most cases the history and physical findings are similar to those in ALL (see above). Bone pain and radiological evidence of bone infiltration are less common in AML, and CNS disease is very unusual at presentation. Lymph node enlargement is also less frequently found than in ALL.

In myelomonocytic (M4, Table 28.1) and monocytic (M5) leukaemia, gum infiltration is common, leading to gum 'hypertrophy'. Skin infiltrates are common in these forms and associated features are a high total WBC and high serum and urinary lysozyme, which are liberated from the tumour.

Pallor, hepatosplenomegaly, purpura and bone tenderness are the most common physical signs. The WBC is often elevated, with myeloblasts usually demonstrable. Confirmation of the diagnosis is made by bone marrow examination and the use of special stains when appropriate (Table 28.3).

Treatment
Remission induction

The aim is to induce a complete marrow and clinical remission. To do this, intensive therapy is normally needed with blood, platelet and antibiotic support during the period of hypoplasia, which is the inevitable accompaniment of the chemotherapy (see Chapter 8). At present, all the subtypes except M3 are usually given induction chemotherapy with combinations of high-dose cytosine arabinoside and daunorubicin (Figure 28.5). Induction chemotherapy usually requires hospitalization of several weeks to receive the chemotherapy and recover from its side-effects. Idarubicin and mitoxantrone, although increasingly widely used, are probably not

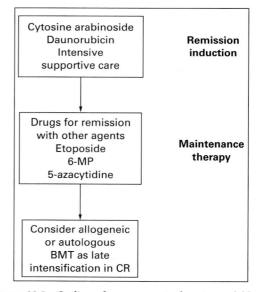

Figure 28.5 Outline of management of acute myeloblastic leukaemia. BMT, bone marrow transplantation; CR, complete response; 6-MP, 6-mercaptopurine.

substantially more effective than the now-classic anthra-cycline daunorubicin. Addition of a third drug such as etoposide, fludarabine or thioguanine does not seem to improve results. The blast count usually falls rapidly in the blood and bone marrow with suppression of normal haematopoiesis. The mortality of this stage is now about 10% when skilled support is available. During the hypoplastic period further cytotoxic therapy is often needed if the marrow still shows disease, and this intensifies the hypoplasia and increases the risk.

For the M3 form of AML (promyelocytic leukaemia), the use of all-*trans*-retinoic acid (ATRA) has been a major step forward, in addition to standard induction chemotherapy (see below). Great care must be taken to prevent disseminated intravascular coagulation complicating the treatment of M3 leukaemia, when the promyelocytes release the contents of their granules into the peripheral circulation. As pointed out by Chen and Chen [23], this type of leukemia is characterized by a life-threatening bleeding syndrome. It is, however, often now frequently curable with current treatment protocols using idarubicin and ATRA – see Ref. [24], for an excellent account of this dramatic progress in a previously lethal condition. The induction of remission is a highly skilled procedure, best carried out in dedicated leukaemia units where the nursing and medical staff are experienced in the problems of bone marrow failure. For patients with low-to-intermediate-risk APL (i.e. those with a total white-cell count at diagnosis of less than 10×10^9/L), treatment with ATRA plus arsenic trioxide (ATI) may be a more effective and safer alternative – see Ref. [25]. ATI is active even as a single agent, through specific binding of the promyelocytic leukemia protein (PML) moiety of the disease-specific PML-retinoic acid receptor alpha oncoprotein; synergy between ATI and ATRA has been repeatedly demonstrated. During treatment, scrupulous attention to fluid and electrolyte problems is essential, as is prompt diagnosis and treatment of infection (see Chapter 8). Prophylactic treatment of the CNS is not usually given.

Supportive care

Blood product support is essential during the intensive phase of remission induction. As discussed in Chapter 8, platelet transfusion has been a major advance in prevention of death from haemorrhage. The indications for platelet transfusion are discussed on pages 131–132.

Blood transfusions are essential for anaemia but should be avoided if possible if the WBC is very high ($>100 \times 10^9$/L) because leucostasis in cerebral vessels may occur. Chemotherapy and, if necessary, leucopheresis should be used to reduce the WBC before transfusion. The use of haemopoietic growth factors is described in Chapter 8. During intensive treatment an indwelling subcutaneously tunnelled intravenous line (Hickman line) is of great help.

To prevent infection patients should be instructed to wash carefully, with particular attention to the perineal region. Dental and oral sepsis should be treated promptly. Food should be cooked and clean – fresh salads are best avoided. Regular examination of the mouth, skin and perineum are essential and cultures should be taken regularly to detect pathogens such as *Klebsiella* or *Pseudomonas*. Co-trimoxazole is given prophylactically in some units, and it gives protection against the opportunistic pathogen *Pneumocystis carinii*.

Most patients will develop fever at some stage during the period of neutropenia. The management of infection in the neutropenic patient is discussed in Chapter 8. Often no bacteriological diagnosis is made. Most fatal infections are from Gram-negative organisms. Infections occur around Hickman lines, particularly with skin commensals such as *Staphylococcus epidermidis* or *Staphylococcus aureus*. Vancomycin and teicoplanin are very useful antibiotics for treatment of this complication; meropenem and/or piperacillin (Tazocin) are also often employed. See also Chapter 8 for further details of treatment of these common problems.

Opportunistic infections cause considerable diagnostic difficulty in a patient with fever and pulmonary infiltration (see Chapter 8). Fungal infection, *Pneumocystis carinii* and, less commonly, cytomegalovirus and other viral infections must be considered.

After blood cultures have been taken at the onset of fever, broad-spectrum intravenous antibiotic therapy is begun. Such regimens usually include an aminoglycoside and a cephalosporin, and metronidazole is often added, particularly if there is clinical deterioration after 24 hours. If there are pulmonary infiltrates, treatment with high-dose co-trimoxazole for *Pneumocystis*, amphotericin B for fungal infection and aciclovir for herpes simplex should be considered.

Results of treatment and new approaches [22,26–28]

Complete remission occurs in 65% of patients below the age of 60 and in 50% above that age. The development of new approaches to remission induction in poor-risk cases is, therefore, an important area of further investigation, particularly since most patients will relapse even after an apparently successful induction chemotherapy programme. More therapy will therefore be needed to eliminate non-detectable disease and achieve a cure.

The specific type of post-remission therapy will be individualized, based both on the patient's prognostic factors (see above) and general health. For good-prognosis leukaemias, namely those with inv(16), t(8;21) and t(15;17), patients will typically undergo an additional three to five courses of intensive chemotherapy, whereas for those at high risk of relapse (e.g. those with high-risk cytogenetics, underlying MDS, or therapy-related AML), allogeneic BMT is usually recommended if the patient is judged able to tolerate this procedure, and has a suitable donor. The most suitable post-remission therapy for intermediate-risk AML (i.e. with normal cytogenetics or cytogenetic changes falling between the good-risk and high-risk groups) is less clear-cut, and depends on the age and overall health of the patient, the patient's views and priorities, and whether a suitable stem-cell donor is available. New approaches include the use of the anti-CD33 monoclonal antibody gemtuzumab ozogamicin, which improved survival in the recent UK-based AML 15 trial, at least for patients with certain characteristics, generally low-risk, when given as part of the induction chemotherapy regimen – see Ref. [29]. More intensive maintenance or consolidation regimens are of course more difficult to implement in the elderly. A worse outcome is to be expected in patients over 60 years, those with a high WBC and poor performance status, and those who have developed AML after a myelodysplastic t(9;11) syndrome. Cytogenetic changes are also prognostically important: t(q;11), 5q– and inv(3) are adverse and t(8;21) is favourable (Table 28.5). Overall, 10-year disease-free survival is about 30%. Broadly speaking, prognostic factors (such as the patient's performance status, age, and various biochemical features such as albumin, bilirubin and creatinine) can be divided into those associated with treatment-related death prior to response and those associated with resistance to treatment at a later stage [26]. In addition, it is known that treatment-related AML, or AML arising after MDS, is usually more resistant to standard treatment than AML arising *de novo*. Younger patients can clearly tolerate more intensive regimens, with high-dose cytarabine as standard post-remission therapy for certain prognostic groups, such as those related to the karyotypic features t(8;21) or inv(16) regarded as favourable. Many patients with an intermediate prognosis have a normal chromosomal pattern, whereas more adverse cases often have a more complex karyotypic abnormality. In cases such as these, novel investigational agents are currently being assessed,

particularly in patients with a good performance status and no evidence of current infection.

Although the results of intensive conventional chemotherapy in AML have improved, the long-term outlook is still poor for most patients. Approaches using BMT (especially allogeneic) are not appropriate for many patients as AML is mainly a disease of the elderly. Allogeneic BMT is usually carried out in first complete response and, in historical comparisons with conventional treatment, seems to reduce leukaemic relapse by 20% – see Ref. [30] for an excellent recent review. Some of this benefit appears to be due to the graft-versus-leukaemia effect, which may contribute to long-term disease-free survival in about 50% of patients [27]. Against this must be set the acute mortality especially from allogeneic BMT, which is still considerable. Autologous BMT has been shown to reduce the risk of relapse [28]. The procedure is more widely applicable than allogeneic BMT, since matched donors are not needed. In allogeneic BMT, high-dose cyclophosphamide and TBI are usually used. Complications are of course severe, including prolonged neutropenia, graft-versus-host disease and oromucositis. This last complication, often distressing and painful, may require prolonged opiate treatment. One recent study has suggested that use of the recombinant keratinocyte growth factor (KGF) receptor-binding agent palifermin may help to alleviate this troublesome complication [31]. Using this agent, the frequency of severe mucositis (WHO grade III) was reduced from 98% to 68%, with a consequent reduction in morphine requirement. With autologous BMT, regimens are generally based on chemotherapy alone [32]. Haemopoietic growth factors appear to allow increased treatment intensity without stimulating leukaemic proliferation.

For elderly patients, the majority of cases, there are additional problems of comorbidity that do not permit intensive approaches. Nevertheless, many studies have excluded patients over the age of 60 without good reason and a more refined approach to fitness is needed. Lower-intensity autologous or allogeneic transplantation are possible approaches to improving results.

Treatment of relapse

Although induction of a second remission is possible in patients who have relapsed after treatment has been discontinued, these remissions are usually short-lived. For patients below 60 years, a second remission can sometimes be obtained using high-dose cytosine arabinoside. For young adults and those with favourable prognostic indicators, there is a chance of cure by allogeneic or autologous BMT, usually preceded by reinduction chemotherapy. The studies comparing allogeneic and autologous transplantation cannot be randomized except by whether a donor is available or not as a surrogate 'genetic' randomization. For this reason, and the technical and clinical difficulties, it is not clear if either method offers a better outcome. CNS relapse is treated in a similar fashion to ALL (see above). Temporary responses may also be seen with infusion of T lymphocytes from the original donor, following relapse after stem-cell allogeneic transplant.

Treatment of acute promyelocytic leukaemia (M3)

APL accounts for 10% of AML. Induction of remission is complicated by disseminated intravascular coagulation when cytotoxic chemotherapy is given. This seems to be due to release of a procoagulant (cysteine proteinase). The cells differentiate *in vitro* in response to ATRA. When patients with APL are treated with ATRA, the bone marrow slowly (over 2 months) returns to normal, with loss of the typical t(15;17) karyotype, and disseminated intravascular coagulation does not occur [33]. Side-effects include dry skin, headache and potentially fatal hyperleucocytosis (which may cause pulmonary oedema). The combination of idarubicin and ATRA has improved the cure rate in this type of leukaemia to about 80%, with much reduced toxicity compared to older regimens. The breakpoint t(15;17) is near the gene for the retinoic acid α receptor on chromosome 17, and the use of ATRA is only successful when this translocation is present.

Myelodysplastic syndromes and secondary leukaemia

MDS and secondary leukaemia include a range of disorders, usually of unknown aetiology, characterized by one or more peripheral cytopenias, with a cellular marrow showing morphological evidence of disordered haematopoiesis. This may include ring sideroblasts, hypogranular polymorphs with abnormally segmented nuclei, and increased numbers of early myeloid cells. MDS has an inherent tendency to progress to acute leukaemia.

MDS is classified according to the major abnormality present, but there is often more than one abnormality and precise categorization may be difficult and arbitrary. When ring sideroblasts are the prominent abnormality a diagnosis of sideroblastic anaemia is usually made, and when blast cells are present in modest numbers the disease is labelled as refractory anaemia with an excess of blasts. This has a particular propensity to develop into acute leukaemia. Increasing numbers of patients with ALL secondary to MDS are now being seen. Some are the late effects of chemotherapy for a previous cancer. These leukaemias are characteristically difficult to treat. In younger patients, remission may be obtained with cytosine arabinoside and doxorubicin in 60% of cases, but the relapse rate is high and the toxicity of treatment is considerable. The role of allogeneic BMT is not yet fully evaluated.

The chronic leukaemias

There are two main forms of chronic leukaemia: chronic lymphocytic (lymphatic) leukaemia (CLL) and chronic myeloid leukaemia (CML, also often termed chronic granulomatous leukaemia, CGL). The former is exceptionally rare below 40 years, while the latter can occur at any age, although it is commoner in middle and old age.

Chronic lymphocytic leukaemia

CLL is nearly always a chronic neoplastic proliferation of small B lymphocytes, resulting in the accumulation of mature B lymphocytes. These B cells are probably early in the B-cell differentiation pathway [34]. In recent years it has been recognized that diagnosis by conventional criteria should always be complemented by immunophenotyping, using cellular markers such as CD5, CD23, CD79b and FMC7. In fact, the last decade or so has seen a profound alteration in our understanding of this disorder, now viewed as a remarkably diverse group of haematological malignancies, largely as a result of differences in the mutation levels of the V genes and expression of CD38 and ZAP-70. When cases of CLL are categorized on the basis of these cytogenetic differences, widely different clinical behaviour is observed. This allows differentiation into two main groups, the first including patients with a greater than 2% level of mutated rearranged V_H genes ('mutated' CLL) and in the second, patients with few or no mutated V genes. Gene expression profiles show that unmutated CLL cells express more ZAP-70 mRNA than mutated cells, and the increasing use of testing for ZAP-70 is now providing a far better indicator than previously possible for prognostic advice in the individual case. In consequence, both the molecular genetic markers and the patient's clinical state can be used to offer a risk-adapted approach to management (see below). Important recent work from the Harvard group and others have more clearly defined the landscape of somatic mutations in CLL, unexpectedly highlighting pre-RNA splicing as a critical cellular process contributing to the development of this disease – see Ref. [35]. Using the technique of massive parallel sequencing of cancer genomes in 91 patients with CLL, nine novel genes were identified, each mutated at significant frequencies, including five with previously unestablished roles. The most important of these, SF3B1, was mutated primarily in tumours with deletion of chromosome 11q, known to be associated with a poor prognosis.

In many cases, the immunoglobulin classes IgM and IgD are present in small amounts on the cell membrane, but no cytoplasmic immunoglobulin can be detected. Free light chains can be found in the urine in many patients. Since the tumour is a clonal proliferation, each cell bears the same immunoglobulin molecule with the same type of light chain. The phenotype of the B cell is similar to B cells of the mantle zone of lymph nodes. Chromosomal abnormalities (see Table 28.5) include trisomy 12, for which five different probes are currently in widespread use employing fluorescence *in situ* hybridization (FISH) analysis, and deletion of 13q14 (the retinoblastoma gene). Additional studies can also be valuable for confirmation [36], including demonstration of deletions at 6q21, 11q23 and 17p13 (the *p53* locus). These cytogenetic abnormalities are adverse prognostically. The *bcl*-2 gene is overexpressed, resulting in inhibition of apoptosis. These features are well discussed by Chiorazzi and colleagues (see Further reading) and our current understanding of the true nature of CLL is informed by these recent studies.

Clinical features

CLL is the commonest form of leukaemia in adults, about twice as common in men and women, with an incidence of 4.2 per 100 000 population. About three-quarters of new cases are diagnosed in patients over the age of 50 years and the peak age at diagnosis is 71.

Over 25% of patients have no symptoms at the time of diagnosis. The disease is discovered because of lymphocytosis noted on an incidental blood count or because enlargement of lymph nodes or spleen is detected on physical examination. In other patients, the symptoms are due to noticeably enlarged lymph nodes in the neck or elsewhere, fatigue and malaise due to mild anaemia, infection due to immunosuppression, pain from an enlarged spleen or bruising and bleeding due to thrombocytopenia.

Physical examination reveals painless enlarged lymph nodes that are rubbery and mobile. Many node groups are affected (unlike most lymphomas) and the spleen is often palpable. Massive splenomegaly is unusual at presentation and splenic infarction is less frequent than in CGL.

The diagnosis is made on the blood count. This shows a raised total WBC which may even be as high as $500-1000 \times 10^9$/L but is more usually below 100×10^9/L. The diagnosis must be considered when the lymphocyte count is above 10×10^9/L. The differential count shows a great excess of small lymphocytes, which usually have a normal morphology but which are sometimes larger with less mature-looking nuclei. Cleaved nuclei suggest the diagnosis of follicular-centre cell lymphoma rather than CLL (see Chapter 26). Prolymphocytic leukaemia cells (see page 576) are larger with more cytoplasm and a distinct prominent nucleolus. Hairy cell leukaemia (HCL) (see page 576) is usually distinguishable on morphological grounds. Occasionally, it may be necessary to undertake a lymph node biopsy. In CLL, this shows diffuse infiltration with small well-differentiated lymphocytes. A marrow aspiration and biopsy shows a marked diffuse increase in small well-differentiated lymphocytes in CLL. A blood film is all that is necessary for diagnosis in the great majority of cases.

Occasionally, the lymphocytosis is slight and it is then not clear if the patient has a reactive lymphocytosis or CLL. This problem can now often be solved by examining the cell surface for light chain restriction, and the presence of CD5. In CLL, all the cells are identical and are restricted to one light-chain type (κ or λ), while both light-chain types are represented in a reactive lymphocytosis.

Anaemia is variable and, when present, indicates extensive marrow infiltration. Autoimmune haemolytic anaemia sometimes occurs. The platelet count may be low as a result of marrow infiltration, hypersplenism, chemotherapy and, occasionally, autoimmune thrombocytopenia. There is suppression of immunoglobulin synthesis in many patients, with marked hypogammaglobulinaemia which leads to increased susceptibility to infection.

Staging

It may seem contradictory to stage a leukaemia (see Chapter 4). However, it has been shown that a simple staging classification, based on clinical findings and blood count, has prognostic value. This staging notation is shown in Table 28.7. The worse prognostic categories (III–IV) have greater degrees of marrow failure at presentation.

Table 28.7 Staging of CLL.

Stage		Definition	Median survival (months)
0	A	No enlarged nodes or spleen, Hb >11 g/dL, platelets >100 × 10^9/L, lymphocytes <15 × 10^9/L	150
I	B	As stage 0 with enlarged nodes	100
II		As stage 0 with enlargement of spleen or liver	70
III	C	As 0, I or II; Hb <11 g/dL	20
IV		As 0, II, or III; platelets <100 × 10^9/L	20

The staging notation 0–IV was introduced by Rai *et al.* in 1975, and A–C by Binet *et al.* in 1981. The International Workshop on CLL has recommended integrating these two staging systems.

Treatment

There is no cure for CLL. Taking all cases together, treatment [36,37] undoubtedly produces symptomatic benefit and may prolong survival, though patients with early-stage (Stage A) disease have no immediate benefit from chemotherapy, which of course may lead to unwanted and hazardous side-effects. It is often better to "watch and wait" – see Ref. [19] for a good discussion of this point. Stage A patients have a survival expectancy similar to the normal age-matched population, and an overall survival above ten years from diagnosis. Clear indications for treatment include troublesome symptoms of fatigue, night sweats and fever, greatly enlarged nodes especially if causing pressure, splenic discomfort and marrow failure causing anaemia and thrombocytopenia. Most patients requiring treatment will have stage II–IV disease. As mentioned above, both the molecular markers and also the patient's clinical status are now employed to make an intelligent decision about treatment or surveillance. Previously, factors such as clinical stage, pattern and degree of lymphocyte infiltration, and lymphocyte doubling time would be regarded as sufficient; the current approach would still of course include all these important prognostic features but also add the mutational status of the imunoglobulin V_H genes, expression of ZAP-70 and CD38, and FISH cytogenetics. Often but not always there will be close concordance with the clinical state, but careful clinical monitoring in such cases is usually the key to a successful treatment strategy. Since, ultimately, CLL must still be regarded as an incurable disease, close

attention to the patient's quality of life is of fundamental importance, bearing in mind the toxicities of some of the agents now commonly used.

Drug treatment

Alkylating agents (especially chlorambucil) were previously the mainstay of treatment. Chlorambucil is given intermittently, 2 weeks on, 2 weeks off, at a dose of about 0.1–0.2 mg/kg. An alternative is to give 2.5 mg/kg over 2–4 days each month. The treatment is continued until the symptoms and signs of the disease have regressed to a considerable extent, and then discontinued. A prolonged period of stable disease may then follow before progression, which will then require further treatment. Repeated chemotherapy will ultimately contribute to bone marrow failure. Trials have shown no benefit for treatment with cyclophosphamide, vinblastine and prednisolone (CVP) or the combination of cyclophosphamide, doxorubicin, vincristine and prednisolone (CHOP) compared with chlorambucil. Steroids (usually prednisolone) are useful in patients developing marrow failure (anaemia, thrombocytopenia) since they do not suppress haemopoiesis. In a patient with anaemia, prednisolone 30–40 mg can be given daily by mouth for 2–3 weeks followed by an alkylating agent.

Some newer agents have been found to be very effective. Fludarabine, a nucleoside analogue, produces responses in 60% of patients with 40% complete responses [36]. This agent has a unique method of action, affecting both DNA and RNA synthesis, including DNA repair. In terms of response, this is a superior agent to chlorambucil, although using fludarabine early does not appear to improve overall survival [37] and some clinicians still prefer to use the traditional agent first, reserving fludarabine for a later stage. Nonetheless, the authors of this important trial call for the use of fludarabine with cyclophosphamide to become the new treatment of choice, emphasizing the importance of improved response rates and time to progression. These agents are now widely used as initial treatment, even though fludarabine may add to the immunosuppression that is already present. Many authorities are increasingly moving towards a regimen of fludarabine and rituximab (more fully described in Chapter 27) as front-line therapy, and bendamustine has also emerged as an extremely important agent in CLL, also superior to chlorambucil and now widely used – see Ref. [38]. In one large recent study cited by NICE comparing bendamustine to chlorambucil in over 300 patients in whom fludarabine-based therapy was judged as inappropriate, the overall response rates were dramatic: 68% versus 31%, respectively, including a very much higher complete clinical response rate. Progression-free survival was 21.6 versus 8.3 months (Stages B and C patients were included in this study). See also Ref. [39] – a landmark study. As they pointed out 'Bendamustine should be considered as a preferred first-line option over chlorambucil for CLL patients ineligible for fludarabine, cyclophosphamide and rituximab'.

2-Chlorodeoxyadenosine also produces responses (but is myelosuppressive), and so does the purine antimetabolite pentostatin (deoxycoformycin), an inhibitor of the enzyme adenosine deaminase, which is frequently used for HCL as well (see below). Further exploration of the use of these drugs, alone and in combination, is in progress. The monoclonal antibody alemtuzumab (directed against CD52) has been used for refractory disease. Exploration of the use of autologous and allogeneic BMT has also begun, in younger patients in whom complete remission has been obtained.

Radiotherapy

Splenic irradiation is sometimes used palliatively for painful splenomegaly, often to a dose of 10 Gy in six to eight fractions over 2 weeks. The lymphocyte count falls and the spleen shrinks. Peripheral nodes may diminish in size. Myelosuppression can be troublesome particularly if the spleen (and, therefore, the treatment field) is very large. Splenectomy is then preferable if the patient is fit enough. If there are painful enlarged lymph nodes, these can also be treated effectively by irradiation.

Treatment of infection

The hypogammaglobulinaemia renders patients highly susceptible to bacterial infection. Febrile illnesses such as upper respiratory infections should be treated promptly with antibiotics and patients warned of their susceptibility. Immunoglobulin is sometimes given prophylactically to patients who have recurrent infections. Penicillin is usually given prophylactically to patients who have been splenectomized or who have had an episode of pneumococcal infection.

Prognosis

In this elderly population, death frequently occurs from other causes. Infection contributes to mortality, and as the disease progresses marrow failure develops, increasing the likelihood of infection and bleeding. Survival is closely related to the initial stage of disease (Table 28.7).

Second cancers are possibly more common in CLL than in the general population. A small proportion of patients die from an aggressive malignant transformation with fever, weight loss and rapidly increasing tumour containing large undifferentiated cells. This disorder, Richter's syndrome, is unusual.

Prolymphocytic leukaemia

This uncommon disease occurs in the elderly. The presentation is like CLL but without much lymph node enlargement and with marked splenomegaly. The WBC is high ($>100 \times 10^9$/L). The white cells are larger than CLL cells, with more cytoplasm and a single prominent nucleolus. The cells are B cells with bright staining for surface immunoglobulin, although occasional T-cell variants have been described.

Treatment is with chemotherapy and splenic irradiation. Combination chemotherapy is usually used, with regimens similar to those used in high-grade non-Hodgkin's lymphoma (see Chapter 26).

Hairy cell leukaemia [40]

HCL occurs more commonly in men (male to female ratio 4:1), mostly diagnosed around the ages of 50–70, and is characterized by anaemia, thrombocytopenia and neutropenia, together with splenomegaly and the presence of cells in the blood that have unusual cytoplasmic villi, the so-called hairy cells. In a minority of cases, the white cell count is elevated, not suppressed. B-cell markers (surface immunoglobulin) are usually present, and the current view is that the cell is an activated clonal B lymphocyte. Diagnosis is assisted by the presence on immunostaining of antiannexin A1 antibody, which is highly specific for hairy-cell leukaemia. Increase in the probability of BRAF V600E mutation has also been reported, and there is also coexpresssion of CD11c, CD25 and CD103 antigens though these are less specific. The cells contain cytoplasmic tartrate-resistant acid phosphatase, and are usually morphologically distinct to the experienced observer. Sometimes also known as 'histiocytic leukaemia', it is one of the rarest B-cell neoplasms, with fewer than 2000 cases diagnosed annually, in the whole of the USA and western Europe combined. Apart from the 'classic' HCL, there are two additional major variants, one of which, HCL-V (the V stands simply for 'variant'), is most probably a prolymphocytic type of leukaemia, usually diagnosed in males over the age of 70 years, and more aggressive and more resistant to treatment than classic HCL. The other variant, the Japanese type, is generally easier to treat.

The symptoms are usually those of bone marrow failure, partly due to physical crowding out of the marrow space by disordered and disrupted hairy cells. Persistent fatigue is common. There is little enlargement of lymph nodes and constitutional symptoms (fever, night sweats) are very unusual unless there is an intercurrent infection due to the neutropenia. Pyrexia may be caused by intercurrent mycobacterial infection, again related to the characteristic neutropenia.

Interferon is an effective form of medication, and both recombinant interferon alfa-2a and interferon alfa-2b have been used. Recommended schedules have varied in frequency (daily or twice weekly), duration (6–18 months) and dose. The complete response rate is about 8% and the partial response rate 75%. When selected as the appropriate treatment, it should generally be given for about 1 year. However, interferon can be difficult to tolerate, and over the past few years chemotherapy with either deoxycoformycin (pentostatin) or 2-chlorodeoxyadenosine (leustatin) has increasingly been preferred. Deoxycoformycin was initially isolated from the bacterium *Streptomyces antibioticus* and is technically a natural product. It is well tolerated, generally administered as an infusion every 2 weeks, and has myelosuppression as its main side-effect. The complete response rate is about 70%, with a further 25% showing a useful partial response, often durable for several years. In the large study from the Royal Marsden Hospital [40], the overall response to pentostatin was 96%, with complete responses in 81%, and a median disease-free survival of 15 years. Response to first-line 2-chlorodeoxyadenosine was 100%, with a complete response in 82% and disease-free survival of 11 years or more. The relapse rates at 5 years and 10 years were 24% and 42%, respectively, with pentostatin, and 33% and 48% with 2-chlorodeoxyadenosine. Survival at 10 years was respectively 96% and 100%. These agents can be given with interferon, but it is not clear if this improves results. Myelosuppression and fever are the main toxicities. The advent of these drugs has led to a reappraisal of the role of splenectomy, which was traditionally offered before the advent of effective chemotherapy but is now mainly performed in cases where there is no bone marrow infiltration. The 5-year survival is now over 80% but the prognosis is worse in patients with either massive splenomegaly or abdominal lymphadenopathy.

Large granular lymphocytic (T-cell) leukaemia

One of the rare neoplasms of peripheral (post-thymic) T cells, this accounts for just 2% of all CLL but in other respects, especially in clinical behaviour and treatment, resembles it. Morphologically, the cells are larger and more granular than B-cell CLL. Splenomegaly is commoner and lymph node enlargement is unusual. The cells are CD8 (suppressor) and CD3. There is often neutropenia and hypergammaglobulinaemia. About 30% of patients have co-existing rheumatoid arthritis. The aetiology of T-cell LGL leukemia has not been fully elucidated, but chronic antigenic stimulation with exogenous antigens such as human T-cell lymphotrophic virus (HTLV) or endogenous auto antigens may be responsible for inducing the activation and clonal expansion of effector CD8+ LGLs. The diagnosis of T-cell LGL leukemia is based on the presence of an LGL lymphocytosis, characteristic immunophenotype, and confirmation of clonality using TCRβ and γ gene rearrangement studies. Characteristically, LGLs are medium-to-large cells containing abundant cytoplasm, coarse azurophilic granules, and eccentric nuclei. T-cell LGL leukemic cells typically co-express CD3+CD8+CD57+ markers. Treatment is as for B-cell CLL.

Chronic myeloid (myelogenous) leukaemia

Chronic myeloid leukaemia is, in the majority of patients, associated with a specific acquired chromosomal defect [41,42]. It occurs with a frequency of about 1.6 per 100 000 adults, with about 5000 new cases annually in the USA. The male-to-female ratio is approximately 1.4:1, with a median age at diagnosis of 55 years. After a period of slow progression, the disease transforms into a more malignant variety of leukaemia. It occurs in 1.5 per 100 000 individuals per year. Most importantly, CML was the first malignancy to be linked with a clear genetic abnormality, the Philadelphia chromosome (named after its discovery in 1960 by Nowell and Hungerford in Philadelphia). The chromosomal abnormality (described above) involves a translocation that moves the *C-abl* proto-oncogene from chromosome 9 to 22, producing a *bcr–abl* fusion gene product, a tyrosine kinase. The full notation of the Philadelphia chromosome is t(9;22)(q34;q11). The fused Bcr–Abl protein apparently interacts with the interleukin (IL)-3βc receptor subunit and a casade of proteins that control the cell cycle and, therefore, cellular growth in the malignant product – uncontrolled myeloid proliferation. The Bcr–Abl protein also inhibits DNA repair, causing further genetic instability. This myeloproliferative disease is, therefore, the result of an acquired mutation, and appears equally prevalent around the world and in all racial and ethnic groups which have been studied in detail. The chromosomal characteristics of CML have been outlined on pages 562–564.

These important events render the malignant cells susceptible to targeted therapy designed specially to inhibit the activity of the Bcr–Abl protein, thereby producing lengthy remissions in CML. As Hehlmann and colleagues point out, 'CML was the first neoplastic disease for which knowledge of the genotype has led to a rationally designed therapy' [42].

Clinical features

These are shown in Table 28.8. The patient may be asymptomatic and the diagnosis made on a routine blood count, but fatigue, anaemia, weight loss and splenic pain eventually occur. Bruising and bleeding may develop. Abdominal pain may be due to stretching of the splenic capsule or may be acute and pleuritic if there has been splenic infarction. Peptic ulceration is 10 times more common than in the general population.

On examination there is usually splenomegaly and often sternal tenderness. The spleen is often considerably enlarged. Hepatomegaly and purpura may be present and retinal haemorrhages are not infrequent.

Table 28.8 Clinical and laboratory findings in chronic myeloid leukaemia.*

Symptoms and signs
Malaise and fatigue (80%)
Weight loss (60%)
Bruising and bleeding (40%)
Abdominal discomfort (40%)
Bone tenderness (70%)
Hepatomegaly (50%)
Purpura (25%)
Splenomegaly (95%)

Typical laboratory findings
Anaemia: Hb 9–12 g/dL
White blood cells: $25–1000 \times 10^9$/L
   Granulocytes 40%
   Metamyelocytes 10%
   Myelocytes 30%
   Promyelocytes 5%
   Myeloblasts 3%
Platelets
   $<150 \times 10^9$/L: 10%
   $150–400 \times 10^9$/L: 40%
   $>400 \times 10^9$/L: 50%

*Percentages indicate frequencies.

Investigation

The WBC is grossly elevated, with an increase in all stages of the granulocyte series, particularly myelocytes. Promyelocytes and myeloblasts are present in smaller numbers than myelocytes unless the presentation of the disease is with acute transformation ('blast crisis'). There is a variable degree of anaemia and the platelet count may be high, because of excess production of abnormal platelets, or low, because of hypersplenism or marrow failure. Thrombocytopenia is an indication that blastic transformation may have occurred. The diagnosis can usually be made from the blood film, and the bone marrow examination (although usually performed) does not contribute to diagnosis. It shows an expanded hypercellular marrow with an increase in the myeloid series, with an excess of early forms.

Leucocyte alkaline phosphatase is low or absent, and the Ph[1] chromosome can be demonstrated in metaphases in cultured marrow cells. The greatly increased turnover of myeloid cells leads to hyperuricaemia.

Patients who are Ph[1]-negative usually show more anaemia, a less high WBC, more numerous monocytes in the blood and more abnormal myeloid forms.

Evolution

As the leukaemic mass increases, the spleen enlarges and the patient becomes progressively more anaemic. The WBC doubles every 3–12 months. With treatment (see below) the WBC falls and a stable 'plateau' may then be reached with the patient off treatment. Gradually the 'remissions' become shorter and the recurrences more rapid. Finally, an aggressive disease develops with drug-resistant splenomegaly or rising WBC showing blastic transformation. The clinical picture is now dominated by an acute leukaemia that responds poorly to treatment and with a fatal outcome in a few months.

The transformation is usually accompanied by malaise, splenic enlargement, skin deposits, bone pain which may be localized, and a rising blast count. The median onset of transformation is 44 months. It may be more insidious, the disease showing only progressive loss of control from chemotherapy and sometimes with features of myelosclerosis.

The transformation is usually into AML, but 20% of cases show transformation into ALL in which the blast cells are Ph[1]-positive. About 20% of cases of adult ALL are Ph[1]-positive.

Treatment in chronic phase (Figure 28.6)

Use of the targeted therapy imatinib mesylate, an oral tyrosine kinase inhibitor, has totally revolutionized the management of CML. Imatinib, taken orally at a dose of 400–600 mg/day, is highly effective in CML, with a 95% complete haematological remission rate and major cytogenetic response in over 60%. The elevated WBC has often normalized within 3 weeks but the treatment needs to be given for life. Since the advent of imatinib, CML has become the first cancer in which what is now a standard medical treatment may give the patient a normal life expectancy [43]. It is now thought that this agent not only acts as an inhibitor of tyrosine kinase(s) but also induces cellular 'autophagy'. In this process, the native lysosomal degradation machinery is activated by imatinib-stimulated upregulation, a result that has now been confirmed experimentally in a number of mammalian cell lines. Classic studies showed that it is clearly superior to both interferon alfa and cytarabine the previously well-regarded agents for initial therapy [44,45],

with much improved patient preference. Side-effects of imatinib do occur, including fatigue, muscle pain, diarrhoea, skin rash and nausea, leading to intolerance and cessation of therapy in a small proportion of patients.

Interferon alfa was the previous treatment of choice, with 80% of patients responding and about 20% showing a reduction in marrow Ph[1]-positive cells. In some patients, the blood count remains stable for many months even after discontinuation of treatment. Both progression-free and overall survival are improved compared with hydroxycarbamide (hydroxyurea) and busulfan, which previously had also been widely employed. Effective targeted therapy with imatinib rapidly produces a symptomatic and haematological improvement in almost all patients. The leukaemic mass is reduced, with a fall in the WBC, reduction in splenic size, improvement in marrow function and a rise in haemoglobin. Hydroxycarbamide still occasionally has a place in management, having previously been widely used as initial treatment. The drug acts on the late progenitor cells. The dose is

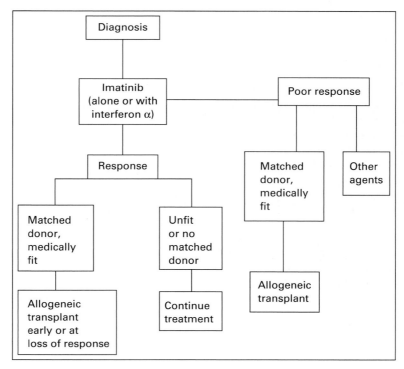

Figure 28.6 A simplified schematic for management of chronic myeloid leukaemia in its chronic phase. As the disease progresses into its accelerated and/or blastic phases, treatment inevitably becomes more aggressive if the patient is sufficiently fit and the bone marrow reserve haematologically adequate. Other targeted therapies for patients no longer responsive to imatinib include dasatinib and nilotinib. In general, these therapies require long-term administration.

1.5–2.0 g daily by mouth, and the response is more rapid than another previously widely used drug, busulfan, and appears to give better survival.

Recent work suggests that successful therapy leads to a biphasic exponential decline of leukaemic cells [46]. The initial slope represents the turnover rate of differentiated leukaemic cells, while the second slope appears to represent the turnover rate of leukaemic progenitors, the model suggesting that imatinib therapy will greatly inhibit the production of differentiated leukaemic cells without necessarily depleting the stem cells. This model is therefore able to calculate the probability of developing imatinib resistance mutations and estimates a time until detection of resistance, also providing the first quantitative insights into the *in vivo* kinetics of a human cancer.

Other targeted therapies (tyrosine kinase inhibitors) have recently been introduced, including dasatinib, which has a similar mechanism of action to imatinib but which appears to inhibit a broader spectrum of tyrosine kinases; it was approved for use in the USA in June 2006. This novel oral agent is active against Bcr–Abl and Src-family kinases, and has been remarkably successful in selected patients with imatinib-resistant disease, in the chronic phase. In an important study of almost 200 patients, a complete haematological response rate of 87% (imatinib-resistant patients) and 97% (imatinib intolerant patients) was achieved, using an oral dose of 140 mg daily given as 70 mg twice daily [47]. Over 50% of patients also had a major cytogenetic response. In addition, nilotinib and ceflatonin are currently under study in CML patients who have become resistant to imatinib. In imatinib-resistant patients, nilotinib was used successfully in a study from centres in the USA and Germany, producing significant responses in chronic or accelerated-phase CML, and even in a proportion of patients (13/33) with the blastic phase [48]. The authors noted that nilotinib is more potent than imatinib against CML cells by a factor of 20–50. Overall, a complete cytogenetic remission is now achievable with modern targeted treatment in over 85% of patients [42], and dasatinib and nilotinib have now both been approved by the FDA in the USA (2010) for first-line use, and more recently nilotinib, as first-line treatment by NICE in the UK as well (2012) – for further details, see also the current NICE guidance 2012 for these newer targeted agents. Several novel agents, including ponatinib, bosutinib and omacetaxine have now been approved by the FDA (though some of these await approval for use elsewhere than the USA) for relapsed or resistant cases no longer treatable with the other tyrosine kinase inhibitors.

Sadly, many of these agents will remain too expensive for routine use in the near future, and the current situation regarding approval remains fluid and somewhat confusing! One important recent study co-ordinated at the MD Anderson Hospital in Houston, Texas, addressing the role of ponatinib, showed remarkable results in heavily pretreated patients – see Ref. [49]. This oral agent appears to be a potent TKI of both mutated and unmutated BCR-ABL, including BCR-ABL with the TKI-refractory threonine-to-isoleucine mutation at position 315 (T315I). Among 267 patients with chronic-phase CML, 56% had a major cytogenetic response, mostly of durable benefit, with responses observed regardless of the baseline BCR-ABL kinase domain mutation status. Finally, in patients where the leukaemia clone(s) has or have acquired a mutation resulting in the substitution of tyrosine for isoleucine in amino acid position 315 in the Bcr-Abl fusion protein, causing resistance to all currently available tyrosine kinase inhibitors, high-dose chemotherapy with BMT is the only active treatment option. The general view remains, however, that wherever possible, further attempts at second- and even third-line therapy should be made after failure of response to imatinib, rather than offering BMT at that point, with its inevitably higher burden of both morbidity and mortality. Patients carrying the T315I mutation are more difficult to treat successfully.

A fascinating development recently reported is the potential use of vaccination, using the Bcr–Abl p210 fusion protein in patients with stable disease, in conjunction with granulocyte/macrophage CSF [50]. This exciting approach clearly has considerable promise but has not yet become established as part of standard management.

Treatment of accelerated and blast phase

As the speed of relapse increases the spleen usually starts to enlarge and marrow failure, due to both the disease and its treatment, becomes apparent. If the patient has not been previously treated with imatinib, this is the next step. Half of all patients will achieve haematological remission and 25% will have a major cytogenetic response. Hydroxycarbamide (1–2 g/day) may also produce temporary benefit.

Blastic transformation is usually to AML and is often treated as such unless the patient is infirm or elderly. Responses to imatinib also occur in blast crisis, but these are usually short-lived with only 30% of patients alive at 1 year. In those cases where ALL supervenes, treatment is as for adult ALL. In both cases the prognosis is very bad.

Remissions may be obtained but median survival is only 3 months.

Bone marrow transplantation

Current advice is that allogeneic BMT [51] should be carried out early in the chronic phase for patients aged less than 60 who have a matched donor. This accounts for only 40% of all patients. The earlier in the chronic phase the transplant is carried out, the better the outcome. The 5-year relapse-free survival is 75% in such patients and it appears to be the only curative treatment for the disease. The greatly improved rates of remission with imatinib are likely to alter the timing and the choice of allogeneic BMT. Recently, less toxic transplant regimens have been introduced, since the graft-versus-host reaction may partly account for the effectiveness of therapy. The extreme discomfort of treatment-induced oral mucositis may to some extent be alleviated by the use of palifermin, which appears to have a useful protective benefit [31]. Palifermin is a modified version of a naturally occurring human protein, KGF, which has the capacity to stimulate growth of cells in tissues such as the skin and the surface layer of the mouth, stomach and colon. In turn this helps maintain the normal structure of the skin and gastrointestinal surface, assisting in repair of the skin and gastrointestinal lining. These newer supportive measures and techniques have widened the range of patients who can be accepted or at least considered for transplantation.

The results of BMT in blastic transformation are usually disappointing although occasional patients have had a return of normal Ph^1-negative haemopoiesis.

Prognosis

Without transplantation less than 5% of patients survive 10 years. The impact of imatinib on prognosis remains to be determined. About 60% of patients undergoing allogeneic BMT in chronic phase remain disease-free. Only 25% survive at 5 years when transplanted in accelerated phase.

Ph^1-negative chronic granulocytic leukaemia

These patients differ from Ph^1-positive CGL in having a greater degree of splenomegaly at presentation, more profound anaemia and a lower WBC. The blood film reveals more abnormal neutrophils and monocytes, and fewer myelocytes. The disease appears to run a more rapid course than Ph^1-positive CGL, with a median survival of only 18 months in some series. Treatment is along the same lines as Ph^1-positive CGL.

Eosinophilic leukaemia

This disease is characterized by eosinophilia sometimes accompanied by anaemia, neutropenia and thrombocytopenia. There may be cough associated with transient pulmonary infiltration, and non-bacterial endocarditis occurs, leading to heart failure.

The disease may be difficult to distinguish from other forms of chronic eosinophilia and the diagnosis of leukaemia may be hard to establish. Acute blastic transformation of the disease occurs in some patients and the response to treatment is poor.

Chronic myelomonocytic leukaemia

This is a disease of the elderly. The onset is insidious with bruising or bleeding, fleeting urticarial skin rash, slight splenomegaly and a history of infections. There is a monocytosis with abnormal forms. Bone marrow shows abnormal nuclear morphology of a monocyte type. Chromosome 3 may show karyotypic abnormalities, t(3;16). The clinical course is often slow. Treatment is usually with hydroxycarbamide but is unsatisfactory and reserved for symptomatic disease.

References

1 Sandier OP. Epidemiology and etiology of leukaemia. *Curr Opin Oncol* 1990; 2: 3–9.

2 Kaldor JM, Day NE, Pettersson F *et al.* Leukaemia following chemotherapy for ovarian cancer. *N Engl J Med* 1990; 322: 1–6. [See also accompanying paper describing risk for Hodgkin's disease. *N Engl J Med* 1990; 322: 7–13.]

3 Morton LM, Dores GM, Tucker MA *et al.* Evolving risk of therapy-related acute myeloid leukaemia following cancer chemotherapy among adults in the United States 1975–2008. *Blood* 2013; 121: 2996–3004.

4 Wintrobe M. *Blood Pure and Eloquent.* New York: McGraw-Hill, 1980: 528.

5 Fialkow PJ, Singer RW, Raskind WH *et al.* Clonal development, stem-cell differentiation and clinical remissions in acute non-lymphocytic leukaemia. *N Engl J Med* 1987; 317: 468–73.

6 Bain BJ. *Leukaemia Diagnosis. A Guide to the FAB Classification.* Philadelphia: JB Lippincott, 1990.

7 MIC Study Group. Morphologic immunologic and cytogenetic (MIC) working classification of the acute myeloid leukaemias. *Br J Haematol* 1988; 68: 487–94.

8 Cancer Genome Atlas Research Network. Genomic and epigenomic landscapes of adult de novo acute myeloid leukemia. *New Engl J Med* 2013; 368: 2059–2074.

9 Pui C-H, Relling MV, Downing JR. Acute lymphoblastic leukaemia. *N Engl J Med* 2004; 350: 1535–48.

10 Schrappe M, Hunger SP, Pui C-H *et al.* Outcomes after induction failure in childhood acute lymphoblastic leukemia. *New Engl J Med* 2012; 366: 1371–1381.

11 Chessels JM, Bailey C, Richards SM. Intensification of treatment and survival in all children with lymphoblastic leukaemia: results of MRC trial UK ALL X. *Lancet* 1995; 345: 143–8.

12 Pieters R, Schrappe M, De Lorenzo P *et al.* A treatment protocol for infants younger than 1 year with acute lymphoblastic leukaemia (Interfant-99): an observational study and a multicentre randomized trial. *Lancet* 2007; 370: 240–50.

13 Freeman AL, Weinberg V, Brecher ML *et al.* Comparison of intermediate-dose methotrexate with cranial irradiation for the post-induction treatment of acute lymphocytic leukaemia in children. *N Engl J Med* 1994; 330: 477–84.

14 Balduzzi A, Valsecchi MG, Uderzo C *et al.* Chemotherapy versus allogeneic transplantation for very-high-risk childhood acute lymphoblastic leukaemia in first complete remission: comparison by genetic randomization in an international prospective study. *Lancet* 2005; 366: 635–42.

15 Barrett AJ, Horowitz MM, Gale RP *et al.* Marrow transplantation for acute lymphoblastic leukaemia: factors affecting relapse and survival. *Blood* 1989; 74: 862–71.

16 Pui C-H, Robison LL and Look AT. Acute lymphoblastic leukaemia. *Lancet* 2008; 371: 1030–43.

17 Rabin KR. Attacking remaining challenges in childhood leukemia. *New Engl J Med* 2012; 366: 1445–1446.

18 Yeoh EJ, Ross ME, Shurtleff SA *et al.* Classification, subtype discovery, and prediction of outcome in pediatric acute lymphoblastic leukaemia by gene expression profiling. *Cancer Cell* 2002; 1: 133–43.

19 Grigoropoulos NF, Petter R, Van't Veer MB *et al.* Leukaemia update. Part 1: diagnosis and management. *Brit Med J* 2013; 346: f1660. Part 2: Managing patients with leukaemia in the community. *Brit Med J* 2013; 346: f1932.

20 Durrant IJ, Prentice HG, Richards SM. Intensification of treatment for adults with acute lymphoblastic leukeamia: results of UK Medical Research Council randomized trial UKALL XA. *Br J Haematol* 1997; 99: 84–92.

21 Czuczman MS, Dodge RK, Stewart CC *et al.* Value of immunophenotype in intensively treated adult acute lymphoblastic leukaemia: CALGB study 8364. *Blood* 1999; 93: 3931–9.

22 Estey E, Döhner H. Acute myeloid leukemia. *Lancet* 2006; 368: 1894–907.

23 Chen S-J and Chen Z. Targeting agents alone to cure acute promyelocytic leukemia. *New Engl J Med* 2013; 369: 186–187.

24 Wang ZY and Chen Z. Acute promyelocytic leukemia: from highly fatal to highly curable. *Blood* 2008; 111: 2505–2515.

25 Lo-Coco F, Avvisati G, Vignetti M *et al.* Retinoic acid and arsenic trioxide for acute promyelocytic leukemia. *New Engl J Med* 2013; 369: 111–121.

26 Ferrara F. Unanswered questions in acute myeloid leukaemia. *Lancet Oncol* 2004; 5: 443–50.

27 Mayer RJ, Davis RB, Schiffer CA *et al.* Intensive postremission chemotherapy in adults with AML. *N Engl J Med* 1994; 331: 896–903.

28 Zittoun RA, Mandell I, Willemze R *et al.* Autologous or allogeneic bone marrow transplantation compared with intensive chemotherapy in acute myelogenous leukaemia. *N Engl J Med* 1995; 332: 217–23.

29 Burnet AK, Hills RK, Milligan D *et al.* Identification of patients with acute myeloblastic leukaemia who benefit from the addition of gemtuzumab ozogamicin: results of the MRC AML 15 trial. *J Clin Oncol* 2011; 29: 369–377.

30 Roboz GJ. Current treatment of acute myeloid leukaemia. *Curr Opin Oncol* 2012; 24: 711–719.

31 Spielberger R, Stiff P, Bensinger W *et al.* Palifermin for oral mucositis after intensive therapy for hematologic cancers. *N Engl J Med* 2004; 351: 2590–8.

32 Burnett AK, Goldstone AH, Stevens RMF *et al.* Randomised comparison of addition of autologous bone-marrow transplantation to intensive chemotherapy for acute myeloid leukaemia in first remission: results of MRC AML 10 trial. *Lancet* 1998; 351: 700–8.

33 Feneaux P, Le Deley MC, Castaigne S *et al.* Effect of all-*trans*-retinoic acid in newly diagnosed promyelocytic leukaemia: results of a multicenter randomized trial. *Blood* 1993; 82: 3241–9.

34 Dohner H, Stilgenbauer S, Benner A *et al.* Genomic aberrations and survival in chronic lymphocytic leukaemia. *N Engl J Med* 2000; 343: 1910–16.

35 Wang L, Lawrence MS, Wan Y *et al.* SF3B1 and other novel cancer genes in chronic lymphocytic leukemia. *New Engl J Med* 2011; 365: 2497–2506.

36 Rai KR, Peterson BL, Applebaum FR *et al.* Fludarabine compared with chlorambucil as primary therapy for chronic lymphocytic leukaemia. *N Engl J Med* 2000; 343: 1750–7.

37 Catovsky D, Richards S, Matutes E *et al.* on behalf of the UK National Cancer Research Institute Haematological Oncology and Chronic Leukaemia Working Groups. Assessment of fludarabine plus cyclophosphamide for patients with chronic lymphocytic leukaemia (the LRF CLL 4 trial): a randomized controlled trial. *Lancet* 2007; 370: 230–9.

38 National Institute for Health and Clinical Excellence (NICE). Bendamustine for the first-line treatment of chronic lymphocytic leukaemia 2011. www.nice.org.uk.

39 Knauf WU, Lissitchkov T, Aldaoud A *et al.* Bendamustine compared with chlorambucil in previously untreated patients with chronic lymphocytic leukaemia: updated results of a randomized phase III trial. *Brit J Haematol* 2012; 159: 67–77.

40 Else M, Ruchlemer R, Osuji N *et al.* Long remissions in hairy cell leukemia with purine analogs: a report of 219 patients with a median follow-up of 12.5 years. *Cancer* 2005; 104: 2442–8.

41 Michor F, Hughes TP, Iwasa Y *et al.* Dynamics of chronic myeloid leukaemia. *Nature* 2005; 435: 1169–70.

42 Hehlmann R, Hochhaus A, Baccarani M for the European LeukemiaNet. Chronic myeloid leukaemia. *Lancet* 2007; 370: 342–50.

43 Druker BJ, Guilhot F, O'Brien SG *et al.* for IRIS Investigators. Five-year follow-up of patients receiving imatinib for chronic myeloid leukemia. *N Engl J Med* 2006; 355: 2408–17.

44 Chronic Myeloid Leukaemia Trialists Collaborative Group. Interferon alfa versus chemotherapy for chronic myeloid leukaemia: a meta-analysis of seven randomized trials. *J Natl Cancer Inst* 1997; 89: 1616–20.

45 O'Brien SG, Guilhot F, Larson RA *et al.* Imatinib compared with interferon and low-dose cytarabine for newly-diagnosed chronic-phase chronic myeloid leukemia. *N Engl J Med* 2003; 348: 994–1004.

46 Campbell PJ, Green AR. Mechanisms of disease: the myeloproliferative disorders. *N Engl J Med* 2006; 355: 2452–66.

47 Hochhaus A, Kantarjian HM, Baccarani M *et al.* Dasatinib induces notable hematologic and cytogenetic responses in chronic-phase chronic myeloid leukemia after failure of imatinib therapy. *Blood* 2007; 109: 2303–9.

48 Kantarjian H, Giles F, Wunderle L *et al.* Nilotinib in imatinibresistant CML and Philadelphia chromosome-positive ALL. *N Engl J Med* 2006; 354: 2542–51.

49 Cortes JE, Kim D-W, Pinilla-Ibarz P, *et al.* A phase 2 trial of ponatinib in Philadelphia chromosome-positive leukemias. *New Engl J Med* 2013; 369: 1783–1796.

50 Bocchia M, Gentili S, Abruzzese E *et al.* Effect of p210 multipeptide vaccine associated with imatinib or interferon in patients with chronic myeloid leukaemia and persistent residual disease: a multi-centre observational trial. *Lancet* 2005; 365: 657–62.

51 Hansen JA, Gooley TA, Martin PJ *et al.* Bone marrow transplantation from unrelated donors for patients with chronic myeloid leukaemia. *N Engl J Med* 1998; 338: 962–8.

Further reading

Andreeva SV, Drozdova VD, Emel'ianenko LA. Chromosome 11 rearrangements in the different haematological neoplasias. *Tsitol Genet* 2007; 41: 42–8.

Appelbaum FR. Hematopoietic-cell transplantation at 50. *N Engl J Med* 2007; 357: 1472–5.

Apperley JF. Mechanisms of resistance to imatinib in chronic myeloid leukaemia. *Lancet Oncol* 2007; 8: 1018–29.

Chiorazzi N, Rai KR, Ferrarini M. Mechanisms of disease: chronic lymphocytic leukemia. *New Engl J Med* 2005; 352: 804–15.

Copelan EA. Medical progress: hematopoietic stem-cell transplantation. *N Engl J Med* 2006; 354: 1813–26.

Deininger M, Druker BJ. Specific targeted therapy of chronic myelogenous leukaemia with imatinib. *Pharmacol Rev* 2003; 55: 401–23.

Druker BJ. Circumventing resistance to kinase-inhibitor therapy. *N Engl J Med* 2006; 354: 2594–6.

Faderl S, Kantarjin HM. Drug insight: emerging new drugs in the treatment of myelodysplastic syndromes. *Nat Clin Pract Oncol* 2005; 2: 348–55.

Fernandez HF, Sun Z, Yao X *et al.* Anthracyclene dose intensification in acute myeloid leukemia. *N Engl J Med* 2009; 361: 1249–59.

Fröhling S, Döhner H. Chromosomal abnormalities in cancer. *N Engl J Med* 2008; 359: 722–34.

Foa R. Changes in the treatment landscape for chronic lymphoid leukemia. *New Engl J Med* 2014; 371: 273–4.

Gilliland DG, Griffin JD. Role of FLT3 in leukemia. *Curr Opin Hematol* 2002; 9: 274–81.

Landgren O, Albitar M, Wanlong M *et al.* B-cell clones as early markers for chronic lymphocytic leukaemia. *N Engl J Med* 2009; 360: 659–67.

Licht JD. Acute promyelocytic leukemia. *N Engl J Med* 2009; 360: 928–30.

Mitchell C, Hall G, Clarke RT. Acute leukaemia in children: diagnosis and management. *Br Med J* 2009; 338: 1491–5.

Mullighan CG, Goorha S, Radtke I *et al.* Genome-wide analysis of genetic alterations in acute lymphoblastic leukaemia. *Nature* 2007; 446: 758–64.

Mullighan CG, Xiaoping S, Zhang J *et al.* Deletion of IKZF1 and prognosis in acute lymphoblastic leukaemia. *N Engl J Med* 2009; 360: 470–80.

National Institute for Health and Clinical Excellence (NICE). Dasatinib, high-dose imatinib and nilotinib for the treatment of imatinib-resistant chronic myeloid leukaemia (CML) 2012. www.nice.org.uk.

Pui C-H, Campana D, Pei D *et al.* Treating childhood acute lymphoblastic leukemia without cranial irradiation. *N Engl J Med* 2009; 360: 2730–41.

Schiffer CA. BCR-ABL tyrosine kinase inhibitors for chronic myelogenous leukaemia. *N Engl J Med* 2007; 357: 258–65.

Schlenk RF, Döhner K, Krauter J *et al.* for the German–Austrian Acute Myeloid Leukemia Study group. Mutations and treatment outcome in cytogenetically normal acute myeloid leukaemia. *N Engl J Med* 2008; 358: 1909–18.

Trivedi AK, Pal P, Behre G, Singh SM. Multiple ways of C/EBPα inhibition in myeloid leukaemia. *Eur J Cancer* 2008; 44: 1516–23.

Vardiman JW, Harris NL, Brumming RD. The World Health Organisation classification of the myeloid neoplasms. *Blood* 2002; 100: 2292–302.

Vaughan WP, Karp JE. The long road to a cure for acute myelocytic leukaemia: from intensity to specificity. *J Clin Oncol* 2008; 26: 3475–7.

Index

Page numbers in *italics* represent figures, those in **bold** represent tables. The index is in letter-by-letter order.

Cancer and its Management, Seventh Edition. Jeffrey Tobias and Daniel Hochhauser.
© 2015 John Wiley & Sons, Ltd. Published 2015 by John Wiley & Sons, Ltd.